INFECTIOUS DISEASES

The Clinician's Guide to Diagnosis, Treatment, and Prevention

INFECTIOUS DISEASES

The Clinician's Guide to Diagnosis, Treatment, and Prevention

Edited by
DAVID C. DALE, M.D.
Professor of Medicine
University of Washington
Medical Center
Seattle, Washington

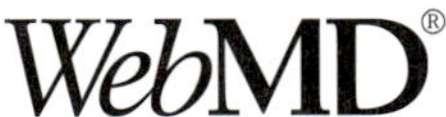

ISBN: 0-9703902-6-2

Vice President and Publisher	Nancy E. Chorpenning
Director, Electronic Publishing	Liz Pope
Sponsoring Editor	Erin Michael Kelly
Development Editor	John Heinegg
Senior Copy Editor	John J. Anello
Copy Editor	Dave Terry
Art and Design Editor	Elizabeth Klarfeld
Electronic Composition	Diane Joiner, Jennifer Smith
Manufacturing Producer	Kelly Mercado
Indexer	Julia Brooks Figures

Printed in the United States of America

Published by WebMD Inc.

WebMD Professional Publishing
224 West 30th Street
New York, NY 10001-4905

Contents

ORGANISMS CAUSING INFECTIOUS DISEASES

ORGANISMS CAUSING INFECTIOUS DISEASES *(continued)*

Contributors

Michael Augenbraun, M.D.
Associate Professor of Medicine, State University of New York Downstate Medical Center

Robert W. Coombs, M.D., Ph.D.
Associate Professor, Department of Laboratory Medicine, University of Washington School of Medicine

Michael S. Donnenberg, M.D.
Professor of Medicine, Professor of Microbiology and Immunology, and Head, Division of Infectious Diseases, University of Maryland School of Medicine

Jeffrey S. Duchin, M.D.
Assistant Professor of Medicine, Division of Allergy and Infectious Disease, University of Washington School of Medicine; and Chief, Communicable Disease Control, Department of Public Health, Seattle and King County, Washington

Layne O. Gentry, M.D.
Clinical Professor of Medicine, Baylor College of Medicine; and Chief, Infectious Disease Section, and Medical Director, Infection Control, St. Luke's Episcopal Hospital

Donald H. Gilden, M.D.
Professor and Chairman, Department of Neurology, University of Colorado Health Sciences Center

Marcia B. Goldberg, M.D.
Associate Physician, Division of Infectious Disease, Massachusetts General Hospital, and Associate Professor of Medicine (Microbiology and Molecular Genetics), Harvard Medical School

Matthew R. Golden, M.D., M.P.H.
Assistant Professor of Medicine, University of Washington School of Medicine

Francisco González-Scarano, M.D.
Professor of Neurology and Microbiology, Department of Neurology, University of Pennsylvania School of Medicine

Duane J. Gubler, Sc.D.
Adjunct Professor, Department of Microbiology, Colorado State University; Adjunct Professor, Department of International Health, Johns Hopkins University School of Public Health; and Director, Division of Vector-Borne Infectious Diseases, National Center for Infectious Diseases, Centers for Disease Control and Prevention

Kalpana Gupta, M.D., M.P.H.
Acting Assistant Professor of Medicine, Division of Infectious Diseases, Department of Medicine, University of Washington School of Medicine

Frederick G. Hayden, M.D.
Stuart S. Richardson Professor of Clinical Virology and Professor of Medicine and Pathology, Departments of Internal Medicine and Pathology, University of Virginia School of Medicine

Martin S. Hirsch, M.D.
Professor of Medicine, Harvard Medical School, and Physician, Massachusetts General Hospital

Jan V. Hirschmann, M.D.
Professor of Medicine, University of Washington School of Medicine, and Assistant Chief, Medical Service, Puget Sound Veterans Affairs Medical Center

Christian E. Huber, M.D.
Post-Doctoral Research Fellow, Infectious Disease Division, Brown University School of Medicine

Michael G. Ison, M.D.
Fellow, Division of Infectious Diseases, University of Virginia School of Medicine

Adolf W. Karchmer, M.D.
Professor of Medicine, Harvard Medical School, and Chief, Division of Infectious Diseases, Beth Israel Deaconess Medical Center

Carol A. Kauffman, M.D.
Professor of Medicine, Department of Internal Medicine, University of Michigan Medical School

Nino Khetsuriani, M.D., Ph.D
Medical Epidemiologist, Respiratory and Enteric Viruses Branch, Centers for Disease Control and Prevention

W. Conrad Liles, M.D., Ph.D.
Associate Professor of Medicine, University of Washington School of Medicine

Brian F. Mandell, M.D., Ph.D.
Education Program Director, Department of Rheumatic and Immunologic Diseases, and Senior Associate Program Director, Internal Medicine Residency Program, Cleveland Clinic Foundation

Jeanne M. Marrazzo, M.D., M.P.H.
Assistant Professor of Medicine, University of Washington School of Medicine

Steven M. Opal, M.D.
Professor of Medicine, Department of Medicine, Brown University School of Medicine

Umesh D. Parashar M.D., M.P.H.
Medical Epidemiologist, Centers for Disease Control and Prevention

Lyle R. Petersen, M.D., M.P.H.
Deputy Director for Science, Division of Vector-Borne Infectious Diseases, Centers for Disease Control and Prevention

David A. Relman, M.D.
Associate Professor, Department of Medicine (Infectious Diseases) and Department of Microbiology and Immunology, Stanford University School of Medicine, and Staff Physician, Veterans Affairs Palo Alto Health Care System

Harvey B. Simon, M.D.
Associate Professor of Medicine, Harvard Medical School; Health Sciences and Technology Faculty, Massachusetts Institute of Technology; and Physician, Massachusetts General Hospital

Shawn J. Skerrett, M.D.
Associate Professor of Medicine, University of Washington School of Medicine

Frederick S. Southwick, M.D.
Professor and Chief, Division of Infectious Diseases, and Associate Chairman, Department of Medicine, University of Florida College of Medicine

David H. Spach, M.D.
Associate Professor of Medicine, Division of Allergy and Infectious Diseases, University of Washington School of Medicine

Walter E. Stamm, M.D.
Professor, Department of Medicine, and Head, Division of Allergy and Infectious Disease, University of Washington School of Medicine

Morton N. Swartz, M.D.
Professor of Medicine, Harvard Medical School; and Chief, James Jackson Firm, Medical Services, and Chief Emeritus, Infectious Disease Unit, Massachusetts General Hospital

Jo-Anne van Burik, M.D.
Assistant Professor, University of Minnesota Medical School

Peter F. Weller, M.D.
Professor of Medicine, Harvard Medical School; and Co-Chief, Infectious Diseases Division, and Chief, Allergy and Inflammation Division, Beth Israel Deaconess Medical Center

Preface

In our ever-changing world, problems with infections remain paramount in medicine—for the generalist and the specialist in every field. New pathogens are continually emerging. The best techniques for diagnosis are constantly evolving, and resistance to antibiotics is a rapidly growing problem. Most textbooks are not updated often enough to be satisfying for current information about diagnosis and management. Too much information in textbooks is another risk, especially if the information you need is not easily accessible. In developing this new clinician's guide, we have tried to address these problems with a well-referenced, concise text, richly illustrated with figures and tables to help you to quickly get to the right answers in the management of most infectious disease problems.

While there are literally hundreds of books on the subject of infectious disease, in my experience very few of them are truly created with the working primary care physician in mind. Therefore, while this book is written by the world's leading infectious disease specialists, we have taken pains to make their recommendations accessible for clinicians practicing outside of the subspecialty. This means not having to wade through extremely rare conditions, or tests and treatments only used by the most specialized infectious disease experts. Instead, you get a focused guide that does not overwhelm with unneeded details and is geared towards the specific needs of primary care practitioners.

To create this book, we have extracted the newly revised and reorganized infectious disease section and a few other key chapters from our internal medicine reference, *WebMD Scientific American® Medicine*—the quarter-century leader in continually updated medical information. The result is a clinic-friendly reference that covers such rapidly evolving subjects as bioterrorism, while still providing practical guidance on the mainstays of infectious disease, such as upper respiratory infections, STDs, and meningitis. Viral, bacterial, and fungal infections; slow viruses; and prions—all the most common and clinically significant forms of infection are represented in these pages.

WebMD Scientific American® Medicine is renowned for its rich illustrations, which enhance learning by distilling text into lucid visual explanations. We take full advantage of images, with liberal use of full color for the 107 figures spread throughout *Infectious Diseases*. And of course we give you rapid access to key decision-making steps by highlighting the most significant of this information in over 130 tables and sidebars. This book is also fully indexed, with over 4,000 entries.

We certainly hope that you find this book helpful in your daily practice of medicine and that it contains the information necessary for you to provide excellent care to your patients.

David C. Dale, M.D.
Editor

Dedication

Dedicated to Morton N. Swartz, who began the Infectious Disease section in Scientific American® Medicine; *my teachers and mentors Sheldon M.Wolff, Robert G. Petersdorf, and William M. Kirby; and my wife, Rose Marie.*

DCD

1 Hyperthermia, Fever, and Fever of Undetermined Origin

Harvey B. Simon, M.D.

Thermoregulation and Abnormal Elevation of Body Temperature

REGULATION OF BODY TEMPERATURE

Like so many biologic functions, human body temperature normally displays circadian rhythmicity, often rising from values of 36.1° C (97.0° F) or lower in the predawn hours to 37.4° C (99.3° F) or higher in the afternoon. This diurnal flux has two important practical consequences. First, fever associated with disease states is superimposed on the normal cycle and tends to peak in the evening; hence, a patient cannot be considered afebrile until his or her temperature has been monitored for at least 24 hours. Second, temperatures exceeding what is mistakenly regarded as the normal value of 37.0° C (98.6° F) are often recorded in perfectly healthy individuals.[1] Unfortunately, many patients with temperature elevations that are entirely physiologic have been subjected to potentially hazardous tests and treatments because their elevated temperatures were incorrectly regarded as pathologic.

Within the limits of the circadian rhythm, however, body temperature is closely regulated by homeostatic mechanisms that strike a balance between heat production and heat dissipation.[2] Heat is a by-product of all metabolic processes. At rest, metabolic activity in the liver and heart produce much of the body's heat; metabolic activity in skeletal muscle accounts for the greatly enhanced thermal load of exercise. Heat is dissipated at the body's surfaces; the skin accounts for about 90% of heat loss, with the lungs contributing most of the remaining 10%. In the basal state, about 70% of the body's thermal load is dissipated by conduction, and 30% is removed by the evaporation of insensible perspiration; radiation and convection are less important mechanisms of heat removal. When the ambient temperature rises or metabolic heat production increases, evaporation accounts for the major share of heat dissipation.

The preoptic nucleus of the anterior hypothalamus functions as the thermal control center and acts to maintain the body temperature at a set value—the so-called hypothalamic thermal set point.[3] In response to elevations in core body temperature (i.e., the temperature of the blood perfusing the internal organs), the hypothalamus stimulates the autonomic nervous system to produce cutaneous vasodilatation and sweating, both of which dissipate heat. In response to either a falling core temperature or a falling skin temperature, the hypothalamus conserves heat by causing cutaneous vasoconstriction. When cold stress is severe, the hypothalamus acts to increase heat production by stimulating muscular activity in the form of shivering; shivering is mediated by the action of somatic nerves, but it is an automatic and involuntary process.

HYPERTHERMIA AND FEVER

Abnormal elevation of body temperature, or pyrexia, can occur in one of two ways: hyperthermia[4] or fever [*see Figure 1*]. In hyperthermia, thermal control mechanisms fail, so that heat production exceeds heat dissipation. In contrast, in fever, the hypothalamic thermal set point rises, and intact thermal control mechanisms are brought into play to bring body temperature up to the new set point. The distinction between fever and hyperthermia is more than academic: hyperthermia is best treated with physical cooling methods that promote heat dissipation, whereas fever is best treated with aspirin, acetaminophen, or other drugs that lower the thermal set point.

Hyperthermia

ETIOLOGY

Numerous clinical disorders can disrupt thermoregulatory homeostasis by causing increased heat production, decreased heat dissipation, or

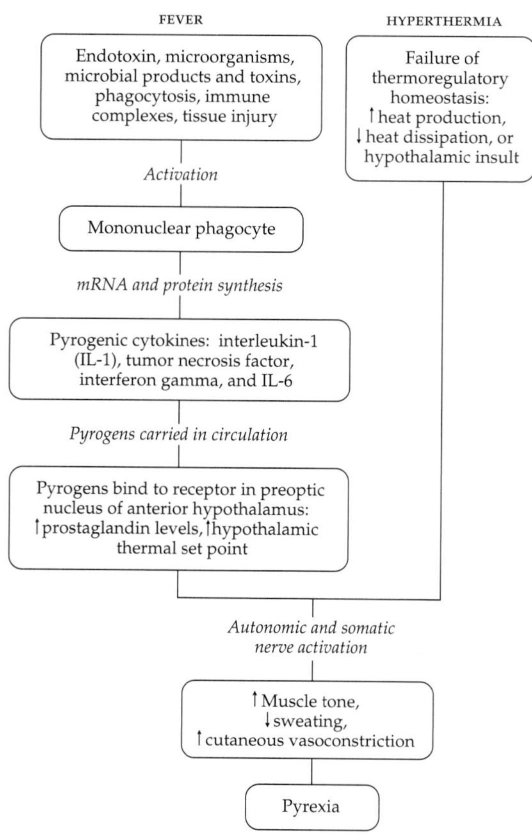

Figure 1 **Body temperature can rise to abnormal levels in one of two ways: hyperthermia or fever. In hyperthermia, thermal control mechanisms fail. In contrast, in fever, the hypothalamic thermal set point rises.**

hypothalamic insult, thereby inducing hyperthermia [*see Table 1*]. Mild forms of hyperthermia are common. In dehydration, for example, cutaneous vasoconstriction and cessation of sweating occur in response to the decrease in intravascular volume as a means of conserving further loss of fluid and of minimizing the consequences of fluid loss. As a result, heat dissipation is impaired and body temperature may rise. The hyperthermia of dehydration is usually mild and is readily corrected by fluid replacement. In some cases, however, thermoregulatory disorders cause extreme pyrexia, in which body temperatures rise to 41.1° C (106.0° F) or higher[5]; examples of these thermoregulatory disorders are heatstroke, malignant hyperthermia of anesthesia, thyroid storm, and hypothalamic insult caused by infection, tumor, or drugs.

Numerous exogenous agents, including cocaine and amphetamine, may cause severe hyperthermia. Because salicylates uncouple oxidative phosphorylation in skeletal muscle, excessive heat production is probably responsible for the hyperthermia seen in some children with severe aspirin toxicity.

The hyperthermia that may accompany thyroid storm and pheochromocytoma crisis also results from increased heat production, triggered in these cases by the calorigenic properties of thyroid hormones and catecholamines.[6] Anticholinergic drugs may impair heat dissipation by reducing sweat production.

Hypothalamic disorders are uncommon causes of hyperthermia. Cerebrovascular accidents, however, may be responsible for sustained hyperthermia; this so-called central fever is easily confused with true fever caused by infection or drug hypersensitivity in patients who are hospitalized for major cerebrovascular accidents.

Because infectious and inflammatory diseases can also cause extreme fever, the magnitude of elevation of a patient's temperature cannot be used to distinguish between hyperthermia and fever.[5]

In most cases, hyperthermia is an acute rather than a recurrent problem, and the underlying disorder can be readily diagnosed by careful clinical examination. Exceptions occur in patients with endocrinologic[6] or hypothalamic disorders who present as diagnostic puzzles in the category of fever of undetermined origin (FUO) [*see* Fever of Undetermined Origin, *below*].

HEATSTROKE

Heatstroke is a medical emergency that occurs in warm, humid conditions: the high ambient temperature impairs heat loss by conduction, and the high ambient humidity limits heat dissipation by the evaporation of sweat. In one form of the syndrome, exertional heatstroke, exercise imposes the additional thermal burden of increased heat production.[7] Although increased heat production does not occur in the other form of heatstroke, classic heatstroke, patients with this more common type of hyperthermic emergency often have impaired heat dissipation caused by a failure of sweating (anhidrosis) as well as more subtle thermoregulatory problems imposed by underlying diseases and the medications used to treat them.

Epidemiology

Heatstroke is far from rare. Between 1979 and 1997, more than 7,046 deaths in the United States were attributed to excessive heat exposure[8]; it seems likely that heatstroke goes unrecognized or

Table 1 Causes of Hyperthermia

Cause	*Example*
Excessive heat production	Delirium tremens Drug abuse (cocaine or amphetamines) Exertional hyperthermia Generalized tetanus Heatstroke (exertional)* Lethal catatonia Malignant hyperthermia of anesthesia Neuroleptic malignant syndrome* Pheochromocytoma Salicylate intoxication Status epilepticus Thyrotoxicosis
Diminished heat dissipation	Anticholinergic drugs Autonomic dysfunction Dehydration Heatstroke (classic)* Neuroleptic malignant syndrome* Occlusive dressings
Hypothalamic dysfunction	Cerebrovascular accidents Encephalitis Idiopathic hypothalamic dysfunction Neuroleptic malignant syndrome* Sarcoidosis and granulomatous infections Trauma Tumors

*Pathogenesis of these disorders is mixed.

unreported in many cases and that hyperthermia also contributes to the morbidity and mortality attributed to underlying diseases.

Classic heatstroke is the most common hyperthermic emergency.[4] Occurring principally during summer heat waves, classic heatstroke is most likely to affect the elderly and patients with serious underlying diseases. The urban poor are particularly vulnerable to classic heatstroke; women are affected more often than men, and infants are also at risk.

Pathophysiology

The crucial pathophysiologic events causing classic heatstroke are excessive ambient heat and humidity and impaired heat dissipation caused by anhidrosis. The typical victim of classic heatstroke is an elderly or debilitated person who is confined to a poorly ventilated room without benefit of an air conditioner or fan during a summer heat wave. Dehydration, which limits heat dissipation, is an important predisposing condition. Other factors that increase risk include neurologic and cardiovascular diseases, obesity, the use of diuretics, and the use of neuroleptics and other medications with anticholinergic properties; alcohol consumption also contributes to some cases.

The second form of heatstroke is triggered by exercising in a warm, humid environment. The major pathophysiologic mechanism responsible for exertional heatstroke is increased heat production from exercising skeletal muscles. Working at maximal intensity, muscle can increase its energy consumption to levels 20 times its basal rate; because the body's efficiency is only about 25%, much of this energy is converted into heat, which is transferred from muscle to blood, raising the core temperature. Patients who suffer exertional heatstroke do not appear to have intrinsic abnormalities of their thermoregulatory mechanisms, but they may have a high proportion of type II skeletal muscle fibers and a lower work efficiency.[9] Whereas classic heatstroke occurs in outbreaks, exertional heatstroke occurs sporadically and typically affects young, healthy individuals who engage in strenuous exercise. Exertional heatstroke is much more common in men than in women. In the United States, military recruits, industrial workers, and athletes such as runners and football players are at greatest risk; in Saudi Arabia, both forms of heatstroke are particularly common during the annual hajj, the pilgrimage to Mecca. In addition to ambient weather conditions and muscular exertion, predisposing factors include inappropriately heavy clothing, exposure to direct sunlight, dehydration,[10] lack of cardiovascular conditioning, and lack of acclimatization to heat. Because all of these factors can be anticipated and corrected, exertional heatstroke is preventable.

Diagnosis

Early diagnosis is critical to prevent life-threatening complications. People who experience weakness or undue fatigue, lack of concentration or confusion, light-headedness or dizziness, headaches, nausea, or muscle cramps in the heat should cease exercise, get to a cool environment, and drink cool fluids to avert more serious heat injury. They should also be sure that medical help is available if symptoms progress.

Clinical features Despite differences in pathophysiology and epidemiology, the major manifestations of the classic and exertional heatstroke syndromes are similar. An abrupt rise in body temperature is universal; most patients with heatstroke have core temperatures in excess of 40.5° C (105° F). Disordered mentation is no less common and may span a spectrum ranging from confusion and lethargy to delirium, stupor, coma, and seizures. Despite the dramatic central nervous system manifestation of extreme hyperthermia, most patients who survive do not exhibit neurologic impairment.[11] Virtually all patients with heatstroke also exhibit cardiovascular abnormalities. Tachycardia is present in most patients, and hypotension is present in many; shock, arrhythmias, myocardial ischemia, and pulmonary edema are most likely to occur early in elderly or debilitated patients with classic heatstroke but are also frequent preterminal events in patients with exertional heatstroke. Most heatstroke victims present with hyperventilation; pulmonary abnormalities may also include pulmonary edema, acute respiratory distress syndrome, and aspiration pneumonia. Other common clinical manifestations of heatstroke include oliguria, vomiting, and diarrhea; hematuria and gastrointestinal bleeding may reflect disseminated intravascular coagulation (DIC). One cutaneous manifestation of heatstroke is hemorrhagic diathesis; the skin is hot and dry in many patients with classic heatstroke but is often moist and clammy in patients with exertional heatstroke.

Laboratory findings Laboratory abnormalities in patients with heatstroke reflect widespread damage to a number of organ systems. Leukocytosis is common, and hemoconcentration may raise the hematocrit in patients who are volume depleted. Thrombocytopenia is frequently present and may be severe; prolonged prothrombin times, depressed fibrinogen levels, and elevated levels of fibrin split products indicate DIC, which is more common in exertional heatstroke than in classic heatstroke. DIC in heatstroke has been attributed to direct thermal injury to vascular endothelium; clinically significant bleeding may result from the coagulopathy, which can persist for 36 hours after the onset of heatstroke.

Renal abnormalities are common in heatstroke. The urine may sometimes be dilute despite hypotension and oliguria; hematuria, myoglobinuria, proteinuria, and casts are frequently observed. The blood urea nitrogen (BUN) and creatinine levels are usually elevated; acute renal failure occurs in about one third of patients with exertional heatstroke but is less common in patients with classic heatstroke.

Elevated bilirubin levels in patients with heatstroke may reflect hepatic injury, hemolysis, or both. Elevated transaminase levels are the rule, reflecting damage to both liver and muscle cells. Elevated creatine phosphokinase (CPK) and aldolase levels indicate muscle injury; severe rhabdomyolysis with myoglobinuria and renal failure is much more common in exertional than in classic heatstroke.

Heatstroke causes numerous metabolic abnormalities. Respiratory alkalosis is common early in the syndrome, particularly in classic heatstroke; lactic acidosis may supervene, particularly in exertional heatstroke. Potassium levels are variable, sometimes being low early and high later in the course of heatstroke. Hypophosphatemia is the rule; hypokalemia may occur, particularly in exertional heatstroke. Hypoglycemia, perhaps reflecting depletion of glycogen stores, has been reported in many patients with exertional heatstroke. Electrocardiographic abnormalities include conduction disturbances and ST-T segment changes.[12] Elevated levels of pyrogenic cytokines have been reported in heatstroke patients,[13] but it is unclear whether the cytokines participate in the pathogenesis of heatstroke or simply reflect a subsequent host response to tissue injury.

Differential Diagnosis

The differential diagnosis of elevated body temperature with numerous clinical and laboratory abnormalities is broad and includes sepsis, the systemic inflammatory response syndrome, and the other causes of hyperthermia. In practical terms, the major challenge is to distinguish classic heatstroke from sepsis and to distinguish exertional heatstroke from less severe exercise-induced abnormalities, such as exertional hyperthermia and heat exhaustion.[7]

Treatment

Heatstroke necessitates prompt and aggressive therapy. Lowering body temperature is the crucial element in management; because the pathogenesis of heatstroke involves thermoregulatory failure rather than an elevated hypothalamic set point, physical cooling is essential, but antipyretic medications are ineffective.

Field management includes removing the patient's clothing, fanning the patient, and bathing the patient's skin with cool water; ice packs should be applied if they are available. Hypothermic mattresses or, in urgent circumstances, ice-water immersion may be employed. These treatments are very uncomfortable and should be used only when the hyperthermia is truly deleterious. The patient should be protected from sunlight and should be moved to a cool environment and evacuated to an emergency ward as soon as possible. First-aid measures to maintain the patient's airway and prevent injury are important. Cool intravenous fluids should be administered as soon as parenteral therapy becomes available, but oral hydration is inadvisable because of the risk of aspiration.

Physical cooling must continue after the patient arrives in the emergency ward; many techniques are available, but choosing among them is problematic. Immersion in ice water has been a standard approach. Another traditional technique is the application of ice packs to the body surface. Both techniques have the disadvantage of producing cutaneous vasoconstriction, which could impede the transfer of heat from the body's surface; ice-water baths may also pose logistic difficulties in heatstroke patients who are combative and in those with seizures, vomiting, or diarrhea. Despite these drawbacks, ice-water baths are effective; there were no fatalities in a series of 252 marine recruits whose therapy for exertional heatstroke included ice-water immersion.[14] A newer technique for cooling relies on evaporation rather than conduction to dissipate heat: the patient is sprayed with water at 15° C, then warm air at 30° to 35° C is blown on the patient. A special body-cooling unit that facilitates evaporative cooling has been used with good results in Saudi Arabia.[15] Although alcohol is more volatile than water, the former should not be used for evaporative cooling because of the risk of alcohol intoxication, especially in children. Many other cooling techniques, ranging from ice-water enemas and gastric lavage to the use of the downdraft from helicopter blades, have been used to treat heatstroke but are of secondary importance. In general, hospitals in the United States should choose a cooling technique on the basis of their experience and facilities.

Body temperature should be monitored continuously during cooling; in most cases, body temperature will decline significantly in 10 to 40 minutes, at which time cooling should be reduced to avoid hypothermic overshoot with shivering and rigors.

The administration of room-temperature intravenous fluids is an important aspect of therapy, helping to lower core temperature and to correct dehydration; meticulous cardiovascular monitoring is essential to prevent fluid overload while ensuring adequate volume replacement. In addition to needing cardiovascular support, patients with heatstroke require careful respiratory monitoring and support, along with fluid and electrolyte monitoring and therapy. Complications such as rhabdomyolysis, renal failure, aspiration pneumonia, DIC, and seizures necessitate additional therapeutic interventions. Despite its efficacy in malignant hyperthermia of anesthesia (see below), dantrolene sodium is ineffective in heatstroke.[13]

Prevention

Even with aggressive therapy, heatstroke has an appreciable mortality. Most patients who recover have normal thermoregulatory mechanisms and heat tolerance, but all should be instructed on ways to reduce the risk of recurrences. Classic heatstroke can be prevented by publicizing community heat-wave alerts; providing cool environments for people at risk; instructing those at risk to limit sun exposure and maintain adequate hydration; and promoting judicious use of diuretics, tranquilizers, antidepressants, and anticholinergic medications.

NEUROLEPTIC MALIGNANT SYNDROME

First described in 1968, the neuroleptic malignant syndrome (NMS) is uncommon, occurring in fewer than 1% of patients receiving neuroleptic agents. NMS usually occurs within the first 30 days of therapy; haloperidol is most often implicated, but various phenothiazines, butyrophenones, and thioxanthenes may also be responsible.[16] NMS may also be precipitated by the withdrawal of amantadine, levodopa, or other dopaminergic drugs used to treat Parkinson disease.[17] In some cases, dehydration and agitation are contributing factors.[18]

NMS is primarily a disorder of excessive heat production. It is probably precipitated by the blockade of dopaminergic receptors in the corpus striatum, leading to uncontrolled contractions of skeletal muscle, which, in turn, produce excessive body heat. There is no genetic predisposition for NMS, nor does it occur as a result of a drug overdose. Physical exhaustion, dehydration, and underlying organic brain syndromes have been cited as predisposing factors. Some patients who have recovered from NMS have subsequently received neuroleptic agents without suffering recurrences of NMS, but recurrent NMS does develop in 30% of patients who are rechallenged with neuroleptics.

Diagnosis

The clinical features of NMS evolve rapidly, usually over a period of 1 to 3 days. Hyperthermia is universal. Other symptoms include severe muscular rigidity; altered sensorium; autonomic dysfunction that produces tachycardia, labile blood pressure, and diaphoresis; and extrapyramidal abnormalities. Laboratory abnormalities include hypernatremia and other electrolyte abnormalities, acidosis, hemoconcentration and leukocytosis, rhabdomyolysis, and abnormal findings on renal and hepatic function tests.

The differential diagnosis of NMS includes infections and lethal catatonia,[19] an uncommon psychiatric disorder in which agitation progresses to muscular rigidity and hyperthermia.

Treatment

The offending neuroleptic agent must be withdrawn in all cases of NMS. Meticulous fluid and electrolyte therapy and careful cardiovascular support are also mandatory. Dantrolene sodium, a muscle relaxant, and bromocriptine, a dopamine agonist, have each been reported to reduce the duration of hyperthermia, but these agents have not been evaluated in controlled trials.[20] Physical cooling as treatment for NMS has not been evaluated in clinical trials but should prove useful in the acute phase of the disorder.

MALIGNANT HYPERTHERMIA OF ANESTHESIA

Like NMS, malignant hyperthermia of anesthesia (MHA) is a high-mortality disorder of involuntary skeletal muscle hyperactivity and excessive heat production triggered by a pharmacologic agent. Unlike NMS, however, MHA is a genetically determined disorder precipitated by anesthetic agents such as halogenated inhalation agents and depolarizing muscle relaxants. Patients who are susceptible to MHA may be identified by a family history of the disorder and by performance of a muscle biopsy and a caffeine-halothane contracture test.[21]

Diagnosis

MHA usually begins shortly after the anesthetic is administered, but it may be delayed for hours. Muscular rigidity and severe hyperthermia are typical; other findings include tachycardia, hypotension, arrhythmias, hyperpnea, hypoxia, hypercapnia, hyperkalemia, lactic acidosis, rhabdomyolysis, and DIC.

Treatment

MHA is an anesthetic emergency. The treatment of choice is intravenously administered dantrolene sodium, which has markedly improved the prognosis of MHA. Discontinuance of anesthesia is mandatory; physical cooling is therapeutically important, as are cardiopulmonary support and correction of the metabolic abnormalities.

Fever

Fever has been recognized as a cardinal feature of disease since antiquity, but only recently has the pathophysiology of fever come to be understood. Only with the work of Dr. Paul Beeson in 1948 did it become clear that the ultimate cause of fever is not a bacterial product (a so-called exogenous pyrogen) but a product of host inflammatory cells (i.e., an endogenous pyrogen). For years, the endogenous pyrogen was thought to be a product of polymorphonuclear leukocytes and was referred to as leukocytic pyrogen. Exciting studies, however, have demonstrated that mononuclear phagocytes are the principal source of endogenous pyrogen and that a variety of mononuclear cell products—cytokines—can mediate the febrile response.[22,23] Cytokines are also important as mediators of the acute-phase response to infection and inflammation.

PATHOGENESIS

The cytokines interleukin-1 (IL-1), IL-6, interferon gamma, and tumor necrosis factor (TNF) function as pyrogens by acting directly on the hypothalamus to elevate the thermal set point. A variety of stimuli, such as microorganisms, exposure to endotoxin and other bacterial toxins or microbial products, phagocytosis, antigen-antibody immune complexes, and various forms of tissue injury, can initiate IL-1 production by mononuclear phagocytes and many other cells. In the pathogenesis of fever, IL-1 acts as a hormone in that it is carried by the circulation from the local inflammatory site of production to the CNS, where it acts directly on the hypothalamic thermal control center. Its mechanism of action appears to involve induction of phospholipases, which in turn cause the release of arachidonic acids from membrane phospholipids. As a result, prostaglandin levels rise, particularly levels of prostaglandin E. Elevated levels of prostaglandins appear to be important in raising the hypothalamic thermal set point; this mechanism accounts for why prostaglandin inhibitors such as aspirin are effective antipyretic agents.

Although this classic model of pathogenesis has been validated by numerous studies of fever, new research suggests that several additional pathways may be involved. For example, pyrogenic cytokines may be produced locally in the CNS as well as systemically,[24] and cytokines may signal the thermal control center by neural as well as hormonal mechanisms.[25]

Once the hypothalamic thermal set point has been elevated, thermoregulatory mechanisms are brought into play to raise the body temperature to the level of the new set point. Autonomic efferents lead to heat conservation through cutaneous vasoconstriction and cessation of sweating. Somatic nerves are responsible for increasing heat production via increased skeletal muscle tone or shivering. The myalgias that accompany many febrile states may in part be caused by this increased muscle tone. Rigor, which is a dramatic precursor of some fever spikes, is nothing more than an exaggerated form of shivering that rapidly elevates body temperature in response to an increased hypothalamic thermal set point.

CONSEQUENCES OF ELEVATED BODY TEMPERATURE

Possible Benefits of Fever

Although fever is a common response to infection in many species, there is no direct evidence that it is beneficial to host defense mechanisms in humans. However, new insights into the immunostimulatory properties of IL-1 and TNF have led to speculation that fever itself may promote recovery from infection.[26] IL-1 and TNF appear to act across species, order, and class barriers and probably evolved 300 million years ago; this evolutionary stability further suggests that fever plays a role in host defense mechanisms.

In humans, fever appears to decrease serum iron levels. Many microbes need iron for growth, and it has been suggested that fever-induced hypoferremia is a helpful host defense mechanism. Fever is also marked by a metabolic shift away from glucose, an excellent substrate for bacteria, to fat and protein as energy sources. In addition, some microbes, including gonococci and *Treponema pallidum,* are quite heat sensitive and can be killed in experimental animals by artificially induced fevers. However, natural infection never produces body temperatures that are high enough to have this effect.

Extreme pyrexia may be surprisingly well tolerated. It seems likely that the widespread tissue damage, multiple laboratory abnormalities, and high mortality observed in disorders such as heatstroke, MHA, thyroid storm, and NMS are caused by the underlying disorder rather than the elevated temperature itself. Indeed, in the preantibiotic era, fever therapy was well tolerated, with little evidence of tissue damage, despite the fact that temperatures as high as 41.7° C (107.1° F) were induced.

Therapeutic hyperthermia is being used to treat noninfectious diseases. Regional hyperthermia is a traditional therapy for many musculoskeletal disorders. Such techniques as heating pads, whirlpools, and ultrasonography have all been used to increase the temperature of injured tissues. Despite widespread endorsements by patients and practitioners, however, heat treatments for musculoskeletal injuries have not been subjected to controlled clinical trials. Hyperthermia is also being investigated for a possible role in treating malignancies. Adjunctive regional hyperthermia often improves the rate of response when compared with radiotherapy or chemotherapy; superficial tumors respond most favorably, but better responses may be obtained with internal malignancies as techniques for deep heating are improved.

Complications

Pyrexia can have deleterious consequences, but complications depend more on the underlying cause of the temperature elevation and the patient's overall condition than on the level of the temperature. Elevated body temperatures are most harmful to the very young and very old. Because pyrexia increases oxygen consumption, it imposes circulatory demands that may precipitate ischemia, arrhythmias, or congestive heart failure in patients with cardiovascular disease. Febrile seizures are a risk in children between 6 months and 6 years of age. Although febrile convulsions are generally benign, they are alarming, and it is always necessary to exclude underlying neurologic illnesses, including meningitis. Both intravenous diazepam and intranasal midazolam are effective in controlling febrile convulsions.[27] In the absence of unprovoked seizures, long-term anticonvulsant therapy is usually unnecessary in children with febrile seizures and may even be deleterious; diazepam, administered orally only when fever occurs, safely and effectively reduces the risk of recurrent febrile seizures.[28] The long-term prognosis is excellent.[29]

Febrile seizures do not occur in adults, but fever often results in decreased concentration and sleepiness; high temperatures commonly produce an altered sensorium, including stupor and delirium. Patients with strokes are at risk for additional brain injury from fever[30]; the result is a marked increase in morbidity and mortality,[31] especially when the pyrexia occurs soon after the stroke.[32] Because of this, even modest elevations in temperature should be suppressed in patients with acute strokes.[33] In addition, moderate induced hypothermia may improve the outcome of strokes, even in patients who are afebrile on presentation.[34,35]

DIAGNOSIS

Body temperature can be measured in several ways. In most clinical circumstances, rectal temperature is an accurate reflection of central (core) temperature. Sublingual temperature measurements are also useful but are more subject to technical variation, especially when patients are unable to fully cooperate. The presence of cerumen may introduce error into tympanic membrane temperature measurements, which are otherwise accurate. Axillary temperature measurements are often inaccurate[36] but are often used in the sickest patients.

TREATMENT

The approach to the febrile patient involves three elements: diagnosis and management of the underlying disorder; cardiac, respiratory, and metabolic support; and, when indicated, lowering of body temperature. Infection is the leading cause of elevated body temperature; all febrile patients should be systematically evaluated for infection, and antibiotics should be administered whenever appropriate.

In patients with extreme pyrexia, additional laboratory studies are important both to screen for hyperthermia caused by thermoregulatory defects and to assess tissue damage. Electrolytes, coagulation parameters, muscle enzymes, and arterial blood gases should all be measured, and renal and liver function should be assessed. Studies of thyroid and adrenal function may be indicated. Cardiac function, blood pressure, urine output, and neurologic status should be monitored closely. Adequate hydration is mandatory, and circulatory or respiratory support may be necessary.

Proper management of the elevated temperature itself depends on the clinical circumstances. Although clinicians usually choose to suppress fever, it is unclear whether elevated body temperatures promote or impede recovery from infection[37]; similarly, the risks and benefits of antipyretic therapy have not yet been defined.[38] Because many patients tolerate high body temperatures very well, antipyretic therapy may actually produce more discomfort than the pyrexia itself. In other patients, myalgias, flushing, fatigue, loss of concentration, shivering, or chills can be very uncomfortable, and antipyretic therapy should be used for symptomatic relief. Significant pyrexia should always be treated in patients with strokes, in young children, in elderly or debilitated patients, and in persons with cardiopulmonary disease, because these patient groups are most likely to suffer adverse consequences. Hyperthermia should be treated in all patients with malignant hyperthermia of anesthesia, heatstroke, NMS, or thyroid storm. Finally, it may be prudent to treat any patient whose temperature exceeds 40.0° C (104.0° F), even a healthy young adult.

The choice of cooling technique depends on the pathogenesis of the temperature elevation [*see Figure 1*]. In patients with fever caused by infection or other inflammatory states, an elevated hypothalamic thermal set point is responsible for the pyrexia. Aspirin or acetaminophen should be used to lower the set point; the drugs seem equally effective as antipyretics, but acetaminophen is preferred in pediatric patients because aspirin may precipitate Reye syndrome in children with influenza or varicella. A broad range of nonsteroidal anti-inflammatory drugs (NSAIDs) can also lower the set point.[39] If physical cooling methods are used before antipyretic drugs are fully effective, homeostatic mechanisms will continue to operate in an attempt to raise body temperature, resulting in intense vasoconstriction and shivering,[40] which produce adverse cardiovascular and metabolic effects as well as intense patient discomfort. To avoid these problems, febrile patients who require physical cooling to rapidly lower body temperature should be heavily sedated and ventilated to prevent shivering in conjunction with physical cooling.[41] In contrast, physical cooling is the treatment of choice for patients with hyperthermia. In all patients, careful attention is required to prevent hypothermic overshoot on the one hand and recurrent fever on the other.[42] Although pyrexia may be the most spectacular symptom, meticulous attention to the underlying disorder is of primary importance in all cases.

Fever of Undetermined Origin

FUO presents one of the most challenging and perplexing problems in clinical medicine. Such fevers may persist for weeks or months in the absence of characteristic clinical findings or clues. Ultimately, most such obscure fevers prove to be caused by common diseases presenting in an atypical fashion rather than by rare and exotic illnesses.

Table 2 Causes of Fever of Undetermined Origin Over 4 Decades

Cause	Study				
	New Haven, 1961[43] (% of 100 Patients)	*Boston, 1973[77] (% of 128 Patients)*	*Seattle, 1982[78] (% of 105 Patients)*	*Leuven, Belgium, 1992[79] (% of 199 Patients*)*	*Rhode Island, 1992[45] (% of 89 Patients)*
Infections	36	35	30	23	33
Neoplasms	19	23	31	7	24
Collagen vascular diseases	13	16	9	18	16
Other specific causes	25	18	18	29	18
Undiagnosed	7	8	12	23	9

*Percentages have been modified to conform to the diagnostic criteria used in the American series.

Petersdorf and Beeson in their classic monograph[43] specified three criteria to define FUO:

1. Duration: at least 3 weeks. This requirement eliminates from consideration most short-lived fevers of indeterminate or viral origin and most postoperative fevers.
2. Magnitude: a temperature that is greater than 38.3° C (101.0° F) on at least several occasions. This criterion eliminates from consideration persons with unusually prominent circadian fluctuations in body temperature with daily readings on the order of 38.0° C (100.4° F). If such persons are not clinically ill, their elevated temperature should not cause too much concern.
3. Obscure nature: perplexing enough to defy diagnosis after 1 week of study. In the past, inpatient study was required to evaluate FUO, but with changing admission practices, intelligent and invasive outpatient study is now considered sufficient.[44]

ETIOLOGIC CLASSIFICATION

Although geographic factors are relevant, the leading causes of FUO are reasonably uniform throughout the United States. The relative frequency of the etiologic categories responsible for FUO have been relatively stable over the past 4 decades [*see Table 2*]. In a community hospital study,[45] noninvasive studies provided the diagnosis in 42% of patients, with serologies and lysis centrifugation blood cultures being the most useful noninvasive techniques. Computed tomography–guided percutaneous biopsies were the most useful invasive procedures. Only 9% of patients remained undiagnosed. With an increasing population of immunosuppressed and chronically ill patients, the relative importance of the disorders that cause FUO may change. As a result, it may be prudent to consider so-called classic FUO separately from FUO in patients with HIV infection, neutropenia, or nosocomial fevers.[46,47] Despite changes in host factors and diagnostic techniques, the basic categorization of the causes of FUO remains valid.

Infections

In the initial evaluation of FUO, the possibility of infection should be carefully considered.

Systemic infections The two major systemic infections to consider in the evaluation of FUO are tuberculosis (usually disseminated but sometimes confined predominantly to the liver and spleen) and infective endocarditis [*see Table 3*]. Most FUO cases caused by miliary tuberculosis arise in elderly patients in whom dissemination has followed activation of quiescent foci. Often, in cases caused by miliary tuberculosis, the intermediate-strength (5 tuberculin units) purified protein derivative skin test is negative, and miliary pulmonary lesions are not present on the chest x-ray. Anemia, leukopenia, or, rarely, a leukemoid reaction caused by bone marrow involvement may be evident; bone marrow biopsy is a very helpful diagnostic test in patients in whom miliary tuberculosis is suspected. An isolated elevation of the serum alkaline phosphatase level may indicate miliary involvement of the liver by tuberculosis, other infection, or neoplasm. The histologic findings on liver biopsy often suggest the diagnosis, and a por-

Table 3 Causes of Fever of Undetermined Origin

Systemic Infections
- Tuberculosis (miliary)
- Infective endocarditis (primarily bacterial endocarditis but also endocarditis with a fungal, Q fever, or chlamydial etiology)
- Bacteremia from an inapparent primary focus
- Chronic meningococcemia
- Brucellosis
- Listeriosis, vibriosis, leptospirosis, relapsing fever (caused by *Borrelia recurrentis*), rat-bite fever (caused by either *Streptobacillus moniliformis* or *Spirillum minus*)
- Miscellaneous
- Psittacosis, toxoplasmosis (disseminated acquired form), Q fever, disseminated deep mycotic infections (e.g., histoplasmosis, blastomycosis, cryptococcosis), cytomegalovirus infection, Whipple disease

Localized Infections and Abscesses
- Hepatic infections
- Liver abscess
- Cholangitis
- Intraperitoneal infections
- Upper abdomen: empyema of gallbladder, pericholecystic and subhepatic abscesses, right or left subphrenic abscesses, lesser sac abscess
- Lower abdomen: periappendiceal and peridiverticular abscesses
- Other intra-abdominal abscesses
- Tubo-ovarian abscess, pelvic inflammatory disease, pelvic abscess
- Retroperitoneal abscess, pancreatic abscess
- Urinary tract infections
- Perinephric abscess
- Renal carbuncle
- Pyelonephritis with ureteral obstruction and pyonephrosis
- Prostatic abscess

Neoplasms
- Hematopoietic malignancies: Hodgkin disease and other lymphomas, leukemias, myeloid metaplasia, malignant histiocytosis
- Other malignancies: renal cell cancer, colon cancer, hepatoma
- Benign neoplasms: left atrial myxoma, pheochromocytoma

Collagen Vascular Diseases
- Temporal arteritis, adult-onset juvenile rheumatoid arthritis, Wegener granulomatosis, polyarteritis, systemic lupus erythematosus, relapsing polychondritis

Granulomatous Diseases
- Sarcoidosis, idiopathic granulomatous hepatitis

Metabolic and Hereditary Disorders
- Familial Mediterranean fever, Fabry disease

Endocrine Disorders
- Adrenal insufficiency, thyrotoxicosis, hyperparathyroidism

Thermoregulatory Disorders
- Hypothalamic dysfunction (e.g., caused by strokes or tumors), encephalitis

Drug Fever
- Antimicrobial agents (β-lactam antibiotics, sulfonamides, nitrofurantoin, isoniazid), antihypertensives (hydralazine), anticonvulsants (phenytoin), allopurinol, and many others

Miscellaneous Conditions
- Pulmonary emboli, alcoholic hepatitis and cirrhosis, inflammatory bowel disease, thrombophlebitis, factitious fever

tion of the specimen should always be cultured for the presence of tubercle bacilli.

Infective endocarditis, usually subacute, is also an important diagnostic consideration. Most patients with subacute bacterial endocarditis have a heart murmur. In about 5% of cases, however, particularly in the elderly, the murmur may be absent or may be considered functional. Blood cultures would be expected to provide the diagnosis in a patient with subacute bacterial endocarditis, particularly because only 5% of patients with endocarditis have negative blood cultures. The leading cause of negative blood cultures in patients with endocarditis is the prior administration of antibiotics. It is therefore very important that a number of blood cultures be obtained, including some as long as 5 to 10 days after antibiotics have been withdrawn. Other causes of culture-negative endocarditis that should be considered in patients with FUO include infection with fastidious bacteria, chlamydial infection, and Q fever. Careful scrutiny for the peripheral stigmas of endocarditis is essential in the evaluation of any patient with FUO. Echocardiography may reveal valvular vegetations in patients with endocarditis; transesophageal studies are more sensitive but more invasive than transthoracic echocardiography. Left atrial myxomas mimic culture-negative endocarditis but may be detected with echocardiography.

Other systemic infections, including bacteremias that occur in the absence of any obvious primary site of involvement, only rarely cause FUO [*see Table 3*]. Viral infections are usually self-limited and do not produce fevers that last longer than 3 weeks. Important exceptions to this generalization are Epstein-Barr virus (EBV)[48] and cytomegalovirus (CMV) infections, which may occasionally present as FUO (often with some mononucleosis-like features) in otherwise well individuals. More frequently, CMV infection develops in patients who have received multiple blood transfusions or who have undergone organ transplantation; CMV is the cause of 50% of all febrile episodes in renal transplant recipients.

Localized infections The more common types of localized infection that present as FUO include hepatic abscess, subphrenic abscess, and subhepatic and pericholecystic abscess [*see Table 3*]. Liver abscesses are often occult; the physician should look for a history that includes symptoms of biliary tract disease, recent blunt abdominal trauma, or travel, which might suggest the diagnosis of amebiasis. Hepatomegaly may be absent initially. The serum alkaline phosphatase level is usually elevated even when the abscess is solitary. Serologic tests for amebiasis are positive in patients with amebic liver abscess. Elevation of the diaphragm, particularly when accompanied by overlying pulmonary atelectasis or a pleural effusion, should raise suspicion of a subphrenic abscess. Ultrasonography and CT are valuable in identifying such collections; gallium scans are less useful for this purpose.

Localized infection in the urinary tract is an important consideration in a patient with FUO; perinephric abscess and renal carbuncle are best diagnosed by ultrasonography or CT. Many other localized infections occasionally present as FUO; occult dental infections are one such example and illustrate the need for thoroughness in the evaluation of patients with obscure fevers.

Neoplasms

Lymphoma, particularly Hodgkin disease, is the most common neoplastic cause of obscure fever. Lymphoma may be difficult to diagnose when the principal site of involvement is the retroperitoneal nodes, but abdominal CT scans greatly facilitate this diagnosis. Although so-called Pel-Ebstein recurrent fevers suggest Hodgkin disease, they are observed in only a minority of patients with this disorder. The development of fever in a patient who has myeloma or chronic lymphocytic leukemia is usually caused by superimposed infection and not by the neoplastic process. In some patients, however, the febrile course appears to be caused by the leukemia itself. Occasionally, a patient with the preleukemia syndrome will present with fever and atypical blood and bone marrow changes, suggesting myeloid metaplasia or a leukemoid response. Only after some months can the hematologic picture be established as leukemia.

Solid tumors can also be associated with fever; hypernephroma is the leading example. As many as 10% of patients with colorectal carcinoma present with fever; either extension of the tumor through the bowel wall, producing a paracolonic abscess, or necrosis and abscess formation in a polypoid intraluminal lesion may be the underlying mechanism. Metastatic cancer may be responsible for continuing fever; hepatic involvement is not necessary for fever to occur. Occasionally, a neuroblastoma involving bone or soft tissues or a pheochromocytoma may have a febrile course. Fevers caused by malignant disease often respond to therapy with NSAIDs; fevers caused by infections may be less likely to respond completely to these agents.[49]

Collagen Vascular Disease

A variety of connective tissue disorders and vasculitides may produce prolonged fevers before the development of articular or other characteristic manifestations. In the elderly, polymyalgia rheumatica and the closely related disorder giant cell arteritis (temporal arteritis) are the most common connective tissue disorders presenting as FUO. Malaise, weight loss, muscle weakness, mild arthralgias without overt arthritis, and a markedly elevated erythrocyte sedimentation rate (often > 100 mm/hr) are usual features. Jaw claudication, visual symptoms, and a tender or thickened temporal artery suggest the diagnosis of giant cell arteritis. As many as 15% of cases of giant cell arteritis present as FUO, and in some patients, the vasculitis itself remains occult. Similarly, virtually all patients with adult-onset Still disease are febrile,[50] and systemic symptoms such as fever and weakness may antedate by weeks or months the evolution of the more characteristic clinical manifestations of adult juvenile rheumatoid arthritis. In other patients, involvement of the paranasal sinuses and mastoid or the rapid excavation of a pulmonary lesion suggests Wegener granulomatosis. Many other connective tissue diseases, ranging from classic vasculitides such as systemic lupus erythematosus to uncommon disorders such as relapsing polychondritis, can also present as FUO.

Less Common Etiologic Categories

Granulomatous disease Granulomatous diseases of noninfectious origin may be responsible for FUO. Prolonged fever is uncommon in sarcoidosis, but when it does occur, prominent hilar adenopathy, ocular involvement, erythema nodosum, and hepatic granulomas are usually also present. Biopsy of involved lymph nodes, muscle, or liver usually shows noncaseating granulomas. In addition to sarcoidosis, there are about 40 diseases that may be associated with hepatic granulomas. Treatable infectious granulomatous diseases (e.g., tuberculosis, brucellosis, histoplasmosis, and cat-scratch disease) must be ruled out by cultures, skin tests, serologic tests, and special stains of tissue biopsy specimens. In rare instances, despite extensive investigation and therapeutic trials with antituberculous drugs, an etiologic diagnosis cannot be made in patients with noncaseating hepatic granulomas who have a febrile illness of many months' duration.[51] Beneficial results have been achieved in such cases by giving corticosteroids after excluding the other specific granulomatous diseases; methotrexate also appears to be helpful.[52] Corticosteroids have been beneficial for other patients with idiopathic granulomatosis and FUO.[53] Starch peritonitis represents a febrile granulomatous response to starch introduced on surgical gloves. The nature of the process may not be appreciated for weeks; the initial supposition is that a doughy abdominal mass and fever are caused by a postoperative abscess.

Inflammatory bowel disease Bowel symptoms are prominent in almost all patients with idiopathic ulcerative colitis, granulomatous colitis, or regional enteritis, and the diagnosis is obvious in such febrile patients. Occasionally, however, bowel symptoms may not be marked or may be of such long duration that they become accepted as the norm. In this setting, FUO may be the presenting complaint in a patient with inflammatory bowel disease.

Alcoholic hepatitis and cirrhosis Fever is occasionally observed in cases of cirrhosis.[54] Attention should first be directed to possible complicating infections—such as spontaneous bacterial peritonitis, enterogenous bacteremias, or tuberculosis—or to an unrelated process. Active hepatocellular necrosis may occur in the course of alcoholic hepatitis and may account for low-grade fever.

Pulmonary emboli In rare instances, a patient may have multiple small pulmonary emboli, but no significant changes in arterial blood gases or on the chest film will be apparent; the patient will present primarily with a problem of unexplained fever. The fever may exceed 39.0° C (102.2° F), but high-grade fevers caused by pulmonary emboli seldom persist longer than 1 week. Thrombophlebitis itself may be a source of protracted fever, even in the absence of pulmonary emboli.

Drug fever Drug fever frequently occurs in the absence of other manifestations of hypersensitivity, such as rash and eosinophilia. Antimicrobial agents (e.g., β-lactams, sulfonamides, nitrofurantoin, or isoniazid), antihypertensives (e.g., hydralazine or methyldopa), anticonvulsants (e.g., phenytoin), and allopurinol are among the most common offenders, but many other drugs have been implicated. In most instances, the diagnosis of drug fever is considered within the first several weeks of onset of FUO, and any recently administered drugs are discontinued. Several drugs, however, such as phenytoin, methyldopa, and isoniazid, may not produce drug fever until weeks or months after their initial use. Drugs such as these may be overlooked just because they have been administered for some time without producing side effects. Intramuscular injections of analgesics can produce FUO, which may or may not be accompanied by the presence of a sterile abscess or other gross evidence of tissue injury.

Factitious fever In rare instances, a patient may simulate illness by deliberately producing false elevations in temperature.[55] Factitious fever is one of the most challenging etiologic categories of FUO. The patients are usually female and are often paramedical personnel. The underlying problem may be malingering or a more complicated emotional disorder. Discordance between the marked temperature elevations and the pulse rate, distortion of the usual diurnal temperature curve, and absence of diaphoresis when the fever abates suggest the diagnosis.

Miscellaneous causes The diagnosis of familial Mediterranean fever is suggested by ethnic background, episodic occurrence of fever in association with abdominal pain or other signs of polyserositis, and well-being between attacks. The diagnosis can be difficult when recurrent fever is the only symptom[56]; molecular techniques can facilitate the diagnosis of various hereditary periodic fever syndromes.[57]

Whipple disease is a multisystem infection caused by the gram-positive actinomycete *Tropheryma whippelii*. It may present as a prolonged febrile illness with weight loss, arthralgias, and weakness. Special tissue culture and immunodiagnostic tests are being studied[58]; a polymerase chain reaction test for the causative organism has been developed,[59] but false positive reactions have been reported.[60] Inflammatory pseudotumor of intra-abdominal lymph nodes may present as FUO[61]; the clinical features of this disorder may resemble those of Whipple disease, but the pathologic findings are distinctive, and surgical excision of the involved nodes may induce prolonged remissions. Kikuchi-Fujimoto disease is another rare cause of fever and lymphadenopathy.[62]

CNS lesions are decidedly uncommon causes of FUO, except in very obtunded patients with extensive brain damage. Endocrinologic abnormalities, such as subacute thyroiditis, or metabolic disorders, such as hypertriglyceridemia, hypercholesterolemia, or glycosphingolipid storage disease (Fabry disease), may occasionally present as FUO. Many other disorders as diverse as pernicious anemia[63] and renal malacoplakia[64] have been identified as rare causes of FUO.

FUO in Patients with AIDS

Fever is extremely common in patients infected with HIV; typically, the diagnostic challenge is not in determining the source of fever but in deciding which of several potentially pyrogenic processes is most important. However, patients infected with HIV can also present with prolonged, diagnostically obscure fevers. Most often, such patients have advanced AIDS, with CD4 cell counts of less than 100/mm^3.[65] Infections account for more than 75% of FUO cases in such patients[66]; in one series, the more common diagnoses were disseminated *Mycobacterium avium* complex (31%), *Pneumocystis carinii* pneumonia (13%), CMV infection (11%), disseminated histoplasmosis (7%), and lymphoma (7%).[67] Other infectious etiologies are toxoplasmosis, cryptococcosis, salmonellosis, and varicella-zoster virus infections. In Europe, leishmaniasis is also an important cause of FUO in patients with AIDS.[66] Among noninfectious etiologies, lymphoma and drug fever are most prominent. HIV itself is an uncommon cause of FUO. Blood cultures are the most useful diagnostic tests; although more invasive, bone marrow,[68] liver,[69] or lymph node biopsies may provide more rapid diagnosis by allowing direct visualization of organisms. Other useful tests include CT of the chest and abdomen and a serum cryptococcal antigen determination.

DIAGNOSIS

With rare exceptions, neither the temperature nor the pattern of fever permits discrimination between the causes of FUO. Detailed review of the history is essential, particularly regarding travel, animal exposure, occupational risks, and other epidemiologic factors; previous trauma or surgery; or features relevant to each of the diagnoses outlined. When physical findings are being evaluated, particular attention should be paid to structures that may be inapparent sources of obscure fever, such as the cardiovascular system, abdominal viscera, and genitourinary tract. Lymph nodes should be examined not only in the usual distribution but also in the epitrochlear areas and along the medial aspect of the upper arm. Search of the skin, nail beds, and mucous membranes for petechiae and vasculitic lesions may provide important clues to the diagnosis of endocarditis or of collagen vascular diseases. Funduscopic examination may reveal choroidal tubercles or signs of vasculitis or endocarditis. Rectal examination is particularly important in elderly or obtunded patients, in whom a perirectal or prostatic abscess may be overlooked.

Common Laboratory Studies

Blood cultures Blood cultures should include aerobic (5% to 10% CO_2 tension) and anaerobic cultures that have been incubated for at least 2 weeks. Newer blood culture techniques, including the use of lysis centrifugation and the BACTEC radiometric mycobacterial culture system, may be helpful, particularly in HIV-positive patients.

Serologic tests Serologic tests often employed in cases of FUO include *Brucella* and *Salmonella* agglutinations (usually not very helpful), antistreptolysin O (ASO) titer if acute rheumatic fever is suspected, Venereal Disease Research Laboratories (VDRL) test for syphilis, serologic tests for less common infections (e.g., psittacosis, toxoplasmosis, and CMV), the test for rheumatoid factor, and antinuclear antibody tests. A serum specimen obtained during an acute-phase host response can be frozen for subsequent comparison with a late-phase or convalescent-phase specimen to look for rising titers to specific pathogens. HIV testing should be performed to evaluate host factors that may predispose to FUO.

Sedimentation rate A sedimentation rate greater than 100 mm/hr suggests vasculitis but does not differentiate between this disorder and neoplasms, tuberculosis, or pyogenic infections.

Serum enzymes and chemistries The results of liver function tests may indicate primary involvement (e.g., caused by hepatitis or a liver abscess) or secondary infiltration (e.g., miliary tuberculosis) of the liver.

Skin tests Skin testing may aid in diagnosis if other positive results are obtained (e.g., a positive tuberculin test result would suggest tuberculosis) or if anergy, a characteristic finding in sarcoidosis, Whipple disease, and Hodgkin disease, is demonstrated.

Spinal fluid examination Examination of the spinal fluid is usually unrewarding unless the patient has CNS signs or symptoms, such as headache or stiff neck.

Radiologic Studies

Various radiologic studies in addition to chest films may assist in making the diagnosis:

1. Ultrasonography and CT scans are valuable for detecting intra-abdominal and pelvic abscesses and retroperitoneal adenopathy. The use of CT scans has led to a decrease in the number of biopsies of normal tissues performed in patients with FUO.[70]
2. Radionuclide scans may also be helpful.[71] Bone scans are considerably more sensitive than bone x-rays in the detection of osseous metastases or

foci of osteomyelitis. Gallium scans are occasionally useful in detecting occult abscesses, but gallium scanning has had mixed results in patients with FUO[72]; scans utilizing indium-111–labeled leukocytes are being investigated, as are scans employing indium-111–labeled human immunoglobulin G[73] and technetium-99m–labeled ciprofloxacin.[74] Positron emission tomography (PET) may also prove helpful in selected cases.[75]

3. Intravenous pyelograms may indicate intrarenal or perirenal abscesses or renal tumors. Some parenchymal lesions can be demonstrated only with the use of a renal angiogram.
4. Upper and lower GI tract x-rays may indicate regional enteritis, ulcerative colitis, or large-bowel neoplasms.
5. Bone x-rays generally are not helpful in the absence of skeletal symptoms.
6. Other radiographic examinations, such as cholangiograms, angiograms, and lymphangiograms, may occasionally be useful but should only be performed on the basis of clinical clues that suggest specific diagnoses.

Biopsies

All biopsied material should be cultured for bacteria, mycobacteria, and fungi and examined histologically. Biopsies that may help determine the diagnosis in patients with FUO include the following:

1. Percutaneous liver biopsy. Neoplastic or granulomatous diseases can generally be detected more easily by percutaneous liver biopsy than by bone marrow biopsy, particularly if hepatomegaly, abnormalities of hepatic function, or both are present.
2. Bone marrow biopsy. This technique may also be used to detect granulomatous diseases or metastatic tumor; it may be rewarding in patients in whom hematologic abnormalities are evident.
3. Lymph node biopsy. Enlarged, matted, or unusually situated nodes are the most favorable for biopsy. Because of the frequent occurrence of chronic inflammation in inguinal lymph nodes, biopsy of these nodes is unsatisfactory.
4. Skin and muscle biopsy. Biopsy of skin and muscle may prove useful in diagnosing collagen vascular disease (e.g., polyarteritis or dermatomyositis); biopsy may also be useful in sarcoidosis.
5. Temporal artery biopsy. Biopsy of the temporal artery may be the only way to establish the diagnosis of giant cell arteritis in an elderly patient who has FUO, an elevated erythrocyte sedimentation rate, and some thickening of the temporal artery.

Therapeutic Trials

Therapeutic trials have generally proved more misleading than helpful when applied to the patient with prolonged FUO. Coincidental temporary defervescence can suggest a specific therapeutic response, thus delaying measures that may provide the correct diagnosis. Occasionally, a therapeutic trial may be reasonable when directed at a specific diagnosis. Thus, a 1- to 2-week trial of a penicillin or vancomycin and an aminoglycoside may be employed when endocarditis is a realistic possibility. Aspirin may be tried in patients who may have adult-type juvenile rheumatoid arthritis. Patients with disseminated tuberculosis presenting as FUO often show a clinical response within 2 weeks after appropriate chemotherapy.

Exploratory Laparotomy

In the past, laparotomy was advocated and employed successfully in the diagnosis of FUO. However, noninvasive radiologic techniques, especially when combined with percutaneous needle biopsies (see above), have generally supplanted laparotomy for the diagnosis of FUO. Laparotomy should be reserved for patients in whom the clinical and laboratory findings point to an intra-abdominal or retroperitoneal source for the fever, particularly when the fever has followed a prolonged and debilitating course.

UNDIAGNOSED FUO

In 10% to 15% of patients with FUO, a detailed workup fails to reveal the diagnosis.[76] In about half these cases, the fever resolves spontaneously. Reevaluation of the patient some weeks or even months later may provide the diagnosis. The prognosis of patients with undiagnosed FUO is surprisingly good[76]; few require empirical corticosteroid therapy, and many can be managed symptomatically with NSAIDs.

References

1. Mackowiak PA, Bartlett JG, Borden EC, et al: Concepts of fever: recent advances and lingering dogma. Clin Infect Dis 225:119, 1997
2. Webb P: The physiology of heat regulation. Am J Physiol 268:R838, 1995
3. Boulant JA: Role of the preoptic-anterior hypothalamus in thermoregulation and fever. Clin Infect Dis 31:S157, 2000
4. Simon HB: Hyperthermia. N Engl J Med 329:483, 1993
5. Simon HB: Extreme pyrexia. JAMA 236:2419, 1976

6. Simon HB, Daniels GH: Hormonal hyperthermia: endocrinologic causes of fever. Am J Med 66:257, 1979

7. Epstein Y, Moran DS, Shapiro Y: Exertional heat stroke: a case series. Med Sci Sports Exerc 31:224, 1999

8. Heat-related illnesses, deaths, and risk factors—Cincinnati and Dayton, Ohio, 1999, and United States, 1979–1997. MMWR Morb Mortal Wkly Rep 49:470, 2000

9. Epstein Y: Predominance of type II fibres in exertional heat stroke. Lancet 350:83, 1997

10. Sawka MN, Montain SJ: Fluid and electrolyte supplementation for exercise heat stress. Am J Clin Nutr 72(suppl):564S, 2000

11. Sminia P, van der Zee J, Wondergem J, et al: Effect of hyperthermia on the central nervous system: a review. Int J Hyperthermia 10:1, 1994

12. Akhtar MJ, al-Nozha M, al-Harthi S, et al: Electrocardiographic abnormalities in patients with heat stroke. Chest 104:411, 1993

13. Duthie DJ: Heat-related illness. Lancet 352:1329, 1998

14. Costrini A: Emergency treatment of exertional heatstroke and comparison of whole body cooling techniques. Med Sci Sports Exerc 22:15, 1990

15. Weiner JS, Khogali M: A physiological body-cooling unit for treatment of heat stroke. Lancet 1:507, 1980

16. Caroff SN, Mann SC: Neuroleptic malignant syndrome. Med Clin North Am 77:185, 1993

17. Ueda M, Hamamoto M, Nagayama H, et al: Susceptibility to neuroleptic malignant syndrome in Parkinson's disease. Neurology 52:777, 1999

18. Sachdev P, Mason C, Hadzi-Pavlovic D: Case-control study of neurologic malignant syndrome. Am J Psychiatry 154:1156, 1997

19. Boeve BF, Rummans TA, Philbrick KL, et al: Electrocardiographic and echocardiographic changes associated with malignant catatonia. Mayo Clin Proc 69:645, 1994

20. Rosenberg MR, Green M: Neuroleptic malignant syndrome: review of response to therapy. Arch Intern Med 149:1927, 1989

21. Loke J, MacLennan DH: Malignant hyperthermia and central core disease: disorders of Ca^{2+} release channels. Am J Med 104:470, 1998

22. Dinarello CA: Cytokines as endogenous pyrogens. J Infect Dis 179 (suppl 2):S294, 1999

23. Mackowiak PA: Concepts of fever. Arch Intern Med 158:1870, 1998

24. Netea MG, Kullberg BJ, Van der Meer JW: Circulating cytokines as mediators of fever. Clin Infect Dis 31:S178, 2000

25. Blattels CM, Sehic E, Li S: Pyrogen sensing and signaling: old views and concepts. Clin Infect Dis 31(suppl 5):S168, 2000

26. Mackowiak PA: Fever: blessing or curse? A unifying hypothesis. Ann Intern Med 120:1037, 1994

27. Lahat E, Goldman M, Barr J, et al: Comparison of intranasal midazolam with intravenous diazepam for treating febrile seizures in children: prospective randomized study. BMJ 321:83, 2000

28. Rosman NP, Colton T, Labazzo J, et al: A controlled trial of diazepam administered during febrile illnesses to prevent recurrence of febrile seizures. N Engl J Med 329:79, 1993

29. Verity CM, Greenwood R, Golding J: Long-term intellectual and behavioral outcomes of children with febrile convulsions. N Engl J Med 338:1723, 1998

30. Albrecht RF II, Wass CT, Lanier WL: Occurrence of potentially detrimental temperature alterations in hospitalized patients at risk for brain injury. Mayo Clin Proc 73:629, 1998

31. Hajat C, Hajat S, Sharma P: Effects of poststroke pyrexia on stroke outcome: a meta-analysis of studies in patients. Stroke 31:410, 2000

32. Castillo J, Davalos A, Marrugat J, et al: Timing for fever-related brain damage in acute ischemic stroke. Stroke 29:2455, 1998

33. De Keyser J: Antipyretics in acute ischaemic stroke. Lancet 352:6, 1998

34. Schwab S, Schwarz S, Spranger M, et al: Moderate hypothermia in the treatment of patients with severe middle cerebral artery infarction. Stroke 29:2461, 1998

35. Kammersgaard LP, Rasmussen BH, Jorgenson HS, et al: Feasibility and safety of inducing modest hypothermia in awake patients with acute stroke through surface cooling: a case-control study. The Copenhagen Stroke Study. Stroke 31:2251, 2000

36. Craig JV, Lancaster GA, Williamson PR, et al: Temperature measured at the axilla compared with rectum in children and young people: systematic review. BMJ 320:1174, 2000

37. Hasday JD, Garrison A: Antipyretic therapy in patients with sepsis. Clin Infect Dis 31:S234, 2000

38. Plaisance KI, Mackowiak PA: Antipyretic therapy: physiologic rationale, diagnostic implications, and clinical consequences. Arch Intern Med 160:449, 2000

39. Simmons DL, Wagner D, Westover K: Nonsteroidal anti-inflammatory drugs, acetaminophen, cyclooxygenase 2, and fever. Clin Infect Dis 31(suppl 5):S211, 2000

40. Lenhardt R, Negishi C, Sessler DI, et al: The effects of physical treatment on induced fever in humans. Am J Med 106:550, 1999

41. Axelrod P: External cooling in the management of fever. Clin Infect Dis 31(suppl 5):S224, 2000

42. O'Donnell J, Axelrod P, Fisher C, et al: Use and effectiveness of hypothermia blankets for febrile patients in the intensive care unit. Clin Infect Dis 24:1208, 1997

43. Petersdorf RG, Beeson PB: Fever of unexplained origin: report on 100 cases. Medicine (Baltimore) 40:1, 1961

44. Arnow PM, Flaherty JP: Fever of unknown origin. Lancet 350:575, 1997

45. Knockaert DC, Vanneste LJ, Vanneste SB, et al: Fever of unknown origin in the 1980s: an update of the diagnostic spectrum. Arch Intern Med 152:51, 1992

46. Trivalle C, Chassaagne P, Bouaniche M, et al: Nosocomial febrile illness in the elderly. Arch Intern Med 158:1560, 1998

47. Marik PE: Fever in the ICU. Chest 117:855, 2000

48. Borer A, Gilad J, Haikin H, et al: Clinical features and costs of care for hospitalized adults with primary Epstein-Barr virus infection. Am J Med 107:144, 1999

49. Mackowiak PA: Diagnostic implications and clinical consequences of antipyretic therapy. Clin Infect Dis 31(suppl 5):S230, 2000

50. Pouchot J, Sampalis JS, Beaudet F, et al: Adult Still's disease: manifestations, disease course, and outcome in 62 patients. Medicine (Baltimore) 70:118, 1991

51. Simon HB, Wolff SM: Granulomatous hepatitis and prolonged fever of unknown origin: a study of 13 patients. Medicine (Baltimore) 52:1, 1973

52. Knox TA, Kaplan MM, Gelfand JA, et al: Methotrexate treatment of idiopathic granulomatous hepatitis. Ann Intern Med 122:592, 1995

53. Telenti A, Hermans PE: Idiopathic granulomatosis manifesting as fever of unknown origin. Mayo Clin Proc 64:44, 1989

54. Singh N, Yu VL, Wagener MM, et al: Cirrhotic fever in the 1990s: a prospective study with clinical implications. Clin Infect Dis 24:1135, 1997

55. Sarwari AR, Mackowiak PA: Factitious fever: a modern update. Curr Clin Top Infect Dis 17:88, 1997

56. Ben-Chetrit E, Levy M: Familial Mediterranean fever. Lancet 351: 659, 1998

57. Drenth JP, van der Meer JW: Periodic fevers enter the era of molecular diagnosis (editorial). BMJ 320:1091, 2000

58. Raoult D, La Scola B, Lecocq P, et al: Culture and immunological detection of *Tropheryma whippelii* from the duodenum of a patient with Whipple disease. JAMA 285:1039, 2001

59. Ramzan NN, Loftus E Jr, Burgart LJ, et al: Diagnosis and monitoring of Whipple disease by polymerase chain reaction. Ann Intern Med 126:520, 1997

60. Ehrbar HU, Bauerfeind P, Dutley F, et al: PCR-positive tests for *Tropheryma whippelii* in patients with Whipple's disease. Lancet 353: 2214, 1999

61. Fisher RG, Wright PF, Johnson JE: Inflammatory pseudotumor presenting as fever of unknown origin. Clin Infect Dis 21:1492, 1995

62. Norris AH, Krasinskas AM, Salhany KE, et al: Kikuchi-Fujimoto disease: a benign cause of fever and lymphadenopathy. Am J Med 171: 401, 1996

63. Mouallem M, Matetzky S, Raichlin E, et al: A man with a prosthetic valve, anaemia, fever, and splenomegaly. Lancet 348:1216, 1996

64. Mitchell MA, Markovitz DM, Killen PD, et al: Bilateral renal parenchymal malacoplakia presenting as fever of unknown origin: case report and review. Clin Infect Dis 118:704, 1994

65. Hirschmann JV: Fever of unknown origin in adults. Clin Infect Dis 24:291, 1997

66. Miralles P, Moreno S, Perez-Tascon M, et al: Fever of uncertain origin in patients infected with the human immunodeficiency virus. Clin Infect Dis 20:872, 1995

67. Armstrong WS, Katz JT, Kazanjian PH: Human immunodeficiency virus–associated fever of unknown origin: a study of 70 patients in the United States and review. Clin Infect Dis 28:341, 1991

68. Benito N, Nunez A, de Gorgolas M, et al: Bone marrow biopsy in the diagnosis of fever of unknown origin in patients with acquired immunodeficiency syndrome. Arch Intern Med 157:1577, 1997

69. Prego V, Glatt AE, Roy V, et al: Comparative yield of blood culture for fungi and mycobacteria, liver biopsy, and bone marrow biopsy in the diagnosis of fever of undetermined origin in human immunodeficiency virus–infected patients. Arch Intern Med 150:333, 1990

70. Rowland MD, Del Bene VE: Use of body computed tomography to evaluate fever of unknown origin. J Infect Dis 156:408, 1987

71. Corstens FH, van der Meer JW: Nuclear medicine's role in infection and inflammation. Lancet 354:765, 1999

72. Knockaert DC, Mortelmans LA, De Roo MC, et al: Clinical value of gallium-67 scintigraphy in evaluation of fever of unknown origin. Clin Infect Dis 18:601, 1994

73. de Kleijn EM, Oyen WJ, Claessens RA, et al: Utility of scintigraphic methods in patients with fever of unknown origin. Arch Intern Med 155:1989, 1995

74. Vinjamuri S, Hall AV, Solanki KK, et al: Comparison of ^{99m}Tc infection imaging with radiolabelled white-cell imaging in the evaluation of bacterial infection. Lancet 347:233, 1996

75. Blockmans D, Knockaert D, Maes A, et al: Clinical value of [^{18}F] fluoro-deoxyglucose positron emission tomography for patients with fever of unknown origin. Clin Infect Dis 32:191, 2001

76. Knockaert DC, Dujardin KS, Bobbaers HJ: Long-term follow-up of patients with undiagnosed fever of unknown origin. Arch Intern Med 156:618, 1996

77. Jacoby GA, Swartz MN: Fever of undetermined origin. N Engl J Med 289:1407, 1973

78. Larson EB, Featherstone HJ, Petersdorf RG: Fever of undetermined origin: diagnosis and follow-up of 105 cases, 1970–1980. Medicine (Baltimore) 61:269, 1982

79. Kazanjian PH: Fever of unknown origin: review of 86 patients treated in community hospitals. Clin Infect Dis 15:968, 1992

2 Chemotherapy of Infection

Harvey B. Simon, M.D.

Guidelines for Antimicrobial Chemotherapy

The essential feature of effective chemotherapeutic agents is the ability to inhibit microorganisms at concentrations tolerable by the host. The most successful antimicrobial agents are those that target anatomic structures or biosynthetic functions unique to microorganisms.

The appropriate choice of chemotherapy for an infection depends on five considerations: (1) the infecting organism and its antimicrobial susceptibilities; (2) the type of infection (e.g., abscess, bacteremia, meningitis, urinary tract infection); (3) host factors (e.g., neutropenia, immune deficiencies, concurrent illnesses, age, drug allergies, renal function); (4) the antimicrobial agents (e.g., dosage, routes of administration, drug interactions, serum levels and tissue penetration, potential toxicities, cost); and (5) public health considerations. The widespread use of antibiotics selects highly resistant organisms that subsequently pose a risk for the patient and the community.

IDENTIFICATION OF THE INFECTING ORGANISM

Prompt identification of the causative organism is essential for the selection of appropriate antimicrobial drugs. A Gram stain of infected body fluids can provide early clues to the etiologic agent. Other relatively simple laboratory procedures, such as immunodiagnostic tests, may provide rapid identification of infecting organisms. If it is not possible to perform a Gram stain, initial decisions are based on the clinical features and the usual bacteriology of the illness, pending results of appropriate cultures. Culture results must be interpreted with full recognition of the indigenous flora on various mucosal surfaces and on the skin. Cultural identification of the infecting organism can offer a clue to the likely antimicrobial susceptibilities [*see Table 1*].

DETERMINATION OF BACTERIAL SUSCEPTIBILITY TO SPECIFIC DRUGS

Determination of the in vitro susceptibility of isolated bacteria is usually necessary. However, susceptibility of certain species (e.g., group A streptococci) to the drug of choice (e.g., penicillin G) has been so uniform that routine in vitro testing is unnecessary.

In vitro susceptibility data provide a necessary, but not sufficient, basis for choosing chemotherapeutic agents. For example, although *Salmonella* isolates are almost always susceptible in vitro to gentamicin, gentamicin is not effective against systemic salmonellosis. Similarly, although viridans streptococci show in vitro susceptibility to chloramphenicol, this drug is ineffective as an alternative to penicillin for subacute bacterial endocarditis. Susceptibility data may not accurately predict the therapeutic outcome for infections caused by other organisms, such as *Staphylococcus epidermidis*, enterococci (especially when enterococci infect the bloodstream or deep tissue), and *Enterobacter* species, which rapidly develop penicillin and cephalosporin resistance because of inducible β-lactamase enzymes.

Most laboratories test antimicrobial susceptibility by the disk diffusion method. When necessary, organisms can be tested by tube dilution techniques to determine the minimal inhibitory concentration (MIC) and the minimal bactericidal concentration (MBC) of various antibiotics. Newer techniques include the gradient diffusion method and various nucleic acid–based tests that can detect genes conferring antibiotic resistance in bacteria.[1]

THE SITE OF INFECTION AND ANCILLARY THERAPY

The efficacy of antibiotic therapy depends on drug delivery to the site of infection. Transport across the blood-brain barrier varies considerably among antibiotics.[2] Intracellular parasites, such as

Table 1 Representative Antimicrobial Susceptibilities of Clinical Isolates at the Massachusetts General Hospital

Organism	*Strains Susceptible to Various Antimicrobials (%)*										
	Pen	*Oxa*	*Cef*	*Eryth*	*Tetra*	*Chlor*	*Clind*	*Vanco*	*Trim-Sulf*	*Levo*	
Staphylococcus aureus	10	63	63	48	88	—*	68	100	92	61	
Coagulase-negative staphylococci	12	34	34	33	84	—*	59	100	56	53	
Pneumococci	65	—*	—*	78	85	87	92	100	65	100	
	Amp		*Pip*	*Cef*	*Ceftaz*	*Imi*	*Gent*	*Amik*	*Levo*	*Trim-Sulf*	*Tetra*
Escherichia coli	66		69	95	99	100	98	100	97	84	76
Klebsiella pneumoniae	0		0	86	90	100	95	99	91	89	77
Proteus mirabilis	91		93	99	98	100	96	100	96	92	0
Proteus vulgaris	0		93	0	100	100	100	100	100	95	51
Pseudomonas aeruginosa	—*		82	—*	84	83	76	81	60	—*	—*
Enterobacter cloacae	0		71	0	76	100	89	99	90	86	74
Acinetobacter (Herellea) calcoaceticus	0		2	0	85	96	81	93	83	87	71
Serratia marcescens	0		90	0	97	100	98	100	93	97	11

*Isolate has not been tested.

Note: This listing represents the results of standard disk susceptibility tests performed on clinical isolates (from both hospitalized and ambulatory patients) and reported routinely at the Massachusetts General Hospital from 2000 to 2001. Drugs selected for testing often represent a class of antibiotics (e.g., oxacillin for the penicillinase-resistant penicillins such as oxacillin and nafcillin; cephalothin for the first-generation cephalosporins such as cefazolin and cephradine). The listing does not routinely include the susceptibilities of all isolates to certain selected antimicrobials. Thus, for example, although many strains of *A. calcoaceticus* appear to be resistant to the drugs for which susceptibility is regularly determined, some of these very resistant strains are susceptible in vitro to minocycline.

Amik—amikacin Amp—ampicillin Cef—cefaxolin Ceftaz—ceftazidime Chlor—chloramphenicol Clind—clindamycin Eryth—erythromycin Gent—gentamicin Imi—imipenem Levo—levoflaxacin Oxa—oxacillin Pen—penicillin Pip—piperacillin Tetra—tetracycline Trim-Sulf—trimethoprim-sulfamethoxazole Vanco—vancomycin

rickettsiae and mycobacteria, require therapy with agents that can reach the intracellular milieu of the organism. Necrotic lesions such as sequestra in bone or large abscesses hinder penetration by antimicrobial agents.

Drainage, debridement, or both, combined with vigorous chemotherapy, are necessary. Antibiotic therapy for infection in or around a foreign body or prosthesis often is ineffective unless these materials are removed or replaced. Infections behind obstructing lesions, such as pneumonia behind a blocked bronchus or cholecystitis caused by biliary obstruction, will not respond to antibiotics until the obstruction is relieved.

FACTORS AFFECTING DOSAGE AND ROUTE OF ADMINISTRATION

Many antibiotics are absorbed sufficiently well via the oral route to provide effective blood levels in patients with normal gastrointestinal function.[3] The enteral absorption of some antimicrobials is impeded by food and some medications (e.g., antacids); these antibiotics, such as tetracyclines, should be administered at least 1 hour before or several hours after meals. Certain antibiotics, such as neomycin, are essentially nonabsorbable and are used primarily for their effects on bowel flora. Many antibiotics cannot be given intramuscularly because of local pain or necrosis at the injection site. Intravenous administration must be used in the treatment of major and life-threatening infections such as septic shock, meningitis, and endocarditis. In many cases, patients are clinically stable during intravenous treatment, and it is often possible to discharge them and to administer parenteral antibiotics on an outpatient basis. Supervision by special teams of physicians, nurses, and pharmacists is required[4]; antibiotics can be administered either in the hospital outpatient department or at home if competent family members are available. New antibiotics with long half-lives can be used with improved intravenous catheters and delivery devices in simplified regimens; this leads to substantial economic benefits, enhanced patient comfort, and good therapeutic results with few complications.[5]

HOST FACTORS

Hypersensitivity to Antibiotics

Because of widespread exposure, many patients develop allergies to antimicrobial agents.[6] A careful history of hypersensitivity should thus be obtained [*see* Hypersensitivity Reactions, *below*].

Concurrent Illnesses

Patients with immunosuppressive illnesses are vulnerable to opportunistic pathogens. These patients may require broader antimicrobial coverage as well as intense therapy for ordinary pathogens. The same is true to a lesser extent for patients with chronic debilitating illness. Patients with renal insufficiency or liver disease may be unusually susceptible to direct drug toxicity [*see* Direct Drug Toxicity, *below*].

Many antimicrobial agents (e.g., penicillins, cephalosporins, aminoglycosides, vancomycin, and fluoroquinolones) are excreted primarily by the kidneys; guidelines for dosage adjustment in patients who have severe renal failure and are undergoing dialysis or peritoneal dialysis are listed elsewhere. Antibiotics with nonrenal metabolism may be preferable in azotemic patients, provided the infecting organism is susceptible. A number of antibiotics, including nafcillin, piperacillin, doxycycline, metronidazole, and rifampin, are excreted by the liver.

Antibiotics in Pregnancy

The administration of antimicrobial agents during pregnancy and in the postpartum period poses several problems. Foremost is the question of safety, both for the mother and for the fetus or neonate. Although most antibiotics cross the placenta and enter maternal milk, the concentrations to which the fetus or neonate is exposed vary widely. Because the immature liver may lack the enzymes required to metabolize certain drugs, pharmacokinetics and toxicities in the fetus are often very different from those in older children and adults. Teratogenicity is a major concern when any drug is administered during pregnancy. Finally, it may be necessary to alter the dosage schedules of drugs that appear to be safe to use during pregnancy; increases in maternal blood volume, glomerular filtration rate (GFR), and hepatic metabolic activity often reduce the maternal serum levels of antimicrobials by 10% to 50%, especially late in pregnancy and in the early postpartum period. In some women, delayed gastric emptying may reduce the absorption of antibiotics that have been administered orally during pregnancy.

Even though 25% to 40% of women receive antibiotics during pregnancy, data regarding safety and efficacy in this setting are often scarce. Some general recommendations have been proposed, but they are intended only as a guide [*see Table 2*]; in all cases, therapy must be individualized, and both the indications for antibiotics and the possible risks to mother and fetus must be considered. Individual decisions are also required for lactating mothers; although most antimicrobials appear safe for breast-fed infants, chloramphenicol and the tetracyclines should be avoided.[7]

Antibiotics in the Elderly

Physiologic changes that occur with age can alter the pharmacokinetics of antimicrobial agents. For example, decreased gastric acidity and intestinal motility can impair drug absorption; increased body fat and decreased serum albumin levels can alter drug distribution; and decreased hepatic blood flow and enzymatic action can delay drug metabolism. Although these factors have not consistently affected antibiotic levels in the elderly, the decrease in GFR that occurs with age can lead to the accumulation of drugs excreted by the kidney. The high therapeutic index of the penicillins and cephalosporins obviates major changes in dosage schedules in elderly patients who have normal serum creatinine levels. However, in the case of aminoglycosides and vancomycin, decreased dosage schedules are often required; ideally, drug levels should be measured and renal function should be monitored when these agents are given. The dosage of amantadine and rimantadine should also be reduced in elderly patients.

Adverse Reactions to Antimicrobial Agents

There are three general types of adverse reactions to antimicrobial agents: hypersensitivity reactions (which are not dose related), direct drug toxicity (which usually is dose related and manifests in a single organ or, occasionally, in several organs), and microbial superinfection. In rare situations, antibiotic therapy can lead to a worse clinical outcome; for example, antibiotic therapy has been associated with gastroenteritis caused by *E. coli* 0157:H7.[8]

HYPERSENSITIVITY REACTIONS

A history of allergies should be taken before antimicrobial therapy is initiated in any patient. More information is available regarding allergies to the penicillins than allergies to other agents, but

Table 2 Antibiotics in Pregnancy

Drug	*Major Toxic Potential*		*Pharmacology*	
	Maternal	*Fetal*	*Maternal Serum Levels*	*Excreted in Mother's Milk*
Considered Safe				
Cephalosporins	Allergies	None known	Decreased	Trace
Erythromycin base	Allergies, GI intolerance	None known	Decreased	Yes
Penicillins	Allergies	None known	Decreased	Trace
Spectinomycin	?	None known	?	?
Use with Caution				
Aminoglycosides	Ototoxicity and nephrotoxicity	Ototoxicity	Decreased	Yes
Clindamycin	Allergies, colitis	None known	Unchanged	Trace
Ethambutol	Optic neuritis	Probably safe	?	?
Isoniazid	Allergies, hepatotoxicity	Neuropathy, seizures	Unchanged	Yes
Rifampin	Hypersensitivity, hepatotoxicity	Probably safe	Unchanged	Yes
Sulfonamides (contraindicated at term)	Allergies, crystalluria	Kernicterus (at term), hemolysis (G6PD deficiency)	Unchanged	Yes
Avoid if Possible				
Metronidazole	Hypersensitivity, alcohol intolerance, neuropathy	None known (teratogenic in animals)	Probably unchanged	Yes
Contraindicated				
Chloramphenicol	Blood dyscrasias	Gray syndrome	Unchanged	Yes
Erythromycin estolate	Hepatotoxicity	None known	Decreased	Yes
Nalidixic acid	GI intolerance	Increased intracranial pressure	?	?
Norfloxacin, ciprofloxacin, ofloxacin, lomefloxacin	GI intolerance	Arthropathies in immature animals	?	?
Nitrofurantoin	Allergies, neuropathy, GI intolerance	Hemolysis (G6PD deficiency)	Decreased	Trace
Tetracyclines	Hepatotoxicity, renal failure	Tooth discoloration and dysplasia, impaired bone growth	Probably unchanged	Yes
Trimethoprim	Hypersensitivity	Teratogenicity	Unchanged	Yes

skin eruptions, drug fever, and even anaphylaxis may be produced by many antibiotics. Allergic reactions occur in 1% to 10% of patients who receive penicillin. Fatal anaphylactic reactions are much less frequent.

DIRECT DRUG TOXICITY

Although antimicrobials can produce damage to virtually all human organ systems, the potential for toxicity varies widely from drug to drug.[9] The principal antibiotics that are directly toxic to the kidney are aminoglycosides, polymyxins, and amphotericin B; azotemia and renal tubular damage may be caused by any of these drugs. Patients with preexisting renal insufficiency are at increased risk for toxic reactions to various antibiotics, including nephrotoxicity, coagulopathies and other hematologic toxicities, seizures, and ototoxicity and other neurotoxicities.

Chloramphenicol can produce bone marrow suppression, which is usually mild and reversible but rarely presents as an irreversible fatal aplastic anemia. Because of the risk of bone marrow depression, a complete blood count and differential blood count should be performed three times weekly in all patients receiving chloramphenicol. Chloramphenicol, sulfonamides, nitrofurantoin, and primaquine can cause hemolytic anemia in patients who have deficiencies of erythrocyte glucose-6-phosphate dehydrogenase (G6PD). Hemolytic anemia, thrombocytopenia, and leukopenia that involve an immune mechanism can be caused by penicillins, cephalosporins, tetracyclines, and rifampin, but these reactions are uncommon. Macrolides and trimethoprim-sulfamethoxazole have been associated with agranulocytosis. Trimethoprim can produce anemia, leukopenia, and thrombocytopenia from folate deficiency; the effect is reversible with folinic acid. Amphotericin B commonly produces a reversible normocytic normochromic anemia, probably secondary to injury to the red cell membrane. Flucytosine causes bone marrow suppression (leukopenia or pancytopenia) when its excretion is reduced by renal failure. Linezolid can also produce myelosuppression; although experience is limited, bone marrow function usually recovers when the drug is discontinued. Neutropenia can occur during therapy with penicillins, cephalosporins, or vancomycin. It may be severe, but it is self-limited; recovery occurs 1 to 7 days after the antibiotic is withdrawn. Penicillins inhibit platelet aggregation by adenosine diphosphate, which may account for the bleeding that occurs in some patients receiving these antibiotics in high doses. Various cephalosporins may produce coagulopathies by prolonging the prothrombin time; the methylthiotetrazole side chain present in cephalosporins such as cefotetan appears to be responsible.

Antibiotics may produce a wide range of toxic effects on the central and peripheral nervous systems. Ototoxicity, either vestibular or auditory, can be produced by any of the aminoglycosides; neuromuscular blockade is much less common. Minocycline has occasionally been reported to produce significant vestibular reactions. Vancomycin can cause auditory neurotoxicity. Intravenous administration of large doses of penicillin and other β-lactams may produce seizures, especially when administered in very high doses or when given to azotemic patients or to patients with underlying epilepsy.

Peripheral neuropathy can occur as a complication of therapy with nitrofurantoin, particularly when renal failure is present. The neuropathy that occurs with isoniazid can be prevented by the daily administration of 50 mg of pyridoxine. Tetracycline may in rare instances produce reversible benign intracranial hypertension with headache and papilledema. Nalidixic acid may also produce intracranial hypertension and seizures in children. Metronidazole can sometimes cause ataxia, encephalopathy, seizures, or peripheral neuropathies. Ofloxacin has been reported to cause seizures; mania has been attributed to clarithromycin. Optic neuritis, usually manifested by decreased visual acuity and decreased perception of the color green, may occur as a side effect of ethambutol.

The principal antimicrobials that produce adverse effects on the liver are those used in the treatment of tuberculosis: isoniazid, rifampin, aminosalicylic acid, and pyrazinamide. Trovafloxacin was restricted for use in seriously ill patients because of hepatotoxicity, but other fluoroquinolones have not been implicated. The tetracyclines can occasionally cause fatty liver; hepatotoxicity is most likely to occur in patients receiving 2 g or more daily by the intravenous route. Patients receiving high-dose β-lactam antibiotics may develop hepatitis or cholestasis, presumably as a result of hypersensitivity reactions. Nitrofurantoin may cause chronic active hepatitis in some patients. Erythromycins and sulfonamides have been associated with acute hepatitis, and a case of fatal hepatic necrosis has been attributed to fluconazole.

GI reactions to antibiotics result either from direct irritation by the drug, the occurrence of which is usually dose related, or from bacterial overgrowth.[10] Irritative GI side effects are usually produced when antibiotics are administered orally rather than parenterally. The predominant site of irritation varies from drug to drug; for example, erythromycin more commonly produces gastric irritation with epigastric distress and nausea, whereas tetracyclines may produce diarrhea as well as upper GI symptoms. Some qualitative and quantitative changes in the intestinal flora occur after antibiotic administration; they may contribute to flatulence and other lower GI symptoms, which are quite common when broad-spectrum antibiotics are administered orally. Selective overgrowth of *Clostridium difficile* can result in antibiotic-induced pseudomembranous enterocolitis [see 17 Anaerobic Infections].

Antibiotics may cause various other toxicities. Erythromycin and other macrolides can cause prolongation of the QT interval and polymorphic ventricular tachycardia; in rare instances, this toxicity occurs in the absence of predisposing factors, but it is more likely to occur in patients with significant heart disease and in patients taking terfenadine, astemizole, or cisapride. Several fluoroquinolones, such as moxifloxacin, gatifloxacin, and sparfloxacin, can have similar effects on cardiac conduction.[11,12] All fluoroquinolones can cause tendinitis. Trimethoprim-sulfamethoxazole can cause hyperkalemia, particularly in azotemic patients. Sulfonamides, fluoroquinolones, and tetracyclines can produce photosensitivity.[13]

MICROBIAL SUPERINFECTION

Antimicrobial therapy reduces susceptible organisms from the normal flora of the skin, oral and genitourinary mucosae, and GI tract and exerts selective pressures that favor survival of drug-resistant organisms. Such resistant organisms can occasionally establish a superinfection either at the site of the original infection or at remote sites.

PUBLIC HEALTH CONSIDERATIONS

Antimicrobial Resistance

The extensive use of antimicrobial agents, especially in intensive care units[14] and other health care facilities, strongly favors the selection of resistant microbial species, particularly bacterial strains harboring plasmids that confer transmissible resistance.[15,16] The widespread use of antibiotics for animals compounds the problem; about 50% of the 25,000 tons of antibiotics that are sold annually in the United States are used in agriculture and aquiculture.[17] Infections from highly resistant strains of *Enterococcus, Pneumococcus, S. aureus, Gonococcus, Salmonella, Serratia, Klebsiella, Acinetobacter, Enterobacter,* and *Mycobacterium* have become important problems. Infections from resistant strains can spread rapidly, first within an institution, then throughout a community, and eventually even globally.[18] Although antibiotic resistance is a worldwide problem, control depends on local measures, beginning with the judicious prescription of antibiotics by individual practitioners[19] and with formulary restrictions that reinforce prudence.[20] Patients harboring resistant strains should be identified rapidly, treated appropriately, and isolated as needed to prevent the spread of infection. New classes of antimicrobials are being developed to deal with drug resistance.

The Choice of Antimicrobial Drugs

The simultaneous use of multiple antibiotics in a shotgun fashion should be avoided because of the problems of drug toxicity and sensitizations, microbial superinfections, and antagonisms between certain agents. Most bacterial infections can be treated satisfactorily with a single antimicrobial agent. There are a limited number of situations, however, in which the simultaneous administration of chemotherapeutic agents is warranted: (1) synergism between two antimicrobials against a specific infecting agent; (2) prevention of emergence of resistance to one or both drugs; (3) treatment of polymicrobial infections for which one antibiotic is not sufficient; and (4) initial treatment of life-threatening infections before isolation of the etiologic agent.

Although the choice of antimicrobial drugs must always be individualized, there are useful guidelines that can be followed [*see Table 3*].[21–23]

PENICILLINS

The penicillins are bactericidal antibiotics that impair synthesis of the bacterial cell wall peptidoglycan by attaching to penicillin-binding proteins located on the inner surface of the cell membrane. At least eight penicillin-binding proteins have been identified; they are the enzymes that are responsible for linking individual elements of the bacterial cell wall together. Penicillins and other β-lactam antibiotics have different affinities for various penicillin-binding proteins.[24]

The penicillins may be classified into subgroups on the basis of their structure, β-lactamase susceptibility, and spectrum of action. Dosages of these agents vary according to the type and severity of infection [*see Table 4*]. The penicillins are generally well tolerated. Hypersensitivity and GI reactions are the most common side effects; granulocytopenia, hemolytic anemia, bleeding, intestinal nephritis, hepatitis, and seizures may occur. The side effects of penicillin are generally shared by all its derivatives; however, broad-spectrum penicillins such as ampicillin are more likely to cause pseudomembranous colitis, and penicillins with α-carboxyl substitutions such as ticarcillin are more likely to impair platelet function. Patients allergic to one penicillin compound are likely to be allergic to other such compounds.

Penicillin G and Penicillin V

Penicillin G, the first antibiotic to be used for systemic infections, is still the drug of choice for various infections.

Resistance to penicillin has not been observed in group A streptococci, meningococci, and *Treponema pallidum* organisms, and penicillin G is highly effective in subacute bacterial endocarditis caused by susceptible bacteria. Penicillin V (phenoxymethyl penicillin) has the same spectrum of activity as penicillin G but is more acid-stable and is thus better absorbed from the GI tract. Although all forms of penicillin introduced since the release of penicillin G are prescribed by weight, penicillin G is still prescribed for parenteral administration by unitage. For interconversion, 1 mg of penicillin G equals approximately 1,600 units. An intramuscular injection of procaine penicillin G is almost painless; because the drug is slowly absorbed, injections are required only every 12 to 24 hours for treatment of highly susceptible infections.

Table 3 Antimicrobial Drugs of Choice for Various Infections in Adults[18]

	Causative Organism	Drug of Choice	Alternative Drugs
Gram-Positive Cocci	*Staphylococcus aureus*		
	Methicillin-sensitive		Linezolid, quinupristin-dalfopristin
	Methicillin-resistant[1]	Vancomycin,[2] with or without rifampin or gentamicin	Trimethoprim-sulfamethoxazole (TMP-SMX),[2] with or without rifampin[2]; a fluoroquinolone[3]; a tetracycline[4]
		Penicillinase-resistant penicillin[5]	A cephalosporin,[6] clindamycin, vancomycin,[7] meropenem or imipenem,[8] ticarcillin–clavulanic acid, ampicillin-sulbactam, amoxicillin–clavulanic acid, piperacillin-tazobactam, a fluoroquinolone[3]
	Coagulase-negative staphylococci[9]	Vancomycin,[7] with or without rifampin[2] or gentamicin	Linezolid, quinupristin-dalfopristin, a cephalosporin, a penicillinase-resistant penicillin, meropenem or imipenem,[8] a fluoroquinolone[3]
	Anaerobic streptococcus *(Peptostreptococcus)*	Penicillin G[10]	Clindamycin, a cephalosporin,[6] vancomycin[7]
	Streptococcus bovis	Penicillin G[10,11]	A cephalosporin,[6] vancomycin[7]
	Groups A, G, and C streptococci	Penicillin G[10,12] or penicillin V	A cephalosporin,[6] vancomycin,[7] an erythromycin,[13] clindamycin, clarithromycin, azithromycin
	Group B streptococcus	Penicillin G[10,12] or ampicillin	A cephalosporin,[6] vancomycin,[7] an erythromycin
	S. pneumoniae (pneumococcus)		
	Penicillin sensitive	Penicillin G[10,12] or penicillin V, amoxicillin	An erythromycin,[12,13] a cephalosporin,[6] meropenem or imipenem,[8] vancomycin,[7,12] azithromycin, clarithromycin, a fluoroquinolone; a tetracycline[4]
	Non–penicillin sensitive	Vancomycin; ceftriaxone or cefotaxime[6]; levofloxacin, moxifloxacin, or gatifloxacin[3]; linezolid; quinupristin-dalfopristin; imipenem or meropenem	—
	Viridans streptococci	Penicillin G,[10,11] with or without gentamicin	A cephalosporin,[6] vancomycin[7]
	Enterococcus		
	Endocarditis or other serious infection	Penicillin or ampicillin, plus gentamicin[14] or streptomycin	Vancomycin,[7] with gentamicin or streptomycin; linezolid; quinupristin-dalfopristin
	Uncomplicated urinary tract infection	Ampicillin or amoxicillin	A fluoroquinolone,[3] nitrofurantoin,[15] fosfomycin
Gram-Positive Bacilli	*Bacillus cereus, B. subtilis*	Vancomycin	Meropenem or imipenem,[8] clindamycin
	Bacillus anthracis	Penicillin G	Ciprofloxacin,[3] a tetracycline,[4] an erythromycin[2]
	Clostridium difficile	Metronidazole[16]	Vancomycin[16]
	C. perfringens	Penicillin G; clindamycin	Metronidazole, meropenem or imipenem,[8] chloramphenicol[7]
	C. tetani	Metronidazole	Penicillin G, a tetracycline[4]
	Corynebacterium diphtheriae	An erythromycin	Penicillin G
	Corynebacterium, JK group	Vancomycin	Penicillin G, with gentamicin; an erythromycin
	Listeria monocytogenes	Ampicillin, with or without gentamicin	TMP-SMX
	Propionibacterium	Penicillin G	Clindamycin, an erythromycin
Gram-Negative Cocci	*Moraxella* (formerly *Branhamella*) *catarrhalis*	Cefuroxime,[6] a fluoroquinolone[3]	TMP-SMX, amoxicillin–clavulanic acid, an erythromycin, a tetracycline, third-generation cephalosporins, clarithromycin, azithromycin
	Neisseria gonorrhoeae[17]	Ceftriaxone or cefixime,[6] ciprofloxacin, ofloxacin, or gatifloxacin	Cefotaxime,[10] penicillin or ampicillin
	N. meningitidis		
	Meningitis, bacteremia	Penicillin G	A third-generation cephalosporin,[6] TMP-SMX, a fluoroquinolone,[3] chloramphenicol[7]
	Carrier state	Rifampin	Minocycline, ciprofloxacin
Enteric Gram-Negative Bacilli	*Bacteroides*		
	GI tract strains (*B. fragilis*)	Metronidazole or clindamycin	Cefoxitin, cefotetan, ceftizoxime, or cefmetazole; chloramphenicol[18]; imipenem or meropenem[8]; ticarcillin–clavulanic acid; ampicillin-sulbactam, piperacillin-tazobactam
	Respiratory tract strains	Penicillin G or clindamycin	Metronidazole, cefoxitin,[6] cefotetan, ceftizoxime, cefmetazole, chloramphenicol[7]
	Campylobacter fetus	Imipenem or meropenem[8]	Gentamicin
	C. jejuni	Azithromycin or an erythromycin	A fluoroquinolone,[3] a tetracycline,[4] gentamicin[7]

Note: all supersccript numbers refer to footnotes that follow table.

Table 3 (continued)

	Causative Organism	*Drug of Choice*	*Alternative Drugs*
Enteric Gram-Negative Bacilli (continued)	*Citrobacter*	Imipenem or meropenem[8]	A fluoroquinolone,[3] amikacin; TMP-SMX; a tetracycline[4]; a third-generation cephalosporin[6]
	Enterobacter	Imipenem or meropenem[8]	A third-generation cephalosporin[6]; for serious infections, use with a fluoroquinolone[3] or gentamicin; gentamicin, tobramycin, amikacin, a fluoroquinolone,[3] a carboxypenicillin or acylaminopenicillin,[19] aztreonam[20]
	Escherichia coli	Ampicillin, a cephalosporin,[6] a fluoroquinolone,[3] TMP-SMX[22]	Gentamicin,[21] tobramycin, amikacin, imipenem or meropenem,[8] aztreonam[20]
	Helicobacter pylori	Tetracycline with metronidazole and bismuth subsalicylate or omeprazole with amoxicillin and clarithromycin	Amoxicillin with metronidazole and bismuth subsalicylate; tetracycline with clarithromycin and bismuth subsalicylate; clarithromycin with omeprazole; amoxicillin with clarithromycin
	Klebsiella	A cephalosporin[6]	Imipenem or meropenem,[9] gentamicin,[23] tobramycin, amikacin, TMP-SMX,[21] a carboxypenicillin or acylaminopenicillin,[21] amoxicillin–clavulanic acid, ampicillin-sulbactam, ticarcillin–clavulanic acid, piperacillin-tazobactam, aztreonam,[20] a fluoroquinolone[3]
	Proteus mirabilis	Ampicillin	A cephalosporin, gentamicin or tobramycin, chloramphenicol,[7] a carboxypenicillin or acylaminopenicillin,[19] imipenem or meropenem,[8] TMP-SMX, aztreonam,[20] a fluoroquinolone[3]
	Non-*mirabilis*, including *P. vulgaris, Morganella morganii,* and *Providencia rettgeri*	A third-generation cephalosporin[6]	Gentamicin, tobramycin, amikacin, a carboxypenicillin or acylaminopenicillin,[19] imipenem or meropenem,[8] aztreonem,[20] ampicillin-sulbactam, ticarcillin–clavulanic acid, piperacillin-tazobactam, amoxicillin–clavulanic acid, a fluoroquinolone[3]
	Providencia stuartii	A third-generation cephalosporin[6]	An aminoglycoside, TMP-SMX,[21] imipenem or meropenem,[8] aztreonam,[20] a carboxypenicillin or acylaminopenicillin,[19] a fluoroquinolone[3]
	Salmonella typhi	Ceftriaxone or a fluoroquinolone[3]	Chloramphenicol or ampicillin,[22] TMP-SMX
	Other *Salmonella* species	Ceftriaxone or a cefotaxime or a fluoroquinolone[3]	Ampicillin or amoxicillin, TMP-SMX, chloramphenicol[7]
	Serratia	Imipenem or meropenem	A third-generation cephalosporin,[6] gentamicin or amikacin, a carboxypenicillin or acylaminopenicillin,[19] chloramphenicol,[7] aztreonam, a fluoroquinolone[3]
	Shigella	A fluoroquinolone[3]	TMP-SMX, ampicillin, ceftriaxone, azithromycin
Other Gram-Negative Bacilli	*Acinetobacter (Herellea)*	Imipenem or meropenem[8]	Tobramycin, gentamicin, amikacin, doxycycline, minocycline, a carboxypenicillin or acylaminopenicillin,[19] TMP-SMX, a fluoroquinolone,[3] ceftazidime
	Aeromonas hydrophilia	TMP-SMX[2]	A fluoroquinolone,[3] gentamicin, tobramycin, imipenem or meropenem[8]
	Bartonella henselae (cat-scratch disease)	Azithromycin	Ciprofloxacin,[3] TMP-SMX, gentamicin; rifampin, erythromycin
	Bartonella henselae (bacillary angiomatosis)	Erythromycin	Doxycycline, azithromycin
	Bordetella pertussis (whooping cough)	Erythromycin	TMP-SMX; azithromycin or clarithromycin
	Brucella	A tetracycline, with rifampin	A tetracycline with gentamicin or streptomycin; chloramphenicol,[7] with or without streptomycin; TMP-SMX[2] with or without gentamicin; ciprofloxacin[3] with rifampin
	Eikenella corrodens	Ampicillin	An erythromycin, a tetracycline,[4] amoxicillin–clavulanic acid, ampicillin-sulbactam, ceftriaxone
	Francisella tularensis (tularemia)	Streptomycin	Gentamicin, a tetracycline,[4] chloramphenicol,[7] ciprofloxacin[3]
	Fusobacterium	Penicillin	Clindamycin, metronidazole, chloramphenicol[7]; cefoxitin
	Gardnerella (formerly *Haemophilus*) *vaginalis*	Metronidazole[2] (oral)	Intravaginal metronidazole, intravaginal or oral clindamycin

Note: all superscript numbers refer to footnotes that follow table.

Table 3 (continued)

	Causative Organism	*Drug of Choice*	*Alternative Drugs*
Other Gram-Negative Bacilli (continued)	*Haemophilus influenzae* Bronchitis, otitis media	TMP-SMX	Ampicillin or amoxicillin; a tetracycline[4]; amoxicillin–clavulanic acid, cefuroxime axetil, ceftizoxime, clarithromycin, azithromycin, a fluoroquinolone[3]
	Meningitis, epiglottitis, life-threatening infections	Cefotaxime or ceftriaxone	Chloramphenicol,[24] meropenem[9]
	Legionella species	Azithromycin or a fluoroquinolone[3]	Erythromycin, rifampin,[25] TMP-SMX,[2] doxycycline[4]
	Pasteurella multocida	Penicillin G	A tetracycline,[4] a cephalosporin,[6] amoxicillin–clavulanic acid, ampicillin-sulbactam
	Calymmatobacterium granulomatis (granuloma inguinale)	TMP-SMX	A tetracycline[4]; ciprofloxacin with or without rifampin
	H. ducreyi (chancroid)	Ceftriaxone or azithromycin	A fluoroquinolone[3]
	Pseudomonas aeruginosa		
	Urinary tract infections	Ciprofloxacin[3]	Levofloxacin; gentamicin or tobramycin; amikacin; ceftazidime,[6] with or without gentamicin or tobramycin; imipenem or meropenem[8]; aztreonam,[20] a carboxypenicillin or acylaminopenicillin[19]
	Other infections	Gentamicin or tobramycin, with or without a carboxypenicillin or acylaminopenicillin[19]; ceftazidime or cefepime; imipenem or meropenem[8]; aztreonam,[20] alone or with gentamicin or tobramycin	Amikacin, with or without a carboxypenicillin cr acylaminopenicillin[19]; ciprofloxacin[7]
	P. cepacia	TMP-SMX	Chloramphenicol,[7] ceftazidime,[2] imipenem[2,8] or meropenem[8]
	Streptobacillus moniliformis (rat-bite fever)	Penicillin G	A tetracycline,[4] streptomycin
	Vibrio cholerae	A tetracycline[4]	TMP-SMX, a fluoroquinolone[3]
	V. vulnificus	A tetracycline[4]	Cefotaxime
	Agents of Vincent stomatitis (trench mouth)	Penicillin G	A tetracycline,[4] an erythromycin
	Stenotrophomonas (formerly *Xanthomonas*) *maltophila*	TMP-SMX	Minocycline, ceftazidime,[6] a fluoroquinolone[3]
	Yersinia enterocolitica	TMP-SMX[2]	A fluoroquinolone, gentamicin,[2] tobramycin,[2] amikacin, cefotaxime[2,6] or ceftizoxime[2,6]
	Y. pestis (plague)	Streptomycin with or without a tetracycline	A tetracycline,[4] chloramphenicol,[7] gentamicin,[2] TMP-SMX
Acid-Fast Bacilli	*Mycobacterium avium* complex	Clarithromycin or azithromycin plus one or more of the following: ethambutol, rifabutin, ciprofloxacin	Rifampin, amikacin
	M. fortuitum	Amikacin[2] with clarithromycin	Rifampin,[2] cefoxitin, a sulfonamide, doxycycline, ethambutol, linezolid
	M. kansasii	Isoniazid with rifampin, with or without ethambutol or streptomycin	Cycloserine, ethionamide, clarithromycin
	M. leprae	Dapsone[7] with rifampin, with or without clofazimine	Minocycline,[4] ofloxacin or sparfloxacin,[3] clarithromycin
	M. marinum (balnei)[26]	Minocycline	TMP-SMX, rifampin, clarithromycin, doxycycline
	M. tuberculosis[27]	Isoniazid with rifampin, and pyrazinamide with or without ethambutol or streptomycin	Ciprofloxacin or ofloxacin; third-line agent
Actinomycetes	*Actinomycetes israelii*	Penicillin G	A tetracycline[4]; an erythromycin; clindamycin
	Nocardia	TMP-SMX	Minocycline, sulfisoxazole, imipenem or meropenem,[8] amikacin,[2] cycloserine, linezolid
Chlamydia	*Chlamydia psittaci* (psittacosis)	A tetracycline[4]	Chloramphenicol[7]
	C. trachomatis		
	Inclusion conjunctivitis	An erythromycin (oral or I.V.)	A sulfonamide (topical plus oral)
	Lymphogranuloma venereum	A tetracycline[4]	An erythromycin

Note: all supersccript numbers refer to footnotes that follow table.

Table 3 (continued)

	Causative Organism	Drug of Choice	Alternative Drugs
Chlamydia (continued)	Pneumonia	An erythromycin	A sulfonamide
	Trachoma	Azithromycin	A tetracycline[4] (topical plus oral), a sulfonamide (topical plus oral)
	Urethritis or pelvic inflammatory disease	Doxycycline or azithromycin	Erythromycin, ofloxacin, amoxicillin
	C. pneumoniae	An erythromycin or clarithromycin or azithromycin; a fluoroquinolone	A tetracycline[4]
Mycoplasma	*Mycoplasma pneumoniae*	An erythromycin, clarithromycin or azithromycin; a fluoroquinolone,[3] doxycycline[4]	—
	Ureaplasma urealyticum	An erythromycin	A tetracycline,[4] clarithromycin, or azithromycin; ofloxacin[3]
Rickettsia	Various rickettsial organisms Rocky Mountain spotted fever, epidemic and endemic (murine) typhus, rickettsial pox, Q fever, scrub typhus	Doxycycline[4]	Chloramphenicol,[7] a fluoroquinolone,[3] rifampin
Spirochetes	*Borrelia burgdorferi* (Lyme disease)	Doxycycline or amoxicillin or ceftriaxone	Penicillin, an erythromycin, clarithromycin, azithromycin, cefuroxime
	B. recurrentis (relapsing fever)	A tetracycline[4]	Penicillin G
	Leptospira	Penicillin G	A tetracycline,[4] an erythromycin
	Treponema pallidum	Penicillin G	A tetracycline,[4] an erythromycin, ceftriaxone

1. Some strains of S. *aureus* and most strains of coagulase-negative staphylococci are resistant to penicillinase-resistant penicillins; these strains are also resistant to cephalosporins.
2. Not approved for this indication by the FDA.
3. See Table 6 for attributes of the various fluoroquinolones. None of these drugs is recommended for children. In 1999, the FDA limited trovafloxacin to inpatient use for limb- or life-threatening infections.
4. Doxycycline is the safest tetracycline for treatment of extrarenal infections in renal insufficiency. Tetracyclines should be avoided in pregnant women and in children younger than 8 yr.
5. For severe infections, I.V. nafcillin or oxacillin should be used. For mild infections, oral cloxacillin, dicloxacillin, or oxacillin may be employed. Between 1% and 2% of *S. aureus* strains are resistant to penicillinase-resistant penicillins (and usually to cephalosporins) but are susceptible to vancomycin. High doses of penicillin G, ampicillin, amoxicillin, carbenicillin, or ticarcillin do not overcome the clinical resistance of penicillinase-producing staphylococci to these drugs.
6. Cephalosporins are sometimes used as alternatives to penicillin in patients with suspected penicillin allergy but not in patients with serious hypersensitivity (especially immediate anaphylactic or accelerated urticarial reactions). Patients allergic to penicillin may be hypersensitive to cephalosporins. Only third-generation cephalosporins are effective in bacterial meningitis.
7. In view of the occurrence of adverse reactions, this drug should be used only for serious infections and when less toxic drugs are ineffective.
8. Imipenem and meropenem are β-lactam antibiotics that should be used with caution in patients who are allergic to penicillins and cephalosporins.
9. In vitro sensitivity testing with cephalosporins or penicillins may be misleading because of heteroresistance and because these antibiotics may be bacteriostatic only. For serious infections, vancomycin is preferred (see text).
10. Crystalline penicillin G is administered parenterally for serious infections. For less severe infections caused by pneumococci, group A streptococci, gonococci, or *T. pallidum*, procaine penicillin is administered I.M. once or twice daily. For mild infections caused by streptococci and pneumococci, oral penicillin V is preferable to oral penicillin G. Benzathine penicillin G is given I.M. (once monthly for the prophylaxis of rheumatic fever, a single injection for the treatment of group A streptococcal pharyngitis) when patients' compliance for oral medication is questionable and for treatment of syphilis, in one to three doses at weekly intervals, depending on the stage of the disease.
11. The combination of penicillin G with streptomycin for the first 2 wk of treatment of endocarditis caused by viridans streptococci is preferred by some.
12. In patients with major allergy to penicillin, erythromycin is the alternative for respiratory tract infections; chloramphenicol is the preferred alternative for meningitis. Occasional strains of pneumococci have high-level resistance to penicillin and to most other antibiotics except vancomycin.
13. Some strains of pneumococci and group A streptococci are erythromycin resistant.
14. Various aminoglycosides have been used in synergistic combination with penicillin or vancomycin. Because of the appearance of enterococcal strains resistant to the synergistic action with streptomycin (but not gentamicin), gentamicin is preferred for use in the combination.
15. Contraindicated in pregnancy or in the presence of renal insufficiency.
16. Antibiotics maybe administered orally for antibiotic-associated pseudomembranous enterocolitis. Vancomycin and metronidazole are equally effective but metronidazole is much less expensive.
17. Large doses of penicillin G or ampicillin (or amoxicillin) may be required because some strains are resistant to these drugs. Penicillinase-producing gonococci, which are more resistant to penicillin, have appeared in the United States; spectinomycin is the treatment of choice for infections with such strains.
18. In CNS infection, metronidazole or chloramphenicol should be used.
19. The carboxypenicillins are carbenicillin and ticarcillin; the acylaminopenicillins are mezlocillin, azlocillin, and piperacillin. When one of these drugs is used for a severe infection, an aminoglycoside is often recommended as well.
20. Aztreonam is a β-lactam antibiotic; cross-sensitivity has not occurred, but use with caution in patients allergic to penicillins, cephalosporins, or imipenem.
21. Principally in treatment of uncomplicated urinary tract infections.
22. Ampicillin or amoxicillin may be effective in milder cases.
23. In severely ill patients, an aminoglycoside is combined with a cephalosporin.

(continued)

24. Some encapsulated *H. influenzae* (type b) strains and some unencapsulated strains are resistant to ampicillin, and rare strains are resistant to chloramphenicol. Chloramphenicol plus ampicillin (or chloramphenicol alone) should be used for initial treatment of meningitis or epiglottitis in children until the organism is identified and its susceptibility is determined. For adults with meningitis of unknown etiology and an indeterminate Gram stain and in whom *H. influenzae* is suspected, chloramphenicol is added to ampicillin (or penicillin G) for the first 24 hr until the results of culture are available. Ampicillin is preferred when the infecting strain of *H. influenzae* is susceptible.

25. Not an FDA-approved use. Evidence for possible efficacy comes only from in vitro susceptibility testing and from treatment of infections in experimental animals. In both cases, *L. pneumophila* is highly susceptible to rifampin.

26. Most infections are self-limited without therapy.

27. Various combination treatments are available.

Penicillinase-Resistant Penicillins

Four penicillinase-resistant penicillins are available in the United States. Oxacillin and nafcillin can be administered parenterally or orally, but cloxacillin and, especially, dicloxacillin, which are available only as oral preparations, are preferred for oral administration because of superior GI absorption.

Penicillinase-Susceptible Broad-Spectrum Penicillins (Second-Generation Penicillins)

Ampicillin has a broader range of activity than penicillin G. Its spectrum encompasses not only pneumococci, meningococci, gonococci, and various streptococci but also several gram-negative bacilli. Like penicillin G, however, ampicillin is readily cleaved by β-lactamase and is useless in the treatment of infections caused by *S. aureus* or other organisms elaborating this enzyme. Plasmids conferring ampicillin resistance have appeared in *S. typhi, Haemophilus influenzae,* and *Neisseria gonorrhoeae*. As use of ampicillin has become more frequent, increasing resistance has appeared among strains of *Escherichia coli* and nontyphoidal *Salmonella* strains.

Amoxicillin has a spectrum of activity that is identical to ampicillin's, but amoxicillin is more efficiently absorbed from the GI tract, and effective concentrations are present in the circulation for twice as long.

Extended-Spectrum Carboxypenicillins (Third-Generation Penicillins)

The change from an amino to a carboxyl substituent on the side chain converts ampicillin to carbenicillin, which is much less active than ampicillin when compared by weight but has an extended spectrum of activity against gram-negative bacilli, including *Pseudomonas aeruginosa, Proteus* species other than *P. mirabilis,* and some strains of *Enterobacter.* The indanyl carbenicillin ester is acid stable and is suitable for oral administration in the treatment of urinary tract infections caused by susceptible gram-negative bacilli, including *Pseudomonas* [*see Table 4*], but blood levels are too low for use in other infections. Ticarcillin is the other carboxypenicillin; it may be administered intravenously to treat serious infections caused by susceptible organisms [*see Tables 3 and 4*]. Ticarcillin has an extended spectrum of activity against gram-negative bacilli, including *P. aeruginosa.* Because of widespread use of the antibiotic, however, many strains of *P. aeruginosa* are now ticarcillin-resistant.[25]

Extended-Spectrum Acylaminopenicillins (Fourth-Generation Penicillins)

Like the carboxypenicillins, the acylaminopenicillins (mezlocillin, piperacillin, and azlocillin) are ampicillin derivatives. They are active against most organisms that are susceptible to ampicillin, including many pneumococci, most streptococci, *N. meningitidis,* most *E. coli* and *P. mirabilis* strains, and non–penicillinase-producing strains of *H. influenzae* and *N. gonorrhoeae;* however, none of these drugs is superior to ampicillin or penicillin in treating infections caused by these organisms. All five drugs are ineffective against penicillinase-producing strains of *S. aureus.*

All five extended-spectrum penicillins differ from ampicillin in their increased effectiveness against many anaerobes, including about 50% of *Bacteroides fragilis* strains. However, the major role of these drugs depends on their spectrum of activity against resistant gram-negative bacilli, which is somewhat broader for the acylaminopenicillins than it is for the carboxypenicillins. Despite these in vitro differences, clinical studies have not demonstrated that the acylaminopenicillins are superior to the carboxypenicillins in treating organisms susceptible to both groups. The newer cephalosporins and carbapenems, however, appear to be preferable for treating infections caused by resistant *Klebsiella* and *Serratia* strains. The emergence of resistance is a concern with the acylaminopenicillins; like the carboxypenicillins, these newer drugs should generally be used with an aminoglycoside to treat seriously ill patients, especially those with neutropenia.

The serum levels, tissue distribution, half-life, and recommended dosage ranges of piperacillin, mezlocillin, and azlocillin are similar to those of

Table 4 Antimicrobial Drug Dosages for Treatment of Bacterial and Fungal Infections in Adults with Normal Renal Function

Class of Drug	Specific Agent	Trade Names	*Mild Infections**				*Uncomplicated Urinary Tract Infections*		*Major and Systemic Infections*†			
			Oral		*Intramuscular*		*Oral*		*Intramuscular*		*Intravenous*	
			Daily Dose	*Interval*	*Daily Dose*	*Interval*	*Daily Dose*	*Interval*	*Daily Dose*	*Interval*	*Daily Dose*	*Interval*
Penicillinase-susceptible penicillins	Penicillin G	Pentids, Crystifor, Pfizerpen, etc.	0.8–3.2 million units	6 hr	1.2 million units	8 hr	—	—	—	—	4–24 million units	2–4 hr
	Penicillin G benzathine	Bicillin	—	—	1.2–2.4 million units	See fn. 1	—	—	—	—	—	—
	Penicillin G procaine	Crysticillin, Duracillin, etc.	—	—	0.6–4.8 million units	6–24 hr	—	—	—	—	—	—
	Penicillin V	Pen-Vee K, V-cillin K, etc.	0.8–3.2 million units (0.5–2.0 g)	6 hr	—	—	—	—	—	—	—	—
Penicillinase-susceptible penicillins with activity against gram-negative bacilli	Amoxicillin	Amoxil, Larotid, etc.	750 mg–1.5 g	8 hr	—	—	750 mg–1.5 g	8 hr	—	—	—	—
	Ampicillin	Omnipen, Polycillin, etc.	1–4 g	6 hr	1–2 g	6 hr	2–4 g	6 hr	—	—	4–12 g	2–4 hr
	Azlocillin	Azlin	—	—	—	—	—	—	—	—	12–18 g	4 hr
	Carbenicillin indanyl sodium	Geocillin	—	—	—	—	4–8 tablets[2]	6 hr	—	—	—	—
	Mezlocillin	Mezlin	—	—	—	—	—	—	—	—	12–18 g	4 hr
	Piperacillin	Pipracil	—	—	See fn. 3	See fn. 3	—	—	See fn. 3	See fn. 3	12–18 g	4 hr
	Ticarcillin	Ticar	—	—	See fn. 4	See fn. 4	—	—	—	—	16–24 g	3–6 hr
Penicillinase-resistant penicillins	Cloxacillin	Tegopen	1–3 g	6 hr	—	—	—	—	—	—	—	—
	Dicloxacillin	Dynapen, Pathocil	1–2 g	6 hr	—	—	—	—	—	—	—	—
	Nafcillin	Nafcil, Unipen	2–4 g[5]	6 hr	2–3 g	4–6 hr	—	—	—	—	4–12 g	4–6 hr
	Oxacillin	Bactocill, Prostaphlin	2–4 g	6 hr	1–2 g	6 hr	—	—	—	—	4–12 g	4–6 hr
Penicillins with β-lactamase inhibitors	Amoxicillin–clavulanic acid	Augmentin	750 mg–1.5 g (amoxicillin)	8 hr	—	—	750 mg (amoxicillin)	8 hr	—	—	—	—
	Ampicillin-sulbactam	Unasyn	—	—	1 g (ampicillin)	6 hr	—	—	1–2 g (ampicillin)	6 hr	1–2 g (ampicillin)	6 hr
	Piperacillin-tazobactam	Zosyn	—	—	—	—	—	—	—	—	12 g (piperacillin)	6 hr
	Ticarcillin–clavulanic acid	Timentin	—	—	—	—	—	—	—	—	12–18 g (ticarcillin)	4–6 hr

Cephalosporins	Cefaclor	Ceclor	750 mg–1.5 g	8 hr	—	—	750 mg–1.5 g	8 hr	—	—	—	—
	Cefadroxil	Duricef	500 mg–2 g	12–24 hr	—	—	500 mg–2 g	12–24 hr	—	—	—	—
	Cefamandole	Mandol	—	—	2–4 g	6 hr	—	—	—	—	4–12 g	2–4 hr
	Cefazolin	Ancef, Kefzol	—	—	750 mg–1.5 g	8 hr	See fn. 6	See fn. 6	2–3 g	6–8 hr	2–6 g	6–8 hr
	Cefdinir	Omnicef	600 mg	24 hr	—	—	—	—	—	—	—	—
	Cefditoren pivoxil	Spectracef	200–400 mg	12 hr	—	—	—	—	—	—	2–6 g	8–12 hr
	Cefepime	Maxipime	—	—	—	—	400 mg	24 hr	—	—	—	—
	Cefixime	Suprax	400 mg	24 hr	—	—	—	—	—	—	2–4 g	12 hr
	Cefmetazole	Zefazone	—	—	—	—	—	—	—	—	4–8 g	6–12 hr
	Cefonicid	Monocid	—	—	See fn. 7, 8	See fn. 7, 8	—	—	—	—	0.5–2.0 g	12–24 hr
	Cefoperazone	Cefobid	—	—	See fn. 7, 8	See fn. 7, 8	—	—	—	—	2–12 g	6–8 hr
	Ceforanide	Precef	—	—	See fn. 7, 8	See fn. 7, 8	—	—	—	—	1–2 g	12 hr
	Cefotaxime	Claforan	—	—	See fn. 7, 8	See fn. 7, 8	—	—	—	—	2–12 g	4–6 hr
	Cefotetan	Cefotan	—	—	See fn. 7, 8	See fn. 7, 8	—	—	—	—	2–6 g	12 hr
	Cefoxitin	Mefoxin	—	—	2–4 g	6 hr	—	—	—	—	4–12 g	4 hr
	Cefpodoxime	Vantin	200–800 mg	12 hr	—	—	200 mg	12 hr	—	—	—	—
	Cefprozil	Cefzil	500 mg–1 g	12–24 hr	—	—	—	—	—	—	—	—
	Ceftazidime	Fortaz, Tazidime	—	—	See fn. 7, 8	See fn. 7, 8	—	—	—	—	2–6 g	8–12 hr
	Ceftibuten	Cedax	400 mg	24 hr	—	—	400 mg	24 hr	—	—	—	—
	Ceftizoxime	Cefizox	—	—	See fn. 7, 8	See fn. 7, 8	—	—	—	—	2–6 g	8–12 hr
	Ceftriaxone	Rocephin	—	—	See fn. 7, 8	See fn. 7, 8	—	—	—	—	1–4 g	12–24 hr
	Cefuroxime	Zinacef, Ceftin (p.o.)	250–500 mg	12 hr	See fn. 7, 8	See fn. 7, 8	—	—	—	—	3–6 g	6 hr
	Cephalexin	Keflex	1–4 g	6 hr	—	—	1–4 g	6 hr	—	—	—	—
	Cephapirin	Cefadyl	—	—	2–3 g	6 hr	—	—	—	—	4–12 g	2–4 hr
	Cephradine	Anspor, Velosef	1–4 g	6 hr	2 g	6 hr	2 g	6 hr	—	—	3–8 g	4–6 hr
	Loracarbef	Lorabid	400–800 mg	12 hr	—	—	400 mg	12 hr	—	—	—	—

Note: all superscript numbers refer to footnotes that follow table.
*Infections of the upper respiratory tract, soft tissues, etc.
†Osteomyelitis, peritonitis, bacteremia, meningitis, endocarditis, etc.

Table 4 (continued)

Class of Drug	Specific Agent	Trade Names	Mild Infections*				Uncomplicated Urinary Tract Infections		Major and Systemic Infections†			
			Oral		Intramuscular		Oral		Intramuscular		Intravenous	
			Daily Dose	Interval	Daily Dose	Interval	Daily Dose	Interval	Daily Dose	Interval	Daily Dose	Interval
Carbapenems	Imipenem-cilastatin	Primaxin	—	—	—	—	—	—	—	—	1–4 g	6–8 hr
	Meropenem	Merrem	—	—	—	—	—	—	—	—	3 g	8 hr
	Ertapenem	Ivanz	—	—	—	—	—	—	—	—	1 g	24 hr
Monobactams	Aztreonam	Azactam	—	—	1–2 g	8–12 hr	—	—	—	—	3–8 g	6–8 hr
Aminoglycosides	Amikacin	Amikin	—	—	—	—	—	—	15 mg/kg[9]	8–12 hr	15 mg/kg[10]	8 hr
	Gentamicin	Garamycin	—	—	3–5 mg/kg[11]	8 hr	—	—	3–5 mg/kg	8 hr	3–5 mg/kg[12]	8 hr
	Kanamycin	Kantrex	—	—	—	—	—	—	15 mg/kg[13]	8–12 hr	15 mg/kg[14]	8 hr
	Neomycin	—	See fn. 15	See fn. 15	—	—	—	—	—	—	—	—
	Netilmicin	Netromycin	—	—	4–6 mg/kg[11,12]	8 hr	—	—	4–6 mg/kg	8 hr	4–6 mg/kg[16]	8 hr
	Streptomycin	—	—	—	1–2 g	12 hr	—	—	1–2 g	12 hr	—	—
	Tobramycin	Nebcin	—	—	3–5 mg/kg[11]	8 hr	—	—	3–5 mg/kg	8 hr	3–5 mg/kg[16]	8 hr
Tetracyclines	Demeclocycline	Declomycin	600 mg	6 hr	—	—	600 mg	6 hr	—	—	—	—
	Doxycycline	Vibramycin, etc.	100–200 mg[17]	12 hr	—	—	100–200 mg[17]	12 hr	—	—	100–200 mg[18]	12 hr
	Minocycline	Minocin	200 mg[19]	12 hr	—	—	200 mg[19]	12 hr	—	—	200 mg[20]	12 hr
	Oxytetracycline	Terramycin	1–2 g	6 hr	See fn. 21	See fn. 21	1–2 g	6 hr	—	—	—	—
	Tetracycline	Achromycin, Panmycin, Sumycin, Tetracyn, etc.	1–2 g	6 hr	See fn. 21	See fn. 21	1–2 g	6 hr	See fn. 21	See fn. 21	750 mg–1 g[22]	6–12 hr
Macrolides	Azithromycin	Zithromax	500 mg day 1 250 mg days 2–5	24 hr	—	—	—	—	—	—	—	—
	Clarithromycin	Biaxin	500 mg–1 g	12 hr	—	—	—	—	—	—	—	—
	Dirithromycin	Dynabac	500 mg	24 hr	—	—	—	—	—	—	—	—

Macrolides (*continued*)	Erythromycin	E-Mycin, Erythrocin, Ilotycin	1–2 g	6 hr	See fn. 21	See fn. 21	—	—	See fn. 21	See fn. 21	2–4 g	6 hr
	Erythromycin estolate[23]	Ilosone	1–2 g	6 hr	—	—	—	—	—	—	—	—
Sulfonamides	Sulfadiazine	—	2–4 g[24]	6 hr	—	—	2–4 g[24]	6 hr	—	—	—	—
	Sulfisoxazole	Gantrisin	2–6 g[24]	6 hr	—	—	2–6 g[24]	6 hr	—	—	100 mg/kg[24]	4–6 hr
	Trimethoprim-sulfamethoxazole	Bactrim, Septra	4 tablets[25]	12 hr	—	—	4 tablets[25]	12 hr	—	—	8–12 mg/kg[25] (trimethoprim)	6 hr[25]
Miscellaneous antibacterial agents	Clindamycin	Cleocin	600 mg–1.8 g	6 hr	600 mg–1.2 g	6–8 hr	—	—	1.2–2.4 g	6–8 hr	1.8–3.0 g	6–8 hr
	Chloramphenicol	Chloromycetin	1.5–3.0 g	6 hr	See fn. 26	See fn. 26	1.5–2.0 g[27]	6 hr	See fn. 26	See fn. 26	2–4 g	6 hr
	Metronidazole	Flagyl	250 mg	8 hr	—	—	—	—	—	—	30 mg/kg	6 hr
	Spectinomycin	Trobicin	—	—	2 g[28]	Single injection	—	—	—	—	—	—
	Trimethoprim	Proloprim, Trimpex	200 mg	12 hr	—	—	200 mg	12 hr	—	—	—	—
	Vancomycin	Vancocin	2 g[29]	6 hr	—	—	—	—	—	—	1–2 g	6–12 hr
Urinary tract disinfectants	Fosfomycin	Monurol	—	—	—	—	3 g	1 dose	—	—	—	—
	Methenamine mandelate	Mandelamine	—	—	—	—	4 g	6 hr	—	—	—	—
	Methenamine hippurate	Hiprex	—	—	—	—	2 g	12 hr	—	—	—	—
	Nalidixic acid	NegGram	—	—	—	—	2–4 g	6 hr	—	—	—	—
	Nitrofurantoin	Furadantin, Macrodantin	—	—	—	—	200–400 mg	6 hr	—	—	Not recommended	—
Antifungal drugs	Amphotericin B	Fungizone	—	—	—	—	—	—	—	—	0.25–1.0 mg/kg[30]	24 hr
	Fluconazole[31]	Diflucan	100–200 mg[32]	24 hr	—	—	—	—	—	—	200 mg[31]	24 hr
	Flucytosine	Ancobon	50–150 mg/kg[33]	6 hr	—	—	—	—	—	—	—	—

Note: all superscript numbers refer to footnotes that follow table.
*Infections of the upper respiratory tract, soft tissues, etc.
†Osteomyelitis, peritonitis, bacteremia, meningitis, endocarditis, etc.

Table 4 (continued)

Class of Drug	Specific Agent	Trade Names	Mild Infections*				Uncomplicated Urinary Tract Infections		Major and Systemic Infections†			
			Oral		Intramuscular		Oral		Intramuscular		Intravenous	
			Daily Dose	Interval	Daily Dose	Interval	Daily Dose	Interval	Daily Dose	Interval	Daily Dose	Interval
Antifungal drugs (continued)	Itraconazole	Sporanox	100–400 mg	12 or 24 hr	—	—	—	—	—	—	—	—
	Ketoconazole	Nizoral	200 mg[33]	24 hr	—	—	—	—	See fn. 32	See fn. 32	See fn. 32	See fn. 32
	Miconazole	Monistat	—	—	—	—	—	—	—	—	600 mg–3.6 g[34]	8 hr
	Nystatin	Mycostatin	1.5–3.0 million units[35]	8 hr	—	—	—	—	—	—	—	—
Fluoroquinolones[36]	Alatrofloxacin[36]	Trovan I.V.	—	—	—	—	—	—	—	—	200 mg	24 hr
	Ciprofloxacin	Cipro	500 mg	12 hr	—	—	250–500 mg	12 hr	—	—	400 mg	12 hr
	Levofloxacin	Levaquin	500 mg	24 hr	—	—	500 mg	24 hr	—	—	500 mg	24 hr
	Lomefloxacin	Maxaquin	400 mg	24 hr	—	—	400 mg	24 hr	—	—	—	—
	Norfloxacin	Noroxin	—	—	—	—	800 mg	12 hr	—	—	—	—
	Ofloxacin	Floxin	400–800 mg	12 hr	—	—	400 mg	12 hr	—	—	800 mg	12 hr
	Sparfloxacin	Zagam	400 mg first day, then 200 mg	24 hr	—	—	—	—	—	—	—	—
	Trovafloxacin[36]	Trovan	See fn. 36	See fn. 36	—	—	—	—	—	—	—	—
	Gatifloxacin	Tequin	400 mg	24 hr	—	—	400 mg	24 hr	—	—	400 mg	24 hr
	Moxifloxacin	Avelox	400 mg	—	—	—	400 mg	24 hr	—	—	—	—
Streptogramins	Quinupristin/dalfopristin	Synercid	—	—	—	—	—	—	—	—	7.5 mg/kg	8 hr
Oxazolidinones	Linezolid	Zyvox	400 mg	12 hr	—	—	—	—	—	—	600 mg (I.V. or p.o.)	12 hr

Note: all superscript numbers refer to footnotes that follow table.

*Infections of the upper respiratory tract, soft tissues, etc.

†Osteomyelitis, peritonitis, bacteremia, meningitis, endocarditis, etc.

1. Benzathine penicillin G is used primarily in three circumstances: (1) treatment of streptococcal pharyngitis in cases in which patient compliance is questionable (a single dose of 1.2 million U I.M.); (2) prophylaxis for rheumatic fever recurrences (1.2–2.4 million U I.M. once monthly); (3) treatment of syphilis: for primary, secondary, or early (less than 1 yr) latent syphilis, a single dose of 2.4 million U I.M.; for late syphilis (late latent, cardiovascular, neurosyphilis, etc.)2.4 million U I.M. weekly for three doses has been recommended, but many physicians now treat neurosyphilis with high-dose I.V. penicillin.

2. Each tablet of carbenicillin indanyl sodium is equivalent to 382 mg of carbenicillin (usual dosage is one to two tablets p.o., q.i.d.).

3. Piperacillin is most often used in the treatment of serious infections caused by susceptible *Pseudomonas, Klebsiella, Enterobacter*, and non-*mirabilis Proteus* strains; the agent is given in maximal dosage (12–18 g daily I.V.). It is commonly used in synergistic combinations with tobramycin or gentamicin for treatment of *Pseudomonas* infections. Occasionally, it is given in smaller dosages (1.0–1.5 g I.M. or I.V. q. 6 hr) to treat an uncomplicated urinary tract infection caused by the same organisms.

4. Ticarcillin, piperacillin, mezlocillin, and azlocillin are usually used in the treatment of serious infections caused by susceptible *Pseudomonas, Enterobacter*, and non-*mirabilis Proteus* strains and are given in maximal dosage (12–24 g daily I.V.). One of these agents is commonly used in synergistic combination with tobramycin or

gentamicin for treatment of *Pseudomonas* infections. Occasionally, they are given in small dosages (1 g I.M. or I.V. q. 6 hr) to treat an uncomplicated urinary tract infection caused by the same organisms.

5. Nafcillin is not reliably absorbed by the oral route.

6. Cefazolin may be used to treat uncomplicated urinary tract infections caused by susceptible gram-negative bacilli (*Escherichia coli, Proteus mirabilis*, and *Klebsiella*). It is administered I.M. in a dosage of 2 g daily (given as aliquots q. 8 hr).

7. Although the second- and third-generation cephalosporins can be used for milder infections at the lower end of their recommended dosage range, these potent but expensive agents should generally be reserved for serious infections or for the treatment of resistant organisms when the alternative is a more toxic antimicrobial drug.

8. The I.M. route is acceptable for milder illnesses, but the I.V. route is recommended for serious infections, including bacteremias and meningitis. The I.M. dosage range is the same as that for the I.V. dosage.

9. Dosage must be reduced in the presence of renal insufficiency. The daily parenteral dose should not exceed 15 mg/kg, and the total daily amount administered should not exceed 1.5 g, regardless of the patient's weight.

10. The I.V. dose should be infused over a period of 30–60 min q. 8 hr.

11. For urinary tract infections caused by resistant organisms.

12. Dosage must be reduced in the presence of renal insufficiency. The I.V. dose should be administered over a period of 30–60 min q. 8 hr. In patients with meningitis caused by susceptible gram-negative bacilli, intrathecal gentamicin (5 mg for adults, 1–2 mg for infants) is often administered once daily along with parenteral gentamicin until CSF cultures are negative.

13. Dosage must be reduced in the presence of renal insufficiency. The daily parenteral dose should not exceed 15 mg/kg (daily dose should not exceed 1.5 g, regardless of weight); the total quantity administered in a therapeutic course should not exceed 15 g.

14. The I.V. route should be employed only when I.M. administration is not possible. The I.V. drug should be administered over a period of at least 60 min q. 8 hr.

15. There are no clinical indications for the parenteral administration of neomycin in view of its marked toxicity and the availability of safer alternative drugs. The drug is given p.o. or by nasogastric tube (4–6 g daily in four divided doses) to reduce the number of ammonia-forming bacteria in the intestine in the short-term treatment of acute hepatic coma. It is also given in a total daily dose of 2–3 g in long-term therapy for chronic hepatic encephalopathy or episodic hepatic coma. Nephrotoxicity and ototoxicity have followed prolonged high-dose therapy in hepatic coma, particularly in patients with some renal impairment.

Neomycin is also used along with vigorous mechanical cleansing of the large bowel as preoperative prophylaxis for bowel surgery. In this situation, it is administered for 1–3 days preoperatively (40 mg/kg p.o. daily in six divided doses).

16. Dosage must be reduced in the presence of renal insufficiency. The intravenous dose should be administered over a period of 30–60 min q. 8 hr.

17. Usually administered as 100 mg p.o. q. 12 hr on the first day of treatment, followed by 50 mg q. 12 hr. For more difficult infections, the dosage may be continued at 100 mg q. 12 hr.

18. Usually administered as 100 mg I.V. q. 12 hr on the first day of treatment. Thereafter, it may be given as 50–100 mg q. 12 hr I.V. Each I.V. dose should be given over a period of 1–4 hr.

19. Usually administered initially as 200 mg p.o., followed by 100 mg q. 12 hr.

20. Usually given initially as 200 mg I.V., followed by 100 mg q. 12 hr. Maximal dose in any 24-hr period is 400 mg.

21. I.M. administration is generally unsatisfactory because of poor absorption and local irritation.

22. In special circumstances, it may be given in higher doses but not in excess of 500 mg q. 6 hr.

23. Cholestatic hepatitis may develop as a hypersensitivity response to erythromycin estolate but not to the other erythromycin preparations. For this reason, erythromycin base or erythromycin stearate is preferable.

24. A loading dose of half the daily dosage is given initially. In severe infections, the dosage of sulfonamide is adjusted to provide a blood level of 10–15 mg/dl. Sulfonamides must be used with caution in patients with renal insufficiency. Sulfisoxazole is the preferred sulfonamide.

25. Each tablet contains 80 mg trimethoprim and 400 mg sulfamethoxazole. Double-strength tablets are also available (usual dosage is one tablet q. 12 hr). Pediatric suspensions contain 40 mg trimethoprim and 200 mg sulfamethoxazole per 5 ml. Trimethoprim-sulfamethoxazole has also been used in the treatment of typhoid fever in the same dosage as recommended for urinary tract infections. It has been used in a dosage of four to eight standard tablets daily in the treatment of brucellosis. For pneumonia caused by *Pneumocystis carinii*, the dosage is 20 mg/kg trimethoprim and 100 mg/kg sulfamethoxazole per 24 hr (equally divided doses q. 6 hr).The I.V. dosage of trimethoprim-sulfamethoxazole ranges from 8 mg/kg trimethoprim and 40 mg/kg sulfamethoxazole per 24 hr to 20 mg/kg trimethoprim and 100 mg/kg sulfamethoxazole per 24 hr. The lower dosage range is used in the treatment of urinary tract infections that require parenteral antimicrobial therapy and in the treatment of shigellosis; the larger dosage is employed in the treatment of *P. carinii* pneumonia.

26. Chloramphenicol sodium succinate, the parenteral preparation, should only be used I.V. It is ineffective when administered I.M.

27. Chloramphenicol should not be used in the treatment of a urinary tract infection that could be managed with another, safer, effective antimicrobial.

28. The only approved indication for the use of spectinomycin is in the treatment of anogenital and urethral gonorrhea in a penicillin-allergic patient or when the infecting organism is highly penicillin resistant. In geographic areas where antibiotic-resistant gonococci are prevalent, treatment with 4 g of spectinomycin (2 g in each gluteal region) may be indicated.

29. Vancomycin is not absorbed through the GI tract. Its use orally is for treatment of staphylococcal enterocolitis or antibiotic-associated enterocolitis.

30. The dry powder is reconstituted by addition of Sterile Water for Injection, USP, *without a bacteriostatic agent*. The solution is then added to a bottle of 5% Dextrose Injection, USP. The pH of the dextrose solution should first be checked to verify that it is above 4.2. If it is not, a buffer solution (as described in package insert) should be added. Amphotericin B solutions should be administered promptly after preparation and should be protected from light during administration. It is given once a day over 6 hr. (Later in the course of administration, double the daily dose is sometimes given on an alternate-day schedule.) Dosage is 1 mg on the first day and then increased in 5 mg increments each day until maintenance dosage is reached. The daily dose is determined by the susceptibility of the organism and the occurrence of toxic side effects. In some instances (e.g., cryptococcal meningitis), combination therapy with flucytosine p.o. may allow employment of smaller daily doses (0.3–0.4 mg/kg) of amphotericin B. In fungal meningitis, intrathecal administration may be necessary (0.1 mg initially, increased gradually to 0.5 mg q. 48–72 hr), depending on the evaluation of the patient's condition.

31. Fluconazole is very useful for the treatment of oropharyngeal, esophageal, and disseminated infections caused by *Candida* and for control of cryptococcus, especially chronic suppression of cryptococcal meningitis in patients with AIDS. To initiate therapy, a loading dose of twice the usual daily dose should be used. A daily dose of 400 mg can be used for cryptococcal meningitis, depending on the patient's response to therapy. The dose should be reduced in patients who have renal insufficiency.

32. Used in the treatment of urinary tract infections and visceral infections caused by *Candida*. Also used in cryptococcal infections in which amphotericin B is not tolerated. Resistance to flucytosine may develop during treatment of candidal and cryptococcal infections. Sometimes used in combination with amphotericin B to treat systemic fungal infections.

33. Ketoconazole is indicated in the treatment of patients with susceptible fungal infections that have failed to respond to amphotericin B or in the treatment of patients unable to tolerate the toxic effects of amphotericin B. In either role, it is generally preferred to therapy with miconazole when the patients can take oral medications. It is also the drug of choice in the long-term treatment of chronic mucocutaneous candidiasis. It has been useful in the treatment of histoplasmosis, coccidioidomycosis, chromomycosis, and paracoccidioidomycosis. In view of its poor penetration of the CSF, it should not be used in the treatment of coccidioidal or cryptococcal meningitis. Ketoconazole requires gastric acidity for dissolution and absorption. Antacids and cimetidine, if needed, should be given at least 2 hr after a dose of ketoconazole. The most frequent side effects have been nausea and vomiting. Several cases of liver injury of varying severity, possibly the result of idiosyncratic reactions, have occurred during ketoconazole therapy. Liver function tests, therefore, should be evaluated before and periodically during treatment, especially in patients who are on prolonged therapy or who have preexisting hepatic disease. Ketoconazole, in daily dosages of 200–1,800 mg p.o., is used in major and systemic fungal infections for which the mycotic agent is susceptible and amphotericin B cannot be employed.

34. Miconazole is available for parenteral therapy for systemic mycoses. Experience is relatively limited, and it should probably be reserved for patients who cannot tolerate or who do not respond to amphotericin B and flucytosine. Miconazole is metabolized by extrarenal mechanisms, and patients with fungal bladder infections require supplementary bladder irrigation with the drug. Side effects of miconazole include phlebitis, fever, rash, nausea and vomiting, anemia, thrombocytopenia, and transient hyperlipidemia caused by the diluent used.

35. Not absorbed from the GI tract. Use only in treatment of intestinal tract colonization by *Candida* species and not for any systemic mycotic infection. Nystatin suspension (400,000–600,000 units q.i.d.) is used as a mouthwash in treatment of oral thrush. The suspension can also be swallowed for use in the treatment of candidal esophagitis.

36. See Table 6 for attributes of the various fluoroquinolones. None of these drugs is recommended for children. In 1999, the FDA limited trovafloxacin to inpatient use for limb- or life-threatening infections.

ticarcillin. Unlike ticarcillin, however, piperacillin, mezlocillin, and azlocillin are excreted in the bile and the urine and do not accumulate in patients with renal failure. The toxicities of these drugs are identical, except that mezlocillin seems less likely to impair platelet function; the major adverse reactions include rash, drug fever, eosinophilia, leukopenia, thrombocytopenia, and abnormalities in liver function.

Penicillin–β-Lactamase Inhibitor Combinations

The major mechanism of resistance to the penicillins is bacterial production of β-lactamase enzymes that hydrolyze the β-lactam ring, rendering the molecule inactive. Clavulanic acid, sulbactam, and tazobactam are β-lactam compounds that have little intrinsic antibacterial activity. They do, however, bind irreversibly to the β-lactamase enzymes that are produced by many bacteria, thus inactivating these enzymes and rendering the organisms sensitive to β-lactamase–susceptible penicillins.

Clavulanic acid is available with amoxicillin in an oral formulation. Ampicillin-sulbactam, ticarcillin–clavulanic acid, and piperacillin-tazobactam are parenteral formulations. In addition to showing activity against ampicillin-susceptible organisms, the combinations are also active against various ampicillin-resistant organisms, including *Moraxella catarrhalis*, β-lactamase–producing strains of *H. influenzae*, *E. coli*, *K. pneumoniae*, some *Proteus* species, and *S. aureus* (except methicillin-resistant strains). The combinations are also active against gonococci, enterococci, and many anaerobes, including *B. fragilis*. However, *P. aeruginosa* and many strains of *Serratia* and *Enterobacter* are resistant to ampicillin–clavulanic acid and ampicillin-sulbactam.

Amoxicillin–clavulanic acid therapy has been used successfully to treat upper and lower respiratory tract infections, urinary tract infections, and human and animal bites. Twice-a-day administration is effective.

The ampicillin-sulbactam combination has been used successfully to treat gynecologic and intra-abdominal infections, as well as infections of the upper and lower respiratory tracts, urinary tract, skin and soft tissues, and bones and joints. Ticarcillin–clavulanic acid has been successful in the treatment of pulmonary, urinary tract, bone, soft tissue, and bloodstream infections. Piperacillin-tazobactam is very similar to ticarcillin–clavulanic acid in its spectrum of activity, pharmacokinetics, toxicities, and expense. The recommended dosage of 3 g of piperacillin and 375 mg of tazobactam every 6 hours for adults with normal renal function is lower than the recommended dosage for piperacillin alone (18 g/day) and is not sufficient for some serious infections caused by *P. aeruginosa*.

CEPHALOSPORINS

The cephalosporins and closely related cephamycins (e.g., cefoxitin and cefotetan) are a large and rapidly expanding group of β-lactam antibiotics. Like the penicillins, the cephalosporins are bactericidal antibiotics that inhibit bacterial cell wall synthesis and have a low intrinsic toxicity. The adverse effects of the cephalosporins are mainly hypersensitivity reactions, local pain (with intramuscular use), and thrombophlebitis (with intravenous use). Less common toxicities include GI symptoms, elevated liver enzyme levels, and renal impairment; third- and fourth-generation cephalosporins may cause seizures, including nonconvulsive status epilepticus, in patients with renal failure.[26] Pseudomembranous colitis may also develop. Because the cephalosporins share immunologic cross-reactivity, patients who are allergic to one cephalosporin are likely to be allergic to others; there is also a possibility of cross-reactivity in penicillin-allergic patients.[27] The cephalosporins are grouped into generations on the basis of their antibacterial spectrum[28] [*see Table 5*]; in general, activity against gram-positive cocci diminishes from the first generation to the third generation, whereas the spectrum of activity against gram-negative organisms increases. Agents in each group exhibit pharmacologic differences that are related to differences in serum levels and half-lives; thus, recommended doses vary substantially. Most cephalosporins are excreted primarily by the kidneys; dosages must be reduced in the presence of renal failure. Probenecid blocks tubular secretion of most cephalosporins, prolonging and enhancing the blood levels achieved. Cephalosporins cross the placenta and penetrate the pericardium and joints. The third-generation cephalosporins display good activity in cerebrospinal fluid; none of the first-generation drugs and only one second-generation agent (cefuroxime) are effective in meningitis. Cefepime is the only drug currently classified as a fourth-generation cephalosporin; it closely resembles the third-generation drugs. Like the newer penicillins, the newer cephalosporins have an extraordinarily broad spec-

Table 5 Properties of Cephalosporin Antibiotics

	Specific Agent	*Trade Names*	*Comments**
First Generation	Oral		
	Cefadroxil	Duricef, Ultracef	Longer half-life
	Cephalexin	Keflex	Most experience with this agent
	Cephradine	Anspor, Velosef	Properties are similar to those of cephalexin
	Parenteral		
	Cefazolin	Ancef, Kefzol	Longer half-life; well tolerated when given I.M.
	Cephapirin	Cefadyl	Properties are similar to those of other first-generation cephalosporins
	Cephradine	Anspor, Velosef	Properties are similar to those of other first-generation cephalosporins
Second Generation	Oral		
	Cefaclor	Ceclor	Moderately active against *Haemophilus influenzae*
	Cefuroxime axetil	Ceftin	Active against *H. influenzae*
	Cefprozil	Cefzil	Active against *H. influenzae*
	Cefditoren pivoxil	Spectracef	Active against *H. influenzae*
	Loracarbef	Lorabid	A carbacephem with properties and spectrum similar to cefuroxime
	Parenteral		
	Cefamandole	Mandol	Active against *H. influenzae*; may cause bleeding
	Cefmetazole	Zefazone	Spectrum and half-life similar to cefoxitin; may cause bleeding
	Cefonicid	Monocid	Spectrum similar to that of cefamandole
	Ceforanide	Precef	Spectrum similar to that of cefamandole
	Cefotetan	Cefotan	Spectrum similar to that of cefoxitin; longer half-life than cefoxitin; may cause bleeding
	Cefoxitin	Mefoxin	Active against *Bacteroides fragilis, Serratia, Neisseria gonorrhoeae*
	Cefuroxime	Zinacef, Kefurox	Active against *H. influenzae*; only second-generation drug approved for meningitis (selected pathogens)
Third Generation	Oral		
	Cefixime	Suprax	More active against gram-negative bacilli, gonococci, *Moraxella catarrhalis*, and *H. influenzae* than other oral cephalosporins but much less active against *Staphylococcus aureus*; not active against *Pseudomonas*
	Cefdinir	Omnicef	Similar to cefpodoxime but administered in a single daily dose
	Cefpodoxime	Vantin	Similar to cefixime but more active against *S. aureus*
	Ceftibuten	Cedax	Similar to cefixime except poor activity against pneumococci and staphylococci
	Parenteral		
	Cefepime	Maxipime	Active against most gram-positive cocci (except enterococci and methicillin-resistant staphylococci), *Neisseria, Haemophilus*, enteric gram-negative bacilli, and *Pseudomonas*
	Cefoperazone	Cefobid	Increased activity against *P. aeruginosa* but less against Enterobacteriaceae; may cause bleeding
	Cefotaxime	Claforan	More active against gram-positive cocci
	Ceftazidime	Fortaz, Tazidime, Tazicef	More active against *Pseudomonas*
	Ceftizoxime	Cefizox	Properties are similar to those of cefotaxime
	Ceftriaxone	Rocephin	Longer half-life; less active against *Pseudomonas, B. fragilis*

Note: detailed information about the various cephalosporins is covered in the text.
*Agents are being compared with other members of the same generation of cephalosporins.

trum of antimicrobial activity but are very expensive.

First-Generation Cephalosporins

The first-generation cephalosporins are active against many gram-positive bacteria, including penicillin-sensitive pneumococci, penicillin-resistant *S. aureus*, most streptococci, and most gram-positive anaerobes, including *Actinomyces*. However, they are ineffective against methicillin-resistant *S. aureus*, coagulase-negative staphylococci, penicillin-resistant pneumococci, enterococci, and *Listeria*. Although the first-generation cephalosporins are active against many strains of *E. coli, K. pneumoniae*, and *P. mirabilis*, they are ineffective against many other gram-negative species because these organisms produce chromosomally determined, membrane-bound β-lactamases.

Second-Generation Cephalosporins

Because they are not vulnerable to the β-lactamases produced by many gram-negative bacteria, the second-generation cephalosporins have enhanced activity against gram-negative bacilli, including many strains of *E. coli, Klebsiella, Serratia,* and *Proteus* that are resistant to first-generation cephalosporins[29]; however, they are not effective against *Pseudomonas* or *Enterobacter* species. The second-generation cephalosporins retain activity against gram-positive organisms that are susceptible to first-generation cephalosporins. Despite these similarities, there are also differences among the members of this group of drugs; only certain agents are active against *H. influenzae,* and only three are active against *B. fragilis* [*see Table 3*]. Cefuroxime is the only second-generation cephalosporin approved for use in bacterial meningitis.

Third-Generation Cephalosporins

The third-generation cephalosporins differ from other cephalosporins in some important respects. Their enhanced ability to resist hydrolysis by the β-lactamase of many gram-negative bacilli gives them an expanded antibacterial spectrum. Pharmacologically, these drugs also have an important advantage: unlike older cephalosporins, they achieve therapeutic levels in the CSF and can be used to treat meningitis. These advantages come at an increased cost.

Although third-generation agents are less active than the older cephalosporins against many gram-positive cocci,[30] they are active against most penicillin-nonsensitive pneumococci. Like the earlier cephalosporins, the third-generation agents are inactive against enterococci, methicillin-resistant *S. aureus,* and *Listeria;* however, they have enhanced potency against many gram-negative bacilli, including *E. coli, Klebsiella, Proteus, Serratia,* and *Citrobacter* organisms. They are also very active against penicillinase-producing and non–penicillinase-producing strains of *H. influenzae* and gonococci. The third-generation cephalosporins are active against most *Salmonella* species and have been clinically effective in the treatment of typhoid fever and other *Salmonella* infections; resistant strains are now beginning to emerge in the United States, however.[31] Although most *Enterobacter* species are initially sensitive to third-generation cephalosporins, they rapidly develop resistance because of inducible cephalosporinase; hence, it may be prudent to avoid using a cephalosporin as the sole therapy for these organisms. A similar resistance has been reported in *Klebsiella* species; results of disk diffusion testing indicate that *Klebsiella* organisms may be sensitive to other third-generation cephalosporins, but these antibiotics are inhibitory rather than bactericidal and may be ineffective clinically. Aztreonam resistance is a useful marker for these strains. Imipenem is usually effective against cephalosporin-resistant *Klebsiella.*

Although third-generation cephalosporins exhibit activity against *B. fragilis* and other anaerobes, cefoxitin, cefotetan, and cefmetazole, which are second-generation cephalosporins, are more active. Ceftazidime and cefepime are the cephalosporins with the greatest activity against *P. aeruginosa;* cefoperazone also demonstrates activity, but the other third-generation cephalosporins have been disappointing. Other nosocomial gram-negative pathogens that are resistant to these drugs include *Acinetobacter* and *Xanthomonas.*

The third-generation cephalosporins seem to have the same relatively low toxicities as the older cephalosporins.

Choosing a Cephalosporin

The clinician who is confronted with 16 parenteral and 12 oral cephalosporins may understandably find such an array of drugs confusing. Although the choice of an antimicrobial agent for any one patient must be individualized, a few general guidelines may be helpful.[28]

In general, the least expensive cephalosporin that will be effective should be prescribed. Similarly, to minimize toxicity (including superinfection) and cost, the lowest effective dose should be used. Finally, when choosing an antibiotic, physicians should compare the cephalosporins with other antibiotics, including β-lactams and aminoglycosides, in terms of effectiveness, toxicity, and cost.

Surgical prophylaxis Cephalosporins are widely used perioperatively to prevent infection. For surgical prophylaxis, the newer cephalosporins provide no advantages over the much less expensive first-generation cephalosporins. A possible exception is in colorectal and abdominal operations, for which the prominence of anaerobes makes cefoxitin, cefotetan, or cefmetazole a rational choice; however, even in such cases, bowel preparation with oral antibiotics may provide a less costly alternative. In general, adequate surgical prophylaxis can be achieved with regimens ranging from a single dose to 48 hours of cephalosporin administration.

Meningitis The third-generation cephalosporins have emerged as the agents of choice for gram-negative bacillary meningitis caused by susceptible organisms. *P. aeruginosa* meningitis has been an exception, but ceftazidime and cefepime, alone or combined with an aminoglycoside or ciprofloxacin, have proved useful in this difficult situation. Penicillin remains the drug of choice for meningococcal meningitis; ampicillin is the drug of choice for meningitis caused by non–penicillinase-producing strains of *H. influenzae.* In penicillin-allergic patients who can tolerate cephalosporins, a third-generation cephalosporin is preferable to chloramphenicol in the treatment of meningitis caused by one of these pathogens. None of the cephalosporins should be used for *Listeria* or enterococcal meningitis. First- and second-generation cephalosporins (except cefuroxime) should never be used as therapy for meningitis.

Gram-negative pneumonia Excellent results have been obtained in the treatment of gram-negative pneumonia with the newer cephalosporins. Because aminoglycosides are likely to be less active in the acid pH of infected lungs, the newer cephalosporins may be preferred for the treatment of nosocomial pneumonias other than those caused by either *Acinetobacter,* which is cephalosporin resistant, or *Enterobacter,* which rapidly develops resistance.

Other infections Ceftriaxone is the drug of choice for Lyme disease involving the CNS and for gonorrhea in geographic regions where the prevalence of penicillinase-producing strains of *N. gonorrhoeae* is 1% or higher. Although cephalosporins have been effective in the treatment of many other infections, they have not been clearly identified as the drug of choice in any of these infections. For example, penicillin remains the preferred drug for group A streptococcal infection, and nafcillin or oxacillin is the drug of choice for infections caused by susceptible *S. aureus* strains, although a first-generation cephalosporin is an excellent alternative in patients who cannot tolerate these drugs. Cephalosporins are ineffective against methicillin-resistant *S. aureus* strains, most coagulase-negative staphylococcal infections, and enterococcal infections. Although cefoxitin, cefotetan, and cefmetazole have been very useful for the treatment of anaerobic infections, penicillin or clindamycin appears to be preferable for the treatment of aspiration pneumonia. Antimicrobial regimens that include clindamycin, metronidazole, ticarcillin–clavulanic acid, ampicillin-sulbactam, piperacillin-tazobactam, or imipenem are reasonable alternatives to cephalosporins for the treatment of abdominal and pelvic infections. For cases of suspected sepsis and for infection in immunologically impaired hosts, the effectiveness of a cephalosporin, with or without an aminoglycoside, must be compared with the effectiveness of carbapenems and various penicillin-aminoglycoside combinations.

OTHER β-LACTAM ANTIBIOTICS

Carbapenems

Imipenem and meropenem were the first carbapenems available for clinical use in the United States; the third, ertapenem, was released in 2002. Like other β-lactam antibiotics, they are bactericidal and act by inhibiting bacterial cell wall synthesis.[32] Three properties account for the extraordinarily broad antibacterial spectrum of the carbapenems: there is no permeability barrier excluding the drugs from bacteria; they have high affinity for penicillin-binding protein 2 (PBP-2), which is a crucial component of cell wall structure; and they are extremely resistant to hydrolysis by β-lactamases.

Imipenem is extensively degraded in the renal tubule, which results in low urinary levels of the drug. This drawback can be prevented by using cilastatin, an inhibitor of the brush-border enzyme dehydropeptidase-1. Cilastatin also appears to prevent the tubular damage that is occasionally observed in animals given imipenem alone in high doses. For clinical use, imipenem is administered simultaneously with cilastatin in equal doses.

Meropenem is pharmacologically similar to imipenem except that it is not susceptible to degradation by dehydropeptidase; as a result, it can be administered without cilastatin. About 70% of both meropenem and imipenem is excreted in the urine; the dosage should be reduced in azotemic patients. Like imipenem, meropenem is active against most clinically active gram-positive and gram-negative bacteria, including anaerobes; however, neither drug is active against methicillin-resistant staphylococci or *E. faecium.* Resistant strains of *P. aeruginosa* have emerged during therapy with each drug.

The clinical efficacy and toxicity of meropenem are similar to those of imipenem, except that meropenem appears more likely to be effective in meningitis and less likely to cause seizures. Both drugs are expensive, but meropenem is more costly.

Because the newest carbapenem, ertapenem, has a longer half-life than the other members of the group, it can be administered in a single daily intravenous dose [*see Table 4*].[33] Like the other carbapenems, ertapenem is excreted in the urine, and the dosage should be reduced in azotemic patients. The antibacterial spectrum of ertapenem is similar to that of meropenem, except that *Pseudomonas* and *Acinetobacter* strains are less susceptible, and *E. faecalis* is resistant.[34] Ertapenem appears effective against community-acquired pneumonias, intra-abdominal infections, complicated skin and soft tissue infections, and complicated urinary tract infections, but experience is limited.

The carbapenems have broader antibacterial spectrums than any other β-lactam antibiotics. They are active against most gram-positive bacteria, both aerobes and anaerobes. Exceptions include some enterococci; many *E. faecalis* strains are sensitive to imipenem and meropenem but not ertapenem, and most *E. faecium* strains are resistant to all three drugs. Some diphtheroids are resistant. Although most *S. aureus* strains are very sensitive, the susceptibility of methicillin-resistant *S. aureus* and coagulase-negative staphylococci is highly variable. Methicillin-resistant *S. aureus* and *Listeria* exhibit carbapenem tolerance. Finally, some strains of *C. difficile* are resistant.

Carbapenems are extraordinarily active against gram-negative bacteria. Whereas imipenem tends to be more active against gram-positive cocci, meropenem appears to be more active against gram-negative bacilli. Virtually all Enterobacteriaceae are susceptible. *Haemophilus* and *Neisseria* species are also susceptible to carbapenems but at concentrations somewhat higher than those of third-generation cephalosporins. Acinetobacter, which is resistant to most other β-lactam antibiotics, is susceptible to imipenem and meropenem, as are *Serratia, Salmonella, Citrobacter, Yersinia,* and *Brucella* species. Gram-negative anaerobes, including *B. fragilis,* are susceptible. *P. aeruginosa* is also susceptible, but some resistant strains have emerged during therapy; as a result, imipenem or meropenem should probably be combined with a second antipseudomonal drug when they are used to treat serious pseudomonal infections. Certain nosocomial pathogens, such as *Stenotrophomonas maltophila* and *P. cepacia,* are resistant, as are *Flavobacterium* species. Ertapenem has a spectrum of activity similar to that of meropenem, except that *Pseudomonas* and *Acinetobacter* strains are much less susceptible, and *E. faecalis* is resistant.

The safety of carbapenems seems comparable to that of other β-lactam antibiotics. Nausea and vomiting, local pain at injection sites, and hypersensitivity are the most common reactions. Seizures, although unusual, are a potential concern with imipenem; they have been observed in 0.9% of patients who have received the drug; risk factors for seizure include excessive dosages of the drugs, preexisting CNS lesions, epilepsy, and renal insufficiency. Meropenem is less likely to provoke seizures.[32] Transient elevations of liver enzymes and leukopenia can occur in patients who are given carbapenems. Antibiotic-associated pseudomembranous colitis has occurred.

Because the structure of the carbapenems resembles that of the penicillins and cephalosporins, there is potential for cross-reactivity in patients allergic to other β-lactam antibiotics. Clinical experience in this situation is limited, but it appears prudent to avoid carbapenems in patients with anaphylactic sensitivity to β-lactam drugs and to use them with caution in patients with milder allergies to penicillins or cephalosporins.[35]

Carbapenems have been used successfully in patients with pneumonia, intra-abdominal infections, urinary tract infections, endocarditis, bacteremia, osteomyelitis, cellulitis, and febrile neutropenia. The broad spectrum and apparent low toxicity of carbapenems is impressive, but they should be used with restraint and selectivity.

Monobactams

The monobactams are monocyclic β-lactam antibiotics that lack the thiazolidine ring found in penicillins and the dihydrothiazine ring found in cephalosporins.[32] The antibacterial activity of aztreonam depends on its ability to penetrate the outer membrane of gram-negative bacilli, on its high affinity for penicillin-binding protein–3, and on its resistance to hydrolysis by the β-lactamases of gram-negative bacilli.

The antibacterial activity of aztreonam is restricted to aerobic or facultatively aerobic gram-negative bacteria. Most strains of *H. influenzae,* gonococci, and meningococci are susceptible to aztreonam, as are most enteric gram-negative bacilli, including *E. coli, Klebsiella, Proteus,* and *Enterobacter*. Most strains of *P. aeruginosa* are also susceptible, but somewhat higher concentrations of aztreonam are required to kill these bacteria. *Acinetobacter, S. maltophila,* and *P. cepacia* are generally resistant to aztreonam, as are all gram-positive bacteria and anaerobes.

Excellent blood levels are achieved after intramuscular or intravenous administration, and the drug is widely distributed in body tissues and fluids, including the CSF. The serum half-life of aztreonam is about 90 minutes; glomerular filtration is the major means by which the drug is eliminated. The dosage of aztreonam must be reduced in azotemic patients; the drug is efficiently removed by hemodialysis but not by peritoneal dialysis.

Aztreonam is well tolerated. Its toxicities resemble those of other β-lactam antibiotics; toxicities include occasional instances of local reactions at the site of injection, rash, diarrhea, nausea, and vomiting. Neither nephrotoxicity nor bleeding disorders have been reported. Aztreonam does not cross-react with serum antibodies of penicillin-allergic and cephalosporin-allergic patients, and the drug has been well tolerated in penicillin-allergic patients.

Aztreonam has been used successfully in the treatment of a wide variety of infections caused by gram-negative bacteria, including pneumonias, skin and soft tissue infections, bone and joint infections, urinary tract infections, and bacteremias. Although aztreonam achieves therapeutic concentrations in the CSF, experience in the treatment of meningitis has been very limited.

Because aztreonam has the spectrum of the aminoglycosides and the low toxicity of the β-lactams, it may eventually replace aminoglycosides for many gram-negative infections. A potential disadvantage of aztreonam is the risk of enterococcal superinfections. Aztreonam is significantly more expensive than gentamicin. Synergy can be demonstrated between aztreonam and aminoglycosides for some gram-negative bacilli. More clinical experience is needed to determine the circumstances in which aztreonam should be a substitute for or a supplement to aminoglycosides.

ALLERGIC REACTIONS TO β-LACTAM ANTIBIOTICS

Hypersensitivity is the most common adverse reaction to β-lactam antibiotics. Most often, it is a delayed reaction characterized by maculopapular eruptions, fever, or both; eosinophilia may also be present. Much less common, but much more serious, is immediate hypersensitivity, mediated by IgE; manifestations may include early-onset urticaria, laryngeal edema, or anaphylaxis. Immune complexes can produce serum sickness in some patients. Hypersensitivity to β-lactam antibiotics can also cause hemolytic anemia or allergic interstitial nephritis.

As many as 10% of all patients report a history of penicillin allergy, but only 10% to 20% of those reporting are actually at risk for immediate hypersensitivity reactions.[36] A careful history is the best way to establish true drug allergy. A patient's recollection of rash, urticaria, arthralgias, wheezing, or anaphylaxis confirms the diagnosis of hypersensitivity, whereas treatment failure, diarrhea, vaginitis or other superinfections, or vague symptoms do not. Skin tests have a limited role in predicting true penicillin allergy, but they can help exclude IgE-mediated (anaphylactic) hypersensitivity.[37,38] To document severe allergy, both benzyl penicilloylpolylysine (a major-determinant antigen) and the so-called minor-determinant antigens should be injected; only the former is available commercially, but both are available to most experienced allergists. A wheal-and-flare reaction signifies IgE-mediated allergies; negative reactions to both major and minor determinants make anaphylaxis unlikely, but small test doses of penicillin may be administered for additional safety. Facilities and equipment necessary for the treatment of anaphylaxis should always be on hand when skin testing is performed. Patients with positive skin tests have a 41% to 67% chance of exhibiting significant penicillin allergy if they are rechallenged with the drug. The risk to patients with negative skin tests is only 1% to 4%, and no life-threatening reactions have been reported.

Patients with penicillin allergy, whether documented by history or by skin testing, should receive other antibiotics for infections; in rare cases in which there is no acceptable alternative to a penicillin, desensitization can be attempted. Desensitization is carried out with the equipment and medications for the treatment of anaphylaxis at bedside: a laryngoscope, oxygen, an endotracheal tube, epinephrine 1:1,000, sodium bicarbonate solution, and a running intravenous infusion. Penicillin doses are administered in graded increases in the forearm at a site low enough for a tourniquet to be applied proximally should a reaction occur. The initial dose of 1 unit of penicillin is applied by scratch test. If there is no wheal-and-flare reaction within 15 minutes, a dose of 2 units is injected intradermally. If no local or systemic reactions occur after another 15 minutes, a dose of 5 units is injected intradermally. If no reactions occur, successive doses that approximately double each previous dose are injected intradermally at 15-minute intervals. When the amount injected becomes large, the penicillin dose is administered subcutaneously. When a dose of 100,000 units has been injected without reaction, penicillin can be given intravenously. If an immediate local or systemic reaction occurs, it can be controlled. Use of an alternative drug is then advisable. Oral desensitization regimens are also available. Neither corticosteroids nor antihistamines will prevent anaphylaxis in an individual who is highly sensitive to penicillin.

Patients who are allergic to one penicillin should be considered allergic to all penicillins; however, this generalization may not be true for some children in whom a rash has developed after taking ampicillin or amoxicillin, particularly in the setting of infectious mononucleosis. Patients who are allergic to penicillin have an 8% likelihood of having an allergic reaction to a cephalosporin antibiotic[27]; cephalosporins are best avoided in patients who have IgE-mediated (anaphylactic) hypersensitivity to penicillin. Although there is much less experience with carbapenems (e.g., imipenem, meropenem, and ertapenem), the same guidelines apply for the use of these drugs in patients who are allergic to other β-lactams. However, monobactams (e.g., aztreonam) have not provoked cross-reactive hypersensitivity reactions. There are no reliable skin tests for cephalosporin, carbapenem, or monobactam allergies.

AMINOGLYCOSIDE ANTIBIOTICS

The aminoglycosides are bacterial drugs that act by binding irreversibly to the 30S ribosomal subunit of susceptible bacteria.[39] Because oxygen is required to transport aminoglycosides across the outer bacterial membrane, these agents are ineffective against anaerobes and may function poorly in the anaerobic milieu of abscesses. Although various aminoglycosides display activity against a wide range of microorganisms, they are used chiefly to treat infections caused by aerobic gram-negative bacilli. Aminoglycosides are also used in combination with cell wall–active antibiotics (e.g., penicillins and vancomycin) for the synergistic treatment of deep tissue infections caused by enterococci and coagulase-negative staphylococci. In addition, streptomycin is still used to treat tuberculosis, tularemia, and plague.[40]

The aminoglycosides are not absorbed from the GI tract and must be administered intravenously or intramuscularly. The drugs penetrate pleural, ascitic, and synovial fluids in the presence of inflammation, but they diffuse poorly into other body fluids, such as the CSF, respiratory tract secretions, and the aqueous humor.[41] The aminoglycosides are excreted by glomerular filtration; their dosages must be reduced in the presence of azotemia. Blood levels may be monitored to ensure proper dosing; peak levels may be lower than anticipated in febrile patients, patients with an expanded extracellular volume, patients with major burns, and patients receiving high-dose ticarcillin. The major toxicities of the aminoglycosides include renal damage and ototoxicity, which may be vestibular or auditory.[42] Other adverse reactions include rash, nausea and vomiting, and neuromuscular blockade (which is rare but may occur in patients with myasthenia gravis or in those receiving succinylcholine or similar drugs). Endotoxinlike reactions to gentamicin have been reported.

Specific Aminoglycosides

Gentamicin is active against most strains of *P. aeruginosa* and other aerobic gram-negative bacilli. Gentamicin is much less expensive than the newer aminoglycosides. As a result, tobramycin and amikacin are used principally for gentamicin-resistant gram-negative bacilli; tobramycin is somewhat more active against *P. aeruginosa*. Kanamycin and netilmicin are used infrequently; streptomycin is used in the multidrug treatment of tuberculosis, in synergistic therapy of gentamicin-resistant enterococci, and in other special circumstances.[40]

Once-Daily Aminoglycoside Dosing

In patients with normal renal function, aminoglycosides were conventionally administered in divided doses at 8- to 12-hour intervals. To improve efficacy and decrease toxicity and cost, once-daily dosing regimens have been widely adapted.[43] In most protocols, the total doses are equivalent in the single-dose and divided-dose regimens. Meta-analyses of such trials concluded that in patients with normal renal function, once-daily dosing is as effective as divided dosing and has a lower risk of toxicity.[44] Although most trials evaluated immunocompetent adults, similar trends were noted for children and for patients with febrile neutropenia. In elderly patients, however, the high peak serum concentrations that occur with once-daily dosing may increase the risk of nephrotoxicity, probably because of diminished renal clearance. Once-daily dosing has not been studied adequately in pregnant women or in patients with renal dysfunction, burns, ascites, or endocarditis.

The Changing Role of Aminoglycosides

The aminoglycosides are extremely active antibiotics that have proved to be clinically effective against many serious infections caused by gram-negative bacilli, and these agents have become inexpensive. These assets, however, must be weighed against the potential of aminoglycosides to produce renal and otovestibular toxicity. New efforts to improve the toxic-to-therapeutic ratio of aminoglycosides include once-daily dosage schedules and reevaluations of the recommended therapeutic ranges. To determine the future role of aminoglycosides, the cost-effectiveness of these agents needs to be compared directly with that of the new β-lactams and the fluoroquinolones.

TETRACYCLINES

Tetracyclines were originally widely employed because of their broad spectrum of activity against both gram-positive and gram-negative bacteria. They are used less extensively now because of the availability of the more effective bactericidal penicillins, cephalosporins, and fluoroquinolones. The emergence of resistance among gram-negative bacilli, group A streptococci, and pneumococci and the frequency of superinfection have also tended to decrease indications for their use.

Tetracyclines are the drugs of choice in the treatment of Rocky Mountain spotted fever and other rickettsioses.[45] They are useful in the treatment of pneumonia caused by *Mycoplasma pneumoniae* or *Chlamydia pneumoniae*[46]; urogenital infections caused by *C. trachomatis;* and other chlamydial diseases, such as psittacosis, trachoma, and lymphogranuloma venereum. They may also be used in the treatment of urinary tract infections caused by susceptible organisms. Other indications for their use include brucellosis, plague, cholera, granuloma inguinale, and Lyme disease; they may also be used in the treatment of syphilis in patients allergic to penicillin. Tetracyclines are used as adjuvant therapy in the treatment of severe cystic acne.

Five tetracycline compounds are available in the United States, but doxycycline has emerged as the favored preparation[47]; it is available in oral and intravenous formulations, its long half-life allows administration in one or two daily doses, and it does not accumulate in the presence of renal failure. Concomitant ingestion of milk and antacids impairs the absorption of all tetracyclines; therapeutic doses cannot be administered by the intramuscular route. The tetracyclines should not be given to children younger than 9 years or to pregnant women, because permanent discoloration of teeth may result. Other potential side effects include phototoxicity, allergic reactions, enterocolitis, negative nitrogen balance resulting in increased blood urea nitrogen (BUN) levels, and hepatic injury, which is a rare consequence of high-dose therapy. Minocycline can cause vestibular reactions.

MACROLIDES

The macrolides are composed of 14, 15, or 16 carbon atoms joined together in a complex, central, circular molecule that is linked to various side chains.[48] In the United States, erythromycin, clarithromycin, and azithromycin are the only available macrolides. At least 10 other macrolides are marketed in several other countries. Several newer macrolides are undergoing clinical trials.

Erythromycin

Erythromycin is active against gram-positive bacteria such as penicillin-sensitive *S. pneumoniae, Corynebacterium diphtheriae,* and diphtheroids. In the United States, most streptococci remain susceptible to erythromycin, but in Finland, erythromycin-resistant group A streptococci have been emerging since 1988. In the United States, the extensive use of erythromycin in hospitals has led to the selection and predominance of *S. aureus* strains that are highly resistant to this drug; most pneumococci that are not sensitive to penicillin are also resistant to erythromycin. Erythromycin remains active against *M. pneumoniae, C. trachomatis,* and some gram-negative bacilli, including *Legionella pneumophila, Campylobacter, Flavobacterium,* and *Bordetella pertussis. Neisseria* and *T. pallidum* are also susceptible to erythromycin, as are occasional strains of atypical mycobacteria.

Erythromycin is excreted to a large extent in the bile and only to a minor degree in the urine. The dosage need not be altered in the presence of renal insufficiency. Erythromycin penetrates pleural and peritoneal fluids; it crosses the placenta and is therefore used to treat syphilis in pregnant women allergic to penicillin.

Because erythromycin is active against *Legionella, Mycoplasma,* and *Chlamydia* species, it is an effective treatment for patients with atypical pneumonia who are not producing sputum [see 6 Pulmonary Infections]. Erythromycin is also effective for *Campylobacter* gastroenteritis, for the treatment of diphtheria, and for chemoprophylaxis in pertussis carriers. In patients who cannot tolerate penicillins and cephalosporins, erythromycin is an effective alternative for the treatment of streptococcal pharyngitis, bronchitis, and pneumonia; infections of skin and soft tissue; and syphilis. Other uses of erythromycin include granuloma inguinale and chancroid (for which it is administered with a sulfonamide), prophylaxis for elective bowel surgery (for which it is administered orally with neomycin), and acne (for which it is administered topically or orally).

Erythromycin is administered orally at a dosage of 0.25 to 0.50 g four times daily. Therapeutic blood levels can be achieved with any of the oral erythromycin preparations. Intravenous preparations of erythromycin are available for the treatment of severe infections, but prolonged therapy is difficult because of the frequent occurrence of thrombophlebitis at infusion sites. GI intolerance is the most common side effect; other adverse reactions shared by the macrolides include rash, stomatitis, pseudomembranous colitis, pancreatitis, and ototoxicity. Because of the occasional occurrence of cholestatic hepatitis after administration of the estolate form, erythromycin base or stearate is preferred for adults.

Clarithromycin

Clarithromycin, a semisynthetic 14-member macrolide, is acid stable and well absorbed from the GI tract; meals do not significantly affect its bioavailability.[48] Like erythromycin, clarithromycin achieves wide tissue penetration; because of its longer half-life, however, clarithromycin may be administered twice a day rather than four times a day. In addition, clarithromycin produces fewer GI side effects than erythromycin. Clarithromycin and other macrolides can produce ventricular arrhythmias when administered with cisapride, astemizole, or disopyramide.

Clarithromycin is highly active against organisms that are sensitive to erythromycin; these include streptococci, pneumococci, staphylococci, *Legionella, Campylobacter, Mycoplasma,* and *C. pneumoniae.* Clarithromycin also exhibits excellent activity against *M. catarrhalis* and *H. influenzae,* which therefore makes it an attractive agent for the treatment of respiratory tract infections, including sinusitis, pharyngitis, bronchitis, and pneumonia caused by susceptible organisms; clarithromycin has been used successfully in patients who have Legionnaires disease. The drug has assumed an important role in the multidrug regimens used to treat disseminated *M. avium* complex infections [see 19 Infections Due to *Escherichia coli* and Other Enteric Gram-Negative Bacilli]. Because it displays in vitro activity against several other pathogens, the drug is being used as monotherapy for *Helicobacter pylori* gastric infections and for disseminated cutaneous infections caused by *M. chelonae.* The usual adult dosage is 250 to 500 mg administered orally twice a day. Doses of 2,000 mg a day are poorly tolerated. Clarithromycin is substantially more expensive than erythromycin.

Azithromycin

Azithromycin, a 15-member macrolide, is active against the same broad range of organisms as those that clarithromycin inhibits.[48] An intravenous preparation is available. Like the other macrolides, azithromycin is well absorbed from the GI tract; however, azithromycin differs from clarithromycin in that the bioavailability of azithromycin is decreased by food. As a result, azithromycin should be taken 1 hour before or 2 hours after meals. Azithromycin clears rapidly from serum and moves promptly into interstitial and intracellular tissue compartments. Tissue levels are extraordinarily prolonged, with an average terminal half-life of 68 hours. Therefore, tissue levels of azithromycin can be expected to remain in the therapeutic range from 4 to 7 days after a 5-day treatment course. These unique pharmacokinetics support the current program of administering azithromycin once daily for 5 days. Like clarithromycin, azithromycin appears to be well tolerated and to have fewer GI side effects than erythromycin. Azithromycin is substantially more expensive than erythromycin.

Azithromycin has been effective in the treatment of pharyngitis, sinusitis, bronchitis and pneumonia, and skin and soft tissue infections. Azithromycin has also assumed an important role in the treatment of Legionnaires disease and other atypical and community-acquired pneumonias [see 6 Pulmonary Infections]. In addition to these indications, for which azithromycin has been approved by the Food and Drug Administration, azithromycin has been used successfully as a single-dose therapy for urethritis and cervicitis caused by *C. trachomatis;* it provides a significant advantage because no other single-dose regimen now exists for these infections. Another important use for azithromycin is in the treatment of difficult-to-treat chronic infections, such as *M. avium* complex and bacillary angiomatosis in patients with AIDS.

Dirithromycin

Dirithromycin is an oral macrolide antibiotic with an antibacterial spectrum similar to that of erythromycin; it can be administered once daily but has no other advantages over erythromycin. The drugs produce similar GI side effects, and dirithromycin is substantially more expensive.

CLINDAMYCIN

Clindamycin is active against the following pathogens: *S. aureus, S. pneumoniae,* group A and other streptococci (except enterococci), *Bacteroides* (including *B. fragilis*) and *Fusobacterium* species, anaerobic streptococci and peptococci, and *C. perfringens* and *C. tetani* (but not other clostridial strains). It is also active against *B. anthracis*,[49] but clinical experience is very limited.

Only about 10% of administered clindamycin is excreted in active form in the urine; the remainder is changed into inactive metabolites. In patients with marked renal insufficiency, the half-life of clindamycin is only slightly prolonged, and little change in dosage is necessary. In patients with severe liver disease, however, dosage should be determined with care; serum levels are helpful.

Clindamycin is indicated in the treatment of serious infections caused by susceptible anaerobes, particularly those originating in the GI and female genital tracts.[50] Clindamycin has also been very effective in the treatment of aspiration pneumonia and lung abscess. Because of its ability to rapidly reduce toxin production, clindamycin may be very helpful in the management of streptococcal toxic-shock syndrome and necrotizing infections caused by *C. perfringens* and *S. pyogenes*, possibly in conjunction with penicillin. Clindamycin should not be used in the treatment of pharyngitis; in penicillin-allergic patients who have streptococcal pharyngitis, erythromycin is the preferred alternative. Clindamycin should be used only topically for acne therapy. Clindamycin has been used to treat protozoan infections, such as toxoplasmosis and babesiosis.[47] Because clindamycin does not readily penetrate the CNS, even when there is marked meningeal inflammation, it should not be used to treat meningitis.

Because severe pseudomembranous colitis can be a complication of clindamycin therapy, the drug should be used only for infections that cannot be treated satisfactorily with other agents. Other potential side effects include nausea and vomiting, hypersensitivity reactions, and reversible neutropenia.

CHLORAMPHENICOL

Although chloramphenicol remains a useful antibiotic, its role has decreased as less-toxic alternatives have become available.[47,50] Because of the rare occurrence of aplastic anemia [*see* Adverse Reactions to Antimicrobial Agents, *above*], clinical use of chloramphenicol should be limited to serious infections in which alternative antibiotics may be less effective: serious infections caused by vancomycin-resistant enterococci; typhoid fever; nontyphoidal salmonelloses caused by ampicillin-resistant strains; meningitis caused by ampicillin-resistant strains of *H. influenzae;* meningitis caused by *H. influenzae, N. meningitidis*, or *S. pneumoniae* in patients who are allergic to penicillin and cephalosporins; and infections caused by *B. fragilis*. Even for these traditional uses, however, chloramphenicol must be evaluated in comparison to other antibiotics. For example, the newer cephalosporins and fluoroquinolones should be considered for salmonellosis; second-generation and third-generation cephalosporins should be considered for ampicillin-resistant strains of *H. influenzae;* and combinations of a penicillin and a β-lactamase inhibitor, imipenem, meropenem, cefmetazole, cefoxitin, cefotetan, clindamycin, or metronidazole can be used to treat infections caused by *B. fragilis*.

Chloramphenicol may be administered orally or intravenously. Chloramphenicol diffuses rapidly into most tissues, CSF, ascitic fluid, and aqueous humor. The drug is lipid soluble and achieves levels in the brain up to nine times higher than in the serum. Chloramphenicol is inactivated in the liver by conjugation with glucuronic acid; blood levels may increase in patients with marked cirrhosis and jaundice.

In view of the risk of aplastic anemia, the following guidelines should be employed in the use of chloramphenicol: (1) it should only be used in the treatment of infections for which it is clearly indicated; (2) repeated courses should be avoided; (3) counts should be checked two to three times weekly; and (4) the patient should be observed closely for evidence of sore throat (granulocytopenia) or other new infections. Other potential adverse effects of chloramphenicol include rash, glossitis, GI intolerance, and neurotoxic reactions.

VANCOMYCIN

Vancomycin is a bactericidal glycopeptide that impairs cell wall synthesis of gram-positive bacteria; its spectrum of action includes staphylococci, streptococci, pneumococci, enterococci, clostridia, *Corynebacterium* species, and other gram-positive bacteria.[51] It is bacteriostatic but not bactericidal against some strains of enterococci, coagulase-negative staphylococci, and corynebacteria.

Vancomycin is poorly absorbed when administered orally. The oral route is employed only for the treatment of staphylococcal enterocolitis and antibiotic-associated pseudomembranous enterocolitis; a dosage of 125 to 250 mg every 6 hours is recommended for this purpose. In adults with severe staphylococcal infection or viridans streptococcal or enterococcal endocarditis who have normal renal function and who are highly allergic to penicillin, vancomycin is administered intravenously at a dosage of 0.5 g every 6 hours or 1 g every 12 hours. To avoid hypotension and histaminelike reactions, the drug should always be infused slowly over a period of 1 hour. Pretreatment with antihistamines can help avert the so-called red-man syndrome; in rare cases, desensitization may be necessary. Other adverse effects may include thrombophlebitis at the infusion site, chills and fever, ototoxicity, and possibly nephrotoxicity.

Vancomycin is the drug of choice in the treatment of infections caused by methicillin-resistant *S. aureus*. Concomitant administration of an aminoglycoside is often necessary when vancomycin is used in the treatment of enterococcal endocarditis. Vancomycin can be very useful in therapy for prosthetic valve endocarditis caused by coagulase-negative staphylococci; in this setting, the agent is frequently administered in combination with either gentamicin or rifampin.

Vancomycin does not penetrate normal meninges but does enter the CSF when the meninges are inflamed; however, experience with vancomycin in the treatment of meningitis is very limited. Most of the drug is eliminated through the kidneys; in the presence of renal failure, the dose must be reduced. Although serum vancomycin levels are often monitored, measurements are not necessary in routine cases. However, determination of serum levels is an important guide to dosage when the drug must be administered in the presence of impaired renal function; peak serum levels of 20 to 30 mg/ml are considered ideal, as are trough levels of 10 mg/ml or less. Particular attention to ototoxicity and nephrotoxicity is required when vancomycin is administered with an aminoglycoside.

The epidemiology of vancomycin use provides a cautionary tale for this drug and for other antimicrobials.[52] Although vancomycin is a valuable and effective drug, it is often used inappropriately; inappropriate use results in substantial financial costs and the emergence of vancomycin-resistant organisms that are very difficult to treat, including enterococci[53] and some staphylococci[54] [see 15 Infections Due to Gram-Positive Cocci].

STREPTOGRAMINS

Quinupristin and dalfopristin are two structurally distinct streptogramins that bind to separate sites on the bacterial 50S ribosomal subunit; they thus act synergistically to inhibit protein synthesis. The drugs are marketed together in a 30:70 ratio as Synercid.[55]

Although quinupristin-dalfopristin is active against a variety of bacteria, its major use is in the treatment of serious infections caused by vancomycin-resistant strains of *E. faecium*. The drugs may also be useful in occasional vancomycin-intolerant patients with severe infections caused by methicillin-resistant *S. aureus* or coagulase-negative staphylococci. Although quinupristin-dalfopristin was first marketed in 1999, resistance is already emerging.[56]

Quinupristin-dalfopristin is administered intravenously; because of a high incidence of phlebitis, a central line should be used. Other adverse effects include arthralgias and myalgias, which may be severe, and elevated bilirubin levels. The antibiotic may elevate levels of drugs that are metabolized by the hepatic enzyme CYP3A4; nifedipine and cyclosporin are examples.

The usual dose of quinupristin-dalfopristin is 7.5 mg/kg given intravenously over 1 hour every 8 hours. The drug is metabolized by the liver, so no dose reduction is required in azotemic patients. Quinupristin-dalfopristin is extremely expensive.

OXAZOLIDINONES

In 2000, linezolid became the first member of the oxazolidinone class to be approved for clinical use in the United States.[57] Linezolid is a synthetic antibiotic that inhibits protein synthesis by binding to a site on the bacterial 23S ribosomal RNA of the 50S subunit, thus preventing function of the initiation complex that is required for ribosomal function.[58] Because no other antibiotic acts in this way, bacteria that have developed resistance to other ribosomally active antimicrobials do not display cross-resistance to linezolid.

Linezolid is active against nearly all aerobic gram-positive cocci at concentrations of 4 mg/ml or less,[59] including penicillin-resistant pneumococci, methicillin-resistant staphylococci, and vancomycin-resistant enterococci; however, resistant strains have been isolated.[60] The drug is bacteriostatic against staphylococci and enterococci, but it is bactericidal against most streptococcal strains. Linezolid is also active against *L. monocytogenes, M. catarrhalis, H. influenzae, N. gonorrhoeae, B. pertussis, Pasteurella multocida,* and *Nocardia* species. *C. difficile, C. perfringens,* and *Bacteroides* species are susceptible, but enteric gram-negative bacilli and *Pseudomonas* species are not.[61]

Intravenous and oral preparations of linezolid are available; the oral form is absorbed rapidly and completely with 100% bioavailability that is not affected by meals. Linezolid is widely distributed in well-perfused tissues. Nonrenal mechanisms account for 65% of the drug's clearance. Patients with mild to moderate renal or hepatic insufficiency do not appear to require reduced doses; linezolid is removed by hemodialysis.

Linezolid is well tolerated. Adverse effects have been reported in about 2.8% of all patients[61]; nausea, vomiting, and headaches are the most common side effects, but reversible marrow suppression, including thrombocytopenia, leukopenia, and anemia, can also occur. Because linezolid is a reversible inhibitor of monoamine oxidase, patients taking linezolid may experience an exaggerated hypertensive response to sympathomimetic agents. In addition to avoiding decongestants, patients taking linezolid should avoid foods or beverages with a high tyramine content; aged cheeses, air-dried meats, tap beer, red wine, soy sauce, and sauerkraut are examples. Monoamine oxidase inhibitors and other antidepressants should not be administered during linezolid therapy.

Linezolid has been used successfully in the therapy of multidrug-resistant gram-positive bacterial infections.[57,58,62] The drug is approved for vancomycin-resistant enterococcal infections and for pneumonias and skin and soft tissue infections. The usual dosage is 600 mg every 12 hours (p.o. or I.V.); uncomplicated skin and soft tissue infections may be treated with 400 mg every 12 hours.

Linezolid is a very promising new antimicrobial agent, but clinical experience is still limited. Although resistance is uncommon, it can develop during therapy. As a result, it may be wise to reserve this unique antibiotic for serious infections in hospitalized patients; in particular, linezolid should be useful for infections caused by methicillin-resistant *S. aureus* or coagulase-negative staphylococci that do not respond to vancomycin, for penicillin-resistant pneumococcal infections that do not respond to other agents, and for vancomycin-resistant enterococcal infection.

SULFONAMIDES

Although the sulfonamides no longer play a major clinical role, they are still helpful antimicrobials. Because of their efficacy and low cost, individual sulfonamides can be useful in treating uncomplicated urinary tract infections caused by *E. coli.* Sulfonamides are also useful for nocardial infections. The emergence of ampicillin-resistant *H. influenzae* has brought about a return to sulfonamides (in combination with erythromycin or trimethoprim) for treating otitis media in children. Topical sulfonamides are still used in a few situations. Sulfacetamide eyedrops are sometimes employed to treat superficial ocular infections. Topical silver-sulfadiazine cream is administered to burn surfaces to suppress bacterial growth and prevent subsequent invasive infection. Both the silver ion and the sulfadiazine components of the compound probably contribute to the antibacterial activity.

TRIMETHOPRIM

Trimethoprim is a pyrimidine analogue that, like the sulfonamides, acts to block bacterial folic acid synthesis. Trimethoprim is well absorbed from the GI tract and is widely distributed in tissues (including the prostate); most of the drug is excreted unchanged in the urine. Its antibacterial spectrum encompasses many aerobic gram-negative bacilli; it is not active against *P. aeruginosa*. Trimethoprim is well tolerated; side effects include skin rash (less common than with sulfonamides) and megaloblastic marrow changes (uncommon). The agent is teratogenic in rats and therefore should not be given to pregnant women. Trimethoprim inhibits renal potassium excretion; reversible hyperkalemia has been observed in AIDS patients receiving high-dose trimethoprim-sulfamethoxazole.

Trimethoprim is approved only for the initial treatment of uncomplicated urinary tract infections; the oral dosage is 100 mg twice daily. As a result of the widespread use of trimethoprim as a single agent in many parts of the world, bacterial resistance is beginning to emerge. If trimethoprim resistance were to become widespread, the usefulness of trimethoprim-sulfamethoxazole, a very valuable antimicrobial agent, would be impaired. Hence, it may be prudent to reserve trimethoprim for situations in which other agents are not effective.

TRIMETHOPRIM-SULFAMETHOXAZOLE

Use of the trimethoprim-sulfamethoxazole combination extended the list of clinical situations in which sulfonamides appear to be of value[47]: recurrent bacteriuria and urinary tract infections, prostatitis, acute otitis media, sinusitis or bronchitis caused by susceptible strains of *H. influenzae* and *S pneumoniae,* systemic infections caused by chloramphenicol-resistant and ampicillin-resistant *Salmonella* strains, and shigellosis. Trimethoprim-sulfamethoxazole can be used to prevent or treat traveler's diarrhea. Trimethoprim-sulfamethoxazole can be useful in the treatment of infections caused by gram-negative bacilli resistant to other antimicrobials; it may be administered intravenously to treat serious infections (including meningitis when other drugs are not effective). It is the treatment of choice for the prevention[63] and treatment of *P. carinii* pneumonia and nocardiosis. With widespread use, trimethoprim-sulfamethoxazole–resistant strains of bacteria are appearing, particularly in HIV-infected individuals.[64]

The trimethoprim-sulfamethoxazole synergistic combination is currently available in oral or intravenous preparations in a 1:5 ratio (80 or 160 mg of trimethoprim and 400 or 800 mg of sulfamethoxazole). Both drugs are excreted primarily by the kidneys. The dosage of trimethoprim-sulfamethoxazole for treatment of urinary tract infection in an adult is two single-strength tablets (or one double-strength tablet) every 12 hours; a similar dosage is effective for the treatment of otitis. For serious systemic infections, the intravenous dosage is 8 to 10 mg/kg (based on the trimethoprim component) in two to four equal doses every 6 to 12 hours. For *Pneumocystis* pneumonia, the dosage is 20 mg/kg (based on the trimethoprim component) in equally divided doses every 6 hours. Reduction in dosage is necessary if renal function is impaired.

Adverse reactions to trimethoprim-sulfamethoxazole are similar to those that are caused by sulfonamides alone. They include hypersensitivity reactions, photosensitivity, and nausea and vomiting; hepatitis, pancreatitis, aseptic meningitis, and megaloblastic anemia are rare. In patients with AIDS, however, there is a very high incidence of adverse reactions to this drug combination; desensitization may be possible.[65]

METRONIDAZOLE

Metronidazole was first approved in 1959 for use as an antiparasitic agent; in 1981, the FDA approved an intravenous preparation of metronidazole for the treatment of serious infections caused by anaerobic bacteria. Orally administered metronidazole is excellent for treating pseudomembranous colitis caused by *C. difficile.* Metronidazole is also useful as part of preoperative prophylactic regimens for elective colorectal surgery. The drug is being studied for use in the treatment of nonspecific vaginitis, which is associated with *Gardnerella vaginalis.*

Metronidazole appears to act by disrupting bacterial DNA and inhibiting nucleic acid synthesis. The drug is bactericidal against almost all anaerobic gram-negative bacilli, including *B. fragilis,* and against most *Clostridium* species.[47,50] Although true anaerobic streptococci are generally susceptible to metronidazole, microaerophilic streptococci and *Actinomyces* and *Propionibacterium* species are often resistant. Metronidazole has cured a variety of infections caused by anaerobes: CNS infections, bone and joint infections, abdominal and pelvic sepsis, and endocarditis. Failures have been reported in the treatment of pleuropulmonary infections.

Side effects of metronidazole include dry mouth (associated with a metallic taste) and nausea. Concurrent use of alcohol may cause a reaction similar to that produced when alcohol is drunk after disulfiram ingestion. Neurologic symptoms, including peripheral neuropathy and encephalopathic reactions, and neutropenia are uncommon. Pancreatitis has been reported. Metronidazole is mutagenic for bacteria and carcinogenic for rats and mice. Carcinogenicity in humans has not been demonstrated but remains a concern.

When metronidazole is administered orally, it is well absorbed and is widely distributed in body tissues, including those of the CNS. For serious anaerobic infections, the drug is administered intravenously; a loading dose of 15 mg/kg is given, followed by 7.5 mg/kg every 6 hours until the patient is well enough to take an oral dosage of 7.5 mg/kg every 6 hours. The dosage need not be reduced in azotemic patients, but it should be reduced in patients with hepatic insufficiency.

Because of its bactericidal action and excellent tissue penetration, intravenous metronidazole may be the treatment of choice for *B. fragilis* endocarditis and *B. fragilis* CNS infections, both of which are uncommon. It has supplanted penicillin as the drug of choice for tetanus. Metronidazole is also excellent for anaerobic infections of the abdomen and pelvis, but alternative drugs are available.

QUINOLONES

The addition of a fluorine group and a piperazine substituent to the first quinolones has greatly improved the antibacterial spectrum of this class of drugs; the addition of a methyl group on the piperazine ring appears to further enhance the bioavailability of these compounds. There are currently 10 quinolones available for clinical use in the United States [*see Table 6*], and many additional fluoroquinolones are actively being studied.

The fluoroquinolones are bactericidal compounds that act by inhibiting DNA gyrase, the bacterial enzyme responsible for maintaining the supertwisted helical structure of DNA; DNA

Table 6 Selected Properties of Fluoroquinolone Antibiotics

Generic Name	Trade Name	Comments*
Ciprofloxacin	Cipro	Twice-daily dosing (p.o., I.V.); moderately active against *Pseudomonas aeruginosa*
Enoxacin	Penetrex	Similar to norfloxacin but more side effects
Gatifloxacin	Tequin	Once-daily dosing (p.o., I.V.); active against pneumococci
Levofloxacin	Levaquin	Once-daily dosing (p.o., I.V.); active against pneumococci; moderately active against *P. aeruginosa* and anaerobes
Lomefloxacin	Maxaquin	Once-daily dosing (p.o.); less active against pneumococci, streptococci, mycoplasmas, and chlamydiae; phototoxicity
Moxifloxacin	Avelox	Once-daily dosing (p.o.); active against pneumococci; hepatic elimination; QT prolongation
Norfloxacin	Noroxin	Twice-daily dosing (p.o.); for intestinal and genitourinary infections only
Ofloxacin	Floxin	Twice-daily dosing (p.o., I.V.); moderately active against *P. aeruginosa*
Sparfloxacin	Zagam	Once-daily dosing (p.o.); active against pneumococci; moderately active against *P. aeruginosa* and anaerobes; phototoxicity; QT prolongation
Trovafloxacin	Trovan	Once-daily dosing (p.o., I.V. as alatrofloxacin); active against pneumococci, *P. aeruginosa,* and anaerobes; hepatic elimination; uncommon, serious incidents of hepatic toxicity reported†

*See text for details. Only properties that distinguish among the fluoroquinolones are listed here.
†In 1999, the FDA limited trovafloxacin to inpatient use for limb- or life-threatening infections. The FDA also recommends that trovafloxacin not be used for more than 14 days and for the drug to be discontinued earlier if any clinical manifestations of liver dysfunction appear (see text).

topoisomerase IV is a secondary target.[66] The fluoroquinolones rapidly kill bacteria, probably by impairing DNA synthesis and possibly by mechanisms involving cleaving of bacterial chromosomal DNA. Bacterial resistance to the fluoroquinolones depends on a change in their DNA gyrase. In the case of nalidixic acid, this single-step mutation occurs with a frequency of 10^{-7}; resistance to the newer fluoroquinolones occurs much less frequently (about 10^{-11}) but is a growing concern.[67,68] Bacterial strains that are resistant to one fluoroquinolone tend to be cross-resistant to related compounds; such resistance is usually mediated by chromosomes, but plasmid-mediated resistance raises the possibility of transferable resistance.

The fluoroquinolones are broad-spectrum antimicrobials. Most enteric gram-negative bacilli, including *E. coli, Proteus, Klebsiella,* and *Enterobacter,* are highly susceptible; common GI pathogens, such as *Salmonella, Shigella,* and *Campylobacter* species, are also very sensitive. Other gram-negative organisms that are killed by low concentrations of the fluoroquinolones are *N. gonorrhoeae* and *N. meningitidis, H. influenzae, P. multocida, M. catarrhalis,* and *Y. enterocolitica. Acinetobacter* and *Serratia* are somewhat less susceptible. *P. aeruginosa* is susceptible to ciprofloxacin and trovafloxacin; ofloxacin and levofloxacin are moderately active, but the other quinolones are not effective. *P. cepacia* and *S. maltophila* are quinolone-resistant. Ciprofloxacin is the drug of choice for *B. anthracis;* oflaxacin and levofloxacin are also active in vitro.[49] Among gram-positive cocci, methicillin-sensitive strains of *S. aureus* and coagulase-negative staphylococci are usually susceptible to quinolones, but methicillin-resistant *S. aureus* and enterococci are not. Lomefloxacin is not active against pneumococci and other streptococci; ciprofloxacin and ofloxacin are moderately active; and levofloxacin, sparfloxacin, gatifloxacin, moxifloxacin, and trovafloxacin are highly effective, even against non–penicillin-sensitive pneumococci. Even fastidious intracellular pathogens can be inhibited by the quinolones; *Chlamydia, Mycoplasma, Listeria, Legionella,* and *M. tuberculosis* are in this category. Only trovafloxacin is highly active against anaerobes. Levofloxacin, gatifloxacin, moxifloxacin, and sparfloxacin demonstrate some activity against anaerobes, but the other quinolones do not. *C. difficile* is resistant to quinolones.

The fluoroquinolones are rapidly absorbed from the GI tract. Penetration into body fluids and tissues is generally excellent; therapeutic concentrations are readily achieved in blister fluid, bile, urine, saliva and sputum, bone, and muscle. Excellent concentrations of these drugs are achieved in the prostate, and stool levels are extraordinarily high. The fluoroquinolones appear to penetrate the CSF in the presence of meningeal inflammation,[69] but experience in treating meningitis is scant.

Although serum protein binding is modest, the fluoroquinolones have long serum half-lives, which range from 3 to 4 hours for ciprofloxacin to 12 hours for moxifloxacin. Most fluoroquinolones are eliminated by glomerular filtration and tubular secretion, and their dosages should be reduced in the presence of moderately severe renal failure. Trovafloxacin and moxifloxacin, however, are excreted chiefly by the liver.

The fluoroquinolones appear to be very well tolerated, with mild GI side effects (nausea, vomiting, or anorexia), CNS side effects (light-headedness, dizziness, somnolence, or insomnia), or rash occurring in fewer than 10% of treated patients. Lomefloxacin and sparfloxacin can cause phototoxicity. Less common side effects include allergic intestinal nephritis, pseudomembranous colitis, and neutropenia. Sparfloxacin and moxifloxacin may cause Q-T prolongation and should not be used by patients who have conditions or are using drugs known to prolong the QT interval or predispose to arrhythmias.[70] Tendinitis has been reported; in severe cases, it has resulted in rupture of the tendons of the shoulder and hand and the Achilles tendon. Crystalluria has been reported after the use of very large doses. Because fluoroquinolones have caused arthropathy in young animals, these drugs should be avoided in children and in women who are pregnant or nursing. Ciprofloxacin is safe in long-term use; there is less long-term experience with the other fluoroquinolones.

The fluoroquinolones have been useful clinically in a variety of infections, including urinary tract, genital, prostatic, GI, respiratory tract, soft tissue, and bone infections. Because of their excellent activity against pneumococci and other bacterial and atypical pathogens, levofloxacin, gatifloxacin, sparfloxacin, and moxifloxacin may emerge as the agents of choice for community-acquired pneumonias [see 6 Pulmonary Infections]. Because of its excellent activity against anaerobes, trovafloxacin was considered useful in abdominal and pelvic infections, but concerns about serious hepatotoxicity have restricted its use to infections deemed life- or limb-threatening and for patients in whom the benefit of trovafloxacin outweighs its potential risks. The drug should not be administered for more than 14 days, and liver function must be monitored carefully.

The fluoroquinolones are effective in preventing gram-negative bacteremia when administered prophylactically to neutropenic patients, but they do not reduce gram-positive bacteremias, febrile episodes, or infection-related mortality. The addition of a second agent such as vancomycin or rifampin reduces gram-positive bacteremias without affecting febrile episodes or infection-related mortality.

The fluoroquinolones, administered in various regimens ranging from one dose to 5 days of therapy, are effective in preventing and treating traveler's diarrhea and shigellosis. They have been highly effective in the treatment of typhoid fever. However, prolongation of the carrier state limits their role in nontyphoidal *Salmonella* enteritis, and the development of resistance limits their role in *Campylobacter* enteritis. The fluoroquinolones may be useful in the empirical treatment of severe community-acquired gastroenteritis, particularly if treatment is started early.

Because of their extraordinarily broad antimicrobial activity, their favorable pharmacokinetics, and their low toxicity,[71] the fluoroquinolones are extremely valuable new drugs. Like all antimicrobials, however, fluoroquinolones should be used judiciously, especially in view of new concerns about resistance[72,73] and toxicity and practical considerations about expense.

NITROFURANTOIN

Nitrofurantoin is readily absorbed from the GI tract and rapidly excreted. Antibacterial levels are not attained in the blood; therapeutic utility results from the high urinary concentrations achieved. This drug should be employed only in the treatment of uncomplicated mild urinary tract infections or for the prevention of urinary tract infections.[74] The spectrum of antibacterial activity includes *E. coli*, enterococci, and some strains of *Klebsiella* and *Enterobacter. Proteus* and *Pseudomonas* species are usually resistant. R factor–mediated resistance to nitrofurantoin has not been observed. Nitrofurantoin is administered orally in a dosage of 50 to 100 mg four times daily. It should not be administered when there is significant impairment of renal function. Nausea and vomiting are common side effects, but their incidence may be decreased by use of the microcrystalline formulation and by taking the drug with food. Less frequent adverse reactions include rash, hypersensitivity pneumonitis, peripheral neuropathy, hepatitis, and hemolytic anemia in association with G6PD deficiency.

FOSFOMYCIN

Fosfomycin is a broad-spectrum antibiotic that inhibits cell wall synthesis in *E. coli, S. saprophyticus,* and many other common urinary tract pathogens.[75] Although it has been used parenterally in Europe for many years, the drug is approved in the United States only for the single-dose treatment of uncomplicated urinary tract infections in women. A 3 g dose is generally effective and well tolerated; diarrhea is the most common side effect. A single dose of fosfomycin is much more expensive than a

3-day regimen of comparably effective trimethoprim-sulfamethoxazole or amoxicillin.

RIFAMPIN

Since its development in the 1960s, rifampin has emerged as a major antituberculous drug [see 19 Infections Due to *Escherichia coli* and Other Enteric Gram-Negative Bacilli]. Rifampin is also active against a variety of bacteria; it is effective in eradicating nasopharyngeal carriage of *N. meningitidis* [see 18 Infections Due to *Neisseria*] and can be combined with vancomycin to treat serious infections caused by coagulase-negative staphylococci [see 15 Infections Due to Gram-Positive Cocci]. Most *S. aureus* strains are susceptible to rifampin, but resistance develops rapidly as a result of a single point mutation in bacterial DNA–dependent RNA polymerase.[76] When rifampin is combined with a second drug, however, resistance is less likely. The combination of rifampin and a fluoroquinolone has shown promise for chemoprophylaxis of neutropenic patients, for long-term oral treatment of infected orthopedic prostheses,[77] and for treatment of osteomyelitis in the diabetic foot.[78] More study is needed to determine the optimal role for rifampin in antibacterial therapy.

POLYMYXIN B AND COLISTIMETHATE

The antibacterial spectrum of polymyxin B and colistimethate (polymyxin E) covers most of the common aerobic gram-negative bacilli. However, because polymyxins do not readily enter body tissues and fluid compartments (e.g., the respiratory tract and CSF) and because they have toxic side effects, they are now rarely used systemically. Polymyxin B is used topically in eyedrops and eardrops.

SPECTINOMYCIN

Although spectinomycin is active in vitro against a variety of gram-negative bacteria, it is less effective than many other drugs. Its one clinical use is for the treatment of gonorrhea. It is used in the treatment of urethral and anogenital gonorrhea in patients allergic to penicillins, cephalosporins, and fluoroquinolones. Spectinomycin is not effective in the treatment of gonococcal pharyngitis but can be used as an alternative drug for pelvic inflammatory disease or the arthritis-dermatitis-bacteremia syndrome. The dose of spectinomycin that is used in treating acute gonococcal urethritis, cervicitis, and proctitis is a single intramuscular injection of 2 g; for the arthritis-dermatitis syndrome, the dosage is 2 g given intramuscularly twice a day for 3 days. Side effects have been minor: pain at the injection site, chills and fever, urticaria, and dizziness.

Antimicrobial Chemoprophylaxis

The term antimicrobial chemoprophylaxis refers to the use of antibiotics for preventing infection either before or very shortly after introduction of pathogenic organisms—for example, after the occurrence of a compound fracture but before the appearance of clinical infection. Chemoprophylaxis is most effective when a specific drug is selected for its activity against a particular organism; postexposure anthrax prophylaxis with ciprofloxacin, doxycycline, or amoxicillin is an example.[79] When prophylaxis is aimed at preventing all possible organisms from initiating infection, it is likely to be unsuccessful because it merely selects out the most drug-resistant organism as the cause of any infection that follows. Thus, prophylaxis is ineffective in the prevention of complicating bacterial or mycotic infections in patients with viral respiratory tract infections, in comatose patients or patients with congestive heart failure, and in patients requiring prolonged use of indwelling urinary catheters. Most uses of chemoprophylaxis fall into three general categories: prevention of infection after exposure to a specific pathogen, prevention of specific types of infection in highly susceptible individuals, and prevention of postoperative infectious complications. In many instances, prophylactic use of antimicrobial agents is widely practiced, but convincing data validating the efficacy of this approach are not available.[80] For detailed discussions of the prophylactic use of antimicrobial agents, readers are referred to subsections devoted to specific infectious targets and diseases.

ANTIMICROBIAL PROPHYLAXIS FOR SURGICAL PROCEDURES

The use of antimicrobial prophylaxis in surgery involves a risk-to-benefit appraisal that varies depending on the nature of the operative procedure.[81] To help prevent wound infections in patients undergoing elective surgery, antibiotics should be administered within 2 hours before the incision is made. If prophylactic antibiotics are to be effective, administration should be timed so that therapeutic levels are attained at surgery but selection of bacteria resistant to the drugs is avoided. Antibiotics should usually be stopped 24 hours after the procedure. The indications for prophylaxis with different operations have been reviewed, but in many instances, the available data are insufficient. For clean elective surgical procedures such as mastectomy and thyroidectomy in which no tissue (other than the skin) carrying an indigenous flora is penetrated, the risks of routine antibiotic prophylaxis outweigh the possible benefits.

When cardiovascular prostheses are employed, vancomycin or a first-generation cephalosporin (e.g., cefazolin) is administered intravenously beginning 2 hours before surgery and continuing for 3 to 5 days. Similar regimens may be employed for major vascular surgery. Because of the grave consequences of infection in a prosthetic joint, vancomycin or a first-generation cephalosporin is used prophylactically when a total hip replacement is performed. In the repair of open fractures, which are commonly contaminated, prophylactic treatment with a cephalosporin for 7 days is warranted. Controlled clinical studies have indicated that the administration of oral antibiotics (enteric-coated erythromycin plus neomycin, or tetracycline plus neomycin) just before colon surgery significantly reduces the incidence of infectious complications. The erythromycin-neomycin combination, 1 g of each administered orally at 1:00 P.M., 2:00 P.M., and 11:00 P.M. on the day before surgery, has been found to reduce the number of aerobic and anaerobic organisms remaining in the colon at the time of surgery. The emergence of tetracycline resistance among intestinal *Bacteroides* organisms may limit the future utility of the tetracycline-neomycin combination. When patients cannot be prepared for surgery with oral antibiotics, parenteral cefoxitin, cefotetan, or cefmetazole prophylaxis may be useful in certain circumstances—for example, for patients undergoing colorectal surgery or repair of a ruptured viscus. Cefazolin prophylaxis is recommended for patients undergoing high-risk gastric or biliary operations; cefotetan or cefoxitin is preferred for pelvic surgery.

References

1. Cockerill FR III: Conventional and genetic laboratory tests used to guide antimicrobial therapy. Mayo Clin Proc 73:1007, 1998

2. Lutsar I, McCraken GH Jr, Friedland IR: Antibiotic pharmacodynamics in cerebrospinal fluid. Clin Infect Dis 27:1117, 1998

3. Sensakovic JW, Smith LG: Oral antibiotic treatment of infectious diseases. Med Clin North Am 85:115, 2001

4. Hoffman-Terry ML, Fraimow HS, Fox TR, et al: Adverse effects of outpatient parenteral antibiotic therapy. Am J Med 106:44, 1999

5. Gilbert DN, Dworkin RJ, Raber SR, et al: Outpatient parenteral antimicrobial-drug therapy. N Engl J Med 337:829, 1997

6. Lee CE, Zembower TR, Fotis MA, et al: The incidence of antimicrobial allergies in hospitalized patients: implications regarding prescribing patterns and emerging bacterial resistance. Arch Intern Med 160:2819, 2000

7. Ito S: Drug therapy for breast-feeding women. N Engl J Med 343:118, 2000

8. Wong CS, Jelacic S, Habeeb RL, et al: The risk of hemolytic-uremic syndrome after antibiotic treatment of *Escherichia coli* O157:H7 infections. N Engl J Med 342:1930, 2000

9. Cunha BA: Antibiotic side effects. Med Clin North Am 85:149, 2001

10. Hogenauer C, Hammer HF, Krejs GJ, et al: Mechanisms and management of antibiotic-associated diarrhea. Clin Infect Dis 27:702, 1998

11. Gatifloxacin and moxifloxacin: two new fluoroquinolones. Med Lett Drugs Ther 42:1, 2000

12. Bertino JS Jr, Owens RC Jr, Carnes TD, et al: Gatifloxacin-associated corrected QT interval prolongation, torsades de pointes, and ventricular fibrillation in patients with known risk factors. Clin Infect Dis 34:861, 2002

13. Vassileva SG, Mateev G, Parish LC: Antimicrobial photosensitive reactions. Arch Intern Med 158:1993, 1998

14. Kollef MH, Fraser VJ: Antibiotic resistance in the intensive care unit. Ann Intern Med 134:298, 2001

15. Virk A, Steckelberg JM: Clinical aspects of antimicrobial resistance. Mayo Clin Proc 75:200, 2000

16. Moellering RC Jr: Antibiotic resistance: lessons for the future. Clin Infect Dis 27 (suppl 1):S135, 1998

17. Tenover FC: Development and spread of bacterial resistance to antimicrobial agents: an overview. Clin Infect Dis 33(suppl 3):S108, 2001

18. Williams RJ: Globalization of antimicrobial resistance: epidemiological challenges. Clin Infect Dis 33(suppl 3):S116, 2001

19. de Man P, Verhoeven BAN, Verbrugh HA, et al: An antibiotic policy to prevent emergence of resistant bacilli. Lancet 355:973, 2000

20. Cunha BA: Effective antibiotic-resistance control strategies. Lancet 357:1307, 2001

21. The choice of antimicrobial drugs. Med Lett Drugs Ther 43:69, 2001

22. Systemic antifungal drugs. Med Lett Drugs Ther 39:86, 1997

23. Henry NK, Hoecker JL, Rhodes KH: Antimicrobial therapy for infants and children: guidelines for the inpatient and outpatient practice of pediatric infectious diseases. Mayo Clin Proc 75:86, 2000

24. Wright AJ: The penicillins. Mayo Clin Proc 74:290, 1999

25. Giamarellou H, Antoniadou A: Antipseudomonal antibiotics. Med Clin North Am 85:19, 2001

26. Martinez-Rodríguez JE, Barriga FJ, Santamaria J, et al: Nonconvulsive status epilepticus associated with cephalosporins in patients with renal failure. Am J Med 111:115, 2001

27. Kelkar PS, Li JT: Cephalosporin allergy. N Engl J Med 345:804, 2001

28. Marshall WF, Blair JE: The cephalosporins. Mayo Clin Proc 74:187, 1999

29. Jones RN, Pfaller MA, Jacobs MR, et al: Cefditoren in vitro activity and spectrum: a review of international studies using reference methods. Diagn Microbial Infect Dis 41:1, 2001

30. Guglielmo BJ, Luber AD, Paletta D Jr, et al: Ceftriaxone therapy for staphylococcal osteomyelitis: a review. Clin Infect Dis 30:205, 2000

31. Dunne EF, Fey PD, Kludt P, et al: Emergence of domestically acquired ceftriaxone-resistant *Salmonella* infections associated with AmpC β-lactamase. JAMA 284:3151, 2000

32. Hellinger WC, Brewer NS: Carbapenems and monobactams: imipenem, meropenem, and aztreonam. Mayo Clin Proc 74:420, 1999

33. Odenholt I: Ertapenem: a new carbapenem. Expert Opin Investig Drugs 10:1157, 2001

34. Livermore DM, Carter MW, Bagel S, et al: In vitro activities of ertapenem (MK-0826) against recent clinical bacteria collected in Europe and Australia. Antimicrob Agents Chemother 45:1860, 2001

35. McConnell SA, Penzak SR, Warmack TS, et al: Incidence of imipenem hypersensitivity reactions in febrile neutropenic bone marrow transplant patients with a history of penicillin allergy. Clin Infect Dis 31:1512, 2000

36. Salkind AR, Cuddy PG, Foxworth JW: Is this patient allergic to penicillin? An evidence-based analysis of the likelihood of penicillin allergy. JAMA 285:2498, 2001

37. Harris AD, Sauberman L, Kabbash L, et al: Penicillin skin testing: a way to optimize antibiotic utilization. Am J Med 107:166, 1999

38. Dodek P, Phillips P: Questionable history of immediate-type hypersensitivity to penicillin in staphylococcal endocarditis: treatment based on skin-test results versus empirical alternative treatment—a decision analysis. Clin Infect Dis 29:1251, 1999

39. Edson RS, Terrell CL: The aminoglycosides. Mayo Clin Proc 74:519, 1999

40. Maurin M, Raoult D: Use of aminoglycosides in treatment of infections due to intracellular bacteria. Antimicrob Agents Chemother 45:2977, 2001

41. Lacy MK, Nicolau DP, Nightingale CH, et al: The pharmacodynamics of aminoglycosides. Clin Infect Dis 27:23, 1998

42. Forge A, Schacht J: Aminoglycoside antibiotics. Audiol Neurootol 5:3, 2000

43. Chuck SK, Raber SR, Rodvoid KA, et al: National survey of extended-interval aminoglycoside dosing. Clin Infect Dis 30:433, 2000

44. Bailey TC, Little JR, Littenberg B, et al: A meta-analysis of extended-interval dosing versus multiple daily dosing of aminoglycosides. Clin Infect Dis 24:786, 1997

45. Smilack JD: The tetracyclines. Mayo Clin Proc 74:727, 1999

46. Ailani RK, Agastya G, Ailani RK, et al: Doxycycline is a cost-effective therapy for hospitalized patients with community-acquired pneumonia. Arch Intern Med 159:266, 1999

47. Klein NC, Cunha BA: New uses of older antibiotics. Med Clin North Am 85:125, 2001

48. Alvarez-Elcoro S, Enzler MJ: The macrolides: erythromycin, clarithromycin, and azithromycin. Mayo Clin Proc 74:613, 1999

49. Swartz MN: Recognition and management of anthrax: an update. N Engl J Med 345:1621, 2001

50. Kasten MJ: Clindamycin, metronidazole, and chloramphenicol. Mayo Clin Proc 74:825, 1999

51. Wilhelm MP, Estes L: Vancomycin. Mayo Clin Proc 74:928, 1999

52. Jarvis WR: Epidemiology, appropriateness, and cost of vancomycin use. Clin Infect Dis 26:1200, 1998

53. Moellering RC Jr: Vancomycin-resistant enterococci. Clin Infect Dis 26:1196, 1998

54. Paradisi F, Corti G, Messeri D: Antistaphylococcal (MSSA, MRSA, MSSE, MRSE) antibiotics. Med Clin North Am 85:1, 2001

55. Quinupristin/dalfopristin. Med Lett Drugs Ther 41:109, 1999

56. Johnson AP, Livermore DM: Quinupristin/dalfopristin, a new addition to the antimicrobial arsenal. Lancet 354:2012, 1999

57. Linezolid (Zyvox). Med Lett Drugs Ther 42:1, 2000

58. Diekema DJ, Jones RN: Oxazolidinone antibiotics. Lancet 358:77, 2001

59. Cercenado E, García-Garrote F, Bouza E: In vitro activity of linezolid against multiply resistant gram-positive clinical isolates. J Antimicrob Chemother 47:77, 2001

60. Tsiodras S, Gold HS, Sakoulas G, et al: Linezolid resistance in a clinical isolate of *Staphylococcus aureus*. Lancet 358:207, 2001

61. Clemett D, Markham A: Linezolid. Drugs 59:815, 2000

62. Chien JW, Kucia ML, Salata RA: Use of linezolid, an oxazolidinone, in the treatment of multidrug-resistant gram-positive bacterial infections. Clin Infect Dis 30:146, 2000

63. El-Sadr WM, Luskin-Hawk R, Yurik TM, et al: A randomized trial of daily and thrice-weekly trimethoprim-sulfamethoxazole for the prevention of *Pneumocystis carinii* pneumonia in human immunodeficiency virus-infected patients. Clin Infect Dis 29:775, 1999

64. Huovinen R: Resistance to trimethoprim-sulfamethoxazole. Clin Infect Dis 32:1608, 2001

65. Demoly P, Messaad D, Sahla H, et al: A new protocol for TMP-SMX desensitization in HIV-infected patients is safe and effective. J Allergy Clin Immunol 102:1033, 1998

66. Hooper DC: Mechanisms of action of antimicrobials: focus on fluoroquinolones. Clin Infect Dis 32(suppl 1):S9, 2001

67. Piddock LJV: Fluoroquinolone resistance: overuse of fluoroquinolones in human and veterinary medicine can breed resistance. BMJ 317: 1029, 1998

68. Hooper DC: New uses for new and old quinolones and the challenge of resistance. Clin Infect Dis 30:243, 2000

69. Lipman J, Allworth A, Wallis SC: Cerebrospinal fluid penetration of high doses of intravenous ciprofloxacin in meningitis. Clin Infect Dis 31:1131, 2000

70. Gatifloxacin and moxifloxacin: two new fluoroquinolones. Med Lett Drugs Ther 42:15, 2000

71. Mandell LA, Ball P, Tillotson G: Antimicrobial safety and tolerability: differences and dilemmas. Clin Infect Dis 32(suppl 1):S72, 2001

72. Chen DK, McGeer A, de Azavedo JC, et al: Decreased susceptibility of *Streptococcus pneumoniae* to fluoroquinolones in Canada. N Engl J Med 341:233, 1999

73. Thomson CJ: The global epidemiology of resistance to ciprofloxacin and the changing nature of antibiotic resistance: a 10 year perspective. J Antimicrob Chemother 43:31, 1999

74. Brumfitt W, Hamilton-Miller JMT: Efficacy and safety profile of long-term nitrofurantoin in urinary infections: 18 years' experience. J Antimicrob Chemother 42:363, 1998

75. Fosfomycin for urinary tract infections. Med Lett Drugs Ther 39: 66, 1997

76. Zavasky DM, Sande MA: Reconsideration of rifampin: a unique drug for unique infection. JAMA 279:157, 1998

77. Zimmerli W, Widmer AF, Blatter M, et al: Role of rifampin for treatment of orthopedic implant-related staphylococcal infections: a randomized controlled trial. JAMA 279:1537, 1998

78. Senneville E, Yazdanpanah Y, Cazaubiel M, et al: Rifampicin-ofloxacin oral regimen for the treatment of mild to moderate diabetic foot osteomyelitis. J Antimicrob Chemother 48:927, 2001

79. Post-exposure anthrax prophylaxis. Med Lett Drugs Ther 43:91, 2001

80. Osmon DR: Antimicrobial prophylaxis in adults. Mayo Clin Proc 75:98, 2000

81. Antimicrobial prophylaxis in surgery. Med Lett Drugs Ther 41:75, 1999

3 Bioterrorism

Jeffrey S. Duchin, M.D.

Well before the 2001 anthrax outbreak, public health and government leaders in the United States recognized the need for increased preparedness to detect and respond to acts of biologic terrorism. Concern about the vulnerability of the United States to a biologic attack grew with revelations about the offensive biologic weapons programs of the former Soviet Union and Iraq, as well as uncertainty about the whereabouts of and accountability for biologic agents produced through those programs; the successful chemical attack on the Tokyo subway system by the Aum Shinrikyo cult, coupled with information that the cult was actively experimenting with biologic agents; and information about the potential for domestic bioterrorism.[1–5]

In April 2000, the Centers for Disease Control and Prevention (CDC) published a strategic plan for preparedness and response to biologic and chemical terrorism.[6] This subsection describes the clinician's role in recognizing and responding to biologic terrorism, as presented in the CDC plan; summarizes current information on the diagnosis and management of the most likely agents of bioterrorism; and describes current resources for authoritative information and guidelines related to bioterrorism.

The Clinician's Role in Bioterrorism Preparedness and Response

For clinicians, the response to a bioterrorism attack is in many ways the same as the response to naturally occurring outbreaks of communicable disease.[7,8] Both situations typically require early identification of ill or exposed persons, rapid implementation of preventive therapy, special infection control considerations, and collaboration or communication with the public health system. Examples of naturally occurring communicable diseases that require such a response include meningococcal disease[9]; enteric infection with *Escherichia coli* 0157:H7, *Salmonella*, or *Shigella*[10]; pertussis, rubella, measles, or chickenpox occurring in health care facilities and clinics[11–14]; unusual or newly emerging infections such as West Nile virus and hantavirus pulmonary syndrome[15–17]; and the inevitable reappearance of pandemic influenza.[18]

The first indication of an unannounced biologic attack will likely be an increase in the number of persons seeking care from primary care physicians. In the 2001 anthrax outbreak, as well as in the outbreaks of *E. coli* 0157:H7 disease and hantavirus pulmonary syndrome in 1993 and West Nile virus in 1999, alert clinicians initiated the public health response by recognizing an unusual clinical syndrome, ordering appropriate laboratory tests, and notifying public health officials.[10,16,17] Similarly, primary care physicians and subspecialists alike must be familiar with both the specific clinical syndromes associated with agents of bioterrorism and the ways to rapidly notify public health authorities. In addition to identifying cases and treating ill patients, clinicians also play a critical role in managing postexposure prophylaxis and its complications, as well as psychological and mental health problems brought on by the event.

During both bioterrorism attacks and naturally occurring outbreaks, clinicians are faced with the challenge of excluding the outbreak disease in persons who are worried about potential exposure or who are ill with signs and symptoms similar to those of the outbreak disease. The clinician must have knowledge of the modes of transmission, incubation periods, and communicable periods of these diseases, as well as skill in both clinical evaluation and eliciting an appropriate and thorough history, including relevant occupational, social, and travel information. In the 2001 anthrax outbreak, for example, the epidemiologic setting of cases played an important role in guiding diagnostic tests and treatment.[19] The primary care clinician

Table 1 Critical Biologic Agent Categories for Public Health Preparedness

Category	*Biologic Agent*	*Disease*
A (highest immediate risk)	Variola major *Bacillus anthracis* *Yersinia pestis* *Clostridium botulinum* (botulinum toxins) *Francisella tularensis* Filoviruses and arenaviruses (e.g., Ebola virus, Lassa virus)	Smallpox Anthrax Plague Botulism Tularemia Viral hemorrhagic fevers
B (next highest risk)	*Coxiella burnetii* *Brucella* species *Burkholderia mallei* *Burkholderia pseudomallei* Alphaviruses (VEE, EEE, WEE) *Rickettsia prowazekii* Toxins (e.g., ricin, staphylococcal enterotoxin B) *Chlamydia psittaci* Food-safety threats (e.g., *Salmonella* species, *E. coli* 0157:H7) Water-safety threats (e.g., *Vibrio cholerae, Cryptosporidium parvum*)	Q fever Brucellosis Glanders Melioidosis Encephalitis Typhus fever Toxic syndromes Psittacosis
C (potential, but not immediate, risk)	Emerging-threat agents (e.g., Nipah virus, hantavirus)	

EEE—eastern equine encephalitis VEE—Venezuelan equine encephalitis WEE—western equine encephalitis

has the best opportunity to obtain relevant information early in the evaluation; this is important because such information may be more difficult to obtain as time goes on, particularly if the patient's condition deteriorates.

Physicians and other health care providers should have a working knowledge of the basic classes of isolation and infection control measures recommended for patients exposed to agents of potential bioterrorism. Again, these measures are also used in the management of common communicable diseases.[14,20–22]

Recognition of Potential Bioterrorism Agents

The CDC has developed a list of bacteria, viruses, and toxins thought to pose the greatest risk for use in a bioterrorist attack [*see Table 1*].[23] Agents were included in the list on the basis of their ability to cause disease that (1) is easily disseminated or transmitted from person to person; (2) has high mortality, with potential for major public health impact; (3) may result in panic and social disruption; and (4) requires special action for public health preparedness. Category A agents are thought to pose the highest immediate risk for use as biologic weapons; and category B agents, the next highest risk. Category C agents are thought to pose a potential, but not immediate, risk for use as biologic weapons.

As in naturally occurring outbreaks, early recognition of a bioterrorist attack is critical for rapid implementation of preventive measures and treatment. Early recognition can be challenging, however, because patients presenting for medical care after exposure to a biologic agent may initially exhibit nonspecific symptoms, and pathogens that ordinarily occur in the community, particularly enteric organisms, may be used in a biologic attack.[24,25] A heightened level of suspicion, plus knowledge of the relevant epidemiologic clues, should help physicians recognize changes in illness patterns, including clusters and increases in observed cases over the number expected [*see Table 2*].[26] Physicians should also be able to recognize diagnostic clues in single cases of a syndrome of

Table 2 Epidemiologic Clues of a Biologic Attack

- Presence of a large epidemic
- Unusually severe disease or unusual routes of exposure
- Unusual geographic area, unusual season, or absence of normal vector
- Multiple simultaneous epidemics of different diseases
- Outbreak of zoonotic disease
- Unusual strains of organisms or antimicrobial-resistance patterns
- Higher attack rates in persons with common exposures
- Credible threat, as determined by authorities, of biologic attack
- Direct evidence of biologic attack

Internet Resources on Bioterrorism

General

CDC portal to information for laboratory and health professionals
http://www.bt.cdc.gov/healthprofessionals/index.asp

Contact information for U.S. state and local health departments
http://www.cdc.gov/other.htm#states

CDC Emergency Response Hotline (24 hours): 770-488-7100
Program questions: 404-639-0385

American College of Physicians–American Society of Internal Medicine (ACP-ASIM) bioterrorism resources
http://www.acponline.org/bioterro/?hp

Association for Professionals in Infection Control and Epidemiology, Inc.
http://www.apic.org/bioterror/

Bioterrorism Preparedness and Response Program, National Center for Infectious Diseases, Centers for Disease Control and Prevention—information for laboratory and health professionals
http://www.bt.cdc.gov/healthprofessionals/index.asp

Center for Infectious Disease Research & Policy (CIDRAP), University of Minnesota
http://www1.umn.edu/cidrap/content/bt/bioprep

FDA bioterrorism site
http://www.fda.gov/oc/opacom/hottopics/bioterrorism.html

Department of Health and Human Services Preparedness and Response
http://www.hhs.gov/hottopics/healing/biological.html

Infectious Diseases Society of America
bioterrorism: **http://www.idsociety.org/BT/ToC.htm**
practice guidelines: **http://www.idsociety.org/PG/toc.htm**

Johns Hopkins University Center for Civilian Biodefense Strategies
http://www.hopkins-biodefense.org

National Academies' Expert-selected Web Resources for "First Responders" on Bioterrorism
http://www.nap.edu/shelves/first

National Institute of Allergy and Infectious Diseases
http://www.niaid.nih.gov/publications/bioterrorism.htm

National Library of Medicine Specialized Information Services
http://www.sis.nlm.nih.gov/Tox/biologicalwarfare.htm

St. Louis University Center for Study of Bioterrorism
http://bioterrorism.slu.edu

Treatment of Biological Warfare Agent Casualties (July 17, 2000), U.S. Army Field Manual on Treatment of Biological Warfare Casualties
http://www.nbc-med.org/SiteContent/MedRef/OnlineRef/FieldManuals/Fm8_284/fm8_284.pdf

USAMRIID's Medical Management of Biological Casualties Handbook (Blue Book)
http://www.usamriid.army.mil/education/bluebook.html
word format: **http://www.nbc-med.org/SiteContent/HomePage/WhatsNew/MedManual/Feb01/handbook.htm**

JAMA consensus statement series
http://pubs.ama-assn.org/bioterr.html

Specific Agents

Anthrax as a Biological Weapon, 2002. Updated Recommendations for Management
http://jama.ama-assn.org/issues/v287n17/ffull/jst20007.html

Armed Forces Institute of Pathology site on inhalational anthrax, including slides
http://anthrax.radpath.org

Botulinum Toxin as a Biological Weapon. Medical and Public Health Management
http://jama.ama-assn.org/issues/v285n8/ffull/jst00017.html

Hemorrhagic Fever Viruses as Biological Weapons. Medical and Public Health Management
http://jama.ama-assn.org/issues/v287n18/ffull/jst20006.html

Plague as a Biological Weapon. Medical and Public Health Management
http://jama.ama-assn.org/issues/v283n17/ffull/jst90013.html

Smallpox as a Biological Weapon. Medical and Public Health Management
http://jama.ama-assn.org/issues/v281n22/ffull/jst90000.html

Tularemia as a Biological Weapon. Medical and Public Health Management
http://jama.ama-assn.org/issues/v285n21/ffull/jst10001.html

concern (e.g., inhalational anthrax, plague and tularemia, botulismlike illness, and possible smallpox).[27] Familiarity with the clinical features of diseases from potential bioterrorist agents and diseases prevalent in the community will allow recognition of potentially significant differences from naturally occurring cases. One of the most important lessons learned from the 2001 anthrax attack was that clinical illness caused by agents prepared as biologic weapons may differ from typical natural infections.

The identification of a bioterrorist attack requires clinicians to be prepared, alert, and open-minded [see Sidebar Internet Resources on Bioterrorism] Many local and state health departments post current information about communicable diseases on their Web sites and distribute informational newsletters with relevant data. The CDC's weekly bulletin, *Morbidity and Mortality Weekly Report* (*MMWR*), contains current information on medical conditions of public health importance in the United States. Subscriptions to *MMWR* are available online at http://www.cdc.gov/mmwr/mmwrsubscribe.html.

Communication with Authorities

Once a potential outbreak or significant cluster or event has been detected, prompt consultation with appropriate medical specialists and public health authorities is indicated. Clinicians must have reliable, around-the-clock contact information for emergency resources in the geographic area where they practice; these resources include specialist consultants (e.g., consultants in infectious disease, dermatology, or pulmonary medicine) and infection control professionals or hospital epidemiologists.

All clinicians should know how to contact their local or state public health department 24 hours a day to report suspicious or otherwise immediately notifiable cases or for consultation. Many local and state health departments have such contact numbers on their Web sites. Clinicians should have these numbers readily accessible and keep them current.

Clinicians must also ensure that they have a reliable way to promptly receive urgent communications from public health authorities, both for naturally occurring outbreaks of local significance and for a bioterrorist event or outbreak. Increasingly, public health authorities are disseminating health alerts over the Internet, through Web sites and e-mail listserves.

Smallpox

Smallpox is caused by variola virus, an orthopox virus unique to humans. No known animal or insect reservoirs or vectors exist.[28] Related orthopox viruses infecting humans include vaccinia (smallpox vaccine), monkeypox, and cowpox. Smallpox existed in two forms: variola major, which accounted for most morbidity and mortality, and a milder form, variola minor. Variola major is the type of concern in the context of biologic terrorism.

Smallpox was declared eradicated in 1980, 3 years after the last naturally occurring case was reported from Somalia. Stocks of smallpox virus were retained, however, by World Health Organization (WHO) reference laboratories at the Institute of Virus Preparations in Moscow, Russia, and at the CDC in Atlanta, Georgia. In the late 1990s, allegations were published describing the production of large quantities of smallpox virus by the former Soviet Union. These stores, which may have become disseminated after the breakup of the Soviet Union, would presumably be the source for a bioterrorist attack involving smallpox.

Smallpox is stable and highly infectious in the aerosol form. The risk for a smallpox attack currently is considered low but not zero.[1,4,29,30]

CLASSIFICATION

On the basis of a study from India, the WHO has classified smallpox into five clinical forms: ordinary, flat-type, hemorrhagic, modified, and sine eruptione.[31] These forms reflect different host reactions to the same strain of virus.

Ordinary Smallpox

Ordinary smallpox is the most common form seen in nonimmune persons; it accounted for 90% of cases in the WHO study and had an average case-fatality rate of 30%. The incubation period is 7 to 17 days (mean, 10 to 12 days). Symptoms of the prodromal phase include the acute onset of high fever, malaise, headache, backache, and prostration. Other prominent symptoms include vomiting and abdominal pain.

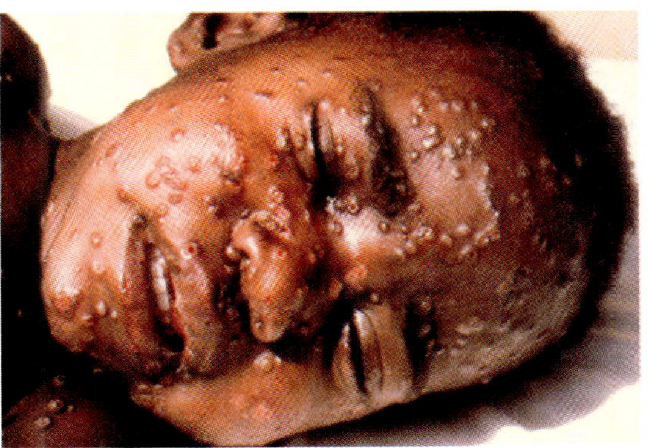

Figure 1 **Lesions of smallpox.**

The characteristic rash occurs 2 to 3 days later, appearing first on the face and forearms. An enanthem involving the oropharyngeal mucosa precedes the rash by a day. The rash progresses slowly, from macules to papules to vesicles and pustules and finally to scabs, with each stage lasting 1 to 2 days. The lesions are firm, discrete vesicles or pustules (4 to 6 mm in diameter) deeply embedded in the dermis; they may become umbilicated or confluent as they evolve [*see Figure 1*]. The patient remains febrile throughout the evolution of the rash, which may become painful as pustules enlarge. A second fever spike 5 to 8 days after onset of the rash may signify a secondary bacterial infection. Pustules remain for 5 to 8 days, after which umbilication and crusting occur. Lesions are in the same stage of development on any given part of the body. They are peripherally distributed, more concentrated on the face and distal extremities than on the trunk, and may involve the palms and soles. Scarring occurs with scab separation from destruction of sebaceous glands.

Experience during the global smallpox eradication program suggests that the onset of communicability coincides with the development of rash, approximately 2 days after the onset of the acute febrile prodrome. However, because the oropharyngeal enanthem and associated release of virus into oral secretions may precede rash onset, it is recommended that for the purposes of postexposure management, anyone who has contact with smallpox patients from the time of onset of fever should be considered potentially exposed [*see* Infection Control, *below*].[32]

Complications of smallpox include fluid and electrolyte disturbances; extensive desquamation that clinically resembles burns; bronchitis and pneumonitis; panophthalmitis and blindness from viral keratitis or secondary infection of the eye; arthritis (developing in up to 2% of children); and encephalitis (less than 1% of cases). Death results from toxemia associated with circulating immune complexes and variola antigens.[33]

Other Forms of Smallpox

Flat-type (or malignant) smallpox occurs in 5% to 10% of cases and is severe, with a 97% case-fatality rate among unvaccinated persons. In this form, lesions are flat and become densely confluent, evolving slowly and coalescing with a soft, velvety texture. Hemorrhagic smallpox was reported in less than 3% of cases, occurring particularly in pregnant women. It is a severe, rapidly progressive, uniformly fatal illness. A dusky erythema develops, followed by hemorrhages into the skin and mucous membranes. Both hemorrhagic and flat-type smallpox have an accelerated and more severe prodromal phase and are thought to be associated with underlying immune dysfunction.

Modified smallpox is a mild form that accounted for 2% of cases in unvaccinated patients and 25% in previously vaccinated patients. This form rarely resulted in death, and these patients had fewer, smaller, more superficial, and more rapidly evolving lesions. Smallpox sine eruptione (without rash) occurs in previously vaccinated persons or children with maternal antibodies to smallpox. It is a mild or asymptomatic illness that has not been documented to be transmissible.[31,33–35]

DIAGNOSIS

A suspected case of smallpox is a public health emergency. Local and state health authorities, the hospital epidemiologist, and other members of a hospital response team for biologic emergencies should be notified immediately (see the CDC Interim Smallpox Response Plan and Guidelines at http://www.bt.cdc.gov/documentsapp/SmallPox/RPG/ContactInfo.asp).

The differential diagnosis of smallpox includes other illnesses that can cause fever and a rash [*see Table 3*]. Severe varicella is the disease most likely to be confused with smallpox. However, familiar-

Table 3 Diagnosis of Smallpox

Incubation Period	*Clinical Presentation*	*Differential Diagnosis*	*Diagnostic Testing*
7–17 days; mean, 10–12 days	Severe, acute febrile prodrome 1–4 days before rash onset, with temperature ≥ 101° F (38.3° C), headache, backache, chills, vomiting, abdominal pain, prostration Enanthem on oropharyngeal mucosa, followed by rash on face, forearms, distal extremities, then trunk; lesions most concentrated on face and distal extremities Lesions evolve slowly from macules to papules to deep-seated, firm, nodular, round, well-circumscribed vesicles or pustules to scabs over 1–2 days per stage; are in same stage of evolution on a given area of the body; may become umbilicated or confluent Hemorrhagic smallpox: bleeding into skin and mucous membranes Flat-type/malignant smallpox: lesions remain soft and flattened, coalesce Modified smallpox: less severe with fewer, more superficial and rapidly evolving lesions	Varicella (chickenpox); disseminated herpes zoster and simplex; drug eruptions; erythema multiforme; enteroviral infections; secondary syphilis; contact dermatitis; impetigo; scabies; molluscum contagiosum Hemorrhagic smallpox: meningococcemia, Rocky Mountain spotted fever, ehrlichiosis, gram-negative bacterial sepsis, severe acute leukemia Malignant smallpox: hemorrhagic chickenpox	Diagnostic testing at BSL-4 laboratory, including skin biopsy, electron microscopic examination of vesicular and pustular fluid, culture, PCR; serology Appropriate infection control precautions

Note: The clinical manifestations of infections acquired during a biologic attack may differ from those of naturally occurring infections. Clinicians should remain alert for compatible syndromes that vary from the descriptions given.
BSL-4—biosafety level 4 PCR—polymerase chain reaction

Table 4 Differentiating Features of Smallpox and Chickenpox

Clinical Feature	*Smallpox*	*Chickenpox*
Prodromal illness	Febrile prodrome lasting 1–4 days; patient appears ill or toxic	No or mild prodrome; patients typically do not appear ill
Appearance of lesions	Firm, round, well-circumscribed, deep-seated lesions; may be umbilicated	Superficial lesions
Stage of lesions on any one part of the body	Lesions are all at the same stage of development on a given area of the body	Lesions occur in crops with various stages of development evident on a given area of the body
Initial lesions	Oral mucosa, face, or forearms	Face, then trunk
Oral lesions	Early; may not be evident	May occur
Severity of illness	Typically severe	Typically not severe
Distribution of rash	Centrifugal: lesions concentrated on the face and extremities, with relative sparing of the trunk	Centripetal: lesions concentrated on the trunk with relative sparing of the face and extremities
Lesions on palms or soles	Lesions on palms and soles in majority of cases	Lesions on palms and soles uncommon
Rate of evolution of rash	Slow evolution of lesions from macules to papules to pustules over days	Rapid evolution from macules to papules to crusted lesions within 24 hours
Presence of pruritus	Lesions may be painful and are not usually pruritic until scabbing occurs	Often pruritic, typically not painful in the absence of secondary infection
Hemorrhagic lesions	Can occur	Can occur

ity with the clinical features of the two diseases, particularly the rash, should help differentiate them [*see Table 4*]. Additional information that may be useful in differentiating smallpox from chickenpox includes a history of exposure to persons with chickenpox, a personal history of chickenpox, a history of vaccination against varicella or smallpox, and the clinical course of illness.

If shingles or disseminated herpes infection is a consideration, direct fluorescent antibody testing for varicella-zoster virus can rapidly confirm varicella-zoster virus and herpes simplex virus infection in patients not considered at high risk for smallpox. Such testing should not be done in patients who are considered at high risk, to avoid exposing laboratory workers to smallpox virus. Certain laboratories can also perform polymerase chain reaction (PCR) testing for herpes simplex virus and varicella-zoster virus. Consultation with an infectious disease specialist, a dermatology specialist, or both is recommended.

Flat-type and hemorrhagic smallpox may be difficult to recognize because of the absence of the characteristic rash of ordinary smallpox, yet these cases are highly infectious. Hemorrhagic smallpox cases may be mistaken for meningococcemia or acute leukemia. All patients with potential smallpox should be asked about their travel history, level of immunocompetence, and current medications.

The local or state health department should be contacted to facilitate specimen collection for smallpox testing (http://www.statepublichealth.org). Protocols for specimen collection for smallpox testing have been published by the CDC and are available at the following Internet address: http://www.bt.cdc.gov/documentsapp/SmallPox/RPG/GuideD/Guide-D.pdf. These protocols are also available through the CDC's smallpox information Web page: http://www.bt.cdc.gov/Agent/Smallpox/SmallpoxGen.asp.

Diagnostic testing is available at designated biosafety level 4 (BSL-4) laboratories and includes electron microscopy, immunohistochemical tests, and viral culture with PCR and restriction fragment length polymorphism (RFLP) testing. Only personnel who have undergone successful smallpox vaccination recently (within 3 years) and who are wearing appropriate barrier protection (gloves, gown, and shoe covers) should be involved in specimen collection for suspected cases of smallpox. Respiratory protection is not needed for personnel with recent, successful vaccination. Masks and eyewear or face shields should be used if splashing is anticipated. If unvaccinated personnel must collect specimens, only those who are without contraindications to vaccination should do so, because they would require immediate vaccination if the diagnosis of smallpox were confirmed. Vesicular or pustular fluid, scabs, punch biopsies of skin lesions, blood, and tissue from autopsy specimens should be obtained, packaged, and transported according to CDC protocol (http://www.bt. cdc.gov/labissues/PackagingInfo.pdf; http://www.bt.cdc.gov/documentsapp/SmallPox/RPG/index.asp).[32,35]

The CDC has developed a protocol in poster format for evaluating patients with an acute vesicular or pustular rash illness and for determining the risk of smallpox. The protocol, including color pictures of smallpox lesions, is available on the Internet at the following address: http://www.bt.cdc.gov/agent/smallpox/index.asp.

INFECTION CONTROL AND POSTEXPOSURE ISOLATION

In the event of a limited outbreak, patients should be admitted to the hospital and confined to rooms that are under negative atmospheric pressure and equipped with high-efficiency particulate air (HEPA) filtration. Standard, contact, and airborne precautions, including use of gloves, gowns, and masks, should be strictly observed. Unvaccinated personnel caring for patients suspected of having smallpox should wear fit-tested N95 or higher-quality respirators. Once successful vaccination is confirmed, care providers are no longer required to wear an N95 mask.[35] Patients should wear a surgical mask and be wrapped in a gown or sheet to cover the rash when they are not in a negative-airflow room. All laundry and waste should be placed in biohazard bags and autoclaved before being laundered or incinerated. Surfaces that may be contaminated with smallpox virus can be decontaminated with disinfectants that are used for standard hospital infection control, such as hypochlorite and quaternary ammonia.

Persons suspected of being infected with smallpox should be immediately isolated, and all their household members and others who have had face-to-face contact with the infected patient after the onset of fever should be vaccinated and placed under surveillance. Because persons who have had contact with an infected patient would not be contagious until the onset of rash, they should take their temperatures at least once daily, preferably in the evening. Any temperature higher than 101° F (38.3° C) during the 17-day period after the last exposure to the infected patient would suggest the possibility of the development of smallpox. This would be cause for immediate isolation until the diagnosis can be determined clinically, by laboratory examination, or both.

In the event of an outbreak, the following high-risk groups should be given priority for vaccination: (1) persons exposed to the initial release of the virus; (2) contacts of suspected or confirmed smallpox patients; (3) personnel who are directly involved in medical or public health evaluation of suspected or confirmed smallpox patients, as well as the care or transportation of such patients; (4) laboratory workers involved in the collection or processing of possible smallpox specimens; (5) other persons who may be in contact with infectious material, such as hospital laundry, medical waste, and mortuary workers; (6) other groups essential to response activities, such as law enforcement, emergency response, or military personnel; and (7) all persons in a hospital where there is a smallpox patient who is not isolated appropriately. Employees for whom vaccination would be contraindicated (see below) should be furloughed.[32,35]

Smallpox Vaccine

Vaccinia vaccine does not contain smallpox (variola) virus. The currently available vaccines were prepared from calf lymph with a seed virus derived from the New York City Board of Health strain of vaccinia virus (Dryvax® vaccine). A supply of licensed Dryvax® vaccine is being used in the first stages of the National Smallpox Vaccination Plan to immunize smallpox healthcare and public health teams. A reformulated vaccine, produced by using cell-culture techniques, is being developed.

The immune status of those vaccinated more than 27 years ago is not clear. Studies have demonstrated persistence of T cell and humoral responses, but absolute levels of neutralizing antibodies decline substantially during the first 5 to 10 years after vaccination. Epidemiologic studies conducted during endemic smallpox outbreaks suggested that remote vaccination can ameliorate disease but does not prevent disease in most persons with high-risk exposures.[30]

Complications of smallpox vaccination Current data on complication rates after primary vaccination are derived from observations made when smallpox vaccine was in routine use in the United States, over 30 years ago.[28] Higher rates of vaccine complications would likely occur today, given the increased number of persons with medical conditions or medications that compromise the immune system. Moderate and severe complications of vaccinia vaccination include eczema vaccinatum, generalized vaccinia, progressive vaccinia, and postvaccinial encephalitis. These complications are rare but are at least 10 times more common after primary vaccination than after revaccination; they occur more frequently in infants than in older children and adults.

The most common complication of smallpox vaccination, occurring in 529.2 cases per million doses, is localized vaccinia infection resulting from inadvertent transfer (autoinoculation) of vaccinia from the vaccination site to other parts of the body. In addition, transmission of vaccinia virus can occur when a recently vaccinated person has contact with a susceptible person; in one study, approximately 30% of eczema vaccinatum cases were persons who had had such contact.[28,36] Inadvertent transfer of vaccinia from the vaccination site to other parts of the body can be prevented by careful hand washing after touching the vaccination site and by keeping the site covered.

Eczema vaccinatum (38.5/million doses) is a localized or systemic dissemination of vaccinia virus that occurs in persons who have eczema or a history of eczema or other chronic or exfoliative skin conditions (e.g., atopic dermatitis). Illness is usually mild and self-limited but can be severe or fatal. Severe cases have also been observed in persons with active eczema or a history of eczema, after contact with recently vaccinated persons.

Generalized vaccinia (241.5/million doses) is characterized by a vesicular rash of varying extent that can occur in persons without underlying illness. The rash is generally self-limited and requires minor or no therapy except in patients whose condition might be toxic or who have serious underlying immunosuppressive illnesses.

Progressive vaccinia (vaccinia necrosum, 1.5/million doses) is a severe, potentially fatal illness characterized by progressive necrosis in the area of vaccination, often with metastatic lesions [*see Figure 2*]. It has occurred almost exclusively in persons with cellular immunodeficiency.

The most common serious complication is postvaccinial encephalitis (12.3/million doses). It occurs mostly in infants younger than 1 year and, less often, in adolescents and adults receiving a primary vaccination. Rates of this complication were influenced by the strain of virus used in the vaccine and were higher in Europe than in the United States. The principal strain of vaccinia virus used in the United States—the New York City Board

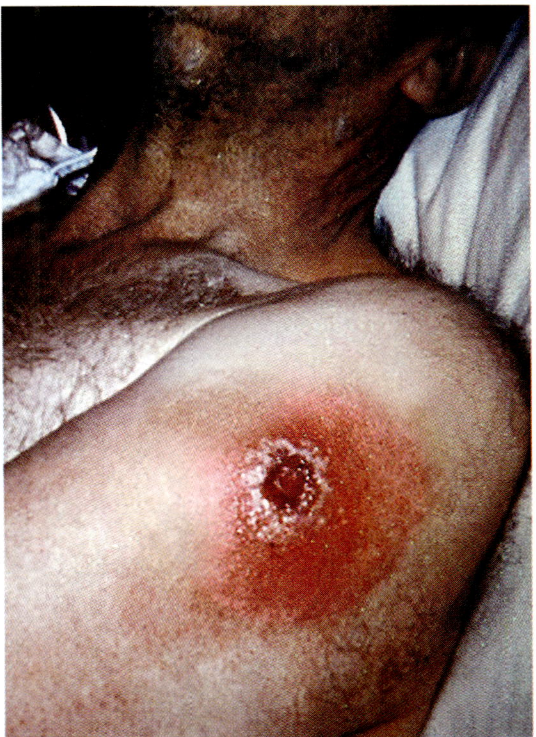

Figure 2 **Progressive vaccinia (vaccinia necrosum) at the site of smallpox vaccination in a 64-year-old man.**

of Health (NYCBOH) strain—was associated with the lowest incidence of postvaccinial encephalitis. Approximately 15% to 25% of affected vaccinees with this complication die, and 25% have permanent neurologic sequelae.

Fatal complications caused by vaccinia vaccination are rare, with approximately one death per million primary vaccinations and 0.25 deaths per million revaccinations. Death is most often the result of postvaccinial encephalitis or progressive vaccinia.

Contraindications Groups at special risk for complications include persons with eczema or other significant exfoliative conditions; patients with leukemia, lymphoma, or generalized malignancy who are receiving therapy with alkylating agents, antimetabolites, radiation, or large doses of corticosteroids; patients with HIV infection; persons with hereditary immune disorders; and pregnant women. In persons with contraindications who require vaccination because of exposure to smallpox virus from a bioterrorist attack, the risk of complications can be reduced by giving vaccinia immune globulin (VIG; see below) simultaneously with vaccination. However, current stores of VIG are insufficient to allow its prophylactic use. Even if VIG is not available, vaccination may still be warranted, given the far higher risk of an adverse outcome from smallpox than from vaccination.

Vaccinia immune globulin Complications of vaccinia vaccination can be prevented or treated with VIG, which is an isotonic sterile solution of the immunoglobulin fraction of plasma from persons vaccinated with vaccinia vaccine. For prophylactic use, in persons with contraindications who require vaccination, VIG is given along with vaccinia vaccine.[28] Very large amounts are required: VIG is administered intramuscularly in a dose of 0.3 ml/kg (e.g., 22.5 ml I.M. for a 75 kg patient) At present, however, supplies of VIG are so limited that its use should be reserved for treatment of patients with the most serious vaccine complications.

For treatment of vaccinia vaccination complications, VIG is administered intramuscularly; 0.6 ml/kg is given in divided doses over a 24- to 36-hour period. A repeat dose may be given 2 to 3 days later if improvement does not occur. VIG is effective for treatment of eczema vaccinatum and certain cases of progressive vaccinia; it might be useful also in the treatment of ocular vaccinia resulting from inadvertent implantation. VIG is contraindicated for the treatment of vaccinial keratitis. VIG is recommended for severe generalized vaccinia if the patient is extremely ill or has a serious underlying disease. VIG provides no benefit in the treatment of postvaccinial encephalitis and has no role in the treatment of smallpox.[28,32]

Anthrax

Anthrax is a zoonotic disease caused by the spore-forming bacterium *Bacillus anthracis,* a large, nonmotile, nonhemolytic, gram-positive rod [see 16 Infections Due to Gram-Positive Bacilli]. The organism is distributed worldwide in soil. Animals, primarily herbivores, become infected through grazing in contaminated areas. Under natural conditions, humans contract the disease after close contact with infected animals or contaminated animal products such as hides, wool, or meat.[37] Hardy spores resistant to heat and environmental degradation are the usual infective form. The spores develop in response to exposure to ambient air. On exposure to favorable, nutrient-rich environmental conditions such as tissues or blood of an animal or human host, the spores germinate, producing vegetative cells.[38]

CLASSIFICATION AND EPIDEMIOLOGY

Anthrax occurs in three clinical forms in humans: inhalational, cutaneous, and gastrointestinal. In a biologic attack, aerosol exposure to anthrax spores would be most likely.[29] Only 18 cases of inhalational anthrax were reported in the United States in the 20th century, none of them after 1976. Sixteen of these cases were attributable to an industrial source of infection, and two cases were laboratory associated.[39] Before 2001, exposure to powdered anthrax spores in an envelope or package was not thought to be an efficient means of causing inhalational disease. However, exposure to anthrax spores sent through the United States mail in the 2001 anthrax attack resulted in 11 cases of inhalational anthrax and 11 cases of cutaneous disease.[19,40,41] Recent research has demonstrated the unanticipated potential for significant dispersion of respirable aerosol particles of spores through opening of a contaminated envelope.[42] In addition, expected clinical findings based on previous experience with naturally occurring anthrax infections did not entirely correspond to the clinical presentation in persons exposed to anthrax in the context of a biologic attack, although there was considerable overlap between the two.

Cutaneous anthrax accounts for the majority of naturally occurring anthrax cases worldwide. It results from inoculation of spores subcutaneously through a cut or abrasion.[43] Given that cutaneous anthrax cases occurred during the 2001 anthrax outbreak, it is possible that a bioterrorist attack could be detected through recognition of cutaneous anthrax cases.[19] Gastrointestinal and oropharyngeal anthrax occur in rural parts of the world where anthrax is endemic. They result from ingestion of meat contaminated with spores or large numbers of vegetative cells.[44] No cases of gastrointestinal anthrax occurred during the 1979 accidental release of anthrax from a military facility in Sverdlovsk, Russia, in which 77 inhalational cases occurred, or during the 2001 outbreak in the United States. Because of the logistic difficulty of effectively contaminating food and water supplies, it is thought that this form of anthrax would be less likely to occur as a result of a biologic attack.[29]

PATHOPHYSIOLOGY

Anthrax is a toxin-mediated disease. In inhalational anthrax, 1 to 5 μm particle–bearing spores are deposited in the terminal airways or alveoli, phagocytized by alveolar macrophages, and transported to mediastinal and peribronchial lymph nodes. Spores may stay in the mediastinal lymph nodes for extended periods and can germinate for up to 60 days or longer.[45] Cases of inhalational anthrax occurred up to 43 days after exposure in the Sverdlovsk outbreak.[46] Spores germinate into vegetative cells, which escape from the macrophages, multiply in the lymphatics, and ultimately gain access to the bloodstream, where they can reach high concentrations (107 to 108 organisms per milliliter of blood). Hemorrhagic meningitis is a complication of bacteremic spread; it develops in up to one half of cases.

In anthrax, tissue damage is mediated by two toxins: edema toxin and lethal toxin. These two toxins are composed of edema factor, lethal factor, and protective antigen. These three components of edema toxin and lethal toxin are produced by vegetative cells. Vegetative cells also produce an antiphagocytic capsule that is necessary for virulence.[47] Lethal toxin is a combination of lethal factor and protective antigen that interferes with cellular protein synthesis; it causes macrophages to release tumor necrosis factor and interleukin-1. In severe cases, it contributes to sudden death from toxemia. Edema toxin is a combination of edema factor and protective antigen that causes increased cellular levels of cyclic adenosine monophosphate (cAMP) and altered water homeostasis, resulting in massive edema. Together, edema toxin and lethal toxin cause edema, hemorrhage, necrosis, and shock. In cutaneous and gastrointestinal anthrax, toxin production results in a similar pathophysiologic process that causes edema and hemorrhagic necrosis in the skin and gastrointestinal mucosa, respectively.

INHALATIONAL ANTHRAX

Clinical Presentation and Diagnosis

Recent information on the clinical manifestations of inhalational anthrax from the 2001 anthrax outbreak both confirms many of the features reported in naturally occurring anthrax cases and reveals unanticipated differences.[39,45,48] The infectious dose of anthrax is not known with certainty. Animal data suggest that the median lethal dose (LD_{50}, which is the dose sufficient to kill 50% of exposed subjects) is 2,500 to 55,000 inhaled spores. Data from naturally occurring cases and from two cases in the 2001 outbreak suggest that the infectious dose may be very low in some persons, particularly those with underlying pulmonary disease.[45,49]

Clinical symptoms develop rapidly after germination of anthrax spores. The incubation period for inhalational disease is most commonly reported as 1 to 6 days but may be prolonged by antibiotic administration or, presumably, a low infectious dose.[50,51] In the 2001 anthrax outbreak, the median incubation period was 4 days (range, 4 to 6 days) for the six cases in which it could be calculated.

Inhalational anthrax has been described as a two-stage disease. The initial stage is a nonspecific, flulike illness lasting from several hours to a few days. In the 2001 bioterrorism-associated anthrax cases, this early clinical presentation included some combination of fever, myalgia, headache, cough, mild chest discomfort, weakness, abdominal pain, and chest pain. Profound malaise, fever, and drenching sweats were prominent symptoms, and nausea and vomiting were frequent. Classically, the initial stage is followed 1 to 3 days later, sometimes after brief improvement, by the rapidly progressive second stage, characterized by fever, dyspnea, diaphoresis, cyanosis, and shock. In the 2001 cases, no brief improvement between stages was observed.

Laboratory studies are nonspecific or unremarkable during the early stage of disease.[48] Chest x-rays were abnormal on initial presentation in all 10 recent cases, although only seven patients had the classic finding of mediastinal widening [*see Figure 3*]. Pleural effusions were present in all cases. These effusions were often small on presentation and were progressive, requiring drainage in the majority of patients. In contrast to previous descriptions, seven patients had pulmonary infiltrates consistent with pneumonia at presentation, and one patient

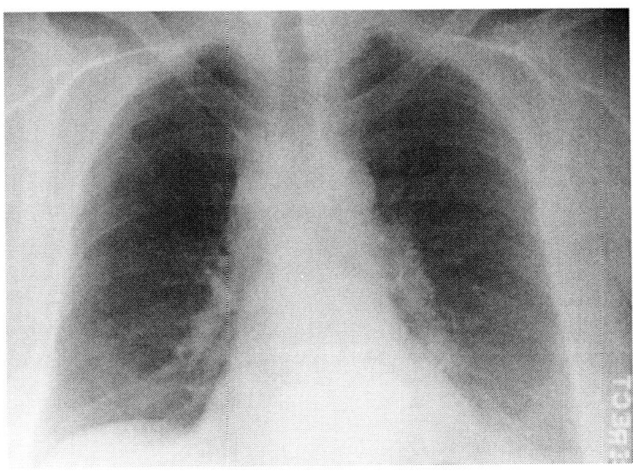

Figure 3 **Chest x-ray of a patient with inhalational anthrax showing mediastinal widening and a small left pleural effusion.**

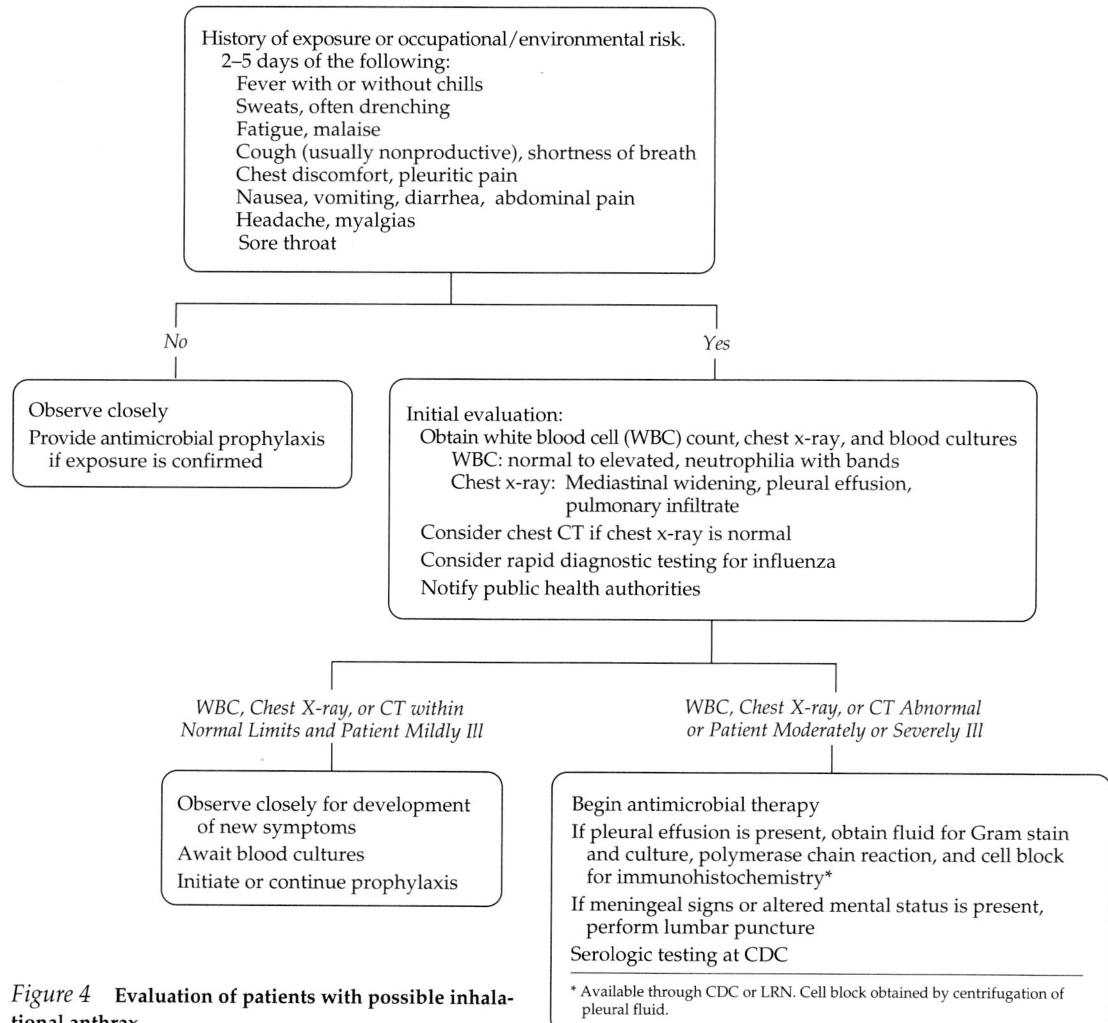

Figure 4 **Evaluation of patients with possible inhalational anthrax.**

was thought to have heart failure with pulmonary congestion. Other abnormalities included paratracheal and hilar fullness. The CT scan was valuable in further characterizing abnormalities in the lungs and mediastinum and was more sensitive than the chest x-ray in revealing mediastinal changes. Blood cultures can be diagnostic, although appropriate antibiotic therapy rapidly reduces the likelihood of isolating the organism. In the 2001 cases, *B. anthracis* was isolated from blood cultures obtained before antibiotic therapy was given, but not from those obtained afterward.

The initial manifestations of inhalational anthrax are nonspecific and are consistent with flulike illnesses caused by a variety of respiratory viruses, as well as with community-acquired bacterial infections. Adults can average one to three episodes of flulike illness a year, and millions of cases occur throughout the United States.[52] Because of the high frequency of flulike illnesses and the low likelihood of inhalational anthrax in a given patient, a combination of epidemiologic, clinical, and (if indicated) laboratory testing should be used to evaluate potential cases of inhalational anthrax [*see Figure 4*]. According to CDC guidelines, consideration of inhalational anthrax hinges on a history of exposure or occupational/environmental risk within 2 to 5 days before illness onset.[19] Whenever possible, exposure and risk determinations should be made in consultation with public health authorities before initiating treatment or preventive therapy.

Diagnostic testing for anthrax should be done in patients whose signs and symptoms are consistent with anthrax and when one or more of the following conditions are present: a history of a recent anthrax case or outbreak in the community; a credible threat of anthrax exposure, as determined by law enforcement and public health authorities; a cluster of anthraxlike cases characterized by rapid deterioration. Anthrax should also be considered in any patient with compatible symptoms and rapid deterioration. All cases of suspected anthrax should be reported immediately to local or state public health authorities and the hospital epidemiologist (http://www.statepublichealth.org). The clinical laboratory should also be alerted when diagnostic specimens of suspected anthrax are submitted to ensure that appropriate precautions are taken to protect laboratory staff, facilitate proper evaluation of the isolate, and expedite confirmatory testing at the nearest laboratory that belongs to the public health Laboratory Response Network.[6]

There is no rapid screening test to diagnose inhalational anthrax in its early stages. In persons with a compatible clinical illness for whom there is a heightened suspicion of anthrax based on clinical and epidemiologic data, the appropriate initial diagnostic tests are a chest x-ray or chest CT scan, or both, and culture and smear of peripheral blood. On chest x-rays, the posteroanterior and lateral view may be more sensitive than the anteroposterior (portable) view in detecting pulmonary abnormalities. Mediastinal widening or hyperdense mediastinal lymphadenopathy (secondary to hemorrhagic lymph nodes) on a nonenhanced CT scan should raise the suspicion of pulmonary anthrax [*see Figure 5*]. Most persons with flulike illnesses do not have radiologic findings of pneumonia; such findings occur most often in the very young, the elderly, and persons with chronic lung disease.

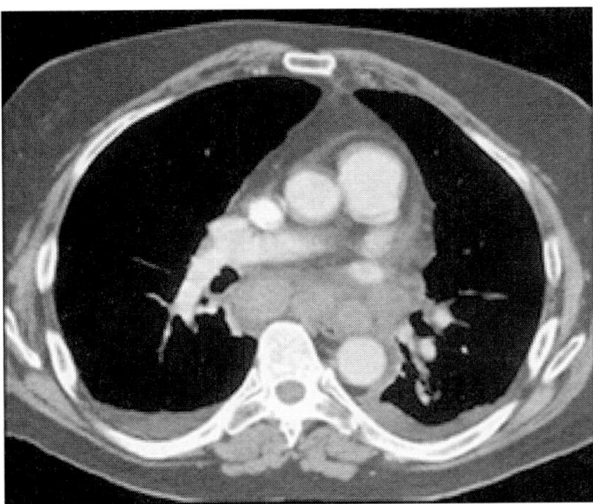

Figure 5 **CT scan of the chest of a patient with inhalational anthrax showing mediastinal lymphadenopathy and small bilateral pleural effusions.**

Pleural fluid and cerebrospinal fluid, as well as biopsy specimens taken from the pleura and lung, are also potentially useful for culture and other testing when disease is present in these sites, whereas sputum culture and Gram stain are unlikely to be useful. In highly suspicious cases, local or state health departments can arrange for additional diagnostic testing, including immunohistochemical staining and PCR at the CDC. Serologic testing is not useful in clinical management but may be used in epidemiologic investigations. Similarly, nasal swabs are of potential value in epidemiologic investigations for determining the route and extent of spread of anthrax in a population, but they have no role in clinical management.

A rapid influenza test can be used when influenza itself is a consideration in a patient with flulike illness, but these kits have limited value because their sensitivity can be relatively low (45% to 90%). However, rapid influenza testing with viral culture can help indicate whether influenza viruses are circulating among certain populations, and this epidemiologic information can be useful in diagnosing flulike illnesses.[52]

Treatment

Early intravenous antibiotic treatment may improve survival in inhalational anthrax.[53] In contrast to the reported case-fatality rate of 85% for 20th-century inhalational anthrax cases, 6 of 11 patients in the 2001 outbreak survived; all the survivors presented during the initial phase of the illness and received treatment the same day with antibiotics active against *B. anthracis*. Fatal cases occurred in patients who had severe disease by the time they first received antibiotics with activity against *B. anthracis*. Aggressive supportive care—including attention to fluid, electrolyte, and acid-base disturbances and drainage of pleural effusions—also played an important role in treatment.[48]

Current CDC treatment recommendations and related guidelines and information can be obtained at http://www.bt.cdc.gov/HealthProfessionals/index.asp. Before initiating treatment, clinicians should review this site to stay informed of revisions and updates. The Working Group on Civilian Biodefense has published similar recommendations with a detailed accompanying text.[45]

At present, intravenous ciprofloxacin or doxycycline plus one or two additional antimicrobials with in vitro activity against *B. anthracis* are recom-

Table 5 Treatment of Inhalational Anthrax

Patients	*Medication and Dosage*	*Comments*
Adults, including pregnant women and immunocompromised persons	Ciprofloxacin, 400 mg I.V., q. 12 hr *or* Doxycycline, 100 mg I.V., q. 12 hr *and* One or two additional antimicrobials*	If meningitis is suspected, doxycycline may be less optimal because of poor central nervous system penetration Modify regimen on the basis of susceptibility testing of isolate; can switch to p.o. after patient is clinically stable; continue treatment for at least 60 days Consider corticosteroids for meningitis, severe edema, or respiratory compromise
Children, including those who are immunocompromised	Ciprofloxacin, 10–15 mg/kg I.V., q. 12 hr, not to exceed 1 g/day *or* Doxycycline If > 8 yr and > 45 kg, give adult dosage If ≤ 8 yr or if > 8 yr but ≤ 45 kg, give 2.2 mg/kg q. 12 hr (maximum, 200 mg/day) *and* One or two additional antimicrobials*	If meningitis is suspected, doxycycline may be less optimal because of poor central nervous system penetration Modify regimen on the basis of susceptibility testing of isolate; can switch to p.o. after patient is clinically stable; continue treatment for at least 60 days Consider corticosteroids for meningitis, severe edema, or respiratory compromise

Note: Treatment recommendations may change over time and according to antimicrobial susceptibility test results during a biologic attack and to availability of selected antimicrobial agents. Before initiating treatment, clinicians should consult with an infectious disease specialist and public health authorities and should check for revisions and updates at http://www.bt.cdc.gov/HealthProfessionals/index.asp. This information is adapted from CDC and Working Group on Civilian Biodefense recommendations and may not represent FDA-approved uses.

*Other agents with in vitro activity anthrax include rifampin, vancomycin, penicillin, ampicillin, chloramphenicol, imipenem, clindamycin, and clarithromycin.

mended for initial empirical treatment [*see Table 5*]. Antibiotic therapy should be modified according to the results of antimicrobial susceptibility testing to ensure that the most effective and least toxic regimen is used. The duration of antimicrobial therapy should be at least 60 days. Once clinical improvement occurs, it may be possible to complete the course of treatment with one or two agents given orally. Corticosteroid therapy has been suggested as adjunct therapy for inhalational anthrax associated with extensive edema, respiratory compromise, and meningitis.[19,43,45]

Prevention

Ciprofloxacin and doxycycline are recommended first-line agents for prophylaxis in persons exposed to inhalational anthrax. In vivo data suggest that other fluoroquinolone antibiotics would have efficacy equivalent to that of ciprofloxacin.[45] High-dose amoxicillin is an option when ciprofloxacin or doxycycline is contraindicated [*see Table 6*]. Postexposure prophylaxis should continue for at least 60 days.[54] Given the uncertainty about the length of time viable spores can persist in the lungs, patients should be instructed to seek prompt medical evaluation if symptoms compatible with anthrax develop after discontinuance of postexposure prophylaxis. Because of uncertainty about the length of time that anthrax spores can remain viable in the lungs, the United States Department of Health and Human Services made two additional options available for preventive treatment for persons exposed to inhalational anthrax in the 2001 outbreak. These options were to follow a 60-day course of antibiotic treatment with either (1) an additional 40 days of antibiotic treatment or (2) an additional 40 days of antibiotic treatment plus three doses of anthrax vaccine over a 4-week period.[55]

Anthrax vaccine The only licensed human anthrax vaccine available in the United States is anthrax vaccine adsorbed (AVA). This is an inactivated, cell-free filtrate of a nonencapsulated attenuated strain of *B. anthracis* (BioPort Corporation, Lansing, Michigan).[51] Primary vaccination consists of three subcutaneous injections at 0, 2, and 4 weeks and three booster vaccinations at 6, 12, and 18 months. To maintain immunity, the manufacturer recommends an annual booster injection. The basis for this recommended schedule of vaccination is not well defined.

Vaccination of adults with the licensed vaccine induced an immune response, as measured by indirect hemagglutination, in 83% of vaccinees 2 weeks after the first dose and in 91% of vaccinees who received two or more doses. Approximately 95% of vaccinees undergo seroconversion after

Table 6 Postexposure Prophylaxis for Anthrax in the Setting of a Bioterrorist Attack

Patients	*Medication*	*Comments*
Adults, including immunocompromised persons	Ciprofloxacin, 500 mg p.o., q. 12 hr *or* Doxycycline, 100 mg p.o., q. 12 hr *or, if strain proved susceptible,* Amoxicillin, 500 mg p.o., q. 8 hr	Give prophylaxis for at least 60 days
Pregnant women	Ciprofloxacin, 500 mg p.o., q. 12 hr *or, if strain proved susceptible,* Amoxicillin, 500 mg p.o., q. 8 hr	Give prophylaxis for at least 60 days
Children, including those who are immunocompromised	Ciprofloxacin, 10–15 mg/kg p.o., b.i.d., not to exceed 1g/day *or, if strain proved susceptible,* Amoxicillin If ≥ 20 kg: 500 mg p.o., q. 8 hr If < 20 kg: 80 mg/kg/day p.o., in divided doses q. 8 hr (maximum, 500 mg/dose)	Give prophylaxis for at least 60 days

Note: Prophylaxis recommendations may change over time and according to antimicrobial susceptibility test results during a biologic attack and to availability of selected antimicrobial agents. Before initiating prophylaxis, clinicians should consult with an infectious disease specialist and public health authorities and should check for revisions and updates at http://www.bt.cdc.gov/HealthProfessionals/index.asp. This information is adapted from CDC and Working Group on Civilian Biodefense recommendations and may not represent FDA-approved uses.

three doses, with a fourfold rise in titers of IgG against protective antigen (the principal antigen responsible for inducing immunity). However, the precise correlation between antibody titer (or concentration) and protection against infection is not defined. The vaccine has shown efficacy in experiments involving animal models of inhalational anthrax in preexposure settings and, in combination with antibiotics, in postexposure settings.[45,52]

Anthrax vaccine is considered acceptably safe by the Advisory Committee on Immunization Practices and the Institute of Medicine.[51,56] Supplies of anthrax vaccine are limited and are held by the United States Department of Defense. A combination of antibiotics and anthrax vaccine, if available, is recommended for exposed persons after a biologic attack.[45,57] At this time, preexposure use of anthrax vaccine is not recommended.

CUTANEOUS ANTHRAX

After an incubation period of approximately 7 days (range, 1 to 12 days), the primary lesion of cutaneous anthrax appears as a nondescript, painless, pruritic papule, usually on an exposed area such as the face, head, neck, or upper extremity. The papule enlarges and develops a central vesicle or bullae with surrounding brawny, nonpitting edema. The central vesicle enlarges and ulcerates over 1 to 2 days, becoming hemorrhagic, depressed, and necrotic and leading to a central black eschar [*see Figure 6*]. Satellite vesicles may be present. The eschar dries and falls off over the next 1 to 2 weeks. The findings of a painless lesion and edema out of proportion to the size of the lesion and the fact that pustules are rarely present in cutaneous anthrax are clinically useful. Tender regional lymphadenopathy, fever, chills, and fatigue may occur. Systemic disease has been reported to have a mortality of 20% if untreated. Cutaneous anthrax of the face or neck may lead to respiratory compromise from massive edema.[43,45,47,58]

The differential diagnosis of cutaneous anthrax includes other causes of eschar and ulceration and the ulceroglandular syndrome.[57] Guidelines for the diagnosis of cutaneous anthrax have been published by the American Academy of Dermatology (http://www.aad.org/BioInfo/anthrax.html).

For patients with the typical appearance and progression of cutaneous anthrax, a Gram stain

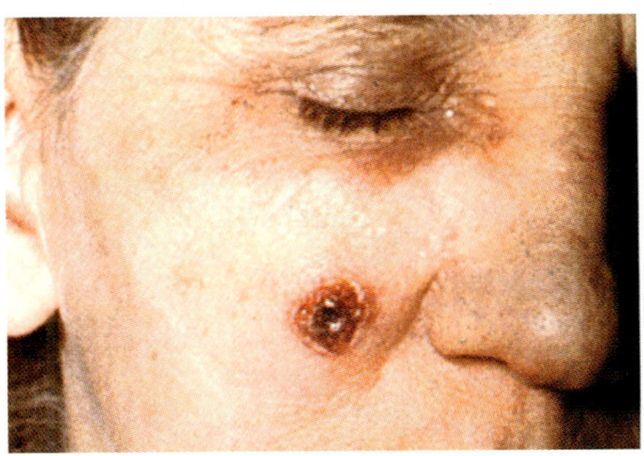

Figure 6 **Cutaneous anthrax lesion, 11 days old.**

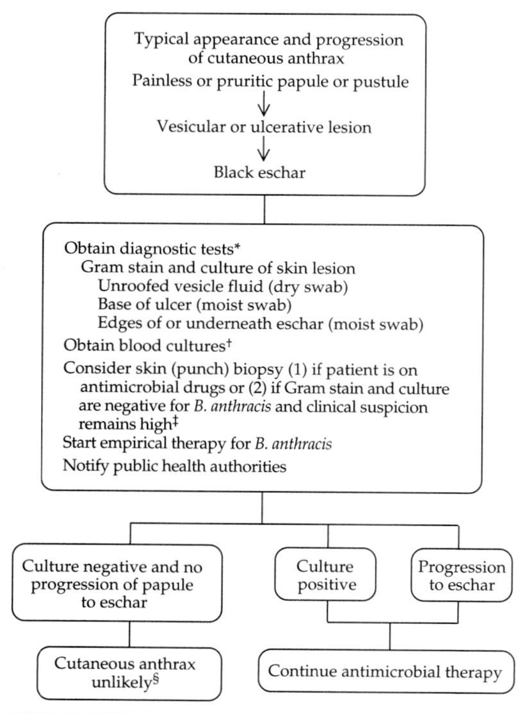

* Serologic testing available at CDC may be an additional diagnostic technique for confirmation of cases of cutaneous anthrax.

† If blood cultures are positive for *B. anthracis*, treat with antimicrobials as for inhalational anthrax.

‡ Punch biopsy should be submitted in formalin to CDC. Polymerase chain reaction can also be done on formalin-fixed specimen. Gram stain and culture are frequently negative for *B. anthracis* after initiation of antimicrobials.

§ Continue antimicrobial prophylaxis for inhalational anthrax for 60 days if aerosol exposure to *B. anthracis* is known or suspected.

Figure 7 **Evaluation of patients with possible cutaneous anthrax.**

and culture of the skin lesion should be obtained using a dry swab for unroofed vesicle fluid and a moist swab for the base of the ulcer and edges underneath the eschar. Blood cultures are also recommended. If the patient is taking antimicrobial drugs or if the Gram stain and culture are negative for *B. anthracis* or clinical suspicion remains high, two punch biopsies for culture (with the specimen placed in saline) and immunohistochemical staining should be performed; PCR (with the specimen placed in formalin) should be performed, or both should be considered [*see Figure 7*]. Immunohistochemical staining and PCR testing at the CDC should be arranged through local public health authorities.[19,45]

Management

Antibiotic treatment is curative in cutaneous anthrax and can be initiated pending confirmation of anthrax infection. Ciprofloxacin and doxycycline are first-line agents for the empirical treatment of cutaneous anthrax and may be administered orally. Intravenous therapy with multiple drugs, as for inhalational anthrax (see above), is recommended for patients with signs of systemic involvement, extensive edema, or lesions of the face and neck.[53]

GASTROINTESTINAL AND OROPHARYNGEAL ANTHRAX

Symptoms appear 2 to 5 days after ingestion of contaminated food and include nausea, vomiting, fever, malaise, and abdominal pain. Severe bloody diarrhea with rebound abdominal tenderness develops. Ulcerative lesions occur primarily in the terminal ileum and cecum. Gastric ulcers with hematemesis, hemorrhagic mesenteric lymphadenitis, and marked ascites may occur. Mediastinal widening has also been reported with gastrointestinal anthrax. Morbidity results from blood loss, fluid and electrolyte imbalances, and shock. The case-fatality rate is reportedly greater than 50%; death results from toxemia or intestinal perforation.[29,44,45]

Oropharyngeal anthrax is characterized by sore throat, fever, dysphagia, and marked edema and lymphadenitis. Ulcerative lesions may have an associated pseudomembrane. Specimens for diagnosis of gastrointestinal anthrax may include ascitic fluid for Gram stain and culture, blood cultures, and tissue samples from affected mucosal sites.

Treatment for gastrointestinal anthrax and oropharyngeal anthrax is the same as that for inhalational anthrax (see above).

INFECTION CONTROL

Person-to-person transmission of anthrax is not known to occur. Patients may be hospitalized in a standard hospital room with standard barrier isolation precautions. No treatment is necessary for contacts of cases.

The microbiology laboratory should be notified upon suspicion of anthrax to ensure that appropriate precautions are taken under BSL-2 conditions when specimens are processed for culture.[59] Sporicidal solutions approved for use in hospitals and commercially available bleach or a 0.5% hypochlorite solution (1:10 dilution of household bleach) are effective for decontamination of contaminated areas. Precautions should be taken during autopsies, and cremation of human remains should be considered to prevent further transmission of disease.[20]

Plague

Plague is caused by the gram-negative coccobacillus *Yersinia pestis*, of the family Enterobacteriaceae. Wild rodents are the animal reservoir for the disease. Under natural conditions, plague is transmitted to humans by the bite of an infectious flea and, less frequently, by direct contact with infectious body fluids or tissues of an infected animal or by inhaling infectious droplets.[60] Plague has a long history of use and development as a biologic weapon, including the catapulting of plague victims' corpses over the walls of a besieged city in the 14th century. The most likely presentation after a biologic attack is primary pneumonic plague.[29] Additional information on plague, including the nonpneumonic forms (bubonic and septicemic plague), microbiology, and pathogenesis, is available elsewhere [see 22 Infections Due to *Brucella, Francisella, Yersinia pestis*, and *Bartonella*].

CLINICAL PRESENTATION

Plague is a severe febrile illness. Pneumonic plague, the most fatal form of the infection, can develop from inhalation of plague bacilli (primary pneumonic plague) or from hematogenous spread secondary to septicemic plague. Approximately 12% of cases of bubonic and primary septicemic plague develop into secondary pneumonic plague. Conversely, septicemic plague can be secondary to primary pneumonic plague.

The incubation period for pneumonic plague is typically 2 to 4 days (range, 1 to 6 days). Presenting symptoms typically include the acute onset of malaise, high fever, chills, headache, chest discomfort, dyspnea, and cough concomitant with or followed rapidly by clinical sepsis. Hemoptysis is a classic sign that should suggest plague in the appropriate clinical context, but sputum may be watery or purulent. Gastrointestinal symptoms may be prominent with pneumonic plague; these include nausea, vomiting, diarrhea, and abdominal pain. A cervical bubo is infrequently present.

The disease is rapidly progressive, with increasing dyspnea, stridor, and cyanosis. Rapidly progressive respiratory failure and sepsis within 2 to 4 days of onset of illness is typical of pneumonic plague. Abnormalities on chest x-ray are variable but frequently show bilateral patchy infiltrates or consolidation. The mortality for pneumonic plague is reported to be 57% and is extremely high when initiation of treatment is delayed beyond 24 hours after symptom onset.[61] Complications of septicemic plague include disseminated intravascular coagulation (DIC), purpuric skin lesions and gangrene of extremities (so-called black death), acute respiratory distress syndrome (ARDS), meningitis, and multiorgan failure with shock.[29,62–64]

DIAGNOSIS

During a confirmed outbreak of pneumonic plague after a biologic attack, a presumptive diagnosis can be made on the basis of symptoms, especially if there is a high index of suspicion. However, other causes of severe pneumonia or rapidly progressive respiratory infection with or without sepsis should be considered. Suspected cases of plague should be immediately reported to the local public health department and the hospital epidemiologist.

There are no widely available, rapid confirmatory tests for *Y. pestis*. Specimens for bacteriologic and serologic testing should be collected before initiating therapy. Sputum, blood, and lymph node aspirate should be submitted for Gram stain and culture. Microscopic examination of clinical specimens or buffy coat may show a gram-negative coccobacillus; Wright, Giemsa, or Wayson stains may show bipolar (safety pin) staining. Sera for acute and convalescent antibody detection should be obtained, but findings are primarily of epidemiologic value. Additional diagnostic testing, including antigen detection, IgM immunoassay, immunostaining, PCR testing, and antimicrobial susceptibility testing, is available through the CDC and designated public health laboratories (http://www.statepublichealth.org). Specimen submission should be arranged through local public health authorities. The laboratory should be notified whenever plague is suspected, to help prevent exposures to staff and to facilitate appropriate testing.[29,61,64]

Laboratory findings are consistent with the systemic inflammatory response syndrome. The leukocyte count is elevated and the differential shows a neutrophil predominance, including immature forms. Platelets may be normal or low. Coagulation abnormalities include increased fibrin degradation products, hypofibrinogenemia, and prolongation of the prothrombin time (PT) and partial thromboplastin time (PTT). Elevated liver function tests and abnormal renal function tests are seen with systemic disease.

TREATMENT

When plague is suspected, antibiotic treatment should begin before laboratory confirmation of the diagnosis [*see Table 7*]. Whenever possible, specimens should be collected for bacteriologic and serologic testing before the start of therapy. Antibiotic resistance is rare with naturally occurring *Y. pestis* but may be present in strains used as biologic weap-

Table 7 Antimicrobial Treatment of Pneumonic Plague

Patients	*Drug*	*Comments*
Adults	Streptomycin, 1 g I.M., b.i.d. *or* Gentamicin, 5 mg/kg I.M. or I.V., q.d., or 2 mg/kg loading dose followed by 1.7 mg/kg I.M. or I.V., t.i.d. *Alternative choices:* Doxycycline, 100 mg I.V., b.i.d., or 200 mg I.V., q.d. Ciprofloxacin, 400 mg I.V., b.i.d. Chloramphenicol, 25 mg/kg I.V., q.i.d.	Treat for 10 days; during a community outbreak of pneumonic plague, all persons developing a temperature ≥ 101.3° F (38.5° C) or greater or a new cough should begin parenteral antibiotic treatment; oral treatment may be given when resources for parenteral treatment are limited; pregnant women should not receive streptomycin or chloramphenicol; tetracycline may be substituted for doxycycline
Children	Streptomycin, 15 mg/kg I.M., b.i.d. (maximum, 2 g/day) *or* Gentamicin, 2.5. mg/kg I.M. or I.V., t.i.d. *Alternative choices:* Doxycycline: if ≥ 45 kg, adult dosage; if < 45 kg, 2.2 mg/kg b.i.d. (maximum, 200 mg/day) Ciprofloxacin, 15 mg/kg I.V., b.i.d. Chloramphenicol, 25 mg/kg I.V., q.i.d.; maintain serum concentration between 5 and 20 μg/ml	Use chloramphenicol in plague meningitis

Note: Treatment recommendations may change over time and according to antimicrobial susceptibility test results during a biologic attack and to availability of selected antimicrobial agents. Before initiating treatment, clinicians should consult with an infectious disease specialist and public health authorities and should check for revisions and updates at http://www.bt.cdc.gov/HealthProfessionals/index.asp. This information is adapted from CDC and Working Group on Civilian Biodefense recommendations and may not represent FDA-approved uses.

ons. Treatment should be continued for 10 days or for 3 days after defervescence and improvement in symptoms. The route of administration can be changed from intravenous to oral after the patient is clinically stable. The choice of antibiotic may be modified after microbial sensitivity testing is completed. The CDC bioterrorism Web site or local public health authorities should be consulted for updated treatment recommendations.[29,61,64]

Postexposure Prophylaxis for Pneumonic Plague

All persons potentially exposed to aerosolized *Y. pestis* and all persons in close contact with pneumonic plague patients (close contact is defined as exposure within 2 m [6.5 ft]) should be treated for 7 days after the last exposure [*see Table 8*]. Persons receiving prophylactic antibiotic treatment should seek medical evaluation immediately if fever or illness with cough develops.

There is no currently available vaccine for pneumonic plague. The previously available licensed plague vaccine in the United States was discontinued in 1999. That vaccine was demonstrated to reduce the severity of illness with bubonic plague but not pneumonic plague.[62]

Table 8 Postexposure Prophylaxis of Pneumonic Plague

Patients	*Drug*	*Comments*
Adults, including pregnant women	Doxycycline, 100 mg p.o., b.i.d. Ciprofloxacin, 500 mg p.o., b.i.d. *Alternative:* Chloramphenicol, 25 mg/kg p.o., q.i.d.	Asymptomatic household contacts, hospital contacts, or other close contacts should receive postexposure prophylaxis for 7 days; contacts who develop fever or cough while receiving prophylaxis should begin antibiotic treatment for plague.
Children	Doxycycline: if ≥ 45 kg, adult dosage; if < 45 kg, 2.2 mg/kg p.o., b.i.d. (maximum, 200 mg/day) Ciprofloxacin, 20 mg/kg p.o., b.i.d. *Alternative:* Chloramphenicol, 25 mg/kg p.o., q.i.d.	Asymptomatic household contacts, hospital contacts, or other close contacts should receive postexposure prophylaxis for 7 days; contacts who develop fever or cough while receiving prophylaxis should begin antibiotic treatment for plague.

Note: Prophylaxis recommendations may change over time and according to antimicrobial susceptibility test results during a biologic attack and to availability of selected antimicrobial agents. Before initiating prophylaxis, clinicians should consult with an infectious disease specialist and public health authorities and should check for revisions and updates at http://www.bt.cdc.gov/HealthProfessionals/index.asp. This information is adapted from CDC and Working Group on Civilian Biodefense recommendations and may not represent FDA-approved uses.

Communicability and Infection Control Considerations

Pneumonic plague is transmitted person to person through respiratory droplets. Aerosol transmission has not been demonstrated. For patients with pneumonic plague, respiratory droplet precautions as well as standard precautions are recommended, including the use of gowns, gloves, eye protection, and surgical masks for the first 48 hours of antimicrobial therapy and until clinical improvement occurs. Hospitalized patients should remain in isolation for the first 48 hours of antimicrobial therapy and until clinical improvement occurs. Hospitalized patients should wear a mask during transport.

Y. pestis is rapidly destroyed by sunlight and drying. Environmental surfaces can be decontaminated with a standard disinfectant. Persons exposed to aerosolized plague bacilli during a biologic attack should shower with warm water and soap. Clothing of persons exposed to an aerosol of *Y. pestis* and linens of plague patients should be washed in hot water.[20,62,63]

Botulism

Botulism is a paralytic illness caused by a potent neurotoxin produced by *Clostridium botulinum,* an anaerobic, spore-forming bacterium. Natural forms of the disease are foodborne botulism, wound botulism, and infant botulism. Foodborne botulism results from ingestion of improperly processed foodstuffs containing preformed toxin produced by *C. botulinum.* Wound botulism results from production of botulinum toxin by *C. botulinum* organisms that contaminate wounds. Infant botulism results from the colonization of the intestinal tract of infants after ingestion of spores. Botulinum toxin has been developed as a biologic weapon. An aerosol attack is considered the most likely use of botulinum toxin for bioterrorism, although intentional contamination of food supplies is possible.[29,65] Additional information about the pathogenesis and epidemiology of noninhalational forms of botulism is available elsewhere [see 17 Anaerobic Infections].

Botulinum toxin is the most potent lethal toxin known. The estimated toxic dose of type A botulinum toxin is 0.001 µg/kg of body weight. There are seven distinct antigenic types of botulinum neurotoxins—types A through G—produced by different strains of *C. botulinum.* Human botulism is caused primarily by toxin types A, B, and E. Botulinum toxin acts to block neurotransmission by binding irreversibly to the presynaptic nerve terminal at the neuromuscular junction and preventing the release of acetylcholine, resulting in bulbar palsies and skeletal muscle weakness. The toxin is colorless, odorless, and presumably tasteless.[29,66,67]

CLINICAL PRESENTATION

The incubation period for foodborne botulism is 2 hours to 8 days; the typical incubation period is 12 to 72 hours. The incubation period for inhalational botulism is not established. Aerosol exposures of monkeys and accidental aerosol exposure of humans have resulted in clinical illness developing 12 to 80 hours after exposure. Type A toxin is associated with more severe disease and a higher fatality rate than type B or E. The neurologic features of all forms of botulism are similar.[29,66,67] Although initial symptoms in foodborne botulism may include nausea, vomiting, abdominal cramps, and diarrhea, these symptoms are thought to result from other bacterial metabolites in contaminated food and may not occur in inhalational botulism.

The so-called classic triad of botulism summarizes the clinical presentation: an afebrile patient, symmetrical descending flaccid paralysis with prominent bulbar palsies, and a clear sensorium.[66–68] Symptoms of cranial nerve abnormalities nearly always begin in the bulbar musculature; patients typically present with difficulty seeing, speaking, or swallowing. Clinical hallmarks include ptosis, blurred vision, and the so-called four Ds: diplopia, dysarthria, dysphonia, and dysphagia. Cranial nerve abnormalities and bulbar weakness are followed by symmetrical descending weakness and paralysis with progression from the head to the arms, thorax, and legs. The extent of paralysis and rapidity of onset of symptoms are proportional to the dose of toxin absorbed into the circulation. Recovery depends on the regeneration of new motor axon twigs to reinnervate paralyzed muscle fibers; recovery may take weeks to months.

Anticholinergic symptoms are common, including dry mouth, ileus, constipation, nausea and vomiting, urinary retention, and mydriasis. Other symptoms include dizziness and sore throat. Sensory findings are not present, with the exception of circumoral and peripheral paresthesias secondary to hyperventilation resulting from anxiety. Botulinum toxin does not cross the blood-brain barrier. Cranial nerve dysfunction and facial nerve weakness may make communication difficult; these symptoms may be mistaken for lethargy and signs of central nervous system involvement.

DIAGNOSIS

Initiation of treatment with botulinum antitoxin should be based on the clinical diagnosis and should not await laboratory confirmation. A clinician who suspects botulism should immediately contact the local or state health department to facilitate procurement of antitoxin for treatment; arrangements should be made for confirmatory diagnostic testing and initiation of an epidemiologic investigation to identify the source of infection. In cases of potential foodborne botulism, any leftover foodstuffs or containers should be held for testing by the public health laboratory.

Demonstration of botulinum toxin in serum samples by mouse bioassay is diagnostic. Samples of serum (in adults, > 30 ml blood in a tiger-top or red-top tube) obtained before administration of botulinum antitoxin should be submitted for testing. For potential foodborne botulism, samples of stool, gastric aspirate, emesis, and suspect foods should also be submitted.[67] The likelihood of finding toxin in the sera of affected patients decreases with time; it is detectable in only 13% to 28% of patients more than 2 days after ingestion.[69]

The possibility of a bioterrorist attack should be considered in any outbreak of botulism. A bioterrorist attack should especially be considered when a cluster of cases occurs; when an outbreak has a common geographic location but there is no common dietary exposure (suggestive of possible aerosol exposure); when there is an outbreak of an unusual botulinum toxin type; or when multiple simultaneous outbreaks occur. A careful dietary and travel history must be taken to help identify the source. Patients should be asked if they know of others with similar symptoms.

The differential diagnosis of botulism includes stroke and other neuromuscular disorders.[66,67] A CT scan of the head may be used to exclude cerebrovascular accident, although it is relatively insensitive in early ischemic stroke. Patients with myasthenia gravis will often have characteristic electromyographic findings and serum antibody tests. A test dose of edrophonium (Tensilon) may briefly reverse paralysis in patients with myasthenia gravis but also, reportedly, in some cases of botulism. Guillain-Barré syndrome typically results in ascending paralysis and sensory abnormalities. Cerebrospinal fluid protein is normal in patients with botulism and is normal or elevated in patients with Guillain-Barré syndrome. The rare Miller-Fisher variant of Guillain-Barré syndrome is characterized by descending paralysis and may be confused with botulism. Other conditions that mimic botulism include tick paralysis; poliomyelitis; Eaton-Lambert syndrome; paralytic shellfish poisoning; pufferfish ingestion; and anticholinesterase intoxication with organophosphates, atropine, carbon monoxide, or aminoglycosides.

The electromyogram (EMG) can help distinguish different causes of paralysis. The EMG in botulism demonstrates normal nerve conduction velocity, normal sensory nerve function, and small amplitude motor potentials with facilitation to repetitive stimulation at 50 Hz.[70]

TREATMENT

The mainstay of treatment for botulism is supportive care, including intensive care, mechanical ventilation, and parenteral nutrition. Morbidity and mortality are usually from pulmonary aspiration secondary to loss of the gag reflex and dysphagia leading to inability to control secretions, respiratory failure secondary to inadequate tidal volume from diaphragmatic and accessory respiratory muscle paralysis, and airway obstruction from pharyngeal and upper airway muscle paralysis. Careful and frequent monitoring of the gag and cough reflexes, swallowing, oxygen saturation, vital capacity, and inspiratory force are critical. Airway intubation is indicated for inability to control secretions and impending respiratory failure. Secondary infections are common and should be sought in patients who develop fever.

Trivalent (ABE) equine antitoxin is available from the CDC through state and local health departments and should be administered as soon as possible after clinical diagnosis. Antitoxin can prevent progression of disease caused by subsequent binding of toxin but does not reverse the effects of already bound toxin. For this reason, antitoxin is not useful if the patient is no longer showing progression of disease or is improving from maximum paralysis. The amount of neutralizing antibody present in the standard treatment dose of antitoxin far exceeds maximum serum toxin concentrations in foodborne botulism patients, and repeat doses are usually not required. In a biologic attack, however, patients may be exposed to unusually high concentrations of toxin, so serum toxin levels should be assessed after initiation of treatment in such cases to determine the need for repeat doses. Botulism caused by toxin types other than A, B, or E would not respond to the trivalent antitoxin. Limited quantities of an investigational heptavalent

(A-G) antitoxin are held by the United States Army. However, because of the time delay involved in typing the toxin, the utility of this product in a biologic attack is probably minimal.[66,68]

Hypersensitivity reactions, including anaphylaxis, have occurred after administration of botulism antitoxin. For that reason, all patients should undergo a skin test before receiving the antitoxin, and resuscitation equipment should be immediately available. Patients showing a positive hypersensitivity reaction on the skin test can be desensitized over several hours.[71,72]

Before administering antitoxin, physicians should carefully review the package insert for dosage and adverse effects. Standard regimens can be used in children, pregnant women, and immunocompromised persons with botulism. Botulism immune globulin intravenous is an investigational human-derived neutralizing antibody that is available only for treatment of infant botulism from the California Department of Health Services, Berkeley. The CDC bioterrorism Web site or local public health authorities should be consulted for updated treatment recommendations.[29,66,67]

Transmissibility and Infection Control

Botulism is an intoxication, not an infection, and thus is not transmitted from person to person. Botulinum toxin does not penetrate intact skin. Standard infection-control precautions are adequate unless meningitis is suspected, in which case droplet precautions are indicated. Clothes of persons exposed to an aerosol release of botulinum toxin should be removed and washed. Exposed persons should shower with soap and hot water. Exposed environmental surfaces can be decontaminated with 0.1% hypochlorite bleach solution.[67]

Tularemia

Tularemia is a zoonotic infection caused by *Francisella tularensis*, a small, nonmotile, gram-negative, pleomorphic coccobacillus. The disease is typically acquired through contact with blood or tissue fluids of infected animals or through the bite of an infected deerfly, tick, or mosquito.[73] Inhalation of organisms aerosolized from the environment and the drinking of contaminated water can also result in human infection.[74] *F. tularensis* was developed for use as a biologic weapon by the United States (before its offensive biologic weapons program was terminated) and other countries.[29] The epidemiology, pathogenesis, and clinical manifestations of the naturally occurring forms of tularemia are discussed in more detail elsewhere [see 22 Infections Due to *Brucella, Francisella, Yersinia pestis*, and *Bartonella*].

CLINICAL PRESENTATION

Tularemia can take several forms in humans, depending on the route of infection. Ulceroglandular, oculoglandular, glandular, typhoidal, and pharyngeal tularemia are discussed elsewhere [see 22 Infections Due to *Brucella, Francisella, Yersinia pestis*, and *Bartonella*]. Inhalational tularemia is a term used to describe infection resulting from an aerosol release of *F. tularensis*.[75] Most patients with inhalational tularemia develop pleuropulmonary tularemia (tularemia pneumonia), but many patients may present with an undifferentiated febrile illness. The infectious dose is as low as one to 50 organisms, and the incubation period is typically 3 to 5 days (range, 1 to 14 days).[29]

The clinical course of inhalational tularemia is less rapidly progressive than that of pulmonary anthrax or plague. Illness onset is acute, with some combination of fever, chills, sweats, myalgias, headache, coryza, and sore throat. Nausea, vomiting, diarrhea, and abdominal pain are common. Anorexia and weight loss may occur as the illness continues. Cough may be dry or mildly productive. Hemoptysis is uncommon. Pleuritic chest pain, substernal chest discomfort, and dyspnea may be present. Chest x-rays may be normal or minimally abnormal or show a variety of abnormalities, including peribronchial patchy infiltrates, effusions, and hilar adenopathy.[76]

F. tularensis infection may be mild and nonspecific or rapidly progressive. Any form of tularemia may result in hematogenous spread with secondary pleuropneumonia, sepsis, and, rarely, meningitis. If left untreated, tularemia can progress to respiratory failure; liver, kidney, and splenic involvement; meningitis; sepsis; shock; and death. There is usually complete recovery with early diagnosis and treatment. Mortality is less than 2% if the patient is treated; it can be as high as 60% for untreated severe disease and pneumonia.[75,77,78]

DIAGNOSIS

A clustering of sudden, severe pneumonias in previously healthy patients should raise the possibility of an intentional aerosolized release of tularemia. Clusters of patients with tularemia and cases in which there is no natural explanation for the disease should be reported immediately to the local or state health department (http://www.statepublichealth.org). There are no rapid confirmatory tests for *F. tularensis*. Gram stain of sputum is not diagnostic but may identify other potential etiologies.[78,79] In the context of a known or suspected outbreak, a presumptive diagnosis can be made on the basis of symptoms. A chest x-ray should be obtained for patients with suspected pleuropulmonary tularemia. The x-ray may show infiltrates, effusion, hilar adenopathy, or subtle abnormalities, or it may be normal. Recent experience with inhalational anthrax suggests that chest CT scans of patients with tularemia may show pulmonary abnormalities, including infiltrates, effusions, and adenopathy, before they are evident on x-ray.[48]

Specimens of respiratory secretions and blood for bacteriologic and serologic testing should be collected before initiating therapy. Pharyngeal washings, sputum specimens, fasting gastric aspirates, and blood can be cultured for *F. tularensis*. Growth may be slow, so cultures should be held for 10 days. Cysteine-enriched culture media should be used to improve yield. Direct examination (by direct fluorescent antibody staining or immunohistochemical testing, antigen detection, microagglutination antibody testing, PCR, and other research tests) is available through designated public health laboratories. Acute and convalescent serologies are valuable for epidemiologic purposes.[75,79]

TREATMENT AND POSTEXPOSURE PROPHYLAXIS

When the index of suspicion is high, antibiotic treatment should be started before diagnosis is confirmed. Streptomycin or gentamicin is the preferred agent. All persons potentially exposed to aerosolized *F. tularensis* should be treated with doxycycline or ciprofloxacin. Close contacts of patients with tularemia pneumonia do not need prophylactic antibiotics. No vaccine for tularemia is currently available. The CDC bioterrorism Web site, local public health authorities, or both should be consulted for updated treatment recommendations.[29,75,80]

Transmissibility and Infection Control

Tularemia is not transmitted from person to person, and isolation of patients with tularemia is not necessary. Standard precautions are recommended for all patients with tularemia. Microbiology staff must be alerted when tularemia is suspected, so they can take precautions to prevent laboratory-acquired infection from culture plates and other infectious materials. Contaminated environmental surfaces can be disinfected with a 10% bleach solution followed by cleansing with 70% alcohol.[75]

Hemorrhagic Fever Viruses

Hemorrhagic fever viruses (HFVs) are RNA viruses classified in several taxonomic families. HFVs cause a variety of disease syndromes with similar clinical characteristics, referred to as acute hemorrhagic fever syndromes [see 34 Viral Zoonoses]. The pathophysiologic hallmarks of HFV infection are microvascular damage and increased vascular permeability. HFVs that are of concern as potential biologic weapons include Arenaviridae (Lassa, Junin, Machupo, Guanarito, and Sabia viruses, which are the causative agents of Lassa fever and Argentine, Bolivian, Venezuelan, and Brazilian hemorrhagic fevers, respectively); Filoviridae (Ebola and Marburg viruses); Flaviviridae (yellow fever, Omsk hemorrhagic fever, and Kyasanur Forest disease viruses); and Bunyaviridae (Rift Valley fever [RVF]). Under natural conditions, humans are infected through the bite of an infected arthropod or through contact with infected animal reservoirs. Hemorrhagic fever viruses are highly infectious by aerosol; are associated with high morbidity and, in some cases, high mortality; and are thought to pose a serious risk as biologic weapons.[29] All suspected cases of HFV infection should be reported immediately to the local or state health department and the hospital epidemiologist.

PATHOPHYSIOLOGY

The exact pathogenesis for HFVs varies according to the etiologic agent. The major target organ is the vascular endothelium. Immunologic and inflammatory mediators are thought to play an important role in the pathogenesis of HFVs. All HFVs can produce thrombocytopenia, and some also cause platelet dysfunction. Infection with Ebola and Marburg viruses, Rift Valley fever virus, and yellow fever virus causes destruction of infected cells. DIC is characteristic of infection with Filoviridae. Ebola and Marburg viruses may cause a hemorrhagic diathesis and tissue necrosis through direct damage to vascular endothelial cells and platelets with impairment of the microcirculation, as well as cytopathic effects on parenchymal cells, with release of immunologic and inflammatory mediators. Arenaviridae, on the other hand, appear to mediate hemorrhage via the stimulation of inflammatory mediators by macrophages, thrombocytopenia, and the inhibition of platelet aggregation. DIC is not a major pathophysiologic mechanism in arenavirus infections.[81,82]

CLINICAL PRESENTATION

The incubation period of HFVs ranges from 2 to 21 days. The clinical presentations of these diseases are nonspecific and variable, making diagnosis difficult. It is noteworthy that not all patients will develop hemorrhagic manifestations. Even a significant proportion of patients with Ebola virus infections may not demonstrate clinical signs of hemorrhage.[83]

Initial symptoms of the acute HFV syndrome may include fever, headache, myalgia, rash, nausea, vomiting, diarrhea, abdominal pain, arthralgias, myalgias, and malaise. Illness caused by Ebola, Marburg, Rift Valley fever virus, yellow fever virus, Omsk hemorrhagic fever virus, and Kyasanur Forest disease virus are characterized by an abrupt onset, whereas Lassa fever and the diseases caused by the Machupo, Junin, Guarinito, and Sabia viruses have a more insidious onset. Initial signs may include fever, tachypnea, relative bradycardia, hypotension (which may progress to circulatory shock), conjunctival injection, pharyngitis, and lymphadenopathy. Encephalitis may occur, with delirium, seizures, cerebellar signs, and coma. Most HFVs cause cutaneous flushing or a macular skin rash, although the rash may be difficult to appreciate in dark-skinned persons and varies according to the causative virus. Hemorrhagic symptoms, when they occur, develop later in the course of illness and include petechiae, purpura, bleeding into mucous membranes and conjunctiva, hematuria, hematemesis, and melena. Hepatic involvement is common, and renal involvement is proportional to cardiovascular compromise.[29,81,83,84]

Laboratory abnormalities include leukopenia (except in some cases of Lassa fever), anemia or hemoconcentration, and elevated liver enzymes; DIC with associated coagulation abnormalities and thrombocytopenia are common. Mortality ranges from less than 1% for Rift Valley fever to 70% to 90% for Ebola and Marburg virus infections.[29,81,83–85]

DIAGNOSIS

The nonspecific and variable clinical presentation of the HFVs presents a considerable diagnostic challenge. Clinical diagnostic criteria based on WHO surveillance standards for acute hemorrhagic fever syndrome include temperature greater than 101° F (38.3° C) of less than 3 weeks' duration; severe illness and no predisposing factors for hemorrhagic manifestations; and at least two of the following hemorrhagic symptoms: hemorrhagic or purple rash, epistaxis, hematemesis, hematuria, hemoptysis, blood in stools, or other hemorrhagic symptom with no established alternative diagnosis. Any suspected case of HFV should result in immediate notification of the hospital epidemiologist, local public health department, and clinical laboratory personnel.[82,86] Laboratory testing is currently available only at the CDC and the United States Army Medical Research Institute for Infectious Diseases. Laboratory techniques for the diagnosis of HFVs include antigen detection, IgM antibody detection, isolation in cell culture, visualization by electron microscopy, immunohistochemical techniques, and reverse transcriptase–polymerase chain reaction. Submission of clinical specimens, including processing and transport, should be arranged through consultation with local public health authorities. The CDC's Packaging Protocols for Biologic Agents/Diseases are available at (http://www.bt.cdc.gov/agent/vhf/index.asp).

TREATMENT

Therapy for HFVs is largely supportive. Treatment of other suspected causes of infection should be administered pending confirmation of HFV infection. Hypotension and shock may require early administration of vasopressors and hemodynamic monitoring with attention to fluid and electrolyte balance, circulatory volume, and blood pressure. HFV patients tend to respond poorly to fluid infusions and rapidly develop pulmonary edema.

Secondary infections may occur and should be diagnosed and treated. Intravenous lines, catheters, and other invasive procedures should be avoided unless they are clearly indicated. The management of bleeding is controversial. Recent recommendations include not treating mild bleeding and use of replacement therapy and heparin for severe bleeding with DIC.[29] Intramuscular injections and medications that interfere with platelet function or coagulation should be avoided.

No treatments of HFVs have been approved by the Food and Drug Administration. Ribavirin is a nucleoside analogue with activity against some Arenaviridae and Bunyaviridae (including the viruses that cause Lassa fever, Argentine hemorrhagic fever, and Crimean-Congo hemorrhagic fever) but not against Filoviridae or Flaviviridae. Ribavirin may be used under an IND protocol for the empirical treatment of HFV patients while awaiting identification of the etiologic agent. Current treatment protocols and dosing recommendations for ribavirin should be obtained through local public health authorities or the CDC's bioterrorism Web site.

Postexposure Prophylaxis

Postexposure prophylaxis is currently recommended only for persons potentially exposed to HFV and for known high-risk contacts or close contacts of HFV patients who develop fever or other clinical criteria of HFV infection with no alternative diagnosis, unless the etiologic agent is known to be a filovirus or a flavivirus.[81]

Infection Control Considerations

Ebola virus, Marburg virus, Lassa fever virus, and the New World arenaviruses are transmissible from person to person through direct contact with blood and body fluids. Airborne transmission of HFVs is unlikely but cannot be completely ruled out. The risk of person-to-person transmission is highest during the latter stages of illness, which are characterized by vomiting, diarrhea, shock, and, often, hemorrhage. The most important step in preventing transmission of HFVs is strict attention to implementation of appropriate barrier infection control measures, including double gloves, impermeable gowns, face shields, eye protection, and leg and shoe coverings.

Airborne precautions are recommended during care of patients with possible HFV infections. Airborne precautions include high-efficiency particulate respirators such as N-95 masks or powered air-purifying respirators (PAPRs) for all persons entering the patient's room. Patients should be placed in a negative-pressure isolation room with 6 to 12 air changes per hour.[82,87]

High-risk contacts of HFV patients include persons having contact with mucous membranes (e.g., through kissing or sexual intercourse) or with secretions, excretions, or blood (through percutaneous injury) of the infected person. Close contacts are persons who have other direct contact with the patient (e.g., shaking hands or hugging), provide medical care to the patient, or process laboratory specimens from a patient with HFV before initiation of infection-control precautions.

Persons potentially exposed to HFVs in a bioterrorist attack and their close and high-risk contacts should be placed under medical surveillance for 21 days from the day of exposure. Temperatures should be recorded twice daily, and any temperature of 101° F (38.3° C) or higher should be reported to the designated clinical or public health authority. Therapy with ribavirin should be initiated promptly unless an alternative diagnosis is established or the etiologic agent is known to be a filovirus or a flavivirus [*see* Treatment, *above*].[81]

HFVs are highly infectious in the laboratory setting through small-particle aerosols generated through procedures such as centrifugation. Laboratory personnel should be alerted when HFV infections are suspected, and appropriate personal-protection precautions and laboratory biosafety procedures should be implemented.

Acknowledgments

Figures 1, 3, 4, and 5 Centers for Disease Control and Prevention Public Health Image Library.
Figure 2 Centers for Disease Control and Prevention Public Health Image Library (Dr Duma).

References

1. Davis CJ: Nuclear blindness: an overview of the biological weapons programs of the former Soviet Union and Iraq. Emerg Infect Dis 5:509, 1999

2. Stern J: The prospect of domestic bioterrorism. Emerg Infect Dis 5: 517, 1999

3. Kortepeter MG, Parker GW: Potential biological weapons threats. Emerg Infect Dis 5:523, 1999

4. Alibek K: Biohazard. Random House, Inc. New York, 1999

5. Henderson DA: The looming threat of bioterrorism. Science 283:1279, 1999

6. Biological and chemical terrorism: strategic plan for preparedness and response. Recommendations of the CDC Strategic Planning Workgroup. MMWR Morb Mortal Wkly Rep 49:1, 2000

7. Gerberding JL, Hughes JM, Koplan JP: Bioterrorism preparedness and response: clinicians and public health agencies as essential partners. JAMA 287:898, 2002

8. Lane HC, Fauci AS: Bioterrorism on the home front: a new challenge for American medicine. JAMA 286:2595, 2001

9. Meningococcal disease and college students. Recommendations of the Advisory Committee on Immunization Practices (ACIP). MMWR Morb Mortal Wkly Rep 49:13, 2000

10. Bell BP, Goldoft M, Griffin PM, et al: A multistate outbreak of *Escherichia coli* 0157:H7-associated bloody diarrhea and hemolytic uremic syndrome from hamburgers: the Washington experience. JAMA 272:1349, 1994

11. Weber DJ, Rutala WA: Pertussis: a continuing hazard for healthcare facilities. Infect Control Hosp Epidemiol 22:736, 2001

12. Measles, mumps, and rubella: vaccine use and strategies for elimination of measles, rubella, and congenital rubella syndrome and control of mumps. Recommendations of the Advisory Committee on Immunization Practices (ACIP). MMWR Morb Mortal Wkly Rep 47:1, 1998

13. Prevention of varicella. Updated Recommendations of the Advisory Committee on Immunization Practices (ACIP). MMWR Morb Mortal Wkly Rep 48:1, 1999

14. Bolyard EA, Tablan OC, Williams WW, et al: Guideline for infection control in healthcare personnel, 1998. Hospital Infection Control Practices Advisory Committee. Infect Control Hosp Epidemiol 19:386, 1998

15. Suspected brucellosis case prompts investigation of possible bioterrorism-related activity—New Hampshire and Massachusetts, 1999. MMWR Morb Mortal Wkly Rep 49:509, 2000

16. Duchin JS, Koster FT, Peters CJ, et al: Hantavirus pulmonary syndrome: a clinical description of 17 patients with a newly recognized disease. The Hantavirus Study Group. N Engl J Med 330:949, 1994

17. Fine A, Layton M: Lessons from the West Nile viral encephalitis outbreak in New York City, 1999: implications for bioterrorism preparedness. Clin Infect Dis 32:277, 2001

18. Pandemic influenza: confronting a re-emergent threat. Proceedings of a meeting. Bethesda, Maryland, 11–13 December 1995. J Infect Dis 176:S1, 1997

19. Update: investigation of bioterrorism-related anthrax and interim guidelines for clinical evaluation of persons with possible anthrax. MMWR Morb Mortal Wkly Rep 50:941, 2001

20. Control of Communicable Diseases Manual 17th ed. Chin JE, Ed. American Public Health Association. Washington DC, 2000

21. Garner JS: Guideline for isolation precautions in hospitals. Infect Control Hosp Epidemiol 17:53, 1996

22. Immunization of health-care workers. Recommendations of the Advisory Committee on Immunization Practices and the Hospital Infection Control Practices Advisory Committee. MMWR Morb Mortal Wkly Rep 46:1, 1997

23. Rotz LD, Khan AS, Lillibridge SR, et al: Public health assessment of potential bioterrorism agents. Emerg Infect Dis 8:225, 2002

24. Torok TJ, Tauxe RV, Wise RP, et al: A large community outbreak of salmonellosis caused by intentional contamination of restaurant salad bars. JAMA 278:389, 1997

25. Kolavic SA, Kimura A, Simons SL, et al: An outbreak of *Shigella dysenteriae* type 2 among laboratory workers due to intentional food contamination. JAMA 278:396, 1997

26. Pavlin JA: Epidemiology of bioterrorism. Emerg Infect Dis 5:528, 1999

27. Recognition of illness associated with the intentional release of a biologic agent. MMWR Morb Mortal Wkly Rep 50:893, 2001

28. Vaccinia (smallpox) vaccine. Recommendations of the Advisory Committee on Immunization Practices (ACIP), 2001. MMWR Morb Mortal Wkly Rep 50:1, 2001

29. Franz DR, Jahrling PB, Friedlander AM, et al: Clinical recognition and management of patients exposed to biological warfare agents. JAMA 278:399, 1997

30. Draft Supplemental Recommendation of the ACIP. Use of Smallpox (Vaccinia) Vaccine, June 2002
http://www.cdc.gov/nip/smallpox/supp_recs.htm

31. Fenner F, Henderson DA, Arita I, et al: Smallpox and its eradication. World Health Organization, Geneva.
http://www.who.int/emc/diseases/smallpox/Smallpoxeradication.html. **32.** Smallpox as a biological weapon: medical and public health management. Working Group on Civilian Biodefense. JAMA 281:2127, 1999

33. Breman JG, Henderson DA: Diagnosis and management of smallpox. N Engl J Med 346:1300, 2002

34. Henderson DA: Smallpox: clinical and epidemiologic features. Emerging Infect Dis 5:537, 1999

35. CDC Interim smallpox response plan and guidelines.
http://www.bt.cdc.gov/agent/smallpox/response-plan/index.asp

36. Lane JM, Ruben FL, Neff JM, et al: Complications of smallpox vaccination, 1968: results of ten statewide surveys. J Infect Dis 122:303, 1970

37. Acha PN, Szyfres B: Zoonoses and Communicable Disease Common to Man and Animals 3rd ed. Vol I. Pan American Health Organization, Washington, DC, 2001

38. Swartz MN: Recognition and management of anthrax: an update. N Engl J Med 345:1621, 2001

39. Brachman PS: Bioterrorism: an update with a focus on anthrax. Am J Epidemiol 155:981, 2002

40. Update: investigation of bioterrorism-related anthrax and adverse events from antimicrobial prophylaxis. MMWR Morb Mortal Wkly Rep 50:973, 2001

41. Cieslak TJ, Eitzen HM Jr: Bioterrorism: agents of concern. J Public Health Manag Pract 6:19, 2000

42. Kournikakis B, Armour SJ, Boulet CA, et al: Risk assessment of anthrax threat letters. Technical Report 2001-048. Defense Research Establishment, Suffield, Canada, 2001

43. Dixon TC, Meselson M, Guillemin J, et al: Anthrax. N Engl J Med 341:815, 1999

44. Sirisanthana T, Brown AE: Anthrax of the gastrointestinal tract. Emerg Infect Dis 8:649, 2002

45. Inglesby TV, O'Toole T, Henderson DA, et al: Anthrax as a biological weapon, 2002: updated recommendations for management. JAMA 287:2236, 2002

46. Meselson M, Guillemin J, Hugh-Jones M, et al: The Sverdlovsk anthrax outbreak of 1979. Science 266:1202, 1994

47. LaForce FM: Anthrax. Clin Infect Dis 19:1009, 1994

48. Jernigan JA, Stephens DS, Ashford DA, et al: Bioterrorism-related inhalational anthrax: the first 10 cases reported in the United States. Emerg Infect Dis 7:933, 2001

49. Brachman PS: Inhalation anthrax. Ann NY Acad Sci 353:83, 1980

50. USAMRIID's Medical Management of Biological Casualties Handbook (USAMRIID Blue Book) 4th ed. United States Army Medical Research Institute of Infectious Diseases. Fort Detrick, Maryland, February, 2001
http://www.usamriid.army.mil/education/bluebook.html

51. Use of anthrax vaccine in the United States. Recommendations of the Advisory Committee on Immunization Practices. MMWR Morb Mortal Wkly Rep 49:1, 2000

52. Considerations for distinguishing influenza-like illness from inhalational anthrax. MMWR Morb Mortal Wkly Rep 50:984, 2001

53. Update: investigation of bioterrorism-related anthrax and interim guidelines for exposure management and antimicrobial therapy, October 2001. MMWR Morb Mortal Wkly Rep 50:909, 2001

54. Update: investigation of anthrax associated with intentional exposure and interim public health guidelines, October 2001. MMWR Morb Mortal Wkly Rep 50:889, 2001

55. Statement by the Department of Health and Human Services regarding additional options for preventive treatment for those exposed to inhalational anthrax. Dec. 18, 2001
http://www.hhs.gov/news/press/2001pres/20011218.html

56. Committee to Assess the Safety and Efficacy of the Anthrax Vaccine. Medical Follow-Up Agency: The Anthrax Vaccine: Is It Safe? Does It Work? Joellenbeck LM, Zwanziger LL, Durch JS, et al, Eds: Institute of Medicine, National Academy Press, Washington, DC, 2002
http://www.iom.edu/iom/iomhome.nsf/Wfiles/Anthrax-8-pager1FINAL/$file/Anthrax-8-pager1FINAL.pdf

57. Additional options for preventive treatment for persons exposed to inhalational anthrax. MMWR Morb Mortal Wkly Rep 50:1142, 2001

58. Carucci JA, McGovern TW, Norton SA, et al: Cutaneous anthrax management algorithm. J Am Acad Dermatol (online), November 21, 2001
http://www.aad.org/BioInfo/Biomessage2.html

59. Biosafety in Microbiological and Biomedical Laboratories (BMBL) 4th Edition. U.S. Department of Health and Human Services Centers for Disease Control and Prevention and National Institutes of Health. May 1999. US Government Printing Office, Washington, DC, 1999
http://www.cdc.gov/od/ohs/biosfty/bmbl4/bmbl4toc.htm.

60. Perry RD, Fetherston JD: *Yersinia pestis*—etiologic agent of plague. Clin Microbiol Rev 10:35, 1997

61. Gage KL, Dennis DT, Orloski KA, et al: Cases of cat-associated human plague in the western U.S., 1977–1998. Clin Infect Dis 30:893, 2000

62. Inglesby TV, Dennis DT, Henderson DA, et al: Plague as a biological weapon: medical and public health management. Working Group on Civilian Biodefense. JAMA 283:2281, 2000

63. Prevention of plague. Recommendations of the Advisory Committee on Immunization Practice. MMWR Morb Mortal Wkly Rep 45: 1, 1996

64. McGovern TW, Friedlander AM: Plague. Medical Aspects of Chemical and Biological Warfare. Textbook of Military Medicine Series. Part I, Warfare, Weaponry and the Casualty. Sidell FR, Takafuji ET, Franz DR, Eds. TMM Publications, Washington, DC, 1997

65. Shapiro RL, Hatheway C, Becher J, et al: Botulism surveillance and emergency response: a public health strategy for a global challenge. JAMA 278:433, 1997

66. Shapiro RL, Hatheway C, Swerdlow DL: Botulism in the United States: a clinical and epidemiologic review. Ann Intern Med 129:221, 1998

67. Arnon SS, Schechter R, Inglesby TV, et al: Botulinum toxin as a biological weapon: medical and public health management. JAMA 285: 1059,2001

68. Cherington M: Clinical spectrum of botulism. Muscle Nerve 21: 701, 1998

69. Woodruff BA, Griffin PM, McCroskey LM, et al: Clinical and laboratory comparison of botulism toxin types A, B and E in the United States, 1975–1988. J Infect Dis 166:1281, 1992

70. Angulo FJ, Getz J, Taylor JP, et al: A large outbreak of botulism: the hazardous baked potato. J Infect Dis 178:172, 1998

71. Eitzen E: Medical management of biological casualties 3rd ed. U.S. Army Medical Research Institute of Infectious Diseases, Fort Detrick, Frederick, Maryland, 1998

72. Black RE, Gunn RA: Hypersensitivity reactions associated with botulinal antitoxin. Am J Med 69:567, 1980

73. Tularemia—United States, 1999–2000. MMWR Morb Mortal Wkly Rep 51:181, 2002

74. Feldman KA, Enscore RE, Lathrop SL, et al: An outbreak of primary pneumonic tularemia on Martha's Vineyard. N Engl J Med 345: 1601, 2001

75. Dennis DT, Inglesby TV, Henderson DA, et al: Tularemia as a biological weapon: medical and public health management. JAMA 285: 2763, 2001

76. Choi E: Tularemia and Q fever. Med Clinics North Am 86:393, 2002

77. Evans ME, Gregory DW, Schaffner W, et al: Tularemia: a 30-year experience with 88 cases. Medicine (Baltimore) 64:251, 1985

78. Gill V, Cunha BA: Tularemia pneumonia. Semin Respir Infect 12: 61, 1997

79. Evans ME, Friedlander AM: Tularemia. Medical Aspects of Chemical and Biological Warfare. Textbook of Military Medicine Series. Part I, Warfare, Weaponry and the Casualty. Sidell FR, Takafuji ET, Franz DR, Eds. TMM Publications, Washington, DC, 1997

80. Limaye AP, Hooper CJ: Treatment of tularemia with fluoroquinolones: two cases and review. Clin Infect Dis 29:922, 1999

81. Borio L, Inglesby T, Peters CJ, et al: Hemorrhagic fever viruses as biological weapons: medical and public health management. JAMA 287:2391, 2002

82. Khan AS, Sanchez A, Pflieger AK: Filoviral hemorrhagic fevers. Br Med Bull 54:675, 1998

83. Bwaka MA, Bonnet MJ, Calain P, et al: Ebola hemorrhagic fever in Kikwit, Democratic Republic of the Congo: clinical observations in 103 patients. J Infect Dis 179:S1, 1999

84. Jahrling PB: Viral hemorrhagic fevers. Textbook of Military Medicine Series. Part I, Warfare, Weaponry and the Casualty. Sidell FR, Takafuji ET, Franz DR, Eds. TMM Publications, Washington, DC, 1997

85. Isaacson M: Viral hemorrhagic fever hazards for travelers in Africa. Clin Infect Dis 33:1707, 2001

86. Acute hemorrhagic fever syndrome. World Health Organization. http://www.who.int/emcdocuments/surveillance/docs/whocd scsrisr992.html/41Acute%20haemorrhagic%20fever%20syndrome.htm

87. Update: management of patients with suspected viral hemorrhagic fever—United States. MMWR Morb Mortal Wkly Rep 44:475, 1995

4 Sepsis

Steven M. Opal, M.D.
Christian E. Huber, M.D.

Sepsis, along with the multiorgan failure that often accompanies the systemic inflammatory response syndrome (SIRS), is a leading cause of mortality in the intensive care unit.[1,2] Sepsis develops in as many as 400,000 patients annually in the United States. Nearly half of these patients manifest severe sepsis and septic shock. The mortality for septic shock remains approximately 35% to 45%, despite a concerted effort to improve the treatment options and outcome.[1-3]

Septic shock has become a major focus of critical care research. Although modest improvements in the prognosis have been made over the past decade, innovations in the management of septic shock are still required. This subsection reviews some of the remarkable advances achieved in the understanding of the molecular pathophysiology of sepsis. This knowledge provides the groundwork for research strategies to improve diagnostic and therapeutic agents for the management of septic shock.

Definitions of Sepsis

Sepsis, septic shock, SIRS, and multiple organ dysfunction syndrome (MODS) were defined at the American College of Chest Physicians/Society for Critical Care Medicine (ACCP/SCCM) Consensus Conference on Definition [*see Table 1*].[4] The definitions take into account the finding that sepsis may result from a multitude of infectious agents and microbial mediators and may or may not be associated with actual bloodstream infection. Despite the clinical logic, intrinsic simplicity, and widespread acceptance of these consensus definitions, their clinical applicability has been justifiably criticized.[5,6] The SIRS definition is so broad and nonspecific that it loses its discriminatory power; many patients admitted to general medical services and most patients in intensive care units meet the definition of SIRS. The current definition of sepsis includes virtually every person within the first 24 hours of an episode of influenza because the SIRS criteria are met and an infectious agent (an orthomyxovirus) causes the syndrome; however, clinicians do not generally regard the flu as sepsis.

One of the tenets on which these definitions are based is that the inflammatory response itself, not the infectious organism, drives the septic process. This hypothesis may be correct, but the patient's host defenses, the antimicrobial susceptibility of the organism, and its ability to generate microbial toxins are also important.[7] Failure to account for the intrinsic differences in microbial virulence limits the utility of current definitions of sepsis.

Physiologic measurements are often used to define the sepsis syndrome, but there is disagreement regarding the level of fluid resuscitation necessary to ensure that the patient is indeed septic rather than hypovolemic. The amount of vasopressor agent necessary to confidently conclude that the patient has true septic shock continues to be debated. Controversy also surrounds the approach to distinguishing preexisting morbidities and organ dysfunction from the morbidity and organ dysfunction induced by the septic process itself. Many patients with sepsis have major underlying organ dysfunction from a variety of diseases. The degree to which sepsis contributes to further disordered organ function may be difficult to determine with accuracy. The same can be said for the degree to which sepsis contributes to the mortality of a given patient who has other serious underlying diseases. All these factors limit the discriminatory value of the consensus definitions of sepsis and jeopardize valid comparisons between different study populations, compromising the ability to pool data and generalize the findings.

Further refinements in sepsis terminology may be possible when rapid diagnostic techniques become available to assess the immune status of

Table 1 The Terminology of Sepsis

Term	*Definition*	*Comments*
ARDS* (acute respiratory distress syndrome)[93]	Acute onset Bilateral infiltrates on chest radiograph Hypoxemia (P_aO_2/F_IO_2 ratio ≤ 200 mm Hg No evidence of left atrial hypertension (pulmonary arterial wedge pressure ≤ 18 mm Hg)	Severity can be scored by use of clinical parameters such as presence of hypoxemia, radiologic evidence of lung consolidation and compliance, and PEEP data from mechanical ventilation (Murray lung injury score)[94]
Bacteremia	Detection of viable bacteria in the bloodstream	Transient bacteremia without clinical symptoms is common; may or may not be found in sepsis
SIRS (systemic inflammatory response syndrome)	Fever (> 38.5° C [101.3° F]) Tachypnea (> 20 breaths/minute) Tachycardia (> 90 beats/minute) Leukocytosis (> 12,000 cells/mm^3 or > 10% immature forms)	Two or more criteria needed; may be caused by infectious and noninfectious etiologies; clinical features may be caused by release of inflammatory mediators into circulation
Sepsis	SIRS caused by an invasive infection	May be caused by viral, bacterial, fungal, or parasitic pathogens; bloodstream infection need not be present
MODS (multiple organ dysfunction syndrome)	Major organ dysfunction from sepsis	A primary determinant of outcome in sepsis
Severe sepsis	Sepsis accompanied by major organ dysfunction (CNS, renal, pulmonary, hepatobiliary, hematologic, or metabolic)	Sometimes referred to as sepsis syndrome
Septic shock	Severe sepsis with hypotension not responsive to fluid challenge	Systolic blood pressure < 90 mm Hg despite adequate fluid resuscitation

* European-American Consensus Committee on ARDS definition.
F_IO_2—fraction of inspired oxygen P_aO_2—arterial oxygen tension PEEP—positive end-expiratory pressure

septic patients. In the meantime, the current consensus definitions will be used despite their limitations.

Epidemiology

The incidence of sepsis has increased over the past 2 decades.[8] This trend will probably continue in the foreseeable future because sepsis has largely become a disease of medical progress. Successful management of a variety of severe medical and surgical diseases has produced a large patient population with critical illness and impaired host defenses; these patients have a greatly increased risk of sepsis. Innovations in organ transplantation, implanted prosthetic devices, and long-term vascular access devices continue to expand this patient population. The gradual aging of the population in many developed countries and the increasing prevalence of antibiotic-resistant microbial pathogens also contribute to the rising incidence of septic shock.

Pathogenesis: Microbial Factors

The microbiology of sepsis has undergone a remarkable transition in the past 25 years. The predominant microbial pathogens responsible for sepsis in the 1960s and 1970s were gram-negative bacilli and *Pseudomonas aeruginosa*, but there has been a progressive increase in the incidence of sepsis caused by gram-positive bacterial[9,10] and opportunistic fungal pathogens. The rapid evolution of antibiotic-resistance genes in gram-positive bacterial pathogens and the frequent occurrence of vascular catheter-related bacterial sepsis may account for the increasing prevalence of gram-positive pathogens as a cause of sepsis.

GRAM-NEGATIVE CAUSATIVE ORGANISMS

The Role of Bacterial Endotoxin

Bacterial endotoxin, which is composed of lipopolysaccharide (LPS), is an intrinsic component of the outer membrane of gram-negative bacteria and is essential for the viability of these bacteria.[11] Humans are one of the species most susceptible to the profound immunostimulant properties of endotoxin, which may be lethal in minute doses. Whether endotoxin is released into the human circulatory system in its free form (released from dead organisms or shed from the membrane of via-

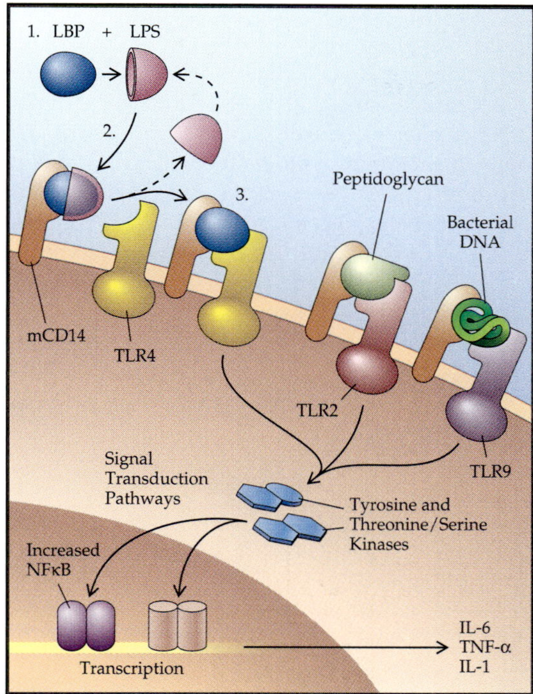

Figure 1 **During lipopolysaccharide (LPS) signaling, (1) plasmatic LPS binds to LPS-binding protein (LPB). (2) This complex is delivered to membrane-bound CD14 (mCD14). (3) The CD14-LPS complex interacts with the transmembranous Toll-like receptor 4 (TLR4), which initiates the intracellular signal transduction pathway. The signal transduction pathway leads to NFκB translocation into the nucleus, with increased transcription of proinflammatory cytokines. TLR2 is known to signal membrane compounds of gram-positive bacteria such as peptidoglycan. TLR9 recognizes bacterial DNA. (IL—interleukin; NFκB—nuclear factor κB; TNF-α—tumor necrosis factor–α)**

ble organisms) or bound to the cell wall of intact bacteria, a vigorous systemic inflammatory response results. It appears that endotoxin functions essentially as an alarm molecule that alerts the host to the presence of invading gram-negative bacteria,[12] a phylogenetically ancient mechanism in eukaryotic organisms.[13]

The Toll-like receptor family The cellular receptor for bacterial endotoxin on the human immune cell has been identified. After decades of research, the Toll-like receptors (TLRs) have been demonstrated to be the transmembrane receptors for endotoxin and many other microbial mediators, such as peptidoglycan, lipopeptides, and lipoteichoic acid [*see Figure 1*].[14] TLR4 is the principal endotoxin receptor,[15] and TLR2 and perhaps other TLRs recognize and signal the presence of a variety of microbial mediators, including endotoxin.[16,17] Comparative genomics in the murine system and *Drosophila* system allowed for the identification of these critical receptors for microbial mediators on human cells.[18] Recently, another TLR has been identified as the cellular receptor for unmethylated CpG motifs (cytosine bases followed by guanines) found in bacterial DNA. Human cells can distinguish bacterial DNA from human DNA, and the recognition of bacterial DNA initiates an intense inflammatory response mediated by TLR9.[19–21]

The TLRs belong to a family of pattern-recognition molecules that alert the innate immune response system to the presence of a microbial invader. Other pattern-recognition molecules include alternative complement components, mannose-binding peptide, and CD14. The innate immune system by nature is a rather nonspecific antimicrobial defense system, lacking the precision of the acquired immune system (B cells and T cells); however, the innate immune response is a critical survival mechanism in its immediate action in phagocytosis and its clearance of pathogens in the initial stages of infection. Activation of the innate immune system and its cellular components (neutrophils, monocytes, macrophages, and natural killer [NK] cells) are primarily responsible for the pathogenesis of septic shock.[13]

LPS signaling LPS is a phosphorylated, polar macromolecule that contains hydrophobic elements in the fatty acids of its lipid A core structure and hydrophilic elements in its repeating polysaccharide surface components. LPS forms microaggregates in biologic fluids and then rapidly interacts with a variety of serum or membrane-bound lipophilic proteins. In humans, there are three recognized receptors for LPS: (1) soluble or membrane-bound CD14 molecules, (2) CD11/CD18 molecules (β2 integrins), and (3) scavenger receptors for lipid molecules. Soluble and membrane-bound CD14 greatly potentiate the host response to small quantities of LPS and other microbial mediators.[22]

In human blood and body fluids, LPS signaling is mediated by interactions with a hepatically derived, acute-phase plasma protein known as LPS-binding protein (LBP).[22] LBP functions primarily as a shuttle molecule that binds to polymeric LPS aggregates and transfers LPS monomers to CD14. CD14 is a glycosyl phosphatidylinositol-linked protein that is found on the cell surfaces of immune effector cells such as the monocyte-macrophage and the neutrophil. After docking to membrane-bound CD14, LPS is delivered to an adjacent cell surface LPS receptor TLR4. This action then triggers a signal to the intracellular space, subsequently activating LPS-responsive genes. CD14 also binds to bacterial peptidoglycan and lipopeptides and delivers these microbial ligands to TLR2 for intracellular signaling.

Through a well-characterized sequence of tyrosine and threonine/serine kinases, intracellular signaling leads to phosphorylation of inhibitory κB (IκB), which releases nuclear factor κB (NFκB) from the cytoplasm, allowing it to translocate into the nucleus. Clotting elements and acute-phase proteins, cytokines, and nitric oxide synthase genes have NFκB binding sites in their regulatory elements. The outpouring of proinflammatory cytokines and other inflammatory mediators after LPS exposure contributes to SIRS and is central to the pathogenesis of septic shock induced by gram-negative bacteria.[23,24]

Bactericidal/permeability-increasing protein Another important endotoxin binding protein found in human plasma is bactericidal/permeability-increasing protein (BPI). This protein is 456 amino acids long, is produced by human neutrophils, and is found in greatest quantities in the azurophilic (primary) granules.[25] It shares a 45% amino acid sequence homology with LBP but has a distinctly antagonistic function with respect to LPS handling. LBP facilitates LPS delivery to CD14, thereby activating cells. BPI has the opposite physiologic effect: it inhibits LPS delivery to CD14. BPI functions as a molecular antagonist and competes with LBP for LPS binding in biologic fluids.[25,26] The relative concentrations of these two endotoxin-binding proteins primarily determine the net effect of LPS release.

In human plasma, the concentration of LBP is two to three orders of magnitude higher than that of BPI. The opposite appears to be true in abscess cavities, where BPI is present in much greater quantities than LBP.[18] This condition favors LPS-activating activity in the plasma and LPS-inhibitory activity in abscess cavities. Thus, BPI functions as an endogenous antiendotoxin molecule; it may become a component of treatment for endotoxin-induced injury.[25]

Endotoxin Tolerance

The phenomenon of endotoxin tolerance has been well characterized in experimental models of sepsis and probably also occurs in human sepsis.[27] Endotoxin tolerance is described as desensitization to endotoxin-induced lethality after administration of a priming (small) dose of endotoxin before an otherwise lethal challenge dose of endotoxin. This phenomenon appears to be mediated primarily at the transcription level, with downregulation of proinflammatory cytokine genes. The precise molecular explanation for endotoxin tolerance is not fully characterized. The desensitizing dose of endotoxin may induce endogenous corticosteroids or anti-inflammatory cytokines such as interleukin 10 (IL-10); decrease cell surface expression of the TLRs; alter nuclear translocation of signal transduction molecules; or decrease the stability of messenger RNA (mRNA) for cytokine genes.

The significance of endotoxin tolerance in humans is unclear, but some degree of endotoxin tolerance has been observed in patients treated with monophosphoryl lipid A.[27] Unquestionably, endotoxin is an important mediator in the pathogenesis of septic shock. Thus, efforts to limit LPS synthesis, prevent activation of host immune response elements, and enhance the clearance of LPS are important therapeutic strategies for the future treatment of septic shock.

BACTERIAL SUPERANTIGENS

Another important microbial mediator in the pathogenesis of septic shock is bacterial superantigen. Superantigens are a diverse group of microbially derived, protein-based exotoxins from streptococci, staphylococci, and other pathogens that share an unusual immunologic property: superantigens have the capacity to activate large numbers of $CD4^+$ T cells in a short period by bypassing the usual mechanism of antigen processing and presentation.[28]

Conventional bacterial antigens are internalized by antigen-presenting cells (APCs), whereby the antigens undergo limited proteolysis and processing within the endosomal component of the macrophage. Appropriate peptide sequences of the microbial antigens (epitopes) are inserted into the central groove of the major histocompatibility class II molecules and are then expressed on the cell surface of APCs. Specific $CD4^+$ T cells that recognize the unique epitope are then activated. Clonal expansion of this small subset of T cells results in a physiologic immune response to the newly introduced antigen. Superantigens, in contrast, do not require intracellular processing by APCs. Superantigens bind directly to class II antigens adjacent to the epitope-specific peptide groove on APCs.

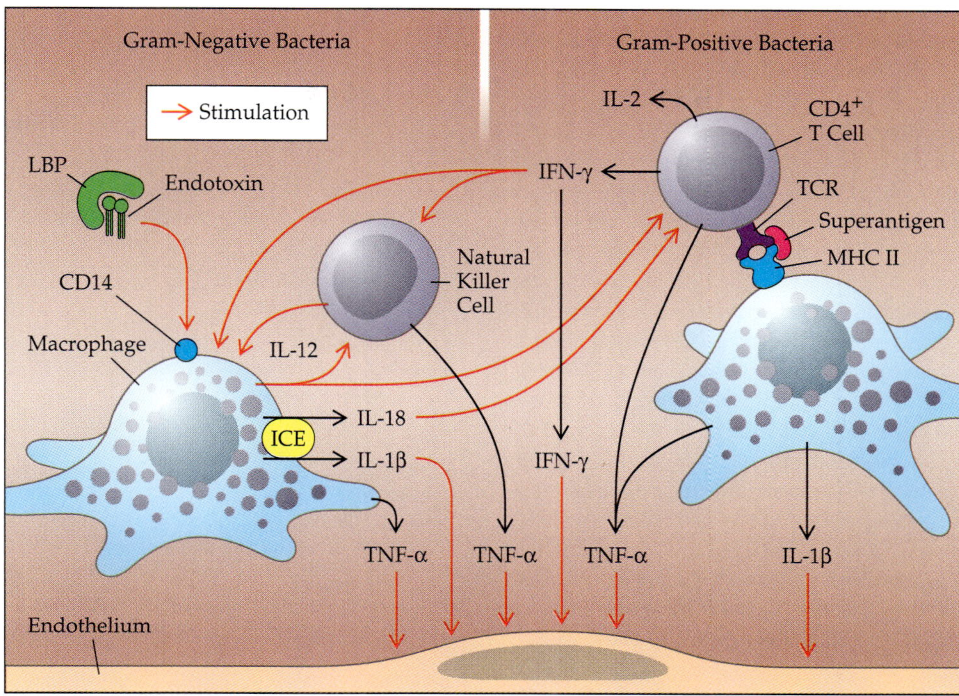

Figure 2 **Interactions between bacterial endotoxin and bacterial superantigens. (ICE—interleukin-1β–converting enzyme; IFN-γ—interferon gamma; IL—interleukin; LBP—LPS-binding protein; TNF-α—tumor necrosis factor–α)**

Superantigens also bind to a limited number of Vβ regions of the T cell receptor on $CD4^+$ T cells. This binding brings $CD4^+$ T cells and macrophages into close proximity, which activates both the monocyte-macrophage and T cell populations. A conventional peptide antigen stimulates only about one in 10^5 circulating lymphocytes that can recognize this unique structural epitope. However, a superantigen (e.g., toxic-shock syndrome toxin-1 from *Staphylococcus aureus*, which binds to the $V\beta_2$ region of T cells) stimulates up to 10% of circulating human lymphocytes. Thus, a single bacterial superantigen can activate as much as 10% of the entire lymphocyte population.[29] This ability results in excessive activation of both lymphocytes and macrophages, and the synthesis and release of proinflammatory cytokines proceed in an uncontrolled fashion.

Superantigen-induced immune activation may terminate in septic shock if the process is left unchecked. Polymicrobial infections that release both bacterial superantigens and endotoxin may be particularly injurious to the host; the toxicity of bacterial endotoxin may be greatly enhanced by superantigens that prime the immune system to react to endotoxin in an overly sensitized manner [*see Figure 2*].

GRAM-POSITIVE AND FUNGAL CAUSATIVE ORGANISMS

Peptidoglycan from the cell wall of bacterial capsular antigens, lipoteichoic acid, lipopeptides, microbial DNA, microbial toxins, and procoagulant substances produced by microbial pathogens may all contribute to the pathogenesis of sepsis. It has been observed that peptidoglycan from gram-positive bacteria interacts with CD14 molecules and activates inflammatory cells via TLR2 in a manner comparable to that observed with bacterial endotoxin.[16,30,31] Although the level of activation is quantitatively less with gram-positive components, CD14-dependent activation of mononuclear cells may occur from either gram-positive or gram-negative bacteria.[30] Bacterial DNA possesses unmethylated CpG motifs not found in eukaryotic DNA. Human inflammatory cells recognize this subtle distinction in actual DNA and react with a vigorous inflammatory response.[19] Recent evidence indicates that this response is mediated by the TLR9 receptor on human cells.[20] CD14-dependent activation of mononuclear cells may occur with components of gram-positive bacteria, although the level of activation is quantitatively less than that observed with gram-negative bacterial components.[32]

Moreover, gram-positive bacterial and fungal pathogens may induce systemic hypotension, resulting in redistribution of blood flow and splanchnic vasoconstriction. The ischemia and reperfusion of blood vessels that supply the gastrointestinal tract may disrupt the intestinal mucosal barrier to bacterial products. Translocation of intact microbial pathogens, as well as bacterial endotoxin, may occur during periods of severe stress and during periods of hypoperfusion of the gastrointestinal mucosa.[33] Bacterial endotoxin may play a pathogenic role in the ongoing inflammatory process after the development of systemic hypotension from infectious and noninfectious insults. Thus, shock states may be potentiated and maintained by the continued release of endotoxin and other microbial mediators from the lumen of the GI tract. This finding has prompted attempts to strengthen the GI mucosal barrier through immunonutrition, epithelial growth factors, and selective decontamination of the GI tract in critically ill patients. These treatments remain potentially viable options and areas of active research in the management of sepsis.

Table 2 Host-Derived Inflammatory Mediators in Septic Shock

Proinflammatory Mediators	*Anti-inflammatory Mediators*
Tumor necrosis factor–α	Interleukin-1 receptor antagonist
Interleukin-1β	Soluble tumor necrosis factor receptor
Interferon gamma	Soluble interleukin-1 receptor
Lymphotoxin-α	Transforming growth factor–β
Interleukin-2	Interleukin-4
Interleukin-8	Interleukin-6
Interleukin-12	Interleukin-10
Interleukin-18	Interleukin-11
Complement	Interleukin-13
Leukotriene B_4	Prostaglandin E_2
Platelet-activating factor	Granulocyte colony-stimulating factor
Bradykinin	Antioxidants
Nitric oxide	Interferon alfa
Granulocyte-macrophage colony-stimulating factor	Interferon beta
Chemokines	
Macrophage inhibitory factor	

Pathogenesis: Host-Derived Mediators

CYTOKINE NETWORKS

Proinflammatory cytokines play a pivotal role in the pathogenesis of sepsis. In animal studies, the administration of human tumor necrosis factor–α (TNF-α), an endogenous monocyte-macrophage–derived protein, was shown to have lethal consequences, and dramatic hemodynamic, metabolic, and hematologic changes were observed after TNF-α was administered to human volunteers.[34,35] The injurious effects of systemic levels of IL-1β have also been demonstrated.[36]

The major proinflammatory cytokines, TNF-α and IL-1β, induce their hemodynamic and metabolic effects in concert with an expanding group of host-derived proinflammatory mediators that work in a coordinated fashion to produce the systemic inflammatory response [*see Figure* 2] and [*see Table* 2].[36] The cytokine system functions as a network of communication signals between neutrophils, monocytes, macrophages, and endothelial cells. Autocrine and paracrine activation results in synergistic potentiation of the inflammatory response once it is activated by a systemic microbial challenge (e.g., endotoxemia). Much of the proinflammatory response is localized and compartmentalized in the primary region of initial inflammation (e.g., lung tissue or GI tract). If left unchecked, the inflammatory response spills over into the systemic circulation, resulting in a generalized reaction and culminating in diffuse endothelial injury and septic shock. The endocrinelike effect of the systemic release of cytokines and chemokines drives the inflammatory process throughout the body.[1-3]

The multitude of inflammatory cytokines and chemokines found in excess quantities in the bloodstream in septic shock is impressive and is matched by an equally daunting group of anti-inflammatory mediators [*see Table* 2]. The proinflammatory mediators tend to predominate in the early phases of sepsis (the first 12 to 24 hours), whereas the endogenous anti-inflammatory components often prevail in the later phases of sepsis.[37] Mice deficient in T and B cells have responded to endotoxin challenge in the same way as normal mice have.[38] Thus, monocyte-macrophage–generated cytokines are sufficient to drive the early septic process. However, lymphocyte-derived cytokines and interferons become important in the regulation of later phases of sepsis and may ultimately determine the outcome for patients with septic shock.

The Role of CD4+ T cells

Important functional differences exist within CD4+ T cells. Activated, yet uncommitted, CD4+ T cells (Th0 cells) have two major pathways of functional differentiation. T cells exposed to IL-12 in the presence of IL-2 are driven toward a Th1-type functional development. These cells produce large quantities of interferon gamma, TNF-α, and IL-2 and promote a proinflammatory, cell-mediated immune response. Uncommitted CD4+ T cells exposed to IL-4 preferentially develop into a Th2-type phenotype; Th2 cells secrete IL-4, IL-10, and IL-13. These cytokines promote humoral immune responses and attenuate macrophage and neutrophil activity.

Interestingly, Th1-type cytokines suppress the expression of Th2-type cytokines; interferon gamma inhibits the synthesis of IL-10. Conversely, IL-10 from Th2 cells is a potent inhibitor of TNF-α and interferon-gamma synthesis by Th1 cells. The nature of the initial lymphocyte response is critical because the system tends to polarize over time into either a Th2-type or a Th1-type response.[39] Recent evidence indicates that similar forms of functional differentiation exist for CD8 cells (CD8+ type 1 and type 2 cells).[40]

This process of functional differentiation is clinically relevant, because sepsis is often accompanied by a late Th2-type response after an initial septic insult. The stress hormone response in septic shock, with expression of adrenocorticotropic hormone, corticosteroids, and catecholamines, promotes a Th2 response after systemic injury. This response may lead to a phase of relative immune refractoriness (immune paralysis), during which the patient may be at increased risk for secondary bacterial or fungal infection.[37] This pathophysiologic state is associated with endotoxin tolerance; anti-inflammatory cytokine synthesis; and deactivation of monocytes, macrophages, and neutrophils. Methods to detect this immunosuppressed state and restore immune competence are under investigation. Patients with depressed expression of major histocompatibility class II antigens (e.g., HLA-DR) on the cell surface of macrophages may be in a functionally immunosuppressed state and may benefit from interferon-gamma treatment.[41]

ROLE OF THE COAGULATION SYSTEM

Activation of the coagulation cascade and generation of a consumptive coagulopathy and diffuse microthrombi are well-recognized complications of severe sepsis. Studies of endotoxin challenge and TNF challenge in normal human volunteers indicate that the extrinsic pathway is the predominant mechanism by which the coagulation system is activated in human sepsis.[42,43] The contact factors in the intrinsic pathway are also activated, secondarily initiating vasodilatation through the generation of bradykinin.[43] Activation of intravascular coagulation results in microthrombi and may contribute to the multiorgan failure that occurs in septic patients. Depletion of coagulation factors and activation of plasmin, antithrombin III, and activated protein C may subsequently lead to a hemorrhagic diathesis. Depletion of these endogenous anticoagulants may secondarily lead to a procoagulant state and portend a poor prognosis.[44]

Current interest in the administration of tissue factor pathway inhibitor, activated protein C, and antithrombin III for treatment of sepsis attests to the potential therapeutic value of regulation of the coagulation system in sepsis.[13,45]

NEUTROPHIL-ENDOTHELIAL CELL INTERACTIONS

The recruitment of neutrophils to an area of localized infection is an essential component of the host inflammatory response. Localization and eradication of invading microbial pathogens at the site of initial infection is the principal objective of the immune response to microbial pathogens. This physiologic process may become deleterious if diffuse neutrophil-endothelial cell interactions occur throughout the circulation in response to systemic inflammation.

The mechanisms responsible for the migration of neutrophils from the intravascular space into the interstitium, where invasive microorganisms may reside, are complex [*see Figure 3*]. Activated neutrophils degranulate and expose endothelial surfaces and surrounding structures to reactive oxygen intermediates, nitric oxide, and a variety of proteases. This process contributes not only to microbial clearance but also to diffuse endothelial injury in the face of generalized systemic inflammatory responses. Regulation of neutrophil activity may represent a new area for therapeutic intervention in the management of sepsis.[46]

ROLE OF NITRIC OXIDE

Nitric oxide is a highly reactive free radical that plays an essential role in the pathophysiology of septic shock. It has a very short half-life (1 to 3 seconds), which tends to limit its activity to local tissues, where it is first generated by one of three isoforms of nitric oxide synthase. Regulation of the nitric oxide synthases is complex. Full expression of inducible nitric oxide synthase requires TNF-α, IL-1, LPS, and probably other regulatory elements.

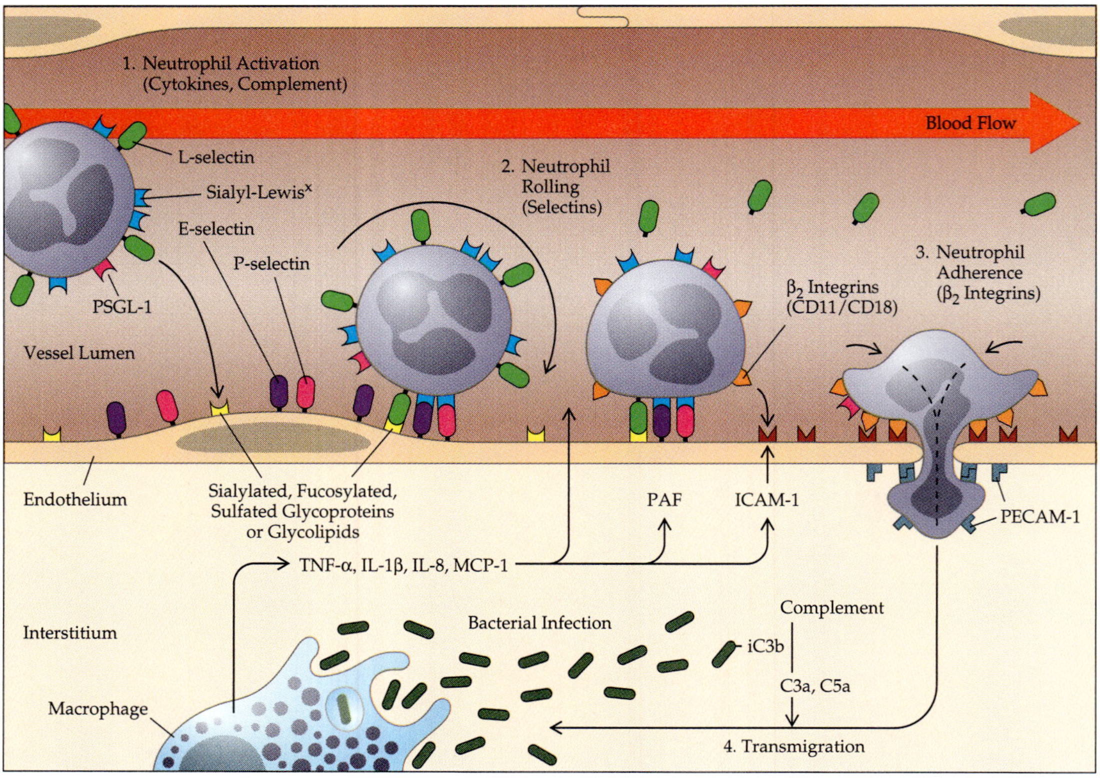

Figure 3 **Neutrophil-endothelial cell interactions in sepsis. (C—complement; ICAM-1—intercellular adhesion molecule-1; IL-1β—interleukin-1β; MCP-1—monocyte chemoattractant protein-1; PAF—platelet-activating factor; PECAM-1—platelet endothelial cell adhesion molecule; PSGL-1—P-selectin glycoprotein ligand-1; TNF-α—tumor necrosis factor–α)**

Nitric oxide is the major endothelial-derived relaxing factor that initiates the vasodilatation and systemic hypotension observed in septic shock patients. Nitric oxide activates guanylate cyclase, which increases cyclic guanosine monophosphate levels inside vascular smooth muscle cells. This condition results in systemic vasodilatation and decreased vascular resistance. Within minutes of administration of an inhibitor of nitric oxide synthesis, however, blood pressure in hypotensive patients in septic shock returns toward normal levels.[47]

The other major physiologic effects of nitric oxide in septic shock are increased intracellular killing and regulation of platelet and neutrophil adherence. Nitric oxide is a highly diffusible gas that does not require specific receptors to enter eukaryotic or prokaryotic cells. In the presence of superoxide anion, nitric oxide leads to the formation of peroxynitrite. The peroxynitrite subsequently decays into such highly cytotoxic molecules as hydroxyl radicals and nitrosyl chloride, which, in turn, initiate lipid peroxidation and cause irreversible cellular damage. Nitric oxide inhibits a variety of key enzymes in the tricarboxylic acid pathway, the glycolytic pathway, DNA repair systems, electron transport pathways, and energy-exchange pathways. Because of its potent reactivity, nitric oxide alters the function of many metalloenzymes, carrier proteins, and structural elements.

It has become apparent that nitric oxide, like many other components of the host inflammatory response, may have both advantageous and disadvantageous properties in sepsis. Nitric oxide regulates microcirculation to vital organs and contributes to intracellular killing of microbial pathogens. However, excess and prolonged release of nitric oxide results in generalized vasodilatation and the systemic hypotension of septic shock. Nitric oxide has become a target for therapeutic strategies in the management of sepsis.[48] Nonselective inhibitors of nitric oxide synthase, for example, have been shown to improve the hemodynamics of septic shock patients.[47] Unfortunately, this finding was not confirmed in a 1999 phase 3 trial.[49]

It has been discovered that at least two additional host-derived mediators contribute to the pathogenesis of septic shock. Macrophage migration inhibitory factor[50] is a late mediator that activates immune cells and contributes to lethal septic shock. This corticosteroid-regulated mediator has proinflammatory actions and has become a target for therapeutic agents in sepsis. High-mobility group-1 (HMG-1) protein also appears to contribute to late-onset inflammatory activity in septic shock patients. Inhibitors of HMG-1 may prove to have a therapeutic role as well.[51]

Diagnostic Approach to Septic Shock

GENERAL CLINICAL FEATURES

In his classic treatise on human nature (*The Prince*, circa 1505), Machiavelli states, "Hectic fever [i.e., sepsis by current consensus definitions] at its inception is difficult to recognize but easy to treat; left untended, it becomes easy to recognize but difficult to treat." This statement is as true today as it was 500 years ago. Fully developed septic shock is a readily apparent clinical syndrome that is seldom confused with other pathologic states. However, the early phases of septic shock may be quite subtle even in carefully monitored patients. Early signs and symptoms may include confusion, apprehension, or decreased sensorium. Although fever is characteristic, hypothermia may be observed and connotes a poor prognosis. An unexplained decrease in urinary output, sudden onset of cholestatic jaundice, unexplained metabolic alkalosis, excess bleeding at venipuncture sites, or even sudden unexplained hypotension may be the presenting finding in septic shock. It is essential that clinicians recognize these early signs and symptoms, because successful management of septic shock depends on early recognition and appropriate intervention.

A variety of clinical, laboratory, and hemodynamic abnormalities are recognized in septic shock [*see Tables 3 and 4*]. Unfortunately, no single clinical or laboratory test is sufficiently specific and sensitive to reliably confirm the diagnosis of septic shock. Blood cultures may or may not be positive, leukocytosis or neutropenia may be seen, hyperglycemia or hypoglycemia may occur, and either respiratory alkalosis or metabolic acidosis may occur. It is the constellation of signs and symptoms that leads to a diagnosis of septic shock.

Table 3 Standard Laboratory Values in Sepsis

Laboratory Study	*Typical Findings*	*Comments*
White blood cell count	Leukocytosis or leukopenia	Stress response, increased margination of neutrophils in sepsis; toxic granulation may be seen; occasionally, bacteria may be found in the peripheral blood smear
Platelet count	Thrombocytopenia	Look for evidence of fragmentation hemolysis in the peripheral blood smear; thrombocytopenia may or may not be accompanied by disseminated intravascular coagulation
Glucose	Hyperglycemia or hypoglycemia	Acute stress response, inhibition of gluconeogenesis
Clotting measurements	Elevated prothrombin time, activated partial thromboplastin time, low fibrinogen levels, and evidence of fibrinolysis	Coagulopathy often seen with systemic endotoxin release
Liver enzymes	Elevated alkaline phosphatase, bilirubin, and transaminases; low albumin	—
Blood cultures	Bacteremia or fungemia	The presence of positive blood culture does not make the diagnosis, and its absence does not exclude the diagnosis
Plasma lactate	Mild elevations (> 2.2 mmol/L)	Hypermetabolism, anaerobic metabolism, inhibition of pyruvate dehydrogenase
C-reactive protein	Elevated	Acute-phase reactant, sensitive but not specific for sepsis
Arterial blood gases	Respiratory alkalosis (early); metabolic acidosis (late)	Measurements of O_2 content and mixed venous O_2 saturation useful in management

Table 4 Hemodynamic Findings in Sepsis

Parameter	*Typical Findings*	*Comments*
Heart rate	> 100 beats/min	Major compensatory mechanism for low systemic vascular resistance
Mean arterial blood pressure	< 65 mm Hg	Hallmark of septic shock
Cardiac index (cardiac output/m^2 [surface area])	> 4 L/min/m^2	Cardiac index elevated in early septic shock; may be depressed in late septic shock
Pulmonary arterial wedge pressure	4–10 mm Hg	Must be sure that hypovolemia is not the cause of hypotension; perform fluid resuscitation until pulmonary arterial wedge pressure returns to normal
Systemic vascular resistance (SVR)	< 800 dyne/sec/cm^{-5}	SVR often low in early septic shock; may become elevated in later phases of septic shock
Oxygen delivery (DO_2) Cardiac index (CI) × arterial O_2 content (A)	< 550 ml/min/m^2	Try to provide sufficient DO_2 to maintain adequate mixed venous O_2 saturation
Mixed venous O_2 saturation	< 70%	Low mixed venous O_2 indicates inadequate O_2 delivery to tissues in sepsis
Oxygen consumption (VO_2) (CI) × (A-VO_2) × 10	> 180 L/min/m^2	Typically increased in early septic shock

The most common hemodynamic findings in early septic shock are a high cardiac output and a low systemic vascular resistance state, with initial maintenance of the systolic blood pressure as the heart attempts to compensate for the loss of systemic vascular tone. Myocardial performance is diminished even in the early phases of septic shock.[52] Without adequate intervention, circulating blood volume is continually lost into the interstitial space and intracellular locations. The heart can no longer compensate sufficiently, and systolic hypotension results. Deterioration of myocardial performance, accompanied by diffuse vasoconstriction, marks the late refractory state of septic shock.

Septic shock may be associated with a loss of normal autoregulation between oxygen delivery and oxygen consumption in the tissues. A supply-dependent dysoxia may contribute to tissue injury in multiorgan failure in sepsis.[53] In clinical studies with septic shock patients, attempts to enhance oxygen delivery to supranormal levels, although theoretically appealing, have not resulted in increased survival.[54] Perhaps a more judicious use of oxygen delivery to tissues would benefit patients in septic shock.

MULTIPLE ORGAN DYSFUNCTION SYNDROME

One of the hallmarks of septic shock is the development of MODS. The development of organ failure at the onset or over the course of sepsis is associated with a poor prognosis and is a primary determinant of outcome [*see Table 5*].[55] The diffuse endothelial injury accompanying septic shock results in organ dysfunction distant from the original site of the septic insult. It is assumed that the signal that results in diffuse endovascular injury is relayed by plasma factors (e.g., proinflammatory cytokines, complement, kinins, and other host-derived inflammatory mediators) or by a cellular element found in one or more of the immune effector cells.

Inadequate blood supply to vital tissues produces MODS. The failure of the microcirculation to support tissue maintenance may be the result of hypoperfusion of capillary beds, redistribution of blood flow within vascular beds, functional arteriovenous shunting, obstruction of blood flow from microthrombi, platelet or white blood cell aggregates, or abnormal deformability of red blood cells. Direct endothelial injury from nitric oxide, reactive oxygen intermediates, proinflammatory cytokines, and inducers of apoptosis may directly damage endothelial surfaces. Endothelial swelling from the movement of intravascular fluid into the extravascular and intracellular spaces may mechanically obstruct the lumina of the capillary beds as well.

Although the origin of multiorgan failure in sepsis is principally related to microvascular effects, myocardial performance and pulmonary function also diminish over the course of septic

Table 5 Multiple Organ Dysfunction Syndrome in Severe Sepsis

Organ System	*Clinical-Metabolic Abnormalities*	*Histopathologic Findings*
CNS	Encephalopathy, decreased sensorium	Cerebral edema, microthrombi
Cardiac	Decreased myocardial performance	Altered calcium influx, interstitial edema
Lung	Acute respiratory distress syndrome	Exudation of fluid into the alveolar spaces, neutrophil plugging, hyaline membrane formation
Kidney	Acute tubular necrosis	Hypoperfusion, focal ischemia, microthrombi
Adrenal	Relative adrenal insufficiency, adrenal hemorrhage	Focal or diffuse hemorrhage, ischemic necrosis
Hepatobiliary system	Cholestatic jaundice, decreased hepatic synthesis of albumin, presence of clotting factors	Zonal necrosis, acalculous cholecystitis
Gut	Translocation of bacterial endotoxin and microorganisms, increased permeability	Diffuse interstitial edema, breaks in the epithelial membrane integrity, mucosal necrosis

shock and may contribute significantly to the development of MODS. Myocardial contractility decreases in response to a variety of myocardial depressant factors found in the plasma of septic patients. TNF-α is a prominent cause of myocardial dysfunction; IL-1, nitric oxide, and other host-derived inflammatory mediators may also be contributing factors.[56]

ACUTE RESPIRATORY DISTRESS SYNDROME

Acute lung injury occurs as a result of damage to the pulmonary vascular circulation and the alveolocapillary membranes. The lung is susceptible to injury in a variety of systemic inflammatory states. Acute respiratory distress syndrome (ARDS) remains a major cause of morbidity and mortality in septic shock. Efforts to prevent lung injury include innovations in respiratory support, avoidance of barotrauma and volutrauma to the alveolocapillary units, avoidance of oxidant-induced lung injury, salvage of functional alveolocapillary units through position change to the prone position, and judicious fluid management.[57] Measurable improvements have been made in the outcome of ARDS patients, but considerable room for improvement remains in sparing the pulmonary function of septic shock patients. A major 1998 finding is the importance of identification of overdistention of airways caused by volume settings being set too high on ventilators during the progression of lung injury and the release of inflammatory mediators into the systemic circulation.[58] The recent ARDS Network study demonstrated conclusively that a lower tidal volume setting (6 ml/kg) is clearly superior to the previously conventional higher tidal volume setting (12 ml/kg).[59] Ventilation with a low tidal volume setting has become the standard of practice in the management of most forms of acute lung injury.

Multiorgan failure is potentially reversible if rapid intervention corrects the hemodynamic and inflammatory abnormalities.

EXPERIMENTAL DIAGNOSTIC TECHNIQUES

The current assays used to diagnose septic shock are cumbersome and are not useful for rapid diagnostic testing; research to develop better assays is ongoing.

Plasma Endotoxin Levels

Measurement of plasma endotoxin levels may prove useful in the diagnosis of sepsis; it has been shown to be of some predictive value in determining which patients are more susceptible to shock.[60] Unfortunately, endotoxin levels are not uniformly elevated in patients with septic shock and may be spuriously elevated in patients with gram-positive infection or other hypotensive disorders. The host response to endotoxin is variable and cannot be determined on the basis of circulating endotoxin levels.

Bacterial Superantigen Levels

Circulating levels of bacterial superantigens have been successfully measured in selected patients with toxic-shock syndrome.[61] Such measurements may prove useful in specific clinical situations.

IL-6 Levels

IL-6 is a multifunctional cytokine with myriad biologic activities, some of which are proinflammatory and others anti-inflammatory. IL-6 has been considered an indicator of cytokine activation because it is reliably present after activation of TNF-α and IL-1β.[57] Patients with elevated IL-6 levels may respond favorably to anticytokine therapies.[62] In several studies,[62–66] elevations of IL-6, as well as failure of IL-6 levels to fall after initiation of treatment for sepsis, were associated with a poor outcome. Unfortunately, IL-6 levels are not specific for sepsis and may be elevated in a variety of inflammatory and infectious states. The lack of specificity limits the reliability of IL-6 measurement as a method for diagnosing septic shock.

Procalcitonin Levels

Procalcitonin is the propeptide of calcitonin, which, under physiologic conditions, is produced by C cells in the thyroid. A specific protease cleaves procalcitonin into calcitonin, katacalcin, and an amino-terminal peptide.[67] Procalcitonin has attributes that make it a potential marker for sepsis. It has a long half-life (approximately 24 hours) and increases from undetectable levels to over 100 ng/ml during the course of septic shock. The precise origin of procalcitonin in sepsis is unclear, but it is extrathyroidal.[67,68] Procalcitonin levels do not rise as rapidly as IL-6 or IL-8 levels; elevated levels of procalcitonin are seen 4 to 6 hours after a systemic challenge with endotoxin or other septic stimuli.[68]

Interestingly, procalcitonin levels are elevated in patients with severe sepsis but not in patients with localized infections,[68] indicating that procalcitonin may be a marker for the systemic inflammatory response. It has also been observed that in patients who have undergone organ transplantation, procalcitonin levels may allow differentiation between the fever associated with rejection and that associated with sepsis.[69] Procalcitonin levels do not appear to be elevated in patients with severe viral infections or inflammatory conditions of noninfectious origin. Although the precise physiologic role of procalcitonin in sepsis has yet to be defined, procalcitonin appears to be the most sensitive and reasonably specific indicator of severe sepsis currently available.[68,70]

Potential Markers for Sepsis

C-reactive protein and plasma lactate have been used as potential markers for sepsis, but the lack of specificity and sensitivity of both of these indicators limits their diagnostic value. IL-8 may prove useful, with or without IL-6, as an indicator of sepsis.[71] Phospholipase A_2 or its precursor, type 1 prophospholipase A_2 propeptide, may become a potential marker for sepsis, but the diagnostic value of measurements of this enzyme needs to be confirmed in clinical studies.[72] Phospholipase A_2 is essential for the generation of platelet-activating factor and arachidonic acid derivatives, including thromboxane, prostacycline, prostaglandins, and leukotrienes.

Management of Septic Shock

There are four goals in the management of septic shock: (1) early recognition and resuscitation, (2) reestablishment of tissue perfusion and arterial blood pressure, (3) provision of optimal supportive care, and (4) timely initiation of treatment to eradicate the causative septic focus. The standard treatment approach has not changed appreciably in the past 2 decades. Changes in treatment may soon occur, however, because activated protein C has been shown to reduce mortality in patients with sepsis.[73]

Despite the lack of changes in standard treatment, there have been modest improvements in outcome because of better nutrition and supportive care and skillful use of vasopressor agents. The key determinants of survival are early recognition of sepsis and initiation of treatment while the process is readily reversible. This approach requires constant vigilance by the clinician caring for patients with a variety of medical and surgical illnesses.

FLUID RESUSCITATION

Fluid resuscitation is a mandatory first step in the treatment of septic shock. The diffuse vascular leak that occurs in septic shock necessitates provision of adequate circulating blood volume to maintain tissue perfusion. Debate continues regarding the appropriateness of colloid versus crystalloid fluids. The lack of clear evidence regarding the benefit of colloid agents (e.g., albumin, dextran, and plasma expanders) and their high cost have generally resulted in the use of saline solutions for volume expansion. A 1998 meta-analysis of studies comparing colloid versus crystalloid fluids in sepsis found a slight worsening of outcome with colloid solutions.[74] The optimal amount of fluid therapy for patients in septic shock remains a source of controversy.

A delicate balance is required between maintenance of tissue perfusion and prevention of fluid overload, with its attendant risk of lung injury. Decreased myocardial performance in patients with sepsis may necessitate a higher filling pressure for adequate cardiac output; however, exudation of fluids into the alveolar space in lung tissue and into the interstitium in other vital organs continues to be a major problem. Maintenance of a pulmonary arterial occlusion pressure of approximately 12 mm Hg is considered a reasonable starting point for patients who have hemodynamic monitors in place.[75] Diligent care and maintenance of central lines reduce the frequency of catheter-related sepsis.[76]

VASOPRESSOR THERAPY

When patients fail to improve hemodynamically with fluids alone, vasopressor agents are often used to reestablish systemic arterial blood pressure.

Dopamine

Dopamine has been the vasopressor agent of choice for the past 2 decades because of its presumed favorable effects on renal vasodilatation and its modest inotropic effects. However, the validity of the privileged status of this choice has been questioned.[77] Dopamine effects are complicated by the fact that this catecholamine has its own receptors (D_1 and D_2 dopaminergic receptors) as well as variable affinities for alpha- and beta-adrenergic receptors. The effects of dopamine depend on the receptor density in specific vascular beds, the blood volume, and the dose used. Higher doses increase the systemic vascular resistance by the effects of dopamine on alpha-adrenergic receptors in the peripheral circulation. Dopamine may have adverse effects on splanchnic blood flow,[69,70] and it has never been shown to be clearly beneficial for septic patients in an adequately controlled clinical trial.

Norepinephrine

Norepinephrine is a potent vasoconstrictor that is being used more frequently to treat the hemodynamic effects of septic shock. Earlier concerns regarding adverse consequences of norepinephrine on renal blood flow may have been overstated; studies suggest that it may actually increase urine output and creatinine clearance in septic patients.[78] Norepinephrine may rapidly restore perfusion pressure within the glomerulus and result in improved glomerular filtration in patients with adequate fluid resuscitation.

Dobutamine

Dobutamine, a beta agonist, may improve cardiac output and oxygen delivery in some patients in septic shock who manifest low cardiac output. However, dobutamine may result in peripheral vasodilatation, which may be harmful for septic patients. Moreover, dobutamine increases myocardial oxygen consumption by its positive inotropic effects, which also may be detrimental. The use of a vasopressor agent in patients with septic shock carries certain risks and should be used only when fluid therapy alone is insufficient to restore hemodynamic stability.

ASSESSMENT OF ADEQUATE TISSUE PERFUSION

The most reliable indicator to assess the adequacy of tissue perfusion in septic shock is not known. It would seem logical to provide adequate oxygen delivery to tissues to meet the metabolic demands of the septic patient. The concept of supply-dependent oxygen consumption was developed by Shoemaker and colleagues.[53] This idea has yet to be proved as a clinical guide in the treatment of septic shock. Numerous methods for measuring tissue oxygenation have been developed to better determine and understand the critical requirements for oxygen delivery to the tissues of septic patients. These methods include gastric tonometry, hepatic venous oxygen measurements, direct tissue oxygen measurements, and other methods. However, the practical value of these measurements in the clinical management of sepsis remains unclear.

BLOOD TRANSFUSIONS

The necessity to improve the oxygen-carrying capacity of blood with blood transfusions has been the subject of considerable debate.[79] It has been demonstrated that humans are remarkably resistant to adverse effects from isovolumetric reduction in hemoglobin values.[80] The lower limit of the transfusion threshold in patients with septic shock has not been defined, but it appears to be considerably lower than the traditional transfusion threshold of less than 10 g/dl. Studies of ICU patients indicate that a conservative transfusion policy set as low as 7 g/dl may in fact be preferable.[81]

MANAGEMENT OF RENAL FAILURE

Expert management of acute renal failure, ARDS, hepatic decompensation, coagulopathy, acid-base disturbances, and disordered hemodynamics is of paramount importance in the management of sepsis.

NUTRITIONAL SUPPORT

Nutritional support in patients with septic shock has changed considerably over the past 2 decades. Reliance on total parenteral nutrition has given way to early and extensive use of enteral hyperalimentation. Enteral feeding of septic patients has been shown to benefit enterocyte function, help maintain the intestinal permeability barrier, and help prevent gut-derived endotoxin and cytokine generation.[82] Nutrition supplementation with glutamine, arginine, and omega-3 fatty acids has experimental support and is increasingly being used in septic patients.[83] The incremental value of such enriched enteral formulations over standard enteral alimentation has not yet been confirmed in large clinical trials.

MANAGEMENT OF FEVER

Fever is commonly present in patients with severe sepsis and appears to be an advantageous response.[84] Heat-shock proteins function as intracellular chaperones to stabilize and prevent denaturation of host proteins. Heat-shock protein induction may actually decrease the mortality associated with experimental endotoxin challenge.[85] Efforts to lower body temperature with cooling blankets are largely ineffective and may not benefit the patient in septic shock. This strategy should generally be avoided unless true hyperthermia is present.[86]

ANTIMICROBIAL THERAPY

The most appropriate antimicrobial therapy for septic shock patients depends on the source of infection, susceptibility patterns of microbial pathogens within a given institution, prior antimicrobial exposure, presence or absence of pregnancy, hepatic and renal function, and history of drug allergy [*see Table 6*]. In septic shock, combinations of bactericidal antimicrobial agents are generally given on an empirical basis. Antibiotic combinations decrease the risk that a multidrug-resistant microbial pathogen will be missed and increase the probability that all important pathogenic microorganisms will be inhibited by at least one of the antimicrobial agents. Concern continues regarding antibiotic-induced endotoxin release in sepsis, but the clinical relevance of this effect has not been demonstrated and should not affect antibiotic choices for septic shock patients.[87]

Table 6 Suggested Empirical Antibiotic Choices in Severe Sepsis

Source of Infection	*Antimicrobial Choice*
Community-acquired pneumonia	Third-generation cephalosporin with a macrolide (alternative: fluoroquinolones)
Hospital-acquired pneumonia	Third- or fourth-generation cephalosporins, extended-spectrum penicillins with or without an aminoglycoside (alternatives: fluoroquinolones, carbapenems, β-lactam–β-lactamase inhibitor)
Urinary tract infections	Extended-spectrum β-lactam agent with or without an aminoglycoside (add ampicillin or vancomycin when enterococci are present)
Intra-abdominal infections	Third- or fourth-generation cephalosporins with or without metronidazole or clindamycin or extended-spectrum penicillins or β-lactam—β-lactamase inhibitor with or without an aminoglycoside (alternative: carbapenem, trovafloxacin)
Biliary tract infections	Extended-spectrum penicillin with or without an aminoglycoside
Neutropenic patients	Extended-spectrum β-lactam agent with an aminoglycoside (add vancomycin when there is evidence of gram-positive infection)

Emerging Therapies for Sepsis

Over the past 15 years, more than 30 double-blind, placebo-controlled, multicenter, phase 2 or phase 3 trials have been conducted to study the efficacy of new experimental agents in the treatment of septic shock.[1,5,88–90] None of these agents has successfully demonstrated convincing evidence of clinical efficacy in septic shock. There are many possible explanations for these failures.[88,89] However, despite these disappointments, work on improved therapies for sepsis continues [*see Table 7*]. Adjuvant strategies to inhibit endotoxin effects, modulate nitric oxide synthesis, attenuate coagulopathy, and regulate the immune response to sepsis indicate that improved therapies for sepsis may be available within the next few years.

Phase 3 clinical trials have shown that activated protein C lowers morbidity in septic patients. The trials were stopped after an interim analysis of approximately 1,500 consecutive patients revealed a survival benefit in the patient group receiving activated protein C over the placebo group.[73] A large (2,300 patients) multicenter trial with antithrombin III did not show any benefit.

Table 7 Experimental Therapies in the Treatment of Septic Shock

Experimental Agent	Treatment Target	Comment
Bactericidal/permeability-increasing protein	Endotoxin	Endotoxin-neutralizing human protein
Anti-CD14 antibody	Endotoxin/peptidoglycan	Endotoxin and peptidoglycan blocker
E5564	Endotoxin	Lipid A antagonist
Polymyxin B–binding columns	Endotoxin	Endotoxin-binding antibiotic
Platelet-activating factor (PAF)–acetylhydrolase	PAF	Rapid metabolism of PAF
FAB 2' anti–tumor necrosis factor (TNF) monoclonal antibody	TNF	Neutralizes TNF in the circulation
Low-dose corticosteroids	Adrenal function	Treat adrenal hypofunction of sepsis
Antithrombin III	Coagulation system	Inhibitors of disseminated intravascular coagulation, microthrombi
Tissue pathway factor inhibitor	Coagulation system	Inhibitors of disseminated intravascular coagulation, microthrombi
Activated protein C	Coagulation system	Inhibitors of disseminated intravascular coagulation, microthrombi
Soluble phospholipase A_2 (PLA_2) inhibitor	PLA_2	Blocks PLA_2-mediated lipid mediators

Positive results with activated protein C therapy (6.1% absolute reduction in mortality),[91] anti-TNF Fab2' antibody therapy (3.11% absolute reduction in mortality),[73,92] and suggestive findings with BPI[90] as an antiendotoxin agent portend a favorable outlook for sepsis therapy in the future.

Acknowledgment

Figures 1, 2, and 3 Seward Hung.

References

1. Bone R: Toward a theory regarding the pathogenesis of the systemic inflammatory response syndrome: what we do and do not know about cytokine regulation. Crit Care Med 24:163, 1996

2. Dellinger RP, Zimmerman J, Opal SM, et al: From the bench to the bedside: the future of sepsis research: executive summary of the American College of Chest Physicians. National Institute of Allergy and Infectious Diseases, and National Heart, Lung, and Bl. Chest 111:744, 1997

3. Opal SM: Lessons learned from clinical trials of sepsis. J Endotoxin Res 2:1, 1995

4. Bone RC, Balk RA, Cerra FB, et al: Definitions for sepsis in organ failure and guidelines for the use of innovative therapies in sepsis. Chest 101:1644, 1992

5. Zeni F, Freeman B, Natanson C: Anti-inflammatory therapies to treat sepsis and septic shock: a reassessment. Crit Care Med 25:1097, 1997

6. Bone RC, Fisher CJ Jr, Clemmer TP, et al: Sepsis syndrome: a valid clinical entity. Crit Care Med 17:339, 1989

7. Cross AS, Opal SM, Sadoff JC, et al: Choice of bacteria in animal models of sepsis. Infect Immun 61:2741, 1993

8. Increase in national hospital discharge survey rates for septicemia: United States, 1979–1987. MMWR Morb Mortal Wkly Rep 39:31, 1990

9. Sands KE, Bates DW, Lanken PN, et al: Epidemiology of sepsis syndrome in eight academic medical centers. JAMA 278:234, 1997

10. Bone RC: Gram-positive organisms in sepsis. Arch Intern Med 154: 26, 1994

11. Rietschel ET, Brade H, Holst O, et al: Bacterial endotoxin: chemical composition, biological recognition, host response, and immunological detoxification. Curr Top Microbiol Immunol 216:39, 1996

12. Horn DL, Opal SM, Lomastro E: Antibiotics, cytokines, and endotoxin: a complex and evolving relationship in gram-negative sepsis. Scand J Infect Dis 101:9, 1996

13. Opal SM: Phylogenetic and functional relationships between coagulation and the innate immune response. Crit Care Med 28:S77, 2000

14. Medzhitov R, Preston-Hurlburt P, Janeway CA Jr: A human homologue of the *Drosophila* Toll protein signals activations of adaptive immunity. Nature 388:394, 1997

15. Poltorak A, He X, Smirnova I, et al: Defective LPS signaling in C3H/HeJ and C57BL/10ScCr mice: mutations in the rlt4 gene. Science 282:2085, 1998

16. Takeuchi O, Hoshino K, Kawai T, et al: Differential roles of TLR2 and TLR4 in recognition of gram-negative and gram-positive bacterial cell wall components. Immunity 11:443, 1999

17. Lien E, Sellati TJ, Yoshimura A, et al: Toll-like receptor 2 functions as a pattern recognition receptor for diverse bacterial products. J Biol Chem 274:33419, 1999

18. Rock FL, Hardiman G, Timans JC, et al: A family of human receptors structurally related to *Drosophila* Toll. Proc Natl Acad Sci USA 95: 588, 1998

19. Hacker H, Vabulas RM, Takeuchi O, et al: Immune cell activation by bacterial CpG-DNA through myeloid differentiation marker 88 and tumor necrosis factor receptor-associated factor (TRAF) 6. J Exp Med 192:595, 2000

20. Akira S: Roles of toll-like receptors in microbial recognition. J Endo Res 6:76, 2000

21. Hemmi E, Takeuchi O, Kawai T, et al: A Toll-like receptor recognizes bacterial DNA. Nature 408:740, 2000

22. Fenton MJ, Golenbock DT: LPS-binding proteins and receptors. J Leuk Biol 64:25, 1998

23. Ulevitch RJ, Tobias PS: Receptor-dependent mechanisms of cell stimulation by bacterial endotoxin. Annu Rev Immunol 13:437, 1995

24. Schumann RR, Leong SR, Flaggs GW: Structure and function of lipopolysaccharide-binding protein. Science 49:1431, 1992

25. Opal SM, Palardy JE, Marra MN, et al: Relative concentrations of endotoxin-binding proteins in body fluids during infection. Lancet 344: 429, 1994

26. von der Mohlen MAM, Kimmings AN, Wedel NI, et al: Inhibition of endotoxin-induced cytokine release and neutrophil activation in humans using recombinant bactericidal/permeability-increasing protein (rBPI23). J Infect Dis 172:144, 1995

27. Astiz ME, Rackow EC, Still JG, et al: Pretreatment of normal humans with monophosphoryl lipid A induces tolerance to endotoxin: a prospective, double-blind, randomized, controlled trial. Crit Care Med 23:9, 1995

28. Florquine S, Goldman M: Immunoregulatory mechanisms of T-cell-dependent shock induced by bacterial superantigen in mice. Infect Immun 64:3443, 1996

29. Choi Y, Lafferty JA, Clements JRL: Selective expansion of T cells expressing Vb2 in toxic shock syndrome. J Exp Med 172:981, 1990

30. Kusunoki T, Hailman E, Juan TS-C, et al: Molecules from *Staphylococcus aureus* that bind CD14 and stimulate innate immune responses. J Exp Med 182:1673, 1995

31. Cleveland MG, Gorham JD, Murphy TL, et al: Lipoteichoic acid preparations from gram-positive bacteria induce interleukin-12 through a CD14-dependent pathway. Infect Immun 64:1906, 1996

32. Opal SM, Cohen J: Clinical gram-positive sepsis: does it fundamentally differ from gram-negative bacterial sepsis. Crit Care Med 27: 1608, 1999

33. Casey LC, Balk RA, Bone RC: Plasma cytokine and endotoxin levels correlate with survival in patients with sepsis syndrome. Ann Intern Med 119:771, 1993

34. Dinarello CA: The proinflammatory cytokines interleukin-1 and tumor necrosis factor and treatment of the septic shock syndrome. J Infect Dis 63:1177, 1991

35. Dinarello CA, Gelfand JA, Wolff SM: Anticytokine strategies in the treatment of the systemic inflammatory response syndrome. JAMA 269:1825, 1993

36. Fantuzzi G, Dinarello CA: The inflammatory response in interleukin-1 beta-deficient mice: comparison with other cytokine-related knockout mice. J Leukoc Biol 59:489, 1996

37. Bone RC: Sir Isaac Newton, sepsis, SIRS and CARS. Crit Care Med 24:1125, 1996

38. Falk LA, McNally R, Perera PY, et al: LPS-inducible responses in severe combined immunodeficiency (SCID) mice. J Endotoxin Res 2:273, 1995

39. Szabo SJ, Dinghe AS, Gubler U, et al: Regulation of the interleukin (IL)-12Rb2 subunit expression in developing T helper 1 (Th1) and Th2 cells. J Exp Med 185:817, 1997

40. Faist E, Kim C: Therapeutic immunomodulatory approaches in the treatment of systemic inflammatory response syndrome and the prevention of sepsis. New Horiz 6:97, 1998

41. Kox WJ, Bone RC, Krausch D, et al: Interferon gamma-1b in the treatment of compensatory anti-inflammatory response syndrome: new approach: proof of principle. Arch Intern Med 157:389, 1997

42. van Deventer SJH, Buller HR, ten Cate JW, et al: Experimental endotoxemia in humans: analysis of cytokine release and coagulation, fibrinolytic and complement pathways. Blood 76:2520, 1990

43. Bauer KA, ten Cate H, Barzegar S, et al: Tumor necrosis factor infusions have a procoagulant effect on the hemostatic mechanism of humans. Blood 74:165, 1989

44. Levi M, ten Cate H, van der Poll T, et al: Pathogenesis of disseminated intravascular coagulation in sepsis. JAMA 270:975, 1993

45. Smith OP, White B, Vaughn D, et al: Use of protein-C concentrate, heparin, and haemodiafiltration in meningococcus-induced purpura fulminans. Lancet 350:1590, 1997

46. Luster AD: Chemokines: chemotactic cytokines that mediate inflammation. N Engl J Med 338:436, 1998

47. Petros A, Bennett D, Vallance P: Effect of nitric oxide synthase inhibitors on hypotension in patients with septic shock. Lancet 338:1557,1991

48. Shenep JL, Toumanen E: Prospective: targeting nitric oxide in the adjuvant therapy of sepsis in meningitis. J Infect Dis 177:766, 1998

49. Grover R, Lopez A, Lorente J, et al: Multicenter, randomized, placebo-controlled, double-blind study of the nitric oxide synthase inhibitor 546C88: Effect on survival in patients with septic shock. Crit Care Med 27:A33, 1999

50. Calandra T, Spiegel LA, Metz CN, et al: Macrophage migration inhibitory factor is a critical mediator of the activation of immune cells by exotoxins of gram-positive bacteria. Proc Natl Acad Sci USA 95:11383, 1998

51. Andersson U, Wang H, Palmblad K, et al: High mobility group 1 protein (HMG-1) stimulates pro-inflammatory cytokine synthesis in human monocytes. J Exp Med 192:565, 2000

52. Parker MN, Suffredini AF, Natanson C, et al: Responses of left ventricular function in survivors and non-survivors of septic shock. J Crit Care 4:19, 1989

53. Shoemaker WC, Montgomery ES, Kaplan E, et al: Physiologic patterns in surviving and non-surviving shock patients. Arch Surg 106:630, 1973

54. Hayes MA, Timmins AC, Yau EHS, et al: Elevation of systemic oxygen delivery in the treatment of critically ill patients. N Engl J Med 330:1717, 1994

55. Pittet D, Thievent B, Wenzel RP, et al: Importance of pre-existing co-morbidities for prognosis of septicemia in critically ill patients. Intensive Care Med 19:265, 1993

56. Finkel MS, Oddis CV, Jacob TD, et al: Negative inotropic effect of cytokines on the heart mediated by nitric oxide. Science 257:387, 1992

57. Milberg JA, Davis DR, Steinberg KP, et al: Improved survival of patients with acute respiratory distress syndrome (ARDS): 1983–1993. JAMA 273:306, 1995

58. Stewart TE, Meade MO, Cook DJ, et al: Evaluation of a ventilation strategy to prevent barotrauma in patients at high risk for acute respiratory distress syndrome. N Engl J Med 338:355, 1998

59. The Acute Respiratory Distress Syndrome Network: ventilation with lower tidal volumes as compared with traditional tidal volume for acute lung injury and the acute respiratory distress syndrome. N Engl J Med 324:1301, 2000

60. Opal SM, Scannon P, Vincent JL, et al: Relationship between plasma levels of lipopolysaccharide (LPS) and LPS-binding protein in patients with severe sepsis and septic shock. J Infect Dis 180:1584, 1999

61. Sriskandan S, Moyes D, Cohen J: Detection of circulating bacterial superantigen and lymphotoxin alpha in patients with streptococcal toxic-shock syndrome. Lancet 348:1315, 1986

62. Damas P, Ledoux D, Nys M, et al: Cytokine serum levels during severe sepsis in humans: IL-6 as a marker of severity. Ann Surg 215:356, 1992

63. Reinhart K, Wiegand-Lohnert C, Grimminger F, et al: Assessment of the safety and efficacy of the monoclonal anti-tumor necrosis factor antibody-fragment, MAK 195F, in patients with sepsis and septic shock: a multicenter, randomized, placebo-controlled, dose-ranging study. Crit Care Med 24:733, 1996

64. Opal SM, Fisher CJ, Pribble JP, et al: The confirmatory interleukin-1 receptor antagonist trial in sepsis: a phase III randomized, double-blind, placebo-controlled, multicenter trial. Crit Care Med 25:1115, 1997

65. Fisher CJ, Dhainaut J-F, Opal SM, et al: Recombinant human interleukin-1 receptor antagonist in the treatment of patients with sepsis syndrome: results from a randomized, double-blind, placebo-controlled trial. JAMA 271:1836, 1994

66. Fisher CJ, Opal SM, Dhainaut J-F, et al: Influence of a murine anti-TNF monoclonal antibody (CB0006) on cytokine levels in patients with sepsis. Crit Care Med 2:318, 1993

67. Gendrel D, Assicot M, Raymond J, et al: Procalcitonin as a marker for the early diagnosis of neonatal infection. J Pediatr 128:570, 1996

68. deWerra I, Jacchard C, Corradin SB, et al: Cytokines, nitrite/nitrate, soluble tumor necrosis factor receptors, and procalcitonin concentration: comparisons in patients with septic shock, cardiogenic shock, and bacterial pneumonia. Crit Care Med 25:607, 1997

69. Staehler M, Hammer C, Meiser B, et al: Procalcitonin: a new marker for differential diagnosis of acute rejection and bacterial infection in heart transplantation. Transplant Proc 29:584, 1997

70. Karzai W, Oberhoffer M, Meier-Helmann A, et al: Procalcitonin: a new indicator of systemic response to severe infections. Infection 6:629, 1997

71. Hack CA, Hart M, van Schijndel RJ, et al: Interleukin-8 in sepsis: relation to shock and inflammatory mediators. Infect Immun 60:2835, 1992

72. Rae D, Porter J, Beechey-Newman N, et al: Type 1-prophospholipase A_2 propeptide in acute lung injury. Lancet 344:1472, 1994

73. Bernard G, Larosa S, Laterre P, et al: The efficacy and safety of recombinant human activated protein C for the treatment of patients with severe sepsis. Crit Care Med 28(suppl):A48, 2000

74. Schierhout G, Roberts I: Fluid resuscitation with colloid or crystalloid solutions in critically ill patients: a systemic review of randomized trials. BMJ 316:961, 1998

75. Rackow EC, Kaufman BS, Falk JL, et al: Hemodynamic response to fluid resuscitation in patients with septic shock: evidence for early depression of cardiac performance. Circ Shock 22:11, 1987

76. Mermel LA: Prevention of intravascular catheter-related infections. Ann Intern Med 132:391, 2000

77. Martin C, Papazian L, Perrin G, et al: Norepinephrine or dopamine for the treatment of hyperdynamic septic shock? Chest 103:1826, 1993

78. Marin C, Eon B, Saux P, et al: Renal effects of norepinephrine used to treat septic shock patients. Crit Care Med 18:282, 1990

79. Hebert PC, Wells G, Marshall J, et al: Transfusion requirements in critical care. JAMA 273:1439, 1995

80. Weiskopf RB, Viely MK, Feiner J, et al: Human cardiovascular and metabolic response to acute, severe isovolemic anemia. JAMA 279:217, 1998

81. Hebert PC, Wells G, Blajchman MA, et al: A multicenter, randomized, controlled clinical trial of transfusion requirements in critical care. N Engl J Med 340:409, 1999

82. Kudsk KA, Croce MA, Fabian TC, et al: Enteral vs. parenteral feeding: effects on septic morbidity after blunt and penetrating abdominal trauma. Ann Surg 215:503, 1992

83. Bower RH, Cerra FB, Bershadshy B, et al: Early enteral administration of a formula (Impact) supplemented with arginine, nucleotides, and fish oil in intensive care unit patients: results of a multicenter, prospective, randomized, clinical trial. Crit Care Med 23: 436, 1995

84. Kluger MJ, Kozak W, Conn C, et al: The adaptive value of fever. Infect Dis Clin North Am 10:1, 1996

85. Ribeiro SP, Chu E, Slutsky AS: Heat stress after injection of LPS in rats decreases mortality. Am J Respir Crit Care Med 153:A252, 1996

86. O'Donnell J, Axelrod R, Fisher C, et al: Use and effectiveness of hypothermia blankets for febrile patients in the intensive care unit. Clin Infect Dis 24:1208, 1997

87. Prins JM, van Deventer SJH, Kuijper EJ, et al: Clinical relevance of antibiotic-induced endotoxin release. Antimicrob Agents Chemother 38:1211, 1994

88. Opal SM, Cross AS: Clinical trials for sepsis: past failures and future hopes. Inf Dis Clin North Am 13:285, 1999

89. Abraham E, Matthay MA, Dinarello CA, et al: Consensus conference definitions for sepsis, acute lung injury, and ARDS: time for reevaluation. Crit Care Med 28:232, 2000

90. Levin M, Quint PA, Goldstein B, et al: Recombinant bactericidal/permeability-increasing protein ($rBPI_{21}$) as adjunctive treatment for children with severe meningococcal disease: a randomized trial. Lancet 356:961, 2000

91. Bernard GR, Vincent J-L, Laterre P-F, et al: Efficacy and safety of recombinant human activated protein C for severe sepsis. N Engl J Med (in press)

92. Marshall J, Panacek E, Barchuk W: Modeling organ dysfunction as a risk factor, outcome and measure of biologic effect in sepsis: result of the MONARC trial. Crit Care Med 28 (suppl):A46, 2000

93. Bernard GR, Artigas A, Brigham KL, et al: The American-European Consensus Conference on ARDS: definitions, mechanisms, relevant outcomes, and clinical trial coordination. Am J Respir Crit Care Med 149:181, 1994

94. Murray JF, Matthay MA, Luce JM, et al: An expanded definition of the adult respiratory distress syndrome. Am Rev Respir Dis 138:720, 1988

5 Bacterial Infections of the Upper Respiratory Tract

Harvey B. Simon, M.D.

Overview of Upper Respiratory Tract Infections

Upper respiratory tract infections range from common, benign processes, such as nasopharyngitis, to uncommon, potentially lethal processes, such as epiglottitis. Pathogens range from pyogenic bacteria [see 15 Infections Due to Gram-Positive Cocci and 23 Infections Due to Mycobacteria] to *Chlamydia* [see 28 Diseases Due to *Chlamydia*], mycoplasmas [see 27 Infections Due to Mycoplasmas], respiratory viruses [see 31 Respiratory Viral Infections], and, on occasion, fungi [see 20 Infections Due to the Enteric Pathogens *Campylobacter, Salmonella, Shigella, Yersinia, Vibrio,* and *Helicobacter*]. Despite this heterogeneity, some general anatomic and physiologic principles apply.

PATHOPHYSIOLOGY

The upper respiratory tract is composed of two distinct types of epithelial surface. A stratified squamous epithelium lines the oropharynx and nasopharynx [*see Figure 1*]. These regions are normally teeming with a varied microbial flora, and many potential pathogens can temporarily colonize these epithelial surfaces without causing true infection [*see Table 1*]. Bacteriologic cultures are easily obtained from these areas. As a result, the microbiology laboratory faces the challenge of isolating potential pathogens from the normal mouth flora, and the clinician faces the challenge of distinguishing between the carrier state and active infection. A respiratory epithelium, composed of ciliated columnar cells, goblet cells, and mucous and serous glands, lines the paranasal sinuses, the middle ear, and the airway below the epiglottis. These regions, in contrast to the oropharynx and nasopharynx, are normally sterile. Because these areas are inaccessible for routine culture, it is often necessary to diagnose and treat infections on the basis of clinical findings and statistical probabilities [*see Table 1*] rather than on the basis of bacteriologic data derived from the patient.

Many host defense mechanisms protect the upper airway from infection. Mechanical defenses tend to prevent penetration by organisms from the nasopharynx and oral cavity into more vulnerable areas. These defenses are the cough, gag, and sneeze reflexes; the viscous mucous secretions, which entrap particulate material; and ciliary action, which propels entrapped particles outward. In addition, local immunologic defenses attempt to deal with organisms that have breached the mechanical barriers; such defenses include abundant lymphoid tissue, secretory IgA antibodies in respiratory secretions, and a rich vasculature that can rapidly deliver phagocytic leukocytes.

ETIOLOGY

Upper respiratory tract infections typically occur after insults to the mechanical defenses—such as allergic rhinitis, chemical irritation, trauma, and, especially, viral respiratory tract infections—that impair ciliary function and produce increased volumes of thin secretions and mucosal edema that block the narrow channels draining the sinuses and middle ear. Barotrauma, which results from a rapid change in atmospheric pressure, can intensify upper respiratory tract problems, particularly in patients with rhinitis, otitis, or sinusitis.

COMPLICATIONS

The complications of upper airway infections stem from several factors. The proximity of upper airway structures to the central nervous system and the presence of abundant vascular channels connecting the two account for some of the most severe complications. In addition, the numerous fascial planes of the head and neck provide potential spaces where infection can become sequestered. Furthermore, the upper airway is narrow, so that infection in the neck may compromise the patency of the airway itself. Finally, immunosuppression renders persons vulnerable to unusual pathogens and unusual complications.

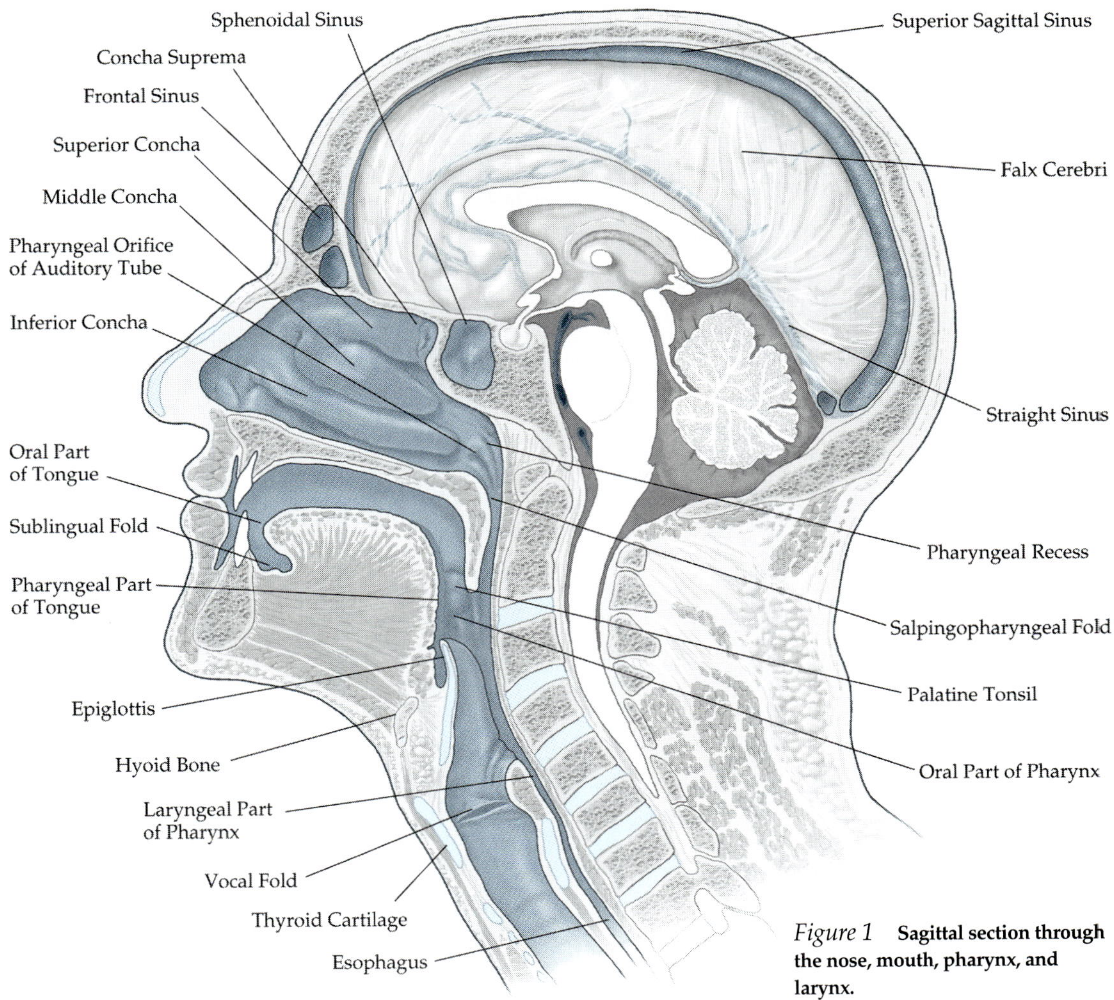

Figure 1 **Sagittal section through the nose, mouth, pharynx, and larynx.**

Sinusitis

Although infections of the paranasal sinuses are common, they are greatly overdiagnosed by patient and physician. Acute sinusitis is characterized by nasal congestion, purulent nasal discharge, fetid breath, facial pain that typically increases when the patient stoops forward, and, often, fever and other systemic symptoms. In most patients, acute sinusitis responds well to medical therapy; in a few persons, however, chronic sinusitis may result. Chronic sinusitis is characterized by purulent discharge, usually without fever, that persists for weeks or months.

ETIOLOGY

Viral, allergic, or vasomotor rhinitis is frequently an antecedent event to sinusitis. Nose blowing propels nasal fluid into the sinuses, potentially introducing viscid fluid and bacteria that could lead to sinusitis.[1] Nasal polyps, deviation of the nasal septum, or hypertrophied adenoids may predispose to purulent sinusitis by obstructing sinus drainage. Cigarette smoke and overuse of topical decongestants impair ciliary action and alter the mucous blanket, predisposing to sinusitis. Contributing factors may also include rapid changes in altitude, trauma, intranasal foreign bodies or tumors, cocaine abuse, and such systemic processes as cystic fibrosis and Kartagener syndrome (situs inversus, bronchiectasis, and sinusitis). Factors that predispose to chronic sinusitis include inadequately treated bacterial infections, long-term impairment of mucociliary clearance, obstruction of sinus drainage, and allergies and asthma. Nosocomial sinusitis occurs as a complication of

Table 1 Major Microbial Flora of the Upper Respiratory Tract

Organism	*Oral Cavity*	*Nasopharynx, Tonsils*	*Epiglottis, Larynx*	*Paranasal Sinuses, Middle Ear*
Gram-positive cocci				
Staphylococcus epidermidis	NF	NF		UP
S. aureus		CC	UP	UP
Pneumococci		CC	UP	CP
Group A streptococci		CC, CP	UP	CP
Groups C and G streptococci		CC, UP		
Other streptococci	NF	NF		CP
Gram-positive bacilli				
Diphtheroids	NF	NF		
Corynebacterium diphtheriae		UC, UP	UP	
Arcanobacterium haemolyticum				
Gram-positive anaerobes				
Anaerobic streptococci	NF	NF		UP*
Anaerobic diphtheroids	NF	NF		
Actinomyces species	NF, UP			
Gram-negative cocci				
Neisseria meningitidis		CC, UP		
N. gonorrhoeae		UC, UP		
Other *Neisseria* species	NF	NF		UP
Moraxella catarrhalis	NF	NF		CP
Gram-negative coccobacilli				
Haemophilus influenzae		CC, UP	CP	CP
Other *Haemophilus* species	NF	NF		
Gram-negative bacilli				
Enterobacteriaceae	UC	UC	UP	
Pseudomonas aeruginosa	UC	UC		
Gram-negative anaerobes				
Bacteroides species	NF, UP			UP*
Fusobacterium species	NF, UP			UP*
Veillonella species	NF			
Mycobacterium				
M. tuberculosis	UP	UP	UP	UP
Spirochetes				
Borrelia species	NF, UP	NF, UP		
Treponema pallidum	UP	UP		
Fungi				
Candida albicans	NF	NF, UP		
Aspergillus species				UP
Mucor species				UP
Chlamydia				
C. pneumoniae (TWAR)		UP		
Mycoplasma				
M. pneumoniae		UC, UP	UP	UC, UP
Viruses				
Epstein-Barr virus		CP, CC		
Herpes simplex virus	CC, CP	UP		
Influenza virus		CP	CP	
Parainfluenza virus		CP	CP	
Adenovirus		CP, UC	CP	
Coxsackievirus	CP	CP	CP	
Rhinovirus		CP	CP	
Respiratory syncytial virus		CP	CP	

*Anaerobic bacteria predominate in the normal flora of the upper respiratory tract. They are uncommon pathogens in acute infections but are common pathogens in chronic sinusitis and otitis, as well as in abscesses, soft tissue infections, and periodontal infections; aerobic pathogens participate synergistically in most of these processes.

CC — Common colonizer: organism present in many individuals, often transiently, without causing disease; CP — Common pathogen: organism frequently causes disease in this location; NF — Normal flora: organism present in most healthy individuals; UC — Uncommon colonizer: organism present without causing disease but relatively uncommon; UP — Uncommon pathogen: organism infrequently causes disease in this location.

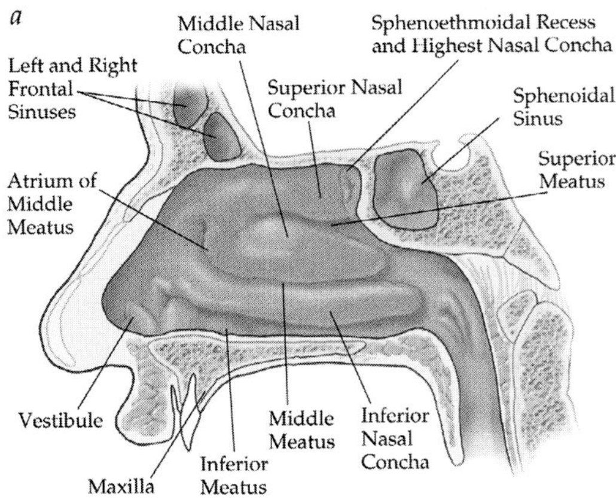

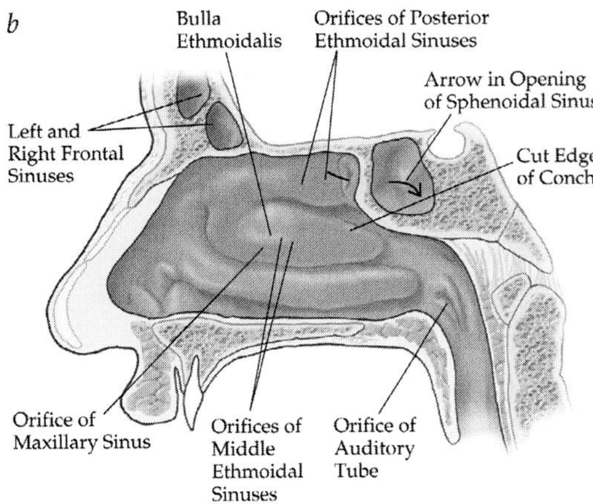

Figure 2 **(*a*) The lateral wall of the right half of the nasal cavity: internal aspect. (*b*) The three nasal conchae have been partially removed.**

nasotracheal intubation or, less often, nasoenteric feeding tubes.[2] Unexplained fever may be the presenting symptom, and computed tomography scanning is often required for diagnosis if the patient cannot localize the pain.

Immunosuppression increases the frequency and severity of sinusitis. Sinusitis is common in patients with AIDS and is often severe and refractory to treatment.[3]

CLINICAL VARIANTS

The sinuses may be involved singly or, more often, in combination [*see Figure 2*]. Frontal sinusitis and maxillary sinusitis are most common in adults; ethmoiditis is most common in children.

Frontal sinusitis produces pain and tenderness over the lower forehead and purulent drainage from the middle meatus of the nasal turbinates. Maxillary sinusitis produces pain and tenderness over the cheeks. Pain is often referred to the teeth, and the hard palate may be edematous in severe cases. Purulent drainage is present in the middle meatus. Patients with ethmoidal sinusitis complain of retro-orbital pain and may have pain, tenderness, and even erythema over the upper lateral aspect of the nose. The anterior ethmoidal cells drain through the middle meatus, whereas the posterior cells drain through the superior meatus. Isolated sphenoid sinusitis, which occurs in only 3% of patients with sinusitis, is often misdiagnosed. This disorder has traditionally been considered to cause pain at the occiput or vertex; in fact, frontotemporal, retro-orbital, or facial pain is more common. Photophobia and tearing may be present. Purulent drainage is present in the superior meatus.

DIAGNOSIS

Clinical Features and Imaging Studies

Acute sinusitis The diagnosis of acute sinusitis can usually be established on clinical grounds. A poor response to decongestants and maxillary toothache are useful criteria.[4] Purulent nasal discharge is not specific for sinusitis and may occur in viral nasopharyngitis.[5] The diagnosis of sinusitis can be confirmed by the finding of opacity when the frontal or maxillary sinuses are transilluminated or by radiographic findings such as mucosal thickening, sinus opacification, or air-fluid levels.

Chronic sinusitis The symptoms of chronic sinusitis are nasal congestion and discharge; pain and headache are usually mild or absent, and fever is uncommon. Bone erosion may be present in chronic sinusitis. CT scans provide much more information than the traditional sinus x-ray series.[6] Radiologic studies are essential in the diagnosis of severe, refractory, nosocomial, or complicated cases of sinusitis but are not necessary in routine cases.

Bacteriology

Because of technical difficulties in obtaining valid cultures, the bacteriology of sinusitis has been incompletely defined. Nasal cultures are unreliable because they correlate poorly with actual sinus fluid. Sinus punctures reveal that the most common pathogens in acute sinusitis are *Haemophilus influenzae*, pneumococci, streptococci, and *Moraxella catarrhalis*.[4,6] *Staphylococcus aureus* has been isolated in nasal cultures from some patients with acute sinusitis, but the organisms are probably contaminants rather than the true causative agents. Nosocomial sinusitis is typically polymicrobial; *S. aureus* and gram-negative bacilli are often present.[7]

Chronic sinusitis is usually a polymicrobial infection. Anaerobic organisms have been isolated in as many as 51% of patients with chronic sinusitis; anaerobic streptococci and *Bacteroides* species predominate. Anaerobes are also important in chronic sinusitis because they predominate in brain abscesses associated with sinus infections. *S. aureus* has been recovered from cultures in as many as 33% of patients with chronic sinusitis; enteric gram-negative bacilli may also be present.

Viruses seldom cause clinical sinusitis. Such fungi as *Aspergillus*, *Mucor*, and *Rhizopus* species produce invasive sinusitis in patients with leukemia or poorly controlled diabetes[8,9] and, occasionally, in normal hosts.[9] In immunocompromised patients, sinusitis may also be caused by *Candida*, *Alternaria*, *Pseudomonas*, *Nocardia*, *Legionella*, atypical mycobacteria, and certain parasites.[10–12]

DIFFERENTIAL DIAGNOSIS

Noninfectious processes must be considered in the differential diagnosis of sinusitis. Allergic or vasomotor rhinitis is by far the most common noninfectious cause of sinus symptoms. However, polyps, tumors, cysts, foreign bodies, and vasculitis (such as Wegener granulomatosis) occasionally produce symptoms of sinusitis.

TREATMENT

Acute sinusitis is treated with analgesics and topical heat for patient comfort. Decongestants are of paramount importance. Pseudoephedrine can be administered orally or by nasal spray. The danger of rebound after short-term use of nasal spray has probably been exaggerated. Patients should spray each nostril once and then wait a minute to allow the anterior nasal mucosa to shrink; a repeat spray will reach the upper and posterior mucosa, including the nasal turbinates and sinus ostia. This procedure can be repeated every 4 hours for several days when needed. Antihistamines may thicken secretions and are therefore less likely to promote drainage. Steroids are not necessary in most patients and may be harmful. Nasal inhalation of warm, humidified vapor may relieve symptoms. Sleeping supine or with the head of the bed elevated 45° promotes sinus drainage; patients with unilateral sinusitis should be encouraged to sleep with the unaffected side on the pillow. Other ancillary measures that may be helpful are nasal saline irrigations and aerobic exercise, which promotes mucous flow. Mucoregulating agents are often recommended but have not been adequately studied.

Many patients with uncomplicated acute sinusitis respond well to decongestants and steam inhalations and do not need antibiotics.[13] Antibiotics should be used in toxic patients, in patients who fail to respond to decongestants, and in patients who have complications. Ampicillin, amoxicillin, amoxicillin–clavulanic acid, and trimethoprim-sulfamethoxazole have produced good results. Other agents that are widely used are cefaclor, cefuroxime, clarithromycin, levofloxacin, and, in children, erythromycin-sulfisoxazole.[4,5] Because both *H. influenzae* and *M. catarrhalis* can produce β-lactamase, the use of antibiotics that resist these enzymes has attracted interest. However, antibiotics that are resistant to β-lactamase have not proved to be superior to those that are susceptible, possibly because comparative studies have been small and because many patients recover without antibiotic therapy; the differences among various antimicrobials is small,[14] and both trimethoprim-sulfamethoxazole and amoxicillin appear to be as effective as newer and much more expensive drugs.[15] The optimal duration of antimicrobial therapy is no more certain than are the indications for therapy or the choice of agents; 7- to 14-day courses of antibiotics are traditional, but one trial found 3 days of trimethoprim-sulfamethoxazole to be as effective as 10 days of therapy.[16] Clinical guidelines for the diagnosis and treatment of sinusitis are available.[17]

Surgical intervention should be avoided in acute sinusitis unless the patient fails to respond to medical therapy and complications are present. Surgical drainage may be necessary in cases of chronic sinusitis or nosocomial sinusitis[7] and is mandatory in invasive fungal sinusitis.[8,9]

Functional endoscopic sinus surgery has provided an important advance in the surgical management of sinusitis. Patients with recurrent or chronic sinusitis who fail to respond to vigorous medical management may be candidates for this procedure. The patient should undergo a detailed preoperative evaluation, which usually includes a sinus CT scan. Surgery is performed using either local anesthesia with sedation or general anesthesia. A fiberoptic nasal endoscope is used to visualize the sinus ostia; when obstruction is present, it can be relieved. This technique restores patency and allows normal ciliary action to transport mucus to the natural ostium. Complications are uncommon when the procedure is performed by a skilled surgeon.

COMPLICATIONS

The potentially life-threatening complications of sinusitis have become uncommon in the antibiotic era. However, frontal sinusitis can lead to osteomyelitis of the frontal bones, especially in children. Patients have headache, fever, and a characteristic doughy edema, termed Pott puffy tumor, over the affected bone.[18] The organisms involved are those responsible for the underlying sinusitis, although *S. aureus* is more common in osteomyelitis than in sinusitis. Treatment should include decongestants for the sinusitis, high-dose intravenous antibiotics for the osteomyelitis, and surgical debridement when bone destruction is substantial. It is important to rule out coexisting brain abscess of the frontal lobe, which may be clinically occult.

Because the orbit is bordered on three sides by the paranasal sinuses, orbital infection can result from sinusitis. This disorder is most frequently a complication of ethmoidal sinusitis; it is caused by direct extension of infection through the lamina papyracea. Orbital cellulitis usually begins with edema of the eyelids and rapidly progresses to ptosis, proptosis, chemosis, and diminished extraocular movements. Patients are usually febrile and acutely ill. Pressure on the optic nerve may lead to vision loss, which can be permanent; retrograde spread can lead to intracranial infection. Therapy with high-dose intravenous antibiotics is mandatory. Unless a specific pathogen can be isolated from the blood or from purulent drainage, antibiotics should cover both staphylococci and gram-negative rods. When an orbital abscess is present, surgical drainage may be necessary; CT and ultrasound studies aid this evaluation.

Retrograde spread along venous channels from the sinuses, the orbit, or the nose can produce septic cavernous sinus thrombophlebitis. Patients have high fever and appear toxic. Lid edema, proptosis, and chemosis are present. In cavernous sinus thrombophlebitis (but not in uncomplicated orbital cellulitis), third, fourth, and sixth cranial nerve palsies are prominent; the pupil may be fixed and dilated, and ophthalmoscopic examination may reveal venous engorgement and papilledema. Although at first the process is usually unilateral, spread across the anterior and posterior intercavernous sinuses makes it bilateral. Patients may exhibit alterations of consciousness, and lumbar puncture may reveal inflammatory changes in the cerebrospinal fluid. CT with a contrast agent or venography may help confirm the diagnosis. High-dose intravenous antibiotics, including antistaphylococcal drugs, are mandatory. Anticoagulants are not of established benefit and may even be harmful.

Sinusitis can lead to intracranial suppuration either by direct spread through bone or by spread through venous channels. Various syndromes, such as epidural abscess, subdural empyema, meningitis, and brain abscess, can result. Clinical findings, which vary greatly, range from the subtle personality changes of frontal lobe abscesses to headache, symptoms of elevated intracranial pressure, alterations of consciousness, visual symptoms, focal neurologic deficits, seizures, and, ultimately, coma and death. These are true medical emergencies requiring high-dose antibiotics and, except for meningitis, neurosurgical intervention [see 13 Bacterial Infections of the Central Nervous System].

Otitis

ACUTE OTITIS MEDIA

Although acute otitis media is common in young children, its incidence declines with age, and it is uncommon in adults. Purulent otitis media results when bacteria ascend from the nasopharynx to the normally sterile middle ear. Abnormal eustachian tube function or obstruction caused by viral or allergic nasopharyngitis is considered important in the pathogenesis; heredity may also play a role.[19]

Etiology

The most common causes of purulent otitis media are the pneumococcus, nontypable strains of *H. influenzae*, and *M. catarrhalis*.[20] Other organisms that can cause acute otitis media are streptococci, *S. epidermidis*, and anaerobic bacteria. Gram-negative bacilli and S. aureus can cause acute otitis media in neonates. Viruses and mycoplasmas are uncommon as the primary pathogens in acute otitis media, but in 41% of children with acute bacterial otitis, respiratory tract viruses are also present; respiratory syncytial virus is the most common, followed by parainfluenza and influenza viruses.[21] Purulent nosocomial otitis is uncommon and occurs in only 4% of patients who have undergone endotracheal intubation; gram-negative bacilli are the responsible agents in this setting.

Diagnosis

Pain and hearing loss are the classic presenting complaints; fever is present in some cases. The cornerstone of the clinical diagnosis is a bulging tympanic membrane, with impaired mobility and obscuration of the bony landmarks. Tympanic membrane perforation and otorrhea may occur.

Needle aspiration of the middle ear can be used to confirm the diagnosis of purulent otitis media and to identify the causative organism, but it is seldom necessary because the bacteriology of otitis media is well defined and the response to antibiotics easy to monitor. Routine nose or throat cultures are not diagnostically reliable.

Differential Diagnosis

The major disorder considered in the differential diagnosis is serous otitis media. Fever and pain are absent in serous otitis media; although fluid is present in the middle ear, the tympanic membrane is usually retracted and the bony landmarks are preserved.

Treatment

Acute otitis media may be treated with analgesics, decongestants, and antibiotics. The utility of antibiotics is being reappraised.[20,22,23] Except in the Netherlands, where only about 30% of patients with otitis media take antibiotics, nearly all affected patients in developed countries are treated with antibiotics. In the United States, 20% of all prescriptions for oral antibiotics are issued for the treatment of otitis media; the average child consumes 3 months' worth of antibiotics in the first two years of life.[24] The benefits of antibiotics appear modest, however; a meta-analysis concluded that to prevent one child from experiencing pain by 2 to 7 days after infection, 17 children must be treated with antibiotics.[25] *H. influenzae*, *M. catarrhalis*, and *S. pneumoniae*, the organisms most frequently responsible for acute otitis media, are manifesting dramatically increased resistance to antibiotics. Further studies are required to determine which patients are most likely to benefit from antibiotics, which drugs are best, and how long therapy should be continued. Until such data are available, clinicians in the United States are likely to continue their traditional use of such drugs as ampicillin, amoxicillin, amoxicillin–clavulanic acid, trimethoprim-sulfamethoxazole, and the newer oral cephalosporins. As in the case of sinusitis, drugs active against β-lactamase–producing bacteria have not proved to be superior to amoxicillin in the treatment of acute otitis media; perhaps because antibiotics are only slightly more effective than placebos,[26] 81% of patients with acute otitis media recover without any antibiotic therapy.[27] Although antibiotics are generally administered for 10 days, 5 days of treatment may be equally effective in uncomplicated cases.[28,29] A single intramuscular dose of ceftriaxone is also as efficacious as 10 days of oral therapy.[30] Antibiotics may be used for chemoprophylaxis of recurrent otitis in children.[20] Myringotomy does not hasten recovery but is indicated for patients with intractable pain, progressive deafness, or early mastoiditis or who respond poorly to medical therapy.

Complications

The prognosis for acute otitis media is excellent. Chronic serous otitis media, hearing loss, and recurrent purulent otitis media are the most common complications. Recurrences are usually caused by reinfection rather than relapse or persistent infection; tympanostomy tubes may be helpful in children with numerous recurrences.

Acute mastoiditis, which is now rare, develops in patients with inadequately treated otitis media. Presenting symptoms consist of fever, otalgia, and postauricular edema and tenderness. The tympanic membrane is abnormal in all cases; perforations and otorrhea are present in about half of cases. Mastoid x-rays are usually abnormal. The species of bacteria responsible for mastoiditis are the same as those that cause acute otitis media. Patients who fail to respond to antibiotic therapy within 48 hours and those with CNS complications should be considered for early mastoidectomy.

Other suppurative complications of acute otitis media are also rare, including purulent labyrinthitis, meningitis, lateral sinus thrombosis, and brain abscess. Bacteremia can be documented in 3% of febrile young children with otitis media, but it does not appear to alter the prognosis or to warrant parenteral antibiotic therapy.

CHRONIC OTITIS MEDIA

Chronic otitis media, which can occur at any age, results from neglected or recurrent acute otitis media. Pain and fever are usually absent but can occur during sporadic flare-ups. Diminished hearing and foul otorrhea are major symptoms.

Physical examination discloses perforation of the tympanic membrane. Central perforations of the pars tensa are associated with benign disease, but peripheral perforations may occur with invasive cholesteatomas. X-rays reveal sclerosis of the mastoid air cells and bone destruction. Various organisms can be cultured from middle-ear drainage, including *P. aeruginosa*, staphylococci, streptococci, and enteric gram-negative bacilli. Anaerobes are present in 16% of cases, almost always in mixed infections with aerobes. Antibiotics are generally of little benefit, and surgery is required in advanced cases. Without therapy, chronic otitis media can cause the same intracranial suppurative complications seen in acute otitis media.

OTITIS EXTERNA

Otitis externa is a common, generally benign inflammatory disorder usually precipitated by excessive moisture in or trauma to the external auditory canal. Patients have pruritus or pain, or both, that may be severe. Crusting, inflammation, and discharge in the canal are typical findings, and pain resulting from movement of the external ear helps distinguish otitis externa from otitis media. A broad range of organisms, including gram-positive cocci, gram-negative bacilli, and fungi, can cause otitis externa. Topical therapy with eardrops containing polymyxin B and neomycin produces excellent results, but patients occasionally acquire true cellulitis of the external ear and then require systemic antibiotics and even debridement of infected cartilage.

Malignant otitis externa, an infection with *P. aeruginosa* that progressively invades the cartilage, soft tissue, and skull, is a rare condition that occurs in diabetic patients. Neurologic complications can be lethal. Prolonged, maximal parenteral therapy with combinations of antipseudomonal agents, such as tobramycin and piperacillin, is generally recommended. Monotherapy with intravenous ceftazidime and prolonged therapy with oral ciprofloxacin have been successful. Other antibiotics that may prove useful alone or in combination are aztreonam and imipenem. Aggressive surgical debridement has been a mainstay of treatment but may be required less often in patients who are treated early and aggressively with antibiotics. CT scans are superior to magnetic resonance imaging for early diagnosis, but either technique can be used to monitor patients for bone destruction and neurologic complications; should these sequelae occur, debridement is required. Mortality is high but has decreased over the past 10 years. *Aspergillus* is a rare cause of malignant otitis externa.

Pharyngitis

Although pharyngitis is one of the most common problems in clinical practice, a surprising number of practical questions remain unanswered. Group A streptococci are the most therapeutically important cause of pharyngitis, although in terms of frequency, they cause as few as 5% of the cases of pharyngitis and as many as 38% of the cases of tonsillitis.

STREPTOCOCCAL PHARYNGITIS

Diagnosis

Because it is impossible to distinguish clinically between streptococcal and viral pharyngitis, laboratory studies are necessary to make a diagnosis of streptococcal pharyngitis.[31] Throat cultures remain the standard method for identifying group A streptococci in the pharynx. In addition, rapid diagnostic tests suitable for office use are available. These procedures entail the extraction of streptococcal antigens from throat swabs so that the antigens can be identified rapidly by immunologic tests such as latex agglutination or enzyme-linked immunosorbent assay (ELISA). The sensitivity of these tests ranges from 77% to 95%, and specificity ranges from 86% to 100%. Thus, these tests are acceptable for clinical practice.

Although the recognition of group A streptococci is straightforward [see 15 Infections Due to Gram-Positive Cocci], it is difficult to determine whether the organisms are responsible for a patient's symptoms. The carrier rate of group A streptococci in healthy persons approaches 20%, and even among patients with symptomatic pharyngitis, only 50% of those with positive throat cultures demonstrate a serologic response to streptococci. Despite the frequency of sore throat, no firm guidelines are available to select patients who should have a throat culture, and except for a serologic determination, there is no proven method for distinguishing between the carrier state and active infection. Similarly, controversy exists about the need for obtaining cultures from asymptomatic family contacts of patients with streptococcal pharyngitis, for treating asymptomatic persons with small numbers of group A streptococci in their throat cultures, and for performing follow-up cultures after therapy. On balance, all these procedures are probably unnecessary unless the patient is highly susceptible to rheumatic carditis because of previous acute rheumatic fever.

Treatment

Fortunately, no uncertainty exists about the therapy for streptococcal pharyngitis in symptomatic patients. The disease is ordinarily self-limited, but early antibiotic therapy can alleviate symptoms.[32] Antibiotics prevent rheumatic fever and local suppurative complications and limit droplet spread. Because rheumatic fever can be prevented even when therapy is delayed as long as 9 days after the onset of symptoms, treatment need not be started until throat culture results are available. The goal of therapy is the eradication of group A streptococci from the nasopharynx. In more than 80% of patients, this result can be achieved with oral penicillin V, 250 mg four times a day for 10 days. Twice-a-day dosing is also effective and may improve compliance.[33] When patient compliance is in doubt, a single injection of 600,000 to 1.2 million units of benzathine penicillin G will be at least as effective. In patients who are allergic to penicillin, oral erythromycin is an excellent alternative, but it must be continued for 10 days. Tonsillectomy was once widely performed on children to prevent recurrent pharyngitis, but it has been largely abandoned.

OTHER FORMS OF BACTERIAL PHARYNGITIS

Other bacterial causes of pharyngitis are uncommon. Groups C and G streptococci can cause pharyngitis, but complications are rare. Gonococci transmitted by oral sex can produce sore throat, erythema, exudates, and lymphadenopathy; or asymptomatic colonization of the pharynx may occur. Meningococci sometimes cause symptomatic pharyngitis but are more commonly found in throat cultures of asymptomatic persons. *H. influenzae* pharyngitis can be extremely painful but is rare in adults; epiglottitis is a life-threatening complication of this type of pharyngitis. In patients who have not been immunized, *Corynebacterium diphtheriae* can cause painful membranous pharyngitis, often characterized by dysphagia and prominent edema of the neck. *Arcanobacterium haemolyticum*, formerly known as *Corynebacterium haemolyticum*, can cause pharyngitis and scarlatiniform rash, particularly in teenagers and young adults; administration of penicillin or erythromycin produces rapid relief of symptoms. *Yersinia enterocolitica* is an uncommon cause of pharyngitis; the pharyngitis may be present without enteritis, particularly in adults.

Many other bacterial species can be cultured from the pharynges of both symptomatic and asymptomatic patients [*see Table 1*], but they almost never cause pharyngitis. In particular, although pneumococci and staphylococci commonly reside in the nasopharynx and can cause severe disease in other parts of the respiratory tract, they do not cause pharyngitis. *Mycoplasma pneumoniae* causes pharyngitis in children and adults, but this diagnosis is seldom made in the absence of pneumonitis. *Chlamydia pneumoniae* can also cause pharyngitis, which may be protracted.[34]

Treponema pallidum, a spirochete that is not part of the normal flora, can cause pharyngitis in primary or secondary syphilis. Among the other causes of pharyngitis, *Mycobacterium tuberculosis* is very rare. *Candida albicans*, which is part of the normal mouth flora, can produce painful oropharyngeal moniliasis, or thrush, if antibiotics or debilitating illnesses (particularly HIV infection) upset microbial interactions and host defenses. This disease is characterized by a white, cheesy exudate that can be scraped off to demonstrate yeast forms by smear and culture. Nystatin oral suspension is therapeutically effective, but frequent, large doses may be required. Clotrimazole troches are also effective. Patients with HIV infection may require systemic therapy with fluconazole. Other forms of fungal pharyngitis are rare.

Deep Tissue Infections

Infections originating in the pharynx may extend by contiguous spread to the deep tissues of the pharynx and neck. In the neck, numerous fascial planes create a variety of potential spaces where infection can become loculated to form a phlegmon or a full-fledged abscess. Although these processes are now uncommon, prompt recognition is mandatory because antibiotics and surgical drainage are required to control infection and to prevent obstruction of the airway, invasion of vital neurologic and vascular structures, and spread of infection to the mediastinum and bloodstream.

PERITONSILLAR ABSCESS

Peritonsillar abscess, also called quinsy throat, is a complication of streptococcal tonsillitis most often seen in adolescents and young adults. Group A streptococci are the primary cause of the condition, although most peritonsillar abscesses also harbor mixed oral bacteria, with a predominance of anaerobes. Patients have fever and sore throat, often with pain referred to the ear. Dysphagia prevents the patient from swallowing saliva, commonly causing drooling; edema and pain produce a characteristic muffled, so-called hot-potato voice. The affected tonsil is visibly displaced forward, downward, and toward the midline; the soft palate may be edematous. Trismus occurs in some patients. CT scans are helpful in diagnosis and management. Treatment consists of parenteral penicillin and surgery. The tra-

a

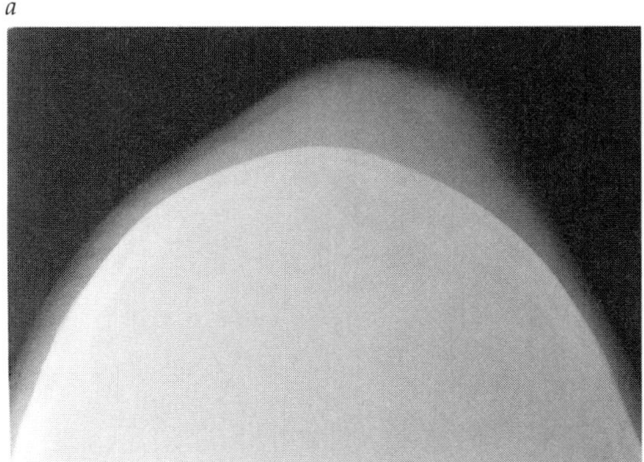

b

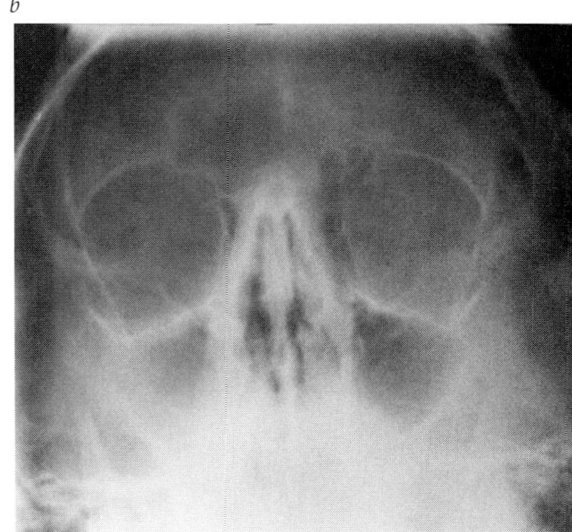

c

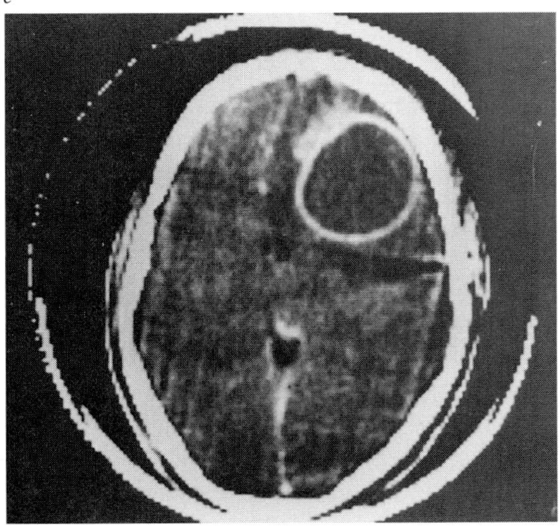

Figure 3 **(*a*) An oblique-view x-ray of the skull of a 16-year-old boy with fever, headache, and doughy edema of the forehead shows soft tissue swelling and a small area of underlying cortical irregularity indicative of osteomyelitis. (*b*) Sinus film reveals severe pansinusitis. (*c*) Because of subtle personality changes, a CT scan was taken; it revealed a large frontal lobe abscess. At surgery, 45 ml of pus was evacuated. Anaerobic streptococci were isolated from the subperiosteal collection and the brain abscess. Prolonged penicillin therapy and surgical management led to recovery.**

ditional approach consists of immediate incision and drainage, followed by tonsillectomy 4 to 6 weeks later; early tonsillectomy has also produced excellent results. Treatment with needle aspiration and oral antibiotics has also been successful; 80% to 92% of patients with peritonsillar abscess can be cured with this approach, thereby obviating hospitalization and surgery.

RETROPHARYNGEAL AND PARAPHARYNGEAL INFECTIONS

Retropharyngeal infections are most common in childhood because the lymph nodes in this region atrophy during adult life. Patients have fever and systemic toxicity as well as neck pain, dysphagia, muffled voice, and respiratory stridor. Physical findings include erythema and bulging of the posterior wall of the pharynx. CT scans and lateral-view x-rays of the neck are extremely useful, invariably demonstrating soft tissue swelling and forward displacement of the larynx [*see Figure 3a, 3b, and 3c*]. Although the bacterial agent of retropharyngeal infections is not determined in many patients, streptococci and other mouth flora predominate. Penicillin is the traditional antibiotic of choice, but agents that provide a broader spectrum of antibacterial coverage may be justified until culture data are available. Surgical drainage is vital to prevent asphyxiation and extension of infection to the mediastinum. Infections of the retropharyngeal space must be distinguished from infections of the prevertebral space.

The prevertebral space lies posterior to the retropharyngeal space and is separated from it by the prevertebral fascia. Infection of the prevertebral space often originates from osteomyelitis of the cervical vertebrae. This infection is frequently caused by staphylococci and may lead to spinal cord damage unless treated by an approach that combines immobilization, antistaphylococcal antibiotics, and external drainage.

The parapharyngeal space is demarcated by the parotid gland and internal pterygoid muscle laterally and by the superior constrictor muscle medially. The internal jugular vein, carotid artery, and cranial nerves IX, X, and XII pass through the space. Infection can reach the parapharyngeal space from the pharynx or from parotid or dental foci. Patients have severe trismus, externally visible inflammation behind the angle of the jaw, and inflammation in the lateral wall of the pharynx with medial displacement of the tonsil. Treatment consists of intravenous penicillin and drainage; CT-guided needle aspiration may be effective in some patients, but surgical drainage from behind the angle of the jaw is required in others.

Infections of the parapharyngeal space occasionally spread to the jugular vein and cause the syndrome of postanginal sepsis (Lemierre syndrome), which is characterized by the presence of septic phlebitis, septic pulmonary emboli, and anaerobic bacteremia. Pharyngitis and dental infections may also lead to postanginal sepsis. Facial swelling is an early diagnostic clue to this syndrome. CT is important for detecting abscesses, and ultrasonography is helpful for identifying jugular vein thrombosis. Anaerobic gram-negative bacilli, such as *Fusobacterium* species, are typically responsible for the condition. Management requires intravenous administration of penicillin; metronidazole and clindamycin are useful alternatives. Heparin, venous ligation, and surgical thrombectomy have also been advocated, but data do not allow firm guidelines to be established for these interventions.

LUDWIG ANGINA

Ludwig angina is a cellulitis of the submandibular, sublingual, and submental regions. In 86% of patients, the infection originates from a dental focus. Clinical features include fever, marked toxicity, and a rapidly progressive brawny edema in the floor of the mouth and the anterior neck. Elevation of the tongue impedes swallowing, and airway obstruction may be lethal. Streptococci and mouth flora are the most common etiologic agents, but *H. influenzae*, staphylococci, and gram-negative bacilli have also been implicated, so that initially broad antibiotic coverage may be necessary. Because endotracheal intubation can provoke laryngeal spasm, tracheostomy may be necessary to preserve the airway. Surgical decompression may be required.

Acute Epiglottitis (Supraglottitis)

No infection of the upper respiratory tract is more rapidly progressive or more lethal than acute epiglottitis, also known as supraglottitis. Acute epiglottitis occurs most commonly in children between 2 and 8 years of age and is more frequent in boys. The incidence of epiglottitis in childhood is declining rapidly in populations that have received *H. influenzae* type b vaccinations. Cases in adults appear to be increasing, however, perhaps because of improved diagnosis.[35]

ETIOLOGY

The major cause of acute epiglottitis in children and adults is *H. influenzae* type b. Other pathogens, including pneumococci, streptococci, staphylococci, and *Klebsiella pneumoniae*, can produce an identical syndrome. Although viral epiglottitis is rare, this syndrome can occur secondary to infection with herpes simplex virus type 1.[36] In the immunocompromised host, additional organisms may be responsible, including *Candida* and *Kingella kingae*; fortunately, such cases are rare.

DIAGNOSIS

The illness begins with startling rapidity; severe sore throat and fever progress rapidly to dysphagia, with retention of secretions and drooling. Systemic toxicity is marked; if the illness is not treated, dyspnea and progressive respiratory obstruction occur in a matter of hours.

Although uncommon, acute epiglottitis in adults is being recognized with increasing frequency. In adults, involvement often extends to the supraglottic structures, and edema may be more prominent than acute inflammation. Whereas children with acute epiglottitis usually present with respiratory distress, adults may first complain of pharyngeal symptoms (severe pain and odynophagia) before developing respiratory symptoms.[37] The course of the disease in adults is slower than in children, often extending over several days because of the larger diameter of the adult airway.

Acute epiglottitis is a medical emergency. The key to the diagnosis is a swollen, edematous, cherry-red epiglottis. Simple inspection of the pharynx is usually unrewarding. Furthermore, any instrumentation, even a tongue blade, can provoke spasm and total airway obstruction, although adults are at lower risk for this complication. Therefore, unless acute respiratory distress is present, a lateral-view x-ray of the neck should be taken immediately. If the film does not demonstrate epiglottal edema, indirect laryngoscopy can be undertaken; if edema is present, however, the diagnosis is confirmed, and instrumentation is unnecessary. In all cases, patients must be monitored continuously for signs of respiratory obstruction.

DIFFERENTIAL DIAGNOSIS

In the differential diagnosis in children, it is important to distinguish between epiglottitis and croup caused by viral laryngitis with laryngeal and subglottal edema and airway obstruction. Croup usually affects younger patients and progresses more slowly than epiglottitis, and patients with croup present with hoarseness and a characteristic cough. In addition, in croup the epiglottis is normal or only minimally inflamed on physical or radiographic examination. Cold, humidified oxygen is the mainstay of treatment of croup, and close observation is vital because emergency intubation or tracheostomy may be necessary. In children, bacterial tracheitis or membranous croup may present as severe laryngotracheitis, requiring antibiotic therapy as well as respiratory support. In patients of all ages, angioneurotic edema of the larynx, foreign bodies lodged in the upper airway, or impingement on the airway by various mass lesions may initially be confused with epiglottitis, but these conditions should be readily recognizable on physical examination and radiographic findings.

TREATMENT

Although tracheostomy is the traditional means of securing a patent airway in these patients, nasotracheal intubation is safe and effective. As a result, direct laryngoscopy by an experienced observer who is prepared to proceed with intubation (or, if necessary, tracheostomy) can be relied on for diagnosis when taking x-rays would produce excessive delay.

Because there is no margin for error, initial therapy with high-dose intravenous antibiotics effective against *H. influenzae* (including penicillinase-producing strains), other gram-negative bacilli, and staphylococci is warranted. Many regimens are available, including cefuroxime or cefamandole, ampicillin-sulbactam, imipenem-cilastatin, and a third-generation cephalosporin combined with a penicillinase-resistant penicillin. The choice of drugs depends on the results of throat and blood cultures and on ampicillin-sensitivity testing of *H. influenzae* isolates. A mist tent may be helpful. Steroids are sometimes advocated to reduce the edema, but their effectiveness has not been tested in controlled clinical trials. Above all, preservation of the airway is critical; nasotracheal intubation or tracheostomy is required in about half of all cases. If the airway can be protected while antibiotics take effect, most patients can be saved.

Miscellaneous Upper Respiratory Tract Infections

Many other infectious processes can invade the upper respiratory tract and adjacent regions of the head and neck. Common viral infections of the oropharynx are primary herpes simplex gingivostomatitis and adenovirus and coxsackievirus infections. Spirochetes play a role in ulcerative gingivitis and periodontitis. *Actinomyces israelii* can produce chronic burrowing infections of the gums and jaw, occasionally with secondary involvement of the respiratory tract. Although rare in the United States, rhinoscleroma, believed to be caused by *Klebsiella rhinoscleromatis*, can occur in immigrants from developing countries or in HIV-infected persons. *S. aureus* may produce acute bacterial sialadenitis or suppurative parotitis; less commonly, gram-negative bacilli or even anaerobes produce parotitis in hospitalized patients.

Many bacterial species have been implicated in a variety of dental infections. Mixed infections with normal mouth flora can occur in debilitated patients. Fusobacteria and spirochetes can cause gingivitis (trench mouth) or necrotic tonsillar ulcers (Vincent angina); patients have foul breath, pain, and dirty-gray membranous inflammation that bleeds easily. Oral irrigations and penicillin are effective therapy. A similar combination of spirochetes and other bacteria can produce a rare but extremely serious invasive gangrene of the mouth, cancrum oris, which occurs only in malnourished infants or in patients with advanced malignant disease or immunosuppression. Anaerobes may play a role in chronic or recurrent tonsillitis.[38] Dental infection is the leading cause of necrotizing cervical fasciitis.[39]

Many noninfectious processes in these regions can produce symptoms that mimic bacterial infection. Aphthous stomatitis may be the most common example. Drug reactions and primary dermatologic diseases cause oral and pharyngeal ulcerations. Vasculitis, carcinomas, lymphomas, and sarcoidosis of the upper airway can also mimic bacterial infection. Even subacute thyroiditis, which may produce fever and referred pain, may be mistaken for pharyngitis or otitis.

Acknowledgment

Figures 1 and 2 Tom Moore.

References

1. Gwaltney JM Jr, Hendley JO, Phillips CD, et al: Nose blowing propels nasal fluid into the paranasal sinuses. Clin Infect Dis 30:387, 2000

2. George DL, Falk PS, Meduri GU, et al: Nosocomial sinusitis in patients in the medical intensive care unit: a prospective epidemiological study. Clin Infect Dis 27:463, 1998

3. Mofenson LM, Korelitz J, Pelton S, et al: Sinusitis in children infected with human immunodeficiency virus: clinical characteristics, risk factors, and prophylaxis. Clin Infect Dis 21:1175, 1995

4. Low DE, Desrosiers M, McSherry J, et al: A practical guide for the diagnosis and treatment of acute sinusitis. Can Med Assoc J 156(6S):S1, 1997

5. Gonzalez R: Purulent secretions and antibiotics for URI. J Gen Intern Med 14:151, 1999

6. Gwaltney JM Jr: Acute community-acquired sinusitis. Clin Infect Dis 23:1209, 1996

7. Talmor M, Li P, Barie PS: Acute paranasal sinusitis in critically ill patients: guidelines for prevention, diagnosis, and treatment. Clin Infect Dis 25:1441, 1997

8. Iwen PC, Rupp ME, Hinrichs SH: Invasive mold sinusitis: 17 cases in immunocompromised patients and review of the literature. Clin Infect Dis 24:1178, 1997

9. DeShazo RD, Chapin K, Swain RE: Fungal sinusitis. N Engl J Med 337:254, 1997

10. Roberts SA, Bartley J, Braathredt G: *Nocardia asteroides* as a cause of sphenoidal sinusitis: case report. Clin Infect Dis 21:1041, 1995

11. Teh W, Matti BS, Marisiddaiah H, et al: *Aspergillus* sinusitis in patients with AIDS: report of three cases and review. Clin Infect Dis 21:529, 1995

12. Dunand VA, Hammer SM, Rossi R, et al: Parasitic sinusitis and otitis in patients infected with human immunodeficiency virus: report of five cases and review. Clin Infect Dis 25:267, 1997

13. van Buchem FL, Knottnerus JA, Schrijnemaekers VJJ, et al: Primary-care–based randomised placebo-controlled trial of antibiotic treatment in acute maxillary sinusitis. Lancet 349:683, 1997

14. de Bock GH, Dekker FW, Stolk J, et al: Antimicrobial treatment in acute maxillary sinusitis: a meta-analysis. J Clin Epidemiol 50:881, 1997

15. de Ferranti SD, Ioannidis JPA, Lau J, et al: Are amoxycillin and folate inhibitors as effective as other antibiotics for acute sinusitis? A meta-analysis. BMJ 317:632, 1998

16. Williams JW Jr, Holleman DR Jr, Samsa GP, et al: Randomized controlled trial of 3 vs 10 days of trimethoprim/sulfamethoxazole for acute maxillary sinusitis. JAMA 273:1015, 1995

17. The evidence base for diagnosis and treatment of uncomplicated acute bacterial sinusitis. ACP-ASIM Online (www.acponline.org/governors/sci-policy/sinusitis.htm)

18. Verbon A, Husni RN, Gordon SM, et al: Pott's puffy tumor due to *Haemophilus influenzae*: case report and review. Clin Infect Dis 23:1305, 1996

19. Casselbrant ML, Mandel EM, Fall PA, et al: The heritability of otitis media: a twin and triplet study. JAMA 282:2125, 1999

20. O'Neill P: Acute otitis media. BMJ 319:833, 1999

21. Heikkinen T, Thint M, Chonmaitree T: Prevalence of various respiratory viruses in the middle ear during acute otitis media. N Engl J Med 340:260, 1999

22. Froom J, Culpepper L, Jacobs M, et al: Antimicrobials for acute otitis media? A review from the International Primary Care Network. BMJ 315:98, 1997

23. Culpepper L, Froom J: Routine antimicrobial treatment of acute otitis media: Is it necessary? JAMA 278:1643, 1997

24. Hirschmann JV: Methods for decreasing antibiotic use in otitis media. Lancet 352:672, 1998

25. Del Mar C, Glasziou P, Hayem M: Are antibiotics indicated as initial treatment for children with acute otitis media? A meta-analysis. BMJ 314:1526, 1997

26. Damoiseaux RAMJ, van Balen FAM, Hoes AW, et al: Primary care based randomized, double blind trial of amoxicillin versus placebo for acute otitis media in children aged under 2 years. BMJ 320:350, 2000

27. Rosenfeld RM, Vertrees JE, Carr J, et al: Clinical efficacy of antimicrobial drugs for acute otitis media: meta-analysis of 5400 children from thirty-three randomized trials. J Pediatr 124:355, 1994

28. Kozyrskyl AL, Hildes-Ripstein GE, Longstaffe EA, et al: Treatment of acute otitis media with a shortened course of antibiotics. JAMA 279:1736, 1998

29. Pichichero ME: Changing the treatment paradigm for acute otitis media in children. JAMA 279:1748, 1998

30. Barnett ED, Teele DW, Klein JO, et al: Comparison of ceftriaxone and trimethoprim-sulfamethoxazole for acute otitis media. Pediatrics 99:23, 1997

31. Carroll K, Reimer J: Microbiology and laboratory diagnosis of upper respiratory tract infections. Clin Infect Dis 23:442, 1996

32. Zwart S, Sachs APE, Ruijs GHM, et al: Penicillin for acute sore throat: randomized double blind trial of seven days versus three days treatment or placebo in adults. BMJ 320:150, 2000

33. Lan AJ, Colford JM Jr: The impact of dosing frequency on the efficacy of 10-day penicillin or amoxicillin therapy for streptococcal tonsillopharyngitis: a meta-analysis. Pediatrics 105(2):E19, 2000

34. Falck G, Engstrand I, Gad A, et al: Demonstration of *Chlamydia pneumoniae* in patients with chronic pharyngitis. Scand J Infect Dis 29:585, 1997

35. Mayo-Smith MF, Spinale JW, Donskey CJ, et al: Acute epiglottitis: an 18-year experience in Rhode Island. Chest 108:1640, 1995

36. Bengualid V, Keesari S, Kandiah V, et al: Supraglottitis due to herpes simplex virus type 1 in an adult. Clin Infect Dis 22:382, 1996

37. Kucera CM, Silverstein MD, Jacobson RM, et al: Epiglottitis in adults and children in Olmstead County, Minnesota, 1976 through 1990. Mayo Clin Proc 71:1155, 1996

38. Nord CE: The role of anaerobic bacteria in recurrent episodes of sinusitis and tonsillitis. Clin Infect Dis 20:1512, 1995

39. Mathieu D, Nevière R, Teillon C, et al: Cervical necrotizing fasciitis: clinical manifestations and management. Clin Infect Dis 21:51, 1995

6 Pulmonary Infections

Harvey B. Simon, M.D.

Pulmonary infections span a wide spectrum, ranging from self-limited processes to life-threatening infections and from acute illnesses to chronic inflammatory diseases. This subsection details the pathophysiology, epidemiology, general features, and treatment of pulmonary infections, particularly bacterial pneumonia, and discusses the diagnosis and treatment of Legionnaires disease, chlamydial pneumonia, and aspiration pneumonia [*see Table 1*].

Pneumonia

Although overall hospitalization rates are declining, hospitalizations for acute lower respiratory tract infections have increased steadily since 1980.[1] Taken together, pneumonia and influenza rank as the sixth leading cause of death in the United States and lead all other infectious diseases in this respect. Antibiotics have greatly modified the natural history of pneumonia and have sharply reduced the overall case-fatality rate. At the same time, the widespread use of antimicrobial agents has led to the emergence of drug-resistant strains, thereby altering and expanding the range of pathogens responsible for pneumonia, especially in hospitalized patients. The growing population of patients with chronic obstructive pulmonary disease (COPD) and other debilitating illnesses and the use of respiratory therapy and immunosuppressive drugs have contributed to the increasing incidence of nosocomial and opportunistic pneumonias, which have a very high mortality.

PATHOPHYSIOLOGY

Host Defense Mechanisms

The lung is normally sterile. In healthy people, an intricate series of defense mechanisms maintain that sterility in the face of heavy bacterial colonization of the upper respiratory tract, inhalation of thousands of bacteria in droplet nuclei each day, and nearly universal aspiration of upper airway secretions during normal sleep each night. Defects in host defense mechanisms account for most cases of pneumonia [*see Table 2*].

Transmission of Organisms to Lungs

Inhalation of aerosolized droplets accounts for the transmission of respiratory viruses, such as influenza, which is highly contagious and often occurs in epidemics. Similar means of spread produce pneumonias caused by other nonbacterial agents, including mycoplasmas that are transmitted from person to person and cause primary atypical pneumonia, rickettsias that are transmitted

Table 1 Major Causes of Pulmonary Infection

Gram-positive cocci: *Streptococcus pneumoniae, S. pyogenes,* other streptococci, staphylococci

Gram-positive bacilli: *Bacillus anthracis*

Gram-negative cocci: *Neisseria meningitidis, Moraxella catarrhalis*

Gram-negative coccobacilli: *Haemophilus influenzae*

Gram-negative bacilli: *Klebsiella pneumoniae, Pseudomonas* species, *Escherichia coli, Proteus, Serratia* species, *Acinetobacter, Yersinia pestis, Francisella tularensis, Enterobacter* species, *Bacteroides, Legionella* species

Mixed flora (aspiration pneumonia)

Mycobacteria: *Mycobacterium tuberculosis, M. avium* complex

Fungi: *Histoplasma, Coccidioides, Blastomyces, Cryptococcus, Candida, Aspergillus,* Mucoraceae

Parasites: *Pneumocystis carinii, Toxoplasma gondii*

Mycoplasmas: *Mycoplasma pneumoniae*

Chlamydiae: *Chlamydia psittaci, C. trachomatis, C. pneumoniae*

Rickettsias: *Coxiella burnetii*

Viruses: influenza virus, parainfluenza virus, adenovirus, respiratory syncytial virus, rhinovirus, measles virus, varicella-zoster virus, cytomegalovirus

Table 2 Host Defense Mechanisms

Mechanism	*Modifying Factors*
Normal flora of upper respiratory tract	Antibiotic therapy, respiratory therapy, hospitalization
Aerodynamic properties of upper respiratory tract	Tracheal intubation
Protective reflexes (e.g., cough, sneeze, gag, bronchoconstrictor)	Sedatives and hypnotics, alcohol and drug abuse, neurologic disorders, age and debility, tracheal intubation (gastrointestinal disorders)
Mucous carpet that entraps particles	Viral infections, smoking, chemical irritants, dehydration
Ciliary action, mucociliary transport	Smoking, viral infections, advanced age, aspirin (?)
Antibacterial substances in respiratory secretions (e.g., lysozyme, lactoferrin, α-antitrypsin, IgA)	None
Fibronectin in respiratory secretions (competitively inhibits adherence of gram-negative bacilli)	Decreased fibronectin levels in seriously ill patients
Free drainage of tracheobronchial tree	Foreign bodies, obstructing tumors, bronchostenosis
Rich blood supply	Vascular obstruction (e.g., emboli)
Alveolar macrophages	Viral infections, smoking (both increase macrophage numbers but impair function)
Lymphatic tissue	Cytotoxic therapy
Humoral immunity (B cells, IgG and IgA antibodies, complement, polymorphonuclear neutrophils)	Immunosuppressive disorders and therapy
Cellular immunity (T cells, lymphokines, mononuclear phagocytes)	Immunosuppressive disorders and therapy

from livestock and cause Q fever, and chlamydiae that are transmitted from birds (*Chlamydia psittaci*) or humans (*C. pneumoniae*). Mycobacterium tuberculosis is spread from person to person by aerosolized droplets. The organisms that are responsible for causing the systemic mycoses are probably inhaled from sources in nature. Among bacteria that cause pneumonia, *Legionella pneumophila* is the species most likely to be spread by inhalation of aerosolized organisms that originate in contaminated freshwater.

Pneumococci are spread from person to person by aerosolized droplets, but pneumococcal pneumonia is not highly contagious and is caused in many cases by aspiration of nasopharyngeal organisms, the second major mechanism of infection. Aspiration of nasopharyngeal organisms occurs in nearly all persons during sleep and is probably responsible for most bacterial pneumonias, including staphylococcal and gram-negative bacillary pneumonias; it certainly accounts for the necrotizing pneumonitis that results from the aspiration of mixed mouth flora.

Hematogenous seeding, the third and least common mechanism that causes pneumonia, accounts for occasional cases of staphylococcal pneumonia in patients with tricuspid valve endocarditis or septic thrombophlebitis. This mechanism is also responsible for various gram-negative bacillary pneumonias in patients with bacteremia.

Tissue Responses

Once organisms succeed in bypassing host defense mechanisms to arrive at the alveoli, a variety of tissue responses may ensue, depending on the nature of the pathogen and on the integrity of the host inflammatory response. Although the inflammatory response is essential for the control of infection, it can produce tissue damage, impair ciliary action, and impede phagocytosis.[2]

The inflammatory response to *Streptococcus pneumoniae* or *Haemophilus influenzae* often produces lobar consolidation, but tissue necrosis is rarely present. In contrast, staphylococci and many gram-negative bacilli often produce necrosis, which can lead to cavitation and even frank abscess formation; a peribronchial distribution is characteristic, but lobar consolidation may occur. Viruses generally produce interstitial inflammation rather than air-space exudates. The infection is usually bilateral and causes diffuse alveolar damage and interstitial edema. Similar tissue responses may be initiated by *Mycoplasma*, *Chlamydia*, and *Legionella* species; by gram-negative bacteremia (shock lung); and by other causes of the acute respiratory distress syndrome (ARDS). Mycobacteria and fungi typically evoke a slow granulomatous response.

EPIDEMIOLOGY AND ETIOLOGY

Community-Acquired Pneumonias

Like other respiratory tract illnesses, pneumonia is most common in the winter because of the seasonal increase in viral infections and the close contact of persons confined indoors. Community-acquired pneumonias are a major problem in the United States, with at least 924,000 cases reported annually.

About 485,000 cases require hospitalization,[3] and at least 50,000 result in death. The mortality of community-acquired pneumonia ranges from less than 1% in patients who are not ill enough to require hospitalization to 13.7% for hospitalized patients, 19.6% for bacteremic patients, and 36.5% for patients admitted to intensive care units.[4] Clinical and laboratory data can be used to determine which patients are at greatest risk for death and thus require hospitalization and aggressive therapy. Comorbidity is the strongest risk factor, with neoplastic disease, neurologic disease, and alcoholism being particularly worrisome.[5–7] Advanced age is another predictor of risk, in part because older patients often underreport symptoms.[8,9] Physical findings of high fever, tachypnea, confusion, hypoxia, and hypotension also portend an adverse result.[10] The presence of extensive radiographic abnormalities, especially bilaterally pleural effusions,[9] is associated with higher risk, as are laboratory abnormalities such as hypoxia, azotemia, acidosis, hyponatremia, and hypophosphatemia. Patients with postobstructive, aspiration, gram-negative, and staphylococcal pneumonias have a high mortality; patients lacking these adverse prognostic indicators have a low risk of death and can usually be treated successfully as outpatients.[6] Patients hospitalized for pneumonia have a greater than fivefold likelihood of requiring subsequent hospitalization for pneumonia than patients with other serious illnesses.

In the preantibiotic era, pneumonia was nearly synonymous with *S. pneumoniae* infection. Pneumococci still account for 30% to 60% of all community-acquired pneumonias for which an etiology can be determined.[4,11] Pneumococci are particularly likely to be responsible for community-acquired pneumonias severe enough to require hospitalization and for pneumonia in persons older than 60 years.[12]

The second most common bacterial cause of community-acquired pneumonia is *H. influenzae*,[4] which accounts for about 10% of cases; patients with COPD are particularly vulnerable. Although infection with *Moraxella catarrhalis* is much less common than infection with *H. influenzae*, it is being recognized increasingly as a cause of community-acquired pneumonia. Like *H. influenzae*, *M. catarrhalis* has a predilection for patients with cardiopulmonary disease.[13] In rare cases, *M. catarrhalis* causes fulminant pneumonia, bacteremia, or both.

Staphylococci and gram-negative bacilli are much less common but more serious causes of community-acquired respiratory infections. Significant predisposing conditions are required for these organisms to produce pneumonia. In the community setting, staphylococcal pneumonia usually follows influenza. *Klebsiella* and other gram-negative pneumonias in the community setting are most common in alcoholics; meningococcal pneumonia is rare.[14] A variety of other bacteria, including *L. pneumophila*, can cause pneumonia in the community setting. Aspiration of mixed mouth flora is responsible for infection in some patients.

In more than half the patients with community-acquired pneumonia, the etiologic agent cannot be identified.[15] Nonbacterial (so-called atypical) agents are responsible for many of these infections, especially in younger patients. In a study of patients with a mean age of 41 years, for example, *M. pneumoniae* accounted for 22.8% of community-acquired pneumonias, *C. pneumoniae* for 10.7%, and influenza A for 2.7%.[15] *C. pneumoniae* is also increasingly being recognized as a cause of community-acquired pneumonia in adults with COPD. Respiratory tract viruses, including respiratory syncytial virus,[16] adenoviruses, and those that cause influenza or parainfluenza, can also cause community-acquired pneumonias in persons of all ages.[1]

Hospital-Acquired Pneumonias

Pneumonia is the second most common nosocomial infection in the United States[17]; about 200,000 cases occur annually, accounting for 17.8% of all hospital-acquired infections and 40,000 to 70,000 deaths. Risk factors for nosocomial infections include aspiration, COPD or other chronic severe illnesses, thoracic and upper abdominal surgery, and treatment in the intensive care unit. Patients who require mechanical ventilation are particularly at risk; pneumonia develops in 6.5% of such patients after 10 days of ventilation and in 28% after 30 days of ventilation. Ventilated patients who acquire nosocomial pneumonia have a much higher mortality (54%) than comparably poorly ventilated patients who do not acquire pneumonia (27%).

The bacterial etiologies of hospital-acquired pneumonias are very different from those of community-acquired pneumonias. Many nosocomial pneumonias are polymicrobial, with gram-negative bacilli isolated in 47% of patients, anaerobes in 35%, and *Staphylococcus aureus* in 26%. In contrast, pneumococci account for no more than 10% of hospital-acquired pneumonias. Other organisms that are associated with community-acquired infections can occasionally cause pneumonia in the hospital setting; such organisms include *Legionella* species, *M. pneumoniae*,[18] and *C. pneumoniae*.[19]

Pseudomonas, *Klebsiella*, and *Escherichia coli* are the most commonly implicated causes of gram-negative pneumonias.[20] Nosocomial gram-negative pneumonias often occur in patients with serious underlying diseases; as a result, mortality is as high as 30% to 50%. Prior antibiotic administration, respiratory therapy, chronic illness, and confinement to bed predispose to oropharyngeal colonization with gram-negative bacilli, which occurs in up to 45% of ICU patients and precedes pneumonia in most cases. Upper intestinal colonization has also been implicated, but its importance is still uncertain.[20] However, although nursing home residents are usually elderly and chronically ill, only 14% of these persons become colonized with gram-negative bacilli; oropharyngeal colonization in this population is transient and does not appear to predispose to gram-negative pneumonia. Hence, pneumonia in these patients can be approached as a community-acquired infection rather than a hospital-acquired infection.[21,22]

Although more invasive techniques are sometimes required for diagnosis of ventilator-associated pneumonias, the treatment, for most patients, can be based on Gram stains and cultures of tracheal aspirates.[23,24] Because of the high mortality associated with pneumonias in the ICU, strategies to prevent them have been studied,[25,26] and comprehensive guidelines are available.[27]

Pneumonias in Immunosuppressed Patients

Immunosuppressed patients, particularly those with AIDS,[28,29] are vulnerable to a broad range of pulmonary pathogens. In addition to being susceptible to the many organisms that produce community- and hospital-acquired pneumonias, these patients are susceptible to many opportunistic microbes that are unlikely to cause pneumonia in immunologically competent hosts. Such organisms include bacteria[30] (e.g., *Pseudomonas*, *Nocardia*, and *Legionella* species), mycobacteria (e.g., *Mycobacterium avium* complex), viruses (e.g., cytomegalovirus and herpesvirus), fungi (e.g., *Candida*, *Aspergillus*, and *Mucor* species), and protozoa (e.g., *Pneumocystis carinii* and *Toxoplasma gondii*). As a result, immunosuppressed patients require an aggressive approach to diagnosis and therapy [see 21 Infections Due to *Haemophilus*, *Moraxella*, *Legionella*, *Bordetella*, and *Pseudomonas*; 22 Infections Due to *Brucella*, *Francisella*, *Yersinia pestis*, and *Bartonella*].

DIAGNOSIS

Clinical Features

Classic symptoms of pneumonia include cough, sputum production, chest pain, fever, chills, hypoxia, and dyspnea. Although physical examination of patients with typical pneumonias is often nonspecific,[31] it may reveal rales, rhonchi, or bronchial breath sounds, as well as percussion dullness over the involved segments of the lung. Pleural effusions may accompany pneumonia. The chest x-ray reveals the presence of infiltrates.

Nonbacterial and bacterial pneumonias have differing clinical presentations. Although both types of pneumonia can affect persons of all ages, nonbacterial pneumonias are most common in older children and young adults. Patients with viral, mycoplasmal, or chlamydial pneumonias will often complain of a severe hacking cough, but substantial sputum production is unusual.

Patients with bacterial pneumonias are more likely to have copious sputum production—as well as an abrupt onset of illness, high temperatures, chills, and development of significant pleural effusions—than are patients with nonbacterial pneumonias.

On physical examination, the patient with bacterial pneumonia generally looks sicker than the patient with nonbacterial pneumonia, and chest examination of patients with bacterial pneumonia usually reveals signs of consolidation or at least localized rales and rhonchi. In contrast, the chest examination of patients with nonbacterial pneumonias typically shows only fine rales, and often, the physical findings are less extensive than the radiologic abnormalities.

Laboratory Studies

Patients with bacterial pneumonias are more likely to have a polymorphonuclear leukocytosis. If the chest x-ray reveals lobar or segmental consolidation, abscess formation, or significant pleural effusion, bacterial pneumonia is more likely. A patchy infiltrate can occur in either process, but a true interstitial infiltrate suggests a nonbacterial etiology. Computed tomography is extremely helpful in patients with complex infections.[32]

The sputum examination is central to the etiologic diagnosis of pneumonia. The sputum of patients with bacterial pneumonia is typically thick and either green or brownish and is sometimes blood tinged. A good sputum specimen for microscopic examination and culture is crucial. If the patient cannot expectorate spontaneously, pulmonary physiotherapy, intermittent positive pressure ventilation with humidified air, or nasotracheal suction may be used to obtain the specimen. The Gram stain of sputum from patients with bacterial pneumonia usually reveals abundant polymorphonuclear leukocytes and will often disclose the primary pathogens. Patients with nonbacterial pneumonias or Legionnaires disease generally produce only scant quantities of thin sputum. In influenzal pneumonia, the sputum may be bloody. The Gram stain of sputum from patients with nonbacterial pneumonia reveals an absence of bacteria and a scant cellular response; in patients with mycoplasmal pneumonia, mononuclear cells may predominate.[33] It can be difficult to determine the etiology in patients with nosocomial pneumonias; prolonged hospitalization, antibiotic administration, and ventilatory therapy predispose to colonization with organisms that contaminate sputum specimens but can also cause pneumonia. Bronchoalveolar lavage is effective in identifying the responsible pathogen.[34]

Kits for the detection of nucleic acids from *Legionella*, *Mycoplasma*, and mycobacterial species in sputum are currently available, and similar tests may soon be available for the detection of other pathogens.

Invasive Studies

In immunocompromised patients, numerous opportunistic agents can cause pneumonia, and aggressive techniques may be required to obtain a satisfactory specimen. Although invasive procedures rarely are necessary in immunocompetent patients, they may be required in patients who present with unusual features, are critically ill, or fail to respond to conventional therapy. Procedures such as transtracheal aspiration, bronchoscopy (sometimes including transbronchial biopsies), bronchial brushing, or percutaneous lung taps may be necessary [see 21 Infections Due to *Haemophilus*, *Moraxella*, *Legionella*, *Bordetella*, and *Pseudomonas*]; bronchoalveolar lavage is a particularly useful technique and is generally well tolerated. If these less invasive techniques fail to produce a diagnosis, open lung biopsy should be considered.

DIFFERENTIAL DIAGNOSIS

Noninfectious diseases can be mistaken for infections of the respiratory tract. Asthmatic bronchitis and hypersensitivity pneumonitis are common examples. COPD, including emphysema and bronchiectasis, may be misleading if previous x-rays are not available. Atelectasis, pulmonary infarction, pulmonary edema, and lung tumors may also be confused with pneumonia. Hypersensitivity reactions and toxins—in the form of aerosols, systemic drugs, or chemicals—produce clinical illnesses and pulmonary infiltrates simulating those of infectious pneumonia. Radiation pneumonitis, sarcoidosis, vasculitis, uremic pneumonitis, pulmonary hemorrhage, eosinophilic pneumonia, organizing pneumonia,[35] and lipoid pneumonitis are included in the differential diagnosis.

One of the primary considerations in patients with a lower respiratory tract infection is to distinguish between acute bronchitis and pneumonia. The distinction is anatomic rather than etiologic because the same basic range of organisms can cause the two syndromes. As a result, these conditions often overlap clinically.

TREATMENT

Certain general principles are useful in the care of all patients with pneumonia. Adequate hydration is important to help clear secretions; hydration can be achieved by systemic administration of fluids and local airway humidification. Expectorants such as guaifenesin may be helpful in loosening the sputum. Although clinical trials have demonstrated that chest physiotherapy does not hasten the resolution of pneumonia, this traditional therapeutic modality may provide symptomatic benefit to patients with copious airway secretions. In general, the cough reflex should not be suppressed in patients with bacterial infections, because coughing is an important mechanism for clearing secretions. If severe paroxysms of coughing produce respiratory fatigue or harsh pain, however, temporary relief may be obtained with small doses of codeine. Chest pain should be treated with analgesics that do not suppress cough. If hypoxia is present, oxygen should be administered. Persons who have COPD and retain carbon dioxide must be monitored very closely because oxygen therapy can lead to respiratory depression.

Specific antimicrobial therapy depends on the etiologic agent. Whereas culture and sensitivity testing require at least 24 to 48 hours to provide definitive information, the clinical setting, chest x-ray, and Gram stain of sputum usually enable the physician to make a reasonable presumptive diagnosis and to initiate therapy at once. Treatment can then be modified as necessary on the basis of culture results. Because antibiotics penetrate sputum by passive diffusion, it is important to maintain adequate blood levels of these drugs. The administration of antibiotics by aerosol is not indicated for most cases of pneumonia but may help patients with cystic fibrosis and endobronchial *Pseudomonas* infections.

It is best to choose an antibiotic regimen directed specifically at organisms seen on Gram stain and, after 24 to 48 hours, identified from sputum or blood cultures. Even if these data are lacking, however, a reasonable choice of initial antimicrobial therapy can be made on the basis of the patient's epidemiologic setting and clinical features.

Community-Acquired Pneumonia

Several factors are responsible for rapid changes in the empirical treatment of community-acquired pneumonias: the emergence of drug-resistant pneumococci; the increasing population of elderly or chronically ill patients who are vulnerable to infections caused by *H. influenzae* and *M. catarrhalis*; the increased importance of atypical pathogens such as *M. pneumoniae*, *C. pneumoniae*, and *L. pneumophila*; and the availability of new fluoroquinolones with enhanced activity against gram-positive cocci (including penicillin-nonsensitive pneumococci) and anaerobes (including mouth flora). For patients who do not require hospitalization, several options are available. Erythromycin is cost-effective,[36] but the macrolides clarithromycin and azithromycin may be preferable because of their better gastrointestinal tolerance and their activity against *Haemophilus* and *Moraxella* species. Doxycycline is an effective and inexpensive alternative.[37] However, because of the increasing prevalence of drug-resistant pneumococci, use of one of the newer fluoroquinolones (e.g., levofloxacin, sparfloxacin, gatifloxacin, or moxifloxacin) is recommended.[38,39] These agents have excellent activity against the major causes of community-acquired pneumonia; prospective trials have been favorable.[40] The newer fluoroquinolones may also emerge as drugs of choice for patients with community-acquired pneumonia who require hospitalization; levofloxacin and gatifloxacin are available in preparations for I.V. administration. Alternative approaches include use of cefotaxime or ceftriaxone alone or with a macrolide or use of azithromycin alone.[41] In communities with a lower prevalence of drug-resistant pneumococci, a second-generation cephalosporin such as cefuroxime may still be useful, either alone or with a macrolide. When aspiration is suspected, penicillin, clindamycin, or metronidazole is useful; newer fluoroquinolones, such as gatifloxacin, moxifloxacin and levofloxacin, also appear active against oral anaerobes.

In all cases, antibiotic therapy should be tailored according to the results of culture and sensitivity, the clinical response, and the occurrence of side effects. Many patients who require intravenous antibiotics initially can be switched to oral therapy within 3 days,[42] facilitating early hospital discharge.[43,44] In most patients with uncomplicated pneumococcal pneumonia, antibiotics can be discontinued after 3 afebrile days; most patients with other bacterial pneumonias are treated for 7 to 14 days, and most with atypical pneumonias are treated for 10 to 21 days.

Hospital-Acquired Pneumonia

Because nosocomial pneumonias are often caused by gram-negative bacilli and *S. aureus*, patients with hospital-acquired pneumonias require broad antimicrobial coverage until the results of Gram stains, cultures, and sensitivity tests permit focused therapy. Options for the initial treatment of hospital-acquired pneumonia include ticarcillin–clavulanic acid or piperacillin-tazobactam, meropenem or imipenem-cilastatin, a third-generation cephalosporin with nafcillin or vancomycin, a first-generation cephalosporin with an aminoglycoside, or vancomycin with an aminoglycoside. The prevalence of resistant bacteria in a particular hospital or patient care unit should help guide the initial therapy; for example, if methicillin-resistant staphylococci are common, vancomycin is a desirable component of the initial therapy, and when multidrug-resistant *Klebsiella* organisms are common, meropenem or imipenem-cilastatin should be considered.

Infections Caused by *Legionella* Species

LEGIONNAIRES DISEASE

Epidemiology and Etiology

Since it was first recognized in 1976, Legionnaires disease has become recognized as a common cause of both community-acquired and hospital-acquired pneumonias. Worldwide, it accounts for between 2% and 15% of all community-acquired pneumonias severe enough to require hospitalization.[45] It is estimated that 10,000 to 25,000 cases occur in the United States each year.

Legionnaires disease is caused by *L. pneumophila*, a fastidious, filamentous, flagellated, aerobic gram-negative bacillus. The organism can be grown on charcoal–yeast extract agar; optimal growth occurs at 35° C in 5% carbon dioxide, but growth is slow, and a period of 3 to 6 days is required for colonies to form.

At least nine serogroups of *L. pneumophila* exist; most clinical isolates belong to serogroup 1. By special staining techniques, large numbers of the organism can be identified in tissue sections of alveoli, both within macrophages and extracellularly. Virulence factors of *L. pneumophila* and various extracellular enzymes that the organism secretes have been identified. *L. pneumophila* is able to survive intracellularly in host leukocytes. Antibody is not protective, but cell-mediated immunity does promote recovery and prevent reinfection.

In nature, *L. pneumophila* survives principally in water and, to a lesser extent, in soil. Human disease is acquired primarily by inhalation of aerosols contaminated with organisms; person-to-person transmission has not been documented. Contaminated water systems have been responsible for both community-acquired and hospital-acquired outbreaks.

The attack rate for Legionnaires disease appears to be higher in elderly persons and persons with underlying conditions such as COPD, neoplastic disease, organ transplants, and renal failure.[46] Although *L. pneumophila* is a relatively uncommon pathogen in persons infected with HIV, it can cause severe disease in these patients.[47]

Diagnosis

Clinical features Legionnaires disease is characterized by a 1-day prodrome of myalgias, malaise, and slight headache after an incubation period of 2 to 10 days. Acute onset of high fever, shaking chills, nonproductive cough, tachypnea, and, often, pleuritic pain ensues. The cough may subsequently become slightly productive, but the sputum is not purulent. Obtundation or toxic encephalopathy is common, but frank meningitis is not a feature. Abdominal pain, vomiting, and, especially, diarrhea may be present. Signs of consolidation on physical examination are present infrequently, but rales are commonly heard. Chest radiographs show patchy or interstitial infiltrates, which often progress to areas of nodular consolidation in a single lobe or multiple lobes; minimal effusions are present in up to one third of cases. Abscess formation is uncommon but has been observed. Pulmonary fibrosis may occur in some survivors.

Although pneumonia is present in nearly all patients with Legionnaires disease, extrathoracic symptoms can be the presenting or predominant features. Central nervous system, GI, and renal manifestations are especially common. *L. pneumophila* has been isolated from blood cultures, and the organism can be found in many organs both in immunosuppressed patients and in previously normal patients who are afflicted with severe disease. Extrapulmonary manifestations include ocular and pericardial involvement, perirectal abscess, wound infection, peritonitis, cellulitis, rhabdomyolysis and acute renal failure, neutropenia, hemolytic anemia, and thrombotic thrombocytopenic purpura. Implanted devices such as heart valves and hemodialysis fistulas can become infected.

A nonpneumonic form of legionellosis called Pontiac fever has a short incubation period and a low mortality. It has been responsible for at least four outbreaks of illness, including several related to whirlpools and hot tubs.

Laboratory studies The peripheral white blood cell count is mildly elevated to between 8,000 and 16,000/mm^3. Cold agglutinins are negative. Other laboratory findings may include an elevated erythrocyte sedimentation rate, hypoxia, abnormal liver function test results, and elevated creatine phosphokinase levels.[48] Proteinuria and microscopic hematuria have been observed, and acute renal failure may complicate the course on occasion.

Gram stains of the sputum or tracheal secretions fail to reveal *L. pneumophila*. The organism can be isolated from sputum and other specimens by using charcoal–yeast extract agar. The diagnosis can be established rapidly in about 20% of cases by demonstrating the organism with direct immunofluorescent staining of sputum specimens; bronchoalveolar lavage may be helpful in immunosuppressed patients. A kit that uses radiolabeled complementary DNA is commercially available, but clinical experience is still limited. A polymerase chain reaction assay has been developed.[49]

Another method of rapid diagnosis involves detection of *L. pneumophila* antigen in the urine[50]; the radioimmunoassay test is highly specific and has a sensitivity of about 90%. However, this test is available only for *L. pneumophila* serogroup 1, which is the most common cause of Legionnaires disease. Most often, however, the diagnosis is established by an indirect fluorescent antibody technique involving staining of the causative bacterium. With this technique, a fourfold or greater rise in titer during the illness or a stable titer of 1:256 or greater is considered diagnostic.

The clinical picture and radiologic findings in Legionnaires disease are not specific. The diagnosis should be considered in patients with segmental, lobar, or interstitial pneumonia in which the etiologic agent is not evident on Gram stains of sputum or tracheal secretions. A mild case may resemble *Mycoplasma* pneumonia or other types of atypical pneumonia.

Treatment

On in vitro susceptibility testing, *L. pneumophila* is susceptible to a variety of antimicrobial agents, including erythromycin, clarithromycin, azithromycin, tetracycline, rifampin, and the fluoroquinolones. Current evidence indicates that azithromycin or levofloxacin is the treatment of choice.[51] Occasionally, patients may experience a relapse if antibiotics are discontinued prematurely; recovery occurs during a second, more prolonged course of treatment. A combination of rifampin and either azithromycin or levofloxacin may be considered in patients who fail to respond to monotherapy alone and in immunologically impaired patients with overwhelming disease.

INFECTIONS CAUSED BY OTHER *LEGIONELLA* SPECIES

Since 1943, unusual, fastidious rickettsia-like organisms have been identified as causes of isolated cases of pneumonia. Long considered medical curiosities, these organisms were named after their discoverers or the patients from whom they were isolated. Such obscure nomenclature (e.g., TATLOCK, OLDA, HEBA, and WIGA) reflected the absence of knowledge concerning these agents. Since then, studies of these organisms have led to their reclassification as *Legionella* species. Of the more than 30 *Legionella* species that have been identified, at least 19 have been recognized as causes of pneumonia, particularly in immunosuppressed hosts.

The clinical picture is not distinctive. Fever is the most common feature, cough is variable in severity, and sputum production is absent or scant. Pleurisy or dyspnea may develop, and chest x-rays show a patchy or nodular, progressive bronchopneumonia. *L. micdadei* is the most important of these organisms. Previously known as TATLOCK and HEBA, this organism was rediscovered as the Pittsburgh pneumonia agent that caused acute suppurative pneumonia in 13 immunosuppressed patients from two centers. *L. midadei* can also cause pneumonia in immunologically intact hosts and extrathoracic infections in immunologically impaired hosts. It has been isolated from hospital water supplies and can cause nosocomial infections in immunosuppressed patients.[52]

In the first 13 patients with Pittsburgh pneumonia, the diagnosis was established through a lung biopsy or autopsy that revealed acute alveolar inflammation and short, weakly acid-fast gram-negative bacilli. More recent cases have been diagnosed by culturing the agent on charcoal–yeast extract agar or by serologic means. Erythromycin has been used with success. Unlike *L. pneumophila*, *L. micdadei* is susceptible to penicillins and cephalosporins in vitro; however, there are no data on the use of these drugs in clinical *L. micdadei* infection.

Many other *Legionella* species have been identified as causes of pneumonia. These organisms grow on charcoal–yeast extract agar. Some cases in which *Legionella* species have been implicated share common features: patients have been exposed to infected water and have COPD or are immunosuppressed.[53] Therapy with erythromycin, alone or with rifampin, has been suggested.

CHLAMYDIA PNEUMONIAE

C. pneumoniae, initially known as the Taiwan acute respiratory disease (TWAR) agent is an important pathogen, accounting for up to 10% of all pneumonias in the United States.[54] Serologic surveys suggest that a majority of adults have been infected at some point, indicating that most cases are mild or subclinical.

Unlike psittacosis, which is a true zoonosis that spreads only from animals to humans, *C. pneumoniae* spreads from person to person via respiratory droplets. The incubation period of *C. pneumoniae* is long. Unlike *C. trachomatis*, which causes neonatal pneumonia, *C. pneumoniae* affects mainly older children and young adults; however, older patients (especially those with COPD) can also be affected.[55] The clinical features of *C. pneumoniae* pneumonia in young patients resemble those of *M. pneumoniae* pneumonia: after a prodrome of pharyngitis that lasts no more than 2 weeks, nonproductive cough and fever occur. Pulmonary infiltrates are mild. The infection is usually self-limited. In older patients with underlying COPD, *C. pneumoniae* can cause bronchitis that may be mild or very persistent. Bronchospasm may be prominent.[56] These organisms can sometimes cause severe pneumonia in patients with COPD, and fatalities have been reported in debilitated patients. A macrolide, a tetracycline, or a fluoroquinolone is recommended for therapy.

Recurrent Pneumonia

Patients with recurrent pneumonia present a diagnostic and therapeutic challenge. Anatomic abnormalities should be carefully sought in all such patients and should be suspected particularly when the infections recur in one bronchopulmonary segment. Examples of anatomic abnormalities include cysts, blebs, abscess cavities, bronchiectasis, and bronchial obstruction by tumors, foreign bodies, or bronchiostenosis. If shifting locations are involved, systemic abnormalities may be present. Examples include defects of leukocyte function, immunoglobulin deficiencies, α_1-antitrypsin globulin deficiency, and cystic fibrosis. Recurrent aspiration may be responsible, in which case a carefully performed neurologic examination and a barium swallow may reveal the proper diagnosis. It is important to remember that noninfectious processes may produce recurrent pulmonary infiltrates that may be accompanied by cough and fever. Examples of such processes include organizing pneumonia,[35] eosinophilic pneumonia, hypersensitivity pneumonitis, vasculitis, pulmonary hemosiderosis, and pulmonary emboli.

Chronic Pneumonia

Often, bacterial pneumonias exhibit delayed resolution, in which radiographic abnormalities persist for weeks or even months after clinical recovery. Infrequently, pyogenic infection pursues a slow but progressively destructive course despite antibiotic therapy; *K. pneumoniae* and other gram-negative bacilli have been implicated in some patients with such chronic bacterial pneumonias. Mycobacteria and *Actinomyces* are common causes of chronic pulmonary infection; fungi are particularly common in patients treated with corticosteroids. Persistent infiltration caused by neoplasia, sarcoidosis, pulmonary hemorrhage, vasculitis, fibrosing alveolitis, alveolar proteinosis, lipoid pneumonia, toxins, and other processes may mimic chronic pulmonary infection. Fiberoptic bronchoscopy is very useful for diagnosis, but lung biopsy may be needed.

Aspiration Pneumonia

EPIDEMIOLOGY AND ETIOLOGY

Seventy percent of patients with depressed consciousness have demonstrable pharyngeal aspiration, often involving much larger volumes of material than that aspirated by healthy persons. Because of the larger volumes of aspirated material, underlying diseases impairing host defenses, and alterations in oropharyngeal flora, patients with altered consciousness are most prone to aspiration pneumonia. In clinical practice, alcoholism, drug abuse, administration of sedatives or anesthesia, head trauma, and seizures or other neurologic disorders are most often responsible for the development of aspiration pneumonia. In addition, patients with abnormalities of deglutition or esophageal motility resulting from placement of nasogastric tubes, esophageal carcinoma, bowel obstruction, or repeated vomiting from any cause are prone to aspiration of GI contents. Poor oral hygiene and periodontal disease predispose to aspiration pneumonia because of the increased bacterial flora in these patients.

The clinical results of pulmonary aspiration depend in large part on the nature and volume of material aspirated. Aspiration of gastric contents is a common problem that may produce Mendelson syndrome, a fulminating illness, if a large volume of acid gastric juice is aspirated. Aspiration of particulate material can produce acute airway obstruction and death by asphyxiation; aspiration of smaller particles may produce atelectasis of a pulmonary segment or even an entire lung with dyspnea, wheezing, and cyanosis. Characteristic pulmonary injuries and distinctive clinical syndromes are produced by aspiration of smoke, freshwater or saltwater, and fats or oils (lipoid pneumonitis).

Whereas aspiration is probably the mechanism responsible for most bacterial pneumonias, the term aspiration pneumonia is best reserved for infection caused by mixed mouth flora.

DIAGNOSIS

Clinical Features

Patients with mixed aspiration pneumonia may present with either an acute febrile illness or a more indolent course extending over many days or even weeks. Fever, cough, and sputum production are the dominant symptoms; the sputum may be copious, foul smelling, or both. Physical examination typically discloses rales and signs of pulmonary consolidation. An evaluation of dental hygiene and of the gag reflex is helpful; disordered pharyngeal sensation is a better predictor of vulnerability than is an absent gag reflex.

Laboratory Studies

Radiographically, infiltrates are most common in dependent areas of the lung, especially the apical segments of the lower lobes and the posterior segments of the upper lobes. Tissue necrosis can occur, and without treatment, aspiration pneumonia may produce multiple small cavities, which reflect a necrotizing pneumonitis. Lung abscesses or empyemas may ensue.

The sputum of patients with classic aspiration pneumonia contains abundant polymorphonuclear leukocytes and a mixed mouth flora. If specimens are obtained by transtracheal aspiration or other procedures that avoid contamination of sputum by organisms from the oral cavity, aerobic and anaerobic bacteriologic techniques can reveal the specific causative bacteria. Because anaerobes are the dominant flora of the upper respiratory tract (outnumbering aerobic or facultative bacteria by 10 to 1), it is not surprising that anaerobes are the dominant organisms in aspiration pneumonia. Of particular importance are *Bacteroides melaninogenicus* and other *Bacteroides* species (slender, pleomorphic, pale gram-negative rods), *Fusobacterium nucleatum* (slender gram-negative rods with pointed ends), and anaerobic or microaerophilic streptococci and *Peptostreptococcus* (small gram-positive cocci in chains or clumps). As expected, multiple organisms are recovered from most patients.

TREATMENT

With the exception of *B. fragilis*, which can be identified along with other anaerobic species in 17% of patients with classic aspiration pneumonia, all the anaerobes found are penicillin sensitive. Penicillin is effective when *B. fragilis* is present in combination with penicillin-sensitive organisms, suggesting that aspiration pneumonias are synergistic infections that can be treated successfully by elimination of most but not necessarily all of the organisms involved. Penicillin dosages of 2.4 to 6.0 million units daily are generally effective. Parenteral therapy is advisable initially, but a 10- to 14-day course of treatment can be concluded with orally administered antibiotics if the patient responds well. Clindamycin represents an excellent alternative agent and may even be superior to penicillin for treatment of necrotizing aspiration pneumonias and lung abscesses.

Hospitalization or antibiotic therapy alters the usual oropharyngeal bacterial flora, so that staphylococci, facultative gram-negative bacilli, or both may be identified in patients. As a result, aspiration pneumonia in hospitalized patients often involves pathogens that are uncommon in community-acquired pneumonias. Gram stains and cultures of sputum are especially important for identifying gram-negative bacilli and staphylococci in the hospital setting. Broad antimicrobial coverage is required until specific pathogens have been identified by culture and sensitivity testing. Although tube feedings are often recommended to prevent aspiration pneumonia, there is no evidence that they are effective.[57]

Other Pulmonary Infections

CHRONIC BRONCHITIS

Patients with chronic bronchitis characteristically produce sputum on most days for at least 3 months each year for more than 2 years. The sputum is frequently colonized by *H. influenzae* (nontypable), *S. pneumoniae*, or *Moraxella catarrhalis*, singly or in combination.[58] The role of long-term prophylactic antibiotic therapy in such patients is controversial. Long-term antibiotic therapy may provide symptomatic relief in certain patients who experience multiple exacerbations of bronchitis during the winter, but it is not useful in improving or preserving pulmonary function. A meta-analysis of randomized, controlled trials demonstrated that antibiotic therapy is effective in treating acute exacerbations of chronic bronchitis.[59] Although physicians often use antibiotics to treat acute bronchitis in patients without underlying lung disease, there is little evidence that this practice is beneficial.[60,61] Currently, 60% to 85% of patients diagnosed with acute bronchitis in the United States receive antibiotics,[62] an unfortunate practice that has contributed to the emergence of antibiotic-resistant bacteria.

BRONCHIECTASIS

True saccular, or cystic, bronchiectasis involves both dilatation of the bronchi and destruction of the bronchial walls. Bronchiectasis results most often from neglected or recurrent pneumonia, especially in childhood, and therefore, bronchiectasis has become much less common since the introduction of antibiotics. Aggressive medical therapy has greatly improved the prognosis.

Symptoms include cough that may be dry or productive of copious foul sputum, recurrent lower respiratory tract infection, and hemoptysis. In rare instances, bronchiectasis can present as pleuritic chest pain. In advanced cases, fibrosis can lead to cor pulmonale and respiratory failure. The chest x-ray may show increased lung markings, honeycombing, atelectasis, or pleural changes, but thin-section or helical chest computed tomography is required for definitive diagnosis.[63]

Lung Abscess

EPIDEMIOLOGY AND ETIOLOGY

In the antibiotic era, lung abscesses have become less common and less serious. The most common variety has been termed the primary, simple, nonspecific, or putrid abscess. Primary lung abscess accounts for about 60% of all lung abscesses and originates from a necrotizing suppurative bronchopneumonia caused by the aspiration of mixed oropharyngeal bacteria. Thus, both the predisposing factors and the causative organisms are similar to those identified in aspiration pneumonia. Patients with primary lung abscesses typically have alterations of consciousness because of underlying problems such as alcoholism and neurologic disorders; periodontal disease is often present. The organisms causing the abscess are much more reliably identified by transtracheal aspirates than by sputum cultures, which are invariably contaminated with anaerobes and other mouth flora. Percutaneous lung aspiration and bronchoalveolar lavage may also be useful for bacteriologic diagnosis. Mixed anaerobic bacteria are seen in most cases; *Fusobacterium nucleatum*, *Bacteroides melaninogenicus*, *Peptostreptococcus*, and anaerobic or microaerophilic streptococci predominate. *B. fragilis* is recovered with other organisms in 15% of cases.

Many other conditions can lead to lung abscess. Necrotizing bacterial pneumonias caused by *S. aureus*, *K. pneumoniae*, or other gram-negative bacilli can lead to abscess formation. In other patients, abscess develops as a result of bronchial obstruction caused by tumors, foreign bodies, or bronchial stenosis. Septic pulmonary embolization is a cause of abscess formation. Pulmonary tuberculosis, fungal infection, or actinomycosis often leads to cavity formation. In the immunosuppressed host, *Nocardia* and other opportunistic organisms may also produce cavitation. Lung abscesses in patients with AIDS occur in the setting of advanced HIV infection; they are caused by a wide array of organisms and respond poorly to therapy.[64]

Noninfectious processes can produce cavitary lung lesions. Primary and metastatic tumors, bullae, cysts, intralobar pulmonary sequestration, pulmonary infarcts, vasculitis (including Wegener granulomatosis), and rheumatoid lung disease must be considered in the differential diagnosis of lung abscess.

DIAGNOSIS

Clinical Features

The clinical presentation of the patient with a lung abscess depends on the type of abscess. Patients with abscesses resulting from necrotizing staphylococcal or gram-negative bacillary pneumonias are usually acutely ill and exhibit clinical features of the underlying pneumonia. Although patients with primary lung abscess may also present acutely with aspiration pneumonia, they more often experience insidiously progressive symptoms for weeks or even months before diagnosis. Cough is present in almost all patients; when the abscess drains into the bronchial tree, production of copious foul-smelling sputum is characteristic. Hemoptysis is present in approximately one third of cases and may occasionally reach life-threatening proportions. Chest pain consisting of either a dull ache or a true pleurisy is common. Most patients have fever, but frank rigors are unusual. In patients with a chronic course lasting many weeks, anorexia, weight loss, and debility are often seen.

Physical Examination and Imaging

Physical examination of a patient with a lung abscess may disclose pulmonary rales, signs of consolidation, or, rarely, clubbing of the nails. These findings are not diagnostic, however, and chest x-rays or CT scans are required to establish the presence of an abscess. Although any lung segment may be involved, abscesses are most common in the posterior segments of the upper lobes and the apical segments of the lower lobes, because these areas are dependent when the patient is recumbent. Abscesses may be single or, less often, multiple. The finding of air-fluid levels signifies rupture into the bronchial tree.

Laboratory Studies

As is the case with other pulmonary infections, examination of the sputum is crucial to diagnosis. In patients with primary lung abscesses, the sputum is often putrid and contains numerous polymorphonuclear leukocytes and an abundant mixed microbial flora. Sputum cultures reveal only normal mouth flora. Meaningful anaerobic bacteriology depends on obtaining, either by transtracheal aspiration or by bronchoscopy, specimens that have not traversed the oropharynx. Percutaneous needle aspiration can also be very helpful, both diagnostically and therapeutically. In a typical case of aspirational putrid lung abscess, these invasive procedures may not be necessary. They are important, however, if the diagnosis is uncertain. The indications for bronchoscopy in patients with lung abscess are debatable. Although some physicians advocate bronchoscopy in all such patients, others reserve the procedure for patients in whom there is a suspicion of bronchial obstruction by a foreign body or tumor, for patients who fail to respond to medical therapy, and for patients from whom specimens are required to rule out tuberculosis, fungal infection, or carcinoma. Bronchoscopy may be helpful therapeutically by promoting bronchial drainage from cavities that incompletely communicate with the bronchial tree.

TREATMENT

If specific pathogens such as *S. aureus* or *Klebsiella* are present in reliable specimens, therapy should be directed at the causative pathogen. In primary lung abscesses caused by mixed oral flora, penicillin has been the drug of choice. Prospective studies comparing penicillin therapy with clindamycin therapy in 66 patients with lung abscess found clindamycin to be the superior agent[61]; however, the long clinical experience with penicillin warrants retaining penicillin as the drug of choice, with clindamycin an excellent alternative for patients who are allergic to penicillin or who respond poorly to that drug. Despite its excellent bactericidal activity against anaerobic bacteria, metronidazole appears less effective in treating lung abscess. Most centers initiate treatment with I.V. penicillin in a dosage range of 6 to 12 million units a day or with I.V. clindamycin in a dosage of 600 mg every 8 hours. After a clear-cut clinical response is observed, oral penicillin V in a dosage of 750 mg four times a day or oral clindamycin in a dosage of 300 mg every 6 hours can be substituted. Two to 4 weeks of parenteral therapy is often required before defervescence, diminished sputum production, and reduction in cavity size occur. The duration of therapy depends on the clinical course, but prolonged treatment for 4 to 8 weeks is usually required.

In addition to antibiotics, adequate drainage is essential and can usually be achieved with intensive pulmonary physiotherapy and postural drainage. Bronchoscopy can be very useful in promoting drainage and for excluding the diagnosis of cancer. Although surgery was once the mainstay of treatment, antibiotics are now almost always able to control infection, and surgery is needed only when complications occur. Massive hemoptysis is an indication for lung resection. Uncontrolled sepsis may occasionally require lobectomy. CT-guided percutaneous tube drainage may be very helpful in patients who are too ill to tolerate thoracotomy and may be the treatment of choice for lung abscesses that are refractory to medical management. Empyema, another complication of lung abscess, requires external drainage by thoracentesis, chest tube, or rib resection. The persistence of a thin-walled cavity after otherwise successful medical treatment, however, is not an indication for surgery. Recurrent or persistent infection, recurrent hemoptysis, or the suspicion of tumor may mandate operative intervention. Shaggy thick-walled cavities may be suggestive of tumor. Complications of lung abscess that have become uncommon because of antibiotic therapy include bronchogenic spread of infection to other pulmonary segments, bronchiectasis, and bacteremia with metastatic infection such as brain abscess.

Whereas patients with gram-negative or staphylococcal bacillary pneumonias or serious underlying diseases have a substantial mortality, the prognosis for patients with primary lung abscess is quite good. It is important to prevent recurrent pulmonary infection by treating dental disease and by avoiding factors that predispose to pulmonary aspiration.

Empyema

ETIOLOGY

Bacteria can reach the pleural space by many routes. Most often, empyema results from the direct spread of bronchopulmonary infections, including pneumonias, lung abscesses, and bronchiectasis.[65] Less often, empyema develops as a complication of thoracotomy or, rarely, thoracentesis. Open chest trauma provides another means for the direct introduction of microorganisms. Intra-abdominal infections, especially subphrenic abscesses, can penetrate the diaphragm to cause empyemas. Uncommonly, esophageal rupture can cause spread of infection from the mediastinum to the pleural space. Finally, hematogenous seeding is an infrequent mechanism of empyema formation.

S. aureus is the most common cause of empyema; various gram-negative bacilli, including *Pseudomonas aeruginosa*, *K. pneumoniae*, and *Escherichia coli*, are next in frequency. Many infections are mixed. Anaerobes have been recognized in 25% to 76% of empyemas and may occur in pure culture or in combination with aerobic or facultative organisms.[66] *Bacteroides* species, *Fusobacterium*, and anaerobic gram-positive cocci are the anaerobes most often seen. *Mycobacterium tuberculosis* has become a relatively uncommon cause of pleural space infections, and fungi are implicated only rarely. Transdiaphragmatic rupture of a liver abscess occasionally produces amebic empyema.

DIAGNOSIS

In most patients, the clinical presentation of empyemas includes fever, dyspnea, chest pain, and cough. Hemoptysis is less common than these other symptoms. If diagnosis and treatment are delayed, weight loss and debility may be prominent. The physical findings in patients with empyemas are no different from those in other patients with pleural effusions. In addition, chest wall tenderness may be present, and there may be signs of an underlying pneumonia or intra-abdominal infection. Tachypnea and respiratory distress may occur, and septic shock may complicate advanced cases. Polymorphonuclear leukocytosis is common; other laboratory findings may include anemia and hypoxia. Chest x-rays reveal pleural effusions that are free flowing in early disease but frequently loculated in late cases. Ultrasonography may be necessary to distinguish fluid from pleural fibrosis. Unless surgery or thoracentesis has been performed, air-fluid levels in the pleural space suggest a bronchopleural fistula.

DIFFERENTIAL DIAGNOSIS

In the differential diagnosis of empyema, it is important to consider the many causes of noninfected pleural effusions. Most important is the distinction between sterile parapneumonic effusions and true empyemas. Thoracentesis is mandatory for the diagnosis of empyema. Several thoracenteses may be needed if the fluid is loculated; CT or ultrasound guidance is very helpful in these circumstances. Gross purulence is diagnostic for empyema, but the absence of frank pus does not rule out infection. Like other inflammatory effusions, empyema fluids have the characteristics of exudates: protein levels greater than 3 g/dl and lactic dehydrogenase values in excess of 550 units. Pleural fluid acidosis is characteristic of empyemas, but alkalosis can occur if the infection is caused by a urea-splitting organism such as *Proteus*. Pleural fluid glucose levels are depressed in empyemas, and although white cell counts are variable, counts above 5,000/mm^3 are common, with polymorphonuclear leukocytes predominating. Gram stains of the pleural fluid will often reveal the causative organisms. Both aerobic and anaerobic cultures are mandatory; a foul odor suggests anaerobic infection. Stains and cultures for mycobacteria and fungi are important in selected cases.

TREATMENT

Treatment of empyemas involves two elements. Antibiotics should be selected on the basis of the causative pathogens. High-dose parenteral therapy is required, and prolonged antibiotic courses of 3 weeks or more are often needed. Adequate drainage is of paramount importance. In acute empyemas, the pleural cavity is lined by acute fibrinous inflammation, and percutaneous drainage of free-flowing fluid may be possible by repeated thoracentesis or tube thoracostomy. Closed chest tube drainage is the traditional method for draining empyemas, but image-guided catheter drainage is also effective, particularly when the fluid is loculated. Resolution of fever generally signifies satisfactory drainage. If complete drainage cannot be achieved with chest tubes, video-assisted thoracoscopic surgery (VATS) can often disrupt intrapleural adhesions and achieve excellent drainage of loculated effusions[67]; although VATS requires endotracheal intubation and general anesthesia, it is less invasive than the next alternative, rib resection with thoracotomy for decortication. Enzymatic debridement with streptokinase may enable some patients to avoid surgery.[68]

Septic Pulmonary Embolism

Although once uncommon, septic pulmonary embolism is now encountered because of narcotic addiction, which accounts for more than 75% of cases; tricuspid valve endocarditis and direct injection of infected material cause most of these cases. *S. aureus* and gram-negative bacilli are the predominant etiologic agents in addiction-related septic pulmonary embolism. Septic pulmonary embolism may also develop in patients with septic phlebitis of peripheral veins (especially phlebitis related to I.V. lines or pelvic infections), abscesses, or other bacteremic infections.

Unlike bland emboli, septic pulmonary emboli produce pulmonary infarction in most instances. Small emboli produce flame-shaped or patchy infiltrates that may shift in location; these manifestations generally resolve with antibiotic therapy. Larger emboli often cavitate and may lead to lung abscess, empyema, or bronchopleural fistula formation. In addition to antibiotics, surgical drainage may be required for such complications. Operative intervention may be needed to control the source of emboli in some patients. Heparin can be useful in patients with septic phlebitis.

References

1. Glezen WP, Greenberg SB, Atmar RL, et al: Impact of respiratory virus infections on persons with chronic underlying conditions. JAMA 283:499, 2000

2. Stockley RA: Role of inflammation in respiratory tract infections. Am J Med 99 (suppl 6B):8S, 1995

3. Marston BJ, Plouffe JF, File TM Jr, et al: Incidence of community-acquired pneumonia requiring hospitalization: results of a population-based active surveillance study in Ohio. Arch Intern Med 157:1709, 1997

4. Brown PD, Lerner SA: Community-acquired pneumonia. Lancet 352:1295, 1998

5. Fine MJ, Smith MA, Carson CA, et al: Prognosis and outcomes of patients with community-acquired pneumonia. JAMA 275:134, 1996

6. Fernandez-Sola J, Junque A, Estruch R, et al: High alcohol intake as a risk and prognostic factor for community-acquired pneumonia. Arch Intern Med 155:1649, 1995

7. Fine MJ, Auble TE, Yealy DM, et al: A prediction rule to identify low-risk patients with community-acquired pneumonia. N Engl J Med 335:243, 1997

8. Conte HA, Chen Y-T, Mehal W, et al: A prognostic rule for elderly patients admitted with community-acquired pneumonia. Am J Med 106:20, 1999

9. Koivula I, Sten J, Makela PH: Prognosis after community-acquired pneumonia in the elderly. Arch Intern Med 159:1550, 1999

10. Leroy O, Devos P, Guery B, et al: Simplified prediction rule for prognosis of patients with severe community-acquired pneumonia in ICUs. Chest 116:157, 1999

11. Ruiz-Gonzalez A, Falguera M, Nogues A, et al: Is *Streptococcus pneumoniae* the leading cause of pneumonia of unknown etiology? A microbiologic study of lung aspirates in consecutive patients with community-acquired pneumonia. Am J Med 106:385, 1999

12. Rello J, Rodriguez R, Jubert P, et al: Severe community-acquired pneumonia in the elderly: epidemiology and prognosis. Clin Infect Dis 23:723, 1996

13. Wood GM, Johnson BC, McCormack JG: *Moraxella catarrhalis*: pathogenic significance in respiratory tract infections treated by community practitioners. Clin Infect Dis 22:632, 1996

14. Winstead JM, McKinsey DS, Tasker S, et al: Meningococcal pneumonia: characterization and review of cases seen over the past 25 years. Clin Infect Dis 30:87, 2000

15. Marrie TJ, Peeling RW, Fine MJ, et al: Ambulatory patients with community-acquired pneumonia: the frequency of atypical agents and clinical course. Am J Med 101:508, 1996

16. Simoes EA: Respiratory syncytial virus infection. Lancet 354:847, 1999

17. Guidelines for prevention of nosocomial pneumonia. MMWR Morb Mortal Wkly Rep 46(RR-1):1, 1997

18. Casalta JP, Piquet P, Alazia M, et al: *Mycoplasma pneumoniae* pneumonia following assisted ventilation. Am J Med 101:165, 1996

19. Dalhoff K, Maass M: *Chlamydia pneumoniae* pneumonia in hospitalized patients: clinical characteristics and diagnostic value of polymerase chain reaction detection in BAL. Chest 110:351, 1996

20. Bonten MJM, Gaillard CA, de Leeuw PDW, et al: Role of colonization of the upper intestinal tract in the pathogenesis of ventilator-associated pneumonia. Clin Infect Dis 24:309, 1997

21. Muder RR: Pneumonia in residents of long-term care facilities: epidemiology, etiology, management, and prevention. Am J Med 105:319, 1998

22. Loeb M, McGeer A, McArthur M, et al: Risk factors for pneumonia and other lower respiratory tract infections in elderly residents of long-term care facilities. Arch Intern Med 159:2058, 1999

23. Bregeon F, Papazian L, Visconti A, et al: Relationship of microbiologic diagnostic criteria to morbidity and mortality in patients with ventilator-associated pneumonia. JAMA 277:655, 1997

24. Kirland SH, Corley DE, Winterbauer RH, et al: The diagnosis of ventilator-associated pneumonia: a comparison of histologic, microbiologic, and clinical criteria. Chest 112:445, 1997

25. Drakulovic MB, Torres A, Bauer TT, et al: Supine body position as a risk factor for nosocomial pneumonia in mechanically ventilated patients: a randomized trial. Lancet 354:1851, 1999

26. Cook D, De Jonghe B, Brochard L, et al: Influence of airway management on ventilator-associated pneumonia: evidence from randomized trials. JAMA 279:781, 1998

27. Kollef MH: The prevention of ventilator-associated pneumonia. N Engl J Med 340:627, 1999

28. Hirschtick RE, Glassroth J, Jordan MC, et al: Bacterial pneumonia in persons infected with the human immunodeficiency virus. N Engl J Med 333:845, 1995

29. Baril L, Astagneau P, Nguyen J, et al: Pyogenic bacterial pneumonia in human immunodeficiency virus–infected inpatients: a clinical, radiological, microbiological and epidemiological study. Clin Infect Dis 26:964, 1998

30. Afessa B, Green B: Bacterial pneumonia in hospitalized patients with HIV infection: the Pulmonary Complications, ICU Support, and Prognostic Factors of Hospitalized Patients with HIV (PIP) Study. Chest 117:1017, 2000

31. Wipf JE, Lipsky BA, Jirschmann JV, et al: Diagnosing pneumonia by physical examination. Relevant or relic? Arch Intern Med 159:1082, 1999

32. Wheeler JH, Fishman EK: Computed tomography in the management of chest infections: current status. Clin Infect Dis 23:232, 1996

33. Reimer LG, Carroll KC: Role of the microbiology laboratory in the diagnosis of lower respiratory tract infections. Clin Infect Dis 26:742, 1998

34. Veber B, Souweine B, Gachot B, et al: Comparison of direct examination of three types of bronchoscopy specimens used to diagnose nosocomial pneumonia. Crit Care Med 28:962, 2000

35. Lohr RH, Boland BJ, Douglas WW, et al: Organizing pneumonia: features and prognosis of cryptogenic, secondary, and focal variants. Arch Intern Med 157:1323, 1997

36. Gleason PP, Kapoor WN, Stone RA, et al: Medical outcomes and antimicrobial costs with the use of the American Thoracic Society guidelines for outpatients with community-acquired pneumonia. JAMA 278:32, 1997

37. Ailani RK, Agastya G, Ailani R, et al: Doxycycline is a cost-effective therapy for hospitalized patients with community-acquired pneumonia. Arch Intern Med 159:266, 1999

38. Bartlett JG, Breiman RF, Mandell LA, et al: Community-acquired pneumonia in adults: guidelines for management. Guidelines from the Infectious Diseases Society of America. Clin Infect Dis 26:811, 1998

39. Gatifloxacin and moxifloxacin: two new fluoroquinolones. Med Lett Drugs Ther 42:15, 2000

40. File TM Jr, Segreti J, Dunbar L, et al: Levofloxacin is highly effective for treating community-acquired pneumonia. Antimicrob Agents Chemother 41:1965, 1997

41. Vergis EN, Indorf A, File TM Jr, et al: Azithromycin vs cefuroxime plus erythromycin for empirical treatment of community-acquired pneumonia in hospitalized patients: a prospective, randomized, multicenter trial. Arch Intern Med 160:1294, 2000

42. Ramirez JA, Vargas S, Ritter GW, et al: Early switch from intravenous to oral antibiotics and early hospital discharge: a prospective observational study of 200 consecutive patients with community-acquired pneumonia. Arch Intern Med 159:2449, 1999

43. Stahl JE, Barza M, DesJardin J, et al: Effect of macrolides as part of initial empiric therapy on length of stay in patients hospitalized with community-acquired pneumonia. Arch Intern Med 159:2576, 1999

44. McCormick D, Fine M, Coley CM, et al: Variation in length of hospital stay in patients with community-acquired pneumonia. Are shorter stays associated with worse medical outcomes? Am J Med 107:5, 1999

45. Stout JE, Yu VL: Legionellosis. N Engl J Med 337:682, 1997

46. Pedro-Botet ML, Sabria-Leal M, Sopena N, et al: Role of immunosuppression in the evolution of Legionnaire's disease. Clin Infect Dis 26:14, 1998

47. Blatt SP, Dolan MJ, Hendrix CW, et al: Legionnaires' disease in human immunodeficiency virus–infected patients: eight cases and review. Clin Infect Dis 18:227, 1994

48. Sopena N, Sabria-Leal M, Pedro-Botet ML, et al: Comparative study of the clinical presentation of *Legionella* pneumonia and other community-acquired pneumonias. Chest 113:1195, 1998

49. Weir SC, Fischer SH, Stock F, et al: Detection of *Legionella* by PCR in respiratory specimens using a commercially available kit. Am J Clin Pathol 110:295, 1998

50. Plouffe JF, File TM, Breiman RF, et al: Reevaluation of the definition of Legionnaire's disease: use of the urinary antigen assay. Clin Infect Dis 20:1286, 1995

51. Edelstein RH: Antimicrobial chemotherapy for Legionnaire's disease: time for a change. Ann Intern Med 129:328, 1998

52. Knirsch CA, Jakob K, Schoonmaker D, et al: An outbreak of *Legionella micdadei* pneumonia in transplant patients: evaluation, molecular epidemiology, and control. Am J Med 108:290, 2000

53. Harris A, Lally M, Albrecht M: *Legionella bozemanii* pneumonia in three patients with AIDS. Clin Infect Dis 27:97, 1998

54. Kauppinen M, Saikku P: Pneumonia due to *Chlamydia pneumoniae*: prevalence, clinical features, diagnosis, and treatment. Clin Infect Dis 21:S244, 1995

55. Troy CJ, Peeling RW, Ellis AG, et al: *Chlamydia pneumoniae* as a new source of infectious outbreaks in nursing homes. JAMA 227:1214, 1997

56. Miyashita N, Kubota Y, Nakajima M, et al: *Chlamydia pneumoniae* and exacerbations of asthma in adults. Ann Allergy Asthma Immunol 80:405, 1998

57. Finucane TE, Brynum JPW: Use of tube feedings to prevent aspiration pneumonia. Lancet 348:1421, 1996

58. Campbell GD Jr: The role of antimicrobial therapy in acute exacerbations of chronic bronchitis. Am J Med Sci 318:84, 1999

59. Saint S, Bent S, Vittinghoff E, et al: Antibiotics in chronic obstructive pulmonary disease exacerbations: a meta-analysis. JAMA 273:957, 1995

60. MacKay DN: Treatment of acute bronchitis in adults without underlying lung disease. J Gen Int Med 11:557, 1996

61. Bent S, Saint S, Vittinghoff E, et al: Antibiotics in acute bronchitis: a meta-analysis. Am J Med 107:62, 1999

62. Gerberding JL: "Sputum aeruginosa": time to rewrite the textbooks on virus-induced airway inflammation. Am J Med 108:91, 2000

63. Lucidarme O, Grenier P, Coche E, et al: Bronchiectasis: comparative assessment with thin-section CT and helical CT. Radiology 200:673, 1996

64. Furman AC, Jacobs J, Sepkowitz KA: Lung abscess in patients with AIDS. Clin Infect Dis 22:81, 1996

65. Bryant RE, Salmon CJ: Pleural empyema. Clin Infect Dis 22:747, 1996

66. Civen R, Jousimies-Somer H, Marina M, et al: A retrospective review of cases of anaerobic empyema and update of bacteriology. Clin Infect Dis 20(suppl 2):S224, 1995

67. Landreneau RJ, Keenan RJ, Hazelrigg SR, et al: Thoracoscopy for empyema and hemothorax. Chest 109:18, 1995

68. Muers MF: Streptokinase for empyema. Lancet 349:1491, 1997

7 Infective Endocarditis

Adolf W. Karchmer, M.D.

Definition

Infective endocarditis is a microbial infection of a cardiac valve or the mural endocardium caused by bacteria, fungi, rickettsiae, or chlamydiae. Analogous infections called infective endaortitis and infective endarteritis occur on the endothelial surface of the aorta and large arteries. On the basis of its clinical course, endocarditis has been classified as either acute (having a duration of less than 6 weeks) or subacute (having a duration of more than 6 weeks). Prosthetic valve endocarditis (PVE) and endocarditis associated with I.V. drug abuse also have acute and subacute forms.

Etiology and Epidemiology

Streptococci and *Staphylococcus aureus* are the predominant causes of community-acquired bacterial endocarditis (BE) involving native valves [*see Table 1*]. Enterococci, coagulase-negative staphylococci (many of which are species other than *S. epidermidis*), and fastidious gram-negative HACEK organisms (HACEK is an acronym for *Haemophilus* species, *Actinobacillus actinomycetemcomitans, Cardiobacterium hominis, Eikenella* species, and *Kingella* species) are other important causes of BE.

Nosocomial BE is a complication of bacteremia associated with intravascular devices, genitourinary tract manipulation, and wound infection; it is caused primarily by *S. aureus,* enterococci, and coagulase-negative staphylococci, most of which are methicillin-resistant *S. epidermidis.* In I.V. drug abusers, *S. aureus* (often methicillin resistant) causes almost 50% of BE [*see Table 1*].

Fungal endocarditis is caused primarily by *Candida* species; it occurs in I.V. drug abusers and as a complication of intravascular devices, particularly in patients with prosthetic valves. Endocarditis caused by mycelial fungi is very rare but occasionally occurs in immunocompromised patients. In rare cases, endocarditis is caused by *Brucella* species, *Legionella* species, *Coxiella burnetii, Chlamydia psittaci,* and *Corynebacterium* species.[1,2] *Bartonella* was recently recognized as a cause of BE and may account for 3% of cases in some areas.[3] *B. quintana* endocarditis occurs more commonly among the homeless, and BE caused by *B. henselae* may be associated with cats.[3–5]

Although the incidence of infective endocarditis, which ranges from 1.7 to 3.8 cases per 100,000 person-years, has remained relatively stable over the past 4 decades, other aspects of the epidemiology of this disease have changed. The ages of patients with endocarditis have increased; in recent series, 50% of patients were older than 50 years.[6] Rheumatic heart disease is now a relatively uncommon predisposing factor for endocarditis, and degenerative valvular diseases, such as calcified aortic stenosis, calcified mitral valve annulus, and mitral

Table 1 Causes of Native Valve Endocarditis[6,8,79–82]

Microorganism	Percentage of Cases		
	Community Acquired	*Nosocomial*	*Addicts*
Staphylococcus aureus	35	55	48
Streptococci	32	7	8
Enterococci	8	16	15
Polymicrobial miscellaneous	6	1	9
Culture-negative	6	2	5
Gram-negative bacilli	4	5	8
HACEK	3	—	—
Pneumococci	1	—	—
Fungi	1	4	7

HACEK—*Haemophilus* species, *Actinobacillus actinomycetemcomitans, Cardiobacterium hominis, Eikenella* species, and *Kingella* species valve prolapse, are far more common predispositions.[7,8] Additionally, endocarditis associated with I.V. drug abuse and prosthetic cardiac valves and endocarditis acquired in nosocomial settings have emerged as severe problems.

SUBACUTE BACTERIAL ENDOCARDITIS

Subacute bacterial endocarditis (SBE) may be caused by a variety of relatively avirulent bacteria, the most common being streptococci that are part of the indigenous flora. These organisms lack sufficient invasiveness to infect normal heart valves or endocardium but can infect deformed heart valves or sites of congenital cardiac lesions.

Many of the streptococci that cause endocarditis can be categorized according to Lancefield serogrouping. About 40% are group D, about 10% are group H (*S. sanguis*), and about 15% are other serogroups (including B, C, G, and K). About 5% are anaerobic streptococci, and the remaining 30% to 35% are nongroupable viridans streptococci. The viridans streptococci, which enter the bloodstream from the oral cavity mucosa and gingival sulci, are strains loosely grouped together because of their capacity to produce an alpha reaction, or incomplete hemolysis, when grown on blood agar.

Enterococcus faecalis, E. faecium, and the nonenterococcal group D streptococcus, *S. bovis,* are often important causes of SBE coming from the GI and genitourinary tracts. The portal of entry for *S. bovis* is often a malignant or premalignant colonic lesion.[9] Consequently, colon evaluation is mandated for patients with *S. bovis* SBE.

The HACEK organisms, coagulase-negative staphylococci, and *Bartonella* species cause SBE. *S. aureus* usually causes acute endocarditis but may in rare instances cause the subacute form. Corynebacteria (diphtheroids) usually involve prosthetic heart valves. Endocarditis caused by *C. burnetii* occurs in the setting of preexisting valvular disease and is a particularly indolent infection.[10]

ACUTE BACTERIAL ENDOCARDITIS

Acute bacterial endocarditis (ABE) is commonly caused by organisms that are more invasive than the agents of SBE. These organisms can infect both normal and abnormal heart valves and mural endocardium and can rapidly destroy cardiac valves and establish suppurative foci at sites of embolic deposition. *S. aureus* is the most frequent cause of ABE; other agents are *S. pneumoniae,* group A streptococcus, *N. gonorrhoeae, Salmonella* species, other members of the family Enterobacteriaceae, and *Pseudomonas aeruginosa. Salmonella* is more frequently implicated as a cause of aortitis in the elderly, who may have a continuous salmonella bacteremia in the absence of a cardiac murmur.

Pathogenesis

High-velocity and turbulent blood flow across a defective valve or through a congenital defect predisposes to the development of SBE. When blood is driven from a high-pressure area through such a defect into a low-pressure sink, the endothelium in this low-pressure sink or on the abnormal valve is a site for platelet adherence and the formation of a platelet-fibrin aggregate.[11] During transient bacteremia, avirulent organisms adhere to the platelet-fibrin aggregate that overlies the abnormal endocardium. Virulent organisms, such as those associated with ABE, may adhere to these sites or to normal valve endocardium. Dense colonies of bacteria grow within the platelet-fibrin aggregate to form a macroscopic vegetation, the prototypical pathologic lesion of endocarditis. The platelet-fibrin mass is a relatively effective physical barrier between polymorphonuclear leukocytes and deeply embedded bacteria. The bacteria that cause endocarditis contribute further to vegetation growth. Extracellular material from some organisms initiate further platelet aggregation, and *S. aureus* can elicit procoagulant tissue factor from the endothelial substrate and local monocytes.[12]

The streptococci that most frequently cause SBE—*Streptococcus mutans* and *S. mitior* (viridans streptococci), *S. sanguis* (group H), and *S. bovis* (group D)—readily adhere to platelet-fibrin thrombi, owing to the presence of dextran on their surface. Streptococcal species that are not dextran producers cause endocarditis much less frequently than these four species. Fibronectin receptors and clumping factor, which occur on the surface of *Staphylococcus aureus,* appear to facilitate the adherence of these organisms to cardiac valves.[13]

Although platelets generally contribute to vegetation growth, they do contain microbicidal proteins that may inhibit bacterial growth in vegetations.[14,15]

Clinical Presentations

SUBACUTE BACTERIAL ENDOCARDITIS

The constitutional symptoms of SBE usually begin insidiously and may persist for months. Feverishness, sweats, weakness, myalgias, arthralgias, malaise, anorexia, and fatigability are prominent. Fewer than 5% of patients are afebrile, and such patients are often elderly, markedly malnour-

a

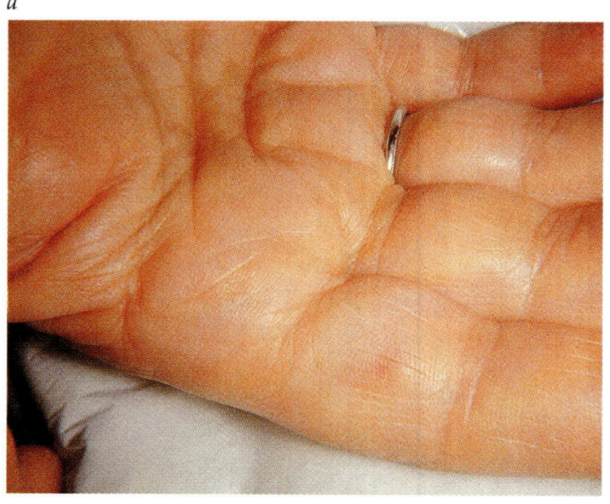

b

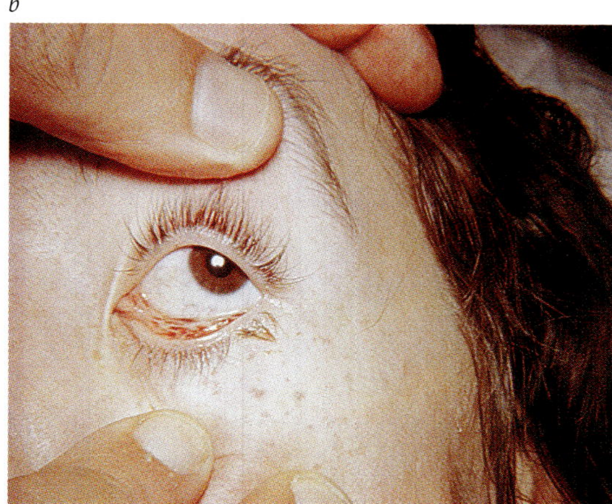

c

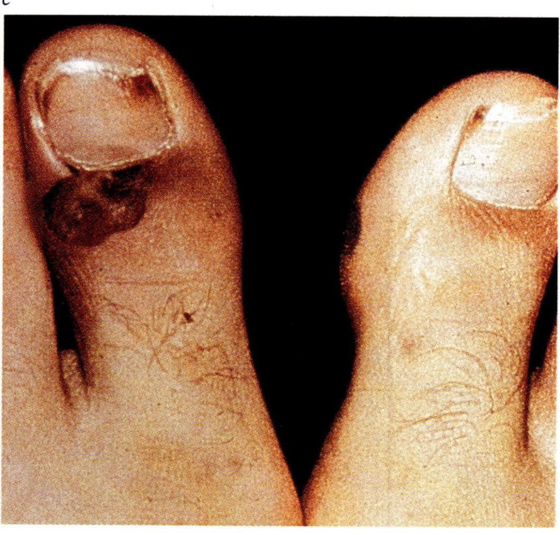

Figure 1 **Findings on physical examination of patients with endocarditis. (*a*) Shown here is an erythematous, palpable, nontender lesion at the base of the first finger consistent with a Janeway lesion. (*b*) Shown here is a patient with conjunctival petechiae. (*c*) Shown here are pustulonecrotic septic embolic lesions at the base of the nail of the right great toe and at the medial aspect of the left great toe at the level of the distal interphalangeal joint.**

ished, or azotemic. Chilly sensations are not uncommon, but frank rigors are unusual.

Because of greater awareness of this disease and the frequent use of blood cultures in the evaluation of febrile illnesses, the diagnosis is now made earlier than in the past; consequently, many of the classic features of SBE, such as clubbing and Osler's nodes, are seldom noted. Fever and nonspecific symptoms in the presence of a predisposing cardiac lesion may be the only clinical manifestations of SBE in some patients. Organs other than the heart may be the source of the patient's presenting symptoms, which may obscure the diagnosis. For example, if there are signs of meningitis, cerebral emboli, or glomerulonephritis, the physician's attention may be focused on the central nervous system or kidneys as the primary site of the illness. Similarly, a patient with left-sided SBE may occasionally present with a nonproductive cough of sufficient prominence to suggest that the lung is the primary disease site. Although it has been suggested that the presentation of native valve endocarditis in the elderly (persons older than 65 years) is muted when compared with that in younger patients (excluding cases involving I.V. drug abuse), recent data do not confirm differences and do suggest that the clinical features are similar across age groups.[16]

Cutaneous Manifestations

Petechiae occur in the conjunctivae [*see Figure 1a, 1b, and 1c*], in the oropharynx, and on the skin; they are particularly common on the lower extremities. Petechiae may continue to appear for some weeks during successful antibiotic treatment. Linear subungual splinter hemorrhages in the middle of the nail bed are a feature of SBE, whereas hemorrhages in the distal nail bed are more likely to have been induced by trauma. Osler's nodes—tender purplish subcutaneous nodules that develop in the pulp of the fingers and disappear within several days—occur in 5% of patients with endocarditis. Osler's nodes may be embolic or result from an immunologically mediated small-vessel vasculitis. Small, slightly nodular, nonpainful erythematous or hemorrhagic areas on the palms or soles, called Janeway lesions, may occur in SBE or, more commonly, in ABE [*see Figure 1a, 1b, and 1c*].

Musculoskeletal Features

Myalgias, arthralgias, arthritis, or low back pain occurs in 40% to 50% of patients with SBE; in about half of these patients, such symptoms represent either initial or prominent manifestations of the disease. Painful, warm, red, tender joints may be noted, but joint effusions are rare. Immunologic mechanisms may be at work in the genesis of articular symptoms. Rheumatoid factor is present in 50% of patients with endocarditis of more than 6 weeks' duration, antinuclear antibody is found in some patients, and circulating immune complexes occur in 75% to 90% of patients. Clubbing of the fingers is now seen in only 15% of patients.

Ocular Findings

Petechial, flame-shaped hemorrhages, Roth's spots, and cotton-wool exudates occur in the retina of patients with endocarditis. Roth's spots are oval white areas surrounded by a zone of hemorrhage; they are noted in 3% to 5% of patients. Ocular findings are not pathognomonic of endocarditis and may be observed in patients with such disorders as severe anemia or collagen vascular diseases.

Splenic Abnormalities

Splenomegaly occurs in 15% to 30% of patients with endocarditis. Splenic infarcts and abscesses occur in 40% and 5% of patients, respectively; they are not linked to splenomegaly. Infarcts occasionally cause local pain but are commonly asymptomatic. Splenic abscess may manifest itself as left shoulder, left upper quadrant, or pleuritic left chest pain; fever that persists during antibiotic therapy; or a relapse of bacteremia. Splenic abscesses occur in association with endocarditis of all etiologies. Splenic lesions are best imaged by computed tomography and magnetic resonance techniques and, to a lesser degree, by ultrasonography; however, the differentiation of abscesses from infarcts by imaging is difficult. Radionuclide scanning is no longer used to detect splenic abscesses.

Renal Manifestations

Microscopic hematuria is observed in about 50% of patients. Embolic renal infarction may cause flank pain and hematuria but rarely causes renal failure. Diffuse membranoproliferative glomerulonephritis results from the deposition of IgG, IgM, and complement in a granular or nodular, lumpy-bumpy fashion in the glomerular basement membrane or on the basement membrane in subepithelial or subendothelial locations. Bacterial antigen may be identified in these glomerular deposits. In patients with this immune complex nephritis, serum complement levels are reduced. Diffuse membranoproliferative glomerulonephritis may cause renal failure, which generally resolves after treatment of the infection.[11] Focal embolic glomerulonephritis was originally thought to result from small bacterial emboli that destroyed segments of the glomerulus. However, it is now recognized as an anatomic variation of immune complex disease. It is occasionally associated with renal failure.

Embolic Phenomena

Significant embolic episodes occur in 25% to 50% of patients with endocarditis. Symptoms and signs include stroke; monocular blindness with occlusion of the central retinal artery; acute abdominal pain, ileus, and melena with mesenteric arterial occlusion; and pain and gangrene in the digits. Most clinical emboli affect the CNS, particularly the middle cerebral artery. Coronary emboli, which are found in as many as 50% of autopsied endocarditis patients, are generally asymptomatic but occasionally result in frank myocardial infarction.

The risk for embolization is difficult to determine because of inconsistencies in findings among studies. Factors associated with increased risk of embolization include vegetations of 10 mm or more in size as seen on transesophageal echocardiography; vegetations on the mitral valve, particularly the anterior leaflet; vegetations that increase in size during therapy; and endocarditis caused by *S. aureus*.[17–21] The incidence of arterial emboli decreases 10-fold during the initial 2 weeks of antimicrobial therapy.[17] Nevertheless, emboli may occur late during therapy or after therapy and do not necessarily indicate failed antimicrobial treatment.

Pulmonary emboli occur in right-sided endocarditis and frequently cause pulmonary infarcts and pneumonia, which may progress to lung abscess, empyema, and pyopneumothorax when invasive organisms such as *S. aureus* are involved.

Mycotic Aneurysms

Mycotic aneurysms, which can form in any artery but are particularly prominent in cerebral arteries, may complicate 2% to 10% of endocarditis cases. These may become symptomatic during active endocarditis or even after valvular infection has been eradicated. The clinical features include pain, a pulsatile mass, evidence of pressure on adjacent structures, or the sudden development of an expanding hematoma or signs of major blood loss. Surgical excision to prevent rupture is usually indicated for extracranial aneurysms of significant size.

Neurologic Manifestations

Neurologic complications develop in 30% to 40% of patients with endocarditis and are associated with increased mortality.[22] Stroke caused by cerebral embolism, commonly in the middle cerebral artery or one of its branches, is the most frequent neurologic complication, occurring in about 15% of patients. Cerebral embolism may be the initial manifestation of endocarditis. Some patients have multiple microscopic embolic infarcts, which are manifested by an altered level of consciousness, seizures, fluctuating focal neurologic signs, or a combination of these symptoms.

Cerebral mycotic aneurysms occur in 1% to 5% of patients with BE and most commonly affect the distal branches of the middle cerebral artery. Multiple aneurysms occur in some patients. In patients with an aneurysm, the overall mortality is 60%.

Mycotic aneurysms present as a sudden cerebral or subarachnoid hemorrhage or as an embolic stroke followed by an intracerebral hemorrhage. Focal neurologic findings or persistent focal headaches may signal the presence of an aneurysm before rupture. A slowly leaking aneurysm may cause mild meningeal irritation. In such cases, the cerebrospinal fluid, although sterile, may contain erythrocytes, leukocytes, and increased levels of protein.

In the search for an aneurysm, contrast-enhanced CT may provide localizing information by detecting intracerebral bleeding. Magnetic resonance angiography is insufficiently sensitive to detect aneurysms that are 5 mm or less; hence, cerebral angiography is the optimal diagnostic test.[23,24] Cerebral angiography for the detection of aneurysms has been advised for patients with focal neurologic signs (especially patients with ABE), persistent unexplained headache, or mild meningeal irritation, particularly if anticoagulant therapy is planned. Treatment of a mycotic aneurysm that has been detected by angiography depends on its location, the presence or absence of hemorrhage, and changes in its size that occur during antimicrobial therapy. Healing of mycotic aneurysms (resolution) during the treatment of endocarditis has been demonstrated by angiography.[25] However, a leaking aneurysm, an aneurysm that is progressively enlarging, or one that persists after antibiotic therapy should be removed surgically, provided it is accessible. These complex cases should be managed with the assistance of infectious disease and neurosurgical consultants.

Large brain abscesses are very uncommon in BE, although septic emboli in patients with *S. aureus* BE may give rise to multiple small abscesses.

Seizures, which are usually triggered by emboli, and toxic encephalopathy may also complicate endocarditis. A CSF pleocytosis with polymorphonuclear leukocytes predominating is observed in some patients with ABE caused by a pyogenic organism. Patients with SBE may have an aseptic CSF profile.

Cardiac Findings

The cardiac features in SBE are primarily those of the underlying valvular or congenital lesion. Murmurs are present in more than 90% of patients. Mild changes in the intensity of a systolic murmur are associated with the development of anemia, high fever, or tachycardia and are often of little significance. The appearance of a new murmur of valvular regurgitation is an important diagnostic event and may have implications for therapy as well. A new aortic diastolic murmur suggests dilatation of the aortic annulus or eversion or fenestration of an aortic leaflet. The sudden onset of a loud mitral pansystolic murmur suggests rupture of a chorda tendineae or fenestration of a mitral valve leaflet. Congestive heart failure resulting from valvular dysfunction may be progressive and severe in some patients. Extension of infection into the annulus, particularly if the infection progresses through the right and noncoronary leaflet portion of the aortic annulus into the membranous septum and the area of the atrioventricular node, may result in cardiac rhythm disturbances.[26] Occasionally, annular infection extends to the pericardium and causes pericarditis [*see* Cardiac Complications of Endocarditis, *below*].

ACUTE BACTERIAL ENDOCARDITIS

The onset of ABE is usually abrupt, and rigors are common. Temperatures reach 39.4° to 40.6° C (102.9° to 105.1° F) and are often remittent. Cutaneous manifestations, particularly petechiae, may be prominent, especially when ABE is caused by *S. aureus*. Occasionally, the clinical features in a patient with acute *S. aureus* endocarditis mimic those of acute meningococcemia: grossly similar skin lesions, including petechiae, purpura, and focal gangrene; similar hematologic changes, including disseminated intravascular coagulation; and the common neurologic findings of nuchal rigidity and CSF pleocytosis. Pustular petechiae or purulent purpura should strongly suggest *S. aureus* endocarditis, rather than meningococcemia [*see Figure 1a, 1b, and 1c*]. A Gram's stain and culture of material from a skin lesion can promptly reveal the etiologic agent and direct antibiotic therapy.

Emboli are common in ABE. Metastatic infections in the spleen, bones (particularly the vertebrae), joints, kidneys, brain, eye (specifically, endophthalmitis), and lungs may arise from either septic embolization or the sustained bacteremia. These metastatic infections may cause organ-specific symptoms or persistent fever in spite of antimicrobial therapy and may require drainage or surgical intervention. Osler's nodes may occur but less often than in SBE. Janeway lesions occur in 5% to 10% of patients who have *S. aureus* endocarditis.

ABE may be present even if the patient does not have a cardiac murmur. The appearance of a new murmur, particularly one characteristic of valvular insufficiency, strongly suggests valvular destruction and confirms the diagnosis of ABE. Valvular damage can lead to severe congestive heart failure and necessitate cardiac surgery.

ENDOCARDITIS ASSOCIATED WITH DRUG ABUSE

Between 0.2% and 2.0% of I.V. drug abusers develop endocarditis annually. At the time of their initial attack of endocarditis, 70% to 80% of drug addicts have no history or findings of preexisting valvular heart disease. In addicts, the tricuspid valve is infected more frequently (55%) than the aortic valve (35%) or mitral valve (30%), and multiple episodes of endocarditis are common.

S. aureus is responsible for approximately 50% of addiction-associated endocarditis [*see Table 1*].[27] Although polymicrobial endocarditis, such as simultaneous infection by *P. aeruginosa* and *S. aureus*, is extremely rare among nonaddicts with native valve endocarditis, 6% of cases in addicts involve multiple organisms. In cases of addiction-associated endocarditis, enterococci, streptococci, and *Candida* primarily infect the aortic and mitral valves. *S. aureus* and *P. aeruginosa* infect valves on both the right and the left side of the heart. *S. aureus*, however, accounts for almost 80% of right-sided endocarditis in addicts. Methicillin-resistant *S. aureus* is often encountered in these patients and may be associated with self-administration of nonprescribed antibiotics. Blood cultures generally reveal the causative organism, even when the endocarditis is exclusively right sided. Microbiologic evaluation of surgically removed arterial emboli may be required to identify the cause in selected cases.

Although the manifestations of endocarditis in addicts are generally similar to those in nonaddicts, there are noteworthy differences caused by variations in the frequency of tricuspid involvement (pulmonic valve infection is rare) and the nature of the infecting organisms in the two groups. Fever, chills, malaise, cough, and pleuritic chest pain are the most common presenting complaints in right-sided endocarditis in addicts. Septic pulmonary emboli occur in about 75% of cases, particularly in patients with *S. aureus* infection, and cause sputum production, hemoptysis, and initial radiologic findings that may suggest pneumonia. Cavitation of embolic pulmonary lesions is common. Significant cardiac murmurs are heard in most patients at some time during their illness, but these may not be detected initially. The murmur of tricuspid regurgitation, a short ejection systolic murmur that is louder on inspiration, may be difficult to detect. Hemodynamically significant tricuspid insufficiency is manifested by jugular vein V waves and a pulsating liver.

Because *S. aureus* and other pyogenic bacteria are the predominant causes of infective endocarditis in addicts, metastatic infections are a frequent complication. Neurologic manifestations and peripheral emboli frequently occur. Peripheral emboli may occlude major vessels and require surgical removal.

PROSTHETIC VALVE ENDOCARDITIS

The cumulative incidence of PVE is estimated at 3% and at 4.0% to 5.5% at 1 and 4 years, respectively, after valve implantation.[28,29] Infection may develop at the time of valve placement or from transient bacteremia anytime thereafter. The overall risk of infection is similar for mechanical and porcine bioprosthetic valves and for aortic and mitral valve prostheses.[29]

The predominant organisms causing PVE during the first year after surgery are methicillin-resistant coagulase-negative staphylococci, predominantly *S. epidermidis* [*see Table 2*]. Coagulase-negative staphylococci are still significant causes of PVE that occurs a year or more after surgery; however, these staphylococci are often species other than *S. epidermidis*, and only 20% to 30% are methicillin resistant. *S.*

Table 2 Etiology of Prosthetic Valve Endocarditis[30,83,84]

Organism	Time of Onset after Valve Implantation and Percentage of Cases		
	≤ 2 months	2–12 months	> 12 months
Coagulase-negative staphylococci	54	56	15
Staphylococcus aureus	8	9	13
Gram-negative bacilli	12	3	1
Streptococci	—	3	34
Enterococci	—	6	11
Corynebacteria	8	—	1
HACEK	—	3	14
Fungi	6	6	3
Miscellaneous	6	6	1
Culture-negative	6	9	6

aureus, streptococci, enterococci, and fastidious gram-negative coccobacilli (organisms frequently associated with native valve endocarditis) cause 72% of PVE beginning a year or more after valve replacement.[29] Coagulase-negative staphylococci, which are often resistant to methicillin, are responsible for at least 35% of cases of PVE and therefore cannot be easily dismissed as contaminants when they are isolated from the blood of a patient with a prosthetic valve.

Infection of prosthetic valves is often associated with invasion of perivalvular tissues, valvular dysfunction, and myocardial abscesses.[30] Necrosis of the annulus that occurs as a result of invasive infection causes partial dehiscence of the prosthesis and hemodynamically significant valvular regurgitation. These pathologic changes are not common when infection involves either porcine or mechanical prosthetic valves, particularly when the valves are in the aortic position or when infection occurs during the first postoperative year.[29,31] Occasionally, vegetations may partially obstruct the valve orifice or restrict valve movement, causing functional stenosis. Such changes are more likely when the prosthesis is in the mitral position. When infection is restricted to the leaflets of a porcine bioprosthetic valve, leaflet destruction, obstructing vegetations, and the delayed onset of leaflet stiffness may cause clinically significant valvular dysfunction.[31]

The dominant clinical feature of prosthetic valve endocarditis that occurs during the first 60 days after surgery (early prosthetic valve endocarditis [EPVE]) is fever; this is the case either with or without a prosthetic regurgitant murmur. Prosthetic valve dysfunction with resulting congestive heart failure is seen in some patients. Petechiae occur in about half of patients with EPVE, but Roth's spots, Osler's nodes, and Janeway lesions are common. Emboli are common in EPVE; emboli that occlude large peripheral arteries suggest fungal endocarditis. Because blood cultures are often negative in patients with fungal endocarditis, this diagnosis must often be made on the basis of histologic examination or culture of the vegetation recovered at embolectomy.

The clinical features of late PVE (PVE that occurs more than 60 days after surgery) may include splenomegaly, petechiae, Roth's spots, Janeway lesions, Osler's nodes, and systemic emboli; these features are quite similar to those of subacute endocarditis on native valves.

Special Diagnostic Considerations

The clinical diagnosis of PVE is made on the basis of findings on physical examination and echocardiography and the demonstration of a continuous bacteremia [*see* Diagnosis, *below*].

Not all patients with a prosthetic heart valve who experience culture-documented nosocomial bacteremia have or subsequently develop PVE. Of bacteremic patients with a prosthetic valve in whom the initial positive blood culture is not sentinel evidence of active PVE, 15% to 20% will develop PVE caused by the blood culture isolate.[32]

A transient gram-negative bacillus bacteremia from an extracardiac source does not necessarily result in early PVE; however, recrudescent or sustained bacteremia that occurs after the extracardiac focus of infection has been eradicated suggests PVE, as does sustained gram-negative bacillus bacteremia with no identifiable extracardiac source, even if a new regurgitant murmur or other signs of endocarditis are lacking. High-grade coagulase-negative staphylococcal bacteremia in a patient with a prosthetic valve strongly suggests PVE. Similarly, PVE is likely when the coagulase-negative staphylococci that have been isolated sporadically from among many blood cultures are shown by molecular techniques to derive from a single clone. Cultures are negative in 6% of cases. Negative cultures are usually the result of previous antibiotic therapy or unique characteristics of the infecting organisms [*see* Diagnosis, *below*].

Diagnosis

Although the diagnosis of endocarditis is readily evident in patients with the classic syn-

Table 3 Duke Criteria for the Diagnosis of Infective Endocarditis[33]

Definite

Pathologic criteria

1. Microorganisms: demonstrated by culture or histologically in a vegetation, in a vegetation that has embolized, or in an intracardiac abscess specimen

or

2. Pathologic lesions: vegetation or intracardiac abscess confirmed by histologic examination showing active endocarditis

Clinical criteria*

1. Two major criteria

or

2. One major and three minor criteria

or

3. Five minor criteria

Possible

Findings consistent with infective endocarditis that fall short of "definite" but are not "rejected"

Rejected

1. Firm alternative diagnosis for manifestations of infective endocarditis

or

2. Resolution of endocarditis syndrome with antibiotic therapy for ≤ 4 days

or

3. No pathologic evidence of infective endocarditis at surgery or autopsy, with antibiotic therapy for ≤ 4 days

*See Table 4 for definitions of major and minor criteria.

drome—fever, typical peripheral signs, systemic emboli, a murmur associated with valvular dysfunction, and bacteremia—the diagnosis is less evident in most patients. A diagnostic approach has been designed by the Duke Endocarditis Service (Duke criteria) [*see Tables 3 and 4*].[33] With these criteria, the diagnosis of endocarditis can be established definitively by pathologic or clinical criteria. The latter require the use of combinations of clearly specified information: microbiologic data (culture or serologic), anatomic evidence of infection by echocardiogram, findings on physical examination, the presence of rheumatoid factor, and the presence of conditions that predispose to endocarditis [*see Table 4*]. In retrospective evaluations of pathologically proven cases of native valve endocarditis and PVE, these clinical criteria were found to be highly sensitive and capable of identifying the cases as definite or possible endocarditis.[33-36] Misdiagnoses rarely resulted when these clinical criteria were used to reassess previously pathologically confirmed cases. The specificity and negative predictive values of these criteria have been reported as 99% and 92%, respectively.[37,38] Use of these clinical criteria very rarely results in the rejection of cases considered to be endocarditis on independent expert evaluation.[39] Thus, if applied judiciously throughout a patient's evaluation (rather than at a single point in time), the Duke criteria identify those patients who merit therapy for endocarditis (i.e., those considered to have definite or possible endocarditis).

ECHOCARDIOGRAPHY

In development of the Duke criteria, recognition was given to the high sensitivity and specificity of echocardiography in defining the anatomic features of endocarditis, especially when experienced echocardiographers apply specific criteria. In patients with pathologically proven native valve endocarditis, vegetations can be detected in 60% by use of transthoracic echocardiography and in 87% to 94% with transesophageal echocardiography; the specificity of both techniques is extraordinarily high.[40-42] In addition, echocardiography is the preferred technique whereby perivalvular infection (abscesses) and other intracardiac complications of endocarditis are identified. For abscess detection, a transesophageal study is significantly more sensitive than transthoracic imaging (and equally specific), with sensitivities of 76% to 87% and 18% to 28%, respectively.[43,44] Also, transesophageal echocardiography is notably superior to transthoracic echocardiography in the evaluation of patients with suspected PVE [*see* Prosthetic Valve Endocarditis, *above*].

Although virtually all patients in whom endocarditis is suspected should undergo echocardiography, it is not a screening test for patients with fever and a positive blood culture. Given its high sensitivity, a negative transesophageal echocardiogram is strong evidence against the possibility of endocarditis in patients at low or intermediate risk of this infection. Conversely, the false negative rate for transesophageal echocardiography is 6% to 11%; hence, if the likelihood of endocarditis is high, a negative echocardiogram does not exclude the diagnosis.[41,45] A repeat transesophageal study in patients with endocarditis reduces the false negative results to approximately 5%.[45] Finally, echocardiography cannot reliably distinguish an infected vegetation from a sterilized vegetation, a nonbacterial thrombotic vegetation of marantic endocarditis, or a thrombus as seen in the antiphospholipid antibody syndrome.

Table 4 Definitions of Terms Used in Duke Criteria for the Diagnosis of Infective Endocarditis[33]

Major criteria

1. Positive blood cultures for the following:

   Typical microorganism consistent with diagnosis from two separate blood cultures

   a. Viridans streptococci, *Streptococcus bovis*, or HACEK organisms

   or

   b. Community-acquired *Staphylococcus aureus* or enterococci, in the absence of a primary focus

   or

   Persistently positive blood cultures, defined as microorganisms consistent with diagnosis from the following:

   a. At least two blood samples drawn > 12 hr apart

   or

   b. Three of three or a majority when more than three blood cultures are drawn, with first and last samples drawn at least 1 hr apart

2. Evidence of endocardial involvement

   Positive echocardiogram for IE

   a. Oscillating intracardiac mass on valve or supporting structures, in the path of regurgitant jets, or on implanted material, in the absence of an alternative anatomic explanation

   or

   b. Abscess

   or

   c. New partial dehiscence of prosthetic valve

   or

   d. New valvular regurgitation (changing of preexisting murmur not sufficient)

Minor criteria

1. Predisposition: predisposing heart condition or I.V. drug use
2. Fever: temperature ≥ 38° C (100.4° F)
3. Vascular phenomena: major arterial emboli, septic pulmonary infarcts, mycotic aneurysm, intracranial hemorrhage, conjunctival hemorrhages, Janeway lesions
4. Immunologic phenomena: glomerulonephritis, Osler's nodes, Roth spots, rheumatoid factor
5. Microbiologic evidence: positive blood culture but not meeting a major criterion (see above)* or serologic evidence of active infection with organism consistent with IE
6. Echocardiogram consistent with infective endocarditis but not meeting a major criterion (above)

*Excludes single positive cultures for coagulase-negative staphylococci, diphtheroids, and organisms that do not commonly cause endocarditis.
IE—infective endocarditis

Transthoracic echocardiography has limited usefulness in the diagnosis of PVE because the prosthesis itself produces echoes that obscure vegetations and abscesses. In contrast, transesophageal two-dimensional and Doppler echocardiography more effectively assess the prosthetic valve and perivalvular tissue, especially when a mitral valve prosthesis is present.[46,47] With PVE, the transesophageal technique identified vegetations in 82% of patients, compared with a 36% identification rate with transthoracic echocardiography.[43] Similarly, detection of paravalvular abscesses in patients with PVE is markedly increased by use of transesophageal rather than transthoracic echocardiography.[47]

BLOOD CULTURES

For patients with putative endocarditis, the determination of a microbial etiology and the antimicrobial susceptibility of that organism are of paramount importance in diagnosis and therapy. In most patients with SBE, all blood cultures taken before initiation of antibiotic therapy are positive, reflecting the sustained bacteremia associated with an infected endothelial surface. Three or four sets of cultures taken before the start of therapy are adequate for demonstrating the bacteremia. Cultures should be taken in both aerobic and anaerobic media and should be incubated in 5% to 10% carbon dioxide; this procedure allows isolation of anaerobic organisms and strains whose growth is enhanced in the presence of carbon dioxide.

Blood cultures are negative in 5% to 14% of patients with endocarditis [*see Tables 1 and 2*].[2,48] In 50% of these cases, cultures are negative as a consequence of previous antimicrobial therapy (even if that therapy was ineffective). Recovery of the causative organism from the blood of these previously treated patients may often be accomplished by repeat blood cultures several days after the antibiotics have been discontinued. Blood cultures may also be negative in cases of right-sided endocarditis caused by relatively noninvasive organisms. At present, however, most cases of right-sided endocarditis occur among I.V. drug abusers and are caused by pyogenic bacteria, such as *S. aureus* and *P. aeruginosa*, which are readily isolated from the blood. Culture of bone marrow or arterial blood does not provide more information than can be obtained from culture of venous blood.

Several additional factors can thwart isolation of the infecting agent from blood and lead to a diagnosis of apparent culture-negative infective endocarditis. Prolonged incubation (3 to 4 weeks) or subculture of blood on special media, such as buffered charcoal–yeast extract agar for *Legionella,* is necessary because of the fastidious growth requirements of HACEK organisms; *Legionella, Bartonella,* and *Brucella* species; diphtheroids; strict anaerobes; and other bacteria. Although the lysis centrifugation technique for blood cultures is recommended when fungal endocarditis is suspected, the particular properties of certain fungal organisms, such as *H. capsulatum* and *Aspergillus* species, make them difficult to isolate. Finally, *C. burnetii* and *C. psittaci* require isolation techniques beyond the capabilities of most laboratories.[1,10,49] Endocarditis caused by *Bartonella* species, *Legionella* species, *Brucella* species, *C. psittaci,* and *C. burnetii* can be presumptively diagnosed with serologic tests; these serologic tests should be performed in the evaluation of apparent culture-negative endocarditis, particularly when negative cultures cannot be attributed to prior antimicrobial therapy. Direct culture on special media, histopathologic examination with special stains, and molecular techniques to recover DNA or 16S ribosomal RNA can be used to determine etiology when vegetations from valves or those embolized to peripheral arteries are available.[50,51]

ADDITIONAL TESTS

In patients with endocarditis, the results of many laboratory tests are abnormal because of the systemic impact of the infection and because of injury to various end organs. Such tests include complete blood count, urine analysis, creatinine level, liver function tests, quantitative immunoglobulins, complement, sedimentation rate, and others. Although these tests may be important in the management of patients with endocarditis, they are not important in establishing the diagnosis.

Differential Diagnosis

The diagnosis of infective endocarditis must be considered in any patient with a heart murmur and fever. The physician must be particularly alert to atypical cases in which the most prominent clinical findings are endocarditis-associated complications in organs other than the heart.

A variety of noninfectious illnesses can mimic infective endocarditis. Acute rheumatic fever can cause fever, cardiac murmurs, and congestive heart failure, but acute rheumatic fever can be distinguished from BE on clinical grounds and by blood cultures, anti–streptolysin O antibody titer, and response to salicylates [see 15 Infections Due to Gram-Positive Cocci]. Marantic endocarditis, which can give rise to multiple embolic episodes and fever, is usually associated with underlying neoplasm or chronic wasting disease. The presence of fever, anemia, and renal involvement in polyarteritis nodosa may suggest a diagnosis of SBE, and the findings on biopsy of a lesion in a large artery may even resemble those of a mycotic aneurysm. In patients with both systemic lupus erythematosus and antiphospholipid antibody syndrome, the manifestations of fever, nonbacterial thrombotic vegetations, systemic emboli, and spontaneous thrombotic events can resemble BE.

A cardiac myxoma, usually in the left atrium, may mimic infective endocarditis in both clinical and laboratory features. Low-grade fever, weight loss, arthralgias, cutaneous lesions (petechiae, Osler's nodes, Janeway lesions), clubbing of the fingers, emboli to major arteries, and the auscultatory findings of mitral stenosis and regurgitation can occur in patients with a cardiac myxoma. Cardiac myxoma syndrome may further parallel infective endocarditis by giving rise to cerebral aneurysms at the sites of myxomatous emboli. Negative blood cultures and echocardiography can help establish the diagnosis.

Neoplasms may mimic infective endocarditis by inducing marantic endocarditis or by their hemodynamic effects. For example, a richly vascular hypernephroma may be associated with cardiomegaly, a flow murmur, anemia, and fever. In addition, on physical examination, a left renal mass may be mistaken for the spleen. Carcinoid tumors occasionally mimic endocarditis when they produce endocardial and valvular fibrosis that leads to tricuspid insufficiency and pulmonary stenosis.

Cardiac Complications of Endocarditis

Congestive heart failure is the most frequent cardiac complication of infective endocarditis. Damage to the aortic valve by infection causes more rapidly progressive and severe hemodynamic consequences than does comparable damage to the mitral valve. A mycotic aneurysm of a sinus of Valsalva or an aortic annulus abscess may rupture through the membranous septum into the right atrium or ventricle [*see Figure* 2]. Flow through the resulting fistula causes a sudden rise in the jugular vein pressure and a continuous or to-and-fro murmur and thrill along the left sternal border. The lungs remain relatively clear. Valvular damage and

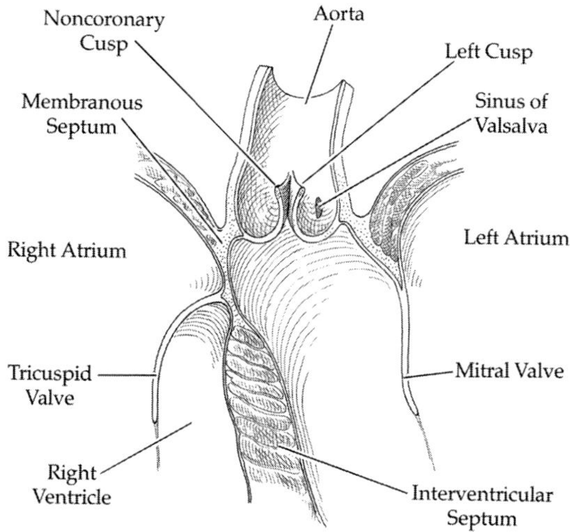

Figure 2 **Anatomic relations between the noncoronary cusp and left cusp of the aortic valve, interventricular septum, membranous septum, tricuspid valve, and mitral valve are shown schematically at the level of the aortic root.**

subsequent dysfunction, as well as intracardiac fistula formation, can be accurately defined with two-dimensional and Doppler echocardiography from a transthoracic or transesophageal approach.

The development of new conduction abnormalities may signal the extension of infection to the septum and its major conduction tissues.[49,52] The proximity of the weakest area of the aortic valve annulus to the membranous septum and conduction system accounts for the development of these conduction abnormalities [*see Figure 3*]. Similarly, extension of infection from the mitral annulus, which is close to the bundle of His and to the atrioventricular (AV) node, may also produce conduction defects, but such extension occurs less frequently than extension from the aortic valve. New PR interval prolongation, a new left bundle branch block, or a new right bundle branch block with left anterior hemiblock suggests the extension of infection from the aortic valve. In the absence of digitalis toxicity or a recent inferior myocardial infarction, the development of nonparoxysmal junctional tachycardia, a Wenckebach block, or complete heart block with a narrow QRS complex serves as a clue to the spread of infection from the mitral annulus into the AV node and proximal bundle of His.[26] Some conduction abnormalities are an indication for pacing. Ventricular premature beats in patients with endocarditis who do not have electrolyte abnormalities or digitalis toxicity may reflect myocarditis, myocardial abscesses, or small coronary emboli.

Annular abscesses, which are most commonly associated with infection of the aortic valve, may be suggested by the recent onset of aortic regurgitation, persistent fever during appropriate antimicrobial therapy, and the development of pericarditis.[53–55] Pericarditis caused by extension of a valve ring abscess into the epicardium is more often hemorrhagic and fibrinous than purulent. Occasionally, pericarditis in the course of infective endocarditis is the result of transmural myocardial infarction secondary to coronary emboli. Transesophageal echocardiography is the most sensitive and preferred noninvasive test for detecting myocardial abscesses in both native valve endocarditis and PVE.[31,44]

Treatment

Two major modalities are used to treat endocarditis: (1) antibiotic therapy and (2) surgical debridement of infected perivalvular tissue and replacement or repair of the infected valve. Effective treatment requires identification of the etiologic agent and determination of its antimicrobial susceptibility. Therefore, in the evaluation of a patient with indolent disease, antibiotic therapy should be delayed until the results of blood cultures are obtained. If recently administered antibiotics have rendered the initial cultures negative, this delay provides an opportunity to obtain additional blood cultures after the effects of the antibiotics have dissipated. Conversely, if the infection is fulminant or if there is valvular dysfunction that may require urgent surgical intervention, empirical antibiotic therapy must be initiated promptly after blood cultures have been obtained. Bactericidal antibiotics are used parenterally in high doses. With the exception of PVE caused by staphylococci, antimicrobial therapy for PVE caused by a specific organism consists of the same regimens recommended for native valve endocarditis, although therapy is administered over a longer period (a minimum of 6 weeks). Patients must be evaluated frequently to assess the efficacy of antimicrobial therapy and the development of complications of therapy or infection.

ANTIMICROBIAL TREATMENT FOR SPECIFIC ORGANISMS

Enterococci

Enterococci are relatively resistant to penicillin, ampicillin, and vancomycin and are overtly resis-

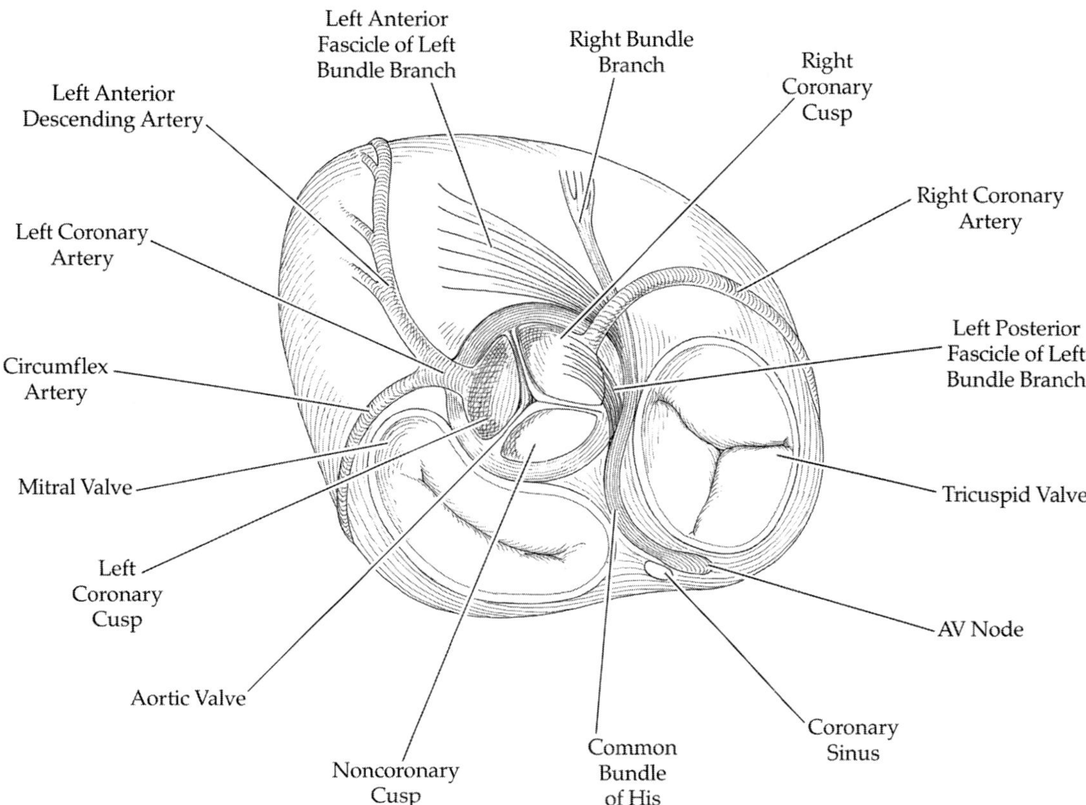

Figure 3 **The close relation of the three cardiac valves and the cardiac conduction system, as seen in this superior schematic view, accounts for the appearance of conduction defects in endocarditis. (AV—atrioventricular)**

tant to cephalosporins. Furthermore, enterococci are resistant to standard therapeutic concentrations of aminoglycosides. Nevertheless, they may be killed by the synergistic interaction of penicillin, ampicillin, or vancomycin (but not cephalosporins) in combination with streptomycin or gentamicin. To achieve the bactericidal synergism that is essential for optimal antimicrobial treatment of enterococcal endocarditis, the enterococcus must simultaneously be exposed to a cell wall–active antibiotic (penicillin, ampicillin, or vancomycin) at a concentration at or above the organism's minimum inhibitory concentration (MIC) and to an aminoglycoside that will exert a lethal effect.[56–58] The ability of enterococcus to grow in the presence of streptomycin at 2,000 μg/ml or gentamicin at 500 to 2,000 μg/ml is indicative of high-level resistance to the respective aminoglycoside and correlates with the inability of the aminoglycoside to exert a lethal effect in combination therapy regardless of the cell wall–active antimicrobial agent employed. High-level resistance to gentamicin is the consequence of an aminoglycoside-modifying enzyme that inactivates gentamicin and all other available aminoglycosides except streptomycin. Accordingly, high-level gentamicin resistance indicates that these other aminoglycosides do not produce bactericidal synergy when combined with a cell wall–active agent. High-level resistance to streptomycin results from an enzyme that is genetically independent of the one mediating high-level gentamicin resistance.

Previously, synergistic bactericidal therapy could be reliably anticipated when gentamicin was combined with penicillin, ampicillin, or vancomycin. Furthermore, for strains that were inhibited by streptomycin at 2,000 μg/ml, streptomycin could be used in lieu of gentamicin in combination therapy, with resultant bactericidal synergy. The predictability of antimicrobial susceptibility among enterococci led to standard regimens for treatment of enterococcal endocarditis [*see Table 5*].[56] In the absence of high-level resistance to streptomycin and gentamicin, considerations of aminoglycoside

Table 5 Antimicrobial Therapy for Endocarditis in Adults

Infectious Agent	*Drug*	*Dosage and Route of Administration*	*Duration of Therapy* (wk)*
Penicillin-susceptible viridans and other nonenterococcal streptococci (minimum inhibitory concentration [MIC] < 0.2 µg/ml)	*Preferred Regimen*		
	Penicillin G	12–18 million units I.V. daily (in divided doses q. 4 hr)	4
	or		
	Penicillin G	12–18 million units I.V. daily (in divided doses q. 4 hr)	2
	plus		
	gentamicin	3 mg/kg I.M. or I.V. daily (in divided doses q. 8 hr)†	2
	or		
	Ceftriaxone	2 g I.V. daily (as a single dose)	4
	Alternative Regimen‡		
	Vancomycin	30 mg/kg I.V. daily (in divided doses q. 12 hr)	4
Relatively penicillin-resistant streptococci	*Preferred Regimen*		
MIC 0.2–0.5 µg/ml	Penicillin G	20–30 million units I.V. daily (in divided doses q. 4 hr)	4
	plus		
	gentamicin§	3 mg/kg I.M. or I.V. daily (in divided doses q. 8 hr)†	2
MIC > 0.5 µg/ml	Penicillin G	Dosages same as in previous regimen	4
	plus		
	gentamicin		
	Alternative Regimen‡		
	Vancomycin§	30 mg/kg I.V. daily (in divided doses q. 12 hr)	4
Enterococci‖	*Preferred Regimen*		
	Penicillin G	20–30 million units I.V. daily (in divided doses q. 4 hr)	4–6
	plus		
	gentamicin	3 mg/kg I.M. or I.V. daily (in divided doses q. 8 hr)†	4–6
	or		
	Ampicillin	12 g I.V. daily (in divided doses q. 4 hr)	4–6
	plus		
	gentamicin	3 mg/kg I.M. or I.V. daily (in divided doses q. 8 hr)†	4–6
	Alternative Regimen‡		
	Vancomycin	30 mg/kg I.V. daily (in divided doses q. 12 hr)	4–6
	plus		
	gentamicin	3–5 mg/kg I.M. or I.V. daily (in divided doses q. 8 hr)†	4–6
Staphylococci (methicillin susceptible) in the absence of prosthetic material	*Preferred Regimen*		
	Nafcillin or oxacillin	12 g I.V. daily (in divided doses q. 4 hr)	4–6
	plus		
	gentamicin (optional; see text)	3 mg/kg I.M. or I.V. daily (in divided doses q. 8 hr)†	3–5 days
	Alternative Regimens‡		
	Cephapirin	12 g I.V. daily (in divided doses q. 4 hr)	4–6
	plus		
	gentamicin (optional; see text)	3 mg/kg I.M. or I.V. daily (in divided doses q. 8 hr)†	3–5 days
	or		
	Vancomycin	30 mg/kg I.V. daily (in divided doses q. 12 hr)	4–6
Staphylococci (methicillin resistant) in the absence of prosthetic material	Vancomycin	30 mg/kg I.V. daily (in divided doses q. 12 hr)	4–6
Staphylococci (methicillin susceptible) in the presence of prosthetic material	Nafcillin or oxacillin	12 g I.V. daily (in divided doses q. 4 hr)	6–8
	plus		
	rifampin	300 mg p.o., q. 8 hr	6–8
	plus gentamicin#	3 mg/kg I.M. or I.V. daily (in divided doses q. 8 hr)	2

(continued)

Table 5 (continued)

Infectious Agent	*Drug*	*Dosage and Route of Administration*	*Duration of Therapy* (wk)*
Staphylococci (methicillin resistant) in the presence of prosthetic material	Vancomycin plus rifampin plus gentamicin#	30 mg/kg I.V. daily in divided doses, q. 12 hr) 300 mg p.o., q. 8 hr 3 mg/kg I.M. or I.V. daily (in divided doses q. 8 hr)	6–8 6–8 2
HACEK organisms	Ceftriaxone**	2 g I.V. daily (as a single dose)	4

*Treatment programs are longer for prosthetic valve endocarditis (6–8 wk).
†Peak serum gentamicin concentration should be approximately 3 µg/ml and trough concentrations < 1 µg/ml. Some authorities prefer a gentamicin dosage of 1.5 mg/kg q. 8 hr, which results in peak concentrations of approximately 5 µg/ml.
‡Alternative regimen is for use in patients with a history of penicillin hypersensitivity.
§Some investigators recommend omission of gentamicin if the MIC is > 0.2 but < 0.5 µg/ml; the role of gentamicin in combination with vancomycin has not been fully established.
||Enterococci have become increasingly antibiotic resistant (see text).
#Administer during the initial 2 weeks (see text).
**Cefotaxime or another third-generation cephalosporin at a comparable dosage could be used.

toxicities and ease of monitoring therapy are pivotal in the choice of an aminoglycoside for combination therapy.[57,58]

Currently, antimicrobial resistance in enterococci is complex and must be carefully considered in the selection of therapy for enterococcal endocarditis.[57,58] For selection of an aminoglycoside that will result in bactericidal therapy, the causative strain must be screened for high-level resistance to gentamicin and streptomycin. Use of gentamicin or streptomycin in combination therapy in the face of high-level resistance exposes the patient to potential toxicity and is without therapeutic benefit. Resistance to cell wall–active agents has become increasingly prevalent among enterococci as well. Intrinsic resistance to penicillin and ampicillin (MIC ≥ 32 µg/ml) is prevalent in *E. faecium*. Penicillin and ampicillin resistance caused by β-lactamase production, which is not detectable with MIC tests but requires screening with the chromogenic cephalosporin nitrocefin, is occasionally seen in *E. faecalis*. Finally, vancomycin resistance (MIC > 16 µg/ml) is being encountered increasingly in *E. faecalis* and *E. faecium*. If an enterococcus is resistant to a cell wall–active agent, that agent cannot participate in the synergistic killing of the strain. Vancomycin is a suitable cell wall–active agent for combination therapy when organisms have intrinsic or β-lactamase–mediated resistance to penicillin or ampicillin; ampicillin-sulbactam is suitable when enterococci have resistance that is mediated by β-lactamase. Enterococci that are resistant to vancomycin may be susceptible to penicillin and ampicillin but more often are resistant to these antibiotics as well. For some of these enterococci, teicoplanin, a glycopeptide antibiotic that has not been approved for use in the United States but is available elsewhere, remains an effective cell wall–active antimicrobial.[57,58]

All enterococci that cause endocarditis must be tested for susceptibility to antimicrobials that have therapeutic potential. Thereafter, a bactericidal synergistic combination of a cell wall–active agent (penicillin, ampicillin, vancomycin, ampicillin-sulbactam, or teicoplanin) and an effective (no high-level resistance) aminoglycoside (gentamicin or streptomycin) can be selected. Single daily dosing of aminoglycosides should not be used in treating enterococcal endocarditis. If a synergistic combination is not possible because of high-level resistance to both gentamicin and streptomycin, prolonged therapy (8 to 12 weeks) with high doses of an effective cell wall–active agent should be administered.

Bactericidal synergistic therapy for enterococcal endocarditis is associated with cure rates approaching 85%. Treatment with an effective cell wall–active agent alone results in cure rates of 40% to 50% at best.[56–59] If bactericidal synergistic therapy is not available, patients with enterococcal endocarditis who fail treatment with a cell wall–active agent alone (i.e., those who experience persistent fever during treatment or who relapse after prolonged treatment) should undergo excision of the infected valve.[57,58]

Streptococci

Viridans streptococci have demonstrated increasing resistance to penicillin and the cephalosporins.[60] Accordingly, in treatment planning, all streptococci that cause endocarditis must be evaluated for susceptibility to penicillin (i.e., by determining the MIC). Various regimens provide comparable effective treatment of endocarditis caused by viridans streptococci and other types of penicillin-sensitive streptococci (i.e., MIC of penicillin mg/ml) [*see Table 5*].[56] One regimen employs parenteral penicillin alone in high doses for 4 weeks. A second regimen brings to bear the synergism achieved against most strains of nonenterococcal streptococci by the combination of penicillin and gentamicin. This synergism allows effective therapy with only 2 weeks of combination therapy.[56,61] The short-duration treatment should be considered only for those cases of native valvular endocarditis with the most favorable prognoses: those without complicating hypotension, renal failure, thrombocytopenia, mycotic aneurysms, or congestive heart failure caused by valvular dysfunction. The streptococci should not be nutritionally variant organisms (i.e., pyridoxal dependent or cysteine dependent) and should be highly susceptible to penicillin (MIC mg/ml). PVE should not be treated with the 2-week regimen. Ceftriaxone, given in a single daily dose for 4 weeks, is now recommended for treatment of endocarditis caused by penicillin-sensitive streptococci; this regimen is easily adapted for outpatient treatment.[56] Although short-duration combination therapy for penicillin-susceptible streptococcal endocarditis using single daily doses of both ceftriaxone and an aminoglycoside has been successful, experience with this regimen is limited, and the regimen is not recommended for general use.[62] *S. bovis* is highly penicillin sensitive, and the endocarditis it causes can be treated with regimens recommended for other penicillin-sensitive streptococci. When combination penicillin-gentamicin therapy is used to treat endocarditis caused by nonenterococcal streptococci, particularly when short-duration therapy is planned, the streptococcus should be screened for high-level resistance to gentamicin. High-level resistance would preclude bactericidal synergy and thus indicate the need for an alternative regimen.

Endocarditis caused by relatively penicillin resistant (MIC 0.2 to 0.5 μg/ml) viridans or other nonenterococcal streptococci is treated with an increased dosage of penicillin G, combined with gentamicin. If the strain is even more resistant to penicillin (MIC > 0.5 μg/ml), the infection is treated with one of the standard regimens for enterococcal endocarditis [*see Table 5*]. Nutritionally variant streptococci (previously called *S. adjacens* or *S. defectivus* and now named *Abiotrophia* species) are often relatively penicillin resistant; cases of endocarditis caused by these organisms should be treated with the standard regimen for enterococcal endocarditis.[56,63] Endocarditis caused by pneumococci or group A streptococci is treated with I.V. penicillin G in a dosage of 20 million units daily for 4 weeks.[56] Pneumococci that are found to be the cause of endocarditis must be tested for susceptibility to penicillin. Vancomycin is the preferred treatment of endocarditis caused by penicillin-resistant strains (MIC > 1.0 μg/ml). The β-hemolytic streptococci belonging to groups B, C, and G have slightly reduced susceptibility to penicillin; when found to be the cause of endocarditis, they should be treated as if they were relatively penicillin resistant (MIC 0.2 to 0.5 μg/ml).[56,64]

Staphylococci

A penicillinase-resistant penicillin (e.g., nafcillin or oxacillin) should be the initial agent used to treat *S. aureus* native valve endocarditis, unless a methicillin-resistant *S. aureus* strain is suspected.[56] In the latter instance, vancomycin should be used until the susceptibility of the strain has been clarified. Penicillin G (20 to 30 million units daily) is substituted only if the particular isolate has been shown to be penicillin susceptible by tube dilution testing and has been demonstrated not to produce penicillinase. To utilize bactericidal synergism, gentamicin is added to a penicillinase-resistant penicillin. Combination therapy reduces the duration of bacteremia. However, in limited retrospective and prospective studies, combination therapy with a penicillinase-resistant penicillin and gentamicin has not resulted in higher cure rates than therapy with a penicillinase-resistant penicillin alone. If gentamicin is used, it should be restricted to the first 3 to 5 days to minimize the risk of nephrotoxicity. Neither experimental nor clinical data provide support for combining rifampin with a penicillinase-resistant penicillin or vancomycin in the treatment of *S. aureus* native valve endocarditis.[65]

Although antibiotic therapy for endocarditis in addicts generally follows the pathogen-specific regimens used for treatment for nonaddicts, methicillin-susceptible *S. aureus* endocarditis restricted to the tricuspid valve (right-sided) without complicating metastatic infection has been successfully treated with a penicillinase-resistant penicillin plus an aminoglycoside (i.e., nafcillin plus gentamicin or tobramycin) given for 2 weeks.[66] Patients who do not respond promptly and completely should receive longer courses of treatment.

Endocarditis caused by coagulase-negative staphylococci is usually engrafted on a prosthetic valve.

More than 80% of the coagulase-negative staphylococci that cause PVE within 1 year after valve implantation are resistant to methicillin and to all β-lactam antibiotics, including cephalosporins.[26,29,56] Only when the onset of this form of PVE occurs more than a year after surgery does the frequency of β-lactam resistance in the coagulase-negative staphylococci fall below 30%.[29,30] Moreover, the β-lactam resistance may not be detected by standard antimicrobial susceptibility testing, particularly that which is automated or performed with the use of microsystems. Most of these coagulase-negative staphylococci are sensitive to vancomycin, gentamicin, and rifampin, although plasmid-mediated resistance to gentamicin has often been noted in some hospitals. For PVE caused by methicillin-resistant organisms that are susceptible to rifampin and gentamicin, the most effective treatment combines vancomycin with rifampin and gentamicin [*see Table 5*].[30,56] If the infecting strain is resistant to gentamicin, either a fluoroquinolone or another aminoglycoside to which the strain is susceptible should be substituted for gentamicin. If the staphylococci are susceptible to methicillin, a penicillinase-resistant penicillin should be used in lieu of vancomycin [*see Table 5*]. The antimicrobial therapy for PVE caused by *S. aureus* should adhere to the regimens outlined above for coagulase-negative staphylococcal PVE [*see Table 5*].

Rigorous susceptibility testing is required, but the coagulase-negative staphylococci that cause native valve endocarditis are usually sensitive to β-lactam antibiotics unless the infection has been acquired nosocomially. Native valve endocarditis caused by coagulase-negative staphylococci can be treated with the regimens that are employed to treat native valve endocarditis caused by *S. aureus*.[56,67]

HACEK Organisms

Some HACEK organisms that cause endocarditis have been found to produce β-lactamase, which causes those organisms to be resistant to ampicillin. Accordingly, endocarditis caused by HACEK organisms should be treated with a third-generation cephalosporin for 4 weeks [*see Table 5*].[56]

Corynebacteria (Diphtheroids)

The combination of penicillin and gentamicin in vitro acts synergistically to kill corynebacteria (diphtheroids) that are susceptible to gentamicin (MIC $\leq$ 4 μg/ml). Synergism is not achieved against strains that are resistant to gentamicin. For PVE caused by gentamicin-sensitive strains, therapy with I.V. penicillin G (20 million units daily) and gentamicin (1.3 mg/kg I.M. or I.V. every 8 hours) is recommended. Vancomycin, which is bactericidal against diphtheroids, is recommended as the initial treatment of diphtheroid PVE, with subsequent treatment determined on the basis of antibiotic susceptibility test results. Vancomycin is also the drug of choice if the infecting strain is resistant to gentamicin or if the patient is allergic to penicillin.[30]

Gram-Negative Bacilli

Endocarditis caused by gram-negative bacilli should be treated with one of the potent β-lactam antibiotics, such as a third-generation cephalosporin, with or without an aminoglycoside, depending on the susceptibility of and the published experience for the specific gram-negative bacillus involved. Effective treatment of endocarditis caused by *P. aeruginosa* requires the synergistic combination of ticarcillin or piperacillin (either drug at a dosage of 3 g I.V. every 4 hours), plus tobramycin, 2.7 mg/kg I.M. or I.V. every 8 hours (8 mg/kg daily), for at least 6 weeks. Because pseudomonal endocarditis is often destructive and is associated with perivalvular abscesses, aggressive early surgical intervention is recommended.[27]

Fungi

The response of fungal endocarditis to therapy is discouraging. Prompt valve debridement and replacement and the use of antifungal chemotherapy are recommended for treatment of native valve endocarditis or PVE caused by fungi.[68] Recent data suggest that medical therapy that includes long-term (possibly indefinitely long) suppressive therapy with oral fluconazole may be effective in patients with candidal PVE in the absence of intracardiac complications.[69] Amphotericin B is the drug of choice for initial treatment for most patients with fungal endocarditis. Synergism in vitro between flucytosine and amphotericin B has been reported with some strains of *Candida*, and the combined use of these two agents in this life-threatening situation seems warranted. Serum levels of flucytosine should be followed if it is employed. The drug, which is cleared by the kidney, should not be given in the presence of renal failure, because excessive serum concentrations can induce severe bone marrow depression.

Culture-Negative Endocarditis

When blood cultures are negative or culture results are not available, the selection of empirical therapy requires careful consideration of the clinical clues and factors predisposing to endocarditis that might suggest the identity of the causative organism. In the absence of information suggesting a probable cause of native valve SBE, treatment as for enterococcal endocarditis, with ampicillin and gentamicin, is advised. If the course is fulminant or if *S. aureus* is an etiologic consideration, the addition of vancomycin to this regimen is recommended. Because blood cultures rarely remain negative in patients with fulminant endocarditis, such empirical therapy can usually be revised later on the basis of the culture results. The spectrum of microorganisms causing PVE differs from that implicated in native valve endocarditis, and culture-negative PVE should be treated with a combination of vancomycin, gentamicin, and a third-generation cephalosporin. The third-generation cephalosporin is directed against the HACEK organisms, which are important causes of late PVE and difficult to isolate from blood cultures. When one is embarking on therapy for culture-negative endocarditis, it is important to consider the possibility that the endocarditis is caused by a fastidious bacterial or nonbacterial organism or that one of the conditions that mimics this disease is present. Appropriate special cultures and serologic studies should be pursued [*see* Diagnosis, *above*].[48]

MONITORING CLINICAL RESPONSE AND SERUM BACTERICIDAL ACTIVITY

A decrease in fever is usually evident within 1 week of the start of appropriate antibiotic therapy; patients with SBE caused by avirulent, highly antibiotic-susceptible organisms may become afebrile 24 to 48 hours after the start of therapy.[54] Fever that persists during the second week of appropriate antimicrobial therapy suggests the possibility of intracardiac abscess, metastatic foci of infection, or nosocomial complications of therapy. Aggressive evaluation is indicated.[54,55] Petechiae and embolic phenomena may occur for several weeks after initiation of recommended treatment; such findings do not necessarily indicate that therapy is ineffective, particularly if other signs indicate that the patient is getting better. If the patient does not become afebrile within a few days after antibiotic therapy is initiated, repeat blood cultures should be obtained. To assess possible relapse, blood cultures should be obtained if fever recurs during the first 2 months after treatment.

The serum bactericidal test, in which dilutions of the patient's serum are tested for bactericidal activity against the organism causing the endocarditis, is no longer recommended for assessment of therapy in patients receiving standard antimicrobial regimens with established efficacy.[56] This test may be useful when endocarditis is treated with regimens for which previous experience is limited. It is important to realize that the serum bactericidal test serves to indicate only whether antibiotic activity in the blood is satisfactory; it does not ensure that the patient will survive the infection.

ANTITHROMBOTIC THERAPY

A decision regarding the use of antithrombotic therapy in patients with native valve endocarditis or PVE should be based on whether the patient has cardiac or extracardiac disease that would warrant use of such therapy in the absence of endocarditis. In endocarditis patients with prosthetic valves who require antithrombotic therapy or who have cardiac disease that requires long-term warfarin therapy, such therapy should be continued during endocarditis unless there are specific contraindications. Excessive warfarin therapy, however, carries a significant risk of intracranial hemorrhage; thus, the prothrombin time should be maintained at an international normalized ratio (INR) of 2.0 to 3.0. In infective endocarditis, antithrombotic therapy to prevent an initial or subsequent systemic embolus is not indicated for patients with normal sinus rhythm who have uncomplicated infective endocarditis involving a native valve or a bioprosthetic valve that does not otherwise require anticoagulation. Two factors that militate against use of anticoagulation to prevent an embolic vegetation in these endocarditis patients are an increased risk of hemorrhage and lack of evidence that antithrombotic therapy will prevent embolization of vegetations. Anticoagulation therapy should be carefully administered to patients with endocarditis when it is indicated for treatment of coexisting conditions (e.g., atrial fibrillation, cardiomyopathy, mural thrombus, and deep vein thrombophlebitis). Anticoagulation should be reversed immediately in the event of CNS complications, especially intracranial hemorrhage.

SURGICAL INTERVENTION

Operative intervention to debride infected perivalvular tissue or to replace or reconstruct a dysfunctioning valve is important in the management of complicated infective endocarditis that involves either a native or a prosthetic valve.[30,56,70–73] Several observations have prompted the increased use of surgery in the treatment of active endocarditis: (1) the mortality of patients undergoing valve surgery during active endocarditis is not greater than that of patients treated medically; (2) the risk that endocarditis from the initial infecting organism will develop on the newly implanted prosthesis is low[70,71]; and (3) some intracardiac complications of endocarditis can be corrected only with surgery. Early aggressive surgical treatment is an essential element of therapy in 45% of patients with PVE. Survival rates for patients who undergo valve replacement during active endocarditis are satisfactory.[30,70–73]

The indications for surgical treatment of active native valve endocarditis and PVE have been developed through a retrospective analysis of therapy. Moderate to severe congestive heart failure from valvular dysfunction is the most widely accepted indication for valve replacement and accounts for 90% of the decisions to operate.[71] Bulky vegetations that obstruct the valve orifice may also produce congestive heart failure and are an equally compelling indication for surgery. Surgical intervention should also be considered when there is clinical evidence of perivalvular invasion and abscess formation and when infection remains uncontrolled despite maximal antimicrobial therapy. Fungal endocarditis, especially in patients with intracardiac complications, is commonly treated surgically.[68] Similarly, PVE that occurs within a year after valve implantation and is caused by coagulase-negative staphylococci frequently results in perivalvular invasion.[30,70] Regardless of the causative agent, if there is evidence that PVE is complicated by perivalvular extension of the infection, particularly if the valve is unstable, the PVE should be managed surgically.[30] Because left-sided native valve endocarditis and particularly PVE caused by *S. aureus* are frequently invasive, early surgery should be considered for patients with these infections who do not show prompt and sustained improvement during antibiotic therapy.[30,71,74] Endocarditis caused by *P. aeruginosa* or other gram-negative bacilli that has not responded after 7 to 10 days of maximal antibiotic therapy should be treated surgically. Although patients with native valve endocarditis who are in relapse after appropriate antibiotic therapy can often be cured by repeat courses of antibiotics, outcome is improved if patients with PVE in relapse are treated surgically.[30,70]

The occurrence of an arterial embolus, particularly to the cerebrum, is another factor to be considered in the decision to operate. Occasionally, systemic embolization itself is an indication for surgery, especially if the risk of further emboli is high, as would be the case if the embolization occurred early in the course of therapy and there existed a residual vegetation of more than 10 mm in diameter on the anterior leaflet of the mitral valve [*see* Embolic Phenomena, *above*].[17–21] Surgery may be beneficial if the vegetations are unusually large and mobile.[21] Occasionally, a single clinical or microbiologic finding constitutes an absolute indication for surgery; more often, however, the decision to operate requires a consideration of relative risks and benefits in light of multiple clinical, echocardiographic, and microbiologic observations, as would be the case when attempting to prevent systemic emboli.

Among surgically treated patients with endocarditis, operative mortality is proportional to the degree of preoperative hemodynamic impairment. If surgery is indicated, it should generally be performed promptly. Delaying surgery to administer additional antibiotic therapy in the presence of uncontrolled infection or deteriorating hemodynamic status may result in a less favorable outcome.[30,71] When cardiac surgery is considered in patients who have sustained a previous neurologic complication, delaying surgery, when hemodynamic status permits, may be desirable. If, after cerebral infarction, surgery is delayed for at least 15 days, the exacerbation rate for cerebral complications is reduced to 10% (< 3% if the delay is 28 days). If cerebral hemorrhage has occurred, cardiac surgery should ideally be delayed 28 days or more.[75] Exclusion of a complicating cerebral mycotic aneurysm should be considered in this setting [*see* Neurologic Manifestations, *above*].

Although implantation of a prosthetic valve in an active drug addict may occasionally be lifesaving, this approach is problematic: endocarditis is likely to recur if I.V. drug abuse continues, and it is more difficult to eradicate an infection involving a prosthetic valve than it is to cure native valve endocarditis. To avoid these problems, tricuspid or pulmonary valvulectomy (without valve replacement) has been employed in the treatment of antibiotic-resistant right-sided endocarditis. However, in addicts with isolated right-sided *S. aureus* endocarditis, surgery should be postponed and antibiotic therapy continued for a prolonged period, despite persistent fever and pulmonary emboli, in an effort to achieve a medical cure. Most I.V. drug addicts with isolated *S. aureus* tricuspid valve endocarditis can be cured medically.[76]

Prophylaxis

Patients who are at higher risk for developing endocarditis than the general population should be given prophylaxis when they undergo procedures

Table 6 Cardiac Conditions and Endocarditis Prophylaxis[75]

Prophylaxis Recommended	*Prophylaxis Not Recommended*
High risk All prosthetic valves Prior infective endocarditis Complex cyanotic congenital heart disease (e.g., single ventricle conditions, transposition of great arteries, tetralogy of Fallot) Surgically constructed systemic pulmonary shunts Moderate risk Other congenital cardiac malformations Acquired valvular dysfunction Hypertrophic cardiomyopathy Mitral valve prolapse with valvular regurgitation and/or thickened valves	Isolated ostium secundum atrial septal defect Surgical repair, without residua, of arterial septal defect, ventricular septal defect, patent ductus arteriosus, pulmonary valve stenosis Previous coronary artery bypass graft Previous Kawasaki disease or rheumatic fever without valvular dysfunction Cardiac pacemaker or implanted defibrillators

likely to lead to bacteremia with organisms that commonly cause endocarditis. These patients have been stratified according to the combined risk of development of endocarditis and the potential morbidity and mortality [*see Table 6*].[77] The need for prophylaxis in all patients with mitral valve prolapse is controversial. Nevertheless, prophylaxis is recommended when mitral valve prolapse is accompanied by an audible murmur, when there is echocardiographic evidence of mitral regurgitation, or when there are thickened valves. Prophylaxis is advised for men older than 45 years with mitral valve prolapse who experience mitral regurgitation during exercise but whose regurgitation is only sometimes present or is wholly absent at rest. After successful repair of a secundum atrial septal defect, a patent ductus arteriosus, a ventricular septal defect, or a stenotic pulmonary valve, patients are no longer at increased risk for endocarditis.[77,78] Repair of other congenital defects, however, is associated with continued risk of endocarditis. Prophylaxis is recommended for patients with such conditions.[77,78] Patients who are not at increased risk relative to the general population do not require prophylaxis.

When patients at high or moderate risk for endocarditis undergo procedures involving the oral cavity, the respiratory tract, or the esophagus that are likely to cause streptococcal bacteremia, prophylaxis is recommended. When these patients undergo procedures involving the genitourinary tract, the GI tract distal to the stomach, or the biliary tract that are likely to cause bacteremia with enterococci, prophylaxis is indicated [*see Table 7*]. For patients who are at unusually high risk, some physicians elect to use prophylaxis in conjunction with procedures entailing a low risk of bacteremia (i.e., procedures for which prophylaxis is generally not recommended).

Antibiotic regimens for prophylaxis have been designed to cover streptococci or enterococci and are assigned to procedures in accordance with the anticipated bacteremic organism [*see Tables 8 and 9*]. When urinary tract manipulation is anticipated, an evaluation for urinary tract infection should be undertaken, and infection, if confirmed, should be treated before the manipulation. If procedures are of necessity performed on infected tissues, prophylaxis is directed at the likely pathogen causing the infection. Such prophylaxis would include use of an antistaphylococcal penicillin or first-generation cephalosporin when the infection involves skin and adjacent soft tissue, joints, or bone.

If a patient who is at risk for endocarditis is receiving or has recently received one of the agents

Table 7 Procedures and Endocarditis Prophylaxis[77]

Prophylaxis Recommended	*Prophylaxis Not Recommended*
Dental procedures likely to produce gingival bleeding (includes professional cleaning and intraligamentary local anesthesia) Surgery on upper respiratory tract (adenoidectomy, tonsillectomy, bronchoscopy with a rigid bronchoscope) Sclerotherapy of esophageal varices Dilation or esophageal stricture Endoscopic retrograde cholangiography with biliary obstruction Biliary tract surgery Surgery involving the intestinal mucosa Prostatic surgery Cystoscopy Urethral dilation Surgery involving infected tissues	Placement of tympanotomy tubes Transesophageal endocardiography GI endoscopy with or without biopsy Vaginal hysterectomy Vaginal delivery, cesarean section If uninfected: urethral catheterization, uterine dilation and curettage, therapeutic abortion, insertion or removal of intrauterine devices, sterilization Cardiac catheterization or angioplasty/stent placement Implantation of pacemaker or defibrillator Clean surgery, including circumcision

Table 8 Prophylactic Antibiotics Recommended for Adults Undergoing Oral Cavity, Respiratory Tract, or Esophageal Procedures[77]

Standard Oral Regimens (Given as single dose 1 hr before procedure)	*Regimens for Patients Unable to Take Oral Medication (Given as single dose within 30 min before procedure)*
Amoxicillin, 2 g	Ampicillin, 2 g I.M. or I.V.
Clindamycin, 600 mg	Cefazolin,* 1 g I.M. or I.V.
Cephalexin,* 2 g	Clindamycin, 600 mg I.V.
Cefadroxil,* 2 g	
Clarithromycin, 500 mg	

*Cephalosporins should not be used in persons with immediate-type hypersensitivity to penicillins.

recommended for prophylaxis, it is prudent to choose for prophylaxis an antibiotic from a different class, rather than increase the dosage of the current regimen. The dosage of penicillin used to prevent recurrences of acute rheumatic fever is insufficient to prevent BE. However, patients taking oral penicillin (or a cephalosporin) for this reason or other reasons may harbor relatively penicillin resistant strains of bacteria in their oral cavity. Prophylaxis with clarithromycin or clindamycin is suggested when relatively penicillin resistant streptococci are anticipated.

Most cases of endocarditis are not related to defined events or procedures. It is likely that these infections arise from bacteremias associated with ordinary activities (e.g., vigorous chewing in patients with gingival disease, use of oral irrigating jets, or minor unrecognized infections). Maintaining optimal dental health is essential if the risk of endocarditis is to be minimized among patients with vulnerable cardiac lesions. Dental evaluations, including extractions and other necessary work, should be performed under appropriate antibiotic prophylaxis several weeks before the insertion of prosthetic heart valves.

Table 9 Prophylactic Antibiotics Recommended for Adults Undergoing Gastrointestinal,* Biliary, or Genitourinary Procedures[77]

High-Risk Patients	*Moderate-Risk Patients*
Ampicillin, 2 g I.M. or I.V., plus gentamicin, 1.5 mg/kg (not to exceed 120 mg) I.M. or I.V., within 30 min of starting the procedure; 6 hr later, ampicillin, 1 g I.M. or I.V., or amoxicillin, 1 g p.o. Vancomycin,† 1 g I.V., plus gentamicin, 1.5 mg/kg (not to exceed 120 mg) I.M. or I.V.; complete infusion within 30 min of starting the procedure	Amoxicillin, 2 g p.o. 1 hr before the procedure Ampicillin, 2 g I.M. or I.V. within 30 min of starting the procedure Vancomycin,† g I.V.; complete infusion within 30 min of starting the procedure

*Except esophageal procedures; for esophageal procedures, see Table 8.
†Infuse vancomycin over 1 hr.

Prognosis

Overall survival for patients with infective endocarditis is about 75% to 80%. The rate depends in large measure on the promptness of initiation of therapy, the nature of the infecting organism, the presence of comorbid conditions, and development of complications of endocarditis. Survival approaches 90% when the infecting organism is a viridans-type streptococcus or *S. bovis* but is about 50% among nonaddicts with endocarditis caused by *S. aureus*. Although outcomes are more guarded for early PVE, recent experience suggests that survival rates for patients with late PVE are similar to those anticipated for native valve infection.[68,50] With the incorporation of earlier surgical intervention into the therapy for endocarditis, cardiac failure is no longer associated with increased mortality. However, major CNS complications (embolic strokes and intracerebral hemorrhage) and uncontrolled infection continue to be associated with increased mortality.[22] The short-term outlook is relatively good for I.V. drug addicts with right-sided endocarditis. Endocarditis caused by fungi or gram-negative bacilli, such as Enterobacteriaceae or *Pseudomonas* species, is extremely difficult to cure despite optimal antimicrobial therapy and aggressive surgical intervention.

Acknowledgments

Figures 2 and 3 Carol Donner.

References

1. Shapiro DS, Kenney SC, Johnson M, et al: Brief report: *Chlamydia psittaci* endocarditis diagnosed by blood culture. N Engl J Med 326:1192, 1992

2. Hoen B, Selton-Suty C, Lacassin F, et al: Infective endocarditis in patients with negative blood cultures: analysis of 88 cases from a one-year nationwide survey in France. Clin Infect Dis 20:501, 1995

3. Raoult D, Fournier PE, Drancourt M, et al: Diagnosis of 22 new cases of *Bartonella* endocarditis. Ann Intern Med 125:646, 1996

4. Drancourt M, Mainardi JL, Brouqui P, et al: *Bartonella (Rochalimaea) quintana* endocarditis in three homeless men. N Engl J Med 332:419, 1995

5. Spach DH, Kanter AS, Dougherty MJ, et al: *Bartonella (Rochalimaea) quintana* bacteremia in inner-city patients with chronic alcoholism. N Engl J Med 332:424, 1995

6. Watanakunakorn C, Burkert T: Infective endocarditis at a large community teaching hospital, 1980–1990: a review of 210 episodes. Medicine (Baltimore) 72:90, 1993

7. Harris SL: Definitions and demographic characteristics. Infective Endocarditis 2nd ed. Kaye D, Ed. Raven Press, New York,1992, p 1

8. Sandre RM, Shafran SD: Infective endocarditis: review of 135 cases over 9 years. Clin Infect Dis 22:276, 1996

9. Ruoff KL, Miller SI, Garner CV, et al: Bacteremia with *Streptococcus bovis* and *Streptococcus salivarius*: clinical correlates of more accurate identification of isolates. J Clin Microbiol 27:305, 1989

10. Stein A, Raoult D: Q fever endocarditis. Eur Heart J 16(suppl B): 19, 1995

11. Weinstein L, Schlesinger JJ: Pathoanatomic, pathophysiologic and clinical correlations in endocarditis (pts 1 and 2). N Engl J Med 291:832, 1122, 1974

12. Bancsi MJ, Thompson J, Bertina RM: Stimulation of monocyte tissue factor expression in an in vitro model of BE. Infect Immun 62:5669, 1994

13. Moreillon P, Entenza JM, Francioli P, et al: Role of *Staphylococcus aureus* coagulase and clumping factor in pathogenesis of experimental endocarditis. Infect Immun 63:4738, 1995

14. Dankert J, van der Werff J, Zaat SA, et al: Involvement of bactericidal factors from thrombin-stimulated platelets in clearance of adherent viridans streptococci in experimental infective endocarditis. Infect Immun 63:663, 1995

15. Dhawan VK, Bayer AS, Yeaman MR: In vitro resistance to thrombin-induced platelet microbicidal protein is associated with enhanced progression and hematogenous dissemination in experimental *Staphylococcus aureus* infective endocarditis. Infect Immun 66:3476, 1998

16. Gagliardi JP, Nettles RE, McCarty DE, et al: Native valve infective endocarditis in elderly and younger adult patients: comparison of clinical features and outcomes with use of the Duke criteria and the Duke endocarditis data base. Clin Infect Dis 26:1165, 1998

17. Steckelberg JM, Murphy JG, Ballard D, et al: Emboli in infective endocarditis: the prognostic value of echocardiography. Ann Intern Med 114:635, 1991

18. Mugge A, Daniel WC, Frank G, et al: Echocardiography in infective endocarditis: reassessment of prognostic implications of vegetation size determined by the transthoracic and transesophageal approach. J Am Coll Cardiol 14:631, 1989

19. Rohman S, Erbel R, Darius H: Prediction of rapid versus prolonged healing of infective endocarditis by monitoring vegetation size. J Am Soc Echocardiogr 4:465, 1991

20. Rohman S, Erbel R, George G, et al: Clinical relevance of vegetation localization by transesophageal echocardiography in infective endocarditis. Eur Heart J 13:446, 1992

21. Sanfilippo AJ, Picard MH, Newell JB, et al: Echocardiographic assessment of patients with infectious endocarditis: prediction of risk for complications. J Am Coll Cardiol 18:1191, 1991

22. Mansur AJ, Grinberg M, Lemos da Luz P, et al: The complications of infective endocarditis: a reappraisal of the 1980s. Arch Intern Med 152:2428, 1992

23. Camarata PJ, Latchow RE, Rufenacht DA, et al: Intracranial aneurysms. Invest Radiol 28:373, 1993

24. Huston JH III, Nichols DA, Luetmer PH, et al: Blinded prospective evaluation of sensitivity of MR angiography to known intracranial aneurysms: importance of aneurysm size. AJNR Am J Neuroradiol 15: 1607, 1994

25. Moskowitz MA, Rosenbaum AE, Tyler HR: Angiographically monitored resolution of cerebral mycotic aneurysms. Neurology (Minneapolis) 24:1103, 1974

26. Hutter AM, Moellering RC: Assessment of the patient with suspected endocarditis. JAMA 235:1603, 1976

27. Sande MA, Lee BL, Mills J, et al: Endocarditis in intravenous drug users. Infective Endocarditis 2nd ed. Kaye D, Ed. Raven Press, New York, 1992, p 345

28. Ivert TSA, Dismukes WE, Cobbs CG, et al: Prosthetic valve endocarditis. Circulation 69:223, 1984

29. Calderwood SB, Swinski LA, Waternaux CM, et al: Risk factors for the development of prosthetic valve endocarditis. Circulation 72:31, 1985

30. Karchmer AW, Gibbons GW: Infections of prosthetic heart valves and vascular grafts. Infections Associated with Indwelling Medical Devices, 2nd ed. Bisno AL, Waldvogel FA, Eds. American Society for Microbiology, Washington, DC, 1994, p 213

31. Sett SS, Hudon MPJ, Jamieson WRE, et al: Prosthetic valve endocarditis: experience with porcine bioprostheses. J Thorac Cardiovasc Surg 105:428, 1993

32. Fang G, Keys TF, Gentry LO, et al: Prosthetic valve endocarditis resulting from nosocomial bacteremia: a prospective, multicenter study. Ann Intern Med 119:560, 1993

32a. Bayer AS, Bolger AF, Taubert KA: Diagnosis and management of infective endocarditis and its complications. Circulation 98:2936, 1998

33. Durack DT, Lukes AS, Bright DK: New criteria for diagnosis of infective endocarditis: utilization of specific echocardiographic findings. Am J Med 96:200, 1994

34. Bayer AS, Ward JI, Ginzton LE, et al: Evaluation of new clinical criteria for the diagnosis of infective endocarditis. Am J Med 96:211, 1994

35. Hoen B, Selton-Suty C, Dauchin N, et al: Evaluation of the Duke criteria versus the Beth Israel criteria for the diagnosis of infective endocarditis. Clin Infect Dis 21:905, 1995

36. Nettles RE, McCarty DE, Corey RG, et al: An evaluation of the Duke criteria in 25 pathologically confirmed cases of prosthetic valve endocarditis. Clin Infect Dis 25:1401, 1997

37. Hoen B, Beguinot I, Rabaud C, et al: The Duke criteria for diagnosing infective endocarditis are specific: analysis of 100 patients with acute fever or fever of unknown origin. Clin Infect Dis 23:298, 1996

38. Dodds GA III, Sexton DJ, Durack DT, et al: Negative predictive value of the Duke criteria for infective endocarditis. Am J Cardiol 77: 403, 1996

39. Sekeres MA, Abrutyn E, Berlin JA, et al: An assessment of the usefulness of the Duke criteria for diagnosing active infective endocarditis. Clin Infect Dis 24:1185, 1997

40. Mugge A: Echocardiographic detection of cardiac valve vegetations and prognostic implications. Infect Dis Clin North Am 7:877, 1993

41. Shively BK, Gurule FT, Roldan CA, et al: Diagnostic value of transesophageal compared with transthoracic echocardiography in infective endocarditis. J Am Coll Cardiol 18:391, 1991

42. Shapiro SM, Young E, De Guzman S, et al: Transesophageal echocardiography in diagnosis of infective endocarditis. Chest 105:377, 1994

43. Daniel WG, Mugge A, Martin RP, et al: Improvements in the diagnosis of abscesses associated with endocarditis by transesophageal echocardiography. N Engl J Med 324:795, 1991

44. Karalis DG, Bansal RC, Hauck AJ, et al: Transesophageal echocardiographic recognition of subaortic complications in aortic valve endocarditis: clinical and surgical implications. Circulation 86:353, 1992

45. Sochowski RA, Chan K-L: Implication of negative results on a monoplane transesophageal echocardiographic study in patients with suspected infective endocarditis. J Am Coll Cardiol 21:216, 1993

46. Vered Z, Mossinson D, Peleg E, et al: Echocardiographic assessment of prosthetic valve endocarditis. Eur Heart J 16(suppl B):63, 1995

47. Daniel WG, Mugge A, Grote J, et al: Comparison of transthoracic and transesophageal echocardiography for detection of abnormalities of prosthetic and bioprosthetic valves in the mitral and aortic positions. Am J Cardiol 71:210, 1993

48. Tunkel AR, Kaye D: Endocarditis with negative blood cultures. N Engl J Med 326:1215, 1992

49. Fournier PE, Casalta JP, Habib G, et al: Modification of the diagnostic criteria proposed by the Duke endocarditis service to permit improved diagnosis of Q fever endocarditis. Am J Med 100:629, 1996

50. Hamed KA, Dormitzer PR, Su CK, et al: *Haemophilus parainfluenzae* endocarditis: application of a molecular approach for identification of pathogenic bacterial species. Clin Infect Dis 19:677, 1994

51. Goldenberger D, Kunzli A, Vogt P, et al: Molecular diagnosis of bacterial endocarditis by broad-range PCR amplification and direct sequencing. J Clin Microbiol 35:2733, 1997

52. Blumberg EA, Karalis DA, Chandrasekaran K, et al: Endocarditis-associated para-valvular abscess: do clinical parameters predict the presence of abscess? Chest 107:898, 1995

53. Arnett EN, Roberts WC: Valve ring abscess in active infective endocarditis: frequency, location, and clues to clinical diagnosis from the study of 95 necropsy patients. Circulation 54:140, 1976

54. Lederman MM, Sprague L, Wallis RS, et al: Duration of fever during treatment of infective endocarditis. Medicine (Baltimore) 71: 52, 1992

55. Blumberg EA, Robbins N, Adimora A, et al: Persistent fever in association with infective endocarditis. Clin Infect Dis 15:983, 1992

56. Wilson WR, Karchmer AW, Dajani AS, et al: Antibiotic treatment of adults with infective endocarditis due to streptococci, enterococci, staphylococci, and HACEK microorganisms. JAMA 274:1706, 1995

57. Eliopoulos GM: Enterococcal endocarditis. Infective Endocarditis 2nd ed. Kaye D, Ed. Raven Press, New York, 1992, p 209

58. Eliopoulos GM: Aminoglycoside resistant enterococcal endocarditis. Infect Dis Clin North Am 7:117, 1993

59. Rice LB, Calderwood SB, Eliopoulos GM, et al: Enterococcal endocarditis: a comparison of prosthetic and native valve disease. Rev Infect Dis 13:1, 1991

60. Doern GV, Ferraro MJ, Brueggemann AB, et al: Emergence of high rates of antimicrobial resistance among viridans group streptococci in the United States. Antimicrob Agents Chemother 40:891, 1996

61. Roberts SA, Lang SDR, Ellis-Pegler RB: Short-course treatment of penicillin-susceptible viridans streptococcal infective endocarditis with penicillin and gentamicin. Infectious Diseases in Clinical Practice 2:191, 1993

62. Francioli P, Ruch W, Stamboulian D, et al: Treatment of streptococcal endocarditis with a single daily dose of ceftriaxone and netilmicin for 14 days: a prospective multicenter study. Clin Infect Dis 21:1406, 1995

63. Bouvet A: Human endocarditis due to nutritionally variant streptococci: *Streptococcus adjacens* and *Streptococcus defectivus*. Eur Heart J 16(suppl B):24, 1995

64. Baddour LM: Infective endocarditis caused by β-hemolytic streptococci. Infectious Diseases Society of America Emerging Infections Network. Clin Infect Dis 26:66, 1998

65. Levine DP, Fromm BS, Reddy BR: Slow response to vancomycin or vancomycin plus rifampin in methicillin-resistant *Staphylococcus aureus* endocarditis. Ann Intern Med 115:674, 1991

66. Torres-Tortosa M, de Cueto M, Vergara A, et al: Prospective evaluation of a two-week course of intravenous antibiotics in intravenous drug addicts with infective endocarditis. Eur J Clin Microbiol Infect Dis 13:559, 1994

67. Caputo GM, Archer GL, Calderwood SB, et al: Native valve endocarditis due to coagulase-negative staphylococci: clinical and microbiologic features. Am J Med 83:619, 1987

68. Melgar GR, Nasser RM, Gordon SM, et al: Fungal prosthetic valve endocarditis in 16 patients: an 11-year experience in a tertiary care hospital. Medicine (Baltimore) 76:94, 1997

69. Nguyen MH, Nguyen ML, Yu VL, et al: *Candida* prosthetic valve endocarditis: prospective study of six cases and review of the literature. Clin Infect Dis 22:262, 1996

70. Calderwood SB, Swinski LA, Karchmer AW, et al: Prosthetic valve endocarditis: analysis of factors affecting outcome of therapy. J Thorac Cardiovasc Surg 92:776, 1986

71. D'Agostino RS, Miller DC, Stinson EB, et al: Valve replacement in patients with native valve endocarditis: what really determines operative outcome? Ann Thorac Surg 40:429, 1985

72. Jault F, Gandjbakhch I, Chastre JC, et al: Prosthetic valve endocarditis with ring abscesses: surgical management and long-term results. J Thorac Cardiovasc Surg 105:1106, 1993

73. Croft CH, Woodward W, Elliott A, et al: Analysis of surgical versus medical therapy in active complicated native valve infective endocarditis. Am J Cardiol 51:1650, 1983

74. John MVD, Hibberd PL, Karchmer AW, et al: *Staphylococcus aureus* prosthetic valve endocarditis: optimal management and risk factors for death. Clin Infect Dis 26:1302, 1998

75. Eishi K, Kawazoe K, Kuriyama Y, et al: Surgical management of infective endocarditis associated with cerebral complications: multi-center retrospective study in Japan. J Thorac Cardiovasc Surg 110:1745, 1995

76. Bayer AS, Blomquist IK, Bello E, et al: Tricuspid valve endocarditis due to *Staphylococcus aureus*: correlation of two-dimensional echocardiography with clinical outcome. Chest 93:247, 1988

77. Dajani AS, Taubert KA, Wilson W, et al: Prevention of bacterial endocarditis: recommendations by the American Heart Association. Committee on Rheumatic Fever, Endocarditis, and Kawasaki Disease, Council on Cardiovascular Diseases in the Young. JAMA 277:1794, 1997

78. Morris CD, Reller MD, Menashe VD: Thirty-year incidence of infective endocarditis after surgery for congenital heart defect. JAMA 279:599, 1998

79. DiNubile MJ, Calderwood SB, Steinhaus DM, et al: Cardiac conduction abnormalities complicating native valve active infective endocarditis. Am J Cardiol 58:1213, 1986

80. Kazanjian PH: Infective endocarditis: review of 60 cases treated in community hospitals. Infectious Diseases in Clinical Practice 2:41, 1993

81. Fernandez-Guerrero ML, Verdejo C, Azofra J, et al: Hospital-acquired infectious endocarditis not associated with cardiac surgery: an emerging problem. Clin Infect Dis 20:16, 1995

82. Terpenning MS, Buggy BP, Kauffman CA: Hospital-acquired infective endocarditis. Arch Intern Med 148:1601, 1988

83. Tornos P, Sanz E, Permanyer-Miralda G, et al: Late prosthetic valve endocarditis: immediate and long-term prognosis. Chest 101:37, 1992

84. Grover FL, Cohen DJ, Oprian C, et al: Determinants of the occurrence of and survival from prosthetic valve endocarditis: experience of the Veterans Affairs Cooperative Study on Valvular Heart Disease. J Thorac Cardiovasc Surg 108:207, 1994

8 Peritonitis and Intra-abdominal Abscesses

Harvey B. Simon, M.D.
Morton N. Swartz, M.D.

Peritonitis

Peritonitis is a diffuse or localized inflammatory process affecting the peritoneal lining.[1,2] Peritonitis has acute and chronic forms and may have a variety of causes, including pyogenic bacteria (such as *Escherichia coli*), tuberculosis, fungi, parasites (such as those from ruptured hepatic amebic abscesses or hydatid cysts), carcinomatosis, chemical irritation (such as that from bile), drug hypersensitivity reaction (such as that induced by practolol), foreign-body reaction (such as starch peritonitis), and certain systemic illnesses (such as familial Mediterranean fever and systemic lupus erythematosus). Only acute peritonitis caused by bacteria or fungi is discussed here, including primary and secondary peritonitis. Primary peritonitis has no underlying intra-abdominal disorder. Secondary peritonitis has an intra-abdominal focus that initiates the infection. Tuberculous peritonitis is considered elsewhere [see 19 Infections Due to *E. coli* and Other Enteric Gram-Negative Bacilli].

SPONTANEOUS BACTERIAL PERITONITIS

Epidemiology

Spontaneous bacterial peritonitis (SBP) is being recognized with increasing frequency in patients with advanced chronic liver disease and concomitant ascites.[3] In children and young adults, the liver disease is usually postnecrotic cirrhosis; in older patients, it is alcoholic cirrhosis. SBP is common, occurring in 8% to 27% of patients with cirrhosis and ascites; it is also serious, with a mortality between 48% and 57%.[2] *E. coli* is the most common cause of SBP and is isolated in about half of patients. Pneumococcal and streptococcal species are each responsible for 15% to 20% of cases, *Klebsiella* for about 10%, and anaerobic or microaerophilic organisms for about 5%. *Staphylococcus aureus* is an infrequent cause of SBP but a major cause of peritonitis in cirrhotic patients with LeVeen peritoneovenous shunts. A variety of other organisms, including *Listeria monocytogenes*, *Campylobacter coli*, and *Aeromonas*, have been responsible for isolated cases of SBP. In most instances in which the causative organism is aerobic, a single organism is involved, and concurrent bacteremia is frequent.

Although primary peritonitis occurs most often in children, it can develop in adults; nearly all patients are female.[4] Although many patients have had nephrosis, most have not had preexisting ascites. The source of infection is usually occult but may involve the female genital tract. The infecting organisms are almost always pneumococci or group A streptococci; gram-negative bacilli are only rarely implicated. For reasons that are unclear, primary peritonitis has decreased strikingly in incidence in the past several decades.

Occasionally, SBP develops in patients with systemic lupus erythematosus and lupus nephritis without detectable ascites, most of whom have been receiving corticosteroid therapy. The most common etiologic agents in this form of SBP are gram-positive cocci such as *Streptococcus pneumoniae* and group B streptococci.

Etiology

The most likely route of infection is bacteremic seeding of the ascitic fluid, precipitated by portal hypertension, intrahepatic shunting, intestinal bacterial overgrowth, and impaired host defense mechanisms, including diminished bactericidal activity in ascitic fluid.[3] Less often, SBP results from transmural migration of enteric bacteria (possibly associated with diarrhea, a common symptom in cirrhosis). Severe liver disease, gastrointestinal bleeding, and a focus of infection in the urinary tract or elsewhere in the body increase the risk of SBP. Prior paracentesis may be contributory in a few instances. Penetrating lesions of the biliary tract, peptic ulcer disease, and overt bowel inflammation (such as appendicitis or diverticulitis) do not appear to be sources of infection.

Diagnosis

Clinical features The clinical presentation of SBP is often subtle.[5] Although ascites is always present, the volume of fluid may occasionally be small enough to necessitate ultrasonography for confirmation. Fever is the most common symptom but is absent in more than 30% of cases. Abdominal pain and hepatic encephalopathy are present in most patients. However, only half of the patients with SBP have abdominal tenderness, and as many as one third may be free of signs and symptoms of infection. Hence, SBP should be suspected in any cirrhotic patient who presents with unexplained clinical deterioration or hypotension.

Laboratory tests The key to diagnosis is examination of the ascitic fluid for bacteria and white blood cells. The polymorphonuclear leukocyte (PMN) count of the ascitic fluid is the best indicator of SBP; counts of more than 250 cells/mm^3 suggest a diagnosis of SBP, and counts above 500 cells/mm^3 are considered specific enough to mandate treatment of SBP in cirrhotic patients in whom no other evidence of infection is present.

Because the bacterial counts are often very low, the Gram stain of ascitic fluid in SBP is typically negative. However, a Gram stain is always useful because visualization of a single bacterial type would be consistent with SBP, whereas the presence of multiple bacterial forms would suggest secondary peritonitis. Because of the low concentration of bacteria, cultures are best performed by inoculation of 10 to 20 ml of ascitic fluid into a blood culture or BACTEC bottle at the bedside.

Three variants of SBP have been recognized on the basis of ascitic fluid PMN counts and cultures. In typical SBP, the PMN count is 250 cells/mm^3 or higher and cultures are positive. When the PMN count is 500 cells/mm^3 or higher but cultures are negative, the syndrome is called culture-negative neutrophilic ascites (CNNA). When the PMN count is below 250 cells/mm^3 but cultures are positive, the syndrome is termed bacterascites (BA). The clinical features and prognosis of SBP and CNNA are indistinguishable, and the two variants should be managed identically. In contrast, BA can be self-limited; if patients are asymptomatic, they can be managed with careful observation and repeat paracentesis after 48 hours, and antibiotic therapy can be initiated if clinical symptoms develop or if the PMN count of the ascitic fluid rises.

It is important to distinguish SBP from secondary peritonitis resulting from intra-abdominal disease, such as a perforated viscus. An ascitic fluid white blood cell count above 10,000/mm^3 suggests secondary peritonitis, as does the presence of multiple bacterial species or of anaerobes or fungi. Patients should, of course, always be evaluated clinically and radiologically to exclude evidence of an underlying intra-abdominal process that might give rise to secondary peritonitis. Peripheral blood leukocytosis and positive blood cultures are common in both SBP and secondary peritonitis.

Differential Diagnosis

Bacterial peritonitis may be closely mimicked by acute pancreatitis, particularly in a patient with cirrhosis [*see also* Pancreatic Abscesses, *below*]. Abdominal pain, fever, rebound tenderness, hypotension, and peripheral leukocytosis are common in both bacterial peritonitis and acute pancreatitis. In a patient with pancreatitis, a diagnostic abdominal aspiration may even reveal cloudy fluid, but the turbidity is caused by floating fat globules derived from fat necrosis. Very high serum amylase levels are present in acute pancreatitis, but elevated levels also occur in peritonitis after intestinal perforation or obstruction and in the presence of renal failure.

In a patient with cirrhosis and ascites, a number of conditions may be mistaken for peritonitis, including acute peptic ulcer, cholecystitis, mesenteric artery occlusion, and other intra-abdominal processes. Paracentesis is helpful in arriving at a diagnosis in these circumstances.

Acute bacterial peritonitis may be distinguished from tuberculous peritonitis by several features, including a more indolent course for tuberculous peritonitis, the absence of a peripheral leukocytosis, radiologic evidence of pulmonary tuberculosis, and a mononuclear response in the peritoneal fluid. In the patient with tuberculous peritonitis who does not have cirrhosis and ascites, the abdomen may have the characteristic so-called doughy feeling.

Peritonitis may be superficially suggested by the abdominal pain of acute porphyria, by lead colic, by diabetic acidosis, and by tabetic crisis, but the other features of these illnesses serve to distinguish them from peritonitis. Bacterial peritonitis is suggested by the high temperature, abdominal pain, abdominal rigidity, and peripheral leukocytosis of familial Mediterranean fever. The periodicity of familial Mediterranean fever and its occurrence predominantly in persons of Sephardic, Armenian, and Arab ancestry are helpful in differentiating it from bacterial peritonitis.

SBP may be difficult to diagnose in a patient with systemic lupus erythematosus who experiences acute abdominal pain and fever. These symptoms may stem from a variety of independent surgical problems, such as perforated ulcer, intestinal obstruction, and mesenteric occlusion, that must be distinguished from abdominal problems directly related to lupus, such as vasculitis, pancreatitis secondary to vasculitis or corticosteroid therapy, and SBP. Examination of peritoneal fluid obtained by paracentesis, by culdocentesis, or during laparotomy may be the only way to determine the presence of bacterial peritonitis.

Treatment

Until culture results are available, broad coverage should be directed against enteric organisms. Nephrotoxic drugs should be avoided whenever possible. Cefotaxime (2 g I.V. q 8 hours) has emerged as the favored agent for the empirical treatment of SBP[6]; other useful agents are ampicillin-sulbactam, ticarcillin–clavulanic acid, cefotetan, cefoxitin, meropenem, and imipenem-cilastatin, as well as combination therapies such as clindamycin and aztreonam.[7] Traditionally, intravenous antibiotics have been administered for 10 to 14 days, but 5 days of therapy appears to be as effective, provided that the patient is doing well clinically and that the ascitic fluid is sterile, with a PMN count that is below 250 cells/mm^3 before discontinuance of antibiotics.

Renal failure is a frequent complication of SBP; peripheral vasodilation and renal vasoconstriction are probably responsible.[8] A recent trial demonstrated that infusions of albumin (1.5 g/kg at the time of diagnosis and 1 g/kg on day 3) can substantially reduce the incidence of renal failure and mortality of patients with SBP.[9]

Recurrences of SBP are common, occurring in 43% of patients within 6 months and 69% within 1 year after the initial episode. Prophylaxis with norfloxacin (400 mg/day)[3] or with trimethoprim-sulfamethoxazole (one double-strength tablet containing 160 mg of trimethoprim and 800 mg of sulfamethoxazole, 5 days a week)[10] substantially reduces the recurrence rate, but the long-term effects of prophylaxis on survival are unclear.

SECONDARY PERITONITIS

Etiology

Secondary peritonitis occurs as a complication of intra-abdominal disease. It may occur as a result of appendicitis, diverticulitis, penetrating abdominal wounds, blunt trauma to the abdomen, perforation of the gastrointestinal tract (e.g., by a peptic ulcer or bowel neoplasm), or rupture of an intra-abdominal abscess. Most of these infections are polymicrobial. They involve both anaerobic species (principally *Bacteroides fragilis*, peptococci, and peptostreptococci) and aerobic species (*E. coli, Proteus* and *Klebsiella* species, and various streptococci and enterococci).[11] Bacteremia is common in such infections, particularly with *Bacteroides* organisms and *E. coli*. The prognosis of secondary peritonitis depends on the underlying cause; mortality is lowest in patients with appendicitis or perforated duodenal ulcer (10%) and highest in those with other intra-abdominal processes (50%) or postoperative peritonitis (60%).

Diagnosis

The clinical features of secondary peritonitis may at first be overshadowed by the manifestations of the underlying condition. In addition to peritoneal signs and a silent abdomen, the findings in a case of perforated peptic ulcer may include free air in the peritoneal cavity that can be demonstrated on upright or left lateral decubitus films of the abdomen. Ileus, edema of the small bowel wall, and obliteration of the normal properitoneal lines may be observed on supine films of the abdomen.

In the absence of ascites, the peritoneum has a remarkable capacity to wall off and localize infection to a portion of the abdomen. Thus, in situations such as rupture of the appendix, a localized peritonitis develops and results in a periappendiceal or pelvic abscess.

In generalized peritonitis secondary to bowel disease or after trauma or surgery, paracentesis in several quadrants is needed to aid in diagnosis. Culdocentesis may be helpful when there is only a small amount of fluid or when the patient has pelvic peritonitis. The leukocyte count of the abdominal aspirate in peritonitis secondary to bowel disease is often higher than it is in spontaneous peritonitis associated with cirrhosis. Because of the origin of infection and its polymicrobial anaerobic nature, the exudate may be malodorous.

Treatment

Peritonitis secondary to bowel perforation, ruptured gangrenous appendix, or penetrating trauma requires prompt surgical intervention in addition to antimicrobial therapy. Surgical therapy should be directed at correction of the underlying disease, debridement of the surrounding tissues, and prevention of recurrent microbial soilage. In general, this requires draining, resecting, excluding, or patching the diseased viscus during laparotomy; in selected cases, laparoscopy may prove useful.[12] Intraoperative saline lavage and radical peritoneal debridement have not proved useful; postoperative peritoneal lavage and planned repeat laparotomy have been suggested but are not of established benefit.

The choice of antimicrobial agent depends on the organisms involved in the peritonitis. Initial selection, however, is made before culture results are available, and it must take into consideration the organisms that are predominant in the colon: *B. fragilis*, enteric gram-negative bacilli, streptococci, and enterococci. Animal studies and clinical experience have shown the importance of using antibiotics that are effective against both aerobic and anaerobic bacteria to treat patients with polymicrobial peritonitis, but clinical trials have failed to establish the superiority of any particular regimen. Newer antibiotics that provide broad-spectrum coverage of many aerobic and anaerobic species allow single antibiotic therapy in many cases. Useful single agents include ampicillin-sulbactam, ticarcillin–clavulanic acid, cefoxitin, cefotetan, cefmetazole, meropenem, and imipenem-cilastatin. Effective multidrug regimens include (1) gentamicin with one of the agents noted above, (2) clindamycin and gentamicin or aztreonam, (3) ampicillin and metronidazole, and (4) ampicillin, metronidazole, and gentamicin [see 2 Chemotherapy of Infection]. Although they provide broader antimicrobial coverage, multidrug regimens do not appear to be more effective than single-drug programs. In all cases, the final choice of antibiotics should be determined by the results of culture and sensitivity testing and the clinical course.

Most antibiotics attain concentrations in ascitic fluid that are at least half of the simultaneous serum levels and exceed the minimum inhibitory concentration for the infecting organism. For this reason, systemic therapy alone is generally adequate in the management of bacterial peritonitis in patients with ascites; routine intraperitoneal instillation of antibiotics does not appear necessary.

PERITONITIS IN DIALYSIS PATIENTS

Epidemiology

Infection has been termed the Achilles heel of peritoneal dialysis. Peritonitis develops in as many as 60% of patients undergoing continuous ambulatory peritoneal dialysis during the first year of treatment, and the infection recurs in 20% to 30% of these patients; elderly patients are the most vulnerable.

Diagnosis

Clinical features The development of fever, abdominal pain or tenderness, and leukocytosis and the isolation of a bacterial or mycotic agent from the effluent fluid in a patient on peritoneal dialysis indicate peritonitis. In the absence of inflammatory cells and accompanying clinical signs, bacteria may be isolated from the dialysate; in this situation, bacteria often signal contamination rather than infection. Turbidity of the dialysate from neutrophils occurs in 2% to 3% of dialyses. Although turbidity itself does not necessarily indicate peritonitis, it should be considered an indication of infection until the results of the culture are available. Because of the extensive dilutions required, the absence of bacteria on a Gram stain of the dialysate sediment cannot be relied on to discriminate between infection and sterile inflammation.

Bacteriology The principal organisms in peritonitis that complicate peritoneal dialysis are coagulase-negative staphylococci, *S. aureus, Pseudomonas aeruginosa, E. coli* and other enteric organisms, and *Candida* species. Their entrance into the peritoneal cavity may occur exogenously (i.e., after colonization of the abdominal wound area or by contamination of the dialysate) or endogenously (i.e., by bacteremia or by transmural migration of bowel flora, perhaps enhanced by catheter-induced trauma). Patients who do not respond to antibiotic therapy within 96 hours are often infected with gram-negative bacilli—most often *Pseudomonas*—and their prognosis is worse than that of patients who respond rapidly. Removal of the dialysis catheter may be necessary to control the infection.

Treatment

Peritonitis caused by *Candida* species occurs most frequently as a complication of peritoneal dialysis, gastrointestinal surgery, or perforation of an abdominal viscus. Candidal peritonitis that complicates peritoneal dialysis is treated with intravenous amphotericin B, intraperitoneal amphotericin B, or both at a final dialysate concentration of 2 to 4 µg/ml. Fluconazole may also prove useful in cases of peritonitis caused by *C. albicans*.

Whereas the addition of peritoneal lavage, with or without antibiotics, does not appear to improve on the results achieved by intravenous antibiotics and conventional surgical therapy, intraperitoneal administration of antibiotics may be useful in patients who require peritoneal dialysis. For example, different antibiotics can be added directly to the dialysate in specific concentrations, such as ampicillin in a concentration of 50 mg/L or gentamicin in a concentration of 5 to 10 mg/L. Because bacteremia may occur, antibiotics should also be administered intravenously in these patients in a dosage appropriate to the patient's level of renal function. If aminoglycosides are being given, serum levels should be monitored. In patients in whom peritonitis develops as a complication of peritoneal dialysis or peritoneovenous shunting, it is often necessary to remove or replace the catheter during administration of antibiotics to control the peritonitis.

Intra-abdominal Abscesses

Intra-abdominal abscesses may present as complications of abdominal surgery, intra-abdominal conditions (e.g., diverticulitis, appendicitis, biliary tract disease, pancreatitis, perforated viscus), or penetrating abdominal trauma; as fever of obscure origin; or as dysfunction of neighboring organs (e.g., so-called lower lobe pneumonia related to a subphrenic abscess). Bacteremic spread of infection from a distant focus to an intra-abdominal site is a less common cause of intra-abdominal abscesses.

Historically, mortality from intra-abdominal abscesses has been high—about 25%. Major advances have been made, however, in the radiologic diagnosis of abscesses, the use of radiologically guided percutaneous drainage procedures, and the recognition and treatment of anaerobic bacteria. New approaches to antibiotic prophylaxis for postoperative and posttraumatic infections have also been developed.

Intra-abdominal abscesses are conveniently classified according to the anatomic location in which they occur: intraperitoneal, retroperitoneal, or visceral. Intraperitoneal abscesses are areas of localized peritonitis in which infection has progressed but has been walled off by omentum, peritoneum, and adjacent viscera. Retroperitoneal infections include perinephric abscesses and paravertebral abscesses. Visceral abscesses develop within abdominal viscera, predominantly the liver and less often the pancreas, spleen, and other organs.

GENERAL APPROACH TO INTRA-ABDOMINAL ABSCESSES

Diagnosis

Although the location of the abscess determines its particular features, many intra-abdominal infections share common elements. Fever, for example, is almost invariable; it often recurs in a spiking pattern and may be accompanied by rigors. Hypotension and even septic shock may develop. Abdominal pain is a major clue to the presence of an intra-abdominal abscess: when present, it can predominate; when it is absent, the diagnosis can be very difficult. Geriatric patients, in particular, may present atypically, without abdominal pain or fever. Leukocytosis and abnormalities of liver function and serum amylase are very common. Bacteremia, which may be polymicrobial, can occur.

Intra-abdominal abscesses characteristically contain multiple bacterial species. Anaerobic bacteria can be isolated from 60% to 70% of such abscesses; the bacteria most commonly isolated include *B. fragilis*, peptostreptococci and peptococci, *Clostridium* species, and aerobes such as *E. coli, Enterobacter, Klebsiella*, and enterococci. The specific organisms isolated do not generally provide clues to the nature of the underlying process. However, the presence of *Citrobacter* organisms strongly suggests a biliary or upper gastrointestinal source. *S. aureus*, otherwise uncommon in intra-abdominal abscesses, suggests the presence of bacteremic seeding or vertebral osteomyelitis, which can lead to retroperitoneal or perinephric abscesses.

Plain radiography (kidneys and upper bladder, upright, and lateral decubitus views) may afford important clues to the diagnosis of intra-abdominal abscesses. For example, air-fluid levels may indicate an intra-abdominal collection, free air may point to perforation of a viscus as the underlying problem, displaced loops of bowel may signify an abscess, and a so-called soap-bubble appearance or loss of the normal psoas shadow may suggest a retroperitoneal collection. Because of their simplicity, speed, and low cost, plain radiographs should always be the initial radiographic step in evaluating patients suspected of having an intra-abdominal abscess.

Ultrasonography and computed tomographic scanning, however, are much more sensitive and specific than plain radiography and are now the standard radiologic techniques for evaluating intra-abdominal abscesses.[13] Both are excellent for diagnosis, and both can be used to guide percutaneous abscess drainage [*see* Treatment and Prevention, *below*].[14] CT scanning is the more accurate study; its specificity and sensitivity rates can exceed 90%. Compared with ultrasonography, CT scanning has the additional advantages of allowing simultaneous administration of contrast, of not requiring skin contact (hence, surgical dressings do not interfere with the study), and of producing accurate results even in the presence of ileus and abdominal gas collections. Ultrasonography, however, is less expensive, is often more readily available, can sometimes be done with portable equipment at the bedside, and does not involve exposure to radiation. Ultrasonography is the most accurate method for detecting abscesses in the left or right upper quadrant of the abdomen and in the true pelvis; it is also sensitive and specific for identifying ascites.

The most significant new development in abdominal imaging is the helical (or spiral) CT.[13] In conventional CT scanning, the patient is moved a predetermined distance on the CT table, then halted to obtain an image. This process is repeated until the scan is complete. In helical CT scanning, images are obtained as the CT table moves the patient continuously during a single breath hold. Although it reduces scanning time and enhances image quality, helical scanning may require additional radiation to obtain the extra images needed to compensate for artifacts caused by the continuous motion. As in conventional CT scanning, intravenous or gastrointestinal contrast material can be administered to improve the accuracy of helical scanning. With intravenous contrast, helical scanning allows detailed evaluation of the intra-abdominal vasculature[13]; with gastrointestinal contrast, it has proved valuable in the diagnosis of appendicitis.[15]

Magnetic resonance imaging plays a negligible role in the evaluation of intra-abdominal infections. Nuclear medicine studies are also less helpful than CT and ultrasonography. Although early results appeared promising, gallium-67 scanning is often disappointing. Indium-111 scanning is also less helpful than CT and ultrasonographic techniques; however, a newer technique, indium-111–labeled IgG scanning, appears to be promising. Cholescintigraphy scans using technetium-99m–labeled HIDA (lidofenin) are useful in evaluating the gallbladder. Arteriography and barium contrast studies are seldom used to diagnose intra-abdominal abscesses. If fistulous tracts are present, however, sinograms may occasionally be helpful.

Treatment and Prevention

The choice of antibiotics depends on the organisms isolated from cultures of blood or abscess material. Until this information is available, the choice of drugs should be guided by the same principles that apply to the treatment of peritonitis. Although the use of antibiotics is essential, especially because of the risk of bacteremia, such therapy alone will not eradicate intra-abdominal abscesses and is therefore secondary to prompt, effective abscess drainage.

Until the mid-1970s, surgical drainage was mandatory for the treatment of intra-abdominal abscesses. However, treatment changed dramatically within just a few years of the introduction of percutaneous abscess drainage under ultrasonographic or CT guidance. Ultrasonography may be used to guide drainage of large or superficial collections, but CT is preferable for smaller or deeper abscesses.[16] Many studies have demonstrated that percutaneous abscess drainage is safe and effective for a broad range of intra-abdominal collections; success rates range from 47% to 92%, with most studies reporting better than 80% success. Failure of treatment is more common in immunosuppressed patients and in those with poorly defined phlegmons, multilocular abscesses, thick hematomas or organized infections, or abscesses with associated fistulous tracts.

Radiographic features alone cannot indicate which abscesses will respond to percutaneous drainage. Hence, it seems reasonable to institute percutaneous drainage in all patients who have a safe access route, provided that skilled personnel are available and that the patient does not otherwise require surgery. Surgical drainage may then be used in patients with recurrences, failures, or complications. Even in the case of abscesses that usually require surgery, such as periappendiceal and diverticular abscesses, percutaneous drainage can provide temporary control of sepsis, allowing surgery to be delayed until conditions are optimal.

Antibiotics can reduce the incidence of wound infection, peritonitis, and intra-abdominal abscesses after various abdominal and pelvic operations.[17] One regimen involves a cathartic such as polyethylene glycol, as well as the oral administration of 1 g each of neomycin and erythromycin at 1:00 P.M., 2:00 P.M., and 11:00 P.M. on the day before the surgical procedure. Programs involving the oral administration of metronidazole plus neomycin (or kanamycin) or neomycin plus a tetracycline are also effective. In addition, parenteral antibiotic prophylaxis has been shown to be effective after colon surgery, appendectomy, hysterectomy, and surgery for penetrating abdominal trauma. An effective regimen entails the use of intravenous cefoxitin, 2 g every 6 hours for 24 hours; in patients who cannot tolerate β-lactam antibiotics, prophylaxis with clindamycin and gentamicin is a reasonable alternative.

INTRAPERITONEAL ABSCESSES

Intraperitoneal abscesses may form in either of two ways: (1) from diffuse peritonitis in which loculations of pus have developed in anatomically dependent areas such as the pelvis, paracolic gutters, and subphrenic areas or (2) by spread of infection from a localized inflammatory process to contiguous peritoneum. About one third of intra-abdominal abscesses are intraperitoneal, and almost one half of intraperitoneal abscesses occur in the right lower quadrant.

Subphrenic Abscesses

About 60% of subphrenic abscesses develop after initially clean intra-abdominal surgery involving the duodenum and stomach, biliary tract, or appendix; 20% to 40% develop after rupture of a hollow viscus (such as perforated peptic ulcer or acute appendicitis), in which the infection is subsequently sealed off. A variable percentage of subphrenic abscesses develops after penetrating, close abdominal trauma, and less than 5% develop without predisposing circumstances.

Clinical features The manifestations of a subphrenic abscess range from a severe acute disorder to an insidious chronic process characterized by intermittent fever, weight loss, anemia, and nonspecific symptoms. The chronic syndrome is most often observed in patients who have previously received antibiotics; such an abscess may smolder subclinically for months or even years before diagnosis. In any patient with fever of undetermined origin who has had an abdominal operation—even if the operation was performed many months earlier—a chronic intra-abdominal abscess must be suspected.

Spiking fever, abdominal pain and tenderness (most often at the lower costal margin), and weight loss are common manifestations. Features of an intrathoracic process, such as shoulder pain, chest pain, cough, dyspnea, rales, and pleural effusion, are more commonly observed than features of an intra-abdominal condition. Leukocytosis of 15,000 to 25,000/mm^3 is almost always present. Occasionally, patients will have prolonged obscure febrile illness complicated by the sudden development of an empyema when the subphrenic abscess ruptures through the diaphragm. Although pleural fluid is present in about 80% of patients with a subphrenic abscess, it is usually a sympathetic transudate. In some cases, a subphrenic abscess penetrates through the diaphragm and empties directly into a bronchus without producing a pleural effusion or empyema; a cough suddenly develops, and the patient produces thick, foul-smelling sputum and may become markedly dyspneic. The acute onset of pulmonary symptoms may be mistaken for the onset of a primary pneumonia, but the character of the sputum and the history of obscure febrile illness should raise the suspicion of a subphrenic abscess.

Imaging tests CT scanning and ultrasonography are the best radiologic techniques for establishing the diagnosis. The plain x-ray changes in subphrenic abscess include pleural effusion, limitation of diaphragmatic movement, elevation of a hemidiaphragm, and lower-lobe pneumonia or atelectasis.

Treatment The primary treatment of a subphrenic abscess is drainage, and percutaneous drainage is usually successful. However, if surgical drainage is necessary, the transperitoneal approach is favored because it allows adequate exploration of several potential abscess sites and drainage of coexistent purulent collections (e.g., a subphrenic abscess with subhepatic extension). Antibiotic therapy is initially aimed at the spectrum of organisms that might be involved in the abscess. Such therapy is later modified on the basis of the results of culture.

RETROPERITONEAL ABSCESSES

Pyogenic infections of the retroperitoneum may occasionally be confused with intra-abdominal sepsis. Indeed, many retroperitoneal abscesses arise from disorders of the abdominal viscera; more than two thirds of patients with retroperitoneal abscesses also have underlying debilitating conditions, including malignancies, corticosteroid use, alcoholism, and diabetes. More than 80% of these infections are polymicrobial, involving aerobic and anaerobic enteric organisms.[18] CT scanning is the key to diagnosis of retroperitoneal abscesses. The same is true for primary psoas abscesses, which are often caused by *S. aureus*,[19] and for perinephric abscesses, which usually originate in the urinary tract. As with other abscesses, successful management requires prompt percutaneous or surgical drainage and the administration of appropriate antibiotics.

Pancreatic Abscesses

Most pancreatic abscesses occur as a complication of pancreatitis, which can occur as a result of alcoholism (38%), gallstones (11%), surgical trauma (16%), or other factors (35%). A pancreatic abscess may also represent secondary infection of an established pseudocyst. Pancreatic abscesses are often polymicrobial, typically containing three or four species of bacteria.[20] Most are enteric organisms, including *E. coli*, enterococci, *Klebsiella* species, and anaerobes such as *Bacteroides, Peptococcus, Fusobacterium*, and *Clostridium* species. Nonenteric organisms, including staphylococci, *Pseudomonas*, and, less often, *Candida*, may be involved. Bacteremia occurs in about 26% of cases.

Clinical features Pancreatic abscess should be suspected in a patient with pancreatitis if fever and ileus persist or if clinical deterioration occurs 1 to 4 weeks after improvement has begun. Nausea, vomiting, and abdominal pain and tenderness are typically present. An abdominal mass may be palpable. A leukocytosis of 15,000 to 20,000/mm^3 is present. In less than half of cases, the serum amylase level is elevated and liver function test results are abnormal. Hypocalcemia and hypoalbuminemia are common features. In some cases, however, pancreatic abscesses may have an indolent presentation or may be clinically indistinguishable from a noninfected pancreatic phlegmon.

Complications of pancreatic abscess include perforation of the peritoneal cavity, which is usually lethal; perforation of the stomach, duodenum, or transverse colon, which frequently produces gastrointestinal bleeding; and formation of satellite intra-abdominal abscesses.

Imaging tests In most patients, the abdominal CT scan is the key to diagnosis. CT-guided percutaneous needle aspiration is a safe and effective way to establish the presence of pancreatic infection and should be performed promptly when the diagnosis is suspected. Ultrasonography helps define a pancreatic mass but cannot reliably distinguish between a pseudocyst and an abscess. Chest films commonly show an elevated hemidiaphragm, atelectasis, and a pleural effusion.

Treatment Pancreatic abscesses are highly lethal: without drainage, mortality is 100%. Surgical drainage is often required; percutaneous drainage may be helpful for diagnosis, for some recurrent abscesses, or for well-circumscribed abscesses. Vigorous antibiotic therapy is important; broad coverage of enteric organisms should be provided until cultures of the abscess or bloodstream reveal the etiologic agents.

VISCERAL ABSCESSES

Liver Abscesses

Pyogenic liver abscesses occur in several settings, including biliary tract infection, direct extension from a contiguous site of infection, portal bacteremia from intra-abdominal septic foci, and nonpenetrating trauma. Liver abscesses may occur as a result of systemic bacteremia or as complications of abdominal surgery or penetrating abdominal trauma. They may also occur as complications of hepatocellular carcinoma[21] or percutaneous transhepatic biliary drainage procedures in patients with cancer and obstructive jaundice. Pyogenic abscesses may be single or multiple.

Clinical features Fever is the most common symptom and is present in nearly 90% of patients. Chills and weight loss occur in about half of cases. Because abdominal pain, abdominal tenderness, or hepatomegaly is present in only half of cases, many of these patients present with fever of undetermined origin. Leukocytosis is present in most cases. Jaundice is infrequent, but the serum alkaline phosphatase level is elevated in almost all patients. Rupture of a liver abscess, although uncommon, is often accompanied by diffuse abdominal pain and septic shock.[22]

Bacteriology Like other intra-abdominal abscesses, pyogenic liver abscesses principally involve enteric bacteria; two thirds of the abscesses have polymicrobial origins, and at least one third involve anaerobes. *S. aureus* may be the causative organism in patients with bacteremia and in children. *Klebsiella* is often responsible for gas-forming liver abscesses, which typically occur in patients with diabetes.[23] Blood cultures are positive in about half of patients with a pyogenic liver abscess, and metastatic infections may occur.

Imaging tests CT scanning is the most accurate diagnostic technique [*see Figure 1a and 1b*], yielding positive results in up to 95% of confirmed cases; ultrasonography is also helpful, yielding positive results in up to 80% of confirmed cases. The initial clue to the diagnosis may come from plain x-rays, which may show an elevated right hemidiaphragm, a right pleural effusion, or an air-fluid level.

The major differential diagnosis is amebic liver abscess [see 39 Protozoan Infections]. Amebic abscesses are more likely to be solitary and confined to the right lobe of the liver; a history of travel or diarrhea may help suggest the diagnosis. A stool examination revealing *Entamoeba histolytica* is very suggestive, but the stool examination is often negative in patients with hepatic amebiasis. However, most patients with amebic liver abscesses have positive amebic serologies. Less often, hepatic cysts or neoplasms may be confused with liver abscesses.

a

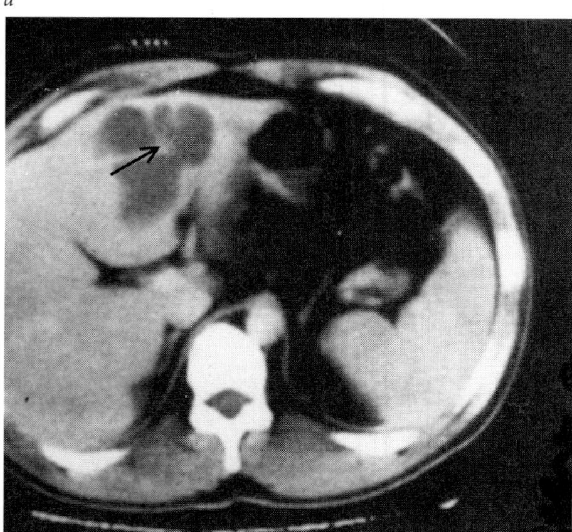

b

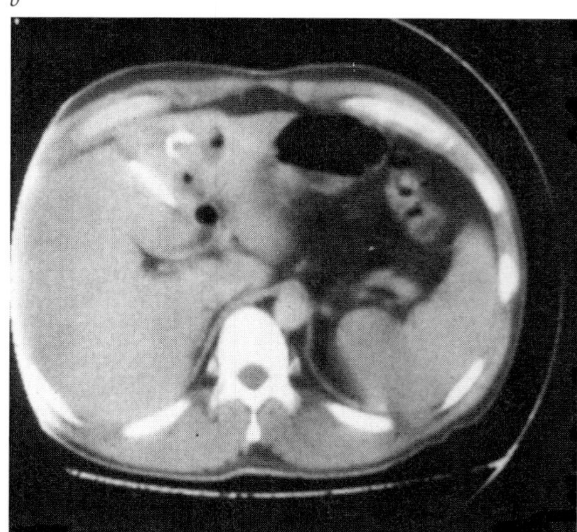

Figure 1 **(*a*) CT scan shows multilobular liver abscess (arrow). (*b*) Four days after percutaneous abscess drainage, CT scan shows resolution of the abscess cavity.**

Treatment Whereas surgery was formerly the mainstay of therapy, percutaneous drainage should now be the initial drainage procedure in most patients with pyogenic liver abscesses. Antibiotics should be administered intravenously, with broad coverage of enteric organisms and staphylococci until specific pathogens have been isolated from the abscess or the bloodstream. Mortality depends largely on the underlying disease and is highest in patients with cancer.[24] Surgical therapy is required for ruptured abscesses, but the mortality is high, approaching 44%.[22]

Splenic Abscesses

Splenic abscesses are uncommon[25]; unlike other intra-abdominal abscesses, they are often bacteremic in origin, especially in patients with endocarditis. In other patients, hemoglobinopathy, vasculitis with splenic infarction, trauma, and immunosuppression may be predisposing factors. Fever and chills and left upper quadrant pain are common. If the upper pole of the spleen is affected, diaphragmatic and pleural and pulmonary symptoms may predominate, but peritoneal symptoms are more common if the lower pole is the site of infection. Responsible organisms include *S. aureus*, streptococci, *Salmonella*, and enteric bacteria; fungi are important causes in immunocompromised patients. CT scans and ultrasonography are the most useful radiographic studies. Appropriate antimicrobial therapy is essential. Splenectomy has been considered mandatory, but operative or percutaneous drainage or even antibiotics alone may suffice in selected cases. More experience is needed before the optimal management of these uncommon infections can be determined.

References

1. Johnson CC, Baldessarre J, Levison ME: Peritonitis: update on pathophysiology, clinical manifestations, and management. Clin Infect Dis 24:1035, 1997

2. Hall JC, Heel KA, Papadimitriou JM, et al: The pathology of peritonitis. Gastroenterology 114:185, 1998

3. Such J, Runyon BA: Spontaneous bacterial peritonitis. Clin Infect Dis 27:669, 1998

4. Hemsley C, Eykyn SJ: Pneumococcal peritonitis in previously healthy adults: case report and review. Clin Infect Dis 27:376, 1998

5. Gilbert JA, Kamath PS: Spontaneous bacterial peritonitis: an update. Mayo Clin Proc 70:365, 1995

6. Dalmau D, Layrargues GP, Fenyves D, et al: Cefotaxime, desacetylcefotaxime, and bactericidal activity in spontaneous bacterial peritonitis. J Infect Dis 180:1597, 1999

7. Farber MS, Abrams JH: Antibiotics for the acute abdomen. Surg Clin North Am 77:1395, 1997

8. Runyon BA: Albumin infusion for spontaneous bacterial peritonitis. Lancet 354:1838, 1999

9. Sort P, Navasa M, Arroyo V, et al: Effect of intravenous albumin on renal impairment and mortality in patients with cirrhosis and spontaneous bacterial peritonitis. N Engl J Med 341:403, 1999

10. Singh N, Gayowski T, Yu VL, et al: Trimethoprim-sulfamethoxazole for the prevention of spontaneous bacterial peritonitis in cirrhosis: a randomized trial. Ann Intern Med 122:595, 1995

11. Wilson SE, Hopkins JA: Clinical correlates of anaerobic bacteriology in peritonitis. Clin Infect Dis 20(suppl 2):S251, 1995

12. Navez B, Tassetti V, Scony JJ, et al: Laparoscopic management of acute peritonitis. Br J Surg 85:32, 1998

13. Gupta H, Dupuy DE: Advances in imaging of the acute abdomen. Surg Clin North Am 77:1245, 1997

14. Sheafor DH, Paulson EK, Simmons CM, et al: Abdominal percutaneous interventional procedures: comparison of CT and US guidance. Radiology 207:705, 1998

15. Rao PM, Rhea JT, Novelline RA, et al: Effect of computed tomography of the appendix on treatment of patients and use of hospital resources. N Engl J Med 338:141, 1998

16. Montgomery RS, Wilson SE: Intraabdominal abscesses: image-guided diagnosis and therapy. Clin Infect Dis 23:28, 1996

17. Nichols RL, Smith JW, Garcia RY, et al: Current practices of preoperative bowel preparation among North American colorectal surgeons. Clin Infect Dis 24:609, 1997

18. Brook I, Frazier EH: Aerobic and anaerobic microbiology of retroperitoneal abscesses. Clin Infect Dis 26:938, 1998

19. Santaella RO, Fishman EK, Lipsett PA: Primary vs secondary iliopsoas abscess. Arch Surg 130:1309, 1995

20. Brook I, Frazier EH: Microbiological analysis of pancreatic abscess. Clin Infect Dis 22:384, 1996

21. Rintoul R, O'Riordan MG, Laurenson IF, et al: Changing management of pyogenic liver abscess. Br J Surg 83:1215, 1996

22. Chou F-F, Sheen-Chen SM, Lee TY: Rupture of pyogenic liver abscess. Am J Gastroenterol 90:767, 1995

23. Chou F-F, Sheen-Chen SM, Chen YS: The comparison of clinical course and results of treatment between gas-forming and non-gas-forming pyogenic liver abscess. Arch Surg 130:401, 1995

24. Yeh TS, Jan YY, Jen LB, et al: Hepatocellular carcinoma presenting as pyogenic liver abscess: characteristics, diagnosis, and management. Clin Infect Dis 26:1224, 1998

25. Ooi LL, Leong SS: Splenic abscesses from 1987 to 1995. Am J Surg 174:87, 1997

9 Infections of the Urinary Tract

Kalpana Gupta, M.D., M.P.H.
Walter E. Stamm, M.D.

Definitions

Urinary tract infection (UTI) is the most common of all bacterial infections; it affects persons throughout their life span [*see Table 1*]. The term urinary tract infection encompasses a variety of clinical entities, ranging from asymptomatic bacteriuria to cystitis, prostatitis, and pyelonephritis. It may be further characterized as complicated (associated with a wide variety of structural and functional abnormalities of the urinary tract and kidney) or uncomplicated (occurring without an anatomic or predisposing reason for infection) and as nosocomial (generally, catheter-associated) or community-acquired.

Epidemiology

In general, UTI occurs more commonly in females than in males, except at the extremes of age, when the incidence is higher in males. A greater frequency of congenital anomalies of the urinary tract in male infants and a high prevalence of prostatic hypertrophy and disease in men older than 50 years account for the increased incidence of UTI in males of these age groups. In persons between 1 and about 50 years of age, UTI is predominantly a disease of females.

As many as 50% to 80% of women in the general population acquire at least one UTI during their lifetime; most of these infections are uncomplicated.[1] Among nuns, the frequency of bacteriuria is significantly reduced in the 4 decades from 15 to 54 years of age; this suggests a role for sexual intercourse in the development of UTI in women. Indeed, in a prospective cohort study of sexually active healthy women, the incidence of UTI was 50 to 70 episodes per 100 person-years.[2] Recent use of a diaphragm with spermicide, frequency of sexual intercourse, and a history of UTI were identified as independent risk factors for UTI in this study. UTI has also been temporally related to recent sexual intercourse.

The incidence of UTI in young men is very low and has traditionally been attributed to the presence of urologic abnormalities. However, it is apparent that uncomplicated UTI can occur in men who (1) have unprotected anal intercourse with men, (2) are not circumcised (lack of circumcision is associated with an increased incidence of *Escherichia coli* colonization of the glans and prepuce and the subsequent migration of *E. coli* to the urinary tract), (3) have unprotected intercourse with a woman whose vagina is colonized with uropathogens, or (4) have AIDS and a CD4+ T cell count less than 200/mm^3.[3–6]

About 20% to 30% of women who have had one episode of UTI will have recurrent episodes.[7] Recurrence may result from relapse or reinfection. Relapse in either sex is caused by the reappearance of an organism from a sequestered focus, usually within the kidney or prostate, shortly after completion of therapy. In reinfection, the course of therapy has successfully eradicated the infection and there is no sequestered focus, but organisms are reintroduced from the fecal reservoir. At least 90% of all recurrences are from reinfection.[8] Studies of the natural history of women with recurrent UTI have found that the rate of recurrence ranges from 0.3 to 7.6 infections per patient per year, with an average

Table 1 Incidence of Urinary Tract Infection According to Age and Sex

Age Group	*Incidence (%)*	*Approximate Sex Ratio (Male:Female)*
Neonatal	1.0	1.5:1.0
Preschool age	1.5–3.0	1:10
School age	1.2	1:30
Reproductive age	3–5	1:50
Geriatric	10–30	1:1.5

rate of 2.6 infections per year.[9] Clustering of episodes occurs; it is not uncommon for multiple recurrences to follow an initial infection. The likelihood of a recurrence decreases with increasing time since the last infection. A recent case-controlled study of women with recurrent UTI identified frequency of sexual intercourse, use of spermicide, having a new sexual partner, a history of first UTI occurring before 15 years of age, and a maternal history of UTI as independent risk factors for recurrent UTI.[10]

The incidence of asymptomatic bacteriuria in pregnant women is 4% to 10%, at least double the incidence in similarly aged nonpregnant women.[11] If not treated, 25% of pregnant women with bacteriuria will acquire acute pyelonephritis later in pregnancy. Premature births and perinatal mortality are increased in pregnancies complicated by UTI.[12] In addition, women who are bacteriuric during pregnancy have a higher rate of UTIs on long-term follow-up than women who are not bacteriuric. About 30% of women with a history of bacteriuria during pregnancy have abnormalities on intravenous pyelograms that suggest chronic pyelonephritis; these abnormalities most likely result from damage by infections in childhood. There is little evidence that the infections that develop during pregnancy have long-term effects.

Susceptibility of diabetic patients to UTI has been studied intensively. The rates of asymptomatic bacteriuria and UTI in diabetic women are twofold to threefold higher than in nondiabetic women; these differences have not been observed in men.[13] In hospitalized diabetic patients, particularly those with multiple-organ complications, the incidence of infection and true pyelonephritis also appears to be increased, partly because of poor bladder function and urinary catheterization. Other clinical conditions causing obstruction in urinary flow or incomplete voiding also predispose diabetic patients to infection. In addition, impaired cytokine secretion may contribute to asymptomatic bacteriuria in diabetic women.[14]

Etiology

The spectrum of organisms causing UTI varies by clinical syndrome. In acute uncomplicated cystitis, the etiologic agents are highly predictable: *E. coli* accounts for 75% to 90% of isolates; *Staphylococcus saprophyticus* accounts for 5% to 15% of isolates (particularly in younger women); and *Klebsiella* species, *Proteus* species, enterococci, and other organisms account for 5% to 10% of isolates. The spectrum of agents that cause uncomplicated pyelonephritis is less well studied but is similar to that of acute cystitis. In complicated UTIs, *E. coli* remains the predominant organism, but other aerobic gram-negative rods, such as *Klebsiella* species, *Proteus* species, *Citrobacter* species, *Acinetobacter* species, *Morganella* species, and *Pseudomonas aeruginosa* are also frequently isolated. Gram-positive bacteria, such as enterococci and *S. aureus,* as well as yeast, are also important pathogens in complicated UTI.

Pathogenesis

Bacteria establish infection in the urinary tract either through the bloodstream or by traveling from the urethra to the bladder and then up the ureter to the kidney. Hematogenous spread accounts for fewer than 2% of documented UTIs and usually results from bacteremia caused by relatively virulent organisms, such as *Salmonella* and *S. aureus*. Focal abscesses or areas of pyelonephritis within a kidney may be established in hematogenous infections and result in positive urine cultures.

More than 98% of UTIs occur via the ascending route. However, introduction of bacteria into the bladder does not make sustained infection inevitable. For example, bacteria often enter the bladder after sexual intercourse, but normal micturition eliminates these organisms. The bladder mucosal surface has antibacterial properties that eliminate some organisms, presumably because of mucus trapping and a polymorphonuclear leukocyte response. In addition, urine that has a low pH, high or very low osmolarity, high urea concentration, or high organic acid content inhibits bacterial growth. Abnormal micturition, a significant residual urine volume, or both will promote true infection. There are also acquired and intrinsic host factors, as well as bacterial virulence factors, which increase the likelihood of developing UTI.[1]

VAGINAL ECOLOGY AND UTI

In women, colonization of the vaginal introitus with organisms from the fecal flora, usually *E. coli,* is the critical initial step in the pathogenesis of UTI. Sexual intercourse and the use of a diaphragm with spermicide or of spermicide alone are strongly associated with an increased risk of *E. coli* vaginal colonization and bacteriuria, probably because of alterations in the normal vaginal microflora.[15] In addition, the diaphragm may have adverse urodynamic effects.

In postmenopausal women, there is an increased incidence of gram-negative vaginal colonization and bacteriuria. These changes correlate with the disappearance of the normally predominant lactobacilli from the vaginal microflora and a rise in pH. Estrogen repletion reverses these effects. In a randomized, placebo-controlled trial, topical estrogen therapy resulted in restoration of the normal vaginal flora and a decrease in both the prevalence of vaginal *E. coli* colonization and the incidence of UTI in postmenopausal women with a history of recurrent UTI.[16]

GENETIC FACTORS

There is increasing evidence that genetically determined factors may influence susceptibility to recurrent UTI. Women with recurrent UTI demonstrate a propensity for persistent vaginal colonization with *E. coli,* even during asymptomatic periods. Vaginal and periurethral mucosal cells from women with recurrent UTI bind threefold more uropathogenic bacteria than do mucosal cells from women without recurrent infection. These observations suggest that epithelial cells from susceptible women may possess specific types or greater numbers of receptors for *E. coli* binding, facilitating colonization. This increased susceptibility is determined in part by Lewis blood group type and whether the woman is a secretor or a nonsecretor of blood group antigens into bodily fluids. Vaginal epithelial cells from nonsecretors of blood group antigens bind significantly greater numbers of bacteria, and nonsecretors are particularly at risk for recurrent UTI.[17,18] Mutations in host response genes (e.g., Toll receptors and interleukin-8 receptor) have recently been linked to severity of UTIs in animals, although they have not yet been linked in humans.[19]

BACTERIAL VIRULENCE

Certain strains of *E. coli* possess chromosomally encoded virulence determinants that confer the ability to infect the anatomically normal urinary tract and produce acute inflammatory disease (e.g., cystitis and pyelonephritis). Characteristics that have been associated with uropathogenicity are the presence of certain O and K surface antigens (the O antigen is the outer polysaccharide portion of the bacterial envelope, and the K antigen is the antiphagocytic capsular antigen), the presence of the siderophore protein aerobactin, resistance to the bactericidal activity of serum, the ability to produce toxins such as hemolysin and cytotoxic necrotizing factor, and certain intracellular metabolic capabilities.[20]

Also important is the presence of adhesins on the surface of uropathogenic bacteria that mediate binding to specific receptors on the surface of uroepithelial cells [*see Figure 1*]. The best-studied form of adhesion is that mediated by P fimbriae, which are hairlike protein structures found on the surface of certain pathogenic strains of *E. coli.* These complex organelles consist of 11 different proteins, the most important being the PapA protein, which makes up the stalk, and the PapG protein, which makes up the tip adhesin. P fimbriae interact with a specific receptor on epithelial cells. This epithelial cell receptor contains the carbohydrate moiety α-D-galactopyranosyl-(1→4)-β-D-galactopyranoside, which is found in the P blood group antigens. The prevalence of P-fimbriated *E. coli* correlates with severity of disease: there is a low prevalence (10% to 20%) in *E. coli* strains from the fecal flora of asymptomatic persons; there is a higher prevalence (50% to 60%) in strains that cause cystitis; and the highest prevalence (70% to 100%) is found in strains that cause pyelonephritis.[19,20] P fimbriae also appear to be important in the pathogenesis of bloodstream invasion from the kidney. About 75% to 100% of *E. coli* strains isolated from the blood of otherwise healthy patients with pyelonephritis express P fimbriae. In contrast, *E. coli* strains that cause urosepsis in persons with compromising medical conditions are much less likely to have P fimbriae.[20,21] Type 1 pili (made up of the FimA shaft and FimH adhesin proteins, as well as other proteins) mediate binding to uroplakins, which are mannosylated glycoproteins on the surface of bladder uroepithelial cells; type 1 pili are also thought to play a key role in initiating *E. coli* bladder infection.[20] All *E. coli* strains possess type 1 pili and activate gene expression in the environment of the urinary tract. In addition to P and type 1 fimbriae, other adhesins are present on uropathogenic strains of *E. coli* that may play a role in mediating attachment of uropathogenic strains to the uroepithelium in selected circumstances. The binding of uropathogenic *E. coli* to receptors on uroepithelial cells initiates a complex series of intracellular signals that alters epithelial cell function. Chemokines and cytokines are synthesized and secreted, and cells undergo apoptosis and exfoliation, carrying attached *E. coli* away in the urine.

ANATOMIC AND FUNCTIONAL ABNORMALITIES

Persons who have major anatomic and functional abnormalities, including vesicoureteral reflux, ureteral obstruction, or a foreign body (e.g., a stone, a catheter, or a tumor), are markedly predisposed to UTI, particularly infections involving

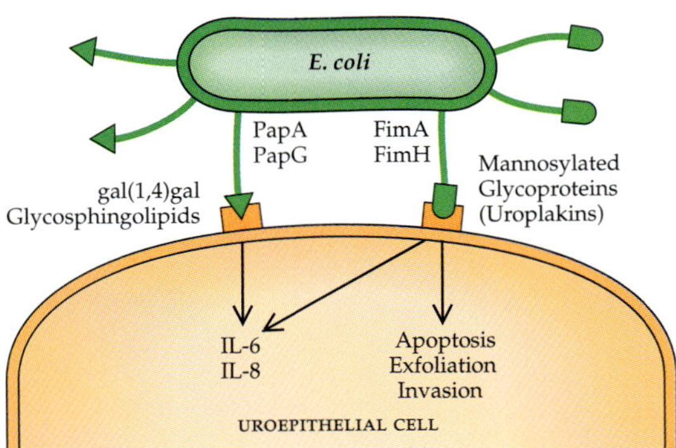

Figure 1 **The consequences of adherence of uropathogenic *Escherichia coli* to epithelial cells. (IL-6 — interleukin-6; IL-8 — interleukin-8)**

the kidney. In such persons, UTI can develop as a result of infection with bacteria, including *E. coli* strains, that are not normally uropathogenic.[20–22] Not surprisingly, infection with nonuropathogenic strains of bacteria is also common in hospitalized patients, presumably because they have anatomic and functional abnormalities.[23,24] Bacterial invasion of the prostate and incomplete bladder emptying caused by bladder outlet obstruction are the primary predisposing factors in men with UTI. Instrumentation and incomplete bladder emptying are important predisposing factors for UTI in patients with spinal cord injury or diabetes. Inhibition of ureteral peristalsis leading to vesicoureteral reflux is important in the pathogenesis of pyelonephritis in pregnant women.

Vesicoureteral reflux plays a key role in the pathogenesis of renal infection and, more important, in the evolution of chronic renal damage. It is commonly associated with UTI in children but also occurs because of anatomic abnormalities in children without UTI. Reflux provides a direct route for infection to reach the pelvicalyceal system of the kidney; severe reflux may occur intrarenally. The urine gains access to the kidney parenchyma via the ducts of Bellini at the papillary tips and then spreads outward along the collecting tubules. Renal scars caused by chronic pyelonephritis are often associated with such reflux. Most reflux-associated renal damage occurs in infancy, because with growth there is a tendency for self-correction of at least mild degrees of reflux. The long-term effects of reflux on kidney structure and function are a major justification for an aggressive radiologic approach in infants and young children with UTI [*see* Management, *below*].[25]

Clinical Presentations

The clinical presentation of UTI is quite variable, ranging from asymptomatic bacteriuria to typical symptomatic cystitis to acute pyelonephritis. In addition, clinical symptoms do not always correlate with the site of infection (bladder versus kidney) or with the degree of bacteriuria. Studies have demonstrated that approximately 30% of patients with lower urinary tract symptoms also have silent infection of the kidney.[8] A great deal of effort has thus been devoted to the development of a noninvasive technique for differentiating renal infections from bladder infections. Unfortunately, we are still lacking such a test. The best noninvasive test to delineate the anatomic site of infection appears to be the response to short-course antibiotic therapy [*see* Management, *below*].

CYSTITIS

The typical symptoms of cystitis are dysuria, urinary frequency, and urgency. Nocturia and suprapubic or back discomfort are also often present. In addition, the urine may be cloudy, malodorous, or bloody. Urine microscopy reveals pyuria in nearly all cases and hematuria in about 30% of cases. Bacteriuria is demonstrable on Gram stain of unspun urine in over 90% of cases when colony counts of 10^5 bacteria/ml or higher are present. However, approximately one third of women presenting with typical symptoms of cystitis do not have significant bacteriuria (defined as $> 10^5$ bacteria/ml); yet, most of these women have pyuria and lower colony counts of typical uropathogens and respond to short-course antimicrobial therapy. Thus, the definition of so-called significant bacteriuria in women with symptoms of cystitis has been reevaluated in recent studies, and a colony count of greater than 10^2 bacteria/ml has been found to have greater sensitivity (95%) and specificity (85%) for the diagnosis of acute cystitis in women.[8] Women with dysuria and pyuria who have less than 10^2 bacteria/ml may have urethritis caused by *Chlamydia trachomatis, Neisseria gonorrhoeae,* or herpes simplex virus or vulvovaginitis caused by *Trichomonas vaginalis* or *Candida* species. Clinical and laboratory criteria can help differentiate these conditions [*see Table 2*]. Women with dysuria but without significant bacteriuria were previously regarded as having the so-called acute urethral syndrome. However, this term is now less useful because most of these women have a definable condition with a specific diagnosis rather than an undefined syndrome.

Table 2 Acute Dysuria in Women[7]

Condition	Pathogen	*Laboratory Findings*			Symptoms, Onset, and Factors
		Pyuria	*Hematuria*	*Urine Culture (cfu/ml)*	
Cystitis	*Escherichia coli*, *Staphylococcus saprophyticus*, *Proteus* species, *Klebsiella* species	Usual	Occasional	10^2 to $\geq 10^5$	Abrupt onset, severe symptoms, multiple symptoms (dysuria, increased frequency, and urgency), suprapubic or low back pain, suprapubic tenderness on examination
Urethritis	*Chlamydia trachomatis*, *Neisseria gonorrhoeae*, herpes simplex virus	Usual	Rare	$< 10^2$	Gradual onset, mild symptoms, vaginal discharge or bleeding (caused by concomitant cervicitis), lower abdominal pain, new sexual partner, cervicitis or vulvovaginal herpetic lesions on examination
Vaginitis	*Candida* species, *Trichomonas vaginalis*	Rare	Rare	$< 10^2$	Vaginal discharge or odor, pruritus, dyspareunia, external dysuria, no increased frequency or urgency, vulvovaginitis on examination

PYELONEPHRITIS

Acute Uncomplicated Infection

The acute onset of fever, shaking chills, nausea, vomiting, and loin pain, with or without symptoms of cystitis, suggests pyelonephritis.[26] Patients typically have a temperature of 102° F (38.9° C) or higher, tachycardia, and costovertebral angle tenderness on deep palpation. Pyuria, white blood cell casts, and significant bacteriuria are usually demonstrable on urine microscopy and Gram stain. Bacteremia may complicate the course of pyelonephritis; but in patients with pyelonephritis, bacteremia is seldom associated with the more serious sequelae of gram-negative infection (i.e., triggering of the complement, clotting, and kinin systems), which may lead to septic shock, disseminated intravascular coagulation, or both. When shock or disseminated intravascular coagulation occurs, the possibility of obstruction must be considered. In a particularly serious form of obstructive uropathy associated with acute papillary necrosis, the sloughed papillae may obstruct the ureter. This form of the disease should be suspected in diabetic patients who have severe pyelonephritis and high-grade bacteremia, particularly if their response to antibiotic therapy is delayed. In some cases of pyelonephritis complicated by diabetes, obstruction, sickle cell disease, analgesic nephropathy, or combinations of these conditions, papillary necrosis may be evident. Emphysematous pyelonephritis, which is a particularly severe form of pyelonephritis associated with production of gas in renal and perinephric tissues, occurs almost entirely in diabetic patients.

Chronic Infection

Although earlier epidemiologic studies suggested that bacteriuria, whether symptomatic or asymptomatic, was associated with increased mortality, more recent findings suggest that bacteriuria does not itself cause an increase in mortality.[27] Rather, bacteriuria appears to be a marker for poor health, particularly in elderly patients. Not surprisingly, then, antimicrobial therapy for asymptomatic bacteriuria in the elderly is of no demonstrable clinical benefit.[28,29]

The relations between recurrent UTI, chronic pyelonephritis, and renal insufficiency have been widely studied. In the absence of anatomic abnormalities, recurrent infection in children and adults does not lead to chronic pyelonephritis or to renal failure. Also, infection does not play a primary role in chronic interstitial nephritis; in this condition, analgesic abuse, obstruction, reflux, and toxic exposure are the primary injurious factors. In the presence of underlying renal abnormalities, infection as a secondary factor can accelerate renal parenchymal damage in experimental and clinical settings. In children, the common combination of reflux, congenital anomalies, and infection appears to lead to significant renal parenchymal damage; moreover, kidneys in growing children appear to be more susceptible to damage than kidneys in adults.

RENAL AND PERIRENAL ABSCESSES

Two unusual forms of UTI are macroscopic renal and perirenal abscesses. In the past, most of these abscesses were secondary to hematogenous infection with *S. aureus.* Today, most of them are secondary to ascending UTI with the usual Enterobacteriaceae organisms. Such infections are often complicated by renal calculi and obstruction of urinary flow from either the kidney or the ureter. Less commonly, preexisting renal cysts become infected and develop into abscesses. In rare instances, there is contiguous spread from a neighboring site of suppuration, such as the colon or overlying rib. The usual presentation of such infections is insidious, with chronic symptoms of fever, weight loss, night sweats, and anorexia, often associated with flank or back pain. When the abscess is under pressure, usually because of obstruction, a more acute presentation with associated bacteremia may occur. Symptoms specific to the urinary tract, such as dysuria, hematuria, and urinary retention, are sometimes noted but are often absent. On physical examination, costovertebral angle tenderness or even a palpable mass may be found; in 30% to 50% of patients, however, the finding is absent.

Routine laboratory tests are of variable value in patients with renal or perirenal abscesses: leukocytosis may be present, anemia is not unusual, and urinalysis may reflect signs of inflammation (e.g., pyuria or proteinuria). In more than half of patients with renal or perirenal abscesses, the organism in the abscess may be isolated on urine culture. Definitive diagnosis, however, depends on radiographic detection of a mass lesion. Gallium and ultrasound scans may be helpful, but computed tomography is considered the diagnostic test of choice.[30] If prompt drainage and antibiotic therapy are not provided, renal or perirenal abscesses may extend to the peritoneal cavity, chest, or skin.

PROSTATITIS

A common complication of UTI in men is prostatitis. Bacterial prostatitis is usually caused by the same gram-negative bacilli that cause UTI in females; 80% or more of such infections are caused by *E. coli.* The pathogenesis of this condition is poorly understood. Antibacterial substances in prostatic secretions probably protect against a higher incidence of such infections. Acute bacterial prostatitis is a febrile illness associated with a number of symptoms: chills, dysuria, urinary frequency and urgency, and perineal, back, or pelvic pain. There may be bladder outlet obstruction. On physical examination, the prostate is found to be enlarged, tender, and indurated. Chronic prostatitis may be more occult and may be manifested only as recurrent bacteriuria or variable low-grade fever with back or pelvic discomfort. Urinary symptoms usually relate to the reintroduction of infection into the bladder; a chronic prostatic focus is the most common cause of recurrent UTI in men.[31]

Diagnostic Guidelines

The correlation between clinical symptoms and the presence of infection is imprecise. It is also frequently difficult to obtain a urine specimen that is uncontaminated by the normal microbial flora of the distal urethra, vagina, or skin. Therefore, the following guidelines are necessary for more accurate evaluation of urine cultures[1,3]:

1. In more than 95% of UTIs, a single bacterial species causes the infection. Thus, whenever mixed bacterial species are grown out on culture, the likelihood of contamination is quite high, and the culture should be repeated. Polymicrobial infection may be present when long-term catheterization is being employed, when the bladder does not completely empty because of neurologic dysfunction, or when a fistulous communication exists between the GI or genital tract and the urinary tract.
2. There is a narrow and predictable spectrum of agents that cause acute uncomplicated cystitis in young women; 80% to 90% of infections are caused by *E. coli,* 5% to 15% are caused by *S. saprophyticus,* and a small percentage are caused by other organisms. *E. coli* is also the predominant pathogen in complicated UTIs, but other gram-negative bacilli, enterococci, and *Candida* species are also frequently found. *S. epidermidis,* diphtheroids, and lactobacilli, on the other hand, are commonly found in the vaginal introitus and distal urethra but seldom cause UTI.
3. The presence of squamous epithelial cells in a urine specimen strongly suggests contamination, and another clean voided specimen should be obtained. Pyuria is highly associated with inflammation of the urinary tract, the most common cause of which is infection.
4. The number of organisms per milliliter of a clean voided urine specimen is a useful indicator of bacterial infection. The growth of 10^5 or

Table 3 Treatment Regimens for Acute Uncomplicated Cystitis[7]

Characteristic Pathogens	*Host Considerations*	*Empirical Treatment Regimens**
Escherichia coli (85%–90%) *Staphylococcus saprophyticus* (5%–15%) Other organisms (< 5%) *Proteus mirabilis* *Klebsiella pneumoniae* *Enterococcus* species	Otherwise healthy woman	3-day regimens: oral trimethoprim-sulfamethoxazole, trimethoprim, fluoroquinolone (ciprofloxacin, gatifloxacin, levofloxacin, ofloxacin, lomefloxacin, temafloxacin), cefixime, or cefpodoxime proxetil† 7-day regimens: nitrofurantoin monohydrate/macrocrystals or nitrofurantoin macrocrystals†
	Male sex, diabetes symptoms for > 7 days, recent antimicrobial use, age > 65 yr	Consider 7-day regimen: oral trimethoprim-sulfamethoxazole, fluoroquinolone, cefixime, or cefpodoxime proxetil†
	Pregnancy	Consider 7-day regimen: oral amoxicillin, nitrofurantoin monohydrate/macrocrystals or nitrofurantoin macrocrystals, cefixime, cefpodoxime proxetil or trimethoprim-sulfamethoxazole†

*Treatments listed are those to be prescribed before the etiologic agent is known (Gram stain can be helpful); they can be modified once the agent has been identified. The recommendations are limited to drugs currently approved by the Food and Drug Administration, although not all the regimens listed are approved for these indications. Optimal empirical regimens may differ among settings because of differences in the antimicrobial susceptibility profiles of uropathogens. Fluoroquinolones should not be used in pregnancy. Although trimethoprim-sulfamethoxazole is classified as pregnancy category C, it is widely used; avoid use of this drug in the third trimester of pregnancy.
†See Table 4.

more colonies of a single bacterial species per milliliter of urine in two consecutive urine cultures is the criterion used to evaluate female patients with asymptomatic bacteriuria.[1] In women with acute dysuria, the presence of at least 10^2 organisms/ml of a single coliform species appears to be a better indication of infection than a finding of 10^5 organisms/ml.[2] In men, the minimal level indicating infection appears to be 10^3 organisms/ml. In general, probably 70% of persons with true bacterial UTI will have more than 10^5 organisms/ml; 30% will have lower concentrations of bacteria.

5. The demonstration of organisms on Gram stain of unspun urine is highly suggestive of significant UTI; however, a negative Gram stain does not rule out infection. The Gram stain has excellent sensitivity for demonstrating bacteriuria when the urine colony count exceeds 10^5 organisms/ml but has poor sensitivity at lower colony counts.

Management

ANTIMICROBIAL THERAPY

In general, antimicrobial therapy is warranted for any symptomatic infection of the urinary tract. The choice of antimicrobial agent, dose, and duration of therapy depends on the site of infection and the presence or absence of complicating conditions. Therefore, each category of UTI merits a different approach on the basis of the particular clinical syndrome that is present.[3,32,33]

Treatment of Women with Acute Uncomplicated Cystitis

Antimicrobial therapy for healthy reproductive-age women with uncomplicated UTI should have the dual objective of eradicating the infection and eliminating uropathogenic clones of bacteria from the vaginal and GI reservoirs to prevent early recurrences. In general, the species and antimicrobial susceptibilities of the bacteria that cause acute uncomplicated cystitis are highly predictable. Thus, in otherwise healthy women presenting with typical symptoms of acute cystitis (dysuria and frequency without signs or symptoms of vaginitis), it is safe and cost-effective to omit the urine culture and use empirical short-course therapy. Three-day therapy seems to be optimal; single-dose therapy results in higher relapse rates (probably because of failure to eradicate the uropathogen from the vaginal reservoir), and 7-day therapy offers no additional benefit but costs more and leads to more side effects. Therapy for 7 days should be considered in women with a history of recent UTI, symptoms of more than 7 days' duration, or diabetes.

There are several effective therapeutic regimens available [*see Tables 3 and 4*]. Traditionally, trimethoprim-sulfamethoxazole has been recommended

Table 4 Oral Regimens for the Treatment of Cystitis

Oral Regimen	*Dosage*
Trimethoprim-sulfamethoxazole	160/800 mg every 12 hr
Trimethoprim	100 mg every 12 hr
Ciprofloxacin	100 to 250 mg every 12 hr
Levofloxacin	250 mg once daily
Ofloxacin	200 mg every 12 hr
Norfloxacin	400 mg every 12 hr
Lomefloxacin	400 mg once daily
Temafloxacin	400 mg once daily
Gatifloxacin	200 mg once daily
Cefixime	400 mg once daily
Cefpodoxime proxetil	100 mg every 12 hr
Nitrofurantoin monohydrate/macrocrystals	100 mg every 12 hr
Nitrofurantoin macrocrystals	50 to 100 mg four times a day
Amoxicillin	250 mg every 8 hr

as the first-line treatment of acute uncomplicated cystitis in women.[34] However, resistance of uropathogens to trimethoprim-sulfamethoxazole is increasing and now approaches 15% to 20% in some communities.[35] In such settings, an alternative first-line agent should be considered for empirical therapy.[36] Many strains of *E. coli* that are resistant to trimethoprim-sulfamethoxazole are also resistant to amoxicillin and cephalexin; thus, these drugs should not be used. Other β-lactams, such as cefixime or cefpodoxime, can be used but are expensive and may be associated with higher relapse rates, probably because they fail to eradicate the uropathogen from the vaginal reservoir. Nitrofurantoin remains highly active against *E. coli* and most non–*E. coli* isolates (except for *Proteus* species, which are intrinsically resistant to the drug); however, 7 days of therapy may be required to achieve reasonable cure rates with this drug. There is accumulating evidence that low doses of fluoroquinolones are effective for short-course therapy of cystitis. In a recent randomized trial, 3-day regimens of ciprofloxacin (100 mg twice daily), trimethoprim-sulfamethoxazole (160/800 mg twice daily), and ofloxacin (200 mg twice daily) were equally effective in the treatment of acute uncomplicated cystitis in women.[37] In separate studies, it was found that 3-day regimens of trimethoprim-sulfamethoxazole and ofloxacin were equally cost-effective.[38,39] Higher costs were associated with 3-day regimens of ampicillin, cefadroxil, and nitrofurantoin because of lower efficacy and higher rates of side effects.[38,39]

If a patient is still symptomatic after therapy, both urinalysis and urine culture are necessary [*see Figure* 2]. If the symptomatic patient has negative results on urinalysis and culture, treatable infection is not present and no antimicrobial therapy is indicated. If the patient is pyuric but not bacteriuric, an alternative diagnosis such as chlamydial, gonococcal, or herpetic infection should be considered. If the patient is both pyuric and bacteriuric, the antimicrobial susceptibility of the infecting strain should be assessed for resistance and an alternative agent should be given. Finally, a patient who is symptomatic after a short-course regimen and has persistent infection with a uropathogen that is sensitive to the antibiotic used should be regarded as having covert renal infection. In this circumstance, a 14-day course of a fluoroquinolone or trimethoprim-sulfamethoxazole is indicated.[8]

The antimicrobial approach for older women with symptomatic cystitis is similar to that for younger women—namely, short-course therapy with trimethoprim-sulfamethoxazole or a fluoroquinolone initially; longer courses of therapy should be reserved for patients who do not respond to short-course therapy. In a randomized clinical trial of the treatment of acute cystitis in postmenopausal women, 3-day therapy with ofloxacin was more cost-effective than 7-day therapy with cephalexin.[40] The major difference in the management

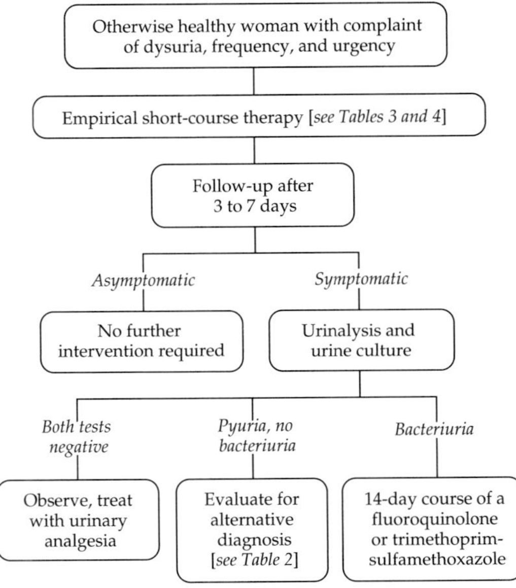

Figure 2 **Clinical approach to the woman with acute uncomplicated cystitis.**

of older women with UTI is the recognition that topical or systemic estrogen replacement can markedly decrease the incidence of recurrent UTI in postmenopausal women.[16]

Treatment of recurrent UTI Recurrence of uncomplicated cystitis in reproductive-age women is common, and some form of preventive strategy is indicated if three or more symptomatic episodes occur in 1 year. A variety of antimicrobial strategies are available, but before embarking on one of them, the patient should try such simple interventions as voiding immediately after sexual intercourse and using a contraceptive method other than a diaphragm and spermicide. Ingestion of cranberry juice has been shown to be effective in decreasing both bacteriuria and pyuria in an elderly population and in decreasing the rate of recurrent UTI in younger women when combined with lingonberry.[41,42] This effect appears to be independent of any urinary acidification; rather, it is postulated that cranberry juice contains substances that inhibit the attachment of bacterial adhesins to the uroepithelium.[43]

If simple nondrug measures are ineffective, continuous or postcoital (if the infections are temporally related to intercourse) low-dose antimicrobial prophylaxis with one of several regimens should be considered. A single dose of trimethoprim-sulfamethoxazole (one half of a single-strength tablet containing 40 mg of trimethoprim and 200 mg of sulfamethoxazole), a fluoroquinolone (one tablet), or nitrofurantoin (50 mg; or 100 mg of nitrofurantoin macrocrystals) can safely and effectively decrease the rate of recurrent infections.[44] Typically, a prophylactic regimen is initially prescribed for 6 months and then discontinued. If the infections recur, the prophylactic program can be instituted for a longer period. Antimicrobial prophylaxis has been effectively used for as long as 5 years in preventing recurrence of infection.[9] An alternative approach to antimicrobial prophylaxis for women with less frequent recurrences (fewer than four recurrences a year) is to provide a supply of trimethoprim-sulfamethoxazole or fluoroquinolone to the patient and allow her to self-medicate with short-course therapy at the first symptoms of infection. The patient is directed to keep track of the number of such episodes and to contact the physician if more than four episodes occur over a 12-month period or if symptoms persist on such therapy. This approach has been shown to be safe and effective in two separate studies of women with recurrent UTI.[45,46]

Treatment of relapsing infection The approach to the minority of patients with relapsing infection, as evidenced by the recurrence of the same strain of UTI within 2 weeks of completion of antimicrobial therapy, is very different. Two factors may contribute to the pathogenesis of relapsing infection in women: deep tissue infection of the kidney that is suppressed but not eradicated by a 14-day course of antibiotics, and a structural abnormality of the urinary tract, particularly calculi. Patients with true relapsing UTIs should undergo radiologic or urologic evaluation and should be considered for longer-term therapy.

Acute Uncomplicated Pyelonephritis

Patients with clear-cut symptomatic pyelonephritis have deep tissue infection, have or are at risk for bacteremia, and merit intensive antimicrobial therapy. The therapeutic regimen for these patients has two components: (1) the immediate delivery to the bloodstream and urinary tract (often with parenteral therapy) of effective concentrations of an antimicrobial agent to which the invading organism is susceptible and (2) the completion of the therapy, aimed at eradicating residual infection in the tissues, with an oral regimen.

Initial antimicrobial programs to obtain control of systemic sepsis are prescribed so that the infecting organism has at least a 99% probability of being sensitive to the chosen regimen and so that adequate blood levels of the drug or drugs can be quickly achieved in the patient. At present, there is no evidence to suggest that, provided the two requirements are fulfilled, any particular antibiotic program is inherently superior to another for control of systemic sepsis. Similarly, the merits of I.V. therapy stem from the reliability of drug delivery rather than from any inherent desirability of I.V. drugs. In patients with milder disease who are free of nausea and vomiting, advantage can be taken of the excellent antimicrobial spectrum and bioavailability (and the easy achievement of high blood levels, provided the GI tract is functioning adequately) of such drugs as trimethoprim-sulfamethoxazole and the fluoroquinolones by prescribing oral administration for the entire therapeutic course.[8] A recent randomized clinical trial demonstrated that 7 days of therapy with oral ciprofloxacin was highly effective for the initial management of pyelonephritis in the outpatient setting.[47]

When parenteral therapy is required, various regimens can be used, such as ampicillin plus gentamicin, parenteral trimethoprim-sulfamethoxazole or fluoroquinolones, or the third-generation cephalosporins (e.g., ceftriaxone). β-Lactam–β-lactamase inhibitor combinations (ampicillin-sulbactam, ticarcillin-clavulanate, and piperacillin-tazobactam) or imipenem-cilastatin can be used in patients with more complicated histories, previous episodes of pyelonephritis, or recent urinary tract manipulations. After the patient has been afebrile for 24 hours (usually within 72 hours of initiating therapy), there is no benefit in maintaining parenteral therapy. Currently, prescription of oral trimethoprim-sulfamethoxazole or a fluoroquinolone to complete a 14-day course of therapy appears to be the most effective means of eradicating both tissue infection and residual clones of uropathogens present in the GI tract that could cause early recurrence if left in place.[3]

Treatment during Pregnancy

There are three major differences between the approach to UTI in pregnant women and that in nonpregnant women. First, in pregnant women, asymptomatic bacteriuria is actively sought and is as aggressively treated and followed as symptomatic infection; this is clearly not the case in nonpregnant women, for whom screening for asymptomatic bacteriuria is not recommended. Second, although short-course therapy is also the cornerstone of treatment during pregnancy for patients with uncomplicated cystitis (as well as asymptomatic bacteriuria), the drugs that can be safely used are far more limited for pregnant women. Third, follow-up of patients with bacteriuria during pregnancy is more intense, with a more rapid deployment of prophylactic strategies in pregnant women with recurrent bacteriuria.[12,48]

Sulfonamides, nitrofurantoin, ampicillin, and the cephalosporins have been considered relatively safe in early pregnancy, with sulfonamides avoided near term because of a possible role in the development of kernicterus. Trimethoprim is usually avoided because of evidence of fetal toxicity at high doses in animals, although it has been used successfully in humans during pregnancy without evidence of toxicity or teratogenicity. Fluoroquinolones are avoided because of possible adverse effects on fetal cartilage development. Nitrofurantoin, ampicillin, and the cephalosporins have been used most extensively in pregnancy and are the regimens of choice for the treatment of asymptomatic or minimally symptomatic UTI [*see Tables 3 and 4*]. For pregnant women with overt pyelonephritis, admission to the hospital for parenteral therapy should be the standard of care; β-lactams with or without aminoglycosides are the cornerstone of therapy.[12,49]

Effective prevention of UTI, including pyelonephritis, can be accomplished during pregnancy with nitrofurantoin or cephalexin taken prophylactically after coitus or at bedtime without relation to coitus. Those who should be considered for such prophylaxis during pregnancy are patients who have had acute pyelonephritis during pregnancy, patients with bacteriuria during pregnancy who have had a recurrence after a course of treatment, and patients who had recurrent UTI before pregnancy that required prophylaxis.[50,51]

Treatment of Men with UTI

As previously noted, it is uncommon for men to have UTI that is analogous to acute uncomplicated cystitis in women. When it does occur, men should never be treated with short-course therapy because of a high rate of early relapse. Instead, 7- to 14-day regimens of trimethoprim-sulfamethoxazole or a fluoroquinolone should be prescribed.[52]

In men older than 50 years with UTI, tissue invasion of the prostate and possibly the kidneys should be considered, even in the absence of overt signs of infection at these sites. Acute bacterial prostatitis should be treated with trimethoprim-sulfamethoxazole for at least 4 weeks or a fluoroquinolone for 2 weeks. However, relapse is common. Recurrent infection in men usually connotes a sustained focus in the prostate that has not been eradicated by previous courses of therapy. Several factors make eradication of prostatic foci difficult. Many antimicrobial agents do not diffuse well across the prostatic epithelium into the prostatic fluid, where the infection lies. The prostate may harbor calculi, which can block drainage of portions of the prostate gland or act as foreign bodies in which persistent infection can reside. An enlarged (and inflamed) prostate gland can cause bladder outlet obstruction, resulting in pools of stagnant urine in the bladder that are difficult to sterilize.[52]

As a result of these factors, intensive therapy for at least 4 to 6 weeks is recommended for chronic bacterial prostatitis. The drugs of choice for this purpose, assuming the invading organisms are susceptible, are the fluoroquinolones. The best alternative agent is trimethoprim-sulfamethoxazole. Prolonged treatment with any of these drugs has a greater than 60% probability of eradicating infection. Most of the failures result from either the anatomic factors listed above or infection by *E. faecalis* or *P. aeruginosa;* these two organisms cause a particularly high rate of relapse after treatment with the antimicrobial agents currently recommended. Relapses should be treated for 12 weeks. If this therapy fails, a choice has to be made among three therapeutic approaches: long-term antimicrobial suppression, repeated treatment courses for each relapse, or surgical removal of the infected prostate gland under coverage of systemic antimicrobial therapy. The approach chosen depends on the patient's age, sexual activity, general condition, and degree of bladder outlet obstruction.[52]

Complicated UTI

Complicated UTI occurs in a heterogeneous group of patients with a wide variety of structural and functional abnormalities of the urinary tract and kidney. The range of antimicrobial species and their susceptibility to antimicrobial agents is likewise heterogeneous. As a consequence, therapy for patients with complicated UTI requires individualization, although the following guidelines appear to be useful[3]:

1. As a general rule, only symptomatic UTI requires therapy. The major exceptions arise when asymptomatic bacteriuria occurs in the setting of pregnancy, neutropenia, or renal transplantation. Asymptomatic bacteriuria in a patient who is scheduled for instrumentation of the urinary tract should also be treated. In this instance, sterilization of the urine before manipulation and continuation of antimicrobial therapy for 3 to 7 days after manipulation can prevent life-threatening urosepsis.
2. If the antimicrobial susceptibilities of the infecting organism are not known and symptomatic infection requires immediate therapy, broad-spectrum regimens such as ampicillin plus gentamicin, imipenem-cilastatin, and piperacillin-tazobactam should be considered until the susceptibilities of the invading organism are known. In patients with subacute infection, a fluoroquinolone or trimethoprim-sulfamethoxazole is an appropriate alternative.
3. Whenever possible, every effort should be made to correct the underlying complicating factor in conjunction with the antimicrobial therapy.

RADIOLOGIC EVALUATION TO RULE OUT FUNCTIONAL ABNORMALITIES

A final consideration in the management of UTI is the role of radiologic evaluation. To rule out obstruction, intravenous pyelography, ultrasonography, or CT should be carried out expeditiously in any patient with acute pyelonephritis who does not respond to an effective antimicrobial agent and in any patient in whom a persistent bacteremia has been demonstrated. Contrast-enhanced helical CT is the radiologic study of choice for imaging and evaluation of renal infections. Noncontrast images should be obtained when renal calculi are suspected.[30]

For ambulatory patients who have UTI, guidelines are less clear. Radiographic evaluation, usually intravenous pyelography and voiding cystourethrography, is carried out for delineation of surgically correctable lesions that might predispose patients to recurrent infection or progressive renal disease. Because congenital anatomic anomalies are particularly prevalent in young children who have a first or second UTI, such studies are obligatory for patients in this age group. In addition, careful prostatic examination and assessment of postvoiding residual urine volume should be considered in males with UTI at any stage of life because such infection is highly unlikely in this population unless anatomic anomalies are present.[53] In women with uncomplicated UTI, the incidence of correctable anatomic lesions is so low that radiologic and urologic evaluation should be restricted to patients who have rapid recurrence of infection or recurrent pyelonephritis despite having undergone adequate therapy.[5,54]

Catheter-Associated UTI

The most common nosocomial infections (representing 40% of all nosocomial infections) are UTIs. Nosocomial UTIs are associated with a threefold increase in mortality. Such infections caused by *Serratia marcescens* are a particular problem: 16% result in bacteremia, an incidence four times higher than that seen with other nosocomial uropathogens.[55] The occurrence of nosocomial diarrhea while a catheter is in place is a risk factor for the development of UTI.[56]

Most nosocomial UTIs are related to bladder catheterization.[55,57] Several guidelines can be followed to minimize the occurrence of catheter-related infection [*see Table 5*]. Most important, the catheter should be inserted with strict aseptic technique by trained persons. In addition, a closed system should be used at all times. Even with optimal care, however, long-term catheter use will eventually result in bladder infection. Apparently, little additional protection is provided by antibiotic rinses for the bladder, antibiotic ointments applied to the urethral meatus, and

Table 5 Guidelines for Bladder Catheter Care

Use catheters only when absolutely necessary; remove as soon as possible.

Insert catheters aseptically and maintain by trained personnel only; the use of catheter teams is preferable.

A sterile closed drainage system is mandatory. The catheter and drainage tube must never be disconnected except when irrigation is necessary to relieve obstruction. Strict aseptic technique is employed under these circumstances.

Obtain urine for culture by aspirating the catheter with a 21-gauge needle after the catheter is prepared with povidone-iodine.

Maintain downhill, nonobstructed flow, with the collection bag always below the level of the bladder and emptied at frequent intervals.

Replace indwelling catheters when obstruction or concretions are demonstrated.

Separate catheterized patients from each other whenever possible; in particular, a patient with a sterile bladder catheter system should always be kept separate from a patient with infected urine, and strict hand-washing precautions should be observed by staff caring for these patients.

Obtain postcatheterization urine for culture.

Administer prophylactic antibiotics during catheter insertion and removal to patients with cardiac disease (particularly prosthetic valves) that predisposes to bacterial endocarditis.

instillation of disinfectants such as hydrogen peroxide into the urinary collection bag. Although systemic antibiotics are of no value when the closed system is to be in place for an extended period, antibiotics may be protective when the catheter is in place for only a few days.[55,57] However, this advantage should be balanced against the risk of selecting for resistant flora if catheterization must be prolonged unexpectedly. In women not receiving antibiotics, use of a silver oxide–coated urinary catheter may offer some protection against infection.[58] In a recent randomized study of hospitalized patients, use of a silver-coated urinary catheter resulted in a lower rate of UTIs and a significant cost savings.[59] A nitrofurazone-impregnated catheter also has been shown to decrease the incidence of UTIs caused by gram-negative organisms.[60]

Treatment of catheter-associated UTI requires good clinical judgment. If a patient is symptomatic (exhibiting, for example, fever, chills, dyspnea, and hypotension), immediate antibiotic therapy is indicated [*see* Management, *above*]. When therapy is given, it may be useful to also remove and replace the urinary catheter if it has been in place for a week or longer. This eliminates difficult-to-eradicate organisms in the biofilm on the catheter. In an asymptomatic patient, therapy should be postponed until the catheter can be removed. Patients with persistent asymptomatic bacteriuria and those with lower urinary tract symptoms who have had the catheter removed respond well to short-course therapy.[61] Patients with long-term indwelling catheters seldom become symptomatic unless the catheter is obstructed or is eroding through the bladder mucosa. In patients who do become symptomatic, appropriate antibiotics should be administered, and close attention should be directed to either changing the catheter or changing the type of urinary drainage by substitution of a suprapubic tube. Therapy for asymptomatic catheterized patients leads to the selection of increasingly antibiotic-resistant bacteria.[55,57] Thus, although long-term bladder catheterization carries a significant risk of chronic pyelonephritis (10% or more if the catheter is in place for more than 90 days), there is no method for avoiding this event other than catheter removal.[62]

Kalpana Gupta, M.D., M.P.H., has received grant or research support from Bayer Corp. and Procter & Gamble Pharmaceuticals, Inc.; is a consultant for Bayer Corp.; and has received speaking honoraria from Bayer Corp.

Walter E. Stamm, M.D., has received grant or research support from Procter & Gamble Pharmaceuticals, Inc., Medimmune, Inc., and Ortho-McNeil Pharmaceutical, Inc., and is a consultant for Ortho-McNeil Pharmaceutical, Inc.

Acknowledgment

Figure 1 Seward Hung.

References

1. Kunin CM: Urinary tract infections in females. Clin Infect Dis 18:1, 1994

2. Hooton TM, Scholes D, Hughes J, et al: A prospective study of risk factors for symptomatic urinary tract infection in young women. N Engl J Med 335:468, 1996

3. Stamm WE, Hooton TM: Management of urinary tract infections in adults. N Engl J Med 329:1328, 1993

4. To T, Agha M, Dick PT, et al: Cohort study on circumcision of newborn boys and subsequent risk of urinary-tract infection. Lancet 352:1813, 1998

5. Spach DH, Stapleton AE, Stamm WE: Lack of circumcision increases the risk of urinary tract infection in young men. JAMA 267:679, 1992

6. Hoepelman AI, van Buren M, van den Broek J, et al: Bacteriuria in men infected with HIV-1 is related to their immune status (CD4+ cell count). AIDS 6:179, 1992

7. Foxman B, Gillespie B, Koopman J, et al: Risk factors for second urinary tract infection among college women. Am J Epidemiol 151 1194, 2000

8. Hooton TM, Stamm WE: Diagnosis and treatment of uncomplicated urinary tract infection. Infect Dis Clin North Am 11:551, 1997

9. Stamm WE, McKevitt M, Roberts PL, et al: Natural history of recurrent urinary tract infections in women. Rev Infect Dis 13:77, 1991

10. Scholes D, Hooton TM, Roberts PL, et al: Risk factors for recurrent urinary tract infection in young women. J Infect Dis 182:1177, 2000

11. Hooton TM, Scholes D, Stapleton AE, et al: A prospective study of asymptomatic bacteriuria in sexually active young women. N Engl J Med 343:992, 2000

12. Patterson TF, Andriole VT: Detection, significance, and therapy of bacteriuria in pregnancy: update in the managed health care era. Infect Dis Clin North Am 11:593, 1997

13. Patterson JE, Andriole VT: Bacterial urinary tract infections in diabetes. Infect Dis Clin North Am 11:735, 1997

14. Geerlings SE, Brouwer EC, Van Kessel KC, et al: Cytokine secretion is impaired in women with diabetes mellitus. Eur J Clin Invest 30: 995, 2000

15. Hooton TM, Roberts PL, Stamm WE: Effects of recent sexual activity and use of a diaphragm on the vaginal microflora. Clin Infect Dis 19:274, 1994

16. Raz R, Stamm WE: A controlled trial of intravaginal estriol in postmenopausal women with recurrent urinary tract infections. N Engl J Med 329:753, 1993

17. Stapleton A: Prevention of recurrent urinary tract infection in women. Lancet 353:7, 1999

18. Stapleton A, Hooton TM, Fennell C, et al: Effect of secretor status on vaginal and rectal colonization with fimbriated *Escherichia coli* in women with and without recurrent urinary tract infection. J Infect Dis 171:717, 1995

19. Mulvey MA, Schilling JD, Martinez JJ, et al: Bad bugs and beleagured bladders: interplay between uropathogenic *Escherichia coli* and innate host defenses. Proc Natl Acad Sci USA 97:8829, 2000

20. Johnson JR: Virulence factors in *Escherichia coli* urinary tract infection. Clin Microbiol Rev 4:80, 1991

21. Otto G, Sandberg T, Marklund BI, et al: Virulence factors and pap genotype in *Escherichia coli* isolates from women with acute pyelonephritis, with or without bacteremia. Clin Infect Dis 17:448, 1993

22. Garin EH, Campos A, Homsy Y: Primary vesicoureteral reflux: review of current concepts. Pediatr Nephrol 12:249, 1998

23. Ikaheimo R, Siitonen A, Karkkainen U, et al: Virulence characteristics of *Escherichia coli* in nosocomial urinary tract infection. Clin Infect Dis 16:785, 1993

24. Ulleryd P, Lincoln K, Scheutz F, et al: Virulence characteristics of *Escherichia coli* in relation to host response in men with symptomatic urinary tract infection. Clin Infect Dis 18:579, 1994

25. Ross JH, Kay R: Pediatric urinary tract infection and reflux. Am Fam Physician 15:1472, 1999

26. Pinson AG, Philbrick JT, Lindbeck GH: Fever in the clinical diagnosis of acute pyelonephritis. Am J Emerg Med 15:148, 1997

27. Bengtsson C, Bengtsson U, Bjorkelund C, et al: Bacteriuria in a population sample of women: 24-year follow-up study: results from the prospective population-based study of women in Gothenburg, Sweden. Scand J Urol Nephrol 32:284, 1998

28. Abrutyn E, Mossey J, Berlin JA, et al: Does asymptomatic bacteriuria predict mortality and does antimicrobial treatment reduce mortality in elderly ambulatory women? Ann Intern Med 120:827, 1994

29. Abrutyn E, Berlin J, Mossey J, et al: Does treatment of asymptomatic bacteriuria in older ambulatory women reduce subsequent symptoms of urinary tract infection? J Am Geriatr Soc 44:293, 1996

30. Kaplan DM, Rosenfield AT, Smith RC: Advances in the imaging of renal infection: helical CT and modern coordinated imaging. Infect Dis Clin North Am 11:681, 1997

31. Lipsky BA: Urinary tract infections in men: epidemiology, pathophysiology, diagnosis, and treatment. Ann Intern Med 110:138, 1989

32. Warren JW, Abrutyn E, Hebel JR, et al: Guidelines for antimicrobial treatment of uncomplicated acute bacterial cystitis and acute pyelonephritis in women. Infectious Diseases Society of America (IDSA). Clin Infect Dis 29:745, 1999

33. Saint S, Scholes D, Fihn SD, et al: The effectiveness of a clinical practice guideline for the management of presumed uncomplicated urinary tract infection in women. Am J Med 106:636, 1999

34. Huang ES, Stafford RS: National patterns in the treatment of urinary tract infections in women by ambulatory care physicians. Arch Intern Med 162:41, 2002

35. Manges AR, Johnson JR, Foxman B, et al: Widespread distribution of urinary tract infections caused by a multidrug-resistant *Escherichia coli* clonal group. N Engl J Med 345:1007, 2001

36. Gupta K, Hooton TM, Stamm WE: Increasing antimicrobial resistance and the management of uncomplicated community-acquired urinary tract infections. Ann Intern Med 135:41, 2001

37. McCarty JM, Richard G, Huck W, et al: A randomized trial of short-course ciprofloxacin, ofloxacin, or trimethoprim-sulfamethoxazole for the treatment of acute urinary tract infection in women. Am J Med 106:292, 1999

38. Hooton TM, Johnson C, Winter C, et al: Single-dose and three-day regimens of ofloxacin versus trimethoprim-sulfamethoxazole for acute cystitis in women. Antimicrob Agents Chemother 35:1479, 1991

39. Hooton TM, Winter C, Tiu F, et al: Randomized comparative trial and cost analysis of 3-day antimicrobial regimens for treatment of acute cystitis in women. JAMA 273:41, 1995

40. Raz R, Rozenfeld S: 3-day course of ofloxacin versus cephalexin in the treatment of urinary tract infections in postmenopausal women. Antimicrob Agents Chemother 40:2200, 1996

41. Avorn J, Monane M, Gurwitz JH, et al: Reduction of bacteriuria and pyuria after ingestion of cranberry juice. JAMA 271:751, 1994

42. Kontiokari T, Sundqvist K, Nuutinen M, et al: Randomised trial of cranberry-lingonberry juice and *Lactobacillus* GG drink for the prevention of urinary tract infections in women. BMJ 322:1571, 2001

43. Howell AB, Vorsa N, Der Marderosian A, et al: Inhibition of the adherence of *Escherichia coli* to uroepithelial-cell surfaces by proanthocyanidin extracts from cranberries. N Engl J Med 339:1085, 1998

44. Stapleton A, Latham RH, Johnson C, et al: Postcoital antimicrobial prophylaxis for recurrent urinary tract infection: a randomized, double-blind, placebo-controlled trial. JAMA 264:703, 1990

45. Gupta K, Hooton TM, Roberts PL, et al: Patient-initiated treatment of uncomplicated recurrent urinary tract infections in young women. Ann Intern Med 135:9, 2001

46. Schaeffer AJ, Stuppy BA: Efficacy and safety of self-start therapy in women with recurrent urinary tract infections. J Urol 161:207, 1999

47. Talan DA, Stamm WE, Hooton TM, et al: Comparison of ciprofloxacin (7 days) and trimethoprim-sulfamethoxazole (14 days) for acute uncomplicated pyelonephritis in women: a randomized trial. JAMA 283:1583, 2000

48. Rouse DJ, Andrews WW, Goldenberg RL, et al: Screening and treatment of asymptomatic bacteriuria of pregnancy to prevent pyelonephritis: a cost-effectiveness and cost-benefit analysis. Obstet Gynecol 86:119, 1995

49. Wing DA, Hendershott CM, Debuque L, et al: A randomized trial of three antibiotic regimens for the treatment of pyelonephritis in pregnancy. Obstet Gynecol 92:249, 1998

50. Pfau A, Sacks TG: Effective prophylaxis for recurrent urinary tract infections during pregnancy. Clin Infect Dis 14:810, 1992

51. Sandberg T, Brorson JE: Efficacy of long-term antimicrobial prophylaxis after acute pyelonephritis in pregnancy. Scand J Infect Dis 23: 221, 1991

52. Lipsky BA: Prostatitis and urinary tract infection in men: what's new; what's true? Am J Med 106:327, 1999

53. Andrews SJ, Brooks PT, Hanbury DC, et al: Ultrasonography and abdominal radiography versus intravenous urography in investigation of urinary tract infection in men: prospective incident cohort study. BMJ 324:454, 2002

54. Fowler JE Jr, Pulaski ET: Excretory urography, cystography, and cystoscopy in the evaluation of women with urinary-tract infection: a prospective study. N Engl J Med 304:462, 1981

55. Warren JW: Catheter-associated urinary tract infections. Infect Dis Clin North Am 11:609, 1997

56. Lima NL, Guerrant RL, Kaiser DL, et al: A retrospective cohort study of nosocomial diarrhea as a risk factor for nosocomial infection. J Infect Dis 161:948, 1990

57. Saint S, Veenstra DL, Sullivan SD, et al: The potential clinical and economic benefits of silver alloy urinary catheters in preventing urinary tract infection. Arch Intern Med 160:2670, 2000

58. Johnson JR, Roberts PL, Olsen RJ, et al: Prevention of catheter-associated urinary tract infection with a silver oxide–coated urinary catheter: clinical and microbiologic correlates. J Infect Dis 162:1145, 1990

59. Karchmer TB, Giannetta ET, Muto CA, et al: A randomized crossover study of silver-coated urinary catheters in hospitalized patients. Arch Intern Med 160:3294, 2000

60. Tambyah PA, Halvorson KT, Maki DG: A prospective study of pathogenesis of catheter-associated urinary tract infections. Mayo Clin Proc 74:131, 1999

61. Harding GM, Nicolle L, Ronald AR, et al: How long should catheter-acquired urinary tract infection in women be treated? A randomized controlled study. Ann Intern Med 114:713, 1991

62. Warren JW, Muncie HL Jr, Hebel JR, et al: Long-term urethral catheterization increases risk of chronic pyelonephritis and renal inflammation. J Am Geriatr Soc 42:1286, 1994

10 Sexually Transmitted Diseases

Matthew R. Golden, M.D., M.P.H.

Sexually transmitted diseases (STDs) are among the most common causes of infectious illness in the world. The United States leads industrialized nations in the occurrence of STDs, with an estimated 12 million new cases annually, three million of them in teenagers.[1] The situation in much of the developing world is direr still. In many developing nations, STDs (excluding HIV infection) are the second greatest cause of disability-adjusted years of life lost,[2] and highly prevalent bacterial and viral STDs are thought to play an important role in facilitating HIV transmission.[3]

STD is an emerging infectious disease problem. Of the more than 30 sexually transmitted pathogens that are currently recognized, eight have been identified since 1980, and it seems likely that the full spectrum of STD remains undefined.[4] Antimicrobial resistance has made treatment of some well-established infections (e.g., gonorrhea) more difficult. Finally, decreasing age of menarche, declining median age of populations in developing countries, delayed marriage, increased global travel and trade, urbanization, migration, war and associated social upheaval, and the dissolution of socially restrictive political systems in the former Soviet Union and, to a lesser extent, China all ensure that STDs will remain a major and probably increasing health problem in coming decades.[5]

For the clinician, the increasing recognition of viral STDs and the emergence of screening for chlamydial infections as a population-based STD control strategy has heightened the importance of familiarity with the management of these common infections. This subsection presents general concepts in the epidemiology and approach to patients with STD and reviews important STD syndromes, including urethritis, vulvovaginitis, mucopurulent cervicitis, pelvic inflammatory disease, and genital ulcer disease. Finally, the approach to STD in men who have sex with men and to sexually transmitted enteric infections will be presented. Specific pathogens, including *Chlamydia*, *Neisseria gonorrhoeae*, herpes viruses, and *Treponema pallidum*, are discussed in other subsections. The Centers for Disease Control and Prevention (CDC) issues guidelines for STD/HIV testing and counseling, as well as STD treatment (http://www.cdc.gov/hiv/dhap.htm). Clinicians are advised to refer to these guidelines for updated recommendations.[6–8]

Epidemiology and Transmission Dynamics

The transmission of an STD through a population can be conceptualized mathematically with the formula $R_0 = \beta c D$, in which R_0 is the average number of secondary cases generated by each primary infection in a population (i.e., the reproductive number); β is the average probability of transmission with each sexual contact; c is the average number of sexual partnerships formed per unit of time; and D is the mean duration of infection.[9] For diseases in which each case generates an average of one additional case, R_0 equals 1 and the prevalence remains stable; values less than 1 and greater than 1 are associated with a declining or rising prevalence, respectively.

Although each of the terms in this equation is complex, the simplification that the equation offers can explain a great deal about the distribution of different STDs in a population and provides a framework for conceptualizing STD epidemiology. For example, gonorrhea is thought to be efficiently transmitted ($\beta = 0.5$), but it has a relatively short duration of infection, especially in settings in which medical care and therapy are readily available.[9,10] Consequently, for the reproductive number to remain 1 or greater, c must be relatively high. Thus, infection tends to concentrate in a population of highly sexually active persons, sometimes referred to as a core group.[11] In part because young people tend to be more sexually active than older people, the incidence of gonorrhea, like that of chlamydial infection, is highest among teenagers and persons in their early 20s. (This is less true of men who have sex with men, in whom gonorrhea incidence is less concentrated in the young.) In contrast, herpes simplex virus type 2 (HSV-2) has a very long duration of infection, and R_0 may exceed 1 even in populations with very low rates of partnership change. As a result, the prevalence of genital herpes rises with age, peak incidence likely occurs at a somewhat older age than with *Chlamydia* infection or gonorrhea, and the infection is widely disseminated throughout the population.[12]

This simple model of STD transmission dynamics focuses on average behavior in a population and the host-parasite relationship as determinants of STD epidemiology. However, it neglects the critical role played by variance in sexual behavior and patterns of sexual mixing (i.e., sexual networks) in defining transmission dynamics. The prevalence of STD in a population is in part a function of the extent to which persons who are more sexually active mix primarily with one another (assortative mixing) versus mixing in a more random way with others, including persons who are less sexually active.[13] The frequency of concurrent multiple partnerships in a population also exerts a profound influence on STD prevalence; such partnerships act as bridges, allowing infections to spread in two directions, connecting groups of people and facilitating rapid transmission of infection.[14,15]

Recognition of the role that sexual networks play in STD epidemiology should inform clinicians' thinking about STD risk. In eliciting a sexual history, clinicians have traditionally focused on the patient's behavior, asking about the number of sexual partners the patient has had and about the use of condoms. In many cases, however, self-reported behavior is not associated with risk of STD; sexual network factors may be more important in defining risk. For example, virtually all studies of selective screening for chlamydial infection have found that self-reported behavior is an insensitive predictor of infection,[16–18] whereas demographic factors such as age, race, socioeconomic status, source of clinical care, and geography are strongly associated with a variety of STDs.[19–21] These factors, which reflect the organization of human society and dictate sexual mixing patterns, play a critical role in defining an individual's risk of infection.[22] STDs exist within a social context; therefore, clinicians should base their assessment of risk on their practice setting and the patient's social milieu. Persons whose behavior would suggest a low risk of STD can in fact be at elevated risk simply by virtue of their sexual network, a population that is often socially determined rather than individually chosen. This knowledge should temper any tendency to entertain stigmatizing stereotypes related to sexual behavior and STD.

STD Prevention

SEXUAL HISTORY AND COUNSELING

What is the best way to elicit a sexual history? Although relatively little research has been done on this question, some general principles can be articulated. In eliciting a sexual history, the clinician must balance the need to collect specific information with the desire to engage the patient in a conversation about sexual risk. Whenever possible, questions should be open ended, allowing the patient to define factors that may have placed him or her at risk for STD (e.g., "What are you doing now, or what have you done in the past, that you think may have put you at risk for a sexually transmitted disease?"). Subsequent questions may be more specific, but the questions should be clear, direct, and phrased nonjudgmentally (e.g., "Do you have sex with men, women, or both men and women?"). Typically, a sexual history should include questions about sexual orientation, the number of sexual partners, the use of condoms, any history of STD, and the sexual repertoire (oral, insertive or receptive anal, and vaginal sex). Persons with HIV or those at high risk for HIV should be asked if they know the HIV status of their sexual partners. Persons with HIV should be asked whether they have informed their partners of their own HIV status.

Clinicians should seek to integrate elicitation of the sexual history with STD prevention counseling. The CDC recommends a client-centered approach to counseling. This approach involves an effort to help patients assess the circumstances and behaviors that place them at risk for STD and then help them commit to a single, defined plan for reducing their risk. Risk-reduction plans should be specific rather than general. For example, a specific goal might be to carry condoms when going out on a date or to ask a specific partner about his or her HIV status, rather than the general goals of using condoms all the time or having safe sex all the time.[23] Client-centered counseling has been shown (in a randomized trial of heterosexual STD clinic patients) to reduce the risk of STDs.[6,24]

STD REPORTING AND SEXUAL PARTNER MANAGEMENT

By law, gonorrhea, syphilis, chancroid, lymphogranuloma venereum (LGV), donovanosis (granuloma inguinale), and, in most parts of the

United States, chlamydial infections must be reported to local health departments. In general, health departments in the United States routinely attempt to ensure the treatment of sexual partners of persons with syphilis; they only sometimes attempt to contact persons reported to have HIV to offer them assistance in notifying their sexual and needle-sharing partners; and they seldom make any routine effort to notify the partners of persons with gonorrhea or chlamydial infection. Some health departments will provide such services if specifically asked to do so by a clinician or a person diagnosed with an STD. Although clinicians should make their patients aware that they may be contacted by public health authorities regarding partner notification, in most instances, it is the responsibility of the diagnosing clinician and the patient to ensure that sexual partners are evaluated and treated. Several recent studies have suggested that giving patients medication to give to their sexual partners is feasible and may reduce chlamydial reinfection rates.[25–27] However, at present, there are no guidelines that define the circumstances in which this approach to partner management should be employed.

STD SCREENING

Because STDs are often asymptomatic, screening is a critical component of prevention. Recommendations for screening vary according to population [*see Table 1*].[8] Data in support of STD screening are strongest for chlamydial infection; a randomized trial has demonstrated that chlamydial screening reduces the rate of PID.[28]

Table 1 Recommended STD Screening[8]

Population	*Screening Measures*
All men and women	Retest all patients diagnosed with gonorrhea or *Chlamydia* infection 10–18 wk after initial treatment
Women Sexually active, age ≤ 24 yr Age > 24 yr with a new sexual partner or multiple sexual partners	Annual chlamydial screening
Pregnant woman	Test for *Chlamydia trachomatis, Neisseria gonorrhoeae,* hepatitis B virus infection, and syphilis; offer HIV testing and counseling Test for bacterial vaginosis in women at high risk (e.g., those with history of preterm delivery) Perform Pap smear if none was performed in the past year
Men who have sex with men (MSM)*	Perform the following at least annually: Serologic testing for HIV and syphilis Rectal culture for gonorrhea and chlamydial infection Pharyngeal culture for gonorrhea Consider serologic testing for HSV-2, particularly in HIV-negative MSM Serologic testing for hepatitis A and B antibodies†

*Screening guidelines apply to both HIV-positive and HIV-negative MSM. HIV and hepatitis testing should be performed only for susceptible patients. Current data are insufficient for a recommendation of technologies other than culture to test for rectal gonorrhea or chlamydial infection or pharyngeal gonorrhea. Because herpes simplex virus type 2 (HSV-2) increases the risk of HIV acquisition, HSV-2 screening should be considered to aid in HIV risk assessment and counseling. More frequent screening should be considered for those at highest risk of STD.
†Vaccinate for hepatitis A and B if negative.

Urethritis in Men

EPIDEMIOLOGY

Urethritis is one of the most common STD syndromes in men, resulting in an estimated 200,000 initial physician visits in the United States in 2000.[28] The syndrome is typically divided into urethritis resulting from infection with *N. gonorrhoeae* and nongonococcal urethritis (NGU). Rates of gonococcal urethritis in most developed nations have declined dramatically over the past 20 years, although rates in the United States and Europe now appear to be rising again, particularly among men who have sex with men.[29,30]

ETIOLOGY AND MICROBIOLOGY

Since the mid-1970s, *Chlamydia trachomatis* has been recognized as the most common cause of NGU; *C. trachomatis* has typically been isolated in 30% to 40% of cases of NGU, although the prevalence of *C. trachomatis* in men with NGU may now be declining,[31] and chlamydial infection is less common in older men with NGU than in younger ones. In areas of the United States where the prevalence of *C. trachomatis* has declined in recent years, most patients with symptomatic urethritis have no evidence of either gonorrhea or chlamydial infection.[32] Other established causes of NGU include *Trichomonas vaginalis,* HSV-2, and, in men who engage in insertive anal intercourse, enteric pathogens. Approximately one third of men with primary genital herpes have dysuria and a urethral discharge. *T. vaginalis* is a more common cause of NGU in older men. However, HSV and *Trichomonas* combined are probably responsible for fewer than 10% of all cases of NGU. *Ureaplasma urealyticum* and *Mycoplasma genitalium* have been associated with NGU in case-control studies, but at present no tests for these organisms are commercially available.[33–35]

DIAGNOSIS

Clinical Manifestations

Clinical manifestations of urethritis include urethral discharge, dysuria, and itching at the distal urethra. Inguinal adenopathy is unusual. Likewise, fever, chills, perineal pain, scrotal mass, genital pain, and other urinary symptoms (e.g., hematuria, frequency, hesitancy, nocturia, or urgency) are unusual and should prompt consideration of alternative diagnoses, such as urinary tract infection (UTI), epididymitis, orchitis, or prostatitis. Although gonorrhea is generally associated with a more abrupt onset of symptoms and a more copious and purulent discharge than NGU, these distinctions are not reliable.

Asymptomatic and subclinical gonococcal and chlamydial urethral infections probably play an important role in sustaining endemic levels of these STDs, but their incidence is uncertain. A prospective study of gonococcal urethritis found that only 2% of infections remained asymptomatic in the 14 days after acquisition.[36] However, cross-sectional studies have demonstrated that asymptomatic infection is common among the sexual partners of infected women[37] and, at least in some parts of the United States that have a high prevalence of gonorrhea, in the general population of young adults.[38] Prospective data on the frequency of asymptomatic chlamydial urethritis are not available, but as with gonorrhea, cross-sectional studies have demonstrated that asymptomatic or subclinical chlamydial urethritis is common.[38,39]

Physical Examination

Objective evidence of urethral inflammation should be sought in men presenting with dysuria or urethral discharge. Physical examination should include a genital examination, preferably conducted several hours after the patient last urinated; the examination should include a search for purulent or mucopurulent discharge. If no discharge is observed, the examiner should strip the urethra from the base of the penis to the urethral meatus to elicit a discharge.

Laboratory Tests

A urethral Gram stain should be performed on all men with symptoms of urethritis, even those with no discharge evident on physical examination. Urethral specimens for Gram stain are obtained by inserting a thin calcium-alginate–tipped swab 3 to 4 cm into the urethra, then rolling the swab over a glass slide. A diagnosis of urethritis is established by the presence of five or more polymorphonuclear neutrophils (PMNs) per 1,000× oil-immersion field. Alternatively, the diagnosis can be made through use of a centrifuged 10 to 15 ml first-void urine specimen; the diagnosis is established by the finding of 10 or more PMNs per 400× field on at least one of five randomly selected fields. A positive urine leukocyte esterase test is also sufficient for establishing the diagnosis. Among experienced microscopists, the finding of gram-negative intracellular diplococci (GND) is 90% to 95% sensitive and over 95% specific in detecting urethral gonorrhea in symptomatic men,[40,41] and the presence of GND establishes the diagnosis of gonorrhea [*see Figure 1*]. The Gram stain should be considered equivocal if only extracellular organisms are seen. Regardless of Gram stain findings, specific microbiologic testing should be performed for *N. gonorrhoeae* and *C. trachomatis*.

Because it provides data on antimicrobial susceptibility, culture remains the preferred microbiologic test for gonorrhea. Nonamplified DNA probes offer the advantage of simplified specimen

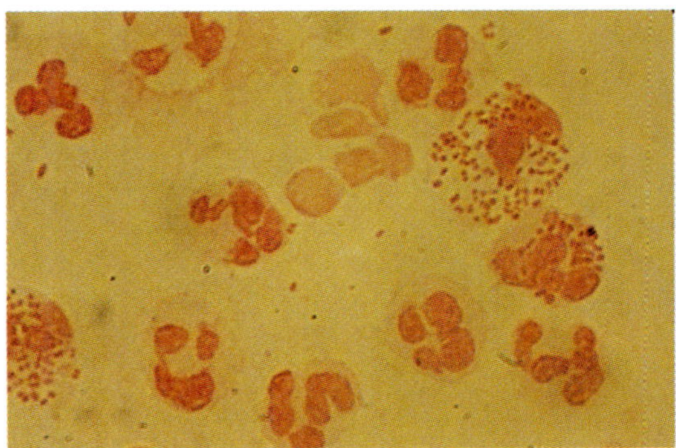

Figure 1 **This figure shows a Gram stain of a urethral discharge from a man with gonorrhea. The gram-negative intracellular diplococci are *Neisseria gonorrhoeae* organisms.**

handling and the ability to perform both gonococcal and chlamydial testing on a single specimen. These tests have a specificity of approximately 99%, and their sensitivity is comparable to that of culture for gonorrhea.[42]

Nucleic acid amplification tests (NAATs) of urethral specimens or urine (e.g., ligase chain reaction [LCR], polymerase chain reaction [PCR], transcription-mediated amplification [TMA], and strand displacement amplification [SDA]) have sensitivities comparable or superior to that of culture; although typically more costly, these assays offer the advantage of testing without urethral swabs. In low-prevalence populations, positive NAAT results may require confirmatory testing. The sensitivities of tests for *C. trachomatis* vary widely. Although test performance varies, depending on organism burden and anatomic site of collection, culture has a sensitivity of between 50% and 90%; enzyme immunoassays and nonamplified genetic probes have a sensitivity of 40% to 75%; and NAATs have a sensitivity of more than 90%.[43,44] For that reason, NAATs are preferred, when available.

TREATMENT

Initial Management

Patients with evidence of gonococcal infection on urethral Gram stain should be treated for gonorrhea. Recommended regimens include single doses of the following agents: (1) cefixime, 400 mg orally; (2) ceftriaxone, 125 mg intramuscularly; (3) ciprofloxacin, 500 mg orally; (4) ofloxacin, 400 mg orally; and (5) levofloxacin, 250 mg orally. Quinolone-resistant *N. gonorrhoeae* has recently emerged as a problem in Asia, the Pacific Islands, and, most recently, California. Consequently, quinolones are no longer recommended for the empirical treatment of gonorrhea in persons in these areas or in their contacts. Because of the high chlamydial coinfection rate, all patients with gonorrhea should also be treated for *Chlamydia,* unless that diagnosis has been microbiologically excluded. Treatment for presumptive chlamydial infection in men with NGU is with azithromycin in a single 1 g oral dose or doxycycline, 100 mg orally twice a day for 7 days.

Treatment of Recurrent or Persistent Urethritis

Although recognition of the pathogenic role of *C. trachomatis* has reduced a major cause of persistent or recurrent urethral symptoms after treatment for gonococcal urethritis, such symptoms continue to affect a minority of patients. Management should include questions regarding adherence to medical therapy and partner treatment, a urethral Gram stain to document evidence of urethral inflammation, and repeat testing for gonorrhea and chlamydial infection. Consideration should be given to possible trichomonal or herpes infection. Erythromycin, 500 mg four times a day for 7 days, with or without a single 2 g dose of metronidazole, is the recommended empirical treatment in patients who are believed to have adhered to their initial regimen and who have not been reexposed to gonorrhea or chlamydial infection.[8]

Lower Genital Tract Infections in Women

Women with STDs involving the lower genital tract may present with dysuria, urethritis or vulvovaginitis, and abnormal or altered vaginal discharge. The initial evaluation of women with these complaints seeks to differentiate urethritis, cystitis, vulvovaginitis, and cervicitis and to identify women with upper genitourinary tract infections (e.g., pyelonephritis or salpingitis). Subsequent microbiologic testing and treatment are guided by this evaluation.

SYNDROMES CAUSING DYSURIA AND URETHRITIS

STDs that can cause dysuria in women include vulvitis resulting from candidal infection and genital herpes and urethritis caused by *C. trachomatis* or *N. gonorrhoeae*. Dysuria and sterile pyuria (the presence of leukocytes and the absence of more than 10^2 organisms/ml of conventional urinary pathogens in a midstream urine specimen) in a woman are consistent with a diagnosis of urethral infection.[45] Other factors suggesting urethral infection include the absence of other symptoms and signs typical of UTI; risk factors or risk markers for chlamydial infection (young age, new or multiple sexual partners, failure to consistently use condoms, African-American race); symptoms lasting 7 days or longer; purulent vaginal discharge; pelvic pain or tenderness; and evidence of mucopurulent cervicitis.

Women presenting with a syndrome of dysuria and sterile pyuria should be tested for gonorrhea and chlamydial infection. Because HSV-2 can cause urethritis in women, particularly in women with primary HSV infection, the possibility of genital herpes should also be considered. HSV or candidal vulvitis typically causes external, as opposed to internal, dysuria, which occurs when urine comes in contact with the introitus or labia. Women with these infections typically have vulvar irritation or

Table 2 Clinical Features and Management of Vulvovaginitis

Feature	*Normal Vaginal Examination*	*Vulvovaginal Candidiasis*	*Trichomonal Vaginitis*	*Bacterial Vaginosis*
Etiology	Uninfected; lactobacilli predominate	*Candida albicans* most common; candidiasis caused by species other than *C. albicans* may be increasing	*Trichomonas vaginalis*	Loss of normal vaginal lactobacilli; associated with *Gardnerella vaginalis*; increased anaerobic bacteria and mycoplasmas
Symptoms	None	Abnormal vaginal discharge, external dysuria, vulvar itching, pain and/or irritation	Yellow vaginal discharge, external dysuria, vulvar itching	Increased, abnormal, or malodorous vaginal discharge
Discharge				
Amount	Variable	Scant	Profuse	Moderate
Color	Clear or white	White	Yellow	White or gray
Consistency	Nonhomogeneous, patchy (floccular)	Clumped; adherent plaques	Homogeneous or frothy	Adherent, homogeneous discharge that uniformly coats vagina
Inflammatory findings	None	Vulvar erythema, edema, or fissure; erythema of vaginal epithelium; introitus	Erythema of vaginal and vulvar epithelium; colpitis macularis	None
pH of vaginal fluid*	Usually ≤ 4.5	Usually ≤ 4.5	Usually > 4.5	Usually > 4.5
Amine (fishy) odor with 20% KOH	None	None	May be present	May be present
Microscopy	Normal epithelial cells; lactobacilli predominate	Leukocytes, epithelial cells; mycelia or pseudomycelia† (50%–85% of cases)	Leukocytes; trichomonads seen in 50%–70% of culture-positive cases	Clue cells (81%–94% of cases); few leukocytes; lactobacilli outnumbered by mixed flora
Recommended treatment	—	Intravaginal imidazole (butoconazole, clotrimazole, miconazole, terconazole, tioconazole) for 3–7 days; fluconazole, 150 mg p.o. (single dose)	Metronidazole, 2 g p.o. (single dose); metronidazole, 500 mg p.o., b.i.d., for 7 days	Metronidazole, 500 mg p.o., b.i.d., for 7 days; metronidazole gel, 0.75%, 5 g intravaginally each night for 5 nights; clindamycin cream 2%, 5 g intravaginally each night for 7 days
Sexual partner treatment	—	None if asymptomatic; topical treatment if candidal dermatitis of the penis or balanitis is detected	Metronidazole, 2 g orally (single dose)	None

*pH determination is not useful if blood is present.
†To detect fungal elements, vaginal fluid is digested with 10% KOH before microscopic examination; to examine for other features, fluid is mixed (1:1) with normal saline. Culture may be necessary if microscopy results are negative and the suspicion of *Candida* is high.

lesions; vaginal discharge; or a history of either HSV or candidal vaginitis.

In the differential diagnosis of dysuria in women, particular attention should be given to bacterial UTI, which is the most common cause of dysuria. Symptoms, signs, and laboratory findings that support the diagnosis of bacterial cystitis include urinary frequency or urgency, a history of UTI, duration of symptoms of less than 4 days, gross or microscopic hematuria, the patient's belief that she has a UTI, suprapubic tenderness, a positive urine nitrite test, and evidence of typical urinary tract pathogens on Gram stain or urine culture.[46–48] Fever or flank pain in a woman with dysuria and other findings consistent with UTI suggests pyelonephritis. Vaginal discharge or irritation is not typical of UTI.

Diagnostic testing for gonococcal and chlamydial urethritis in women should be based on specific tests [*see* Laboratory Tests, *above*]. In women with no evidence of pelvic inflammatory disease (PID), treatment is identical to that for men [*see* Treatment, *above*].

SYNDROMES CAUSING VULVOVAGINITIS AND VAGINAL DISCHARGE

Abnormal vaginal discharge is one of the most common reasons for women to seek medical attention. Since the 1960s, the number of women receiving care for vulvovaginal infections increased approximately threefold. In 2000, an estimated three million initial physician office visits in the United States were prompted by vulvovaginal infections.[28]

The most common causes of an abnormal vaginal discharge are bacterial vaginosis (BV), vulvovaginal candidiasis (VVC), and trichomonal vaginitis (TV) [*see Table 2*]. Both BV and trichomoniasis have been associated with preterm labor.[49,50] However, to date, treatment of these infections has not definitively been shown to decrease preterm delivery.[51–54] BV has been identified as a risk factor for PID, and both BV and trichomoniasis may increase the risk of HIV acquisition and transmission.[55–59] Consequently, these diagnoses have assumed new importance in HIV prevention.

Evaluation of women with vaginal complaints should include a pelvic examination and a directed laboratory evaluation. Although these infections tend to have different clinical features, a study of patients triaged and selectively treated after a telephone assessment found poor agreement between the diagnosis made by nurses and other providers and the diagnoses obtained after examination and testing.[60] Similarly, a study of women purchasing over-the-counter antifungal therapies found that only one third had vaginal candidiasis, and 53% had a diagnosis other than vulvovaginal candidiasis.[61] These findings emphasize the need for a complete evaluation in women complaining of vaginal discharge or discomfort. Less frequent causes of vaginitis include atrophic vaginitis with secondary bacterial infection, vaginitis associated with foreign bodies or toxins, *Staphylococcus aureus* vaginitis associated with toxic-shock syndrome, group A *Streptococcus*–associated vaginitis, desquamative vaginitis (clindamycin responsive), erosive lichen planus, allergic vaginitis, vaginitis associated with autoimmune disease, and idiopathic vaginitis.[62]

Bacterial Vaginosis

BV is the most common cause of vaginal discharge in women of reproductive age. Prevalence studies have found BV in 10% to 40% of women tested, with higher rates of infection in women tested in STD clinics and in African Americans. Douching and use of intrauterine devices (IUDs) have also been associated with BV.[63]

Pathophysiology and transmission The etiology of BV is unknown. The syndrome constitutes a disturbance in normal vaginal bacterial flora characterized by a reduction in the concentration of hydrogen peroxide–producing lactobacilli[64] and increased growth of mixed bacterial flora that include *Gardnerella vaginalis,* anaerobes, and *Mycoplasma hominis*. There is evidence that BV can be transmitted sexually. This evidence includes the following: studies have demonstrated that the inoculation of women with vaginal fluid from another woman with BV can induce the syndrome[65,66]; there is a high prevalence of BV in patients being treated at STD clinics; there are high rates of concordant BV among lesbian sexual partners[67]; longitudinal studies have associated BV with having higher numbers of sexual partners and with having new sexual partners[68–70]; and most studies have found that BV is absent in virgins.[71] Evidence against sexual transmission includes the lack of benefit from treating sexual partners[72–74] and inconsistent associations with levels of sexual activity.

Diagnosis Physical examination of women with BV typically reveals a homogeneous, white, uniformly adherent vaginal discharge.[63] The Amsel criteria for diagnosis of BV include the following: (1) presence of a homogeneous, thin vaginal discharge; (2) vaginal pH greater than 4.5; (3) clue cells (bacteria attached to vaginal epithelial cells on wet mount); and (4) presence of an amine (fishy) odor when vaginal fluid is mixed with 10% potassium hydroxide (KOH).[71,75–77] The presence of three of the four criteria establishes the diagnosis [*see Table 3*].

Treatment BV is treated with metronidazole. A meta-analysis found higher cure rates with a dosage of 1 mg a day for 7 days than with a single 2 g dose (82% versus 73%).[63] Intravaginal metronidazole and intravaginal clindamycin offer efficacy comparable to 7-day courses of metronidazole, with fewer side effects, but are not effective in the treatment of trichomoniasis and are typically more costly. Recurrence of BV is common, occurring in

Table 3 Amsel Criteria for the Diagnosis of Bacterial Vaginosis[71,75,77]

Criterion	*Sensitivity (%)*	*Specificity (%)*
Homogeneous, thin vaginal discharge	52–65	71–97
Vaginal pH > 4.5	92–97	53–62
Clue cells on vaginal wet mount	81–94	94–98
Amine odor when vaginal fluid is mixed with 10% potassium hydroxide (KOH)	43–84	98–99

Note: the presence of three of these four criteria establishes the diagnosis of bacterial vaginosis.

50% to 70% of cases. Multiple randomized trials have failed to demonstrate any benefit from treating male partners.[72–74]

Trichomoniasis

T. vaginalis is a sexually transmitted protozoan. In the United States, the number of women seeking care for trichomonal vaginitis declined by over 50% from 1966 to the mid-1980s; in 2000, physicians in the United States saw an estimated 200,000 patients with TV.[28] A cross-sectional study of 13,816 pregnant women in the United States found TV in 13%; the vast majority of those infections were subclinical or asymptomatic. Risk factors for TV included African-American ethnicity, cigarette smoking, unmarried status, and lower educational level.[77] Untreated infections in women are thought to persist for a median of 3 to 5 years.[78]

Diagnosis Clinical manifestations of trichomonal infection include yellow vaginal discharge and vulvar itching. Neither is highly sensitive or specific. On physical examination, signs associated with *Trichomonas* infection include frothy or purulent vaginal discharge, which is sometimes profuse; vulvar or vaginal erythema; and cervical mucopus.[79,80] All of these signs have far greater specificity than sensitivity. The finding of colpitis macularis—punctate cervical hemorrhages and ulcers, sometimes referred to as strawberry cervix—has a specificity of 99% for TV but is seen in fewer than 5% of patients on unaided physical examination; colpitis macularis is much more readily visible on colposcopy.[79] In expert hands, a finding of motile *Trichomonas* on wet-mount examination has a sensitivity of 50% to 70%, although in clinical practice, wet-mount examination is usually considerably less sensitive. Culture on Diamond medium is the traditional diagnostic gold standard, but this technique is not available in most practice settings. Recently, InPouch, a relatively simple and inexpensive culture method, became available. The sensitivity of InPouch is comparable to that of Diamond medium and superior to that of wet mount.[81] PCR has been successfully used in research settings, but no NAAT is commercially available at present. Antigen detection tests are also under investigation.

Treatment A single 2 g dose of metronidazole is the treatment of choice for TV. Reported cure rates are 82% to 88%.[80] Sexual partners should be treated concurrently, and couples should be advised to abstain from sex for 1 week after treatment. Topical metronidazole is not effective.[82] Resistance to metronidazole occurs infrequently, and most cases respond to prolonged courses of metronidazole therapy. Some authors have reported successful treatment of metronidazole-resistant cases using either tinidazole or paromomycin cream.[83]

Vulvovaginal Candidiasis

Because VVC is not a reportable infection, only limited epidemiologic data are available. In the United States, a study of female university students found that over half experienced at least one episode of VVC by 25 years of age,[84] and 6.5% of women who participated in a national random-digit–dialing survey reported that a health care provider had told them they had candidal vaginitis at least once in the preceding 2 months.[85] Higher rates of VVC have been observed in African Americans and in users of oral contraceptives, vaginal sponges, or IUDs.[86] Although VVC is not clearly identified as an STD, it has been associated with the onset of sexual activity in young women and with cunnilingus.[84,86] Other predisposing factors include recent use of antibiotics; diabetes mellitus; pregnancy; and immunodeficiency, including that from HIV infection.

Diagnosis Vulvovaginal pruritus is generally the most common symptom of VVC.[87] Other findings sometimes associated with VVC include a cottage-cheese–like discharge; external dysuria; external genital burning or pain; perineal edema or erythema; and vulvar erythema, edema, and fissures.[87,88] However, several studies have reported the absence of any signs or symptoms significantly associated with VVC.[4,89] As a result, the diagnosis requires microscopic and, at times, microbiologic assessment. A 10% KOH preparation of fluid taken from the vagina has a sensitivity of 50% to 85% in the diagnosis of VVC[90,91]; if this test is negative but the clinical picture is consistent with VVC and there is no alternative diagnosis, culture for yeast should be performed.

Treatment Topical azoles (e.g., butoconazole, clotrimazole, miconazole, econazole, tioconazole, and terconazole) are 80% to 90% effective in treating VCC [*see Table 2*]. Most of these agents are available over the counter. No clear advantage favors one azole over another. Oral azoles (fluconazole or itraconazole) are comparably or slightly more effective and may be more convenient, but these agents also pose a small risk of systemic reactions. Because there are no compelling data favoring any one agent or route of administration, patient preference should guide the choice of treatment. Immunosuppressed patients and those with candidal infections caused by a species other than *Candida albicans* may require more prolonged therapy (e.g., 14 days).

Long-term therapy is indicated for patients with recurrent VVC, which is defined as four or more episodes of VCC in a year. Approximately 5% of women with VVC experience recurrences. Treatment may require 14 days of induction therapy followed by once-weekly maintenance therapy. Patients with *C. glabrata* VVC who do not respond to prolonged courses of azole therapy may benefit from topical boric acid (600 mg once a day for 2 weeks) or topical flucytosine.[92]

Mucopurulent Cervicitis

Mucopurulent cervicitis (MPC) is an inflammatory process affecting the columnar epithelium and subepithelium of the endocervix and adjacent exocervix. As with NGU in men, MPC is common and has most frequently been associated with *N. gonorrhoeae* or *C. trachomatis* and, less frequently, with HSV or *T. vaginalis*. Unlike NGU, MPC typically produces no symptoms; or it may produce nonspecific symptoms, such as a yellow vaginal discharge, that often do not prompt women to seek treatment. In recent years, as the prevalence of gonorrhea and chlamydial infections have decreased in some settings, MPC with no defined microbiologic etiology has come to constitute the majority of cases.[4] MPC is important because of its association with known infections and because patients with MPC have an elevated risk of PID and adverse pregnancy outcome.

Diagnosis Different diagnostic criteria have been used for MPC. According to current CDC guidelines, the diagnosis of MPC is made on the basis of a finding of a visible purulent or mucopurulent exudate on cervical examination or on endocervical swab. The finding of cervical mucopus is 28% to 52% sensitive and 82% to 94% specific for the presence of either *C. trachomatis* or *N. gonorrhoeae*.[88,93,94] Some investigators use additional criteria for MPC, including a finding of from 20 to 30 PMNs per high-power field (hpf) on cervical Gram stain or easily induced cervical bleeding.[4,94] These factors have been associated with the likelihood of *C. trachomatis* or *N. gonorrhoeae* infection, but they have not consistently been included as diagnostic criteria of MPC; with regard to the use of cervical Gram stain, these findings have not consistently been useful in defining a population in need of empirical therapy.

Treatment The decision to treat MPC is based largely on the local prevalence of *C. trachomatis* or *N. gonorrhoeae* and on the patient's risk. In areas where both gonorrhea and chlamydial infection are common, empirical therapy should be directed at both pathogens. In areas where gonorrhea rates are low, treating for *Chlamydia* infection alone is reasonable. Recent evidence suggests that in areas where the prevalence of both infections is low, older patients (i.e., those older than 30 years) suspected of having MPC need not be treated until microbiologic test results are available, provided follow-up care is ensured.[94]

Pelvic Inflammatory Disease

PID is an inflammatory process involving a variable combination of endometritis, salpingitis, tuboovarian abscess, and pelvic peritonitis. PID can be blood-borne (e.g., tuberculosis) or result from extension of an intra-abdominal process. At present, however, PID most often develops when bacteria ascend from the vagina or cervix into the endometrium, fallopian tubes, and pelvic peritoneum. Although the number of women seeking care for PID has declined by over 25% since the 1980s, 8% of participants in the 1995 National Survey of Family Growth, a national representative sample of United States women, reported a history of PID.[95] Identified risk factors for PID include a previous history of PID, higher numbers of lifetime sex partners, douching, and a history of bacterial STD. In the past, IUD use was identified as a risk factor, but its importance beyond the first 30 days after insertion is now controversial; a recent case-control study found no association between the use of currently available copper IUDs and the occurrence of PID.[96] Gynecologic procedures that disrupt the protective cervical barrier (e.g., pregnancy termination, IUD insertion, dilatation and curettage, and hysterosalpingography) elevate the risk of PID and may lead to PID in the absence of classic sexually transmitted pathogens.

MICROBIOLOGY

Studies of PID conducted in the United States and Europe in the 1980s typically implicated *C. trachomatis, N. gonorrhoeae,* or both as a cause of PID in approximately half of cases.[97] Frequently, these bacteria were part of a polymicrobial infection involving diverse normal vaginal flora, including anaerobic bacteria, facultative anaerobes, and genital mycoplasmas. *M. genitalium* has been associated with endometritis and PID.[98] *Actinomyces israelii* is a cause of PID in women with IUDs.

DIAGNOSIS

The diagnosis of PID is difficult. To date, studies have been unable to identify any single clinical finding or constellation of findings that allow accurate identification of women with PID.[99,100] Moreover, PID studies have typically enrolled only women with overt disease and, consequently, have not provided an accurate picture of the full spectrum of the clinical entity. Indeed, most cases of PID probably go undiagnosed. Approximately two thirds of women with postinfectious fallopian tube occlusion report no history of PID, although many have sought care for abdominal pain.[101] When the diagnosis is made clinically, it may not be supported by surgical findings. Only 60% to 70% of women with clinically diagnosed PID typically have laparoscopic evidence of PID.[102]

In clinically detected cases, the cardinal symptom of PID is pelvic or abdominal pain. The pain is typically dull or aching. Onset can be acute or subacute and frequently occurs at the beginning of menses. Typically, patients present after having symptoms for less than 2 weeks. In a Swedish study of 623 patients with PID, all had pelvic or abdominal pain, cervical motion tenderness, and increased inflammatory cells in vaginal or cervical secretions. Other symptoms and laboratory findings included an erythrocyte sedimentation rate (ESR) of 15 mm/hr or higher (75%), leukocytosis greater than 10,000/ml (60%), abnormal vaginal discharge (55%), fever higher than 38° C (100.4° F) (41%), abnormal vaginal bleeding (36%), dysuria (19%), vomiting (10%), and anorectal symptoms (anorectal pain, tenesmus, or rectal bleeding or discharge) (7%).[103] A large study showed that only temperatures higher than 38° C (100.4° F) had a specificity of more than 90% for the diagnosis of PID, although its sensitivity was only 11%.[103]

The differential diagnosis of PID includes other causes of abdominal or pelvic pain. Depending on the clinical circumstances, the physician may need to consider such disorders as appendicitis, endometriosis, bleeding corpus luteum, pelvic adhesions, gastroenteritis, and ectopic pregnancy.

Although laparoscopy has been the traditional gold standard for diagnosing PID, many women with abnormal fimbrial biopsies have normal results on laparoscopy. Moreover, some women have histologic evidence of endometritis without salpingitis,[104] which suggests that laparoscopy may be insensitive for the detection of milder cases or of PID that is restricted to the uterus.

Transvaginal ultrasound (TVUS) should be performed when symptoms are severe, when the physical examination reveals a pelvic mass, or when the diagnosis of PID is uncertain. Studies assessing the performance of different imaging modalities in the diagnosis of PID have been small, with no single study enrolling more than 50 patients with the diagnosis.[102] Small studies of TVUS have reported sensitivities of 81% to 93%, but specificities have been highly variable, ranging from 5% to 100%, with the test performing best in patients with more severe infection.[102] A case-control study of power Doppler TVUS reported a sensitivity of 100% and a specificity of 80%,[105] suggesting it may offer advantages over conventional TVUS. In women with tubo-ovarian abscess, repeat TVUS is often indicated to assess response to therapy. Small studies of CT and pelvic MRI have also reported high sensitivity and specificity. Laparoscopy should be performed if appendicitis, ectopic pregnancy, or ruptured abscess is suspected; laparoscopy should also be considered in women who do not respond to antibiotics.

TREATMENT

Because the diagnosis of PID can be challenging, the sequelae of PID can be severe, and treatment is safe and inexpensive, all patients suspected of having PID should undergo treatment for PID. The CDC recommends initiating treatment of PID in all sexually active young women with adenexal tenderness or cervical motion tenderness.[8] These criteria are likely to be sensitive, but they are also quite nonspecific.[100]

Treatment for PID is directed against *C. trachomatis, N. gonorrhoeae,* gram-negative facultative anaerobes, vaginal anaerobes, and streptococci.

Table 4 Treatment Regimens for Pelvic Inflammatory Disease

Route	*Regimen*
Parenteral	Cefotetan, 2 g I.V. q. 12 hr *or* Cefoxitin, 2 g I.V. q. 6 hr *plus* Doxycycline, 100 mg p.o. or I.V. q. 12 hr
	Clindamycin, 900 mg I.V. q. 8 hr *plus* Gentamicin, 2 mg/kg I.V. or I.M. once, then 1.5 mg/kg I.V. q. 8 hr (single daily dose may be used)
	Ofloxacin, 400 mg I.V. q. 12 hr *or* Levofloxacin, 500 mg I.V. q.d. *plus* Doxycycline, 100 mg p.o. or I.V. q. 12 hr *with or without* Metronidazole, 500 mg I.V. q. 8 hr *or* Ampicillin-sulbactam, 3 g I.V. q. 6 hr
Oral	Ofloxacin, 400 mg p.o., b.i.d. *or* Levofloxacin, 500 mg I.V. q.d. for 14 days *with or without* Metronidazole, 500 mg p.o., b.i.d., for 14 days
	Ceftriaxone, 250 mg I.M. once *or* Cefoxitin, 2 g I.M. once with probenecid, 1 g p.o. *plus* Doxycycline, 100 mg b.i.d. for 14 days *with or without* Metronidazole, 500 mg p.o., b.i.d., for 14 days

*Parenteral therapy can be discontinued after the patient improves clinically, but doxycycline should be continued for 14 days.

Numerous regimens have been found acceptable [*see Table 4*]. A recent randomized trial in women with mild to moderate PID found no advantage of inpatient therapy with intravenous cefoxitin and doxycycline over outpatient therapy with a single intramuscular dose of cefoxitin and probenecid followed by oral doxycycline.[106] Indications for hospitalization include the following: (1) inability to exclude a possible surgical emergency (e.g., appendicitis), (2) pregnancy, (3) failure to respond to oral antibiotics, (4) inability to tolerate or adhere to outpatient oral therapy, (5) tubo-ovarian abscess, and (6) inability to reliably ensure follow-up. Patients should show significant improvement within 3 days after starting therapy. Those receiving oral therapy should be reevaluated within 72 hours. Treatment should include efforts to ensure that sexual partners also receive therapy. In addition, patients with *Chlamydia* or *N. gonorrhoeae* infections should be rescreened for those infections 10 to 18 weeks after treatment.

COMPLICATIONS

Although the vast majority of women with PID in developed nations recover fully, long-term sequelae are common; these sequelae include tubal infertility, ectopic pregnancy, and chronic pelvic pain. In the largest study of PID sequelae performed to date, Swedish investigators performed laparoscopy on 1,730 women with suspected PID and then followed them for a mean of 6.9 years. After a single episode of PID, 8% of patients suffered tubal infertility, compared with 1% of control subjects in whom there was no laparoscopic evidence of PID. Of PID patients who subsequently became pregnant, 10% had an ectopic pregnancy, compared with 1% of women without PID. Similarly, pelvic pain lasting longer than 6 months occurred in 17% of women with PID but in only 2% of control subjects.[107] Recurrent episodes of PID multiplied the risk of sequelae [*see Figure 2*], as did more severe PID and longer duration of symptoms before treatment.

Genital Ulcer Disease

Genital ulcers are a frequent presentation of STDs. Epidemiologic studies, as well as studies

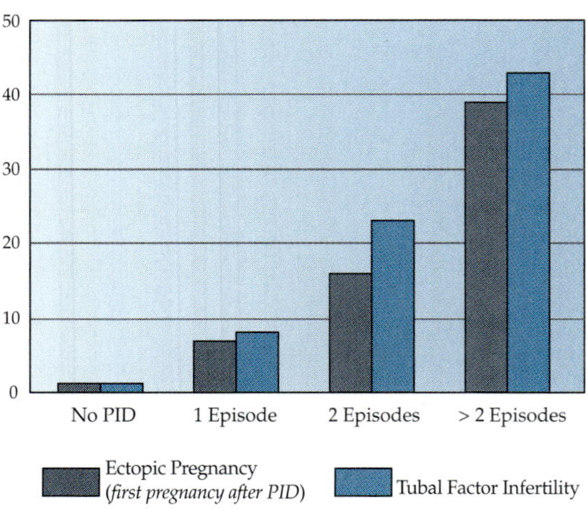

Figure 2 **Proportion of women experiencing an ectopic pregnancy or tubal infertility by number of episodes of pelvic inflammatory disease (PID) among 1,282 patients with PID and 448 control subjects.[97,107]**

measuring HIV shedding, suggest that genital ulcer disease (GUD) increases the risk of both HIV acquisition and HIV transmission.[3,108] As a result, the prevention and treatment of GUD is a high public health priority.

ETIOLOGY

Herpes, syphilis, and chancroid are the major causes of genital ulcer disease. Less common causes of GUD include lymphogranuloma venereum (infection with L-serotypes of *C. trachomatis*), donovanosis (infection with *Calymmatobacterium granulomatis*), superinfection of ectoparasitic infections, trauma, neoplasm, Behçet syndrome, Reiter syndrome, and fixed drug eruptions (e.g., from doxycycline or sulfonamides).

Herpes is the most common cause of GUD in developed nations. In the United States in 2000, over two million people sought care for genital herpes. In contrast, a total of 5,979 cases of primary and secondary syphilis and 82 cases of chancroid were reported to the CDC.[28] A 1996 study of 516 STD clinic patients with genital ulcers found that 62% had HSV, 10% had syphilis, 3% had both syphilis and herpes, 3% had chancroid, and 22% had no identified pathogen.[109]

Traditionally, chancroid and syphilis have been the most common cause of genital ulcers in most developing nations. However, recent studies undertaken in sub-Saharan Africa have documented the increasing importance of herpes as a cause of GUD, particularly in areas where HIV is highly prevalent.[110]

DIAGNOSIS

Clinical Manifestations

When examining patients with genital ulcers, clinicians should note the number and depth of lesions; the presence of vesicles, induration, necrotic material on the ulcer bed, or an undermined ulcer border (i.e., the ulcer invades beneath the superficial edges); the presence or absence of pain; and any associated adenopathy [*see Table 5*]. Although physical findings can be helpful, different GUD etiologies cannot be reliably distinguished by physical examination alone.[111]

Laboratory Tests

Because physical findings are unreliable, clinical assessment should be supported by laboratory evaluation. The laboratory evaluation of GUD typically concentrates on herpes and syphilis. Chancroid, donovanosis, or LGV should be considered if the patient lives in or has traveled to an area where one of those infections is common or if the physical findings are highly suggestive of one of those infections.

When possible, laboratory evaluation should include dark-field microscopy, serologic testing for syphilis (e.g., rapid plasma reagin [RPR] or venereal disease research laboratory [VDRL]; and fluorescent treponemal antibody [FTA] or microhemagglutination assay for antibody to *T. pallidum*), and culture for herpes. If available, RPR should be performed. Dark-field microscopy is 70% to 95% sensitive in detecting treponemes, but sensitivity is highly dependent on the expertise of the technician. Culture should seek to distinguish between HSV-1 and HSV-2, because the former typically produces a less severe infection with fewer recurrences. This is particularly important in light of recent data that suggest that HSV-1 is an increasingly common cause of genital herpes.[112] If initial evaluation does not establish a cause of genital ulcers and the clinician's suspicion for chancroid, LGV, or donovanosis remains low, further diagnostic efforts should focus on ruling out genital herpes. Several type-specific serologic tests that target the HSV glycoprotein G-2 (gG-2) are now available.[113] Patients who have no serologic evidence of HSV-2 may have primary infections. Only limited data are available on how soon seroconversion can be detected by commercially available type-specific tests, but the median time from exposure to seroconversion appears to be 2 to 3 weeks. Patients with a clinical syndrome consistent with genital herpes who test negative for HSV-2 should be retested after 6 to 12 weeks if an intervening recurrence of genital ulcers does not establish the diagnosis of HSV infection and the clinical suspicion for genital herpes is high. Older HSV serologic tests are neither sensitive nor specific and should not be used. Clinicians should be aware that type-specific serologic tests have not been studied extensively for HSV-2 screening. Given the imperfect specificity of these tests, it is likely that widespread testing in populations in which the prevalence of HSV-2 is low will result in large numbers of false positive test results. Because of poor specificity, a positive HSV-2 serologic test result in a patient without signs or symptoms of genital herpes or definite exposure to HSV-2 should be interpreted with caution.

TREATMENT

Treatment of patients with genital ulcers is usually empirical [*see Table 6*]. If patients have physical findings suggestive of syphilis, are residents of or recent travelers to areas where syphilis remains

Table 5 Clinical Features and Laboratory Diagnosis of Genital Ulcers

Disease	*Etiology*	*Incubation Period*	*Number of Lesions*	*Primary Lesion Type*	*Ulcer Diameter*	*Ulcer Characteristics*	*Pain or Tenderness*	*Lymphadenopathy*	*Laboratory Diagnosis*
Syphilis	*Treponema pallidum*	9–90 days	Usually one	Papule	5–15 mm	Superficial or deep; sharply demarcated; indurated; nonvascular, purulent base	Uncommon	Firm, nontender, bilateral	Darkfield microscopy, RPR/VDRL and FTA, MHA-TP
Herpes	HSV-1 or -2	2–7 days	Multiple, may coalesce	Vesicle	1–2 mm	Superficial; erythematous edges, no induration	Frequently tender	Firm, tender, small, often bilateral with first episode	DFA, culture, serology
Chancroid	*Haemophilus ducreyi*	1–14 days	Multiple, may coalesce	Pustule	Variable	Deep; irregular, undermined edges; purulent base bleeds easily	Usually tender	Tender, may be fluctuant, loculated; usually unilateral	Culture of ulcer base,* NAAT (e.g., PCR, LCR, TMA, SDA)
LGV	L-serotypes of *Chlamydia trachomatis*	3 days to 6 wk	Usually one	Papule, pustule, or vesicle	2–10 cm	Very rarely seen, because of rapid healing; can be superficial, deep, elevated, round, or oval	Variable	Tender, may suppurate or form sinus tracts; loculated, usually unilateral, more common in men than women	Culture, PCR, microimmunofluorescent antibody
Donovanosis	*Calymmatobacterium granulomatis*	1–4 wk (up to 6 mo)	Variable	Papule	Variable	Extensive, indolent ulcer with granulation tissue; elevated, rolled irregular edges on raised ulcer; beefy-red vascular base bleeds easily†	Uncommon	None; pseudobuboes	Giemsa or Wright stain of tissue smear

*Culture of material from bubo seldom positive.

†Less common variants can be hypertrophic, necrotic, or sclerotic.

DFA—direct fluorescent antibody HSV—herpes simplex virus LGV—lymphogranuloma venereum LCR—ligase chain reaction MHA-TP—microhemagglutination assay–*T. pallidum* NAAT—nucleic acid amplification test PCR—polymerase chain reaction RPR—rapid plasma reagin SDA—strand displacement amplification TMA—transcription-mediated amplification VDRL—Venereal Disease Research Laboratory

Table 6 Treatment of Genital Ulcers

Disease	*Regimen*
Syphilis	Benzathine penicillin G, 2.4 million U I.M.*
Chancroid	Azithromycin, 1 g p.o. once *or* Ceftriaxone, 250 mg I.M. once *or* Ciprofloxacin, 500 mg p.o., b.i.d., for 3 days *or* Erythromycin, 500 mg p.o., b.i.d., for 7 days
Lymphogranuloma venereum	Doxycycline, 100 mg p.o., b.i.d., for 21 days
Donovanosis	Doxycycline, 100 mg p.o. for at least 3 wk or until lesion is healed *or* Trimethoprim-sulfamethoxazole, double strength (800 mg/160 mg), one tablet p.o., b.i.d., for at least 3 wk or until lesion is healed
Herpes	See Table 7

Note: treatment should always include evaluation and treatment of sexual partners.
*For primary or secondary syphilis.

common, or are members of groups at high risk for syphilis (e.g., men who have sex with men, as well as commercial sex workers or their clients), treatment should include benzathine penicillin G, 2.4 million units intramuscularly, and a regimen for genital herpes [*see Table 7*]. If the suspicion for syphilis is low and follow-up can be ensured, initial empirical treatment can focus on genital herpes alone. The treatment and follow-up of patients with genital herpes and syphilis are discussed in other subsections.

Patients with genital herpes should be counseled about the recurrent nature of the infection and advised that subclinical viral shedding is common. The median recurrence rate in the first year after HSV-2 acquisition is 0.33 recurrences monthly.[114] During the first 6 months after HSV-2 acquisition, virus can be isolated by culture on 6% of days and by PCR on 20% to 35% of days.[115] It is not known to what extent HSV can be transmitted by patients whose cultures are negative and whose PCR results are positive. The American Social Health Association Web site (http://www.ashastd.org) is an excellent source of information on STD in general and genital herpes in particular, and it has information on support services for persons with genital herpes.

STDs in Men Who Have Sex with Men and Anorectal STDs in Women

Although surveillance data on STDs in men who have sex with men (MSM) are limited, cases of gonorrhea and syphilis in MSM in selected cities in the United States declined by more than 10-fold in the decade following the first recognition of AIDS.[116] Numerous cities in the United States and Europe have reported rising rates of STDs in MSM.[30,117] Limited data suggest that HIV transmission may also be increasing.[118] Because STDs can enhance HIV transmission, the control of STDs in MSM is a public health priority. Moreover, an STD can be a sentinel event, alerting the clinician to a patient's risk of acquiring HIV infection or transmitting it to others.

GENERAL CONSIDERATIONS IN MSM

Several aspects of the care of MSM merit consideration. First, it is imperative that clinicians adopt a nonjudgmental, direct approach when discussing sexual behavior. In addition to the questions typically included in a sexual history, clinicians should ask patients about the HIV status of their sexual partners and about their anal sexual exposure. The latter can be determined by asking, "Are you a top, a bottom, or both a top and a bottom?" The term top refers to a man who practices insertive anal sex; a bottom practices receptive anal sex.

Second, the spectrum of STD is wider in MSM than in heterosexuals. Several pathogens that are

Table 7 Treatment of Genital Herpes in Immunocompetent Patients

Primary herpes	Acyclovir, 400 mg p.o., t.i.d., for 7–10 days *or* Valacyclovir, 1 g p.o., b.i.d., for 7–10 days *or* Famciclovir, 250 mg p.o., t.i.d., for 7–10 days
Recurrent herpes	Acyclovir, 800 mg p.o., b.i.d., for 5 days *or* Acyclovir, 800 mg p.o., t.i.d., for 2 days *or* Valacyclovir, 1 g p.o., q.d., for 5 days *or* Valacyclovir, 500 mg p.o., b.i.d., for 3–5 days *or* Famciclovir, 125 mg p.o., t.i.d., for 5 days

rarely sexually transmitted among heterosexuals are relatively common causes of STD in MSM. These include hepatitis A virus, *Shigella* species, *Salmonella* species, *Campylobacter* species, *Giardia lamblia*, and *Entamoeba histolytica*. *Strongyloides stercoralis* and *Enterobius vermicularis* are occasionally transmitted sexually in MSM.

Third, the anus is a more common sexual organ for MSM than it is for heterosexuals. Consequently, STD should figure prominently in the differential diagnosis of MSM who present with anorectal symptoms, and rectal screening should be part of standard STD screening in MSM.[24] Finally, although there are no guidelines for regular STD screening of heterosexual men, the CDC currently recommends annual STD screening for MSM [*see Table 1*].[8]

PROCTITIS, PROCTOCOLITIS, AND ENTERITIS

Although anorectal STD occurs in both men and heterosexual women, anal STD syndromes are more common in MSM. The symptoms of anorectal infection vary, depending on the level and extent of anatomic involvement and on the microbiologic etiology.[119] Proctitis is limited to the rectum. It results from direct inoculation of pathogens through anal sex and presents as some combination of rectal pain, constipation, hematochezia, tenesmus, and mucopurulent rectal discharge. Sexually transmitted proctitis is caused by gonorrhea, chlamydial infection (non-LGV), syphilis, or HSV. In proctocolitis, the inflammatory process extends to the colon. As a result, in addition to the symptoms of proctitis, patients may complain of diarrhea, abdominal pain, and bloating or nausea. Most cases of proctocolitis result from oral-genital or oral-anal sex (anilingus, or so-called rimming) and are caused by *Shigella*, *Salmonella*, or *Campylobacter* species; *E. histolytica*; or LGV serovars of *C. trachomatis*. *G. lamblia* infection involves the small bowel alone (enteritis) and typically presents as diarrhea, abdominal pain, and bloating or nausea in the absence of rectal symptoms. The differential diagnosis in patients presenting with symptoms of colitis or proctocolitis should include *Clostridium difficile* infection and inflammatory bowel disease. In persons with HIV infection and $CD4^+$ T cell counts less than 50/mm^3, cytomegalovirus infection is also a possibility. Depending on their level of immunosuppression, HIV-infected patients presenting with enteritis should also be evaluated for *Mycobacterium avium* complex, cryptosporidium, *Isospora belli*, *Cyclospora cayetanensis*, and *Microsporidia* organisms.

DIAGNOSIS

History and Physical Examination

Evaluation of a patient with anorectal symptoms should include questions about anal, oral-genital, and oral-anal sex and condom use. In the evaluation, an attempt should be made to differentiate symptoms of proctitis, proctocolitis, and enteritis. Physical examination should include a careful anal examination, digital rectal examination, and anoscopy directed toward finding ulcers consistent with HSV or syphilis, condylomata lata, or rectal discharge or bleeding.

Laboratory Tests

If a rectal exudate is present, a Gram stain should be performed to look for gonorrhea. The reported sensitivity of Gram stain is highly variable (30% to 79%).[120] In one study, rectal Gram stain specimens obtained by anoscopy were more sensitive in detecting gonorrhea than were those obtained blindly (53% versus 79%).[120] In men without rectal symptoms, however, anoscopically obtained rectal cultures do not appear to be more sensitive in detecting gonorrhea than those obtained by blindly inserting a swab 2 to 3 cm into the rectum.[121]

Laboratory evaluation in patients with suspected proctitis or proctocolitis should include cultures for gonorrhea and chlamydial infection, a serologic test for syphilis, and a rapid syphilis test. Rectal ulcers or lesions should be cultured for HSV; when possible, a specimen should be obtained for dark-field evaluation. If symptoms suggest proctocolitis, stool specimens should be obtained for enteric pathogens and *E. histolytica*. Patients with recent antibiotic exposures should also be tested for *C. difficile*. Stool *Giardia* antigen testing should be performed if enteritis is suspected.

TREATMENT

In general, treatment should be directed by laboratory findings. If patients with proctitis have severe symptoms or if follow-up cannot be ensured, empirical therapy should be directed against gonorrhea and chlamydial infection. The CDC recommends treatment with ceftriaxone, 250 mg intramuscularly, and doxycycline, 100 mg a day orally for 7 days. Alternative therapies for gonorrhea (cefixime, 400 mg orally or ciprofloxacin, 500 mg orally once) and chlamydial infection (azithromycin, 1 g orally once) are probably effective but have not been studied. Clinicians should have a low threshold for adding empirical therapy for herpes to this regimen.

References

1. Eng TR, Butler WT: The Hidden Epidemic: Confronting Sexually Transmitted Diseases. Committee on Prevention and Control of Sexually Transmitted Diseases, Institute of Medicine (U.S.), National Academy Press, Washington, DC, 1997, p 432

2. Gerbase AC, Rowley JT, Heymann DH, et al: Global prevalence and incidence estimates of selected curable STDs. Sex Transm Infect 74(suppl 1):S12, 1998

3. Fleming DT, Wasserheit JN: From epidemiological synergy to public health policy and practice: the contribution of other sexually transmitted diseases to sexual transmission of HIV infection. Sex Transm Infect 75:3, 1999

4. Holmes KK: Introduction. Sexually Transmitted Diseases, 3rd ed. Holmes KK, Mårdh P-A, Sparling PF, et al, Eds. McGraw-Hill, New York, 1999, p xi

5. Holmes KK: Human ecology and behavior and sexually transmitted bacterial infections. Proc Natl Acad Sci U S A 91:2448, 1994

6. Revised guidelines for HIV counseling, testing and referral. MMWR Recomm Rep 50(RR-19):1, 2001

7. Revised recommendations for HIV screening of pregnant women. MMWR Recomm Rep 50(RR-19):63, 2001

8. Sexually transmitted diseases treatment guidelines 2002. MMWR Recomm Rep 51(RR-6):1, 2002

9. Anderson RM: Transmission dynamics of sexually transmitted infections. Sexually Transmitted Diseases, 3rd ed. Holmes KK, Mårdh P-A, Sparling PF, et al, Eds. McGraw-Hill, New York, 1999, p 25

10. Brunham RC, Plummer FA: A general model of sexually transmitted disease epidemiology and its implications for control. Med Clin North Am 74:1339, 1990

11. Thomas JC, Tucker MJ: The development and use of the concept of a sexually transmitted disease core. J Infect Dis 174(suppl 2):S134, 1996

12. Fleming DT, McQuillan GM, Johnson RE, et al: Herpes simplex virus type 2 in the United States, 1976 to 1994. N Engl J Med 337:1105, 1997

13. Garnett GP, Anderson RM: Sexually transmitted diseases and sexual behavior: insights from mathematical models. J Infect Dis 174(suppl 2):S150, 1996

14. Morris M: Concurrent partnerships and syphilis persistence: new thoughts on an old puzzle. Sex Transm Dis 28:504, 2001

15. Kretzschmar M: Sexual network structure and sexually transmitted disease prevention: a modeling perspective. Sex Transm Dis 27:627, 2000

16. Handsfield HH, Jasman LL, Roberts PL, et al: Criteria for selective screening for *Chlamydia trachomatis* infection in women attending family planning clinics. JAMA 255:1730, 1986

17. Marrazzo JM, Fine D, Celum CL, et al: Selective screening for chlamydial infection in women: a comparison of three sets of criteria. Fam Plann Perspect 29:158, 1997

18. van Valkengoed IG, Morre SA, van den Brule AJ, et al: Low diagnostic accuracy of selective screening criteria for asymptomatic *Chlamydia trachomatis* infections in the general population. Sex Transm Infect 76:375, 2000

19. Marrazzo JM, White CL, Krekeler B, et al: Community-based urine screening for *Chlamydia trachomatis* with a ligase chain reaction assay. Ann Intern Med 127:796, 1997

20. Laumann EO, Youm Y: Racial/ethnic group differences in the prevalence of sexually transmitted diseases in the United States: a network explanation. Sex Transm Dis 26:250, 1999

21. Sucato G, Celum C, Dithmer D, et al: Demographic rather than behavioral risk factors predict herpes simplex virus type 2 infection in sexually active adolescents. Pediatr Infect Dis J 20:422, 2001

22. Laumann E, Gagnon J, Michaels S: The Social Organization of Sexuality: Sexual Practices in the United States. University of Chicago Press, Chicago, 1994

23. Sexually transmitted disease and HIV screening guidelines for men who have sex with men. Sex Transm Dis 28:457, 2001

24. Efficacy of risk-reduction counseling to prevent human immunodeficiency virus and sexually transmitted diseases: a randomized controlled trial. Project RESPECT Study Group. JAMA 280:1161, 1998

25. Ramstedt K, Forssman L, Johannisson G: Contact tracing in the control of genital *Chlamydia trachomatis*. Int J STD AIDS 2:116, 1991

26. Kissinger P, Brown R, Reed K, et al: Effectiveness of patient delivered partner medication for preventing recurrent *Chlamydia trachomatis*. Sex Transm Infect 74:331, 1998

27. Golden MR, Whittington WL, Handsfield HH, et al: Partner management for gonococcal and chlamydial infection: expansion of public health services to the private sector and expedited sex partner treatment through a partnership with commercial pharmacies. Sex Transm Dis 28:258, 2001

28. Scholes D, Stergachis A, Heidrich FE, et al: Prevention of pelvic inflammatory disease by screening for cervical chlamydial infection. N Engl J Med 334:1362, 1996

29. Gonorrhea among men who have sex with men: selected sexually transmitted disease clinics, 1993–1996. MMWR Morb Mortal Wkly Rep 46:889, 1997

30. Nicoll A, Hamers FF: Are trends in HIV, gonorrhoea, and syphilis worsening in western Europe? BMJ 324:1324, 2002

31. Stamm WE, Hicks CB, Martin DH, et al: Azithromycin for empirical treatment of the nongonococcal urethritis syndrome in men: a randomized double-blind study. JAMA 274:545, 1995

32. Marrazzo JM, Whittington WL, Celum CL, et al: Urine-based screening for *Chlamydia trachomatis* in men attending sexually transmitted disease clinics. Sex Transm Dis 28:219, 2001

33. Bowie WR, Wang SP, Alexander ER, et al: Etiology of nongonococcal urethritis: evidence for *Chlamydia trachomatis* and *Ureaplasma urealyticum*. J Clin Invest 59:735, 1977

34. Tully JG, Taylor-Robinson D, Cole RM, et al: A newly discovered mycoplasma in the human urogenital tract. Lancet 1:1288, 1981

35. Totten PA, Schwartz MA, Sjostrom KE, et al: Association of *Mycoplasma genitalium* with nongonococcal urethritis in heterosexual men. J Infect Dis 183:269, 2001

36. Harrison WO, Hooper RR, Wiesner PJ, et al: A trial of minocycline given after exposure to prevent gonorrhea. N Engl J Med 300:1074, 1979

37. Handsfield HH, Lipman TO, Harnisch JP, et al: Asymptomatic gonorrhea in men: diagnosis, natural course, prevalence and significance. N Engl J Med 290:117, 1974

38. Turner CF, Rogers SM, Miller HG, et al: Untreated gonococcal and chlamydial infection in a probability sample of adults. JAMA 287:726, 2002

39. Klausner JD, McFarland W, Bolan G, et al: Knock-knock: a population-based survey of risk behavior, health care access, and *Chlamydia trachomatis* infection among low-income women in the San Francisco Bay area. J Infect Dis 183:1087, 2001

40. Jacobs NF, Kraus SJ: Gonococcal and nongonococcal urethritis in men: clinical and laboratory differentiation. Ann Intern Med 82:7, 1975

41. Rothenberg RB, Simon R, Chipperfield E, et al: Efficacy of selected diagnostic tests for sexually transmitted diseases. JAMA 235:49, 1976

42. Koumans EH, Johnson RE, Knapp JS, et al: Laboratory testing for *Neisseria gonorrhoeae* by recently introduced nonculture tests: a performance review with clinical and public health considerations. Clin Infect Dis 27:1171, 1998

43. Marrazzo JM, Stamm WE: New approaches to the diagnosis, treatment, and prevention of chlamydial infection. Curr Clin Top Infect Dis 18:37, 1998

44. Black CM, Marrazzo J, Johnson RE, et al: Head-to-head multicenter comparison of DNA probe and nucleic acid amplification tests for *Chlamydia trachomatis* infection in women performed with an improved reference standard. J Clin Microbiol 40:3757, 2002

45. Stamm WE, Wagner KF, Amsel R, et al: Causes of the acute urethral syndrome in women. N Engl J Med 303:409, 1980

46. Hooton TM, Stamm WE: Diagnosis and treatment of uncomplicated urinary tract infection. Infect Dis Clin North Am 11:551, 1997

47. Bent S, Nallamothu BK, Simel DL, et al: Does this woman have an acute uncomplicated urinary tract infection? JAMA 287:2701, 2002

48. Gupta K, Hooton TM, Roberts PL, et al: Patient-initiated treatment of uncomplicated recurrent urinary tract infections in young women. Ann Intern Med 135:9, 2001

49. Association between bacterial vaginosis and preterm delivery of a low-birth-weight infant. The Vaginal Infections and Prematurity Study Group. N Engl J Med 333:1737, 1995

50. *Trichomonas vaginalis* associated with low birth weight and preterm delivery. The Vaginal Infections and Prematurity Study Group. Sex Transm Dis 24:353, 1997

51. Metronidazole to prevent preterm delivery in pregnant women with asymptomatic bacterial vaginosis. National Institute of Child Health and Human Development Network of Maternal-Fetal Medicine Units. N Engl J Med 342:534, 2000

52. Klebanoff MA, Carey JC, Hauth JC, et al: Failure of metronidazole to prevent preterm delivery among pregnant women with asymptomatic *Trichomonas vaginalis* infection. N Engl J Med 345:487, 2001

53. Koumans EH, Kendrick JS: Preventing adverse sequelae of bacterial vaginosis: a public health program and research agenda. Sex Transm Dis 28:292, 2001

54. Gulmezoglu AM: Interventions for trichomoniasis in pregnancy. Cochrane Database Syst Rev (3):CD000220, 2002

55. Martin HL, Richardson BA, Nyange PM, et al: Vaginal lactobacilli, microbial flora, and risk of human immunodeficiency virus type 1 and sexually transmitted disease acquisition. J Infect Dis 180:1863, 1999

56. Taha TE, Hoover DR, Dallabetta GA, et al: Bacterial vaginosis and disturbances of vaginal flora: association with increased acquisition of HIV. AIDS 12:1699, 1998

57. Cu-Uvin S, Hogan JW, Caliendo AM, et al: Association between bacterial vaginosis and expression of human immunodeficiency virus type 1 RNA in the female genital tract. Clin Infect Dis 33:894, 2001

58. Sorvillo F, Smith L, Kerndt P, et al: *Trichomonas vaginalis,* HIV, and African-Americans. Emerg Infect Dis 7:927, 2001

59. Wang CC, McClelland RS, Reilly M, et al: The effect of treatment of vaginal infections on shedding of human immunodeficiency virus type 1. J Infect Dis 183:1017, 2001

60. Allen-Davis JT, Beck A, Parker R, et al: Assessment of vulvovaginal complaints: accuracy of telephone triage and in-office diagnosis. Obstet Gynecol 99:18, 2002

61. Ferris DG, Nyirjesy P, Sobel JD, et al: Over-the-counter antifungal drug misuse associated with patient-diagnosed vulvovaginal candidiasis. Obstet Gynecol 99:419, 2002

62. Sobel JD: Vaginitis. N Engl J Med 337:1896, 1997

63. Hillier S, Holmes K: Bacterial vaginosis. Sexually Transmitted Diseases, 3rd ed. Holmes KK, Mårdh P-A, Sparling PF, et al, Eds. McGraw-Hill, New York, 1999, p 563

64. Eschenbach DA, Davick PR, Williams BL, et al: Prevalence of hydrogen peroxide-producing *Lactobacillus* species in normal women and women with bacterial vaginosis. J Clin Microbiol 27:251, 1989

65. Gardner H, Dukes C: *Haemophilis vaginalis vaginitis*: a newly defined specific infection previously classified as "nonspecific" vaginitis. Am J Obstet Gynecol 69:962, 1955

66. Criswell BS, Ladwig CL, Gardner HL, et al: *Haemophilus vaginalis*: vaginitis by inoculation from culture. Obstet Gynecol 33:195, 1969

67. Marrazzo JM, Koutsky LA, Eschenbach DA, et al: Characterization of vaginal flora and bacterial vaginosis in women who have sex with women. J Infect Dis 185:1307, 2002

68. Avonts D, Sercu M, Heyerick P, et al: Incidence of uncomplicated genital infections in women using oral contraception or an intrauterine device: a prospective study. Sex Transm Dis 17:23, 1990

69. Barbone F, Austin H, Louv WC, et al: A follow-up study of methods of contraception, sexual activity, and rates of trichomoniasis, candidiasis, and bacterial vaginosis. Am J Obstet Gynecol 163:510, 1990

70. Hawes SE, Hillier SL, Benedetti J, et al: Hydrogen peroxide–producing lactobacilli and acquisition of vaginal infections. J Infect Dis 174:1058, 1996

71. Amsel R, Totten PA, Spiegel CA, et al: Nonspecific vaginitis: diagnostic criteria and microbial and epidemiologic associations. Am J Med 74:14, 1983

72. Vejtorp M, Bollerup AC, Vejtorp L, et al: Bacterial vaginosis: a double-blind randomized trial of the effect of treatment of the sexual partner. Br J Obstet Gynaecol 95:920, 1988

73. Vutyavanich T, Pongsuthirak P, Vannareumol P, et al: A randomized double-blind trial of tinidazole treatment of the sexual partners of females with bacterial vaginosis. Obstet Gynecol 82:550, 1993

74. Colli E, Landoni M, Parazzini F: Treatment of male partners and recurrence of bacterial vaginosis: a randomised trial. Genitourin Med 73:267, 1997

75. Eschenbach DA, Hillier S, Critchlow C, et al: Diagnosis and clinical manifestations of bacterial vaginosis. Am J Obstet Gynecol 158:819, 1988

76. Thomason JL, Gelbart SM, Anderson RJ, et al: Statistical evaluation of diagnostic criteria for bacterial vaginosis. Am J Obstet Gynecol 162:155, 1990

77. Demographic and behavioral predictors of *Trichomonas vaginalis* infection among pregnant women. The Vaginal Infections and Prematurity Study Group.Obstet Gynecol 78:1087, 1991

78. Bowden FJ, Garnett GP: *Trichomonas vaginalis* epidemiology: parameterising and analysing a model of treatment interventions. Sex Transm Infect 76:248, 2000

79. Wolner-Hanssen P, Krieger JN, Stevens CE, et al: Clinical manifestations of vaginal trichomoniasis. JAMA 261:571, 1989

80. Krieger J, Alderete J: *Trichomonas vaginalis* and trichomoniasis. Sexually Transmitted Diseases, 3rd ed. Holmes KK, Mårdh P-A, Sparling PF, et al, Eds. McGraw-Hill, New York, 1999, p 587

81. Levi MH, Torres J, Pina C, et al: Comparison of the InPouch TV culture system and Diamond's modified medium for detection of *Trichomonas vaginalis*. J Clin Microbiol 35:3308, 1997

82. Tidwell BH, Lushbaugh WB, Laughlin MD, et al: A double-blind placebo-controlled trial of single-dose intravaginal versus single-dose oral metronidazole in the treatment of trichomonal vaginitis. J Infect Dis 170:242, 1994

83. Sobel JD, Nyirjesy P, Brown W: Tinidazole therapy for metronidazole-resistant vaginal trichomoniasis. Clin Infect Dis 33:1341, 2001

84. Geiger AM, Foxman B, Gillespie BW: The epidemiology of vulvovaginal candidiasis among university students. Am J Public Health 85:1146, 1995

85. Foxman B, Barlow R, D'Arcy H, et al: *Candida* vaginitis: self-reported incidence and associated costs. Sex Transm Dis 27:230, 2000

86. Foxman B: The epidemiology of vulvovaginal candidiasis: risk factors. Am J Public Health 80:329, 1990

87. Abbott J: Clinical and microscopic diagnosis of vaginal yeast infection: a prospective analysis. Ann Emerg Med 25:587, 1995

88. Ryan CA, Courtois BN, Hawes SE, et al: Risk assessment, symptoms, and signs as predictors of vulvovaginal and cervical infections in an urban US STD clinic: implications for use of STD algorithms. Sex Transm Infect 74(suppl 1):S59, 1998

89. Schaaf VM, Perez-Stable EJ, Borchardt K: The limited value of symptoms and signs in the diagnosis of vaginal infections. Arch Intern Med 150:1929, 1990

90. Sobel J: Vulvovaginal candidiasis. Sexually Transmitted Diseases, 3rd ed. Holmes KK, Mårdh P-A, Sparling PF, et al, Eds. McGraw-Hill, New York, 1999, p 629

91. Bertholf ME, Stafford MJ: Colonization of *Candida albicans* in vagina, rectum, and mouth. J Fam Pract 16:919, 1983

92. Sobel JD, Chaim W: Treatment of *Torulopsis glabrata* vaginitis: retrospective review of boric acid therapy. Clin Infect Dis 24:649, 1997

93. Myziuk L, Romanowski B, Brown M: Endocervical Gram stain smears and their usefulness in the diagnosis of *Chlamydia trachomatis*. Sex Transm Infect 77:103, 2001

94. Marrazzo J, Handsfield H, Whittington W: Predicting chlamydial and gonococcal cervical infection: implications for management of cervicitis. Obstet Gynecol 100:579, 2002

95. Miller HG, Cain VS, Rogers SM, et al: Correlates of sexually transmitted bacterial infections among U.S. women in 1995. Fam Plann Perspect 31:4, 1999

96. Hubacher D, Lara-Ricalde R, Taylor DJ, et al: Use of copper intrauterine devices and the risk of tubal infertility among nulligravid women. N Engl J Med 345:561, 2001

97. Westrom L, Eschenbach D: Pelvic inflammatory disease. Sexually Transmitted Diseases, 3rd ed. Holmes KK, Mårdh P-A, Sparling PF, et al, Eds. McGraw-Hill, New York, 1999, p 783

98. Cohen CR, Manhart LE, Bukusi EA, et al: Association between *Mycoplasma genitalium* and acute endometritis. Lancet 359:765, 2002

99. Kahn JG, Walker CK, Washington AE, et al: Diagnosing pelvic inflammatory disease: a comprehensive analysis and considerations for developing a new model. JAMA 266:2594, 1991

100. Peipert JF, Ness RB, Blume J, et al: Clinical predictors of endometritis in women with symptoms and signs of pelvic inflammatory disease. Am J Obstet Gynecol 184:856, 2001

101. Wolner-Hanssen P: Silent pelvic inflammatory disease: is it overstated? Obstet Gynecol 86:321, 1995

102. Munday PE: Pelvic inflammatory disease: an evidence-based approach to diagnosis. J Infect 40:31, 2000

103. Jacobson L, Westrom L: Objectivized diagnosis of acute pelvic inflammatory disease: diagnostic and prognostic value of routine laparoscopy. Am J Obstet Gynecol 105:1088, 1969

104. Eckert LO, Hawes SE, Wolner-Hanssen PK, et al: Endometritis: the clinical-pathologic syndrome. Am J Obstet Gynecol 186:690, 2002

105. Molander P, Sjoberg J, Paavonen J, et al: Transvaginal power Doppler findings in laparoscopically proven acute pelvic inflammatory disease. Ultrasound Obstet Gynecol 17:233, 2001

106. Ness RB, Soper DE, Holley RL, et al: Effectiveness of inpatient and outpatient treatment strategies for women with pelvic inflammatory disease: results from the Pelvic Inflammatory Disease Evaluation and Clinical Health (PEACH) Randomized Trial. Am J Obstet Gynecol 186:929, 2002

107. Westrom L, Joesoef R, Reynolds G, et al: Pelvic inflammatory disease and fertility: a cohort study of 1,844 women with laparoscopically verified disease and 657 control women with normal laparoscopic results. Sex Transm Dis 19:185, 1992

108. Wald A, Link K: Risk of human immunodeficiency virus infection in herpes simplex virus type 2–seropositive persons: a meta-analysis. J Infect Dis 185:45, 2002

109. Etiology of genital ulcers and prevalence of human immunodeficiency virus coinfection in 10 US cities. The Genital Ulcer Disease Surveillance Group. J Infect Dis 178:1795, 1998

110. Korenromp EL, Bakker R, De Vlas SJ, et al: Can behavior change explain increases in the proportion of genital ulcers attributable to herpes in sub-Saharan Africa? A simulation modeling study. Sex Transm Dis 29:228, 2002

111. DiCarlo RP, Martin DH: The clinical diagnosis of genital ulcer disease in men. Clin Infect Dis 25:292, 1997

112. Lafferty WE, Downey L, Celum C, et al: Herpes simplex virus type 1 as a cause of genital herpes: impact on surveillance and prevention. J Infect Dis 181:1454, 2000

113. Ashley RL: Performance and use of HSV type-specific serology test kits. Herpes 9:38, 2002

114. Benedetti J, Corey L, Ashley R: Recurrence rates in genital herpes after symptomatic first-episode infection. Ann Intern Med 121:847, 1994

115. Corey L, Wald A: Genital herpes. Sexually Transmitted Diseases, 3rd ed. Holmes KK, Mårdh P-A, Sparling PF, et al, Eds. McGraw-Hill, New York, 1999, p 285

116. Doll L, Ostrow D: Homosexual and bisexual behavior. Sexually Transmitted Diseases, 3rd ed. Holmes KK, Mårdh P-A, Sparling PF, et al, Eds. McGraw-Hill, New York, 1999, p 151

117. Mayer KH, Klausner JD, Handsfield HH: Intersecting epidemics and educable moments: sexually transmitted disease risk assessment and screening in men who have sex with men. Sex Transm Dis 28:464, 2001

118. Dukers NH, Spaargaren J, Geskus RB, et al: HIV incidence on the increase among homosexual men attending an Amsterdam sexually transmitted disease clinic: using a novel approach for detecting recent infections. AIDS 16:F19, 2002

119. Quinn TC, Stamm WE, Goodell SE, et al: The polymicrobial origin of intestinal infections in homosexual men. N Engl J Med 309:576, 1983

120. William DC, Schapiro CM, Felman YM: Pharyngeal carriage of *Neisseria meningitidis* and anogenital gonorrhea: evidence for their relationship. Sex Transm Dis 7:175, 1980

121. Deheragoda P: Diagnosis of rectal gonorrhoea by blind anorectal swabs compared with direct vision swabs taken via a proctoscope. Br J Vener Dis 53:311, 1977

11 Septic Arthritis

Brian F. Mandell, M.D., Ph.D.

Bacterial infections account for less than 20% of all cases of acute monoarticular and oligoarticular arthritis. Crystal-induced arthritis is approximately four times more common. Because septic arthritis represents a potential threat to life and limb, the possibility of infection dictates the sequence and pace of the diagnostic evaluation. This subsection reviews the clinical presentation, diagnosis, microbiology, and treatment of joint infections. Lyme disease, which can manifest as arthritis of the large joints, is discussed elsewhere [see 25 Leptospirosis, Relapsing Fever, Rat-Bite Fever, and Lyme Disease].

Epidemiology

Case series of patients with septic arthritis include increasing numbers of immunosuppressed and elderly patients with significant comorbidity. Large retrospective studies from Europe indicate a consistent male-to-female ratio of approximately 1:1, a mean age of approximately 55 years, and polyarticular involvement in up to 15% of cases.[1,2] These data are comparable to those reported from the United States,[3–5] although some clinicians' experiences may include younger patients with disseminated gonococcal or HIV infection or older patients with prosthetic joints.[6] Patients with damaged joints are at increased risk. Infection complicates 0.05% to 0.48% of arthroscopies[7]; the higher risk is associated with reconstructive or repeat procedures. In very rare cases, infection complicates arthrocentesis.

Pathogenesis

Presumably, most bacteria reach the joint via the bloodstream and the vascular synovial membrane (and, in children, the epiphyseal plate). Previously damaged joints seem to be at increased risk for infection,[1,6] which may be attributable to unique properties of certain bacteria, the neovascularization of inflamed synovial membranes, or the increased expression of adhesion molecules on activated synovial endothelial cells. Some specific *Staphylococcus* strains exhibit tropism to joints.[8] In rare instances, joints are directly infected by traumatic inoculation; this circumstance may be more common in infections involving small finger joints. Synovial reaction and biochemical changes to cartilage, attributable to products released from inflammatory cells and bacteria, occur within hours after experimental joint infection.[9] Experimental models of bacterial arthritis have shown that even if antibiotic therapy is begun within 24 hours of infection, proteoglycans are by then at least transiently depleted from cartilage. Loss of cartilage and erosion of subchondral bone may begin within days of infection and evolve into destruction of the joint. Polymorphonuclear neutrophils (PMNs) infiltrate the synovium, with subsequent recruitment of mononuclear cells.

Some studies suggest that the degree of damage is determined by several factors, including the type of infecting organism and the accumulation of PMNs and their release of proteolytic enzymes in the joint space. *Neisseria gonorrhoeae* induces only limited PMN activation in vitro, which may partially explain why minimal joint destruction is observed with this infection. Preliminary animal studies suggest that potent anti-inflammatory therapy with corticosteroids, in conjunction with appropriate antimicrobial therapy, may reduce cartilage destruction.[10,11] These observations have not yet been translated into clinical practice. Consistent with animal data, a delay in the initiation of treatment has been found to be a major determinant of poorer outcome in several studies.[1]

Diagnosis of Septic Arthritis

HISTORY

A thorough history remains a key element in the diagnosis of septic arthritis. Pertinent features include acute onset of joint pain or a change in the pattern of chronic joint pain, a history of joint disease or trauma, a history of prodromal extra-articular symptoms suggestive of bacteremia, any comorbid immunosuppression, intravenous drug use or prior intravenous catheterization, presence of sexually transmitted diseases (STDs), and geographic location (e.g., in the case of Lyme disease). A complaint of sudden onset of articular or periarticular pain should never be ignored, especially if the pain is present both when the joint is at rest and when it is in motion. Because joint infections are uncommon, patients and physicians may incorrectly attribute the pain to trauma or overuse syndromes, particularly in the case of shoulder pain.

The presence of fever is not necessary for the diagnosis of septic arthritis in adults [1–4,12] or in children.[13] Fever may be present in fewer than 60% of patients with nongonococcal septic arthritis. Rigors may be present in only 20% of patients.[12] High spiking fevers (> 39° C [102.2° F]) and rigors can also occur in patients with crystal-induced arthritis.[14] Thus, systemic features are neither sensitive enough nor specific enough to warrant a diagnosis of septic arthritis without examination of the synovial fluid.

PHYSICAL EXAMINATION

Detailed physical examination is warranted in all cases of possible septic arthritis, as in any patient with a possible systemic infection. The pattern of joint involvement and the presence of tendinitis or enthesitis should be noted, as should any inflammation of the eyes, skin, or mucosae. The latter finding suggests the possibility of a reactive arthritis. Pain with passive motion of a joint or palpation of the joint capsule, in the absence of trauma, suggests synovitis. Mild to moderate swelling of an infected hip or shoulder is usually not detectable by examination. Septic bursitis, most commonly affecting the prepatellar or olecranon bursae,[15] must be distinguished from arthritis by clinical examination. Septic olecranon and prepatellar bursitis, which are common, are often associated with a peculiar periarticular, often pitting, edema. A complete joint examination should be undertaken, with specific attention paid to the sternoclavicular, sacroiliac, and midfoot joints. In the absence of risk factors for osteomyelitis or stress fractures, exquisite tenderness of the midfoot should raise suspicion for gouty arthritis. Psoriatic arthritis may mimic a septic joint; thus, even trivial skin involvement should be noted. Potential portals of infection (e.g., prior I.V. access sites) should be sought out meticulously.

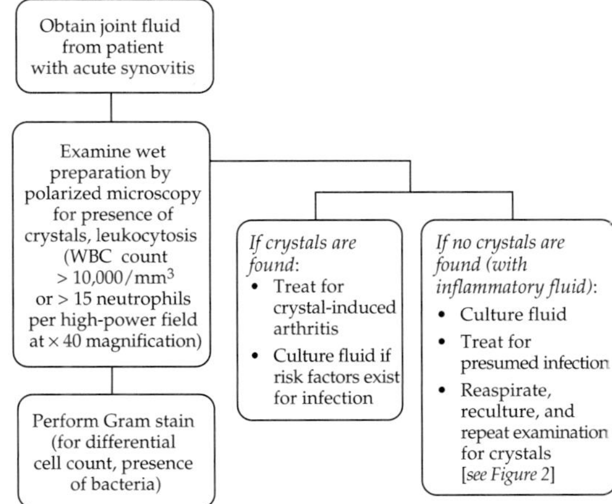

Figure 1 **Algorithm for rapid evaluation of patients with acute monoarticular arthritis on the basis of synovial fluid analysis.**

LABORATORY TESTS

Synovial fluid leukocyte count, polarized microscopy, Gram stain, and culture are the most important laboratory investigations in the diagnosis of septic arthritis. Acutely or painfully swollen joints should be aspirated [*see Figures 1 and 2*]. Peripheral blood leukocytosis[12,14] and neutrophilia, synovial fluid glucose, mucin clot test, and elevated acute-phase reactants are of insufficient sensitivity and specificity to confirm or exclude the diagnosis of septic arthritis. Synovial fluid leukocytosis and neutrophilia are invariably present in septic arthritis, but their presence does not distinguish between infection-induced and crystal-induced arthritis.[16] Most infected joint fluids have a striking degree of leukocytosis. Synovial or bursal fluid may be infected, with a synovial white blood cell (WBC) count of greater than 10,000/mm^3, although on differential counts, more than 85% of cells are almost always neutrophils.[3,16] A rapid approximation of the WBC count can be obtained by microscopic examination of a drop of synovial fluid (magnification: × 40), estimating that each WBC represents 500 WBC/mm^3.

Gram stain and culture of synovial fluid should be performed in all cases of suspected septic arthritis [*see Table 1*]. A Gram stain will permit evaluation of the percentage of PMNs, but it is not sensitive (< 60%) for the presence of bacteria.[2,3,16] Gonococci are observed infrequently. Antibiotic-containing culture plates should not be utilized, and samples must be delivered promptly to the laboratory. In the absence of prior antibiotic therapy, synovial

Reaspirate, reculture, and repeat examination for crystals as often as necessary. At 5 days, perform the following procedures if synovitis persists.

If initial joint cultures are positive:

- Continue drainage and antibiotic therapy on the basis of sensitivities
- Consider surgical drainage, especially if cell count does not diminish, fevers persist without documentation of extra-articular infection, or joint cultures remain positive despite appropriate antibiotic therapy
- Exclude osteomyelitis
- Consider adding anti-inflammatory therapy if some improvement has been documented
- Begin gentle mobilization of joint

If initial joint cultures are negative, with no crystals:

- Exclude osteomyelitis
- Perform *Borrelia* titers and Western blot testing if exposure to Lyme disease is possible
- Consider mycobacterial infection (culture/PCR)
- Consider synovial biopsy if tuberculosis, sarcoidosis, or tumor is suspected
- Administer empirical anti-inflammatory therapy
- Consider diagnosis of psoriasis, inflammatory bowel disease, reactive arthritis, spondylitis, partially treated infection, or gonococcal infection
- Obtain radiographs if symptoms do not respond to anti-inflammatory therapy

If crystals are seen on repeat polarized microscopy:

- Administer anti-inflammatory therapy
- Continue antibiotics until final cultures are negative
- Obtain radiographs if symptoms do not respond to anti-inflammatory therapy

Figure 2 **Approach for patients with persistent monoarticular arthritis on the basis of synovial fluid analysis.**

fluid culture remains the gold standard for the diagnosis of nongonococcal joint infection. Synovial biopsy may have a slightly greater yield of positive cultures, but it is infrequently performed. There is insufficient evidence to recommend routine biopsy.

Blood cultures should be obtained, as should cultures of any other potential extra-articular source of infection. If gonococcal infection is suspected, workup should include rectal, cervical, urethral, and pharyngeal cultures—any of which may be positive, even in the absence of local symptoms.[17] Cultures and Gram stain of any suspicious skin lesions should be obtained, although these are usually sterile.

A wet preparation of synovial fluid should be examined by polarized microscopy for the presence of crystals. Crystal arthropathy and septic arthritis may coexist; thus, the presence of crystals does not rule out septic arthritis.[5,18] A few crystals

Table 1 Likely Causes of Septic Arthritis on the Basis of Gram Stain and Patient Demographics

Findings on Gram Stain	*Patient Characteristics*	*Organism(s) of Concern*
No bacteria	Healthy and young	Gonococci, staphylococci
No bacteria	Presence of rheumatoid arthritis	Staphylococci
No bacteria	Significant immunosuppression, intravenous drug use, or recent hospitalization with possible gram-negative infection	Staphylococci, streptococci, *Pseudomonas* (fungal infection much less likely)
No bacteria	Intermittent synovitis of large joint, in an area endemic for Lyme disease	*Borrelia*
No bacteria or gram-negative bacilli	Recent cat or dog bite	*Pasteurella multocida*
Gram-positive bacilli	No specific features	Staphylococci, streptococci
Gram-negative diplococci	No specific features	Gonococci; consider meningococcemia
Gram-negative bacilli	No specific features	Treat for possible *Pseudomonas* infection
Gram-negative bacilli	Presence of systemic lupus erythematosus or sickle cell anemia	Include coverage for *Salmonella*, as well as for *Pseudomonas*
No bacteria	Patient has a prosthetic joint	*Staphylococcus epidermidis, S. aureus* (possibly methicillin-resistant strains)
No bacteria	Exposure to freshwater or saltwater, especially with any injury; chronic joint swelling	*Mycobacterium marinum*

can be found in synovial fluids from asymptomatic patients with a history of gout. If crystals are observed, patients are generally treated for crystalline arthritis alone, unless there is real suspicion of coexistent infection. Hence, synovial fluid cultures should be obtained even when crystals are observed, especially if there is any suspicion of current or recent infection or if the use of therapeutic intra-articular corticosteroid injections is anticipated. Some clinicians order a bacterial culture for all inflammatory synovial fluids, even if crystals are observed. Local laboratory policy may dictate synovial fluid culture technique, but several preliminary studies suggest that the diagnostic yield may be improved with direct inoculation of fluid into blood culture vials or isolator tubes.

A potential advance in diagnostic testing has been the development of polymerase chain reaction (PCR) techniques for detection of bacterial DNA within synovial fluid and tissue.[19] PCR has been used to diagnose the presence of *Chlamydia* and *Yersinia* organisms and the presence of *Borrelia burgdorferi*, *N. gonorrhoeae*, and *Ureaplasma urealyticum* DNA in synovial fluids. Caution must be used, however, when interpreting the results of PCR analyses. Contamination with minute amounts of DNA can cause false positive results. The test also does not distinguish between the presence of live and dead organisms. Once better standardized, PCR may be useful in diagnosing gonococcal, mycobacterial, and partially treated bacterial infections, which are not rapidly diagnosed by routine culture methods.

The serum uric acid level should absolutely not be used to diagnose or exclude gouty arthritis; the level may be low, normal, or high at the time of a gout attack. Autoimmune serologies (e.g., antinuclear antibody and rheumatoid factor) are of no value in the initial management of patients with acute monoarticular arthritis. The erythrocyte sedimentation rate (ESR) or C-reactive protein (CRP) level may be helpful in monitoring response to treatment in some patients, particularly those with polyarticular or axial joint infections (in whom it can be difficult to assess reduction in local inflammation by physical examination). Although these approaches have not been tested in this setting, CRP has been shown to be of value in monitoring patients with bacterial endocarditis.[20] The ESR may be normal in patients with septic arthritis.[1,2,12]

DIAGNOSTIC IMAGING

In the absence of trauma, radiographs are of limited utility in the diagnosis of acute synovitis. Radiographs are useful when there is clinical suspicion of chronic osteomyelitis, osteonecrosis, or pathologic or insufficiency fracture. Sequential radiographs are useful in evaluating a patient for development of osteomyelitis. Ultrasound imaging is occasionally useful in documenting hip effusions in children or effusions in other joints with abnormal anatomy caused by prior mechanical or inflammatory trauma. Patients with suspected sternoclavicular or sacroiliac joint infections should have a computed tomography or magnetic resonance imaging scan performed to evaluate for mediastinal or pelvic extension. Because of its superior soft tissue imaging properties, MRI is useful for evaluation of periarticular abscesses and soft tissue infections (e.g., psoas abscess mimicking septic arthritis of the hip and subdeltoid bursitis communicating with the shoulder joint). MRI can detect abnormal marrow signal secondary to osteomyelitis or avascular necrosis but may not help in distinguishing between septic and noninfectious inflammatory synovitis.[21]

Radionuclide bone scans are sensitive early indicators of changes in periarticular bone metabolism. In a study comparing the use of a technetium-99 (^{99m}Tc) scan with the clinical gold standard of synovial fluid culture in patients with septic arthritis, ^{99m}Tc scanning had a sensitivity of 100%.[22] Radionuclide scans are not specific enough to establish a diagnosis. Scanning with ^{99m}Tc is helpful in differentiating bone from adjacent soft tissue inflammation.[23]

Gallium-67 (^{67}Ga) localizes to areas of inflammation and increased bone metabolism. In cases of septic arthritis related to intravenous drug use, ^{67}Ga scans show positive results several days before ^{99m}Tc scans do. The ^{67}Ga scan has been largely replaced by the indium-111 (^{111}In) leukocyte scan. Although less sensitive than ^{99m}Tc, ^{111}In is thought to be more specific for joint infection than either ^{99m}Tc or ^{67}Ga, because leukocytes do not normally migrate to areas of increased bone metabolism associated with aseptic processes. No radionuclide scan will reliably distinguish between infection-induced and crystal-induced arthritis.

In the vast majority of patients with septic arthritis, especially those from whom synovial fluid can be obtained, radionuclide imaging studies are unnecessary.

Differential Diagnosis of Acute Arthritis

In the patient with acute monoarticular or oligoarticular arthritis, the clinician must promptly distinguish between crystal-induced arthritis and infection-induced arthritis, because the initial treatment of these two conditions is strikingly different. The diagnostic test of choice is synovial fluid analysis. Acutely inflamed or swollen, painful joints, in the absence of obvious trauma, should be aspirated. A single drop of fluid—even the small amount in the hub of the needle of an apparently unsuccessful arthrocentesis—may be sufficient to establish a diagnosis of crystal-induced arthritis. Wet preparation can provide an initial cell count estimate and a polarized microscopic evaluation for crystals. The fluid sample should then be air-dried and a Gram stain performed to both screen for bacteria and calculate the percentage of PMNs. The inability to demonstrate eosinophils by use of this stain technique is rarely of importance.

Specific Infectious Agents

Causative pathogens are documented by culture in approximately two thirds of presumed septic arthritis cases in most series, and identification rates as high as 93% have been reported. A source of the infection is identified in only half of the cases. In a retrospective study, a portal of entry was identified in 95 of 179 patients; 25% of the infections were iatrogenic, 75% extra-articular. Most were cutaneous, respiratory, and genitourinary infections.[2]

Traditionally, bacterial arthritis is divided into nongonococcal and gonococcal types. The distinction is clinically useful because gonococcal infections have a better prognosis than nongonococcal infections. Viral arthritis, which tends to have a self-limited course (except in some cases induced by parvovirus and hepatitis B or C), will not be discussed in this subsection.

NEISSERIA GONORRHOEAE

In some settings, disseminated gonococcal infection (DGI) is a relatively common cause of septic arthritis and tenosynovitis in healthy, sexually active patients. In a review of 41 cases of gonococcal arthritis, 83% of patients were female, and the mean age was 23 years.[17] Knee synovitis was present in 54% of the patients, followed in frequency by hand and wrist synovitis. Involvement of the hip, but not the spine, is common. Dermatitis (usually sparse peripheral necrotic pustules) and migratory polyarthralgia/polyarthritis were present in 39% and 66% of the patients, respectively. Along with tenosynovitis, these findings constitute the classic triad of DGI. Genitourinary involvement was noted in 63% of the patients but may be asymptomatic in women. Absence of pelvic inflammatory disease does not exclude a diagnosis of DGI. Rectal and pharyngeal colonization are commonly asymptomatic; these sites, as well as blood, should be routinely cultured in all patients suspected of having DGI. Female genital infection may have occurred long before systemic dissemination. The frequency of positive cultures in one study of DGI was as follows: urogenital, 86%; synovial fluid, 44%; rectal, 39%; blood, 13%; and pharyngeal, 7%.[17]

Arthritis and vasculitic skin lesions may reflect local metastatic infection or a sterile inflammation induced by immune complexes. This dual pathophysiology may partially account for both the low frequency of positive joint cultures and the favorable joint outcome. Data compiled by the Centers for Disease Control and Prevention indicate that up to 33% of gonococcal isolates obtained in STD clinics in the United States are resistant to penicillin or tetracycline. Resistant strains are capable of systemic dissemination. There have been no reports thus far of resistance to ceftriaxone or ciprofloxacin; therefore, initial therapy should include parenteral therapy with one of these drugs. Appropriate initial regimens include ceftriaxone (2 g intramuscularly or intravenously once daily), imipenem (0.5 g intravenously every 6 hours), or cefotaxime (1 g intravenously every 8 hours until 24 to 48 hours after resolution of symptoms). Subsequent outpatient therapy should be continued with ciprofloxacin (500 mg orally b.i.d.) or ampicillin (500 to 1,000 mg orally q.i.d.), if sensitivities are available. Documented infection should prompt an evaluation for other STDs, including syphilis and HIV. Empirical treatment for *Chlamydia trachomatis* infection (doxycycline, 100 mg orally b.i.d. for 7 days, or azithromycin, 1 g orally in a single dose) should be given. Dosages may need to be modified in the presence of severe renal insufficiency.

A dermatitis-arthritis syndrome, similar to DGI, can also be associated with *Haemophilus influenzae*, *N. meningitidis*, *Streptobacillus moniliformis* infection, or bacterial endocarditis.

STAPHYLOCOCCUS

Gram-positive bacteria remain the most common cause of septic arthritis, accounting for 70% to 80% of cases. *S. aureus* accounts for more than half of the cases of culture-positive septic arthritis in studies at university hospitals and for even higher percentages of certain patient subgroups: 70% to 80% of patients with polyarticular septic arthritis; more than 80% of infected RA patients[24]; and 82%

of infected hemodialysis patients.[25] Staphylococcal arthritis was particularly frequent in a series of patients with endocarditis related to intravenous drug abuse.[26] The predominance of *S. aureus* in septic arthritis has remained unchanged over the past 40 years,[1] and there is now an increasing prevalence of methicillin-resistant *S. aureus* (MRSA) and *S. epidermidis* in patients with prosthetic joints. *S. aureus* should always be considered when selecting antibiotics in the initial treatment of presumed septic arthritis. Gram stain cannot be relied on to differentiate between *Staphylococcus* and *Streptococcus*, because in biologic smears, *Staphylococcus* may not exhibit the clusters seen when grown in vitro. Bacteremia should be assumed in cases of staphylococcal arthritis, although it cannot always be documented. Endovascular infection with possible metastatic seeding to other areas should be considered in patients with persistent fever, leukocytosis, thrombocytosis, or an elevated ESR or CRP level. Suspected staphylococcal joint infection should be treated initially with vancomycin (1 g intravenously every 12 hours, if renal function is normal) until methicillin resistance can be excluded. On the basis of sensitivities, an appropriate penicillin or a cephalosporin can often be substituted for completion of a 4- to 6-week treatment course.

STREPTOCOCCUS

Non–group A, β-hemolytic streptococci are the second most common cause of septic arthritis, accounting for 10% to 21% of culture-positive cases.[1–3] The number of reported group B (and to a lesser extent, groups C and G) streptococcal infections has been increasing.[27] Group B streptococcal infection may be particularly virulent in diabetic patients and involve axial joints (sacroiliac, sternoclavicular, and manubriosternal) and poor functional outcome. Other manifestations of group B streptococcal sepsis include myositis, fasciitis, and endophthalmitis. Some investigators have expressed concern over development of tolerance to penicillin in these usually penicillin-sensitive organisms and have suggested adding an aminoglycoside to therapy or using alternative antibiotics until sensitivity and bactericidal tests are available. *S. pneumoniae* may account for up to 10% of the cases of septic arthritis. In one study, 11% of patients with septic arthritis requiring transfer to the intensive care unit had pneumococcal infection.[5] Polyarticular pneumococcal infections occur, which is not surprising given the high incidence of bacteremia in patients with pneumococcal pneumonia. Elderly adults may be particularly susceptible, and fever or an extra-articular source of infection may not be evident.[28] Antibiotic therapy must be tailored with knowledge of local resistance patterns. *Enterococci* can occasionally infect native or prosthetic joints.[29]

Initial therapy, on the basis of a Gram stain or preliminary culture showing gram-positive cocci, can reasonably be vancomycin (1 g every 12 hours, with normal renal function). The incidence of penicillin-resistant streptococci, including *S. pneumoniae*, is rising. Definitive therapy can then be determined on the basis of culture results.

GRAM-NEGATIVE ORGANISMS

Gram-negative organisms account for 9% to 20% of septic arthritis cases reported at teaching hospitals and occur most frequently in immunosuppressed patients.[1–4] Although certain pathogens have been associated with specific patient subgroups (e.g., *Salmonella* in patients with systemic lupus erythematosus or sickle cell anemia, *Pseudomonas aeruginosa* in intravenous drug abusers), joint infections with these organisms can occur in immunocompetent patients. In sickle cell patients, *Salmonella* more commonly causes osteomyelitis than septic arthritis and may infect multiple sites.[30]

Comorbid medical conditions, prior antibiotic use, and extra-articular infections (particularly urinary tract infections and decubitus ulcers) predispose to gram-negative septic arthritis. Reviews of septic arthritis in intravenous drug abusers over the past decade report a lower percentage of gram-negative pathogens than were reported in earlier series, in which organisms such as *Enterobacter, Klebsiella, Serratia*, and *P. aeruginosa* accounted for more than 80% of infections.[26] Pathogens and sensitivities associated with intravenous drug abuse are region-specific. This same population is also at risk for HIV and viral hepatitis.

Ampicillin is bactericidal for *Salmonella*; however, an increasing number of *Salmonella* infections are resistant to this drug. Chloramphenicol, trimethoprim-sulfamethoxazole, and especially quinolones are used as alternative agents.[30] For other gram-negative infections, cefotaxime (2 g intravenously every 6 hours) or imipenem (0.5 g intravenously every 6 hours) can be used with or without an aminoglycoside until culture results arrive. If pseudomonal infection is suspected, it is reasonable to initiate dual drug therapy, including an aminoglycoside.

ANAEROBES

Anaerobic joint infections are rare, accounting for at most 7% of cases in reported series; however, they should be considered in patients with deep-tissue or abdominal abscesses. Intra-articular emphysema has been described with anaerobic infection (*Clostridium* species) but is not specific to anaerobes.[31] Empirical treatment for anaerobic septic arthritis is generally not undertaken unless there is a coincident infection with a high likelihood of anaerobic involvement. In those cases, treatment should be based on the suspected organisms and the portal of infection (oral, abdominal, or traumatic).

UREAPLASMA UREALYTICUM

Ureaplasma urealyticum septic arthritis has been reported in hypogammaglobulinemic patients. These patients, who are often already receiving γ-globulin replacement therapy, may develop a destructive monoarthritis, oligoarthritis, or, in rare instances, polyarthritis[32] with fever and subcutaneous nodules. Positive cultures from affected synovial fluid or tissue are notoriously difficult to obtain. PCR now offers the potential for rapid, definitive diagnosis. Eradication of the infection may require several months of tetracycline therapy. Although rapid recognition and treatment have resulted in complete remission,[33] not all patients respond. The microbiology laboratory should be alerted to the possibility of this infection before fluid samples are taken for culture.

This destructive *U. urealyticum* septic arthritis should be distinguished from the rheumatoid-like, but generally nonerosive, sterile polyarthritis associated with hypogammaglobulinemia. Initial treatment of acute-onset arthritis in this setting should include both tetracycline and aggressive intravenous immunoglobulin replacement until *Ureaplasma* infection is excluded.

PASTEURELLA MULTOCIDA

Pasteurella multocida, a pleomorphic gram-negative coccobacillus parasitic to many cats and dogs, is an infrequent cause of septic arthritis.[34] Infection generally follows inoculation from an animal bite, although in one third of cases no trauma is documented. The organism is almost always sensitive to a penicillin; aminoglycosides are generally ineffective. Initial antibiotic coverage after a recent animal bite should include a penicillin or a third-generation cephalosporin. Ampicillin-sulbactam (1.5 g intravenously every 6 hours) and ceftriaxone (2 g intravenously q.d.) are reasonable initial therapies pending final culture results.

MYCOBACTERIUM MARINUM

Mycobacterium marinum is an atypical mycobacterium acquired through exposure to freshwater, saltwater, swimming pools, or fish tanks. *M. marinum* usually causes cutaneous and subcutaneous infection but may result in subcutaneous nodules, tenosynovitis, and septic arthritis.[35,36] Monoarticular, often proliferative, involvement of the metacarpophalangeal and proximal interphalangeal joints is most frequently reported. The arthritis may be only slightly painful with no systemic symptoms. Delays in diagnosis are common (mean, 8 months). Optimal growth of the organism from synovial fluid or tissue requires special attention in the microbiology laboratory. *M. marinum* infection may elicit a positive purified protein derivative (PPD) reaction. Treatment usually consists of prolonged chemotherapy and surgical debridement. There are no evidence-based guidelines to aid in determining the need for initial surgical debridement, although this procedure is frequently utilized, especially when the course of infection is protracted. A reasonable initial therapy is rifampin and ethambutol in combination, although treatment with trimethoprim-sulfamethoxazole or ciprofloxacin may also be effective. Although there are no data demonstrating the superiority of combination therapy, treatment failures with doxycycline monotherapy have been reported. The organisms are usually sensitive to amikacin and clarithromycin.

MYCOBACTERIUM TUBERCULOSIS

Arthritis is an uncommon extrapulmonary complication of tuberculosis[37,38]; osteomyelitis of the low thoracic and lumbar spine occurs more frequently.[39] Recognition of tuberculous peripheral joint and bursa infections are often significantly delayed, partly because of the indolent nature of the inflammation, the rarity of the disease, and the frequent absence of obvious pulmonary disease or a positive PPD test.[37] Although joint motion is frequently maintained, radiographs may show destruction of bone and loss of cartilage. Synovial fluid leukocytosis is modest to marked, usually with a predominance of neutrophils. Acid-fast staining of fluid is usually negative; cultures are usually positive (79%). Limited data suggest that biopsy of synovium yields a higher percentage of positive cultures (94%). Because *M. tuberculosis* is a rare cause of peripheral arthritis, it is not cost-effective to obtain mycobacterial cultures initially from all patients with acute synovitis. Because microbiologic diagnosis takes several weeks, molecular diagnostic tests for *M. tuberculosis* DNA should be requested if there is a significant clinical concern for this infection. No large studies have been undertaken to compare diagnostic approaches or treatment regimens for tuberculous arthritis. The potential for developing drug resistance exists as it does in therapy for pulmonary tuberculosis; thus, initial therapy should include a combination of at least two drugs, including rifampin (600 mg/day), isoniazid (300 mg/day), and perhaps ethambutol (15 mg/kg/day) for the first few months of a planned 18- to 24-month course of treatment.

TREPONEMA PALLIDUM

The arthritis associated with later stages of syphilis is characteristically a chronic, proliferative, symmetrical polyarthritis involving small and large joints.[40] An acute monoarthritis is not typical of syphilis. Synovial fluid usually contains a predominance of mononuclear cells. Treatment should be based on the stage of disease (usually secondary or tertiary) and the presence or absence of HIV infection [see 24 Syphilis and Nonvenereal Treponematoses]. Penicillin remains the antibiotic of choice, although ceftriaxone or doxycycline may be used in some patients without HIV infection.

FUNGAL INFECTIONS

Fungal arthritis is rare and is seemingly more common in immunosuppressed patients. The arthritis is usually subacute or chronic. Osteomyelitis is more common than arthritis in *Cryptococcus, Coccidioides*, and blastomycosis infections.[41,42] Arthritis associated with histoplasmosis may occur with erythema nodosum and clinically mimic sarcoidosis. Arthritis caused by aspergillosis infection has been reported after systemic infection and iatrogenic inoculation at the time of arthrocentesis. Sporotrichosis arthritis can occur after cutaneous inoculation or, in rare cases, through inhalation.[43] Surgical debridement may be helpful; there are limited data, however, to support initial surgery in addition to antifungal therapy. Except in cases of local inoculation (e.g., rose thorn sporotrichosis), the fungal infection is generally assumed to be systemic, and intravenous amphotericin B should be administered. Intra-articular amphotericin B and oral regimens with azole antibiotics have been utilized. These alternative agents and routes of administration should be considered on an individual basis; consultation with an infectious disease specialist should take place early in the treatment program.

Clinical Subgroups at Risk for Septic Arthritis

Several factors predispose certain groups of patients to septic arthritis. Local risk factors include the presence of inflammatory arthritis, prior intra-articular corticosteroid injection, and the presence of implanted synthetic material.[6] Other factors include advanced age, a remote focus of infection, diabetes mellitus, indwelling lines, intravenous drug use, and immunosuppression.

ELDERLY PATIENTS

Age older than 60 years has been repeatedly found to be a risk factor for septic arthritis, perhaps in part because of comorbid conditions.[1,6] Prosthetic joints, which also pose an increased risk of infection, are more common in older patients.

The clinical presentation of septic arthritis tends to be more insidious in elderly patients than in younger patients. The absence of fever is common.[28] Older patients are particularly at risk for septic arthritis as a postoperative complication, often after a bacteremic episode. In a retrospective study of 21 patients older than 60 years with septic arthritis, mortality was 21%.[2]

RHEUMATOID ARTHRITIS PATIENTS

Patients with rheumatoid arthritis (RA) have consistently accounted for a disproportionate percentage of patients with septic arthritis; in some series, 50% of septic arthritis patients had RA. These patients may be predisposed to septic arthritis because of poor clearance of bacteria from abnormal joints or because of phagocytic defects acquired secondary to drugs or disease. Patients with long-standing, severe RA are more likely to develop septic arthritis than patients with less severe disease. The majority of RA patients with septic arthritis present with insidious worsening of joint symptoms, and the diagnosis of infection is often delayed.[24] Although there have been reports of so-called pseudoseptic rheumatoid joints characterized by highly inflammatory, sterile synovial fluids that improve with antirheumatic therapy, any isolated, acutely inflamed joint in a patient with RA should be considered infected until proved otherwise.

With septic arthritis, the outcome is significantly worse for RA patients than nonrheumatoid patients, perhaps because of delays in diagnosis. Reported mortality for RA patients with monoarticular infection has ranged from 15% to 22%. When both monoarticular and polyarticular infections are included, mortality reaches 44% in RA patients, compared with 26% in unselected septic arthritis patients. For patients with a combination of polyarticular septic arthritis and RA, mortality is 50%. Joint outcome is also poor; only 35% of RA patients achieve full functional recovery of the infected joint, compared with 70% of nonrheumatoid patients. A retrospective literature review of 181 RA patients reported recurrence of infection in nonprosthetic joints in 20% of patients.[24]

INTRAVENOUS DRUG ABUSERS

Intravenous drug abusers are at risk for repetitive transient bacteremia as well as direct bacterial inoculation of soft tissue. Bacteremia is thought to be the most common mechanism of infection. Although medium to large joints (such as the wrist and knee) are most commonly involved, fibrocartilaginous joints (sternoclavicular, sacroiliac) and the spine are frequently infected. Gram-positive organisms (especially *S. aureus* and MRSA) are the most common pathogens,[26] followed by gram-negative bacteria (*Enterobacter, Serratia,* and *P. aeruginosa*).

Not all studies of septic arthritis in intravenous drug abusers have specified whether the patients were also HIV positive. Two Spanish studies, one with 25 patients and one with 16 patients, reported no differences in clinical characteristics, infecting organisms, or outcome between intravenous drug abusers with HIV and those without HIV.[44]

HEMODIALYSIS PATIENTS

Hemodialysis patients are at increased risk for septic arthritis because of recurrent vascular infections, intravenous catheterizations, repeated skin trauma, and immune deficits such as decreased clearance of transient bacteremia. Hemodialysis patients are at particularly high risk for *S. aureus* colonization, with reported nasal carriage rates over 40%.

A 10-year review of hemodialysis patients in three tertiary care hospitals identified 11 episodes of septic arthritis, with 82% attributable to *S. aureus.*[25] Almost all of the episodes involved joints above the diaphragm, including one sternoclavicular and one acromioclavicular joint infection.

HIV PATIENTS

Two articular syndromes unique to HIV-infected patients have been reported that can mimic acute septic arthritis. The first, which has been referred to as AIDS-associated arthritis, is characterized by the development over several days of extreme pain and disability involving the knees or ankles, noninflammatory sterile synovial fluid, and an excellent response to nonsteroidal anti-inflammatory drugs (NSAIDs). The reported duration of symptoms is 1 to 6 weeks. The second syndrome, the painful articular syndrome, is characterized by an explosive onset of pain in the shoulders and elbows. The pain resembles gout in its intensity and often requires intravenous narcotics for analgesia. Synovial fluid is noninflammatory, and symptoms last a few hours to several days. The etiology of these syndromes remains unknown.

Despite the multiple immune deficits associated with HIV infection, there have been relatively few reported cases of septic arthritis in patients with HIV. *S. aureus* and *S. pneumoniae* are the most commonly reported organisms.[45] With an increasing degree of $CD4^+$ T cell depletion, infection with *Candida albicans, Cryptococcus neoformans, Histoplasma capsulatum, Nocardia asteroides,* and *Sporothrix schenckii* can occur. HIV patients are also at increased risk for pyomyositis, most commonly secondary to *S. aureus.*[45]

ORGAN TRANSPLANTATION PATIENTS

A review of the University of Pennsylvania renal transplant experience reported the occurrence of septic arthritis in 0.8% of the patient population.[46] All cases occurred within 18 months of transplantation, the period of most intense immunosuppression with high-dose steroids. Infection was caused by bacteria in 66% of cases (half of which were caused by *S. aureus*), mycobacteria in 17%, and disseminated cytomegalovirus infection in 17%. Only three cases of fungal arthritis have been reported in renal transplant patients, but this incidence is likely underreported. With the current ubiquitous use of cyclosporine, gouty arthritis (occasionally polyarticular with atypical joint involvement) is extremely common and may mimic septic arthritis.[47]

INDIVIDUALS WITH PROSTHETIC JOINTS

Prosthetic joint infections, in the absence of wound drainage, are frequently not recognized early and may result in a nonfunctional joint with chronic osteomyelitis. Pain is the predominant or only symptom.[48] Effusions may be small (knee) or impossible to detect clinically (hip or shoulder). Fever and leukocytosis are frequently absent. In studies, *S. epidermidis* was responsible for approximately 40% of both early postoperative and late infections.[48] Although the ESR is usually elevated, it may be normal.[49,50] One study demonstrated a sensitivity of only 60% when an ESR threshold greater than 30 mm/hr was used.[49] The C-reactive protein may be a more sensitive test.[50] Three-phase bone scans are also surprisingly insensitive.[50] If loosening is noted on standard radiographs, bone

Table 2 Initial Empirical Antibiotic Therapy for Acute Septic Arthritis in Adults*

Findings on Gram Stain	*Drug of Choice*	*Alternative Drug*	*Comments*
Gram-positive cocci (small) in pairs and chains	Vancomycin, 1.0 g I.V. every 12 hr†	Cefotaxime, 2.0 g I.V. every 6–8 hr	Smear suggests streptococci or pneumococci; if only single cocci are observed or if cocci are large, treat as for *Staphylococcus aureus* (see next entry)
Gram-positive cocci (large) singly or in small groups	Vancomycin, 1.0 g I.V. every 12 hr	Nafcillin, 2.0 g I.V. every 4 hr, or oxacillin, 2.0 g I.V. every 4 hr‡	Assume that penicillinase-producing *S. aureus* and, possibly, methicillin-resistant strains are present
Gram-negative cocci	Ceftriaxone, 2.0 g I.V. every 24 hr	Imipenem, 0.5 g I.V. every 6 hr	Usually *Neisseria* species; treat with third-generation cephalosporin or imipenem in documented or suspected cases of infections caused by penicillin-resistant *Neisseria* species
Gram-negative bacilli	Cefotaxime, 2.0 g I.V. every 6 hr§	Imipenem, 0.5 g I.V. every 6 hr	Antibiotic susceptibility testing mandatory; fluoroquinolones may be of value
No organisms seen			
Healthy, young patient	Ceftriaxone, 2.0 g I.V. every 24 hr with or without cephalothin, 1 g I.V. every 8 hr; use vancomycin if methicillin-resistant strains are a possibility	Imipenem, 0.5 g I.V. every 6 hr	Probably gonococcal disease, but initial therapy should also treat gram-positive cocci
Patient with underlying disease (e.g., neoplasm, rheumatoid arthritis, intravenous drug use) or immunosuppression	Vancomycin, 1.0 g I.V. every 12 hr, and ciprofloxacin, 400 mg I.V. every 12 hr	Imipenem, 0.5 g I.V. every 6 hr	Broad-spectrum coverage for staphylococci and many types of gram-negative bacilli§

*These recommendations are for nonallergic patients with normal renal function. *Final antibiotic choice should be determined by culture result.* Refer to Table 1 and to text for other special situations.

†Sensitivity of *S. pneumoniae* to penicillin should not be assumed. In geographic areas where penicillin-resistant pneumococcus is not present, a penicillin can be used.

‡It is imperative to document that staphylococci are sensitive to nafcillin or to oxacillin.

§In neutropenic patients or in patients at risk for *Pseudomonas* infection, consider using an aminoglycoside and either ceftazidime or piperacillin.

scanning is of little additional diagnostic value. Arthrocentesis or intraoperative tissue sampling with culture, before antibiotic therapy, remains the gold standard for diagnosis. The value of fluid Gram stain is still debated.[50] Knee replacement can be repeated in some patients as a two-step procedure. Total debridement, followed by 4 to 6 weeks of systemic antibiotic therapy before attempted repeat arthroplasty, is frequently successful.[51]

Treatment for Septic Arthritis

DRAINAGE

Treatment of septic arthritis consists of drainage, parenteral antibiotics (guided by Gram stain, if possible [*see Table 1*]), and initial (not prolonged) joint immobilization for pain control. The controversy surrounding medical versus surgical drainage remains unresolved. A retrospective analysis by Broy and Schmid included pooled data from 80 studies.[52] A slightly larger number of patients who were treated medically (needle drainage) rather than surgically (arthrotomy or arthroscopy) had a good joint outcome (66% versus 57% [$P < 0.05$]) with restoration of normal joint function and minimal residual pain. Perhaps because of increased systemic comorbidity in the medically treated cohort, an inherent problem in nonrandomized studies, medically treated patients had a higher mortality (10% versus 3%; $P < 0.05$). These nonrandomized studies do not permit generation of firm therapeutic guidelines.

Clinicians generally agree that surgical drainage is indicated in the following situations: septic arthritis of the hip or of joints that are difficult to aspirate or monitor for adequate drainage, extensive spread of infection to the soft tissues, and inadequate clinical response to appropriate antibiotics after 5 to 7 days. There is an apparent consensus among rheumatologists that surgical drainage is rarely necessary for patients with gonococcal septic arthritis in whom the response to appropriate antibiotics is characteristically rapid (less than a week) and complete. No prospective or controlled studies support or refute the need to openly drain or lavage an uncomplicated, acutely infected, nongonococcal joint at the initiation of therapy; nonetheless, this orthopedic practice is common in many parts of the country. Surgical drainage should be considered when a previously damaged (e.g., rheumatoid) joint becomes infected because the data indicate a particularly poor outcome for these patients with medical therapy. The data are insufficient to mandate immediate surgical drainage of infected joints in immunosuppressed patients. Initial joint lavage or arthroscopic management does not seem to worsen functional outcome[53]; however, there are no appropriately controlled studies supporting their routine use.

MEDICAL THERAPY

The choice of antibiotics [*see Table 2*] should be guided by patient characteristics and the local microbiologic sensitivity pattern. Intra-articular antibiotics are not required[54] and may cause a chemical synovitis. Parenteral antibiotics are generally administered for approximately 4 to 6 weeks. Acetaminophen and NSAIDs should be avoided until the diagnosis is solid (i.e., through microbiologic identification or by documented defervescence and clinical improvement with antibiotics alone). High-dose NSAIDs can transiently blunt the inflammatory response and may suggest a response to coadministered antibiotics, which might then be construed as evidence for a culture-negative (e.g., gonococcal) infection. There are no data demonstrating that NSAIDs prolong the course of infection, and some animal data suggest that anti-inflammatory therapy may be beneficial.[10,11] Narcotics may be used initially for pain control. Joint immobilization for a short period (1 to 3 days) is appropriate to help with pain control, but daily range-of-motion exercises should be started as soon as possible to hasten return of joint function.[55] Once a definitive diagnosis is made, and if there are no contraindications, NSAID therapy may be initiated to facilitate joint mobilization.

Acknowledgment

The author thanks Dr. Mathilde Pioro for her assistance in the preparation of an initial draft of the manuscript.

References

1. Weston VC, Jones AC, Bradbury N, et al: Clinical features and outcome of septic arthritis in a single UK health district 1982–1991. Ann Rheum Dis 58:214, 1999

2. Le Dantec L, Maury F, Flipo R-M, et al: Peripheral pyogenic arthritis: a study of 179 cases. Rev Rheum Engl Ed 63:103, 1996

3. Goldenberg DL, Cohen AS: Acute infectious arthritis: a review of patients with nongonococcal joint infections (with emphasis on therapy and prognosis). Am J Med 60:369, 1976

4. Rosenthal J, Bole GG, Robinson WD: Acute nongonococcal infectious arthritis: evaluation of risk factors, therapy, and outcome. Arthritis Rheum 23:889, 1980

5. Martens PB, Ho G Jr: Septic arthritis in adults: clinical features, outcome, and intensive care requirements. J Intensive Care Med 10:246, 1995

6. Kanndorp CJE, Krijnen P, Moens HJB, et al: The outcome of bacterial arthritis: a prospective community-based study. Arthritis Rheum 40:884, 1997

7. Mcallister DR, Parker RD, Cooper AE, et al: Outcomes of postoperative septic arthritis after anterior cruciate ligament reconstruction. Am J Sports Med 27:562, 1999

8. Nilsson I-M, Bremell T, Rydén C, et al: Role of the staphylococcal accessory gene regulator (sar) in septic arthritis. Infect Immunol 64:4438, 1996

9. Bremell T, Abdelnour A, Tarkowski A: Histopathological and serological progression of experimental *Staphylococcus aureus* arthritis. Infect Immunol 60:2976, 1992

10. Wysenbeek AJ, Volchek J, Amit M, et al: Treatment of staphylococcal septic arthritis in rabbits by systemic antibiotics and intra-articular corticosteroids. Ann Rheumatic Dis 57:687, 1998

11. Stricker SJ, Lozman PR, Makowski A-L, et al: Chondroprotective effect of betamethasone in lapine pyogenic arthritis. J Pediatr Orthop 16:231, 1996

12. Schlapbach P, Ambord C, Blochlinger AM, et al: Bacterial arthritis: are fever, rigors, leucocytosis and blood cultures of diagnostic value? Clin Rheum 9:69, 1990

13. Yagupsky P, Bar-Ziv Y, Howard CB, et al: Epidemiology, etiology, and clinical features of septic arthritis in children younger than 24 months. Arch Pediatr Adolesc Med 149:537, 1995

14. Ho G Jr, DeNuccio M: Gout and pseudogout in hospitalized patients. Arch Intern Med 153:2787, 1993

15. Garcia-Porrua C, Gonzalez-Gay MA, Ibanez D, et al: The clinical spectrum of severe septic bursitis in northwestern Spain: a 10-year study. J Rheumatol 26:663, 1999

16. Krey PR, Bailen DA: Synovial fluid leukocytosis: a study of extremes. Am J Med 67:436, 1979

17. Wise CM, Morris CR, Wasilauskas BL, et al: Gonococcal arthritis in an era of increasing penicillin resistance: presentations and outcomes in 41 recent cases (1985–1991). Arch Intern Med 154:2690, 1994

18. Ilahi OA, Swarna U, Hamill RJ, et al: Concomitant crystal and septic arthritis. Orthopedics 19:613, 1996

19. Liebling MR, Arkfeld DG, Michelini GA, et al: Identification of *Neisseria gonorrhoeae* in synovial fluid using the polymerase chain reaction. Arthritis Rheum 37:702, 1994

20. Olaison L, Hogevik H, Alestig K: Fever, C-reactive protein, and other acute-phase reactants during treatment of infective endocarditis. Arch Intern Med 157:885, 1997

21. Graif M, Schweitzer ME, Deely D, et al: The septic versus nonseptic inflamed joint: MRI Characteristics. Skeletal Radiol 28:616, 1999

22. Mudun A, Unal S, Aktay R, et al: Tc-99m nanocolloid and Tc-99m MDP three-phase bone imaging in osteomyelitis and septic arthritis: a comparative study. Clin Nucl Med 20:772, 1995

23. Aliabadi P, Nikpoor N: Imaging osteomyelitis. Arthritis Rheum 37: 617, 1994

24. Gardner GC, Weisman MH: Pyarthrosis in patients with rheumatoid arthritis: a report of 13 cases and a review of the literature from the past 40 years. Am J Med 88:503, 1990

25. Slaughter S, Dworkin RJ, Gilbert DN, et al: *Staphylococcus aureus* septic arthritis in patients on hemodialysis treatment. West J Med 163: 128, 1995

26. Sapico FL, Liquete JA, Sarma RJ: Bone and joint infections in

patients with infective endocarditis: review of a 4-year experience. Clin Infect Dis 22:783, 1996

27. Schattner A, Vosti KL: Bacterial arthritis due to beta-hemolytic streptococci of serogroups A, B, C, F, and G. Medicine (Baltimore) 77: 122, 1998

28. Ispahani P, Weston VC, Turner DP, et al: Septic arthritis due to *Streptococcus pneumoniae* in Nottingham, United Kingdom, 1985–1998. Clin Infect Dis 29:1450, 1999

29. Raymond NJ, Henry J, Workowski KA: Enterococcal arthritis: case report and review. Clin Infect Dis 21:516, 1995

30. Anand AJ, Glatt AE: Salmonella osteomyelitis and arthritis in sickle cell disease. Semin Arthritis Rheum 24:211, 1994

31. Roy R, Matei D, Kaufman LD: Emphysematous septic arthritis: case report and review of the literature. J Rheumatol 22:1776, 1995

32. Puechal X, Hilliquin P, Renoux M, et al: *Ureaplasma urealyticum* destructive septic polyarthritis revealing a common variable immunodeficiency. Arthritis Rheum 38:1524, 1995

33. Franz A, Webster AD, Furr PM, et al: Mycoplasmal arthritis in patients with primary immunoglobulin deficiency: clinical features and outcome in 18 patients. Br J Rheumatol 36:661, 1997

34. Kumar A, Kannampuzha P: Septic arthritis due to *Pasteurella multocida*. South Med J 85:329, 1992

35. Alloway JA, Evangelisti SM, Sartin JS: *Mycobacterium marinum* arthritis. Semin Arthritis Rheum 24:382, 1995

36. Harth M, Ralph ED, Faraawi R: Septic arthritis due to *Mycobacterium marinum*. J Rheumatol 21:957, 1994

37. Evanchick CC, Davis DE, Harrington TM: Tuberculosis of peripheral joints: an often missed diagnosis. J Rheumatol 13:187, 1986

38. Wallace R, Cohen AS: Tuberculosis arthritis: a report of two cases with review of biopsy and synovial fluid findings. Am J Med 61:277, 1976

39. Gorse GJ, Pais MJ, Kusske JA, et al: Tuberculous spondylitis: a report of six cases and a review of the literature. Medicine (Baltimore) 62:178, 1983

40. Reginato AJ, Schumacher HR, Jimenez S, et al: Synovitis in secondary syphilis: clinical, light, and electron microscopic studies. Arthritis Rheum 22:170, 1979

41. Bried JM, Galgiani JN: *Coccidioides immitis* infections in bones and joints. Clin Orthop 211:235, 1986

42. Robert ME, Kauffman CA: Blastomycosis presenting as polyarticular septic arthritis. J Rheumatol 15:1438, 1988

43. Perez-Gomez A, Prieto A, Torresano M, et al: Role of the new azoles in the treatment of fungal osteoarticular infections. Semin Arthritis Rheum 27:226, 1998

44. Rivera J, Lopez-Longo J, Sanchez-Atrio A: Septic arthritis in patients with acquired immunodeficiency syndrome with human immunodeficiency virus infection. J Rheumatol 19:1960, 1992

45. Vassilopoulos D, Chalasani P, Jurado RL, et al: Musculoskeletal infections in patients with human immunodeficiency virus infection. Medicine (Baltimore) 76:284, 1997

46. Bomalaski JS, Williamson PK, Goldstein CS: Infectious arthritis in renal transplant patients. Arthritis Rheum 29:227, 1986

47. George T, Mandell BF: Gout in the transplant patient. J Clin Rheum 1:328, 1995

48. Inman RD, Gallegos KV, Brause BD, et al: Clinical and microbial features of prosthetic joint infection. Am J Med 77:47, 1984

49. Levitsky KA, Hozack WJ, Balderston RA, et al: Evaluation of the painful prosthetic joint: relative value of bone scan, sedimentation rate, and joint aspiration. J Arthroplasty 6:237, 1991

50. Spangehl MJ, Masri BA, O'Connell JX, et al: Prospective analysis of preoperative and intraoperative investigations for the diagnosis of infection at the sites of 202 revision total hip arthroplasties. J Bone Joint Surg 81A:672, 1999

51. Hirakawa K, Stulberg BN, Wilde AH, et al: Results of 2-stage reimplantation for infected total knee arthroplasty; J Arthroplasty 13:22, 1998

52. Broy SB, Schmid FR: A comparison of medical drainage (needle aspiration) and surgical drainage (arthrotomy or arthroscopy) in the initial treatment of infected joints. Clin Rheum Dis 12:501, 1986

53. Parisien JS, Shaffer B: Arthroscopic management of pyarthrosis. Clin Orthop 275:243, 1992

54. Hamed KA, Tam JY, Prober CG: Pharmacokinetic optimisation of the treatment of septic arthritis. Clin Pharmacokinet 31:156, 1996

55. Pfeiffenberger J, Meiss L: Septic conditions of the shoulder: an updating of treatment strategies. Arch Orthop Trauma Surg 115:325, 1996

12 Osteomyelitis

Layne O. Gentry, M.D.

Osteomyelitis is an infection of bone characterized by progressive inflammatory destruction of bone, bone necrosis, and new bone formation. Osteomyelitis poses a challenge because it is often difficult to diagnose and treat. Even when appropriate antibiotic therapy is instituted promptly, osteomyelitis can cause serious morbidity. Chronic cases are often refractory to treatment. In diabetic patients, amputation to remove the site of infection is often necessary.

The etiology of osteomyelitis has evolved considerably over the past 2 decades. Twenty years ago, most cases of osteomyelitis were caused by susceptible strains of *Staphylococcus aureus* and were cured with surgical debridement and 4 to 6 weeks of methicillin therapy. Although *S. aureus* is still a common cause of osteomyelitis, an increasing number of infections are caused by gram-negative organisms, such as *Pseudomonas aeruginosa*, or are polymicrobial. Coagulase-negative staphylococci, once regarded as contaminants, are now considered significant pathogens. Increasingly, osteomyelitis is a complication of reconstructive orthopedic surgery. These changes, together with improvements in diagnosis and therapy, indicate a need to reexamine traditional management of osteomyelitis.

Classification

Osteomyelitis is classified on the basis of pathogenesis, duration of disease, extent or type of bone involvement, anatomy of the bone infection, and host characteristics. Osteomyelitis can present as either an acute condition or a chronic infection. Acute osteomyelitis is usually defined as the first clinical episode, complete with the signs, symptoms, and radiographic and histologic findings associated with bone infection. Acute infections often occur soon after an episode of bacteremia and are usually accompanied by fever and bone pain. Chronic osteomyelitis is defined as bone infection that has failed to resolve after one or more treatment attempts. Retained foci of dead bone, or sequestra, are characteristic of chronic osteomyelitis.

Waldvogel and coworkers[1] described three types of osteomyelitis: hematogenous osteomyelitis, osteomyelitis secondary to contiguous focus of disease, and osteomyelitis associated with vascular insufficiency. In hematogenous osteomyelitis, infection is introduced through the bloodstream and usually affects the metaphyses of long bones. Hematogenous osteomyelitis is diagnosed in about 20% of cases of osteomyelitis; it is the most common type of osteomyelitis in children. In osteomyelitis secondary to a contiguous focus of disease, the bone becomes infected from an external source (e.g., penetrating trauma or open fracture) or from the spread of infection from adjacent soft tissue (e.g., abscess or skin infection). Contiguous-focus disease is usually seen in older persons and accounts for 50% of cases of osteomyelitis. Osteomyelitis associated with vascular insufficiency, which is responsible for about 30% of cases, is usually seen in patients with diabetic neuropathy.

Clinical Syndromes

HEMATOGENOUS OSTEOMYELITIS

Hematogenous osteomyelitis is usually seen in children between 1 and 15 years of age and adults older than 50 years or in persons who abuse I.V. drugs. In children, infection usually occurs as a single focus in the metaphyseal area of long bones (particularly the tibia and femur). In older persons, infection of the vertebral bodies is more common. When osteomyelitis is seen in young adults, it is often associated with I.V. drug abuse or sickle cell anemia.

Several predisposing factors are associated with the development of hematogenous osteomyelitis. Children may be predisposed to infection by minor trauma that causes a small hematoma, vessel obstruction, and bone necrosis. Thus, hematogenous osteomyelitis may be seen in teenagers who play contact sports. About one third of patients have a history of trauma to the site of osteomyelitis. Some children with local trauma may have a history of infection at a distant site. In adults, predisposing factors include advanced age, immunodeficiency, chronic bacteremia, I.V. drug abuse, long-term indwelling catheters, and sickle cell anemia.

Etiology

Most cases of hematogenous osteomyelitis are monomicrobial. Although *S. aureus* causes 60% to 90% of cases of hematogenous osteomyelitis, certain organisms tend to cause infections in certain age groups. In newborns, group B streptococci and gram-negative bacilli are common. In children, streptococci and *Haemophilus influenzae* are often seen. Although the incidence of osteomyelitis caused by *H. influenzae* type b might be expected to decrease because of immunization programs, a recent retrospective study in New York State showed that hospital admission rates for children with arthritis and osteomyelitis caused by *H. influenzae* have not declined, especially for high-risk children such as those of minority groups and those living in the inner city.[2] Polymicrobial hematogenous osteomyelitis is usually caused by *S. aureus* and a streptococcus.

The incidence of hematogenous osteomyelitis caused by gram-negative organisms is about 25%. *Escherichia coli* is the most common gram-negative organism isolated from hematogenous bone infections. *P. aeruginosa*, which has a predilection for the cervical vertebrae, and *Serratia* species are common pathogens in I.V. drug abusers. Furthermore, *P. aeruginosa* can be isolated from patients with long-term indwelling catheters.[3] *Salmonella* species are frequently associated with osteomyelitis in patients with sickle cell anemia[4] and may also be seen in patients with AIDS and other hemoglobinopathies.

Tuberculous infection of bone may be seen in patients from areas endemic for tuberculosis and in patients with AIDS. Fungal osteomyelitis, usually caused by opportunistic organisms, is found in patients who are severely immunodeficient or neutropenic or who have indwelling venous catheters. Because of their increasing frequency in all types of infection, *Candida* species may be seen more often in bone infections. Treatment of these infections is difficult, and therapy needs to be individualized against the specific organism.

Clinical Features

Children with acute hematogenous osteomyelitis usually present with fever and localized pain. Leukocytosis may be present. A decreased range of motion and signs of local infection may be seen in the affected area. Drainage is not usually seen. Blood cultures are positive in more than half of patients.[3] Although in most children symptoms are present for 3 weeks or less, some children may present with vague symptoms of 1 to 3 months' duration.

Vertebral osteomyelitis is a form of hematogenous osteomyelitis most commonly seen in older persons and I.V. drug abusers. Most patients present with a constant dull pain that progresses slowly. Percussion over the affected area usually causes intense pain. Neurologic signs are generally absent but, when present, may indicate an epidural abscess. Fewer than half of patients are febrile. Vertebral infection typically involves the vertebral body rather than the spinous or transverse processes; often, two adjacent vertebrae and the disk space between them are affected. The lumbar region is most frequently involved in pyogenic hematogenous osteomyelitis. Thoracic vertebrae are often infected in spinal tuberculosis (Pott disease), and the cervical spine is often the site of infection in patients who abuse I.V. drugs.[5]

In about 10% of patients with acute hematogenous osteomyelitis, the disease progresses to a chronic condition. These patients have recurrent episodes of clinical exacerbations that are usually more indolent than those seen in the acute episode. Patients who are more susceptible to chronic osteomyelitis include those for whom therapy was delayed and those with compound fractures.

Despite the serious nature of hematogenous osteomyelitis, the prognosis is good for most patients. In a retrospective review of 69 children with acute hematogenous osteomyelitis, major sequelae were seen in only 3% of patients and minor problems in 2%. A favorable long-term outcome was associated with early hospitalization and initiation of appropriate antibiotic therapy.[6] Patients with severe underlying conditions have a worse prognosis.

Special Presentations of Hematogenous Osteomyelitis

Brodie abscess In patients with Brodie abscess, the infected portion of bone is completely replaced by pus and forms an intraosseous abscess. The infection, which is contained within a sclerotic membrane, may become quiescent. However, the risk of recurrence is high, and infection may spread. Patients are usually afebrile and may present only with local pain or swelling. Brodie abscess may be misdiagnosed as a bone tumor; the diagnosis of Brodie abscess is confirmed by histologic examination and culture. *S. aureus* is usually the etiologic agent, although *S. epidermidis* is occasionally implicated. Although seemingly benign, Brodie abscess should be aggressively treated. Pus may accumulate and spread through the tissues, causing a draining sinus; if near the joint surface of an intracapsular bone, infection can cause pyogenic arthritis.

Osteomyelitis in patients with sickle cell anemia There are two main differences between hematogenous osteomyelitis in children with sickle cell anemia and that in children who are otherwise healthy. First, infection in children with sickle cell anemia usually localizes in the diaphysis rather than the metaphysis. Second, *Salmonella* species frequently cause infection in this group, although staphylococci are also common.[4] Differentiating between osteomyelitis and thrombotic crisis in patients with sickle cell anemia may be difficult. In both situations, patients may present with bone pain and fever, and the erythrocyte sedimentation rate (ESR) and leukocyte count may be elevated. A bone biopsy is usually required for diagnosis of osteomyelitis. Multiple sites of bone may be infected. Antibiotics for empirical therapy should be effective against both *Salmonella* and staphylococci. A regimen of a semisynthetic penicillin and an aminoglycoside is recommended [*see* Treatment, *below*].

Hematogenous osteomyelitis in I.V. drug abusers In I.V. drug abusers, hematogenous osteomyelitis is associated with subtle clinical signs and symptoms. Patients may present with localized pain, but fever is usually absent. Although vertebral osteomyelitis is common, infection of the pubis and the clavicle is also seen. Culture of the infected site usually yields *S. aureus* or *S. epidermidis*, although *P. aeruginosa* is often seen. Serial radiographs may be necessary, and surgery may be required to confirm the microbiologic diagnosis.

OSTEOMYELITIS SECONDARY TO A CONTIGUOUS FOCUS OF INFECTION

Osteomyelitis in adults almost always derives from a contiguous source of infection. These bone infections are often complex and heterogeneous. Organisms may be inoculated directly into the bone after an open fracture, a penetrating wound, or a surgical procedure; or they may spread from an adjacent soft tissue infection. Because techniques for joint replacements have improved, the number of artificial joints inserted has increased and so has the number of infections associated with prosthetic joints. Osteomyelitis secondary to vascular insufficiency develops in older patients with diabetes or severe vascular impairment, frequently on the small bones of the feet (in patients in whom soft tissue breaks down over weight-bearing or pressure-bearing areas).

Table 1 Common Clinical Associations in Osteomyelitis

Organism	*Common Clinical Associations*
Staphylococcus aureus	Found in 50%–70% of cases
Coagulase-negative staphylococci	Infections of prosthetic devices
Gram-negative bacilli	Decubitus ulcers, vascular insufficiency
Pseudomonas aeruginosa	Puncture wounds
Streptococci and anaerobes	Diabetic foot lesions, decubitus ulcers, bite wounds
Pasteurella multocida	Cat bites
Actinomyces	Periodontal infection or sinusitis
Eikenella corrodens	Mandibular osteomyelitis

Etiology

The cause of osteomyelitis depends, in part, on the route of entry, the phenotypic characteristics of organisms, and the epidemiologic background of the patient. Thus, the bacteriology of osteomyelitis in a diabetic patient who has had multiple hospital admissions and has been treated with multiple antibiotics over several years differs from that in a patient with a community-acquired infection. Organisms with common clinical associations are listed [*see Table 1*].

Because of virulence factors and adherence characteristics, *S. aureus* is the most common single pathogen in contiguous-focus osteomyelitis and accounts for 50% to 70% of cases.[7] In contrast to hematogenous osteomyelitis, contiguous-focus disease is often polymicrobial; multiple organisms may be isolated from 30% to 50% of such patients. The incidence of osteomyelitis caused by gram-negative bacilli (30%) is increasing. Gram-negative pathogens are important in patients who have undergone multiple hospital procedures, have had an extended hospital stay, are in intensive care units, or have had an open fracture. *P. aeruginosa* is often responsible for osteomyelitis associated with comminuted fractures and puncture wounds to the heel.[8] *S. epidermidis* is another common pathogen in contiguous-focus osteomyelitis, particularly in patients who have infected orthopedic prostheses.

Osteomyelitis caused by anaerobic bacteria usually results from contiguous spread of a polymicrobial infection. Anaerobes should be suspected when osteomyelitis is associated with a human bite or is contiguous to a dental infection, intra-abdominal abscess, decubitus ulcer, or otorhinolaryngologic infection.

Clinical Features

In the initial stages of contiguous-focus osteomyelitis, patients may have pain, fever, swelling, and erythema. However, during recurrent episodes of chronic infection, fever subsides, and pain and drainage from a sinus tract or ulcer are often seen. In patients with generalized vascular insufficiency, the disease starts insidiously in an area of traumatized skin. The patient may present with an ingrown toenail, a perforating foot ulcer, cellulitis, or a superficial or deep wound infection. Fever and systemic signs of infection are not usually present.

Osteomyelitis after replacement of the hip joint may occur soon after surgery or later. Often evident within the first few days or weeks after surgery, acute contiguous infections result directly from infected skin, subcutaneous tissue, or muscle. Fever, pain, erythema, edema, and purulent drainage are often present when early infections are caused by pyogenic organisms such as *S. aureus*, streptococci, or enteric gram-negative bacilli. When early infections are caused by less pathogenic organisms, such as *S. epidermidis* or diphtheroids, the disease presents more insidiously. Chronic contiguous infections are usually diagnosed 6 to 24 months after surgery. The patient usually presents with persistent pain. Most infections are probably introduced during surgery but remain quiescent for a long time.

Sternal osteomyelitis, a serious complication of median sternotomy after cardiothoracic surgery, occurs in 1% to 5% of patients. Patients have fever, a slightly erythematous wound, and persistent pain. Frequent pathogens include *S. epidermidis, S. aureus*, and gram-negative bacilli. The presence of sternal wires, used to approximate the sternum, is a major risk factor for chronic recurrent osteomyelitis. Surgical removal of the wires is essential for recovery. The risk of death may be high in complicated cases.[8]

OSTEOMYELITIS ASSOCIATED WITH VASCULAR INSUFFICIENCY

Most patients with osteomyelitis associated with vascular insufficiency have diabetes mellitus or peripheral vascular disease from atherosclerosis. In these patients, osteomyelitis usually develops by contiguous spread of infection from soft tissue to underlying bone. Bone infections develop in about 25% of diabetic patients with superficial mild to moderate foot infections; however, of those patients with serious foot infections, over 50% will have osteomyelitis.[9] Extensive debridement is necessary, and about two thirds of cases require bone resection or partial amputation.[10]

Complex foot lesions in diabetic patients result from a combination of neuropathy, atherosclerotic peripheral vascular disease, and repetitive trauma to the area. Atherosclerosis of the tibial and peroneal arteries of the lower leg is common in diabetic patients.[11] Limb ischemia, combined with poor collateral circulation, impairs wound healing in foot ulcers and allows for the contiguous spread of infection to bone. In addition, this anoxic environment contributes to the development of gangrenous changes and anaerobic infections. Furthermore, peripheral vascular disease may compromise the efficacy of antibiotic therapy by preventing the accumulation of adequate drug levels in the infected tissues.

Osteomyelitis should be considered in all diabetic patients with deep or chronic foot ulcers or infections. Distinguishing between true bone infection and noninfectious destructive neuropathic bone changes in patients with diabetes is challenging and requires diagnostic imaging tests. Although *S. aureus* is the most common pathogen isolated from patients with osteomyelitis associated with vascular insufficiency, multiple organisms, including both anaerobes and aerobes, may be present, especially in hospitalized patients. Mixed gram-positive and gram-negative infections are often seen in patients with chronic or previously treated infections.

Pathogenesis

Pathogens gain access to bone in humans by three methods: direct inoculation, extension from contiguous sites, and hematogenous dissemination. Each type of infection may be further complicated by the presence of a prosthesis.

The sequelae associated with the hematogenous dissemination of bacteria to the bone vary with the age of the patient.[3] In infants, infection can spread via transphyseal vessels to the epiphysis and then to the joint space. Concurrent septic arthritis and epiphyseal destruction may be seen. In children older than 1 year, the growth plate is avascular, and osteomyelitis usually begins in the metaphyseal region of the long bones. Capillary loops do not anastomose in this region, and bacterial emboli can settle in this area and cause a microinfarction. Microscopic metaphyseal hemorrhage and necrosis, caused by insignificant trauma, provide a favorable environment for infection. Once infection is established, it can spread to the periosteum. If pus reaches the subperiosteal space, the periosteum becomes elevated. Osteoblasts beneath the detached periosteum gradually produce new bone.

The pathogenesis of hematogenous osteomyelitis in adults differs from that in children.[6] After growth ceases and the epiphyses close, organisms causing osteomyelitis no longer have a predilection for the metaphyseal area of long bones. The vertebrae, sternoclavicular and sacroiliac joints, and the symphysis pubis are often affected. Infection may spread from the subchondral bone to the joint space. Sites of previous injury or trauma often provide the point of seeding of infectious organisms.

Unlike hematogenous osteomyelitis, contiguous-focus disease may invade any traumatized bone. Local inflammatory response or injury can devitalize bone and tissue. Microbes can multiply in these areas of dead bone. Osteomyelitis often complicates decubitus ulcers or cutaneous ulcerations in diabetic patients. Undetected trauma in diabetic patients with neuropathy provides a portal of entry for bacteria. Moreover, compromised blood flow impairs wound healing and allows unchecked bacterial proliferation.

Histologic findings in acute osteomyelitis include microbes, neutrophils, and congested or thrombosed blood vessels [*see Figure 1a and 1b*]. The local inflammatory reaction contributes to further bone necrosis, which is a distinguishing feature of chronic osteomyelitis. As necrosis progresses, new bone gradually surrounds the infected area of dead bone (sequestrum). The formation of a functionally inert, nonresorbable substratum—either a sequestrum or a foreign body—upon which bacteria can attach and multiply marks the transition from acute to chronic disease.

a

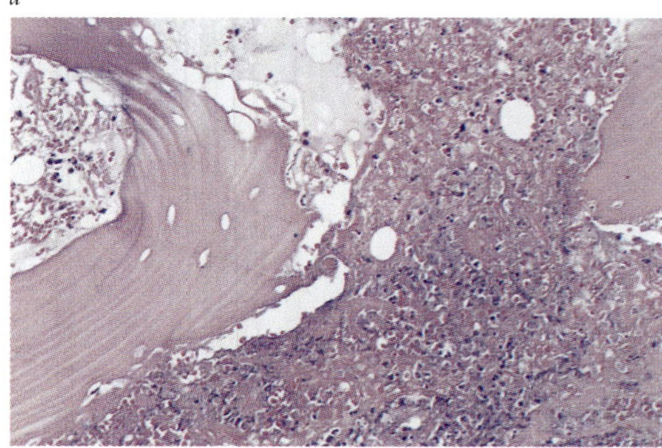

b

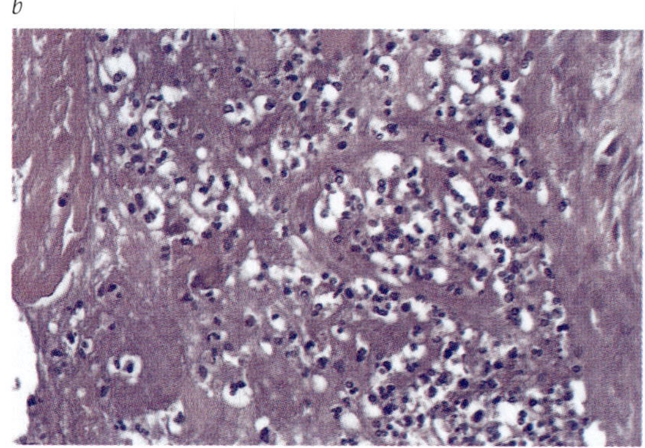

Figure 1 **(*a*) Photomicrograph of a specimen from bone biopsy shows acute osteomyelitis (magnification: × 40). Note missing osteoclastic cells (signifying bone death) and intense inflammatory reaction adjacent to bone fragment. (*b*) Higher magnification (× 100) shows intense polymorphonuclear infiltration at same site.**

Diagnosis

The diagnosis of osteomyelitis should be considered in patients with fever and localized skeletal pain, positive blood cultures, persistently draining wounds, and radiologic findings that suggest a localized inflammatory process. The diagnosis can then be confirmed by the histologic examination and bacteriologic culture of bone specimens obtained either by surgery or by multiple percutaneous needle biopsies. A detailed history with emphasis on previous trauma or surgery is important. Although no laboratory test specifically indicates the diagnosis of osteomyelitis, a complete blood cell count, ESR, and C-reactive protein test may be useful. The white blood cell count is usually elevated only in early stages of the disease. The ESR may be helpful in diagnosing acute hematogenous osteomyelitis in children but is less useful in newborns and children with sickle cell anemia. C-reactive protein is an acute-phase reactant, and although the C-reactive protein test is relatively insensitive and nonspecific, it may be more specific for infection than the ESR.

RADIOLOGIC AND NUCLEAR FINDINGS

There is a plethora of imaging techniques for diagnosing osteomyelitis [*see Table 2*]. The accuracy

Table 2 Radiographic and Radionuclide Techniques for Diagnosing Osteomyelitis

Test	*Sensitivity*	*Specificity*	*Indications/Comments*
Radiograph	Good after 3 weeks	Poor	Initial test for most patients
^{99m}Tc bone scan	Good in first 2 weeks	Poor	Use in patients with suspected osteomyelitis who have a negative result on radiograph
Gallium	Moderate after 2 weeks	Poor	Use in infants and children with a negative result on bone scan
Indium	Moderate	Moderate	May be used in patients with a recent fracture
CT	Excellent	Moderate	Useful in osteomyelitis of the skull, pelvis, and sterno-clavicular junction
MRI	Excellent	Excellent	Reliability distinguishes tumor of infarction from osteo-myelitis; useful in surgical planning for diabetes; good for vertebral disease; very expensive
PET	Excellent	Moderate	May be useful in chronic osteomyelitis in patients with negative results on other tests

CT—computed tomography MRI—magnetic resonance imaging PET—positron emission tomography ^{99m}Tc—technetium-99m

of imaging studies is affected by the extent of inflammation, the duration and site of infection, the vascularity of the site, and associated pathologic conditions. Osteomyelitis cannot be absolutely confirmed or excluded on the basis of results from any one test.

Radiograph

Radiographs, which are relatively inexpensive, should be the initial diagnostic technique for almost all patients suspected of having osteomyelitis. However, findings on conventional radiographs are often normal until at least 2 weeks after the onset of symptoms. Furthermore, radiographic changes can be subtle and nonspecific. In children with hematogenous osteomyelitis, the earliest changes are deep soft tissue swelling, which may be difficult to detect; periosteal elevation; and radiolucent areas of bone destruction, which are not usually detected until 50% to 75% of bone density has been lost.[12] In contiguous-focus disease, the initial radiologic manifestation is periosteal reaction. Radiographs may show the presence of sequestra, sclerosis, and significant bone lysis in patients with chronic disease.

Bone Scan

The technetium-99m (^{99m}Tc) methylene diphosphonate three-phase bone scan is often used to identify osteomyelitis, because it is more sensitive than conventional radiography and can confirm a suspected diagnosis of osteomyelitis within 48 hours after onset of symptoms. The bone scan should be the next imaging study performed in patients with normal radiographs. Classic findings on bone scan are increased blood flow, pooling, and reactive new bone formation. Although sensitivity is good, specificity is poor [*see Table 2*]. Cellulitis and septic arthritis cannot be differentiated from osteomyelitis on bone scan. False positive results may be seen in patients with previous bone injury, tumor, or infarction. Furthermore, bone scans may remain positive for 6 weeks to 6 months after therapy because of bone metabolism and remodeling. In children with uncomplicated hematogenous osteomyelitis, the bone scan has a high sensitivity and specificity; a positive bone scan strongly suggests osteomyelitis, and a negative scan in children older than 3 years excludes the diagnosis.[13] Sensitivity, however, is lower in neonates and in patients with sickle cell anemia.

Gallium Scan

Gallium scans may be useful in infants and in children in whom bone scans are negative. The low specificity of gallium imaging may be improved if it is combined with bone scans. When interpreted in combination with a bone scan, the gallium scan can in some cases be used to differentiate acute cellulitis from acute osteomyelitis. Disadvantages associated with gallium scans include higher doses of radiation and a 1- to 2-day waiting period for results.

Leukocyte Scan

Indium-111–labeled and ^{99m}Tc-labeled leukocyte scans, which are more specific but less sensitive than bone scans, have been used to evaluate patients with osteomyelitis. Leukocyte scans are not useful in patients with chronic, indolent infections. In a patient who is suspected of having osteomyelitis and has recently had a fracture, a leukocyte scan may be the study of choice because results from a bone scan will be equivocal. The cumbersome and expensive technique of leukocyte scanning requires in vitro cell isolation and radiolabeling, which is time-consuming and potentially biohazardous. However, leukocyte scans, especially in combination with bone scans, may be sensitive and specific in detecting osteomyelitis in diabetic patients.[14–16] In a study of 52 diabetic patients with chronic foot ulcers, both specificity and accuracy were significantly higher with leukocyte scans than with bone scans.[14] The combined use of leukocyte scans and bone scans has effectively differentiated osteomyelitis from soft tissue infections in patients with diabetes; the sensitivity of the combination has ranged from 93% to 100%, and the specificity has ranged from 80% to 83%.

Monoclonal Antibody Testing

A ^{99m}Tc-labeled antigranulocyte monoclonal Fab fragment has been used in patients with suspected osteomyelitis. Sensitivity, specificity, and accuracy were comparable or superior to those obtained with leukocyte scanning.[17–19] The monoclonal antibody binds to nonspecific antigens on the surface of leukocytes. This technique is less expensive and simpler to perform than the leukocyte scan. Moreover, results of monoclonal antibody testing are obtained the same day rather than 18 to 24 hours later, as with the leukocyte scan.

Computed Tomography and Magnetic Resonance Imaging

Both CT and MRI have excellent sensitivity and resolution and allow simultaneous evaluation of bone and surrounding soft tissues. CT reliably detects sequestra and devitalized bone and is useful for evaluating patients with osteomyelitis of the skull. However, CT is prone to image degradation and is less specific than other tests. MRI, with its excellent specificity, is helpful in distinguishing bone tumor or infarction from osteomyelitis.[20] Furthermore, MRI is particularly reliable in distinguishing normal areas from abnormal areas when surgery is being planned for diabetic patients with osteomyelitis.[21] In addition, MRI is the technique of choice for detecting and assessing the site and extent of infection in the spine. However, the expense of MRI precludes its use on a routine basis. A limited MRI scan with specialized views and minimal use of gadolinium contrast can be used to control costs.[22] Metallic prostheses exclude the use of MRI and distort image reflection on CT, thereby obscuring early changes of infection.

Positron Emission Tomography

Positron emission tomography (PET) has been used as an imaging tool for infections of the bone and osteosynthetic material.[23] PET with fluorodeoxyglucose (FDG) was shown to be superior to bone scans in diagnosing chronic osteomyelitis of the central skeleton.[24] Because of its excellent sensitivity, FDG PET may be an effective technique for excluding chronic osteomyelitis when a bone scan is negative.[25]

CULTURES

The gold standard for diagnosis of osteomyelitis is aerobic and anaerobic culture of a biopsy specimen obtained under direct vision during surgery. Alternatively, culture of multiple specimens obtained by needle biopsy under ultrasound or radiographic guidance has been a reliable, cost-effective means of diagnosing osteomyelitis at our center. Combining surgical debridement with the obtaining of culture specimens is also cost-effective. Blood cultures should also be obtained, especially from patients suspected of having hematogenous osteomyelitis. Results of swab cultures of the sinus tract are usually inaccurate. Studies have shown that the results of cultures of sinus tract and bone biopsy specimens match in only 44% to 57% of patients with chronic osteomyelitis.[26,27]

Treatment

Optimal management of the patient with osteomyelitis entails microbiologic confirmation of the diagnosis by biopsy and complete surgical debridement, followed by institution of antibiotic therapy that is based on culture and sensitivity results [*see Table 3*]. When debridement is inadequate, therapy often fails, despite appropriate antimicrobial therapy.

HEMATOGENOUS OSTEOMYELITIS

In children with acute hematogenous osteomyelitis, antibiotic therapy alone may be sufficient. When the disease is recognized early and treated promptly, cure can be anticipated. Surgery should be considered for patients who do not respond to antibiotic therapy. For compliant children with a documented microbiologic infection who respond initially to parenteral therapy and who have no

Table 3 Choices for Antibiotic Treatment of Bacterial Osteomyelitis

Organism	*Antibiotic*	*Dosage*	
		Children	*Adults*
Staphylococcus aureus			
Methicillin-sensitive	Nafcillin or oxacillin	150 mg/kg I.V., q. 4 hr	2 g I.V., q. 6 hr
	Cefazolin	—	2 g I.V., q. 8 hr
	Cephalexin	100 mg/kg p.o., q. 6 hr	—
Methicillin-resistant or *S. epidermidis*	Vancomycin*	40 mg/kg I.V., q. 6 hr	1 g I.V., q. 12 hr
Streptococci	Ampicillin	150 mg/kg I.V., q. 6 hr	2 g I.V., q. 6 hr
	Ceftriaxone	50 mg/kg I.V., q. 24 hr	2 g I.V., q. 24 hr
Enterococci	Ampicillin + gentamicin†	—	2 g I.V., q. 6 hr 1 mg/kg q. 8 hr
Enterobacteriaceae	Ciprofloxacin	—	750 mg p.o., q. 12 hr
	Ceftriaxone	50 mg/kg I.V., q. 24 hr	2 g I.V., q. 24 hr
Pseudomonas aeruginosa	Ceftazidime	—	2 g I.V., q. 12 hr
	Ciprofloxacin	—	750 mg p.o., q. 12 hr
	Semisynthetic penicillin‡		
	Piperacillin	—	3 g I.V., q. 6 hr
	with		
	Aminoglycoside‡		
	Amikacin	—	15 mg/kg q.d.
	Gentamicin	—	5 mg/kg q.d.
Mixed infections (diabetic foot)	Ticarcillin-clavulanate§	—	3.1 g I.V., q. 6 hr
	Clindamycin + ciprofloxacin	—	0.9 g I.V., q. 8 hr 750 mg p.o., q. 12 hr
	Imipenem-cilastatin‖	—	1 g I.V., q. 6 hr

*Adding rifampin may increase efficacy.
†Use combination for the first 2 wk, followed by ampicillin alone.
‡Use a semisynthetic penicillin in combination with an aminoglycoside.
§Use in limb-threatening infections.
‖Use in life-threatening infections.

complications, the course of therapy may be completed with oral agents.[28] Cure rates of 95% have been obtained with this regimen. The suggested duration of I.V. therapy ranges from 4 to 14 days, and oral therapy is continued for 14 to 26 days.[29] Although some investigators have suggested that monitoring blood concentrations of antibiotics may be unnecessary,[29] most agree that adequate gastrointestinal absorption of the antibiotic should be confirmed by repeated measurements of serum bactericidal activity.[30] Close outpatient follow-up is essential. In adults with hematogenous osteomyelitis, surgical debridement and drainage of soft tissue abscesses are often necessary. Antibiotic therapy is usually maintained for 4 to 6 weeks.

STAPHYLOCOCCAL INFECTIONS

For infections caused by *S. aureus*, a β-lactamase–resistant semisynthetic penicillin is the drug of choice because most strains of *S. aureus* are resistant to penicillin. At our center, most strains of *S. aureus* isolated from cortical (nonsternal) bone are methicillin-susceptible, but more than 70% of coagulase-negative staphylococci are resistant to methicillin. For methicillin-resistant staphylococci, vancomycin is preferred. In selected cases, after 2 weeks of parenteral therapy, patients can be switched to oral therapy if the appropriate requirements are met. Those requirements include good response to I.V. therapy, strict patient compliance, microbiologic diagnosis, isolated pathogen highly susceptible to the proposed antibiotic, and a high level of bioavailability of the oral agent (serum bactericidal titers may be useful). Although oral therapy with ciprofloxacin has been effective in treating staphylococcal osteomyelitis,[31,32] reports of variable efficacy and the development of resistance indicate that ciprofloxacin should not be used as monotherapy in osteomyelitis caused by staphylococci.[33] However, long-term treatment with the combination of ciprofloxacin and rifampin has been successful in treating implant-related staphylococcal infections in patients who have stable implants and symptoms of short duration.[34] Quinolones are contraindicated in children and pregnant women.

ENTEROCOCCAL AND GRAM-NEGATIVE INFECTIONS

Enterococcus faecalis is an increasingly troublesome pathogen, especially in patients with infected prostheses. Fortunately, *E. faecalis* does not usually cause osteomyelitis of long bones in the absence of prostheses. Because of the serious nature of a possible associated bacteremia in acute infections, aggressive therapy is necessary until acute symptoms resolve and blood cultures become negative.

Treatment of gram-negative osteomyelitis requires an accurate identification of the organism and antimicrobial susceptibility. Oral ciprofloxacin is an effective and inexpensive choice for treating bone infections caused by Enterobacteriaceae.[22,31,32] Furthermore, studies have shown that ciprofloxacin, ofloxacin, and pefloxacin have been effective in treating osteomyelitis caused by multiply resistant gram-negative bacteria.[35] Because of reports of the development of resistance, however, patients should be carefully monitored when ciprofloxacin is used as monotherapy in pseudomonal osteomyelitis. Ceftazidime is another potent antipseudomonal agent. In cases of resistant strains of *Pseudomonas*, a regimen of an extended-spectrum penicillin and an aminoglycoside may be used; however, efficacy is not definitive in cases of osteomyelitis, and the toxicity of an extended regimen of I.V. aminoglycosides is a serious concern.

OSTEOMYELITIS ASSOCIATED WITH VASCULAR INSUFFICIENCY

In addition to traditional culture-directed antibiotic therapy, other methods have been used to improve outcome in patients with osteomyelitis associated with vascular insufficiency. Hyperbaric oxygen therapy, by increasing oxygen levels in ischemic tissues, has improved wound healing and reduced the amputation rate in high risk patients. Revascularization of lesions in the lower extremity vasculature by angioplasty and bypass grafting may help oxygenate tissue with critical ischemia, thereby preventing limb amputations. Prognosis for wound healing improves when the tissue oxygen level is greater than 40 mm Hg and when the popliteal pulse is palpable.[9] Prompt, aggressive surgical and antibiotic therapy and proper wound care are the best means of preserving a functional limb and optimizing outcome in patients with osteomyelitis associated with vascular insufficiency.

GENERAL THERAPEUTIC CONSIDERATIONS

Oral Therapy

Because of rising hospital costs, alternatives to an extended hospital stay for parenteral treatment of osteomyelitis in otherwise healthy patients are being sought. The economic benefits of oral therapy are obvious: decreased hospital stay, reduced pharmacy and supply costs, no need for surgical insertion of a catheter, and decreased catheter-related complications. For patients who require a complete regimen of I.V. antibiotics, outpatient therapy should be considered. Patients should be educated in the care and use of the catheter while they are still in the hospital. Furthermore, drug toxicity and clinical response should be closely monitored. Administration of antibiotics during clinic visits or by a home health agency can substantially reduce costs.

Alternative Delivery of Antibiotics

Antibiotic-impregnated acrylic beads have been used for local treatment of bone infections; however, they have not been approved for use in the United States. Although the beads deliver a high concentration of antibiotic to the area of infection, bactericidal levels of antibiotic are present locally for only 2 to 4 weeks. Thus, the beads should be used in conjunction with systemic antibiotics. Both biodegradable and nonbiodegradable beads have been used. Nonbiodegradable beads, such as the polymethylmethacrylate beads, must be surgically removed after 2 to 4 weeks. Biodegradable antibiotic beads do not require surgical removal and provide local bactericidal concentrations for extended periods.[36,37]

Surgical Therapy

The type of surgical therapy depends on the extent of infection. In children with acute hematogenous osteomyelitis, surgery is usually unnecessary. For patients who do not respond to antimicrobial therapy, surgical decompression may result in the release of intramedullary or subperiosteal pus. In patients with chronic osteomyelitis, surgical debridement of all devitalized bone and soft tissue and removal of foreign bodies are essential for successful treatment. Inadequate surgical debridement, regardless of antibiotic therapy, is the most common cause of treatment failure. Sequestered dead bone can serve as a nidus for persistent infection. In some cases, a two-staged debridement protocol may be necessary to sterilize the wound.[38] Surgical therapy entails filling the dead space created by debridement and reestablishing blood supply to the poorly perfused area. Skin, bone, or muscle grafts are used to cover the wound. Cancellous bone grafts can be used to fill the dead space. Revascularization procedures include the use of local pedicle muscle flaps and myocutaneous flaps. In patients with very large bone defects, the Ilizarov technique has been used to reconstruct large defects in bone and soft tissue. In this procedure, major segmental resections of infected bone are performed, followed by realignment of opposing ends of now noninfected bone so that new bone growth fills in the defect. Each salvage procedure has associated morbidity and expense.

Future Concerns

The problem of methicillin-resistant *S. aureus* is worsening, especially in tertiary medical centers. At our center, the use of vancomycin alone to treat osteomyelitis caused by methicillin-resistant *S. aureus* has failed in the standard 4- to 6-week treatment regimen, and rifampin is now routinely added to the regimen. Similar regimens are used to treat methicillin-resistant *S. epidermidis* infections, especially sternal bone infections after median sternotomy. Unfortunately, because failure of vancomycin alone has been observed with increasing frequency, objective clinical trials to determine efficacy are not likely to be performed, for ethical reasons.

E. faecalis is becoming a problem in postoperative orthopedic patients and in diabetic patients. The isolation of vancomycin-resistant *Enterococcus* species in tertiary medical centers has increased over the past few years. This issue must eventually be confronted in the management of cases of osteomyelitis.

Infection with *C. albicans* and other candidal organisms is most commonly seen in patients who have candidemia with residual bone seeding. Sternal bone infections are also reported. Although these cases are isolated and sporadic, therapy has not been consistently effective.

References

1. Waldvogel FA, Medoff G, Swartz MM: Osteomyelitis: a review of clinical features, therapeutic considerations, and unusual aspects. N Engl J Med 282:198, 1970

2. Liptak GS, McConnochie KM, Roghmann KJ, et al: Decline of pediatric admissions with *Haemophilus influenzae* type b in New York State, 1982 through 1993: relation to immunizations. J Pediatr 130:923, 1997

3. Lew DP, Waldvogel FA: Osteomyelitis N Engl J Med 336:999, 1997

4. Sadat-Ali M: The status of acute osteomyelitis in sickle cell disease: a 15-year review. Int Surg 83:84, 1998

5. Endress C, Guyot DR, Fata J, et al: Cervical osteomyelitis due to I.V. heroin use: radiologic findings in 14 patients. Am J Roentgenol 155:333, 1990

6. Christiansen P, Frederiksen B, Glazowski J, et al: Epidemiologic, bacteriologic, and long-term follow-up data of children with acute hematogenous osteomyelitis and septic arthritis: a ten-year review. J Pediatr Orthop B 8:302, 1999

7. Gentry LO: Osteomyelitis and other infections of bones and joints. The Staphylococci in Human Disease. Crossley KB, Archer GL, Eds. Churchill Livingstone, New York,1997, p 455

8. Laughlin TJ, Armstrong DG, Caporusso J, et al: Soft tissue and bone infections from puncture wounds in children. West J Med 166:126, 1997

9. Lipsky BA: Osteomyelitis of the foot in diabetic patients. Clin Infect Dis 25:1318, 1997

10. Ramsey SD, Newton K, Blough D, et al: Incidence, outcomes, and cost of foot ulcers in patients with diabetes. Diabetes Care 22:382, 1999

11. Hill SL, Holtzman GI, Buse R: The effects of peripheral vascular disease with osteomyelitis in the diabetic foot. Am J Surg 177:282, 1999

12. Jaramillo D, Treves ST, Kasser JR, et al: Osteomyelitis and septic arthritis in children: appropriate use of imaging to guide treatment. AJR Am J Roentgenol 165:399, 1995

13. Sutter CW, Shelton DK: Three-phase bone scan in osteomyelitis and other musculoskeletal disorders. Am Fam Physician 54:1639, 1996

14. Harvey J, Cohen MM: Technetium-99–labeled leukocytes in diagnosing diabetic osteomyelitis in the foot. J Foot Ankle Surg 36:209, 1997

15. Johnson JE, Kennedy EJ, Shereff MJ, et al: Prospective study of bone, indium-111 labeled white blood cell, and gallium-67 scanning for the evaluation of osteomyelitis in the diabetic foot. Foot Ankle Int 17:16, 1996

16. Crerand S, Dolan M, Laing P, et al: Diagnosis of osteomyelitis in neuropathic foot ulcers. J Bone Joint Surg Br 78:51, 1996

17. Kaim A, Maurer T, Ochssner P, et al: Chronic complicated osteomyelitis of the appendicular skeleton: diagnosis with technetium-99m labelled monoclonal antigranulocyte antibody-immunoscintigraphy. Eur J Nucl Med 24:732, 1997

18. Hakki S, Harwood SJ, Morrissey MA, et al: Comparative study of monoclonal antibody scan in diagnosing orthopaedic infection. Clin Orthop 335:275, 1997

19. Becker W, Palestro CJ, Winship J, et al: Rapid imaging of infections with a monoclonal antibody fragment (Leukoscan). Clin Orthop 329: 263, 1996

20. Umans H, Haramati N, Flusser G: The diagnostic role of gadolinium enhanced MRI in distinguishing between acute medullary bone infarct and osteomyelitis. Magn Reson Imaging 18:255, 2000

21. Sammak B, Abd El Bagi M, Al Shahed M, et al: Osteomyelitis: a review of currently used imaging techniques. Eur Radiol 9:894, 2000

22. Gentry LO, Clint B: Adult osteomyelitis. Current Practice of Medicine. Bone RC, Ed. Churchill Livingstone, New York, 1996

p 15.6, **23.** Robiller FC, Stumpe KD, Kossmann T, et al: Chronic osteomyelitis of the femur: value of PET imaging. Eur Radiol 10:855, 2000

24. Guhlmann A, Brecht-Krauss D, Suger G, et al: Fluorine-18-FDG PET and technetium-99m antigranulocyte antibody scintigraphy in chronic osteomyelitis. J Nucl Med 39:2145, 1998

25. Zhuang H, Duarte PS, Pourdehand M, et al: Exclusion of chronic osteomyelitis with F-18 fluorodeoxyglucose positron emission tomographic imaging. Clin Nucl Med 25:281, 2000

26. Patzakis MJ, Wilkins J, Kumar J, et al: Comparison of the results of bacterial cultures from multiple sites in chronic osteomyelitis of long bones: a prospective study. J Bone Joint Surg Am 76:664, 1994

27. Mackowiak PA, Jones SR, Smith JW: Diagnostic value of sinus-tract cultures in chronic osteomyelitis. JAMA 239:2772, 1978

28. Tetzlaff TR, McCracken GH Jr, Nelson JD: Oral antibiotic therapy for skeletal infection of children: II. Therapy of osteomyelitis and suppurative arthritis. J Pediatr 92:485, 1978

29. Peltola H, Unkila-Kallio L, Kallio MJ: Simplified treatment of acute staphylococcal osteomyelitis of childhood. Finnish Study Group. Pediatrics 99:846, 1997

30. Nelson JD: Toward simple but safe management of osteomyelitis. Pediatrics 99:883, 1997

31. Gentry LO, Rodriguez GG: Oral ciprofloxacin compared with parenteral antibiotics in the treatment of osteomyelitis. Antimicrob Agents Chemother 34:40, 1990

32. Lew DP, Waldvogel FA: Use of quinolones in osteomyelitis and infected orthopaedic prosthesis. Drugs 58(suppl 2):85, 1999

33. Trucksis M, Hooper DC, Wolfson JS: Emerging resistance to fluoroquinolones in staphylococci: an alert editorial. Ann Intern Med 114: 424, 1991

34. Zimmerli W, Widmer AF, Blatter M, et al: Role of rifampin for treatment of orthopedic implant-related staphylococcal infections: a randomized controlled trial. Foreign-Body Infection (FBI) Study Group. JAMA 279:1537, 1998

35. Galanakis N, Giamarellou H, Moussas T, et al: Chronic osteomyelitis caused by multi-resistant gram-negative bacteria: evaluation of treatment with newer quinolones after prolonged follow-up. J Antimicrob Chemother 39:241, 1997

36. Calhoun JH, Mader JT: Treatment of osteomyelitis with a biodegradable antibiotic implant. Clin Orthop 341:206, 1997

37. Kanellakopoulou K, Giamarellos-Bourboulis EJ: Carrier systems for the local delivery of antibiotics in bone infections. Drugs 59:1223, 2000

38. Patzakis MJ, Greene N, Holtom P, et al: Culture results in open wound treatment with muscle transfer for tibial osteomyelitis. Clin Orthop 360:66, 1999

13 Bacterial Infections of the Central Nervous System

Jan V. Hirschmann, M.D.

Several barriers protect the central nervous system from bacterial infection. Considerable force is necessary to breach the skull and allow ingress of organisms into the brain or its coverings. Tight junctions between cells in the cerebral vasculature form the blood-brain barrier, limiting access by blood-borne pathogens. The vertebrae and the dura mater enveloping the spinal cord present strong defenses against incursions by microbes from contiguous areas.

Nevertheless, bacteria occasionally overwhelm or bypass these barriers, resulting in CNS infections. They usually arrive by one of three routes: (1) penetration as a result of trauma or surgery, (2) migration from an adjacent site of infection or colonization, or (3) hematogenous spread from another, often distant, location. The major bacterial infections that result are meningitis, brain abscess, epidural abscess, subdural empyema, and septic thrombophlebitis of the cerebral veins.

Acute Bacterial Meningitis

EPIDEMIOLOGY AND ETIOLOGY

Because vaccination has markedly decreased childhood *Haemophilus influenzae* type b infections, acute bacterial meningitis, previously most common in children, has become predominantly a disease of adults.[1] Bacterial meningitis may occur in otherwise healthy people, but it usually afflicts those with significant underlying disorders, such as hypogammaglobulinemia, sickle cell anemia, alcoholism, cirrhosis, and concurrent infections of the ears, paranasal sinuses, lungs, or cardiac valves.[2] Patients with HIV disease have a substantially increased risk of bacterial meningitis, usually when their CD4 count is less than 200 cells/mm^3. The most common organism is *Streptococcus pneumoniae;* bacteremia is nearly always present.[3] Patients with a splenectomy or poor splenic function may develop overwhelming sepsis, often including meningitis, from encapsulated bacteria, primarily *S. pneumoniae*. People with deficiencies of some complement components are susceptible to infections with *Neisseria meningitidis,* and patients with head trauma that disrupts the dura mater can develop meningitis, usually from *S. pneumoniae*. Meningitis that occurs as a complication of neutropenia or cranial surgery is most commonly caused by gram-negative bacilli [*see Table 1*]. A viral upper respiratory tract infection may predispose to meningitis by allowing bacteria that are colonizing the respiratory tract, especially *N. meningitidis,* to enter the bloodstream and invade the meninges.

S. pneumoniae causes approximately 40% to 60% of adult cases of bacterial meningitis in the United States; these cases often occur secondary to bacteremic pneumococcal pneumonia. Other major organisms in community-acquired cases are *N. meningitidis,* primarily in young adults; *Listeria monocytogenes,* especially in immunocompromised or elderly hosts; *H. influenzae;* and group B streptococci (*S. agalactiae*). Usually, the organisms reach the meninges through bacteremia from a mucosal site or a distant infection. Occasionally, the bacteria enter the subarachnoid space from adjacent infectious foci or through direct inoculation via trauma, surgery, or invasive medical procedures, such as lumbar puncture.

Table 1 Causes of Bacterial Meningitis in Adults[1,2]

Organism	*Approximate Frequency*
Streptococcus pneumoniae	40%–60%
Neisseria meningitidis	15%–25%
Listeria monocytogenes	10%–15%
Haemophilus influenzae	5%–10%
Other	5%–20%
Culture negative	10%–15%

DIAGNOSIS

Clinical Features

The duration of symptoms before patients seek medical attention varies from less than 24 hours to more than 1 week. A prodrome resembling a viral upper respiratory tract infection may occur; it is characterized by sore throat, rhinorrhea, and nasal congestion, sometimes accompanied by myalgias. The most common features of bacterial meningitis are headache, fever, nuchal rigidity, and neurologic findings. Fever is present in approximately 95% of patients and typically lasts 4 to 8 days after appropriate therapy has begun.[2,4,5] Stiff neck is apparent in about 90% of patients. Two physical findings that, like nuchal rigidity, arise from meningeal irritation and the neuromuscular response to it are the Kernig sign (when the hip is flexed at 90°, attempted extension of the knee meets resistance at 135°) and the Brudzinski sign (passive flexion of the neck causes knee and hip flexion).[6] Mental changes ranging from lethargy to confusion, stupor, and coma occur in about 80% of patients, somewhat more frequently in the elderly. Seizures, either focal or generalized, occur in about 10% to 30% of patients, usually within 24 hours of admission. Many such seizures arise from alcohol withdrawal. Focal neurologic findings other than seizures develop in about 30% of patients. They include cranial nerve palsies, aphasia, and hemiparesis as a consequence of infection-induced vasculitis or pressure of purulent exudate on neurologic structures. Papilledema occurs only occasionally; its absence does not exclude significantly increased intracranial pressure.

Laboratory Findings

Most patients with acute bacterial meningitis have leukocytosis, and some have hyponatremia, presumably because of inappropriate secretion of antidiuretic hormone. Blood cultures, which are positive in approximately 50% to 60% of cases, are always indicated. The most important diagnostic procedure is a lumbar puncture to obtain cerebrospinal fluid to determine white cell count and differential, to measure protein and glucose levels, and for culture and Gram stain.

Clinicians commonly obtain a CT scan before doing a lumbar puncture, on the basis of two beliefs: that brain herniation is a frequent risk in meningitis and that CT scans can accurately predict its development. Neither belief is correct. Herniation occurs in approximately 1% of patients with bacterial meningitis,[2] sometimes without a preceding lumbar puncture.[7] CT scans are often normal in those who later experience brain herniation, and most patients who develop this complication have focal neurologic findings before the lumbar puncture that suggest that herniation has already begun: dilated, fixed pupils; Cheyne-Stokes respiration; decerebrate posturing; hemiplegia; and coma.[7] In the absence of such findings in patients with suspected bacterial meningitis, clinicians should not delay lumbar puncture to obtain a CT scan.

In approximately 90% of patients, the opening pressure is above 180 mm H_2O; in 20%, it is above 400 mm H_2O; and in about 5%, it is above 500 mm H_2O. The CSF protein level exceeds 40 mg/dl in approximately 85%, and the glucose level is below 40 mg/dl in about 60%.[2] When bacterial meningitis develops in patients with diabetes and hyperglycemia, the CSF glucose level may be normal, but the ratio of CSF glucose to blood glucose in these patients is usually less than 0.31.[8] The CSF white cell count is greater than 100/mm^3 in about 90% of patients and exceeds 1,000/mm^3 in 15% to 20%. Neutrophils nearly always predominate, constituting at least 80% of cells in 80% to 90% of patients. Occasionally, lymphocytes constitute the majority, especially when the white cell count is very low; lymphocytes constitute the majority in about 25% of patients with meningitis caused by *L. monocytogenes*.[9] Several conditions can cause neutrophilia with low CSF glucose levels and can mimic acute bacterial meningitis [*see Table 2*].

Gram stain is positive in approximately 60% to 90% of patients, indicating a concentration of bacteria exceeding 10^5 organisms/ml. Misinterpretation may occur, especially through mistaking pneumococci for *Listeria*. In listerial meningitis, the Gram stain is positive in only 30% of cases.[10]

The CSF culture is positive in approximately 80% of patients. Previous oral antibiotic therapy has little effect on the WBC or differential cell counts, protein level, or glucose level, but it decreases the number of positive Gram stains by about 20% and the number of positive cultures by about 30%.[11] The effect of parenteral therapy is presumably much greater, especially if given more than a few hours before the lumbar puncture. In patients with negative Gram stains and cultures, latex agglutination tests of the CSF are highly specific for *H. influenzae* type b, meningococci, and pneumococci, but their sensitivity ranges from 50% to 80%.

Imaging Studies

Imaging techniques are ordinarily unnecessary in bacterial meningitis unless specific complica-

Table 2 Causes of Neutrophilia with Low Glucose Levels in the CSF

	Infectious Cause	*Noninfectious Cause*
Common	Bacterial meningitis	—
Uncommon	Viral meningitis* (in very early phase only) Certain parameningeal infections Subdural empyema* (usually produces lymphocytic-normal glucose profile) ?Early brain abscess at bacterial cerebritis stage* Cerebral abscess with leakage or rupture into ventricle Embolic cerebral infarction* (bacterial endocarditis) Amebic meningoencephalitis Tuberculous meningitis (only very early in the disease and only in a small percentage of cases) Acute hemorrhagic leukoencephalitis	Chemical meningitis Exogenous (e.g., contrast media, detergents used in cleaning needles) Endogenous (release of material into CSF from tumors: dermoids, craniopharyngiomas) Unusual diseases* Initial phase of Mollaret meningitis Behçet syndrome Hypersensitivity meningitis Drug-induced* (sulfonamides, tolmetin, ibuprofen, isoniazid)

*Glucose level in CSF usually normal.

tions are suspected. The subarachnoid space may be distended on CT or MRI studies; however, this finding is often difficult to interpret in adults, in whom a degree of brain atrophy is common—especially in the elderly. Several days after infection, meningeal enhancement may occur after contrast injection because of meningeal inflammation and vascular congestion. Enhancement of areas in the cerebral cortex usually indicates brain infarction from occlusion of inflamed vessels. Brain edema may occur because of disturbed cerebrovascular autoregulation, dural sinus thrombophlebitis, leakage of fluid from damaged vessels, or cytotoxic edema from injured brain cells. Communicating or noncommunicating hydrocephalus occasionally develops because inflammation obstructs the normal flow of CSF, either at the arachnoid granulations where it is absorbed or at the sites where it leaves the ventricles.

TREATMENT

Intravenous Antibiotics

The most important therapeutic maneuver is prompt initiation of intravenous antibiotics after lumbar puncture, because delay in beginning treatment increases the mortality [*see Table 3*].[12] In the rare situation in which lumbar puncture is justifiably postponed—for example, when signs of brain herniation are present (see above)—blood cultures should be obtained and antibiotics begun, even though they may reduce the yield of the subsequent CSF Gram stain and culture. The antimicrobial agent chosen should be bactericidal against the suspected pathogens and should achieve good CSF levels.

The findings on CSF Gram stain may help guide the choice of antibiotic; when the stain is negative, however, ceftriaxone (2 g I.V. every 12 hours, or 4 g I.V. every 24 hours) is a good choice in adults.[13] Ceftriaxone provides coverage for meningococci, *H. influenzae,* group B streptococci, and *S. pneumoniae,* including many penicillin-resistant strains. With suspected high-level penicillin resistance, use of vancomycin (2 g every 12 hours) is prudent until culture and susceptibility test results are available. If Gram stain of the CSF is negative or if a distinction between pneumococci and *Listeria* is uncertain, the patient should receive, in addition, ampicillin at a dosage of 2 g every 4 hours to treat possible *L. monocytogenes* infection. Although controlled studies have not delineated the optimal length of antibiotic therapy, the duration is usually 7 days for *H. influenzae* and meningococci and 10 to 14 days for most other organisms. Repeat lumbar puncture during or after therapy is usually unnecessary unless treatment seems to be failing.

Systemic Corticosteroids

Some studies, primarily in children infected with *H. influenzae,* have indicated that systemic corticosteroids may help reduce complications of meningitis (especially hearing loss), presumably by decreasing inflammation. Data regarding use of corticosteroids in adults is sparse and unimpressive. Corticosteroids may decrease antimicrobial penetra-

Table 3 Antibiotic Therapy for Bacterial Meningitis in Adults

Organism	*Antibiotic*	*Dose*	*Alternative Antibiotic*
Streptococcus pneumoniae			
Penicillin MIC < 0.1 μg/ml	Penicillin G	4 million units I.V. q. 4 hr	Ceftriaxone, 2 g I.V. q. 12 hr, or chloramphenicol, 1 g I.V. q. 6 hr
Penicillin MIC 0.1–1.0 μg/ml	Ceftriaxone	2 g I.V. q. 12 hr	Vancomycin, 2 g I.V. q 12 hr
Penicillin MIC >1.0 μg/ml	Vancomycin	2 g I.V. q. 12 hr	?Meropenem, 1 g I.V. q. 8hr
Streptococcus			
Groups A and B	Penicillin G	4 million units I.V. q. 4 hr	Ceftriaxone, 2 g I.V. q. 12 hr, or chloramphenicol, 1 g I.V. q. 6 hr
Staphylococcus aureus			
Methicillin sensitive	Nafcillin	2 g I.V. q. 4 hr	Vancomycin, 2 g I.V. q. 12 hr
Methicillin resistant	Vancomycin	2 g I.V. q. 12 hr	No clear alternative
Listeria monocytogenes	Ampicillin	2 g I.V. q. 4 hr	Trimethoprim (TMP)-sulfamethoxazole (SMX): 10–20 mg/kg TMP, 50–100 mg/kg SMX q. day in four divided doses
Haemophilus influenzae			
Ampicillin sensitive	Ampicillin	2 g I.V. q. 4 hr	Ceftriaxone, 2 g I.V. q. 12 hr, or chloramphenicol, 1 g I.V. q. 6 hr
Ampicillin resistant	Ceftriaxone	2 g I.V. q. 12 hr	Chloramphenicol, 1 g I.V. q. 6 hr
Neisseria meningitidis	Penicillin	4 million units I.V. q. 4 hr	Ceftriaxone, 2 g I.V. q. 12 hr, or chloramphenicol, 1 g I.V. q. 6 hr
Escherichia coli, Klebsiella, Proteus, and other enteric gram-negative bacilli	Ceftriaxone	2 g I.V. q. 12 hr	Ceftazidime, 2 g I.V. q. 8 hr
Pseudomonas aeruginosa	Ceftazidime *and* gentamicin	2 g I.V. q. 8 hr 2 mg/kg first dose I.V., then 1.7 mg/kg I.V. q. 8 hr with normal renal function (gentamicin also may be given intrathecally, 4–8 mg q. day)	?Meropenem, 2 g I.V. q. 8 hr *and* intrathecal gentamicin

MIC—minimum inhibitory concentration

tion into the CSF, especially with vancomycin.[14] Accordingly, a reasonable approach is to reserve high-dose systemic corticosteroids for patients with evidence of cerebral edema.

COMPLICATIONS

Many complications may occur in meningitis patients, including secondary nosocomial infections, systemic venous thromboembolism, and adverse effects from the medications administered. The most common systemic complications occur from the initial infection, however, and include septic shock, disseminated intravascular coagulation, and the acute respiratory distress syndrome.[15] The most frequent neurologic complications other than seizures and altered mentation are cerebral edema, hydrocephalus, and cerebrovascular complications.[16] In bacterial meningitis, the internal carotid, basilar, and vertebral arteries and their branches lie within a purulent subarachnoid exudate, which can provoke vascular inflammation and constriction. Smaller arteries may demonstrate vessel wall irregularities, occlusion, narrowing, or widening. Thrombosis of the superior sagittal sinus or the cortical veins can occur. These abnormalities may cause discrete areas of brain damage—evidenced by focal neurologic findings—or increased intracranial pressure produced by leakage of cerebral vessels (vasogenic edema), swelling of damaged neurons (cytotoxic edema), or increased blood volume that occurs when sinus venous thrombosis impedes drainage of blood from the brain.

PROGNOSIS

The mortality associated with meningococcal meningitis is approximately 10% and is typically 20% to 30% in meningitis caused by other organisms. Factors associated with poorer prognoses include advanced age (> 60 years), onset of seizures during the first 24 hours after infection, hypotension, and coma or obtundation on hospital admission.[12] Most survivors recover completely. Approximately 30% of patients with pneumococcal meningitis have moderate to severe sequelae, including dementia, seizures, hearing loss, and gait disturbances; about 20% have mild problems, such as dizziness, slightly impaired memory, headaches, and phonophobia.[17]

Bacterial Meningitis in Special Circumstances

POSTTRAUMATIC BACTERIAL MENINGITIS

Epidemiology and Etiology

Bacterial meningitis develops in about 1% of persons who receive medical attention for blunt cranial injuries, most commonly from motor vehicle accidents.[18] At risk are those in whom the force of impact fractures the base of the skull, tearing the dura mater, the underlying arachnoid, and adjacent soft tissues. The trauma, however, need not be severe: coma or retrograde amnesia is absent or brief in 30% to 40% of cases.

The most common cause of posttraumatic meningitis is *S. pneumoniae,* which accounts for about 65% of cases. In the remainder of cases, the causes are primarily other streptococci, *H. influenzae,* meningococci, and *Staphylococcus aureus* [*see Table 4*]. Enteric gram-negative bacilli are rare causes, except in patients who have previously received antimicrobial therapy.

Pathogenesis

The dural rent resulting from blunt cranial trauma creates a fistula between the subarachnoid space and the nasal cavity, paranasal sinuses, or ear. The most common site for these abnormal communications is the cribriform plate; the disruptions are multiple, however, in about 40% of cases. When these rents are large, they are evident as CSF rhinorrhea; smaller leaks may go unrecognized, and drainage may be delayed or intermittent when tissue occludes the dural laceration. When trauma weakens but does not tear the dura, CSF rhinorrhea may begin abruptly after sudden increases in cerebrospinal pressure from coughing, sneezing, or straining. When the dural fistula occurs in the middle cranial fossa because of a fractured temporal bone, CSF may exit through the ear canal (if the tympanic membrane ruptures) or drain into the pharynx through the eustachian tube and go unrecognized. Evidence of basilar skull fractures may appear shortly after the injury as periorbital bruising, anosmia, hemotympanum, bloody ear drainage, or Battle sign (ecchymoses behind the ear).

Table 4 Causes of Recurrent Meningitis

Bacterial Meningitis*
- Predisposing anatomic defects
  - Congenital: meningomyeloceles, dermal sinuses
  - Traumatic: skull fractures through cribriform plate or petrous ridge
  - Postoperative: craniotomy, transsphenoidal hypophysectomy
  - Tumors: direct invasion through the dura
  - Empty sella syndrome
- Parameningeal infections*
  - Mastoiditis, sinusitis, osteomyelitis of skull
- Immunologic defects*
  - Immunoglobulin deficiencies: congenital or acquired (e.g., myeloma)
  - Asplenic state: splenectomy or functional asplenia (e.g., sickle cell anemia)
  - Complement deficiencies: C6, C7, or C8 deficiency

Endogenous Chemical Meningitis
- Tumors†
  - Craniopharyngioma, epidermoid cyst

Unusual Nonbacterial Recurrent Meningitides
- Mollaret meningitis†
- Behçet syndrome†
- Drug hypersensitivity†
  - Sulfonamides, ibuprofen
- Systemic lupus erythematosus†
- Uveoencephalitides‡ (Vogt-Koyanagi syndrome, Harada syndrome)

*Neutrophilic CSF pleocytosis.
†Either neutrophilic or lymphocytic CSF pleocytosis.
‡Lymphocytic CSF pleocytosis.

Diagnosis

Clinical features The usual clinical features of bacterial meningitis, including fever, headache, and stiff neck, are present in posttraumatic meningitis. Mortality is comparatively low (10%), however, perhaps because the fistula allows drainage of CSF (relieving intracranial hypertension) or because many patients with cranial trauma are young and otherwise healthy. The interval between blunt cranial injury and meningitis is usually less than 1 month, but infection may occur years later; when evaluating patients with unexplained meningitis, clinicians should therefore ask about any significant head trauma, even if such trauma occurred in the remote past.

Recognition of CSF rhinorrhea or otorrhea allows a diagnosis of a dural fistula. The discharge often increases with sudden movement, lowering of the head, performance of the Valsalva maneuver, or jugular vein compression. Unlike normal nasal secretions, the CSF fluid is not sticky, does not stiffen a handkerchief on drying, may taste salty, and has a glucose level greater than 30 mg/dl in the absence of infection. The most sensitive and specific way to identify CSF is by detection of a β_2-transferrin found only in that body fluid.[19]

Imaging studies Several techniques help localize the leak of CSF. CT scans may demonstrate the fistula site by disclosing sinus fractures, displaced bony fragments, or intracranial air (pneumocephalus). Radionuclide-labeled albumin and various dyes injected in the subarachnoid space may leak into the middle and superior meatus of the nose and become detectable on cotton pledgets placed in these locations. Magnetic resonance cisternography, a noninvasive and rapid procedure, seems highly accurate in detecting fistulas.[19] This technology relies on the fact that CSF gives a high signal on T_2-weighted images: demonstration of a continuous high signal through the cribriform plate or the paranasal sinuses that is similar to the signal given by the CSF in the basal cisterns indicates a dural fistula.

Treatment

Because many dural fistulas resolve spontaneously, repair is usually unnecessary unless problems persist for 2 to 3 weeks after the injury. Patients with facial fractures or meningitis are exceptions. Those with fracture sites accessible through the nose typically undergo transnasal closure with fibrin glue, fascia lata, or local flaps. Otherwise, intracranial repair is required. Recurrences may develop if the dural fistula remains uncorrected. Ceftriaxone is a good antibiotic choice for bacterial meningitis after closed head trauma when the CSF Gram stain is negative.

RECURRENT BACTERIAL MENINGITIS NOT CAUSED BY TRAUMA

Although a dural fistula created by blunt cranial trauma is the most common cause of recurrent bacterial meningitis, "spontaneous" leaks of CSF occasionally occur, most of which probably arise from a congenital or acquired weakness in the dura. Defects of the skull or of the floor of the middle cranial fossa are other potential sources of recurrent meningitis, as are bony complications from chronic ear infections. Congenital malformations can lead to dermal sinus tracts, often associated with intradural dermoid tumors, that connect the skin to the CSF. They commonly occur at the lumbodorsal spine but may be present anywhere along the midline. Abnormalities at the cutaneous exit site can include small tufts of hair, a nevus, or a dimple from which purulent drainage may emanate. Other conditions associated with recurrent bacterial meningitis are hypogammaglobulinemia, asplenia, and deficiencies of certain components of complement, which especially predispose to meningococcal meningitis.

CEREBROSPINAL FLUID SHUNT INFECTIONS

CSF shunts, used to relieve hydrocephalus, usually consist of a ventricular catheter; a pressure-regulating valve and reservoir, commonly placed just outside the skull; and distal tubing that drains the CSF, most frequently into the peritoneum but sometimes into the right atrium, pleura, or other sites.

Etiology

Mechanisms of infection of CSF shunts include implantation of microbes during shunt insertion, entry through a break in the overlying skin, hematogenous dissemination from a distant site, and retrograde spread of organisms from the distal end (in the peritoneum or another body cavity).[20] The most common origin is contamination of the device by skin flora at the time of surgery. Most infections become apparent within a few weeks of the shunt's insertion. Entry of microbes into the shunt from overlying skin is probably the next most frequent cause of infection. Retrograde and hematogenous infections seem to be rare except in the case of ventriculoatrial shunts, in which the distal end lies within the bloodstream.

The bacteriology of CSF shunt infections reflects the probable cutaneous source of infection in most cases. The most common isolates are staphylococci, with coagulase-negative species accounting for approximately 50% to 60% of cases and *S. aureus* for approximately 20%. Streptococci, anaerobes, diphtheroids, and polymicrobial infections, primarily from these and other cutaneous species, constitute most of the remaining cases. About 10% of isolates are gram-negative bacilli, and about 5% are the same organisms that commonly cause community-acquired meningitis in patients without shunts: pneumococci, meningococci, and *H. influenzae*.

Diagnosis

Clinical features The manifestations of CSF shunt infections differ from the usual findings of bacterial meningitis and depend on the site involved. Fever is usually present. When ventriculitis occurs, nuchal rigidity rarely develops, because infected CSF typically does not communicate from the ventricle to the meninges. Mental changes, including headache, nausea, lethargy, and confusion, are the most common abnormalities; these may result from infection in the ventricle or from increased intracranial pressure caused by obstruction of the shunt anywhere along its route. Evidence of infection over the shunt may sometimes be detected by the presence of wound dehiscence, cellulitis, or purulent drainage. When the distal end lies within the atrium, bacteremia may occur, sometimes complicated by endocarditis. In chronic bacteremia, usually caused by coagulase-negative staphylococci, renal disease (so-called shunt nephritis) produced by deposition of immune complexes in the kidney may develop. When the distal end lies in the peritoneum, infection may cause peritonitis, manifested by abdominal pain and tenderness, anorexia, and fever. Often, the infection is more insidious, with enlarging cysts developing around the end of the catheter as the inflamed peritoneum fails to absorb the CSF.

Laboratory findings The peripheral white cell count is often normal. Blood cultures are characteristically positive in patients with infected ventriculoatrial shunts but are usually negative when the distal end lies elsewhere. Culturing CSF through use of needle aspiration of the shunt reservoir or of any fluid in contact with the shunt is the best approach to delineating the cause. The CSF will usually show pleocytosis, which is often mild, and an elevated protein level; the glucose level is typically normal or slightly decreased. Gram stain may reveal bacteria, but it is often negative.

Treatment

Treatment of shunt infections usually entails systemic antibiotics, shunt removal, and temporary placement of an external ventricular drain to control intracranial pressure (and to provide a conduit for intraventricular antibiotic administration). The systemic antimicrobials used for the treatment of shunt infections are nafcillin for susceptible strains of *S. aureus* and vancomycin for methicillin-resistant *S. aureus* and coagulase-negative staphylococci, often supplemented by oral rifampin (600 mg daily). Ceftriaxone is used for susceptible gram-negative bacilli; ceftazidime is appropriate for ceftriaxone-resistant organisms, including *Pseudomonas aeruginosa*. Intraventricular antibiotics are commonly employed in patients with ventriculitis (generally, vancomycin at a dosage of 10 to 20 mg daily for gram-positive organisms and gentamicin at a dosage of 4 to 8 mg daily for gram-negative bacilli). Once the infection has resolved (usually after several days), a new shunt can be inserted.

NOSOCOMIAL MENINGITIS AND MENINGITIS AFTER NEUROSURGERY

Epidemiology and Etiology

Nosocomial meningitis is quite rare except in patients who have recently undergone neurosurgery. A study of 51 hospitalized patients who underwent lumbar puncture to exclude bacterial meningitis revealed no cases, despite the presence of mental status changes in 78%, fever in 47%, and meningeal signs or headache in 22%.[21] By contrast, 92% of patients with community-acquired bacterial meningitis had either meningeal signs or headache. The conclusion is that lumbar puncture can be safely withheld in most hospitalized patients who have fever and changes in mental status, unless headache or nuchal rigidity is present or unless the patient has recently undergone neurosurgery.

Even after neurosurgery, bacterial meningitis is very uncommon, especially after spinal surgery or craniotomy; it is somewhat less rare, but still unusual, after transsphenoidal procedures. During neurosurgery, bacteria most commonly enter the subarachnoid space from contiguous sites of colonization on the skin and mucous membranes. Less frequent sources or causes of infection include contaminated instruments or irrigation solutions, airborne organisms, breaches of sterile technique, and organisms from adjacent sites of suppuration. Postoperative sources are wound infections at the operative site, indwelling catheters that allow organisms to enter the ventricle or subarachnoid space, and CSF leaks. A very uncommon cause is hematogenous spread from a distant site of infection, such as the lungs or urinary tract.

Approximately one half of cases of bacterial meningitis after craniotomy or spinal surgery occur in the first postoperative week, approximately 25% in the second week, and the remainder after the second week. After transsphenoidal surgery, about 85% of cases occur in the first week. Because headache, nuchal rigidity, and impaired consciousness are common after cranial surgery, the onset of meningitis may be inconspicuous.

Diagnosis

Clinical features Nearly all infected patients have fever, often accompanied by worsening meningismus, deteriorating mentation, and erythema or purulence at the incision site. CSF rhinorrhea may appear in patients with dural defects.

Laboratory findings The peripheral white cell count is usually elevated; the elevation is accompanied by neutrophilia and increased bands. Blood cultures are positive in about 30% of cases. The most important diagnostic test is sampling of the CSF, usually after obtaining a CT scan to exclude brain abscesses or other fluid collections. In most cases of postoperative meningitis, the CSF protein level is 100 to 500 mg/dl and the white cell count exceeds 1,000/mm^3, with neutrophilic predominance. The CSF glucose level is decreased in 85% of cases; Gram stain discloses the responsible bacteria in 50% to 80%.

The infecting organisms are primarily gram-negative bacilli, including *P. aeruginosa* and species of *Klebsiella* and *Enterobacter*. When ventricular drains are present, coagulase-negative staphylococci predominate. The bacteria isolated in meningitis after transsphenoidal surgery are more diverse, reflecting various nasal mucosal organisms—especially as altered by hospitalization and prior antimicrobial therapy. Causes include gram-negative bacilli, streptococci, staphylococci, diphtheroids, anaerobes, *Haemophilus* species, and, sometimes, polymicrobial isolates. Antimicrobial therapy should be directed by the results of CSF Gram stain and culture. For gram-negative bacilli, ceftazidime (2 g I.V. every 8 hours) is the drug of choice unless the organism is known to be susceptible to ceftriaxone. Often, ceftazidime is combined with intrathecal or intraventricular injection of gentamicin (4 to 8 mg daily). For gram-positive organisms, parenteral vancomycin, supplemented by oral or parenteral rifampin and intrathecal or intraventricular vancomycin (10 to 20 mg daily), is a good regimen. When the Gram stain is negative, a combination of ceftazidime and vancomycin is reasonable until culture results become available.

Differential Diagnosis

A confounding diagnostic problem in patients with a negative Gram stain is that an aseptic meningitis may develop several days after surgery, probably in response to blood in the subarachnoid space. Fever, nuchal rigidity, nausea, vomiting, and altered mentation may all occur, and the findings on lumbar puncture resemble a bacterial infection, including marked pleocytosis, neutrophilic predominance, increased protein, and, sometimes, decreased glucose.

Treatment

When the distinction between bacterial and aseptic meningitis is unclear, a reasonable approach is to initiate appropriate antimicrobial therapy and, if the cultures remain negative, to withdraw the antibiotics and administer systemic corticosteroids, which seem useful in this form of chemical meningitis.[22]

Brain Abscess

EPIDEMIOLOGY AND ETIOLOGY

Brain abscesses are about two to three times more frequent in males than in females. About 50% arise from contiguous infections, such as sinusitis and otitis media, with the organisms arriving in the brain from direct extension or retrograde spread through the venous system. Pathogens from distant areas of suppuration may reach the brain via a hematogenous route through the cerebral arteries. Occasionally, abscesses develop after penetrating trauma or surgery, with organisms directly inoculated into the cerebral tissue. In approximately 20% to 30% of brain abscesses, the source of origin is inapparent.[23]

Chronic otitis media is a common predisposing factor, with the abscesses most frequently forming in the temporal lobe or cerebellum. Those occurring secondary to frontal sinusitis usually develop in the frontal lobe, whereas abscesses originating from the sphenoidal sinus are typically in the temporal lobe. Hematogenous infections from distant sites are commonly multiple and most likely to cause suppuration in the territories supplied by the distal middle cerebral artery. Frequently, these arise when blood-borne organisms bypass the ordinary filtering mechanisms of the lung in such conditions as left-sided endocarditis, pulmonary infections, and right-to-left cardiac or pulmonary shunts. In patients with shunts, concurrent hypoxemia and secondary erythrocytosis may cause brain damage that predisposes them to subsequent infection. Immunocompromised patients, especially patients who have undergone bone marrow transplantation or solid organ transplantation, have an increased risk of developing brain abscesses, usually through hematogenous spread.

Brain abscesses begin as localized—but poorly demarcated—areas of encephalitis, often called cerebritis. At this stage, tissue has not liquefied, and needle aspiration or surgery is unhelpful. Over several days, necrosis occurs, with pus forming in the center of the infection. With time, a capsule of fibrous tissue develops, delimiting the suppuration, but pus may rupture through it into the ventricle or adjacent cerebral tissue, forming satellite abscesses.

The most common organisms isolated from brain abscesses are aerobic, microaerophilic, or anaerobic streptococci; other anaerobic bacteria; staphylococci; and gram-negative bacilli (especially when the abscess arises from chronic ear infection).

DIAGNOSIS

Clinical Features

Most patients have symptoms for several days to weeks before they seek medical attention. Fever is present in only about 40% to 50% of cases. The most common symptom is headache, which may be diffuse or localized to the abscess area. Other frequent findings are altered mental states, such as confusion, aberrant behavior, and somnolence; generalized or focal seizures; and specific neurologic abnormalities, depending on the abscess site. With temporal lobe involvement, contralateral sensory or motor signs, aphasia, and an upper homonymous quadrantanopia may occur. In cerebellar abscesses, ataxia in the ipsilateral extremities, nystagmus, signs of increased intracranial pressure, and ataxic gait are characteristic. In patients with frontal lobe involvement, hemiparesis, aphasia, and impaired mentation are common, whereas the main finding in occipital lobe abscesses is homonymous hemianopsia. Typical features of parietal lobe abscesses include hemianesthesia, homonymous hemianopsia, neglect of one half of the body, alexia, and impaired spatial perception. Papilledema is infrequent, irrespective of the abscess site.

Laboratory Findings

Leukocytosis occurs in approximately 50% of patients, and an elevated erythrocyte sedimentation rate occurs in about 60%. Lumbar punctures are not recommended unless meningitis is strongly suspected, because of the low risk of brain herniation and the low likelihood of positive cultures. Examination of the CSF usually shows a pleocytosis with mixed neutrophils and lymphocytes, elevated protein levels, normal glucose levels, and a negative Gram stain. Blood cultures are positive in about 10% to 20% of patients.

Imaging Studies

During the cerebritis phase, CT scans show low-density abnormalities with mass effect, sometimes with patchy enhancement. On MRI, the characteristic findings are areas of low density on T_1-weighted images and, on proton-density or T_2-weighted images, high-intensity areas surrounded by areas of patchy enhancement with gadolinium. In a mature abscess, the CT scan shows a low-density lesion with uniform ring enhancement and a surrounding area of low density, representing cerebral edema [*see Figure 1a and 1b*]. On T_1-weighted images, the encapsulated abscess appears as a round, low-intensity lesion with mass effect and a surrounding area of low density, signifying edema. On proton-density and T_2-weighted images, the abscess has a high-intensity signal in the center and in the surrounding parenchyma as a consequence of the adjacent cerebral swelling. Ring enhancement occurs with gadolinium.

TREATMENT AND PROGNOSIS

Most patients should undergo prompt stereotactic-guided needle aspiration of pus[24] or craniotomy with excision of the abscess. If possible, antimicrobials should be withheld until a specimen is obtained, to avoid reducing the yield on cultures. Gram stain and culture determine antibiotic choice; appropriate empirical therapy that can be used until the microbiologic results become available include agents effective against anaerobes, streptococci, staphylococci, and gram-negative bacilli.

A good regimen is a combination of ceftriaxone and metronidazole. Patients with significant cerebral edema should receive dexamethasone. Some patients may respond to antibiotic therapy alone—especially those with cerebritis only, those with numerous abscesses that are inaccessible to drainage, or those with small abscesses who have stable neurologic function.

Mortality is approximately 5% to 10%. Many patients have residual neurologic problems, most commonly focal seizures.[25]

Spinal Epidural Abscess

PATHOGENESIS AND PATHOPHYSIOLOGY

The epidural space, an area posterolateral to the spinal cord containing fat and blood vessels, can potentially extend anteriorly to where the dura adheres to the posterior vertebral bodies. Most epidural abscesses occur in midthoracic and lumbar locations, where the space is largest. Cervical abscesses are less common, in part because the epidural space is very small in that area. Because no anatomic barriers prevent superior and inferior

a

b

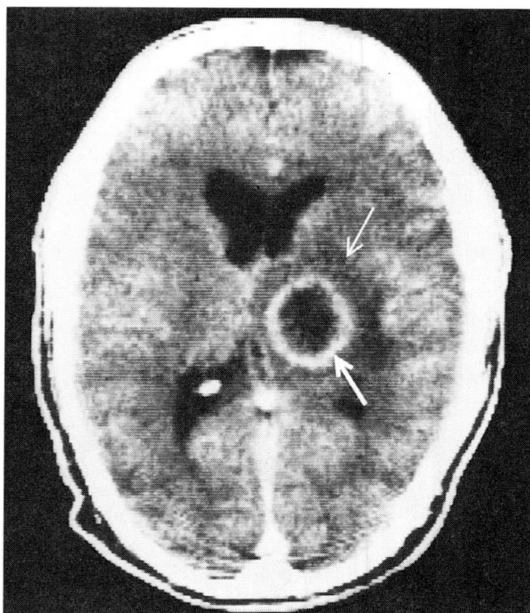

Figure 1 **(*a*) CT scan of a 39-year-old patient reveals a large thalamic abscess. Plain scan demonstrates abscess and surrounding zone of what may be either increased vascularity or an actual capsule formation (arrow). (*b*) Intravenous administration of contrast media enhances definition of the surrounding zone (thick arrow). A wide area of periabscess edema (thin arrow) is also evident. The mass effect can be seen clearly in the asymmetry of the ventricles.**

extension, abscesses typically involve several (an average of four) adjacent vertebral segments.[26]

Organisms may arrive in the epidural space from contiguous infection, especially vertebral osteomyelitis, but also from retropharyngeal, psoas, perivertebral, or perinephric abscess. All these infections are predominantly anterior to the spinal cord. Microbes also enter the epidural space as a result of penetrating trauma, surgery, and epidural catheterization for analgesic administration. Hematogenous spread may occur from distant foci of infection, including the skin and soft tissue, urinary tract, heart valves, and respiratory tract. Patients with frequent or prolonged bacteremias, such as intravenous drug users or those undergoing hemodialysis, are at increased risk.[27] Diabetes mellitus, alcoholism, and underlying disease in the affected spinal area are other predisposing factors. Many patients report recent trauma near the affected location, suggesting hemorrhage at the site with subsequent bacteremic superinfection. Often, the source of infection is inapparent. Males are more frequently affected than females, for unclear reasons.

Pus and granulation tissue in the epidural space can damage the spinal cord, in part by compression, which may impede arterial flow and cause ischemia. Inflammation and increased pressure can also provoke thrombophlebitis or venous thrombosis, which can lead to cord edema and infarction.

ETIOLOGY

S. aureus is the most common isolate from spinal epidural abscess; most of the other isolates are streptococci and gram-negative bacilli. Usually, only a single species of organism is responsible, but polymicrobial infections occur in approximately 5% to 10% of cases. In the United States, *Mycobacterium tuberculosis* is an occasional cause of epidural abscess. In such cases, the infection usually arises from an adjacent vertebral osteomyelitis. Patients may feel back pain for quite some time (weeks to months) before neurologic symptoms appear. Most of these patients have no evidence of pulmonary tuberculosis at the time of epidural infection.

DIAGNOSIS

Clinical Features

The most common symptom is back pain over the infected area. It is typically persistent and unrelieved by altered position or bed rest. Localized tenderness is often present; fever is common but is not invariable. With time, patients may develop radicular pain, primarily along the route of the affected level of the spinal cord. The next stage is usually marked by muscle weakness, typically paraparesis with thoracic involvement or quadriparesis with cervical infection. At this stage, findings of upper motor neuron disease are usually predominant; such findings include spasticity, hyperreflexia, and extensor plantar responses. Bilateral sensory loss and impaired bladder and bowel function may occur. Without treatment, paralysis develops, sometimes abruptly, and is usually irreversible.

Laboratory Findings

Leukocytosis is common in patients with epidural abscess, but white cell counts may be normal, especially in patients with protracted symptoms. The erythrocyte sedimentation rate is usually elevated. A lumbar puncture is not ordinarily recommended, except when needed for myelography; however, when a lumbar puncture is performed, the specimen typically demonstrates pleocytosis of up to a few hundred cells, commonly with a mixture of lymphocytes and neutrophils. The glucose level is normal; the protein level is usually elevated, sometimes by more than 1 g/L when the spinal canal is completely blocked. Gram stain and culture of CSF are usually normal. Blood cultures, which are commonly positive in epidural abscess, are worth obtaining in all suspected cases.

Imaging Studies

When the abscess arises from vertebral osteomyelitis, plain films of the spine may demonstrate erosion of the cortical margins of the vertebrae, narrowed or obliterated intervertebral disk spaces, and bone destruction. Myelograms show evidence of blockage of CSF circulation at the level of the epidural abscess but are rarely necessary when CT or MRI scans are available. CT scans detect vertebral osteomyelitis well; characteristic findings include narrowed intervertebral disk spaces, eroded vertebral end plates, and bony destruction of the vertebral bodies. The epidural abscess is present as a low-density focal epidural mass, which may be better delineated with CT myelography. The best imaging modality, however, is MRI, which discloses a low-intensity or isointense image on T_1-weighted scans (when compared with the spinal cord image) and a high signal on proton-density or T_2-weighted scans. Epidural abscesses typically appear enhanced with gadolinium. Demonstration of the extent of the mass is simple on MRI with both longitudinal and transverse sections, and vertebral osteomyelitis is easily visualized as high-intensity areas on T_2-weighted images.

TREATMENT

Neurosurgery

The most important element of therapy is urgent neurosurgery for removal of pus and granulation tissue—which, rather than purulent material, is sometimes the major or sole finding. Decompressive laminectomies are performed for posterior epidural abscesses, whereas more complicated anterior approaches with bone graft fusion to establish spinal stability may be necessary for ventral collections. Occasionally, patients with absent or minimal neurologic findings respond to antimicrobial therapy alone,[28] but even these patients may benefit from surgery when imaging procedures show significant evidence of spinal cord compression. In such patients, the organism should be identified by blood culture or abscess aspiration, and clinicians should realize that neurologic decline may occur abruptly.[29]

Antimicrobial Therapy

Antimicrobial therapy alone may also be appropriate for patients at high surgical risk because of concurrent medical problems, for those with very extensive spinal involvement, and for patients with paralysis lasting more than 48 hours, after which significant neurologic recovery is highly unlikely. If the infecting organism is unknown, empirical antibiotic therapy should include an agent effective against gram-negative bacilli (e.g., gentamicin or a third-generation cephalosporin) plus one active against *S. aureus* (e.g., a penicillinase-resistant penicillin such as nafcillin). When methicillin-resistant *S. aureus* is a possibility, vancomycin should be used. Results of microbiologic evaluation of surgical specimens or blood cultures can then dictate the appropriate choice. In general, treatment is continued for 3 to 4 weeks in the absence of vertebral osteomyelitis and continued for 6 to 8 weeks when it is present. Patients with tuberculous epidural abscesses should receive antituberculous chemotherapy for at least 6 months.

PROGNOSIS

The prognosis depends on several factors—most important, the extent of neurologic deficiency at the time of surgery. Poor outcomes are common when paresis or, especially, paralysis is present. Other unfavorable prognostic features are advanced age

(> 60 years), substantial thecal sac compression on neuroimaging, and longer duration of symptoms.[30] About 40% of patients recover completely, 25% have residual weakness, 20% have permanent paralysis, and 15% die.

Subdural Empyema

PATHOGENESIS AND PATHOPHYSIOLOGY

A subdural empyema is a collection of pus between the dura mater and the underlying arachnoid. Because this space contains no septations, except where the arachnoid granules lie within the dura, purulent material easily spreads over the surface of the brain. Most cases occur as a complication of sinusitis in older children and young adults, especially males, who account for about 75% of cases.[31] The frontal sinus is nearly always involved, usually along with one or more of the other paranasal sinuses. Another cause is ear infection, either otitis media or mastoiditis; in such cases, the empyema may lie below the tentorium.

In these infections, pathogens probably reach the subdural space via blood draining from the infected sites through the venous sinuses in the dura. Subsequent septic thrombophlebitis of these vessels spreads organisms into the subdural space. Direct extension from contiguous infectious foci through erosion of the bones of the sinus or the ear may also occur. Other possible sources of the organisms causing subdural empyema are bacteremic infection of a preexisting subdural hematoma and direct inoculation of microbes into the area from penetrating head trauma or intracranial surgery.

Once the subdural space is infected, pus may spread widely over the convexities of the ipsilateral cerebrum; it may also travel along the falx separating the two hemispheres. The clinical features arise from pressure exerted on the underlying brain, the systemic effects of infection, and septic thrombophlebitis that spreads to the cortical and subcortical veins, causing brain infarction or infection.

ETIOLOGY

In most cases, only one species of organism is isolated from the pus, but polymicrobial infections can occur. The usual pathogens are aerobic or anaerobic streptococci and other anaerobes, especially with infections arising from sinusitis. Staphylococci and gram-negative bacilli are common causes in postoperative infections. Approximately 20% of cultures are negative, possibly because of inadequate microbiologic techniques (especially in isolating anaerobic bacteria) or previous antimicrobial therapy.

DIAGNOSIS

Clinical Features

Many patients have had a preceding sinusitis or a nonspecific upper respiratory tract illness; in some patients, however, symptoms of subdural empyema arise suddenly. The most common features are fever, stiff neck, and headache, which can be diffuse or localized to the area of empyema or underlying sinusitis. Neurologic abnormalities are usually present, including hemiparesis, seizures, aphasia, hemianesthesia, hemianopsia, and altered mentation, such as confusion, drowsiness, disorientation, and even coma. Papilledema may occur, indicating increased intracranial pressure, which can also cause palsies of the third and sixth cranial nerves. Sinus tenderness and periorbital edema may develop, reflecting the underlying sinusitis. With infratentorial empyema,[32] which usually originates from neglected otic infections, the clinical features include stiff neck, altered consciousness, signs of increased intracranial pressure, otorrhea, and fever. Patients typically deteriorate rapidly.

The presence of fever, headache, nuchal rigidity, and focal neurologic signs, especially in an adolescent or young adult male with sinusitis, should strongly suggest the presence of a subdural empyema and the necessity of immediate neuroimaging with CT or, preferably, MRI.

Laboratory Findings

A peripheral leukocytosis is common. Lumbar puncture is inadvisable because of the risk of brain herniation from increased intracranial pressure, but it is often performed because the clinical features suggest acute bacterial meningitis. Fortunately, serious complications rarely occur. The opening pressure is elevated, and pleocytosis of several hundred white cells or fewer is present. There is commonly a mixture of neutrophils and lymphocytes, with either predominating, but frequently these cells are equal in number. The protein level is typically increased, but the glucose level is almost always normal, and both Gram stain and culture are characteristically negative.

Imaging Studies

CT scans may show the empyema as isodense to low-density collections over one hemisphere and in the interhemispheric space, with a contrast-enhanced rim [*see Figure 2*]. MRI is a more sensitive

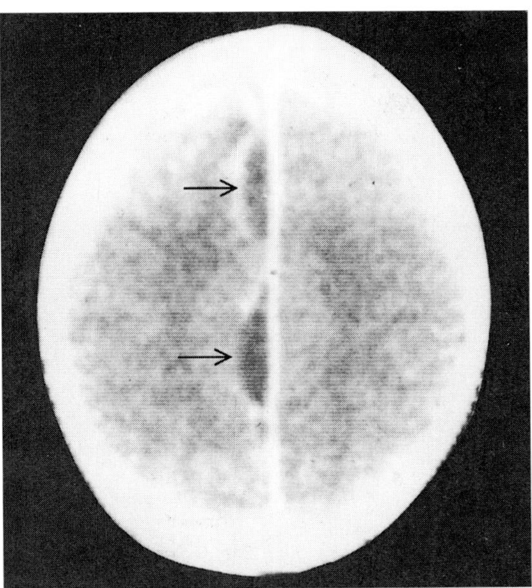

Figure 2 **CT scan of a 17-year-old patient with a subdural empyema shows two loculations (arrows) that are restricted to the interhemispheric area. Contrast-enhanced margins surround the two loculations.**

and accurate imaging technique, however, revealing the empyema as isointense masses on T_1-weighted images but showing high signal on proton density or T_2-weighted images. The rim may be enhanced with gadolinium. These imaging techniques may also demonstrate concurrent complications, which are relatively common and include brain abscess, cranial epidural abscess, cortical thrombophlebitis, and venous infarction.[31]

DIFFERENTIAL DIAGNOSIS

The differential diagnosis for subdural empyema includes bacterial meningitis, brain abscess, and encephalitis. Clinical distinction among these infections may be difficult; however, focal findings are unusual in meningitis, and a stiff neck is uncommon with brain abscesses and encephalitis.

TREATMENT

The most important therapy is removal of the subdural pus through use of multiple bur holes or craniotomy. It is unclear which method is better; the choice may depend on the location of the infection and the patient's neurologic status. With either procedure, but especially with bur holes, multiple operations are often necessary because of inadequate drainage of pus. Antibiotic therapy, usually continued for 3 to 4 weeks after surgery, can be dictated by Gram stain and culture of pus. The combination of ceftriaxone and metronidazole is a reasonable empirical regimen to use until the results of the Gram stain and culture are received.

PROGNOSIS

The prognosis depends greatly on the patient's state of consciousness at the time of surgery, with worsening outcomes accompanying decreasing levels of awareness. Overall mortality is approximately 15%. Significant neurologic sequelae, such as speech abnormalities and hemiparesis, occur in approximately 15% to 20% of survivors, and seizures occur in about 30%. These problems may emerge long after the surgery.

Septic Thrombophlebitis of the Major Cerebral Veins

The dural sinuses drain blood from the brain into the jugular veins. These sinuses lack valves, allowing flow in either direction, depending on the prevailing pressure gradient. Septic thrombophlebitis of these vessels, which may result from intracranial suppuration or spread of infection from extracranial veins, causes increased intracranial pressure, focal cerebral edema, or brain infarction. Usually, the initiating site of infection is clinically obvious in the middle ear, mastoid, paranasal sinuses, or facial skin. The cavernous, lateral, and superior sagittal sinuses are the most commonly involved vessels.[33]

CAVERNOUS SINUS THROMBOPHLEBITIS

Cavernous sinus thrombophlebitis most frequently develops from infections in the paranasal sinuses or the facial skin, especially on the medial third near the eyes and nose. Most cases are caused by *S. aureus*.[34] Other causative pathogens are streptococci, gram-negative bacilli, and anaerobes.

Diagnosis

The earliest symptom is usually headache, which often precedes fever and other findings by several days. The pain typically involves areas innervated by the ophthalmic and maxillary divisions of the trigeminal nerve, which traverse the cavernous sinus. Hyperesthesia or decreased sensation may be demonstrable in the dermatomes served by these nerves. Other focal findings may arise from obstructed ophthalmic veins: unilateral chemosis, proptosis, and edema of the ipsilateral eyelids, nose, and forehead. With time, the findings become bilateral as the phlebitis extends to the opposite cavernous sinus. Compression of the third, fourth, and sixth cranial nerves, which course through the cavernous sinus, leads to varying degrees of ophthalmoplegia. The pupils may dilate and fail to react to light. Retinal veins engorge, visual acuity may lessen, and hemorrhages and papilledema can occur. Lethargy and coma may supervene, reflecting increased intracranial pressure and neuronal damage. Occasionally, bacteremia with metastatic foci of infection develops.

LATERAL SINUS THROMBOPHLEBITIS

Lateral sinus thrombophlebitis is almost always a complication of mastoiditis. Anaerobes, staphylococci, and gram-negative bacilli, especially *Proteus* organisms, are the most common isolates.

The clinical course is usually subacute, with symptoms lasting for several weeks. Earache and drainage are often the first symptoms. Persistent, severe unilateral headache, followed by nausea and vomiting, indicates the development of lateral sinus thrombophlebitis. Fever, chills, and manifestations of increased intracranial pressure, including confusion and papilledema, are commonly present. Postauricular tenderness, venous engorgement, and edema represent involvement of the mastoid emissary vein. Extension into the jugular vein may occur.

Otoscopic examination commonly reveals a perforated or inflamed tympanic membrane. Focal neurologic findings are usually absent except for unilateral sixth nerve palsy, reflecting compression of the inferior petrosal sinus.

SUPERIOR SAGITTAL SINUS THROMBOPHLEBITIS

Superior sagittal sinus thrombophlebitis complicates bacterial meningitis, paranasal sinusitis, contiguous osteomyelitis, and dural infection. The most common organisms are *S. pneumoniae*, other streptococci, and gram-negative bacilli. Thrombosis of only the anterior portion of the sinus is often asymptomatic, but posterior involvement causes increased intracranial pressure. The predominant feature is acute headache, often with nausea and vomiting, followed in a few days by confusion and eventually coma. Focal or generalized seizures are common, and most patients are febrile. Extension of the thrombophlebitis to cortical veins may cause infarction of the underlying cortex, producing such neurologic manifestations as focal seizures and hemiparesis.

DIAGNOSIS

With septic thrombophlebitis in any of the cerebral veins, examination of the CSF may yield normal results or may demonstrate findings consistent with a parameningeal focus of infection: increased protein level, normal glucose level, and a pleocytosis of mixed neutrophils and lymphocytes that rarely exceeds a few hundred cells. Increased opening pressure is also common in all types.

Plain films of the skull are rarely helpful except in cases of septic lateral sinus thrombosis, in which they nearly always reveal mastoiditis. Certain findings on CT scan suggest cerebral venous thrombosis, but MRI provides a much better study. Acutely thrombosed cerebral veins lack a flow void. They are isointense on T_1-weighted images and hypointense on T_2-weighted images. In subacute thrombosis, the methemoglobin in the veins produces areas of high intensity on both images.

TREATMENT

Management of cerebral vein thrombophlebitis includes appropriate antibiotic therapy. For each of these disorders, when the infecting organisms are unknown, a good empirical antibiotic regimen is a combination of ceftriaxone and metronidazole. With cavernous sinus thrombosis in which *S. aureus* is prominent, vancomycin may be added if methicillin-resistant strains are likely.

Occasionally, treatment of cerebral vein thrombophlebitis includes surgery for the areas of purulence from which the infection arose. When paranasal sinusitis is the underlying cause, drainage of the infected sinuses may be necessary to obtain a good clinical response. In lateral sinus thrombophlebitis, radical mastoidectomy and exploration over the lateral sinus are commonly performed to remove purulent material.

Other medical treatment may include mannitol and dexamethasone in superior sagittal thrombophlebitis to help relieve the severe cerebral edema that is often present. The role of anticoagulation in cerebral vein thrombophlebitis remains unsettled; it seems valuable in cavernous sinus thrombosis[35] but appears potentially hazardous in superior sagittal and lateral sinus thrombophlebitis because of the frequent concurrent hemorrhagic venous cortical infarcts that it may exacerbate.

PROGNOSIS

Septic thrombophlebitis of the superior sagittal and cavernous sinuses imposes a high mortality, even with appropriate therapy; however, most patients with involvement of the lateral sinus have a good prognosis.

References

1. Schuchat A, Robinson K, Wenger JD, et al: Bacterial meningitis in the United States in 1995. N Engl J Med 337:970, 1997

2. Durand ML, Calderwood SB, Weber DJ, et al: Acute bacterial meningitis in adults: a review of 493 episodes. N Engl J Med 328:21, 1993

3. Almirante B, Saballs M, Ribera E, et al: Favorable prognosis of purulent meningitis in patients infected with human immunodeficiency virus. Clin Infect Dis 27:176, 1998

4. Sigurdardottir B, Bjornsson OM, Jonsdottir KE, et al: Acute bacterial meningitis in adults: a 20-year overview. Arch Intern Med 157:425, 1997

5. Gorse GJ, Thrupp LD, Nudleman KL, et al: Bacterial meningitis in the elderly. Arch Intern Med 144:1603, 1984

6. Verghese A, Gallemore G: Kernig's and Brudzinski's signs revisited. Rev Infect Dis 9:1187, 1987

7. Rennick G, Shann F, de Campo J: Cerebral herniation during bacterial meningitis in children. BMJ 306:953, 1993

8. Powers WJ: Cerebrospinal fluid to serum glucose ratios in diabetes mellitus and bacterial meningitis. Am J Med 71:217, 1981

9. Powers WJ: Cerebrospinal fluid lymphocytosis in acute bacterial meningitis. Am J Med 79:216, 1985

10. Mylonakis E, Hohmann EL, Calderwood SB: Central nervous system infection with *Listeria monocytogenes*. Medicine (Baltimore) 77:313, 1998

11. Talan DA, Hoffman JR, Yoshikawa TT, et al: Role of empiric parenteral antibiotics prior to lumbar puncture in suspected bacterial meningitis: state of the art. Rev Infect Dis 10:365, 1988

12. Aronin SI, Peduzzi P, Quagliarello VJ: Community-acquired bacterial meningitis: risk stratification for adverse clinical outcome and effect of antibiotic timing. Ann Intern Med 129:862, 1998

13. Cabellos C, Viladrich PF, Verdaguer R, et al: A single daily dose of ceftriaxone for bacterial meningitis in adults: experience with 84 patients and review of the literature. Clin Infect Dis 20:1164, 1995

14. Thomas R, Le Tulzo Y, Bouget J, et al: Trial of dexamethasone treatment for severe bacterial meningitis in adults. Intensive Care Med 25: 475, 1999

15. Pfister HW, Feiden W, Einhaupl KM: Spectrum of complications during bacterial meningitis in adults: results of a prospective clinical study. Arch Neurol 50:575, 1993

16. Pfister HW, Borasio GD, Dirnagl U, et al: Cerebrovascular complications of bacterial meningitis in adults. Neurology 42:1497, 1992

17. Bohr V, Paulson OB, Rasmussen N: Pneumococcal meningitis: late neurologic sequelae and features of prognostic import. Arch Neurol 41:1045, 1984

18. Hirschmann JV: Bacterial meningitis following closed cranial trauma. Bacterial Meningitis. Sande MA, Smith AL, Root RK, Eds. Churchill Livingstone, New York, 1985, p 95

19. Walsh M, Curran AJ: Cerebrospinal fluid rhinorrhoea. Br J Neurosurg 11:189, 1997

20. Morris A, Low DE: Nosocomial bacterial meningitis, including central nervous system shunt infections. Infect Dis Clin North Am 13: 735, 1999

21. Metersky ML, Williams A, Rafanan AL: Retrospective analysis: are fever and altered mental status indications for lumbar puncture in a hospitalized patient who has not undergone neurosurgery? Clin Infect Dis 25:285, 1997

22. Kaufman BA, Tunkel AR, Pryor JC, et al: Meningitis in the neurosurgical patient. Infect Dis Clin North Am 4:677, 1990

23. Mathisen GE, Johnson JP: Brain abscess. Clin Infect Dis 25:763, 1997

24. Shahzadi S, Lozano AM, Bernstein M, et al: Stereotactic management of bacterial brain abscesses. Can J Neurol Sci 23:34, 1996

25. Seydoux C, Francioli P: Bacterial brain abscesses: factors influencing mortality and sequelae. Clin Infect Dis 15:394, 1992

26. Darouiche RO, Hamill RJ, Greenberg SB, et al: Bacterial spinal epidural abscess: review of 43 cases and literature survey. Medicine (Baltimore) 71:369, 1992

27. Obrador GT, Levenson DJ: Spinal epidural abscess in hemodialysis patients: report of three cases and review of the literature. Am J Kidney Dis 27:75, 1996

28. Rigamonti D, Liem L, Sampath P, et al: Spinal epidural abscess: contemporary trends in etiology, evaluation, and management. Surg Neurol 52:189, 1999

29. Hlavin ML, Kaminski HJ, Ross JS, et al: Spinal epidural abscess: a ten-year perspective. Neurosurgery 27:177, 1990

30. Khanna RK, Malik GM, Rock JP, et al: Spinal epidural abscess: evaluation of factors influencing outcome. Neurosurgery 39:958, 1996

31. Dill SR, Cobbs CG, McDonald CK: Subdural empyema: analysis of 32 cases and review. Clin Infect Dis 20:372, 1995

32. Nathoo N, Nadvi SS, van Dellen JR: Infratentorial empyema: analysis of 22 cases. Neurosurgery 41:1263, 1997

33. Southwick FS, Richardson EP Jr, Swarz MN: Septic thrombosis of the dural venous sinuses. Medicine (Baltimore) 65:82, 1986

34. DiNubile MJ: Septic thrombosis of the cavernous sinus. Arch Neurol 45:567, 1988

35. Levine SR, Twyman RE, Gilman S: The role of anticoagulation in cavernous sinus thrombosis. Neurology 38:517, 1988

14 HIV and AIDS

David H. Spach, M.D.

The HIV/AIDS epidemic has dramatically changed in recent years. With each year, the gap between AIDS cases in developed countries and those in developing countries grows ever wider. As developed countries further reap the tremendous benefits of combination antiretroviral therapy, developing countries struggle with minimal resources that cannot prevent the dramatic increases in AIDS-related deaths. In developed countries, aggressive antiretroviral therapy has led to a remarkable decline in the rate of AIDS-related deaths and the incidence of major opportunistic infections,[1,2] but this success has ushered in a new and complicated era of HIV clinical care. This subsection provides an update of key information related to the epidemiology, pathogenesis, and clinical care of the HIV-infected individual. Information regarding HIV serologic tests, HIV quantitative assays (viral load assays), and HIV resistance tests are described in detail elsewhere [see 33 Human Retroviral Infections].

Origin of HIV

Recent research has provided a number of new insights into the origin of HIV in humans. Data suggest that humans acquired HIV type 1 (HIV-1) from *Pan troglodytes troglodytes* chimpanzees infected with simian immunodeficiency virus (SIV), and that HIV-1 was introduced into the human population (as SIV) from these chimpanzees on at least three independent occasions.[3] These conclusions arose primarily from studies that used mitochondrial DNA analysis of available SIV and HIV-1 strains and are based on three important findings: (1) all HIV-1 strains known to infect humans are closely related to the SIV lineage found in the *P. t. troglodytes* chimpanzees; (2) the HIV-1 group is a mosaic of SIV and HIV-1–related sequences, suggesting an ancestral recombination event in a chimpanzee host; and (3) the natural geographical range of *P. t. troglodytes* corresponds with areas endemic for HIV-1 groups M, N, and O. The exact timing and the mechanism for the transmission of HIV-1 remain unknown; given the fact that some peoples in Africa hunt these chimpanzees for food, transmission may have occurred during the capture, preparation, or ingestion of these chimpanzees.

Investigators have identified the origin of HIV-2 as the sooty mangabey monkey (*Cercocebus atys*). Strains of SIV have been discovered in many sooty mangabeys that are genomically indistinguishable from, as well as closely related phylogenetically to, HIV-2.[4] Moreover, the sooty mangabey's natural habitat corresponds with the epicenter of the HIV-2 epidemic. It has been proposed that at least six independent transmission events of SIV from sooty mangabeys to humans have occurred; presumably, these events occurred through the hunting of this animal or through contact with this animal as a pet.

To date, the oldest confirmed isolate of HIV is from a blood sample collected from a patient in the eastern region of central Africa in 1959.[5] Investigators have used supercomputers to analyze HIV-1 phylogenetic relationships through use of maximum-likelihood phylogenetic algorithms and have concluded that HIV-1 originated in humans in Africa in 1931 or earlier.[6] Through use of these methods, it has been suggested that HIV entered the United States in approximately 1967. One investigator has proposed that HIV originated in Africa as a result of contaminated polio vaccines that were widely used in Africa in the late 1950s; this theory proposes that chimpanzee kidney cells were used in preparing the vaccines. However, recent analysis by three independent laboratories of samples of these vaccines stored for more than 40 years failed to show even a trace of HIV or SIV; in addition, these laboratories performed mitochondrial DNA analysis and found no evidence of

Table 1 Centers for Disease Control and Prevention Classification System for HIV Infection[8]

CD4+ T Cell Categories	Clinical Categories: A (asymptomatic, first-degree HIV or progressive generalized lymphadenopathy)	B* (symptomatic, but does not satisfy conditions in categories A or C)	C† (AIDS-indicator conditions)
Category 1: ≥ 500 cells/mm^3	A1	B1	C1‡
Category 2: 200–499 cells/mm^3	A2	B2	C2‡
Category 3: < 200 cells/mm^3	A3‡	B3‡	C3‡

*B conditions include bacterial endocarditis, meningitis, or sepsis; candidiasis (oral); candidiasis (persistent vulvovaginal); cervical dysplasia (or carcinoma in situ); constitutional illness (persistent unexplained fever, diarrhea or weight loss, or disabling weakness); herpes zoster (multidermatomal); listeriosis; myelopathy; nocardiosis; oral hairy leukoplakia; pelvic inflammatory disease; peripheral neuropathy; and thrombocytopenic purpura (idiopathic).

†C conditions include candidiasis (bronchial, esophageal, pulmonary, or tracheal); cervical cancer (invasive); coccidioidomycosis (disseminated or extrapulmonary); cryptococcosis (extrapulmonary); cryptosporidiosis (intestinal, for longer than 1 mo); cytomegalovirus (other than liver, spleen, or nodes); encephalopathy (HIV); herpes simplex virus (ulcers present for longer than 1 mo or esophagitis, bronchitis, or pneumonitis); histoplasmosis (disseminated or extrapulmonary); isosporiasis (intestinal, for longer than 1 mo); Kaposi sarcoma; lymphoma (Burkitt, immunoblastic, or primary in brain); *Mycobacterium avium* complex (disseminated or extrapulmonary), *M. kansasii* (disseminated or extrapulmonary), *M. tuberculosis*, or *Mycobacterium* of other or unidentified species (disseminated or extrapulmonary); *Pneumocystis carinii* pneumonia; recurrent pneumonia (two or more episodes in 1-yr period); progressive multifocal leukoencephalopathy; salmonellosis (recurrent septicemia); toxoplasmosis (brain); wasting syndrome (> 10% weight loss plus either chronic weakness or documented fever for at least 30 days in the absence of a concurrent illness that could explain this finding).

‡AIDS case that satisfies the surveillance definition.

chimpanzee tissue in the vaccines.[7] Furthermore, the phylogenetic studies mentioned above clearly suggest that HIV-1 was in the human population long before the polio vaccine program was introduced and that, by the late 1950s, there was significant diversification of HIV-1. These findings make it highly improbable that HIV was introduced through the polio vaccine.

Classification of HIV and AIDS

In 1982, the Centers for Disease Control and Prevention (CDC) established a surveillance definition of AIDS; persons were classified as having AIDS if they had defects in cell-mediated immunity (without a known cause) and if they had one or more designated opportunistic infections or malignancies. In 1985, the case definition incorporated the newly licensed HIV antibody test. In 1993, the CDC revised the AIDS case definition to include HIV-infected adults and adolescents who had a CD4+ T cell count of less than 200 cells/mm^3 or whose CD4+ T cells constituted less than 14% of total lymphocytes.[8] Because CD4+ T cell counts in children are not comparable to those in adults, the 1993 revised AIDS definition does not apply to pediatric patients. In 1993, the CDC also generated a comprehensive classification system that consists of a matrix of CD4+ T cell status (levels 1, 2, and 3) and clinical manifestations (categories A, B, and C). This system became effective on January 1, 1993, and is still in use [*see Table 1*].

Epidemiology

UNITED STATES EPIDEMIOLOGY

Contemporary estimates of the total number of HIV-infected persons (with or without AIDS) living in the United States generally range from 850,000 to 950,000.[9] As of mid-2000, the cumulative number of AIDS cases in the United States reported to the CDC totaled 753,907 [*see Figure 1*].[1] Of these patients, 83% were male and 17% female. The majority of patients were adults or adolescents; only 1% of the patients were children younger than 13 years. Among men, 48% were white, 33% were African American, and 18% were Hispanic. Among women, 23% were white, 68% were African American, and 7% were Hispanic. Several epidemiologic trends have occurred during the 1990s:

1. An increasing proportion of AIDS patients are African American and Hispanic; since 1996, African Americans have outnumbered whites in the absolute number of new AIDS diagnoses and deaths.
2. The proportion of patients with AIDS who are women has steadily increased; in 1999, 23% of AIDS patients were women.
3. The proportion of persons who acquired HIV heterosexually has increased; in 1994, the proportion of persons who acquired HIV heterosexually surpassed the proportion who acquired HIV through injection drug use.
4. Although men who have sex with men remains the largest group at risk for AIDS, the propor-

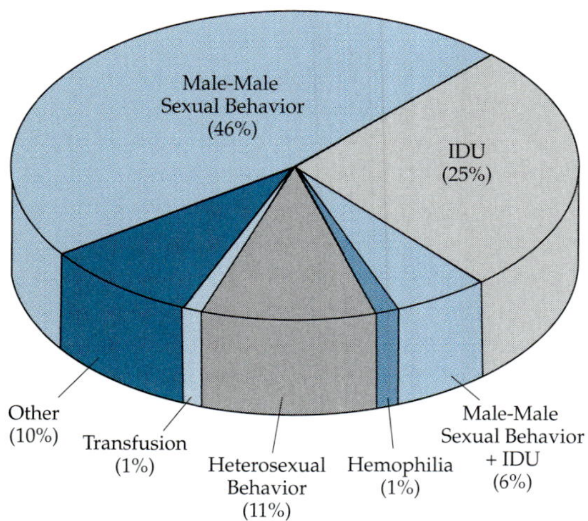

Figure 1 **The percentages of cumulative cases of AIDS of various causes in the United States through December 2000 are depicted in this illustration. These data represent both adult and adolescent AIDS patients.[1] (IDU—intravenous drug use)**

tion of AIDS cases involving this group has decreased in recent years.

As a result of the introduction and widespread use of aggressive antiretroviral therapy, surveillance data have shown a remarkable decline in the number of AIDS-related deaths and in the incidence of AIDS cases.[1,2] In recent years, there has been an increase in the prevalence of AIDS; the number of persons newly diagnosed with AIDS now exceeds the number of persons dying of AIDS. In addition, the number of children with AIDS markedly declined during the 1990s, most importantly as a result of the rapid and widespread implementation of the use of zidovudine (AZT) to prevent perinatal transmission of HIV. With the current approaches, which use more aggressive combination therapy to prevent perinatal transmission of HIV, rates of perinatal transmission of HIV should decline even further.

As of June 2000, 38 states had some type of HIV reporting system (this figure includes Connecticut and Oregon, which provided only for pediatric HIV reporting). In the current HIV/AIDS reporting system, persons who have both HIV and AIDS are counted only once (they are counted as having AIDS). As of June 2000, 130,352 persons were reported as living with HIV (not AIDS); 21,419 new HIV cases were reported in 1999. Women accounted for 32% of the new cases reported in 1999; among these women, 77% were either African American or Hispanic. Of the men with HIV reported in 1999, 59% were African American or Hispanic.

GLOBAL EPIDEMIOLOGY

The Joint United Nations Program on HIV/AIDS (UNAIDS) has estimated that as of December 2000, approximately 36 million persons were living with HIV worldwide, exceeding the World Health Organization (WHO) estimates of 1991 by more than 50%.[9] Of the 36 million, approximately 16 million are women and 1.4 million are children younger than 15 years. During the past year, approximately 5.3 million persons became newly infected with HIV, with women making up 47% of the new adult patients and children constituting about 11% of the overall new patients. The AIDS-related death toll has become astounding: in the year 2000, approximately three million persons died of AIDS, of whom 52% were women and 17% children. Worldwide, cumulative AIDS-related deaths have exceeded 21 million, including more than four million children younger than 15 years.

The global distribution of HIV-infected persons continues to vary widely, with sub-Saharan Africa remaining the hardest hit region, followed by South Asia and Southeast Asia. Although an astounding 25 million persons are living with HIV infection in sub-Saharan Africa, the HIV epidemic in this region has recently shown signs of stabilizing. The exact reason for this favorable trend has not been determined, but it likely relates to two factors: (1) the epidemic has matured, and many of the persons who were most at risk of acquiring HIV have already been infected; and (2) preventive measures have increased. Nevertheless, the impact of the HIV epidemic in this region remains overwhelming: almost 2.5 million people will die in 2000, and the gross domestic product will decline by 17% as a result of the epidemic.

During 2000, the Russian Federation showed explosive growth in their number of HIV-infected persons; in this region, more HIV cases were reported in 2000 than in all previous years combined. This increase reflects the dramatic increase in HIV cases in eastern Europe and central Asia, where the number of cases increased from 420,000 in 1999 to 700,000 in 2000. In the Russian Federation, the epidemic appears to be most heavily driven by injection drug use.

Southern Asia and Southeast Asia continue to attract great attention, mainly because of the massive population in these regions and the fact that more than 5 million persons are already infected. In this region, men make up most of the injection drug users and often drive the earliest waves of HIV infection.

In the Caribbean, although the total number of persons infected with HIV is relatively low compared with the numbers in many other regions of the world, the actual HIV prevalence is second only to the prevalence in Africa. Most wealthy nations have benefited from the widespread use of effective antiretroviral therapy but have recently shown setbacks in prevention efforts.

Transmission of HIV

Person-to-person transmission of HIV can occur through several routes, including sexual contact, sharing contaminated needles used for injecting drugs, receiving a transfusion of a contaminated blood product, transmission from mother to child (either during gestation, at the time of delivery, or post partum via breast-feeding), and occupational exposure. The relative risks of acquiring HIV through these routes is difficult to precisely quantitate, but available data suggest that the highest risk is through receiving contaminated blood products, followed by mother-to-child exposure (assuming the mother is not receiving treatment with antiretroviral therapy) and then by the sharing of needles when injecting drugs. Lower risks are associated with needle-stick injuries and sexual transmission.[10] The risk of sexual transmission is highly dependent on the type of encounter, with receptive anal intercourse posing the highest risk. Globally, sexual contact is by far the most common route of HIV transmission, accounting for at least 75% of HIV infections worldwide.[10]

SEXUAL CONTACT

A number of factors appear to increase the risk of acquiring HIV via sexual contact; these include breaks in the mucosal barrier and increased inflammation in the genital tract caused by either genital ulcer disease, urethritis, or cervicitis.[11] In addition, the source patient probably poses a higher risk of transmission to others during acute HIV infection or when that patient has advanced AIDS. A recent study from Uganda involved 415 couples in which one partner was HIV positive and the other was initially HIV negative; this study found a dose-response relation of increased transmission with increasing HIV RNA levels.[12] Several longitudinal studies have clearly shown that the consistent use of condoms is highly effective in preventing transmission of HIV via heterosexual intercourse.[13] Several studies have suggested that oral-genital sex, although less risky than genital sex, poses a significant risk for HIV transmission, and a number of cases of HIV transmission have now been reported to have occurred via oral-genital sex.[14,15] Human studies have shown that the tissues in the nasopharyngeal tonsils and adenoids have abundant cells of dendritic origin; these cells can serve as an initial target for HIV and can then assist in transmitting HIV to nearby $CD4^+$ T cells.[16]

INJECTION DRUG USE

Although injection drug use accounts for fewer cases of HIV transmission than sexual contact, it does account for a substantial number of cases and represents an important area for efforts at prevention. Although needle-exchange programs are not supported by federal funds in the United States, more than 100 exchange programs have been implemented. Multiple studies have clearly shown that needle-exchange programs decrease the incidence of HIV transmission by an estimated 33% without causing an increase in drug use.[17]

USE OF CONTAMINATED BLOOD PRODUCTS

In the United States, HIV-1 serology testing of blood donations by the American Red Cross began in 1985; in 1992, this program was expanded to include testing for HIV-2. In 1992 and 1993, the risk of transfusion-acquired HIV in the United States was less than one case of HIV for every 450,000 to 600,000 donations of screened blood, with almost all of the risk related to donors who were infected with HIV shortly before donating their blood and who had not yet undergone seroconversion.[18] Using current enzyme immunoassay serologic tests, this so-called window period typically occurs until about day 25 after HIV infection. In 1996, HIV p24 antigen testing was mandated; this test further decreased the risk of HIV transmission. More recent attempts have also used nucleic acid testing as an even more sensitive assay to detect donors during the window period. In an interesting case report, a 13-year-old boy received a blood transfusion 2 days before it was discovered that the donor had acute HIV syndrome. The boy received a three-drug antiretroviral postexposure prophylaxis regimen for 9 months and repeatedly tested negative for HIV RNA antibodies, even when tested 6 months after antiretroviral postexposure prophylaxis was discontinued.[19]

MOTHER-TO-CHILD TRANSMISSION

Mother-to-child transmission of HIV accounts for a substantial proportion of HIV cases in developing countries. Such transmission can occur either during gestation, at the time of delivery, or post partum via breast-feeding. Without the use of antiretroviral therapy, mother-to-child transmission rates generally range from 20% to 30%,[20] with higher rates occurring in developing countries and with women who breast-feed. Multiple studies have clearly shown the presence of HIV RNA in the mother to be a strong predictor of transmission.[21,22] In addition, in mothers with HIV who were not receiving antiretroviral therapy, cesarean section decreased the risk of transmission by about 50%.[23] Although HIV transmission from mother to child can occur early in pregnancy or post partum,[24-26] available data suggest that most perinatal HIV transmission occurs near or at the time of delivery.[25] The widespread use of antiretroviral therapy to prevent mother-to-child HIV transmission has led to a dramatic decline in perinatal HIV transmission in developed countries.[20,25] Current recommendations for the use of antiretroviral therapy to prevent mother-to-child HIV transmission are discussed elsewhere [*see* Antiretroviral Therapy to Prevent Perinatal Transmission, *below*].

OCCUPATIONAL RISKS

As of July 1, 2000, the CDC had reported 56 documented cases of occupational HIV transmission and an additional 138 cases of possible occupational HIV transmission.[1] Among the 56 documented cases, 48 (86%) involved a percutaneous exposure, 5 (9%) involved a mucocutaneous exposure, 2 (4%) involved both percutaneous and mucocutaneous exposures, and 1 (2%) occurred by an unknown route of exposure. In addition, 49 of the 56 cases (88%) involved exposure to blood from an HIV-infected individual. On the basis of available data, the average risk of HIV transmission to a health care worker who experiences a percutaneous exposure to HIV-infected blood but who does not receive postexposure prophylaxis is approximately 0.3%; the risk associated with a mucous membrane exposure to HIV-infected blood is approximately 0.09%.[27] There are no documented cases of HIV transmission in health care workers that resulted from exposure to intact skin. Risk factors associated with increased risk of transmission include deep needle-stick injuries, use of hollow-bore needles, use of a device visibly contaminated with blood, exposure events involving the transference of a large volume of blood, a needle-stick injury in which the needle had been placed directly in an artery or vein of an HIV-infected patient, and the source patient having advanced AIDS.[27] The relative risk of transmission related to the source patient's HIV RNA level has not been established for occupational HIV transmission.

Pathogenesis and Progression of Disease

HIV STRUCTURE AND LIFE CYCLE

HIV is a member of the lentivirus family of retroviruses. When viewed under the electron microscope, HIV appears as spherical particles that are approximately 110 nm in diameter, with knoblike projections on the surface of the virus and a cone-shaped viral core[28] [*see Figure 2*]. HIV particles contain two copies of an RNA genome, each of which is approximately 10,000 base pairs in length and encodes nine genes. Two different HIV species have been identified: HIV-1 and HIV-2. Those isolates of HIV-1 that have been globally identified can be classified into the three major phylogenetic groups: M (main), N (neither M nor O), and O (outlier).[3,29] The M group has predominantly been responsible for the global HIV epidemic. This group can be further subdivided into 10 distinct subtypes or clades, termed subtypes A to J. From the standpoint of pathogenesis, all strains of HIV can be further classified as either R5 or R4, depending on the cellular coreceptor the virus binds to and on whether the virus can cause syncytium induction.[30] The process of syncytium induction refers to the clustering of host T cells, with the potential for a small quantity of HIV to more effectively destroy a larger proportion of host T cells. The R5 strains of virus utilize the CC chemokine receptor–5 (CCR5) coreceptor when binding to a cell. These strains do not cause syncytium induction; accordingly, they are referred to as non–syncytium-inducing viruses. The R4 strains bind to the cellular coreceptor CXC chemokine receptor–4 (CXCR4) and can cause syncytium induction; thus, these strains are referred to as syncytium-inducing viruses.

The life cycle of HIV is similar to that of other retroviruses. Understanding the life cycle is important for understanding both cellular pathogenesis and the targets of current and future anti-HIV therapies. The first step in the viral life cycle involves attachment of the virus to the host target cell. The first point of interaction consists of the binding of the HIV envelope surface protein (gp120) with the host $CD4^+$ T cell receptor [*see Figure 3*]. It has recently been shown that cellular coreceptors (also known as chemokine coreceptors) play a critical role in the second step in the binding process.[31] The

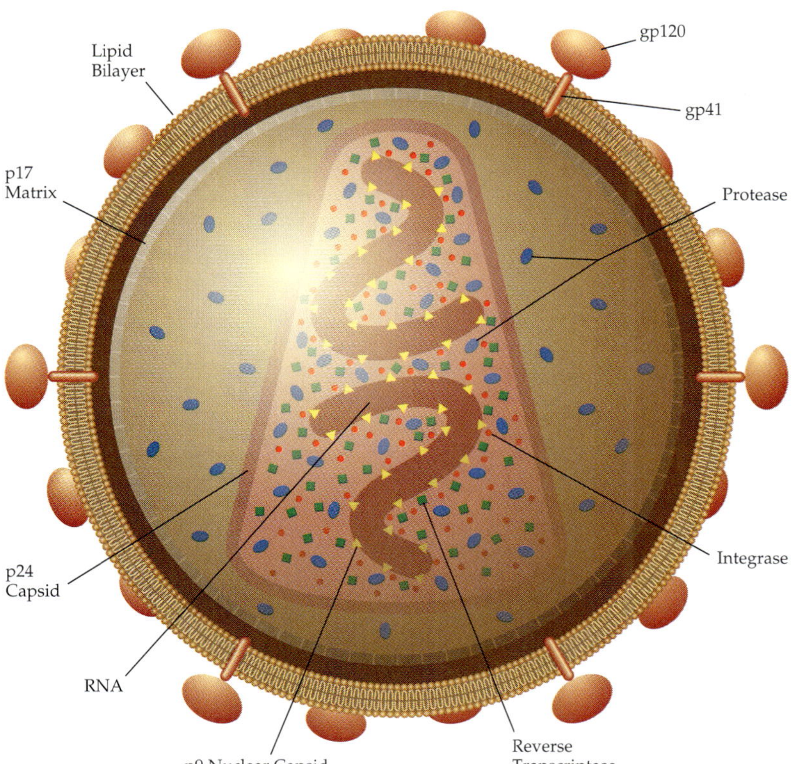

Figure 2 **The structure of HIV.[28]**

third step in the initial binding involves the interaction of the virus with the fusion domain of the host cell; in this step, the HIV and the host cell membranes become fused. Although investigators have discovered numerous coreceptors that can potentially bind HIV, the coreceptors CCR5 and CXCR4 appear to play the most important role.[31] The human $CD4^+$ T cells have both CCR5 and CXCR4 receptors, but the monocyte lines predominantly use CCR5 as the coreceptor. The HIV R5 strains preferentially bind to CCR5 coreceptors, and HIV R4 strains bind to CXCR4 coreceptors [*see Figure 4*]. Available data suggest that initial HIV infection predominantly involves R5 strains of HIV that bind to cells of the monocyte line that express CCR5 coreceptors. Recent studies have shown that there is significant genetic variation in the CCR5 coreceptor and that some individuals are homozygous for a CCR5 deletion mutation (specifically, a 32-base-pair deletion known as Δ32); some of these individuals have been repeatedly exposed to HIV and have not become infected.[32] Individuals who are heterozygous for this Δ32 mutation are not protected against HIV infection, but in these patients, progression of disease appears to be delayed [*see Figure 5*].

Following the fusion of the viral and cellular membranes, the viral capsid enters the cell [*see Figure 6*]. After the virus has entered the cell, the HIV reverse transcriptase enzyme converts the single-stranded HIV RNA into DNA. Through a complex process, some of the viral DNA migrates into the

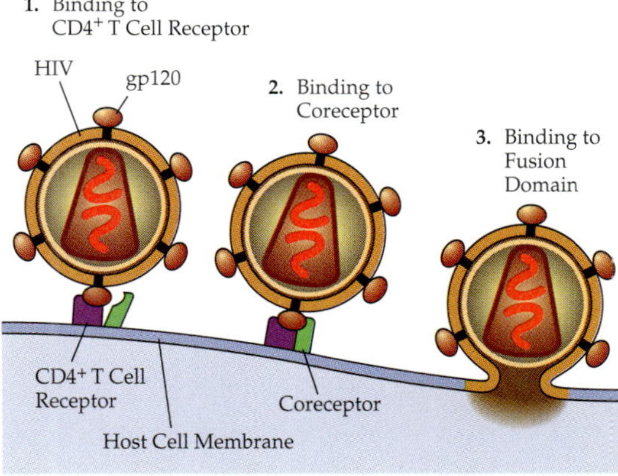

Figure 3 **This illustration shows the major steps involved in HIV binding to and entering the host cell. After binding to the fusion domain, the membranes merge together.**

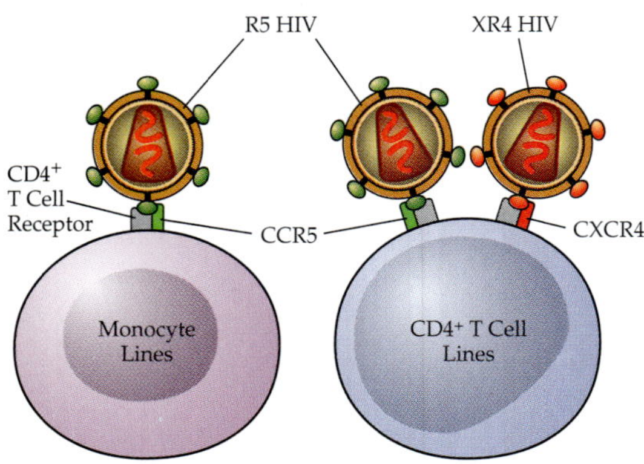

Figure 4 **Schematic illustration showing that R5 strains preferentially bind to CC chemokine receptor–5 (CCR5) coreceptors that are present on both monocytes and CD4+ T cells. R4 strains preferentially bind to CXC chemokine receptor–4 (CXCR4) coreceptors (predominantly on CD4+ T cells).**

nucleus, and the viral enzyme integrase splices the viral DNA into the host cell chromosomal DNA. Once HIV DNA becomes integrated into the human DNA, it is referred to as proviral DNA. Subsequently, the host can transcribe proviral DNA into messenger RNA (mRNA), a process controlled by the interaction of the promoters and enhancers in the viral genome with the Tat protein and cellular factors. Posttranscriptional processing of the viral mRNA takes place in the host cell nucleus. The viral mRNA is transported into the host cell cytoplasm; once there, viral mRNA is translated into viral proteins. The late stages of viral replication involve both the assembly of the viral particles, with each viral core incorporating two copies of the viral RNA genome, and the budding and release of the virus from the surface of the cell. The HIV protease enzyme plays an important role in this late process by cleaving the Env, Gag, and Pol proteins into their smaller functional components, with some of this action occurring shortly after the release of the viral particles from the cell.

DISEASE PROGRESSION

Early studies clearly showed that plasma HIV RNA levels serve as a very strong independent predictor of the progression to AIDS in untreated HIV-infected persons [*see Figure 7*].[33] In essence, the higher the HIV RNA level, the more rapidly the disease will progress. For example, among persons with a CD4+ T cell count greater than 500 cells/mm^3, about 5% of those who have a baseline HIV RNA level of less than 500 copies/ml will develop AIDS within 6 years, compared with 67% of those who have a baseline HIV RNA level of greater than 30,000 copies/ml. In contrast, the CD4+ T cell count provides an accurate way to assess the current immunologic status but does not predict the pace of subsequent decline.

Within 6 months of primary HIV infection, the plasma level of HIV appears to reach a fairly constant level—a level referred to as the set point [*see Figure 8*]. The set point may vary widely from per-

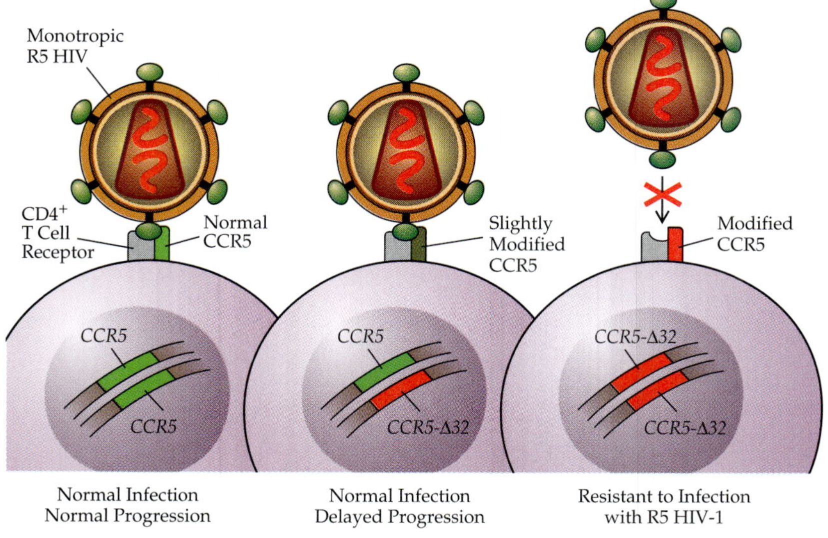

Figure 5 **This diagram shows the relationship of genetic diversity of the CCR5 coreceptor to progression of and susceptibility to HIV infection.**

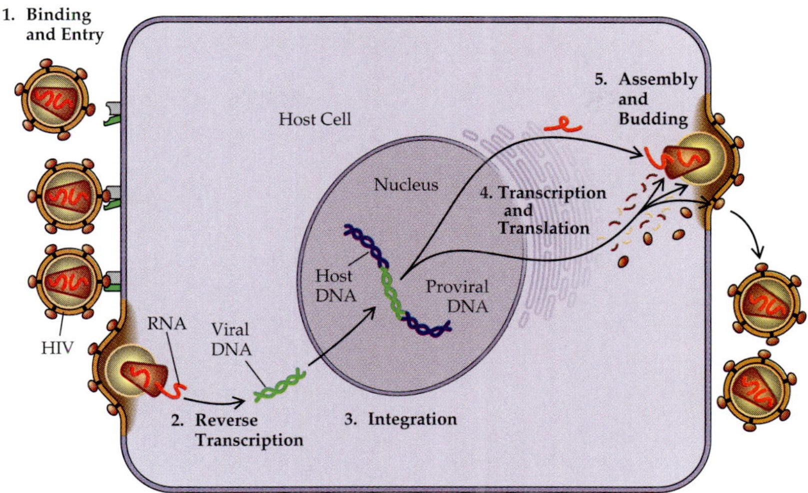

Figure 6 **This illustration depicts the major steps in the life cycle of HIV.**

son to person, and a number of host and viral determinants can influence the set point. Available data suggest that the host cytotoxic T cell response (also known as CTL, for cytotoxic T lymphocyte response) generated by $CD8^+$ T cells is the most important factor in determining the HIV set point.[34] The HIV cytotoxic T cell response occurs before the neutralization of antibodies against HIV and is associated with the initial decline in HIV RNA levels. Those individuals who have a weak cytotoxic T cell response to HIV have a high set point, and the progression of HIV disease is generally rapid; in contrast, those patients with a strong cytotoxic T cell response have a low set point, and therefore, disease progression is slower [*see Figure 9*].[34] The HIV $CD8^+$ cytotoxic T cell response requires a highly coordinated action of multiple cells, including helper T cells.[34] Shortly after acute HIV infection, HIV begins to preferentially destroy HIV-specific helper T cells; this process impairs the critical interaction between host $CD4^+$ T cells and $CD8^+$ T cells and thus weakens the host cytotoxic T cell response.

Genetic variations in the host's HIV coreceptors also may play a significant role in the progression

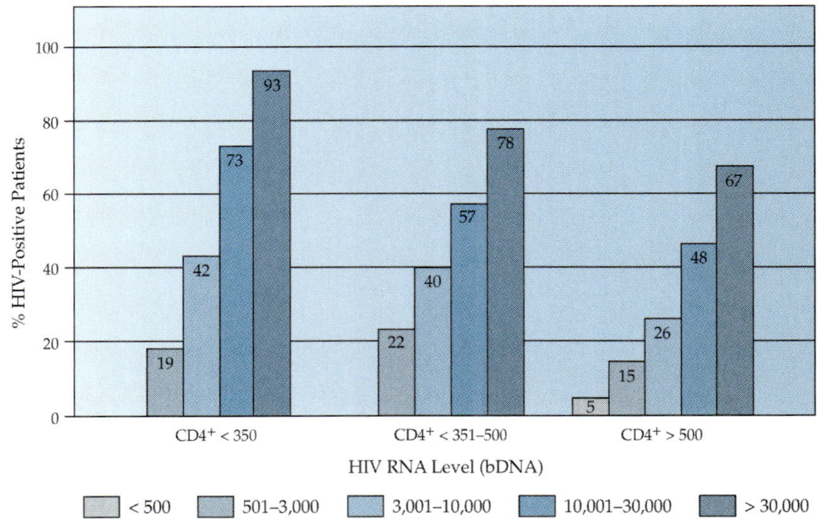

Figure 7 **This graph shows the risk of progression to AIDS at 6 years and the relationship of risk of progression to HIV RNA values and $CD4^+$ T cell counts.[33]**

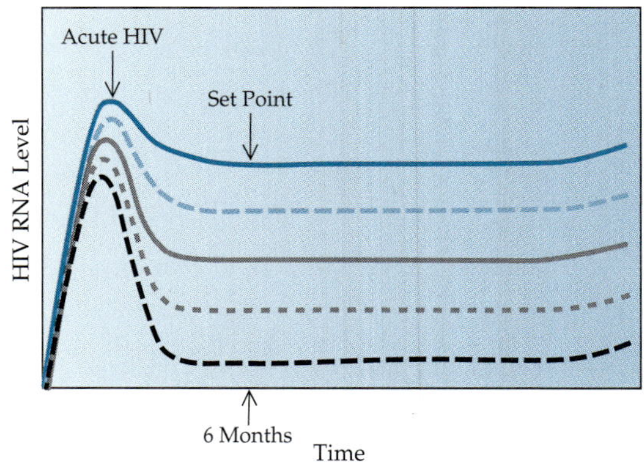

Figure 8 **This conceptual graph depicts the variations that occur over time in HIV-1 RNA levels after acute HIV infection. Each line represents a different HIV-infected individual.**

of HIV disease, most notably with regard to the CCR5-Δ32 heterozygous mutation [*see* HIV Structure and Life Cycle, *above*] and the CCR2-64I mutation.[32] Those individuals with the CCR5-Δ32 or CCR2-64I mutation have coreceptors that do not provide optimal targets for HIV binding, and thus, the rapidity of host cell infection by HIV can be affected. Differences in strains of HIV can also affect the progression of disease. It has been shown that the appearance of the syncytium-inducing strain of HIV correlates with an accelerated rate of CD4+ T cell decline, a rate of decline that may be almost three times more rapid than that seen in persons with the nonsyncytium strains.[30] In a small

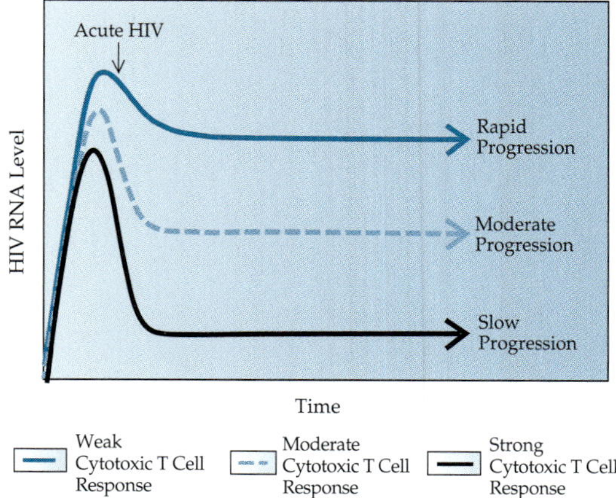

Figure 9 **This diagram shows the relationship of immune cytotoxic T cell response to HIV-1 RNA levels and subsequent progression of HIV disease.[34]**

number of persons, the presence of unusual HIV polymorphisms has been associated with slowed progression or nonprogression of HIV disease; these genetic variations in HIV appear to render the virus less pathogenic.[35,36] Insights into factors that delay disease progression may provide guidance for new and innovative strategies for HIV therapy.

Acute Infection

DIAGNOSIS

Clinical Features

After acquiring HIV, infected persons may develop a nonspecific influenzalike or mononucleosis-like illness. The exact proportion of persons with acute HIV infection whose illness reflects primary HIV infection is difficult to ascertain, but estimates range from 40% to 90%.[37] The most common route for HIV inoculation is via the genital mucosa; after genital inoculation, HIV initially infects Langerhans cells, fuses with local CD4+ T cells, and then infiltrates deeper tissues. Within 48 to 72 hours after inoculation, HIV can spread to adjacent inguinal lymph nodes; systemic dissemination and viremia typically develop after about 7 days after initial infection (range, 4 to 11 days).[38] Once viremia develops, HIV extensively seeds lymphoid organs and the central nervous system. Available data suggest that in this acute phase of infection, persons have very high levels of HIV in the genital tract and are likely to be highly infectious.

If a patient with primary HIV develops a significant clinical illness, it typically begins from 7 to 14 days after the time the patient first acquired HIV. In one study that followed persons considered to be at high risk for HIV, of 23 persons who became infected with HIV, 87% developed an acute HIV illness; of those who developed acute illness, 95% sought medical care, but only 25% were diagnosed as having acute HIV.[15] The correct diagnosis is often missed because of the nonspecific nature of the clinical illness—acute HIV infection may resemble influenza, mononucleosis, secondary syphilis, and more common viral illnesses. The most common signs and symptoms are fever (seen in 80% to 90% of patients), fatigue (70% to 90%), rash (40% to 80%), headache (32% to 70%), lymphadenopathy (40% to 70%), pharyngitis (50% to 70%), and myalgias or arthralgias (50% to 70%).[37] Although the clinical illness caused by acute HIV infection is often nonspecific, clinical findings of a morbilliform rash, acute meningoencephalitis, or mucocutaneous ulcerations may be particularly useful in making the diagnosis. Acute HIV illness typically persists for less than 14 days, but some individuals have had illnesses that have extended for longer than 10 weeks.[15] Several studies have shown that in persons with severe and prolonged symptoms, disease progression is generally more rapid.

Laboratory Studies

Routine laboratory studies are generally nonspecific but may show varying degrees of lymphopenia or thrombocytopenia. Results of the standard recombinant enzyme-linked immunoassay (ELISA) are generally negative at the time a patient presents with acute HIV; these tests do not typically show a positive result until 22 to 27 days after HIV infection.[39] Although the plasma p24 antigen test is the only currently licensed test for diagnosing acute HIV infection, the HIV RNA assay yields positive results 3 to 5 days earlier than the p24 antigen test. The combination of a strongly positive HIV RNA test result and a negative HIV antibody test result confirms the laboratory diagnosis of acute HIV infection. Almost all persons with acute HIV infection have HIV RNA levels that exceed 50,000 copies/ml, and most have levels that exceed 300,000 copies/ml.[37] Persons presenting weeks or months after their acute HIV illness are likely to have significantly lower levels. A low-level positive result on the HIV RNA assay (i.e., a result of less than 3,000 copies/ml) in a person suspected of being recently infected should be viewed with great caution; such a result would most likely be a false positive result. In this situation, if the p24 antigen test or an HIV RNA test cannot be obtained, the HIV serologic test should be repeated 4 to 6 weeks after the clinical illness has resolved.[37]

Implications of Early Diagnosis

Overall, making a diagnosis of acute HIV could have several important ramifications. First, persons with acute HIV are probably highly infectious and more likely to transmit HIV to others if the former are not aware they are infected with HIV. Second, after this initial illness, the person newly infected with HIV may have a very long interval before developing HIV-related or AIDS-related symptoms and thus may go undiagnosed for years. Third, treatment of persons with acute HIV infection may present a unique opportunity to preserve HIV-specific cytotoxic T cell responses.

TREATMENT

At present, there are limited data on the treatment of patients with acute HIV infection. In the only randomized, placebo-controlled trial that has been performed, patients recently infected with HIV received either monotherapy with zidovudine or placebo. After 6 months, those who received zidovudine experienced a mean increase in their $CD4^+$ T cell count of 173 cells/mm^3; those receiving placebo had a mean increase of 6 cells/mm^3.[40]

Several uncontrolled studies involving patients with acute HIV have shown that treatment with two nucleoside reverse transcriptase inhibitors (NRTIs) plus a protease inhibitor can reduce HIV RNA to undetectable levels; this regimen can also decrease HIV proviral levels and increase $CD4^+$ T cell counts.[37] However, patients receiving this regimen continue to have HIV in resting $CD4^+$ T cells and thus are not cured of HIV. Very encouraging data have been reported from a small study of six persons with acute HIV infection who received treatment with potent antiretroviral therapy. In all six patients, HIV RNA was undetectable. In addition, the patients showed vigorous HIV-1–specific responses of helper T cells to HIV p24 protein; such responses were similar to the responses seen in HIV patients in whom the disease did not progress for long periods.[41] This study has generated hope that treatment of patients with acute HIV infection may preserve certain HIV-specific immune responses and thus slow HIV disease progression. The use of structured treatment interruption in patients undergoing treatment for acute HIV infection has also stimulated great interest [*see* Structured Treatment Interruption, *below*]. On the basis of available data, the current Department of Health and Human Services (DHHS) guidelines recommend offering aggressive combination antiretroviral therapy to all patients with acute HIV infection and to those patients who underwent seroconversion within the past 6 months.[42] The optimal duration of treatment of patients with acute HIV infection remains unknown.

Chronic (Established) Infection

INITIAL EVALUATION

The initial evaluation of a patient with HIV who is establishing routine care should include a thorough health history, physical examination, and extensive laboratory studies. This initial evaluation process will require two visits. In the first visit, the health history is obtained, a complete physical examination is performed, and appropriate laboratory studies are ordered. In the second visit, which is conducted several weeks after the first, pertinent laboratory data are reviewed; the patient's disease stage and prognosis are discussed; necessary vaccinations are administered; the need for prophylaxis against opportunistic infection is reviewed; and, if appropriate, antiretroviral therapy is discussed.

Medical History

Particular aspects of the HIV-related medical history that should be emphasized are the risk factors of HIV, the approximate date of acquisition of HIV, results of the first HIV test that indicated the patient had HIV, a history of an acute seroconversion illness, prior $CD4^+$ T and HIV RNA studies, prior HIV-related illnesses, prior and current antiretroviral therapy, and history of other infectious diseases, such as syphilis or hepatitis. Obtaining information regarding the patient's past and current sexual activity and drug use provides insight into original acquisition of HIV and provides insight into current behaviors that may place contacts at risk for HIV. In addition to obtaining a complete medical history, it is important to assess the patient's social and psychiatric situation because social and psychiatric issues can become critical with regard to the patient's adherence to antiretroviral therapy.

Laboratory Studies

The recommended laboratory studies that should be administered at the initial office visit are listed [*see Table 2*].

OVERVIEW OF MANAGEMENT

Vaccines

Most asymptomatic HIV-infected patients who have a $CD4^+$ T cell count greater than 500 cells/mm^3 generally produce good antibody responses to vaccines. Responses are frequently poor in patients with lower $CD4^+$ T cell counts, particularly those with AIDS. Among persons with more advanced immune suppression, the benefit of partial or suboptimal antibody responses remains unknown. Preliminary studies raised concerns that vaccines given to HIV-infected persons could cause significant increases in HIV RNA levels. Further study has shown that although some patients do have a mild to moderate increase in HIV RNA levels after immunization, these increases generally are transient and do not have permanent adverse consequences. Nevertheless, concerns remain regarding use of live virus vaccine in HIV-infected individuals, particularly those persons with advanced immune suppression. Vaccines for HIV-infected adults are listed [*see Table 3*].

Table 2 Laboratory Studies for the Initial Routine Evaluation of an HIV-Infected Adult

Test	*Comment*
HIV antibody test	Need to firmly establish diagnosis; this test can be omitted if HIV RNA test is convincing
$CD4^+$ T cell count	Critical for staging disease and determining need for antiretroviral therapy
HIV RNA level	Critical for predicting progression of disease and determining need for antiretroviral therapy
Complete blood count	Hematologic problems are more common in HIV-infected persons; baseline value is useful because the number of medications used has effects on marrow
Serum chemistries	Useful to have routine serum chemistries as a baseline
Liver function tests	Useful to have as a baseline, considering potential hepatotoxicity of some antiretroviral medications; useful in patients with active hepatitis B virus (HBV) or hepatitis C virus (HCV) infection
Cholesterol panel	Useful as baseline; significant alterations in lipids can occur with antiretroviral therapy
Serologic testing for syphilis	Important with known higher rates of syphilis among HIV-infected persons
Toxoplasma IgG antibody	Useful in determining whether patient is at risk for developing toxoplasmosis; if negative, patient can receive counseling on preventing acquisition of *T. gondii*
Hepatitis A, B, or C antibody; hepatitis B antigen	Useful for identifying patients coinfected with HIV and either HBV or HCV; useful for identifying patients who are seronegative for hepatitis A virus or HBV and who should therefore receive vaccination; if HCV antibody is positive, testing should be performed to determine whether patient has a positive HCV viral load
Purified protein derivative	Considered positive if ≥ 5 mm induration; controls are no longer recommended

Routine Follow-up

How often a patient should return for routine follow-up visits depends on the immune status, clinical status, concomitant medical problems, and whether or not the patient is receiving antiretroviral therapy. In general, patients should have visits at least every

Table 3 Vaccinations for HIV-Infected Adults

Vaccine	*Comment*
Haemophilus influenzae type B vaccine	Not generally recommended for adults
Hepatitis A virus vaccine (Havrix, VAQTA)	Recommended for men who have sex with men, injection-drug users, and persons with chronic liver disease; dosage is 1.0 ml given intramuscularly and repeated 6–12 mo later
Hepatitis B virus (HBV) vaccine (Recombivax HB, Engerix-B)	Recommended; regimen for vaccination is 10–20 µg of recombinant HBV vaccine given in the deltoid muscle at 0, 1, and 6 mo; responses are often suboptimal particularly in those with more advanced immune suppression
Influenza virus vaccine	Recommended; the dosage is 0.5 ml I.M. and should be administered during the period from late October through late December; the goal is to prevent influenza and secondary bacterial pneumonias
Mumps, measles, and rubella vaccine	Recommended, with exceptions; the dosage is 0.5 ml S.C.; patients with severe immunodeficiency should not receive this live vaccine; this vaccine is generally recommended for persons born after 1956 who do not have a documented history of measles or measles vaccination and persons who received the killed vaccine (1963 to 1967) and do not have a documented history of measles or live measles vaccination
Pneumococcal vaccine (polysaccharide 23-valent vaccine)	Recommended if CD4⁺ cell count is > 200 cells/mm³; the dosage is 0.5 ml I.M. repeated every 5 years; consider repeating vaccine if CD4⁺ cell count was less than 200 cells/mm³ but has increased to greater than 200 cells/mm³; there are insufficient data in HIV-infected persons to recommend conjugated 7-valent vaccine
Polio vaccine	Recommended; inactivated vaccine only; live oral polio vaccine is contraindicated in HIV-infected patients; patients who have not been immunized should receive inactivated polio vaccine (trivalent killed poliovirus), 0.5 ml S.C. at 0, 1, and 6 mo
Tetanus-diphtheria toxoid	Recommended; patients previously immunized should receive a booster every 10 years; those never immunized should receive primary vaccination, 0.5 ml I.M. at 0, 1, and 6 mo
Varicella vaccine	Insufficient data to recommend for adults

3 months for monitoring of $CD4^+$ T cell counts, HIV RNA levels, and clinical status. More frequent visits are often needed in patients with significant ongoing HIV-related problems or ongoing concomitant medical problems and in those who have recently begun antiretroviral therapy. Visits every 6 months would be appropriate for patients whose disease will probably not progress in the long term and who have a $CD4^+$ T cell count greater than 500 cells/mm^3 and whose HIV RNA level is less than 10,000 copies/ml.

Antiretroviral Therapy

Careful consideration of both medical and social conditions should take place before antiretroviral therapy is started. In general, HIV-infected individuals should be both interested in and able to consistently take antiretroviral medications. Active social problems, such as ongoing drug use, homelessness, or unstable emotional states, can be major barriers to successful antiretroviral therapy. In addition, if a patient has an active severe medical problem, every attempt should be made to defer antiretroviral therapy until that problem is stabilized. Medical indications for antiretroviral therapy are based on the patient's clinical status, the $CD4^+$ T cell count, and the HIV RNA level [*see* Guidelines for Antiretroviral Therapy, *below*). There is a vast array of possible antiretroviral drug combinations; in choosing a specific regimen, the clinician should take into account the dosing schedule, possible adverse effects, and underlying patient preferences.

Agents Currently, three different classes of medications, comprising a total of 15 drugs, target HIV: (1) NRTIs (abacavir, didanosine, lamivudine, stavudine, zalcitabine, and zidovudine), (2) nonnucleoside reverse transcriptase inhibitors (NNRTIs) (delavirdine, efavirenz, and nevirapine), and (3) protease inhibitors (amprenavir, indinavir, lopinavir plus ritonavir, nelfinavir, ritonavir, and saquinavir) [*see Figure 10*] and [*see Table 4*].[42] The NRTIs—also known as nucleoside analogues—structurally resemble the human nucleosides that HIV uses to make viral DNA. The HIV reverse transcriptase enzyme can mistakenly incorporate the synthetic nucleoside analogue into the elongating strand of viral DNA during the reverse transcriptase process; once incorporated into viral DNA, the nucleoside analogues act as chain terminators because they lack the 3′ hydroxyl group required for chain elongation. The NNRTIs do not act as chain terminators; rather, they directly inhibit the proper functioning of the reverse transcriptase enzyme. The HIV protease inhibitors selectively bind to HIV protease and prevent this

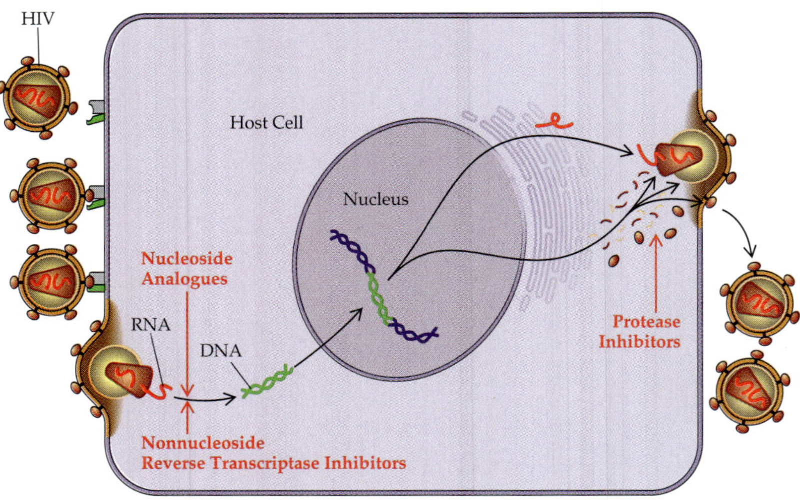

Figure 10 **This illustration depicts the site of action of three major classes of antiretroviral medications.**

enzyme from performing its normal function of cleaving viral polyprotein precursors into individual functional proteins. Successful inhibition of HIV protease causes the formation of deformed HIV particles that generally do not replicate.

Dosing schedules Owing to practical considerations, clinicians have increasingly used antiretroviral regimens that have infrequent dosing schedules, minimal meal restrictions, and the least possible adverse effects. Among the NRTIs, most can be taken twice daily without regard to food consumption except for zalcitabine, which is taken three times daily, and didanosine, which is taken a half hour before a meal or 1 hour after a meal. Although the new enteric-coated didanosine capsule is taken once daily, it should not be taken with meals. Alcohol significantly increases the plasma levels of abacavir. The NNRTIs can be taken without regard to food consumption, with the caveat that efavirenz should not be taken after a meal high in fats, as this will increase the plasma level of efavirenz by approximately 50%. Dosing schedules and food restrictions are more complicated with the protease inhibitors. Nelfinavir, saquinavir, and ritonavir should be taken with food; amprenavir can be taken with or without meals, but it should not be taken with a high-fat meal. Indinavir should be taken 1 hour before or 2 hours after a meal, or it can be taken with a low-fat meal.

Combination therapy Increasingly, pharmacologic boosting of protease inhibitor levels is being used to simplify the dosing schedule, decrease the pill burden, and improve the efficacy of several of the protease inhibitors. Most often, this technique has involved the use of low-dose ritonavir in combination with another protease inhibitor, also at a reduced dosage. Ritonavir significantly increases the trough level of the other protease inhibitor, usually without causing a major increase in the peak levels [*see Figure 11*] and [*see Table 5*]. Long-term data from studies on the combination of ritonavir and saquinavir have shown this combination to be highly effective.[43] The fixed combination of ritonavir and lopinavir (Kaletra) has shown excellent results; this fixed combination has been approved by the Food and Drug Administration. Preliminary data regarding the use of ritonavir in combination with either indinavir or amprenavir are promising. In addition, the use of ritonavir with indinavir eliminates the meal restrictions associated with the use of indinavir alone.

Principles of Antiretroviral Therapy

An expert panel convened by the DHHS and the Henry J. Kaiser Family Foundation has issued antiretroviral therapy recommendations for medical providers in the United States. These guidelines, which are based on data from clinical trials, basic virologic principles, and clinical experience, were last updated February 5, 2001, and will continue to be modified as needed.[42] A second set of recently published guidelines were issued by the International AIDS Society[44]; these guidelines had more international input than the DHHS guide-

Table 4 Antiretroviral Medications

Generic Name	*Trade Name*	*Dosage*
Nucleoside RTIs		
Abacavir (ABC)	Ziagen	300 mg p.o., b.i.d.
Didanosine (ddI)	Videx	400 mg p.o., q.d. (250 mg q.d. if < 60 kg)
Lamivudine (3TC)	Epivir	150 mg p.o., b.i.d.
Stavudine (d4T)	Zerit	40 mg p.o., b.i.d. (30 mg p.o., b.i.d., if < 60 kg)
Zalcitabine (ddC)	Hivid	0.75 mg p.o., t.i.d.
Zidovudine (AZT)	Retrovir	300 mg p.o., b.i.d.; or 200 mg t.i.d.
Zidovudine + lamivudine*	Combivir	One tablet p.o., b.i.d.
Zidovudine + lamivudine + abacavir*	Trizivir	One tablet p.o., b.i.d.
Nonnucleoside RTIs		
Delavirdine	Rescriptor	400 mg p.o., t.i.d.
Efavirenz	Sustiva	600 mg p.o., q.d. (dose can be split and given 200 mg in A.M. and 400 mg in P.M.)
Nevirapine	Viramune	200 mg p.o., q.d. × 14 days, then 200 mg p.o., b.i.d.
Protease inhibitors		
Amprenavir	Agenerase	1,200 mg p.o., b.i.d.
Indinavir	Crixivan	800 mg p.o., q. 8 hr
Lopinavir + ritonavir	Kaletra	3 p.o., b.i.d. (lopinavir, 400 mg b.i.d. + ritonavir, 100 mg b.i.d.)
Nelfinavir	Viracept	1,250 mg p.o., b.i.d. or 750 mg p.o., t.i.d.
Ritonavir	Norvir	600 mg p.o., b.i.d. (dose escalation†)
Saquinavir	Fortovase	1,200 mg p.o., t.i.d.

*Standard dosages are used in fixed combinations.
†Ritonavir dose escalation: 300 mg p.o., b.i.d. × 2 days; 400 mg p.o., b.i.d. × 3 days; 500 mg p.o., b.i.d. × 8 days; 600 mg p.o., b.i.d.
RTI — reverse transcriptase inhibitor

lines. As described in the DHHS guidelines, the goal of antiretroviral therapy is to obtain maximal and durable suppression of HIV, restore and preserve immune function, improve quality of life, and reduce HIV-related mortality.

INITIATION OF THERAPY

The DHHS guidelines recommend that antiretroviral therapy be offered to the following patients: (1) those with acute HIV syndrome, (2) those in whom HIV infection has been diagnosed within 6 months of seroconversion, and (3) those with severe HIV-related symptoms or AIDS. Regarding patients with HIV who do not have HIV-related symptoms, the DHHS guidelines recommend that antiretroviral therapy be offered to those whose CD4+ T cell count is less than 350 cells/mm^3 or whose plasma HIV RNA level is greater than 30,000 copies/ml, as determined by use of the branched-DNA (bDNA) assay, or to those whose plasma HIV RNA level is greater than 55,000 copies/ml, as determined by use of the reverse transcriptase-polymerase chain reaction (RT-PCR) assay. The guidelines note that some experts recommend that therapy be offered to patients whose CD4+ T cell count is less than 200 cells/mm^3, rather than 350 cells/mm^3. These recommendations represent a less aggressive approach in terms of when to initiate therapy; this reflects increasing concerns regarding adverse effects of antiretroviral medications and problems with long-term adherence.

RECOMMENDED REGIMEN

Antiretroviral therapy should consist of a potent regimen that includes a combination of three or more medications [*see Table 6*]. The combination regimens typically consist of (1) two NRTIs plus a protease inhibitor, (2) two NRTIs plus a NNRTI, or (3) two NRTIs plus two protease inhibitors. The International AIDS Society's antiretroviral therapy recommendations, published in 2000, state that for patients without HIV-related symptoms, antiretroviral therapy should be administered if the CD4+ T

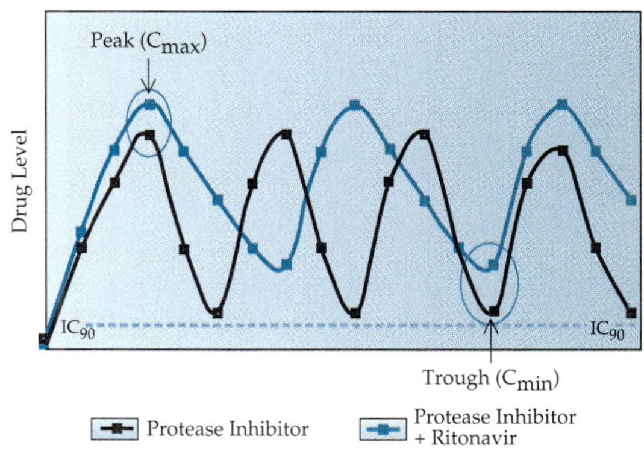

Figure 11 **In this illustration, the drug levels of a protease inhibitor are compared with boosted levels of ritonavir. (IC_{90}—concentration of drug required to inhibit 90% of viral replication)**

Table 5 Ritonavir Boosted Protease Inhibitor Regimens

Ritonavir Dose	*Other Protease Inhibitor*	*Comment*
100 mg b.i.d.	Lopinavir, 400 mg b.i.d.	FDA-approved fixed combination with excellent potency
400 mg b.i.d.	Saquinavir, 400 mg b.i.d.	Combination with best long-term data; highly effective combination, but intolerance to ritonavir common at this dosage
100 mg q.d.	Saquinavir, 1,600 mg q.d.	Possible once-daily combination; minimal data are available
200 mg b.i.d.	Indinavir, 800 mg b.i.d.	Moderate amount of data suggest regimen very potent; can be taken with meals; increased indinavir toxicity at this dosage
400 mg b.i.d.	Indinavir, 400 mg b.i.d.	Moderate amount of data suggest regimen very potent; ideal pharmacokinetics, but intolerance to ritonavir common at this dosage
100 mg b.i.d.	Amprenavir, 600 mg b.i.d.	Moderate amount of data suggest regimen very potent; regimen markedly decreases amprenavir pill burden; preliminary data also suggest ritonavir, 200 mg, plus amprenavir, 1,200 mg, given once daily may also be effective

cell count is less than 350 cells/mm^3 or if the plasma HIV RNA level is greater than 30,000 copies/ml.[44] These guidelines also recommend antiretroviral therapy for persons whose CD4$^+$ T cell count is between 350 and 500 cells/mm^3 and whose HIV RNA level is 5,000 copies/ml or higher.

DRUG SELECTION

Short-term and Long-term Adverse Effects of Drugs

Potentially life-threatening reactions Potential adverse effects can greatly influence the choice of antiretroviral medications and the ability and will-

Table 6 DHHS Recommendations for Antiretroviral Regimens for the Treatment of Established HIV in Adults and Adolescents[42]*

Recommendations	*Column A*	*Column B*
Strongly recommended	Efavirenz Indinavir Nelfinavir Ritonavir + indinavir Ritonavir + lopinavir Ritonavir + saquinavir	Stavudine + didanosine† Stavudine + lamivudine Zidovudine + didanosine Zidovudine + lamivudine
Alternative regimen	Abacavir Amprenavir Delavirdine Nelfinavir + saquinavir-SGC Nevirapine Ritonavir Saquinavir-SGC	Didanosine + lamivudine Zidovudine + zalcitabine
No recommendation (insufficient data)	Hydroxyurea with ARV medications Ritonavir + amprenavir Ritonavir + nelfinavir	
Not recommended (should not be offered)	All monotherapies Saquinavir-HGC	Stavudine + zidovudine Zalcitabine + didanosine Zalcitabine + lamivudine Zalcitabine + stavudine

*Within each category, specific drugs are listed in alphabetical order, not in order of preference. The regimen would consist of one choice from column A and one choice from column B.

†Pregnant women may have increased risk of lactic acidosis and liver damage when taking didanosine plus stavudine.

ARV — antiretroviral DHHS — Department of Health and Human Services HGC — hard gel capsule (Invirase) SGC — soft gel capsule (Fortovase)

Table 7 Adverse Effects Associated with Antiretroviral Medications

Generic Name	*Trade Name*	*Toxicity*
Nucleoside RTIs		
Abacavir (ABC)	Ziagen	Hypersensitivity reaction in 3% of patients; characterized by fever, rash, nausea, vomiting, or malaise; may be fatal; possible lactic acidosis (rare)
Didanosine (ddI)	Videx	Peripheral neuropathy, pancreatitis, nausea; possible lactic acidosis (rare)
Lamivudine (3TC)	Epivir	Few side effects; possible lactic acidosis (rare)
Stavudine (d4T)	Zerit	Peripheral neuropathy; possible lactic acidosis (rare)
Zalcitabine (ddC)	Hivid	Peripheral neuropathy, stomatitis; possible lactic acidosis (rare)
Zidovudine (AZT)	Retrovir	Anemia, neutropenia, gastrointestinal problems, headache; possible lactic acidosis (rare)
Nonnucleoside RTIs		
Delavirdine	Rescriptor	Rash (4%); increased transaminase levels; headache
Efavirenz	Sustiva	Rash seen in 2% of patients; central nervous system side effects (confusion, abnormal dreams, agitation, etc.)
Nevirapine	Viramune	Rash seen in 7% of patients; increased transaminase levels; hepatitis (can be fatal)
Protease inhibitors		
Amprenavir	Agenerase	Gastrointestinal intolerance; lipid abnormalities; perioral paresthesias; possible fat redistribution
Indinavir	Crixivan	Gastrointestinal intolerance; nephrolithiasis; increase of indirect bilirubin; headache; lipid abnormalities; possible fat redistribution
Lopinavir + ritonavir	Kaletra	Gastrointestinal intolerance; lipid abnormalities, including increased triglyceride levels; possible fat redistribution
Nelfinavir	Viracept	Diarrhea; lipid abnormalities; major drug–drug interactions; possible fat redistribution
Ritonavir	Norvir	Gastrointestinal intolerance; perioral and extremity paresthesias; taste perversions; asthenia; hepatitis; major drug–drug interactions; lipid abnormalities, including increased triglyceride levels; possible fat redistribution
Saquinavir	Fortovase	Gastrointestinal intolerance; headache; lipid abnormalities; possible fat redistribution

RTI — reverse transcriptase inhibitor

ingness of a patient to stay on long-term antiretroviral therapy [*see Table 7*]. Possible acute life-threatening reactions include didanosine-induced pancreatitis, abacavir-related hypersensitivity syndrome, lactic acidosis secondary to the use of any of the NRTIs, Stevens-Johnson syndrome secondary to the use of any of the NNRTIs, and nevirapine-associated liver failure.[45] In addition, several reports have described fatalities among persons taking hydroxyurea in combination with didanosine. Unfortunately, the pancreatitis associated with didanosine can occur without warning any time during therapy.

Hypersensitivity syndrome The abacavir hypersensitivity syndrome occurs in approximately 2% to 3% of patients receiving that drug. It typically develops within the first 3 to 4 weeks after abacavir is started. Symptoms of abacavir hypersensitivity syndrome most often consist of rash, fever, nausea, oral lesions, and cough. Patients often describe an accentuation of these symptoms shortly after taking each dose of abacavir. Patients who begin to develop the hypersensitivity syndrome and then stop taking abacavir can have an acute, potentially fatal reaction on resuming abacavir therapy. Treatment of a patient with mild symptoms suggestive of abacavir hypersensitivity should be conducted in consultation with an expert on this matter. Patients can develop a spectrum of abnormalities related to increased serum lactate levels, which result from NRTIs binding to human mitochondrial DNA polymerase gamma.[46] In patients with mild hyperlactatemia, serum lactate levels are from 2 to 5 mmol/L; mild hyperlactatemia is estimated to occur in up to 10% to 20% of patients receiving antiretroviral therapy. In patients with serious hyperlactatemia, lactate levels are 5 mmol/L or greater (but lactic acidosis is not present); serious hyperlactatemia occurs in approximately 1% to 2% of patients.

Lactic acidosis Patients with lactic acidosis have a serum lactate level of at least 5 mmol/L and a serum bicarbonate level of less than 20 mmol/L. Symptoms associated with increased serum lactate levels are generally vague and may include nausea, abdominal pain, malaise, and anorexia. Although severe lactic acidosis rarely develops, patients with serum lactate levels greater than 10 mmol/L have a mortality of approximately 80%.[45]

Increased insulin resistance Several studies have shown that protease inhibitor–based regimens are associated with significant increases in insulin resistance (i.e., increased insulin concentrations and increased C-peptide levels) but do not typically cause an increase in serum glucose or symptoms of diabetes.[47,48] Nevertheless, up to 25% of patients will have an abnormal result on glucose tolerance testing. At present, it is not clear whether protease inhibitor–based therapy causes a significant increase in diabetes.

Increased triglyceride levels In contrast, studies have clearly shown that protease inhibitor–based regimens are associated with increases in total cholesterol and low-density lipoprotein (LDL) cholesterol but not high-density lipoprotein (HDL) cholesterol. In addition, ritonavir has been associated with significant increases in triglyceride levels.[49] Although a few reports have documented cases of premature atherosclerosis among patients taking a protease inhibitor–based regimen who had no or few risk factors for cardiovascular disease, currently there are no data that have been used to estimate the prevalence of cardiovascular disease in persons receiving antiretroviral therapy. Recent recommendations from the Adult AIDS Clinical Trial Group Cardiovascular Disease Focus Group have suggested treating HIV-infected patients who have abnormal lipid profiles in accordance with U.S. National Cholesterol Education Program guidelines.[50] Among the lipid-lowering HMG-CoA (3-hydroxy-3-methylglutaryl coenzyme A) reductase inhibitors, pravastatin has the least severe drug interactions with other protease inhibitors and is often used as a first-line agent. Although atorvastatin has more interactions with protease inhibitors than pravastatin, few adverse events have been reported. In addition, atorvastatin has greater potency than pravastatin, and it has a favorable impact on triglyceride levels.[51] Patients with marked hypertriglyceridemia often require gemfibrozil.

Lipodystrophy Currently, the lipodystrophy syndrome, also known as the fat redistribution syndrome, has become the most problematic long-term complication of antiretroviral therapy. The lipodystrophy syndrome typically presents as either central fat accumulation (i.e., accumulation of fat in the abdomen, breasts, or posterior neck) or as peripheral fat wasting (i.e., wasting in the face, buttocks, and limbs).[48] There are conflicting views on the pathogenesis of the fat redistribution syndrome, but insulin resistance probably plays a major role. It has also been suggested that HIV protease inhibitors play a role by inhibiting lipid and adipocyte regulatory proteins that have partial homology to the catalytic site of HIV protease.[45] Available data suggest that several factors may correlate with the lipodystrophy syndrome, including age greater than 40 years, use of protease inhibitors, use of stavudine, total duration of antiretroviral therapy, and low body weight before starting antiretroviral therapy.[45,52] The fat redistribution syndrome has occurred in a number of patients who had no exposure to a protease inhibitor, which implies that protease inhibitors are one of several factors that play a role. Moreover, one study has shown that NRTIs are specifically associated with lipoatrophy (fat wasting).[53]

Unfortunately, patients with lipodystrophy syndrome who have switched from a protease inhibitor–based regimen to a non–protease inhibitor–based regimen have not consistently experienced major improvement in their lipodystrophy. Studies have shown that lipodystrophy has not been associated with alterations in concentrations of testosterone or sex hormone–binding globulin, and attempts to reduce lipodystrophy using testosterone or anabolic steroids have generally not provided significant benefit. Surgery has been attempted in some patients with fat accumulation, but the fat usually reaccumulates within several months. Although growth hormone has been shown to be of some benefit in a small number of patients with fat accumulation, this approach is not considered practical because of the extreme cost, adverse effects, and the need for continued use to sustain benefit. The most promising results in the treatment of lipodystrophy have been reported from preliminary studies of the insulin-sensitizing agent metformin. In a randomized, double-blind, placebo-controlled trial, use of metformin at a dosage of 500 mg twice daily for 3 months was associated with decreased insulin levels, decreased weight, decreased visceral abdominal fat, and decreased subcutaneous abdominal fat.[54] In this study, patients did not experience an increase in serum lactate levels or hepatic transaminase levels associated with metformin use. These results provide further indirect evidence that insulin resistance plays a central role in the pathogenesis of the fat redistribution syndrome. Further study is needed to better predict which patients will develop fat redistribution syndrome and to identify measures that may prevent this complication of antiretroviral therapy.

MONITORING OF RNA LEVELS AND CD4+ T CELL COUNTS

The HIV RNA level should be checked before antiretroviral therapy is started and then every 4 weeks after that until the level drops to less than 50 copies/ml. Subsequently, the HIV RNA level and $CD4^+$ T cell count should be monitored approximately every 3 months. In most persons, the HIV RNA level should decrease by at least 1 $\log_{10}$ by week 8 and then to less than 50 copies/ml by weeks 16 to 20. Suppressing HIV levels to less than 50 copies/ml diminishes the number of new HIV virions and thus significantly decreases the chance that resistant strains will emerge. The $CD4^+$ T cell counts of patients on antiretroviral therapy should be monitored every 3 to 4 months to assess the impact of antiretroviral therapy on immune function. Despite earlier hopes that treatment with an aggressive antiretroviral regimen for 2 to 3 years could possibly eradicate HIV from an HIV-infected individual, more recent studies have clearly shown that HIV eradication is not a realistic goal of antiretroviral therapy. Although potent antiretroviral therapy does have tremendous impact on the total burden of HIV on the body, several cellular and anatomic reservoirs of virus contribute to the long-term persistence of HIV.[55] Resting $CD4^+$ memory T cells that contain latently integrated HIV DNA are the most important cellular reservoirs; the CNS and the male urogenital tract are the most important anatomic reservoirs. Novel strategies to eliminate the latent HIV reservoirs need to be developed before eradication of HIV becomes a realistic goal.

PATIENT ADHERENCE

Recent data have shown that the degree of adherence with antiretroviral therapy clearly predicts whether or not a patient will sustain long-term viral suppression.[56] Other factors that may affect long-term viral suppression are the inherent potency of the regimen, whether the patient has previously received antiretroviral therapy, the immune status of the patient, absorption of the antiretroviral medications, and drug-drug interactions that may decrease the concentration of the antiretroviral medications. In patients who achieve an HIV RNA level of less than 50 copies/ml, a change in therapy should be considered if there is a significant increase in the HIV RNA level, a persistent decline in the $CD4^+$ T cell count, or evidence of clinical deterioration. The choice of a salvage regimen should take into consideration the patient's prior antiretroviral therapy, resistance testing, the likelihood of adherence with an often complex salvage regimen, and the stage of the patient's HIV disease. The choice of a salvage regimen should be made in consultation with an expert who has experience in antiretroviral therapy.

RESISTANCE AND RESISTANCE TESTING

Antiretroviral therapy can lead to the emergence of resistant strains of HIV, which can render antiretroviral therapy less effective. Indeed, multiple studies have shown that in cases in which HIV suppression fails, there is usually evidence of HIV drug resistance.

Types of Resistance Assays

Two types of resistance assays are now commercially available to test for HIV resistance: genotype and phenotype assays.

The genotype assays identify specific codon mutations associated with resistance by sequencing the reverse transcriptase and protease genes or by using standardized probes to detect mutations known to be associated with resistance. The genotype assays can be performed in 1 to 2 weeks, but interpretation of the results requires expertise and review of current and prior antiretroviral therapy. Phenotype assays generally measure HIV growth in the presence of specific antiretroviral medications; the results are reported as the concentration of drug required to inhibit 50% or 90% of viral replication (IC_{50} and IC_{90}, respectively). As with genotype results, the phenotype results require expertise to interpret and must be interpreted in the context of current and prior antiretroviral therapy. The strains of HIV identified in the patient are compared with reference strains and reported as the "fold" resistance in IC_{50}. In general, phenotype assays require longer periods than genotype assays and are more expensive.

Both testing techniques have inherent problems: the tests may sample only a minority of the HIV strains; the sampled strains from the blood may not adequately represent strains from other body regions (compartments); resistance to medications taken in the past may not be evident; and for resistance to be determined, plasma HIV RNA levels typically must be in the range of at least 500 to 1,000 copies/ml. Nevertheless, several studies have shown that patients who undergo resistance testing in the setting of virologic failure have better virologic outcomes than those who do not undergo resistance testing.[57,58]

To date, no randomized trials have compared genotypic tests with phenotypic tests, and thus, there is no basis for recommending one over the other. The tests generally are better predictors of which drugs will not work than which drugs will likely be successful.

Indications for Resistance Testing

In the DHHS guidelines, resistance testing is recommended for patients who experience virologic failure with an antiretroviral regimen and for patients in whom HIV remains at detectable levels after starting therapy.[42] Virologic failure is constituted by any one of the following three events: (1) there is less than a 0.75 $\log_{10}$ decrease in HIV RNA by week 4 of antiretroviral therapy or there is less than a 1.0 $\log_{10}$ decrease by week 8; (2) there is a failure to suppress the level of HIV RNA to less than 50 copies/ml within 6 months of starting or changing therapy; or (3) a high level of HIV RNA (> 5,000 copies/ml) is repeatedly detected in plasma after initial suppression to less than 50 copies/ml.[42] In addition, some experts consider utilizing resistance testing for those patients with low-level breakthrough viremia (50 to 5,000 copies/ml) if the level was greater than 1,000 copies/ml, a level high enough to obtain a reliable resistance assay.

In addition, multiple recent studies have described the transmission of antiretroviral drug-resistant HIV variants, and a significant proportion of persons newly infected with HIV have been shown to harbor HIV-resistant strains.[59–61] Accordingly, performing resistance testing in persons newly infected with HIV is indicated.[42]

STRUCTURED TREATMENT INTERRUPTIONS

Patients may temporarily discontinue antiretroviral therapy for a number of reasons. Patients who respond well to antiretroviral therapy but whose therapy is interrupted for a month or less have excellent long-term suppression of plasma HIV RNA upon resuming their regimen.[62] In the past several years, investigators have focused great attention on structured treatment interruptions, a process of scheduled starting and stopping of antiretroviral medications that is intended to enhance cytotoxic T cell responses and thus provide better immunologic control of HIV. The interest in structured treatment interruptions arose from studies that showed the importance of cytotoxic T cell responses in controlling HIV[63] and the observation

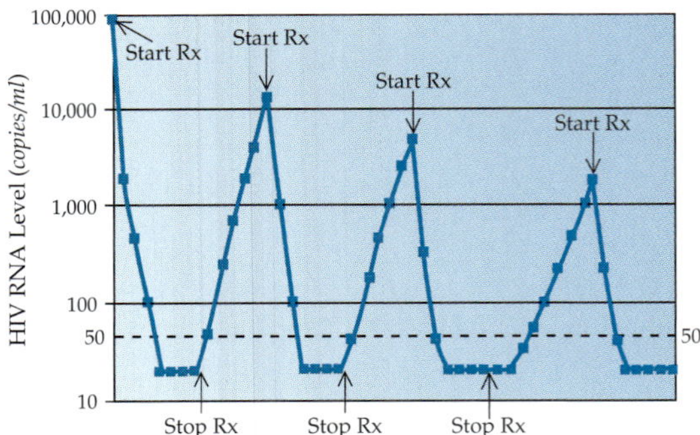

Figure 12 **Conceptual diagram of structured treatment interruption. Medications are started and stopped on several cycles. HIV RNA levels are measured in copies per milliliter. (Rx—therapy)**

that cytotoxic T cell responses become very weak in persons who achieved long-term control of HIV with antiretroviral therapy.[64] The goal of structured treatment interruptions is to intermittently expose the immune system to HIV-1 antigen in an attempt to upregulate HIV-specific cytotoxic T cell activity, thus leading to better immunologic control of HIV [*see Figure 12*].

Treatment Interruptions in Patients with Established HIV Infection

Several small trials of structured treatment interruption have been conducted in persons chronically infected with HIV. In these trials, most of the patients showed good virologic responses each time their antiretroviral regimen was resumed. The desired immunologic responses, however, have generally not been consistently observed, and patients have not had sufficient cytotoxic T cell responses to allow the simplifying or stopping of antiretroviral therapy. In addition, stopping and starting antiretroviral therapy in a chronically infected patient could have several negative effects. First, patients could develop drug resistance when virus rebounds or upon resumption of therapy. The risk of resistance developing as a result of viral rebound would be of particular concern in persons on regimens that included drugs with long elimination half-lives, such as nevirapine or efavirenz. Second, one study has shown that persons who have long-term viral suppression and quiescent lymph nodes will develop hyperplastic and activated lymph nodes within 1 to 2 months after stopping antiretroviral treatment.[65] Third, several reports have now described persons with well-controlled HIV who developed an acute retroviral syndrome after stopping their antiretroviral therapy.[66,67] At present, the use of structured treatment interruptions in persons chronically infected with HIV should not be performed in clinical practice but only in a carefully monitored study.

Treatment Interruptions in Patients with Acute (Primary) HIV Infection

The use of structured treatment interruption in a person who had initially received treatment for acute HIV infection may pose a unique opportunity, mainly because persons treated with aggressive antiretroviral therapy very early after acquiring HIV may preserve excellent HIV-specific cytotoxic T cell responses. In contrast, persons with chronic HIV infection who do not receive antiretroviral therapy in the acute phase likely have permanent impairment of their ability to generate robust HIV-specific cytotoxic T cell responses. Clinical interest in the approach of structured treatment interruption after treatment of acute HIV was sparked by a case report of a single patient known as the Berlin patient.[68] This patient received early aggressive antiretroviral therapy; after several treatment interruptions, excellent control of HIV was achieved when the patient was not receiving antiretroviral therapy, and the patient showed excellent HIV-specific cytotoxic T cell responses.

A subsequent report has shown promising results with structured treatment interruption in a carefully selected group of eight patients who had aggressive antiretroviral therapy at the time that acute HIV was diagnosed; all eight received antiretroviral therapy for longer than 1 year, and in all patients, HIV RNA levels were consistently less than 50 copies/ml as a result of therapy.[69] Patients in this study subsequently had one or two structured treatment interruptions, and all experienced viral rebound with treatment interruption. Despite the initial viral rebound, all eight patients achieved at least a temporary steady state while not receiving therapy, with HIV RNA levels of less than 5,000 copies/ml. Five of the eight remained off antiretroviral therapy; after a median of 6.5 months, their HIV RNA levels were less than 500 copies/ml. Although this study involved only eight patients, these results have generated great interest and should stimulate further study.

Further support for this approach comes from a study of structured treatment interruptions in rhesus macaques infected with SIV.[70] In this randomized, controlled study, 17 animals were infected with SIV; 6 weeks after infection, six of the macaques received continuous potent antiretroviral therapy, six received intermittent potent antiretroviral therapy (subjects underwent a 3-week cycle of therapy in which therapy was administered for 3 weeks, then withheld for 3 weeks, and so on), and five received no antiretroviral therapy. After 21 weeks, none of the animals received antiretroviral therapy. After antiretroviral therapy was discontinued, excellent control of SIV was achieved in all six of the macaques that received intermittent antiretroviral therapy, and these subjects experienced no decline in their $CD4^+$ T cell counts. In contrast, in the animals that received continuous antiretroviral therapy, SIV levels returned to near baseline, and the subjects showed significant declines in $CD4^+$ T cell counts.

Prophylactic Therapy

OCCUPATIONAL POSTEXPOSURE ANTIRETROVIRAL THERAPY

Despite widespread efforts to implement universal precautions, health care workers still occasionally suffer accidental exposures to HIV. Current recommendations for the use of postexposure prophylaxis are based on previous retrospective human data, data from animal studies, and extrapolation of experience with antiretroviral therapy in HIV-infected individuals.

One retrospective case-control study found that use of zidovudine monotherapy for postexposure prophylaxis in health care workers reduced the risk of HIV transmission by approximately 81%.[71] In addition, animal studies have suggested that postexposure prophylaxis decreases the risk of transmission.[27]

Recommendations

In general, after adequately cleaning the site of exposure, the health care worker should initiate postexposure antiretroviral therapy as soon as possible. Although combination therapy for postexposure prophylaxis has not been proven to be more effective than use of zidovudine alone, extrapolations from treatment data in HIV-infected individuals indicate that two- or three-drug regimens are likely to be more effective than zidovudine alone for preventing transmission of HIV. Recommendations on whether to use the basic two-drug regimen or the expanded three-drug regimen depend on the risk of the exposure. For HIV exposures that pose an increased risk of transmission, an expanded regimen that includes the addition of a third drug is recommended. The basic regimen is recommended for circumstances in which there is a recognized risk of occupational HIV transmission, but not to the same degree as noted in the expanded regimen. The expanded regimen is recommended for higher-risk occupational exposures, such as exposures involving larger volumes of blood or exposures in which the source patient has advanced AIDS. The basic regimen for adults consists of either (1) zidovudine (300 mg b.i.d. or 200 mg t.i.d.) plus lamivudine (150 mg b.i.d.); (2) stavudine (40 mg b.i.d.) plus lamivudine (150 mg b.i.d.); or (3) stavudine (40 mg b.i.d.) plus didanosine (400 mg q.d.). For persons who weigh less than 60 kg, the dosage of stavudine should be reduced to 30 mg twice a day, and the dosage of didanosine should be reduced to 300 mg daily. The expanded three-drug regimen consists of the basic regimen plus a potent third drug (either nelfinavir [750 mg t.i.d.] or indinavir [800 mg every 8 hours]). In some circumstances, either abacavir (300 mg b.i.d.), efavirenz (600 mg q.d.), or lopinavir-ritonavir (400 mg b.i.d.) could be considered for use as the potent third drug, but this decision should be made in consultation with an antiretroviral therapy expert.

In addition, the new U.S. Public Health Service guidelines note several special circumstances that warrant consultation with local experts or the National Clinicians' Post-Exposure Prophylaxis Hotline ([PEPline] 1-888-448-4911). These circumstances include cases involving a delayed report of exposure, cases in which the source person is unknown, cases in which the exposed person is pregnant, cases in which the source virus is resistant to antiretroviral agents, and cases in which the health care worker experiences a toxic reaction to the prophylactic regimen.[27]

Regardless of whether the basic regimen or the expanded regimen is used, it should be taken for 28 days. A recent report described two health care workers who developed life-threatening hepatotoxicity associated with the use of nevirapine for postexposure prophylaxis[72]; accordingly, nevirapine should not be used for postexposure prophylaxis. Recent studies have shown that health care workers frequently have adverse effects with postexposure antiretroviral prophylaxis, even to the extent that many could not complete their 28-day course.[73]

Health care workers receiving postexposure prophylaxis should undergo drug-toxicity monitoring at baseline and again 2 weeks after therapy is started. In addition, health care workers with occupational exposure to HIV should undergo serologic testing for HIV on first exposure and at 6 weeks, 3 months, and 6 months after exposure. Because three health care providers experienced seroconversion between months 6 and 12 after exposure, some experts recommend also performing follow-up HIV serologic testing at 12 months. In general, health care workers should use safe sex practices and avoid breast-feeding for at least the first 12 weeks after exposure to HIV.

ANTIRETROVIRAL THERAPY TO PREVENT PERINATAL TRANSMISSION

The Pediatric AIDS Clinical Trials Group Protocol 076 study generated the initial enthusiasm for using antiretroviral therapy to prevent perinatal HIV transmission.[20] In this trial, HIV-infected pregnant women received either placebo or a regimen that consisted of oral zidovudine administered after week 14 of gestation and intravenous zidovudine administered during labor and delivery; in addition, oral zidovudine was given to the newborn until the infant reached 6 weeks of age. The HIV transmission rate among those who received zidovudine was 8.3%, compared with 25.5% among placebo recipients. Longer-term complete results of this study showed transmission rates of 7.6% in the zidovudine group and 22.6% in the placebo group.[74] As perinatal prophylaxis regimens became incorporated into clinical practice, HIV perinatal transmission rates in the United States dramatically declined.[25] Available data have not shown there to be any significant differences with regard to congenital abnormalities, growth rates, or neurologic development, nor have the data uncovered other evidence of long-term toxicity in children exposed to zidovudine, either in utero or post partum, compared with children in the general population.[25]

Subsequent international studies have also shown the benefit of antiretroviral therapy in preventing mother-to-child transmission of HIV. In one study in Thailand in which mothers received zidovudine for 4 weeks before labor and during labor, perinatal transmission was only 9% in the zidovudine group and 19% in the placebo group.[75] In addition, in a study from Uganda that compared nevirapine and zidovudine (a single 200 mg dose of nevirapine was given to the mother at the onset of labor and a single 2 mg/kg dose was given to the infant 48 to 72 hours after birth; or a short course of oral zidovudine was given to the mother during labor and oral zidovudine was given to the infant for 1 week after birth), the HIV infection rate for the newborns at 6 weeks after birth was 12% in the nevirapine group and 21% in the zidovudine group.[76] The enthusiasm for these excellent results with short-course nevirapine was tempered by the discovery of high rates of resistance associated with this therapy: in tests conducted 6 weeks after the conclusion of therapy, 20% of the women were found to have developed resistance to nevirapine.[77] This high rate of resistance after receiving only one dose of nevirapine presumably relates to the very long elimination half-life of this drug.

Recommendations

In its recommendations for reducing perinatal HIV transmission, the Public Health Service Task Force stated that pregnancy should influence the decisions regarding timing and choice of antiretroviral therapy but that antiretroviral therapy should not be deferred on the grounds that the patient is pregnant.[25] Several of the unique and important factors to consider with the use of antiretroviral therapy in pregnancy include the physiologic changes associated with pregnancy, which may require altering dosing of medications; the potential short-term or long-term adverse effects on the fetus and newborn; and the effectiveness of the regimen in reducing the risk of perinatal transmission. In addition, the efficacy of the regimen for treatment of the mother's HIV infection needs to be taken into consideration. Unfortunately, data regarding combination antiretroviral therapy in pregnancy are insufficient to clarify the safety and efficacy of these regimens. Accordingly, medical providers who offer antiretroviral therapy to HIV-1–infected women during pregnancy need to extensively discuss issues related to the potential short-term and long-term risks and benefits of therapy during pregnancy.

If antiretroviral therapy is given during pregnancy, the three-part zidovudine regimen should be used. In general, clinicians are likely to encounter one of four scenarios: (1) the HIV-infected pregnant woman has not received prior antiretroviral therapy; (2) the HIV-infected woman is receiving antiretroviral therapy at the time the pregnancy is discovered; (3) the HIV-infected woman is in labor and has not been receiving antiretroviral therapy during her pregnancy; or (4) the infant is born of an HIV-infected mother who did not receive antiretroviral therapy during pregnancy or labor. Specific considerations and recommendations for each of these scenarios are discussed in detail in the Public Health Service Task Force recommendations.[25] In addition, these recommendations address issues regarding the mode of delivery, with particular consideration to the performance of cesarean section in women who have HIV RNA levels greater than 1,000 copies/ml near the time of delivery. Women who have HIV RNA levels less than 1,000 copies/ml have a very low rate of HIV transmission and thus would be unlikely to receive substantial benefit from cesarean section.

HIV PREVENTIVE VACCINES

In the development of HIV vaccines, major work has been conducted in both the therapeutic and preventive arenas. The goal of HIV therapeutic vaccines is to upregulate the immune system's specific response to HIV and thus delay (or possibly halt) the progression of HIV disease. The leading therapeutic vaccine candidate, HIV-1 immunogen (Remune), produced disappointing results in HIV-infected patients who had $CD4^+$ T cell counts between 300 and 550 cells/mm^3.[78] Other therapeutic vaccines have entered clinical trials, but the data are insufficient to determine whether these vaccines are likely to provide significant benefit to HIV-infected individuals.

The pace of research in HIV preventive vaccines has quickened remarkably in recent years, probably because of a combination of factors that include better understanding of HIV pathogenesis, increased private and federal funding, and a major national commitment to develop an effective preventive vaccine. Different strategies have been attempted to stimulate HIV neutralizing antibodies or cellular responses specific to $CD8^+$ T cells.[79,80] Although earlier research has focused primarily on vaccines that stimulate neutralizing antibodies, recent work has focused on vaccines that stimulate cellular immune responses. One of the biggest hurdles hampering development of an effective vaccine is the lack of knowledge regarding the correlates of immune protection with HIV. Other challenges include developing a vaccine that will produce broad immune responses for the multiple different strains (clades) of HIV present throughout the world. At the time of this writing, no vaccine has been established as being highly effective in preventing HIV infection.

Prevention and Management of Opportunistic Infections

With the widespread use of antiretroviral therapy in developed countries, the incidence of serious opportunistic infections has dramatically declined.[2,81] In the United States, the incidence of development of *Pneumocystis carinii* pneumonia,

Mycobacterium avium complex disease, or cytomegalovirus retinitis in HIV-infected patients declined from 21.9 per 100 persons-years in 1994 to 3.7 per 100 person-years in mid-1997.[2] In addition, a separate study examined the incidence of the most common opportunistic infections in the United States from 1992 to 1998 and found profound declines during that period; the most pronounced reductions occurred from 1996 to 1998, reflecting the widespread use of aggressive antiretroviral therapy.[81] The incidence of Kaposi sarcoma has also markedly declined, with an estimated 50% reduction in persons receiving potent antiretroviral therapy.[82] Despite these advances, major opportunistic infections continue to cause significant morbidity and mortality in HIV-infected persons. Indeed, prevention of major opportunistic infections remains a critical aspect of HIV care.

PREVENTION OF OPPORTUNISTIC INFECTIONS

In 1999, the U.S. Public Health Service, in conjunction with the Infectious Diseases Society of America, issued guidelines for preventing opportunistic infections [*see Table 8*].[83] As the standard of care, these guidelines strongly recommend measures to prevent the first episode of opportunistic disease caused by *M. tuberculosis*, *P. carinii*, *Toxoplasma gondii*, and *M. avium* complex. The guidelines do not recommend the routine use of prophylaxis to prevent a first episode of *Cryptococcus neoformans*, *Histoplasma capsulatum*, or cytomegalovirus infection.

Recently, several studies have addressed the question of whether patients can discontinue opportunistic infection prophylaxis when they have experienced an excellent virologic and immunologic response to antiretroviral therapy, as evidenced by an increase in CD4+ T cell count to a threshold greater than the cut-off level used to start opportunistic infections. Taken together, the available data clearly show that the risk of development of *P. carinii* pneumonia is extremely small in persons who discontinue primary prophylaxis after they maintain CD4+ T cell counts of greater than 200 cells/mm^3 for at least 3 months.[84] Similarly, patients whose lowest recorded CD4+ T cell count is less than 50 cells/mm^3 and who, as a result of potent antiretroviral therapy, sustain a CD4+ T cell count of more than 100 cells/mm^3 can safely discontinue prophylaxis against *M. avium* complex.[85] In addition, preliminary data suggest that patients can discontinue primary prophylaxis against toxoplasmosis when their CD4+ T cell count increases to more than 200 cells/mm^3 in response to potent antiretroviral therapy.[86,87]

MANAGEMENT OF OPPORTUNISTIC INFECTIONS

The following is a brief overview of the typical clinical presentations and treatment of tuberculosis, *P. carinii* pneumonia, toxoplasmosis, cryptococcal meningitis, disseminated *M. avium* complex infection, and cytomegalovirus retinitis.

Tuberculosis

Although tuberculosis can occur in HIV-infected patients regardless of their CD4+ T cell count, the clinical presentation usually varies with the CD4+ T cell count. The clinical picture of HIV-infected patients with active tuberculosis whose CD4+ T cell count is greater than 350 cells/mm^3 is similar to that of persons not infected with HIV—the illness is characterized by gradual onset of weight loss, cough, fever, upper lobe infiltrates, and cavitary lesions. In contrast, patients with advanced AIDS who develop active tuberculosis often have an atypical presentation that may include diffuse pulmonary lesions, lymph node involvement, blood cultures that are positive for *M. tuberculosis*, and an absence of cavitary lesions. A diagnosis is made by isolating *M. tuberculosis* from any body site; most often, the diagnosis is made on sputum staining or from bronchoscopy. It is critical that drug susceptibility testing be performed on the *M. tuberculosis* isolate. Initial therapy for *M. tuberculosis* consists of a minimum of three drugs (isoniazid, rifampin, and pyrazinamide); most experts recommend adding ethambutol until susceptibility results become available [*see Table 9*].

Pneumocystis carinii *Pneumonia*

Patients with *P. carinii* pneumonia generally have a CD4+ T cell count of less than 200 cells/mm^3; the clinical presentation is characterized by a nonproductive cough of gradual onset, dyspnea, fever, and fatigue. Chest radiographs most often show a diffuse, reticulonodular pattern, predominantly in the perihilar region, but up to 30% of patients will have a normal chest radiograph early in the course of their disease. A definitive diagnosis should be established by induced sputum stain or bronchoscopy. For patients with suspected *P. carinii* pneumonia, therapy should not be delayed while the patient undergoes a diagnostic workup. First-line therapy consists of trimethoprim-sulfamethoxazole. Patients whose arterial oxygen tension (P_ao_2) measurement is less than 70 mm Hg or whose alveolar-arterial difference in oxygen (A-aDo$_2$) is greater than 35 mm Hg should also receive corticosteroids as part of their initial therapy. Recent data have suggested that patients who pre-

Table 8 Prophylactic Measures Strongly Recommended as Standard of Care for the Prevention of First Episodes of Opportunistic Disease in Adults and Adolescents Infected with HIV[83]

Pathogen	*Indication*	*First Choice**	*Alternatives**
Pneumocystis carinii†	CD4+ cell count < 200/mm³ *or* Oropharyngeal candidiasis	TMP-SMX, 1 DS q.d. TMP-SMX, 1 SS q.d.	Dapsone, 50 mg b.i.d. or 100 mg q.d. Dapsone, 50 mg q.d. + pyrimethamine, 50 mg q. wk + leucovorin, 25 mg q. wk Dapsone, 200 mg + pyrimethamine, 75 mg + leucovorin, 25 mg q. wk. Aerosolized pentamidine, 300 mg q. mo via Respirgard II nebulizer Atovaquone, 1,500 mg q.d. TMP-SMX, 1 DS t.i.w.
Mycobacterium tuberculosis			
Isoniazid-sensitive‡	TST reaction ≥ 5 mm or previous positive TST result without treatment or contact with case of active tuberculosis	Isoniazid, 300 mg + pyridoxine, 50 mg q.d. × 9 mo Isoniazid, 900 mg + pyridoxine, 100 mg b.i.w. × 9 mo Rifampin, 600 mg + pyrazinamide, 20 mg/kg q.d. × 2 mo	Rifabutin, 300 mg q.d. + pyrazinamide, 20 mg/kg q.d. × 2 mo Rifampin, 600 mg q.d. × 4 mo
Isoniazid-resistant	Same; high probability of exposure to isoniazid-resistant tuberculosis	Rifampin, 600 mg + pyrazinamide, 20 mg/kg q.d. × 2 mo	Rifabutin, 300 mg q.d. + pyrazinamide, 20 mg/kg q.d. × 2 mo Rifampin, 600 mg q.d. × 4 mo Rifabutin, 300 mg q.d. × 4 mo
Multidrug (isoniazid and rifampin)-resistant	Same; high probability of exposure to multidrug-resistant tuberculosis	Choice of drugs requires consultation with public health authorities	None
Toxoplasma gondii§	IgG antibody to *Toxoplasma* and CD4+ cell count < 100/mm³	TMP-SMX, 1 DS q.d.	TMP-SMX, 1 SS q.d. Dapsone, 50 mg q.d. + pyrimethamine, 50 mg q. wk + leucovorin, 25 mg q. wk Atovaquone, 1,500 mg q.d. + pyrimethamine, 25 mg q.d. + leucovorin, 10 mg q.d.
Mycobacterium avium complex‖	CD4+ cell count < 50/mm³	Azithromycin, 1,200 mg q.d. Clarithromycin, 500 mg b.i.d.	Rifabutin, 300 mg q.d. Azithromycin, 1,200 mg q.w. + rifabutin, 300 mg q.d.
VZV	Significant exposure to chickenpox or shingles for patients who have no history of either condition or, if available, have negative antibody to VZV	Varicella-zoster immune globulin (VZIG), 5 vials (1.25 ml each) I.M., administered ≤ 96 hr after exposure, ideally within 48 hr	

*All regimens are oral unless indicated otherwise.

†Prophylaxis should also be considered for persons whose CD4+ cells constitute less than 14% of total lymphocytes, for persons with a history of an AIDS-defining illness, and possibly for those with CD4+ cell counts greater than 200 cells/mm³ but less than 250 cells/mm³. Patients receiving dapsone should be tested for glucose-6-phosphate dehydrogenase deficiency. A dosage of 50 mg q.d. is probably less effective than that of 100 mg q.d. Patients who are being given sulfadiazine-pyrimethamine for toxoplasmosis are protected against *Pneumocystis carinii* pneumonia and do not need additional prophylaxis against that illness.

‡It is recommended that patients receiving isoniazid, 900 mg b.i.w., remain under observation during therapy. Isoniazid regimens should include pyridoxine to prevent peripheral neuropathy. Rifampin should not be administered concurrently with protease inhibitors or nonnucleoside reverse transcriptase inhibitors. Rifabutin may be administered at a reduced dosage (150 mg q.d.) when combined with indinavir, nelfinavir, or amprenavir; at a reduced dosage (150 mg q.o.d. or 150 mg three times weekly) when combined with ritonavir; or at an increased dosage (450 mg q.d.) when combined with efavirenz. Information is lacking regarding coadministration of rifabutin with nevirapine. Exposure to multidrug-resistant tuberculosis might require prophylaxis with two drugs; public health authorities should be consulted. Possible regimens include pyrazinamide plus either ethambutol or a fluoroquinolone.

§Protection against toxoplasmosis is provided by trimethoprim-sulfamethoxazole, dapsone plus pyrimethamine, and possibly atovaquone.

‖As noted in the first footnote above, rifabutin may be administered at a reduced dosage when used in combination with the protease inhibitors indinavir (rifabutin dosage, 150 mg q.d.), nelfinavir (150 mg q.d.), amprenavir (150 mg q.d.), and ritonavir (150 mg q.o.d. or 150 mg three times weekly). It may be administered at an increased dosage with the nonnucleoside reverse transcriptase inhibitor efavirenz (rifabutin dosage, 450 mg q.d.). Information is lacking regarding coadministration of rifabutin with nevirapine.

DS—double-strength tablet SS—single-strength tablet TMP-SMX— trimethoprim-sulfamethoxazole TST—tuberculin skin test VZV—varicella-zoster virus

Table 9 Treatment of Acute Opportunistic Infections

Pathogen	*First Choice**	*Alternatives**	*Comment*
Cryptococcal meningitis	Amphotericin B, 0.7–1.0 mg/kg/day I.V. ± flucytosine, 100 mg/kg/day p.o. × 14 days, followed by fluconazole, 400 mg/day for a minimum of 10 wk	Amphotericin B, 0.7–1.0 mg/kg/day I.V. *or* Fluconazole, 800 mg/day I.V. or p.o. ± flucytosine, 100 mg/kg/day p.o.	Amphotericin is preferred as initial therapy; fluconazole is reasonable as initial therapy only in persons with normal mental status; management of increased intracranial pressure is essential; lumbar punctures should be performed to keep CSF pressure < 200 mm Hg
Cytomegalovirus retinitis	Ganciclovir, 5 mg/kg I.V., b.i.d. × 14–21 days, then 5–6 mg/kg/day I.V.	Foscarnet, 60 mg/kg q. 8 hr I.V. × 14–21 days, then 90–120 mg/kg/day Intraocular ganciclovir pellet + ganciclovir, 1,000 mg p.o. t.i.d. Cidofovir, 5 mg/kg I.V. q. wk × 2, then 5 mg/kg every 14 days	Ganciclovir is much easier to administer than foscarnet; intraocular ganciclovir pellets are very effective, but there is risk involved in administering them and they do not provide protection against disease outside the eye
Mycobacterium avium complex	Clarithromycin, 500 mg b.i.d. + ethambutol, 15 mg/kg/day ± rifabutin, 300 mg/day	Azithromycin, 600 mg q.d. can be substituted for clarithromycin Ciprofloxacin, 500 mg b.i.d. can be substituted for rifabutin	Benefit of adding third drug is unclear; clarithromycin and rifabutin can have significant interactions with antiretroviral medications
Mycobacterium tuberculosis	Isoniazid, 300 mg q.d. + rifampin, 600 mg q.d. + pyrazinamide, 25 mg/kg (maximum, 2 g) q.d. + ethambutol, 15–25 mg/kg (maximum, 2.5 g) q.d. × 9 mo	Rifabutin, 150–450 mg q.d. can be substituted for rifampin and the dose adjusted, depending on interaction	If the isolate is not drug resistant, then pyrazinamide and ethambutol should be discontinued after 2 mo; if the isolate is drug resistant, the regimen should be chosen in consultation with a tuberculosis expert
Pneumocystis carinii	Trimethoprim-sulfamethoxazole, 15–20 mg/kg/day, p.o. or I.V. in three or four divided doses × 21 days	Trimethoprim, 15–20 mg/kg/day in three or four divided doses + dapsone, 100 mg q.d. × 21 days Pentamidine, 3–4 mg/kg I.V. q.d. × 21 days Atovaquone, 750 mg q.d. × 21 days Clindamycin, 450 mg q.i.d. + primaquine, 15 mg base q.d. Trimetrexate, 45 mg/m² I.V. q.d. + folinic acid, 20 mg/m² q.i.d.	Patients with Po_2 < 70 mm Hg or A-a gradient > 35 mm Hg should receive corticosteroids (prednisone, 40 mg b.i.d. × 5 days, then 40 mg q.d. × 5 days, then 20 mg q.d. × 11 days); I.V. pentamidine has been associated with major toxicity
Toxoplasma gondii	Pyrimethamine, 100–200 mg loading dose, then 50–100 1.5–2.0 g q.i.d. + leucovorin, 10–25 mg q.d.	Clindamycin, 600–900 mg q.i.d., can substitute for sulfadiazine Other agents that could substitute for sulfadiazine include azithromycin, 1,200 mg q.d.; clarithromycin, 1.0 g b.i.d.; or atovaquone, 750 mg b.i.d.	After approximately 6–8 wk, patients can change to suppressive regimens that use lower dosages of medications

*All regimens are oral unless noted otherwise.
CSF — cerebrospinal fluid Po_2— oxygen tension

viously developed *P. carinii* pneumonia can discontinue secondary prophylaxis if they have a successful immunologic response to antiretroviral therapy (evidenced by a sustained $CD4^+$ T cell count of greater than 200 cells/mm^3).[88]

CNS Toxoplasmosis

CNS toxoplasmosis typically develops only in patients who have a $CD4^+$ T cell count of less than 100 cells/mm^3; it is characterized by fever, headache, altered thought processes, and, in some instances, seizures. The diagnosis is strengthened by serologic evidence of *Toxoplasma* and findings of multiple enhancing lesions on either computed tomography or magnetic resonance imaging. At 14 days, nearly all patients with *Toxoplasma* encephalitis will show some radiographic improvement in response to therapy. Brain biopsy is rarely performed at the onset of therapy but may be considered in patients who do not respond to therapy. First-line therapy consists of pyrimethamine plus sulfadiazine. There are insufficient data to recommend discontinuing secondary prophylaxis for toxoplasmosis in patients who have a successful immunologic response to antiretroviral therapy.

Cryptococcal Meningitis

Cryptococcal meningitis most often involves patients with a $CD4^+$ T cell count of less than 100 cells/mm^3; the clinical presentation may be very similar to that of *Toxoplasma* encephalitis. Fewer than 25% of patients with cryptococcal meningitis have overt symptoms of meningeal irritation, such as photophobia and neck stiffness. More typically, patients have fever, personality changes, and diminished memory. More than 98% of patients with cryptococcal meningitis have a positive result on serum cryptococcal antigen testing; the definitive diagnosis of cryptococcal meningitis is made by isolating *C. neoformans* from CSF. Recent guidelines have recommended amphotericin B plus flucytosine as initial therapy for the first 14 days, followed by high-dose fluconazole for a minimum of 10 weeks, followed by lower-dose fluconazole.[89] A pretreatment opening CSF pressure of 250 mm H_2O or greater is generally associated with a higher titer of cerebrospinal cryptococcal antigen, increased abnormal focal neurologic findings, and decreased survival.[90] In addition, outcomes are worse among persons whose CSF pressure increases by at least 10 mm H_2O after therapy is started. Accordingly, CSF opening pressure should be measured in all patients with suspected cryptococcal meningitis; those patients whose CSF opening pressure is 250 mm H_2O or greater should undergo large-volume CSF drainage by lumbar puncture. Such drainage should be repeated as often as necessary.

Disseminated Mycobacterium avium *Complex Infection*

Disseminated *M. avium* complex infection is a frequent complication in patients who have a $CD4^+$ T cell count of less than 50 cells/mm^3. This disease is characterized by vague constitutional symptoms, such as fever, night sweats, fatigue, weight loss, abdominal pain, and diarrhea. The preferred method of diagnosis is blood culture, which has a sensitivity of at least 90%; detection of positive growth, however, often takes longer than 7 days. Empirical therapy should generally be discouraged. Therapy for disseminated *M. avium* complex infection consists of clarithromycin (or azithromycin) plus ethambutol; many experts recommend adding either a fluoroquinolone or rifabutin as a third medication, particularly for the first 2 to 3 months of initial therapy.

Cytomegalovirus Retinitis

Cytomegalovirus infection is another common opportunistic infection in patients who have a $CD4^+$ T cell count of less than 50 cells/mm^3. Cytomegalovirus most often causes a retinitis that generates visual symptoms such as floaters, flashing lights, or visual field deficits. The diagnosis is established by characteristic findings on ophthalmologic examination; in general, the patient should be referred to an ophthalmologist for diagnosis. Prompt diagnosis and prompt initiation of therapy are essential to minimize permanent visual loss. Initial therapy should consist of an induction course of either intravenous ganciclovir or intravenous foscarnet, followed by long-term maintenance therapy. Most clinicians prefer ganciclovir as initial therapy because it has fewer adverse effects than foscarnet. Newer therapies include long-term suppression with oral ganciclovir, oral valganciclovir (a ganciclovir prodrug), and implantation of ganciclovir pellets in the affected eye. Cytomegalovirus infection can also occur in the upper or lower gastrointestinal tract, as well as the CNS.

Prevention of Recurrent Disease

The U.S. Public Health Service guidelines include recommendations for preventing recurrent disease after patients have received therapy for acute disease [*see Table 10*]. For patients who have

Table 10 USPHS/IDSA Guidelines for the Prevention of Recurrence of Opportunistic Infections in Adults and Adolescents Infected with HIV after Chemotherapy for Acute Disease[83]

Pathogen or Condition	*Indication*	*First Choice*	*Alternatives*
Cryptococcus neoformans	Documented disease	Fluconazole, 200 mg p.o., q.d.	Amphotericin B, 0.6 mg/kg I.V., q.w. to t.i.w. Itraconazole, 200 mg p.o., q.d.
Cytomegalovirus retinitis	Prior end-organ disease	Ganciclovir, 5–6 mg/kg/day I.V., 5–7 days/wk Ganciclovir, 1,000 mg t.i.d. Foscarnet, 90–120 mg/kg I.V., q.d. For retinitis, sustained-release intraocular ganciclovir pellet, q. 6–9 mo + ganciclovir, 1,000 mg t.i.d.	Cidofovir, 5 mg/kg I.V. every 14 days Fomivirsen, 1 vial (330 µg) injected into the vitreous, then repeated every 2–4 wk
Pneumocystis carinii	Prior *Pneumocystis carinii* pneumonia	TMP-SMX, 1 DS p.o., q.d. TMP-SMX, 1 SS p.o., q.d.	Dapsone, 50 mg b.i.d. or 100 mg q.d. Dapsone, 50 mg q.d. + pyrimethamine, 50 mg q.w. + leucovorin, 25 mg q.w. Dapsone, 200 mg + pyrimethamine, 75 mg + leucovorin, 25 mg q.w. Aerosolized pentamidine, 300 mg q. mo via Respirgard II nebulizer Atovaquone, 1,500 mg q.d. TMP-SMX, 1 DS t.i.w.
Toxoplasma gondii	Prior *Toxoplasma* encephalitis	Pyrimethamine, 25–75 mg q.d. + sulfadiazine, 0.5–1.0 g q.i.d. + leucovorin, 10–25 mg q.d.	Pyrimethamine, 25–75 mg q.d. + clindamycin, 300–450 mg q.i.d. + leucovorin, 10–25 mg q.d. Atovaquone, 750 mg b.i.d. to q.i.d. ± pyrimethamine, 25 mg q.d. + leucovorin, 10 mg q.d.

DS — double-strength tablet IDSA — Infectious Diseases Society of America SS— single-strength tablet TMP-SMX — trimethoprim-sulfamethoxazole USPHS — U.S. Public Health Service

had either toxoplasmosis, cryptococcal meningitis, disseminated *M. avium* complex disease, or cytomegalovirus retinitis, data are insufficient for recommending discontinuance of treatment of these opportunistic infections when the patient has excellent sustained virologic and immunologic responses to antiretroviral therapy.

Additional Resources

As the field of HIV and AIDS continues to change at a very rapid pace, clinicians need easy access to updated material. The resources available in the current electronic era are outstanding, but they are often overwhelming. Several excellent Web sites that provide up-to-date information on treatment guidelines, conference summaries, drug-safety warnings, and summaries of articles are listed [see Sidebar Internet Resources for Information on HIV and AIDS]. In addition, national consultation services provide expert clinical advice

Internet Resources for Information on HIV and AIDS

The AIDS Education and Training Centers (AETC) National Resource Center (NRC)
http://www.aids-ed.org/

HIV Treatment Guidelines
http://www.hivatis.org

Johns Hopkins AIDS Service
http://www.hopkins-aids.edu

UCSF: HIV Insite
http://hivinsite.ucsf.edu

Journal of the American Medical Association (JAMA)
http://www.ama-assn.org/special/hiv

Medscape (Infectious Diseases)
http://www.medscape.com/infectiousdiseases home

The 8th Conference on Retroviruses and Opportunistic Infections
http://www.retroconference.org

The Body
http://www.thebody.com

HIV/AIDS Telephone Consultation Services

WARMLINE

National HIV Telephone Consultation Service

Available from 7:30 AM to 5:00 PM PST; detailed information on the service can be obtained at the following URL: http://www.ucsf.edu/warmline/warmline.html

Telephone: 1-800-933-3413

PEPline

National Clinicians' Post-Exposure Prophylaxis Hotline

Available 24 hrs; detailed information on the service can be obtained at the following URL: http://pepline.ucsf.edu/pepline

Telephone: 1-888-448-4911

and state-of-the-art information [see Sidebar HIV/AIDS Telephone Consultation Services]. These Internet and telephone resources can provide critical information to help practicing clinicians optimally manage their HIV-infected patients.

The author is a consultant for Agouron Pharmaceuticals, Inc., Glaxo Wellcome, Inc., and Merck & Co., Inc., and has received honoraria from Agouron Pharmaceuticals, Inc., Bristol-Myers Squibb Company, Glaxo Wellcome, Inc., Merck & Co., Inc., and Roche Pharmaceuticals.

Acknowledgments

Figures 1, 7, 8, 9, 11, 12 Marcia Kammerer.
Figures 2, 3, 4, 5, 6, 10 Seward Hung.

References

1. National Center for HIV, STD and TB Prevention: HIV/AIDS Surveillance Report. Vol. 12:No. 1. Centers for Disease Control and Prevention. Atlanta, 2000

2. Palella FJ, Delaney KM, Moorman AC, et al: Declining morbidity and mortality among patients with advanced human immunodeficiency virus infection. HIV Outpatient Study Investigators. N Engl J Med 338:853, 1998

3. Gao F, Bailes E, Robertson DL, et al: Origin of HIV-1 in the chimpanzee *Pan troglodytes troglodytes.* Nature 397:436, 1999

4. Hirsch VM, Olmsted RA, Murphey-Corb M, et al: An African primate lentivirus (SIVsm) closely related to HIV-2. Nature 339:389, 1989

5. Zhu T, Korber BT, Nahmias AJ, et al: An African HIV-1 sequence from 1959 and implications for the origin of the epidemic. Nature 391: 594, 1998

6. Korber B, Muldoon M, Theiler J, et al: Timing the ancestor of the HIV-1 pandemic strains. Science 288:1789, 2000

7. Dickson D: Tests fail to support claims for origin of AIDS in polio vaccine. Nature 407:117, 2000

8. 1993 revised classification system for HIV infection and expanded surveillance case definition for AIDS among adolescents and adults. MMWR Morb Mortal Wkly Rep 41(RR-17):1, 1992

9. Pisani E, Schwartlander B, Cherney S, et al: AIDS epidemic update: December 2000. Joint United Nations Programme on HIV/AIDS (UNAIDS). Geneva, 2000

10. Royce RA, Sena A, Cates W, et al: Sexual transmission of HIV. N Engl J Med 336:1072, 1997

11. Mehendale SM, Rodrigues JJ, Brookmeyer RS, et al: Incidence and predictors of human immunodeficiency virus type 1 seroconversion in patients attending sexually transmitted disease clinics in India. J Infect Dis 172:1486, 1995

12. Quinn TC, Wawer MJ, Sewankambo N, et al: Viral load and heterosexual transmission of human immunodeficiency virus type 1. Rakai Project Study Group. N Engl J Med 342:921, 2000

13. de Vincenzi I: A longitudinal study of human immunodeficiency virus transmission by heterosexual partners. European Study Group on Heterosexual Transmission of HIV. N Engl J Med 331:341, 1994

14. Lifson AR, O'Malley PM, Hessol NA, et al: HIV seroconversion in two homosexual men after receptive oral intercourse with ejaculation: implications for counseling concerning safe sexual practices. Am J Public Health 80:1509, 1990

15. Schacker T, Collier AC, Hughes J, et al: Clinical and epidemiologic features of primary HIV infection. Ann Intern Med 125:257, 1996

16. Frankel SS, Wenig BM, Burke AP, et al: Replication of HIV-1 in dendritic cell-derived syncytia at the mucosal surface of the adenoid. Science 272:115, 1996

17. Vlahov D, Junge B: The role of needle exchange programs in HIV prevention. Public Health Rep 113(suppl 1):75, 1998

18. Lackritz EM, Satten GA, Aberle-Grasse J, et al: Estimated risk of transmission of the human immunodeficiency virus by screened blood in the United States. N Engl J Med 333:1721, 1995

19. Katzenstein TL, Dickmeiss E, Aladdin H, et al: Failure to develop HIV infection after receipt of HIV-contaminated blood and postexposure prophylaxis. Ann Intern Med 133:31, 2000

20. Connor EM, Sperling RS, Gelber R, et al: Reduction of maternal-infant transmission of human immunodeficiency virus type 1 with zidovudine treatment. Pediatric AIDS Clinical Trials Group Protocol 076 Study Group. N Engl J Med 331:1173, 1994

21. Garcia PM, Kalish LA, Pitt J, et al: Maternal levels of plasma human immunodeficiency virus type 1 RNA and the risk of perinatal transmission. Women and Infants Transmission Study Group. N Engl J Med 341:394, 1999

22. Mofenson LM, Lambert JS, Stiehm ER, et al: Risk factors for perinatal transmission of human immunodeficiency virus type 1 in women treated with zidovudine. Pediatric AIDS Clinical Trials Group Study 185 Team. N Engl J Med 341:385, 1999

23. The mode of delivery and the risk of vertical transmission of human immunodeficiency virus type 1: a meta-analysis of 15 prospective cohort studies. The International Perinatal HIV Group. N Engl J Med 340:977, 1999

24. John GC, Nduati RW, Mbori-Ngacha DA, et al: Correlates of mother-to-child human immunodeficiency virus type 1 (HIV-1) transmission: association with maternal plasma HIV-1 RNA load, genital HIV-1 DNA shedding, and breast infections. J Infect Dis 183:206, 2001

25. U.S. Public Health Service: Public Health Service Task Force Recommendations for Use of Antiretroviral Drugs in Pregnant HIV-1–Infected Women for Maternal Health and Interventions to Reduce Perinatal HIV-1 Transmission in the United States. Public Health Service and the Perinatal HIV Guidelines Working Group. U.S. Department of Health and Human Services, Hyattsville, Maryland, May, 2001. http://www.hivatis.org/trtgdlns.html#Perinatal

26. Embree JE, Njenga S, Datta P, et al: Risk factors for postnatal mother-child transmission of HIV-1. AIDS 14:2535, 2000

27. Updated U.S. Public Health Service Guidelines for the Management of Health-Care Personnel (HCP) Who Have Occupational Exposure to HBV, HCV, and HIV and Recommendations for Postexposure Prophylaxis. Centers for Disease Control and Prevention MMWR Morb Mortal Wkly Rep 50(RR-11):1, 2000

28. Greene WC: AIDS and the immune system. Sci Am 269:98, 1993

29. Sharp P, Robertson D, Gao F, et al: Origins and diversity of human immunodeficiency viruses. AIDS 265:1193, 1994

30. Koot M, Keet IP, Vos AH, et al: Prognostic value of HIV-1 syncytium-inducing phenotype for rate of CD4+ cell depletion and progression to AIDS. Ann Intern Med 118:681, 1993

31. Kinter A, Arthos J, Cicala C, et al: Chemokines, cytokines and HIV: a complex network of interactions that influence HIV pathogenesis. Immunol Rev 177:88, 2000

32. O'Brien SJ, Moore JP: The effect of genetic variation in chemokines and their receptors on HIV transmission and progression to AIDS. Immunol Rev 177:99, 2000

33. Mellors JW, Rinaldo CR, Gupta P, et al: Prognosis in HIV-1 infection predicted by the quantity of virus in plasma. Science 272:1167, 1996

34. Walker BD, Goulder PJ: AIDS: escape from the immune system. Nature 407:313, 2000

35. Alexander L, Weiskopf E, Greenough TC, et al: Unusual polymorphisms in human immunodeficiency virus type 1 associated with nonprogressive infection. J Virol 74:4361, 2000

36. Learmont JC, Geczy AF, Mills J, et al: Immunologic and virologic status after 14 to 18 years of infection with an attenuated strain of HIV-1: a report from the Sydney Blood Bank Cohort. N Engl J Med 340:1715, 1999

37. Kahn JO, Walker BD: Acute human immunodeficiency virus type 1 infection. N Engl J Med 339:33, 1998

38. Niu MT, Jermano JA, Reichelderfer P, et al: Summary of the National Institutes of Health workshop on primary human immunodeficiency virus type 1 infection. AIDS Res Hum Retroviruses 9:913, 1993

39. Busch MP, Lee LL, Satten GA, et al: Time course of detection of viral and serologic markers preceding human immunodeficiency virus type 1 seroconversion: implications for screening of blood and tissue donors. Transfusion 35:91, 1995

40. Kinloch-De Loes S, Hirschel BJ, Hoen B, et al: A controlled trial of zidovudine in primary human immunodeficiency virus infection. N Engl J Med 333:408, 1995

41. Rosenberg ES, Billingsley JM, Caliendo AM, et al: Vigorous HIV-1–specific CD4+ T cell responses associated with control of viremia. Science 278:1447, 1997

42. Fauci AS, Bartlett J, Goosby E, et al: Guidelines for the Use of Antiretroviral Agents in HIV-Infected Adults and Adolescents. Department of Health and Human Services and the Henry J. Kaiser Family Foundation, San Francisco, 2001. http//www.hivatis.org

43. Paredes R, Puig T, Arno A, et al: High-dose saquinavir plus ritonavir: long-term efficacy in HIV-positive protease inhibitor–experienced patients and predictors of virologic response. J Acquir Immune Defic Syndr 22:132, 1999

44. Carpenter CC, Cooper DA, Fischl MA, et al: Antiretroviral therapy in adults: updated recommendations of the International AIDS Society—USA Panel. JAMA 283:381, 2000

45. Carr A, Cooper DA: Adverse effects of antiretroviral therapy. Lancet 356:1423, 2000

46. Brinkman K: Editorial response: hyperlactatemia and hepatic steatosis as features of mitochondrial toxicity of nucleoside analogue reverse transcriptase inhibitors. Clin Infect Dis 31:167, 2000

47. Carr A, Samaras K, Burton S, et al: A syndrome of peripheral lipodystrophy, hyperlipidaemia and insulin resistance in patients receiving HIV protease inhibitors. AIDS 12:F51, 1998

48. Carr A, Samaras K, Thorisdottir A, et al: Diagnosis, prediction, and natural course of HIV-1 protease-inhibitor–associated lipodystrophy, hyperlipidaemia, and diabetes mellitus: a cohort study. Lancet 353:2093, 1999

49. Periard D, Telenti A, Sudre P, et al: Atherogenic dyslipidemia in HIV-infected individuals treated with protease inhibitors. The Swiss HIV Cohort Study. Circulation 100:700, 1999

50. Dube MP, Sprecher D, Henry WK, et al: Preliminary guidelines for the evaluation and management of dyslipidemia in adults infected with human immunodeficiency virus and receiving antiretroviral therapy: recommendations of the Adult AIDS Clinical Trial Group Cardiovascular Disease Focus Group. Clin Infect Dis 31:1216, 2000

51. Henry K, Melroe H, Huebesch J, et al: Atorvastatin and gemfibrozil for protease-inhibitor–related lipid abnormalities. Lancet 352:1031, 1998

52. Tsiodras S, Mantzoros C, Hammer S, et al: Effects of protease inhibitors on hyperglycemia, hyperlipidemia, and lipodystrophy: a 5-year cohort study. Arch Intern Med 160:2050, 2000

53. Carr A, Miller J, Law M, et al: A syndrome of lipoatrophy, lactic acidaemia and liver dysfunction associated with HIV nucleoside analogue therapy: contribution to protease inhibitor–related lipodystrophy syndrome. AIDS 14:F25, 2000

54. Hadigan C, Corcoran C, Basgoz N, et al: Metformin in the treatment of HIV lipodystrophy syndrome: a randomized controlled trial. JAMA 284:472, 2000

55. Pierson T, McArthur J, Siliciano RF: Reservoirs for HIV-1: mechanisms for viral persistence in the presence of antiviral immune responses and antiretroviral therapy. Annu Rev Immunol 18:665, 2000

56. Paterson DL, Swindells S, Mohr , et al: Adherence to protease inhibitor therapy and outcomes in patients with HIV infection. Ann Intern Med 133:21, 2000

57. Baxter JD, Mayers DL, Wentworth DN, et al: A randomized study of antiretroviral management based on plasma genotypic antiretroviral resistance testing in patients failing therapy. CPCRA 046 Study Team for the Terry Beirn Community Programs for Clinical Research on AIDS. AIDS 14:F83, 2000

58. Durant J, Clevenbergh P, Halfon P, et al: Drug-resistance genotyping in HIV-1 therapy: the VIRADAPT randomised controlled trial. Lancet 353:2195, 1999

59. Boden D, Hurley A, Zhang L, et al: HIV-1 drug resistance in newly infected individuals. JAMA 282:1135, 1999

60. Hecht FM, Grant RM, Petropoulos CJ, et al: Sexual transmission of an HIV-1 variant resistant to multiple reverse-transcriptase and protease inhibitors. N Engl J Med 339:307, 1998

61. Little SJ, Daar ES, D'Aquila RT, et al: Reduced antiretroviral drug susceptibility among patients with primary HIV infection. JAMA 282: 1142, 1999

62. Neumann AU, Tubiana R, Calvez V, et al: HIV-1 rebound during interruption of highly active antiretroviral therapy has no deleterious effect on reinitiated treatment. Comet Study Group. AIDS 13:677, 1999

63. Yang OO, Kalams SA, Trocha A, et al: Suppression of human immunodeficiency virus type 1 replication by CD8+ cells: evidence for HLA class I–restricted triggering of cytolytic and noncytolytic mechanisms. J Virol 71:3120, 1997

64. Kalams SA, Goulder PJ, Shea AK, et al: Levels of human immunodeficiency virus type 1–specific cytotoxic T-lymphocyte effector and memory responses decline after suppression of viremia with highly active antiretroviral therapy. J Virol 73:6721, 1999

65. Orenstein JM, Bhat N, Yoder C, et al: Rapid activation of lymph nodes and mononuclear cell HIV expression upon interrupting highly active antiretroviral therapy in patients after prolonged viral suppression. AIDS 14:1709, 2000

66. Colven R, Harrington RD, Spach DH, et al: Retroviral rebound syndrome after cessation of suppressive antiretroviral therapy in three patients with chronic HIV infection. Ann Intern Med 133:430, 2000

67. Kilby JM, Goepfert PA, Miller AP, et al: Recurrence of the acute HIV syndrome after interruption of antiretroviral therapy in a patient with chronic HIV infection: a case report. Ann Intern Med 133:435, 2000

68. Lisziewicz J, Rosenberg E, Lieberman J, et al: Control of HIV despite the discontinuation of antiretroviral therapy. N Engl J Med 340: 1683, 1999

69. Rosenberg ES, Altfeld M, Poon SH, et al: Immune control of HIV-1 after early treatment of acute infection. Nature 407:523, 2000

70. Lori F, Lewis MG, Xu J, et al: Control of SIV rebound through structured treatment interruptions during early infection. Science 290: 1591, 2000

71. Cardo DM, Culver DH, Ciesielski CA, et al: A case-control study of HIV seroconversion in health care workers after percutaneous exposure. Centers for Disease Control and Prevention Needlestick Surveillance Group. N Engl J Med 337:1485, 1997

72. Serious adverse events attributed to nevirapine regimens for postexposure prophylaxis after HIV exposures—worldwide, 1997-2000. MMWR Morb Mortal Wkly Rep 49:1153, 2001

73. Parkin JM, Murphy M, Anderson J, et al: Tolerability and side-effects of post-exposure prophylaxis for HIV infection. Lancet 355:722, 2000

74. Sperling RS, Shapiro DE, Coombs RW, et al: Maternal viral load, zidovudine treatment, and the risk of transmission of human immunodeficiency virus type 1 from mother to infant. Pediatric AIDS Clinical Trials Group Protocol 076 Study Group. N Engl J Med 335:1621, 1996

75. Shaffer N, Chuachoowong R, Mock PA, et al: Short-course zidovudine for perinatal HIV-1 transmission in Bangkok, Thailand: a randomised controlled trial. Bangkok Collaborative Perinatal HIV Transmission Study Group. Lancet 353:773, 1999

76. Guay LA, Musoke P, Fleming T, et al: Intrapartum and neonatal single-dose nevirapine compared with zidovudine for prevention of mother-to-child transmission of HIV-1 in Kampala, Uganda: HIVNET 012 randomised trial. Lancet 354:795, 1999

77. Jackson JB, Becker-Pergola G, Guay LA, et al: Identification of the K103N resistance mutation in Ugandan women receiving nevirapine to prevent HIV-1 vertical transmission. AIDS 14:F111, 2000

78. Kahn JO, Cherng DW, Mayer K, et al: Evaluation of HIV-1 immunogen, an immunologic modifier, administered to patients infected with HIV having 300 to 549 × 10(6)/L CD4 cell counts: a randomized controlled trial. JAMA 284:2193, 2000

79. Kahn J: Building and testing an effective HIV vaccine. West J Med 171:363, 1999

80. Letvin NL: Progress in the development of an HIV-1 vaccine. Science 280:1875, 1998

81. Kaplan JE, Hanson D, Dworkin MS, et al: Epidemiology of human immunodeficiency virus–associated opportunistic infections in the United States in the era of highly active antiretroviral therapy. Clin Infect Dis 30(suppl 1):S5, 2000

82. Jones JL, Hanson DL, Dworkin MS, et al: Incidence and trends in Kaposi's sarcoma in the era of effective antiretroviral therapy. J Acquir Immune Defic Syndr 24:270, 2000

83. 1999 USPHS/IDSA guidelines for the prevention of opportunistic infections in persons infected with human immunodeficiency virus. U.S. Public Health Service (USPHS) and Infectious Diseases Society of America (IDSA). MMWR Morb Mortal Wkly Rep 48:1, 1999

84. Furrer H, Egger M, Opravil M, et al: Discontinuation of primary prophylaxis against *Pneumocystis carinii* pneumonia in HIV-1–infected adults treated with combination antiretroviral therapy. Swiss HIV Cohort Study. N Engl J Med 340:1301, 1999

85. Currier JS, Williams PL, Koletar SL, et al: Discontinuation of *Mycobacterium avium* complex prophylaxis in patients with antiretroviral therapy–induced increases in $CD4^+$ cell count: a randomized, double-blind, placebo-controlled trial. AIDS Clinical Trials Group 362 Study Team. Ann Intern Med 133:493, 2000

86. Furrer H, Opravil M, Bernasconi E, et al: Stopping primary prophylaxis in HIV-1–infected patients at high risk of *Toxoplasma* encephalitis. Swiss HIV Cohort Study. Lancet 355:2217, 2000

87. Mussini C, Pezzotti P, Govoni A, et al: Discontinuation of primary prophylaxis for *Pneumocystis carinii* pneumonia and toxoplasmic encephalitis in human immunodeficiency virus type I–infected patients: the changes in opportunistic prophylaxis study. J Infect Dis 181:1635, 2000

88. Ledergerber B, Mocroft A, Reiss P, et al: Discontinuation of secondary prophylaxis against *Pneumocystis carinii* pneumonia in patients with HIV infection who have a response to antiretroviral therapy. Eight European Study Groups. N Engl J Med 344:168, 2001

89. Saag MS, Graybill RJ, Larsen RA, et al: Practice guidelines for the management of cryptococcal disease. Infectious Diseases Society of America. Clin Infect Dis 30:710, 2000

90. Graybill JR, Sobel J, Saag M, et al: Diagnosis and management of increased intracranial pressure in patients with AIDS and cryptococcal meningitis. The NIAID Mycoses Study Group and AIDS Cooperative Treatment Groups. Clin Infect Dis 30:47, 2000

15 Infections Due to Gram-Positive Cocci

Harvey B. Simon, M.D.

Pneumococci

Pneumococci are gram-positive organisms that typically appear as lancet-shaped diplococci but may also grow in short chains. When cultured on blood agar plates, they form small, colorless, mucoid colonies with characteristic central depressions. The colonies are surrounded by greenish discoloration of the blood agar, termed α-hemolysis. Laboratories have traditionally identified pneumococci on the basis of sensitivity to surface-active agents such as bile or Optochin; rapid speciation can now be accomplished with a latex agglutination test or a DNA probe.

Although there is only one species of *Streptococcus pneumoniae*, there are 84 distinct serotypes, which are differentiated by the composition of the polysaccharide polymer that forms their outer capsule. Each capsular type is chemically and antigenically unique. The pneumococcal polysaccharide capsule is crucial to virulence. The capsule allows the bacteria to resist phagocytosis by leukocytes unless the organisms have been opsonized by antibody or serum complement components. Antibodies to capsular polysaccharide are essential for recovery from untreated pneumococcal pneumonia. Although such antibodies provide long-lasting immunity, the immunity is strictly type specific. Certain pneumococcal serotypes are particularly virulent; the very heavily encapsulated type 3 pneumococci are perhaps the most virulent. In fact, only 23 serotypes account for about 80% of bacteremic pneumococcal infections in the United States; capsular polysaccharides from these 23 serotypes are incorporated into the polyvalent pneumococcal vaccine that has been available since 1983.

Although the polysaccharide capsule is the critical factor in determining the virulence of pneumococci, several proteins also contribute to the pathogenesis of pneumococcal infections. Surface protein A, neuraminidase, pneumolysin, and IgA protease appear to be the most important of these proteins.[1]

EPIDEMIOLOGY OF PNEUMOCOCCAL INFECTIONS

The nasopharynx is the natural habitat of the pneumococcus; humans are the only known hosts. The nasopharyngeal carrier rate varies widely, from a low of 5% to 10% to a high of up to 60% in closed populations during the winter.[2] Pneumococci are fastidious, nonsporulating bacteria. Because they are rapidly killed by drying or by extremes in temperature, person-to-person spread by droplets requires close contact.

The incidence of infection is not fully determined. The pneumococcus remains the most important cause of bacterial pneumonia; it may account for as many as 500,000 cases each year in the United States. Like other respiratory tract infections, pneumococcal pneumonia is more common in winter. Cigarette smoking is the strongest independent risk factor for invasive pneumococcal disease in immunocompetent, nonelderly adults.[3] Other patients at increased risk include those with cirrhosis, sickle cell anemia, multiple myeloma, chronic lung disease, or cancer. Organ transplantation recipients are also highly susceptible. The pneumococcus accounts for up to 40% of community-acquired pneumonias,[4] causing or contributing to 40,000 deaths annually. The overall case-fatality rate of this pneumonia is 5% to 12%[5]; patients who are very young or elderly, alcoholic, leukopenic, infected with HIV, or infected with certain virulent pneumococcus serotypes (notably type 3) are at the highest risk. Pneumococcal bacteremia develops in about 50,000 Americans annually, with a case-fatality rate of 20%[6]—a figure that has not changed over the past 40 years. Pneumococcal otitis media is one of the most common childhood illnesses; the estimated incidence in the United States is seven million cases a year. Pneumococci cause about 3,000 meningitis cases each year, with a case-fatality rate of about 21%.[7]

Epidemics of pneumococcal disease were common in the preantibiotic era, but sporadic cases are now the rule. Outbreaks have occurred, however, in shelters for the homeless, in jails, and in child care centers. Pneumococcal infection is typically community acquired, but it can occur nosocomially, particularly in chronically ill immunosuppressed patients; because of underlying diseases, the case-fatality rate of nosocomial pneumococcal bacteremia is 40%.[8] The incidence of pneumococcal bacteremia is increased about 40-fold in patients with AIDS.

PATHOGENESIS OF PNEUMOCOCCAL INFECTIONS

Pneumococci produce IgA protease, which cleaves the secretory immunoglobulin IgA1. IgA protease may be partly responsible for the high carrier rate and the respiratory tract pathogenicity of these bacteria. The organisms do not provoke an inflammatory response or cause clinical illness in the nasopharynx. Host defense mechanisms prevent penetration into more vulnerable areas, such as the paranasal sinuses, middle ear, and pulmonary alveoli. Examples of these defenses include the cough, gag, and sneeze reflexes; the viscous mucus lining the respiratory epithelium that traps bacteria; and ciliary action, which expels trapped particles. Pneumococcal infection often follows influenza[9] or other viral infection of the upper respiratory tract, which impair host defenses by increasing the volume and decreasing the viscosity of secretions. Other factors that predispose to pneumococcal infection include dementia, seizure disorders, alcoholism, stupor, and other conditions that increase the likelihood that oropharyngeal contents will be aspirated into the lungs. Air pollution, cigarette smoking, congestive heart failure, chronic obstructive lung disease, and HIV infection increase the risk of pneumococcal infection, but diabetes does not.

Once pneumococci arrive in the alveoli, a vigorous inflammatory response occurs. The earliest manifestations are vasodilatation, increased vascular permeability, and exudation of edema fluid—the classic pathologic stage of congestion. Pneumococci can survive and even proliferate in the edema fluid. The organisms appear to float to adjacent alveoli, producing lobar consolidation. Within hours to days, polymorphonuclear leukocytes arrive and progressively pack the alveoli to produce the traditional stages of red and gray hepatization. However, only a minority of the pneumococci are phagocytosed and killed by the leukocytes in the first days of infection. Capsular polysaccharide antigen is often present in the serum and urine during these early stages.

After 5 to 7 days, type-specific anticapsular antibody appears. As a result, a more efficient and enhanced opsonization that involves anticapsular antibody and the classical complement pathway occurs. As pneumococci are ingested and killed by the polymorphonuclear leukocytes, the patient experiences a clinical crisis marked by an abrupt fall in temperature and an increase in well-being; resolution commences. Because pneumococci only rarely produce significant tissue necrosis, healing is usually complete and residual fibrosis is minimal.

CLINICAL PNEUMOCOCCAL INFECTIONS

Pneumonia

Clinical presentation Sir William Osler's classic description of pneumococcal pneumonia was recorded in 1892,[10] only 10 years after the discovery of the pneumococcus, but it remains lucid and accurate today:

> Abruptly, or preceded by a day or two of indisposition, the patient has a severe chill, lasting from ten to thirty minutes. In no acute disease is an initial chill so constant or so severe. The fever rises quickly. There is pain in the side, often of an agonizing character. A short, dry painful cough soon develops and the respirations are increased in frequency. When seen on the second or third day the patient presents an appearance which may be quite pathognomonic. He lies flat in bed, often on the affected side; the face is flushed, particularly the cheeks; the breathing is hurried; the alae nasi dilate with every inspiration; the eyes are bright, the expression is anxious, and there is a frequent short cough which makes the patient wince and hold his side. The expectoration is blood-tinged and extremely tenacious. The temperature rises rapidly to 104° or 105°. The pulse is full and bounding and the pulse-respiration ratio much disturbed. Examination of the lung shows the physical signs of consolidation-blowing breathing and fine rales. After persisting for from seven to ten days the crisis occurs, and with a fall in the temperature the patient passes from a condition of extreme distress and anxiety to one of comparative comfort.
>
> Pneumonic sputum is viscid, tenacious, and blood-tinged. The gummous viscidity, together with the red blood-corpuscles in various stages of alteration, give pathognomonic characters to the sputa, unknown in any other disease. The rusty tinge becomes more marked as the disease progresses, and so tenacious is the expectoration that it has to be wiped from the lips of the patient, and a spitcup, half full, may be inverted without spilling. Microscopically, the sputum contains red blood-corpuscles in all stages of degeneration, alveolar epithelium, diplococci and other micro-organisms, cell-moulds of the alveoli, and, in some cases, small

fibrinous casts of the bronchioles. The latter are sometimes plainly visible to the naked eye.

It should be emphasized, however, that not all patients with pneumococcal pneumonia present with a viral upper respiratory tract infection followed by abrupt onset of fever, chills, pleurisy, dyspnea, and cough that is productive of purulent or blood-tinged sputum. If the patient has used antipyretics, fever can be modest or absent. The initial rigor may also be absent, but patients may occasionally have recurrent chills. In the elderly or debilitated patient, confusion or stupor may be the presenting feature, far overshadowing pulmonary symptoms. In contrast, patients with chronic pulmonary disease may have rapidly progressive respiratory failure, which is disproportionately more severe than fever, sputum production, or other manifestations of infection. In rare cases, asplenic patients present with shock and hemorrhagic skin lesions that reflect disseminated intravascular coagulation. Because modest hyperbilirubinemia is common in pneumococcal pneumonia, right lower lobe pneumonia may masquerade as acute cholecystitis because of fever, jaundice, and right upper quadrant discomfort.

Laboratory tests The key to the diagnosis of pneumococcal pneumonia is the Gram stain of a sputum smear, which typically reveals many polymorphonuclear leukocytes and abundant lancet-shaped gram-positive diplococci. If the patient cannot spontaneously produce an adequate sputum specimen, chest physiotherapy or nasotracheal suctioning should be considered. Sputum specimens should be promptly cultured on blood agar plates, preferably in 5% CO_2 incubators. Because pneumococci are fastidious and fragile, the sputum culture may be negative in patients with clearly positive Gram stains. It is important to obtain blood cultures in all patients with suspected pneumococcal pneumonia; 25% to 30% of these patients will have positive blood cultures, which confirms the diagnosis even if sputum cultures are negative. An immunochromatographic test can be used to detect pneumococcal polysaccharide in the urine of patients with pneumonia, but pneumococcal nasopharyngeal colonization can produce false positive results.[11]

Imaging tests The classic physical and radiographic findings of lobar consolidation may be absent in patients with pneumococcal pneumonia. In fact, a bronchopneumonic pattern is radiographically more common than lobar consolidation. Dehydration may minimize pulmonary findings, and underlying chronic lung disease may predispose to patchy areas of pulmonary infiltration. Pleural effusions are relatively common and can occasionally obscure the underlying pulmonary parenchymal involvement.

Differential diagnosis In the differential diagnosis, the other bacterial and nonbacterial pneumonias must be considered [see 6 Pulmonary Infections]. Less commonly, pulmonary edema, pulmonary emboli, atelectasis, or lung tumors can be mistaken for pneumonia.

Complications The complications associated with pneumococcal pneumonia have diminished markedly in the antibiotic era. Intrathoracic complications include pleurisy with sterile pleural effusion (common) and empyema (uncommon). Lung abscess is rare; if abscess or empyema occurs, it is likely to be caused by the heavily encapsulated type 3 pneumococcus or by a concomitant anaerobic infection. Purulent pericarditis is even rarer than abscess or empyema. Radiographic abnormalities often resolve slowly. About one third of patients have persistent consolidation at 1 month; although consolidation should resolve in all patients by 8 to 10 weeks, volume loss, pleural disease, and interstitial changes can persist for up to 4 months.

Bacteremia is by far the most common extrathoracic complication. Approximately 90% of patients with pneumococcal bacteremia have pneumonia, but patients occasionally present with pneumococcal bacteremias without an identifiable septic focus. Recurrent pneumococcal bacteremia may develop in patients with underlying diseases. Bacteremia is an adverse prognostic sign. The reported fatality rate is 11% to 36%, but it is probably higher in the elderly and in patients with severe underlying diseases. Metastatic infections such as meningitis, septic arthritis, peritonitis, and endocarditis are relatively uncommon; they appear to be more common and to occur at younger ages in African Americans than in whites.[12]

Pneumococcal Infections in Persons Infected with HIV

The pneumococcus is the leading cause of invasive bacterial respiratory tract infections in HIV-positive persons. The clinical features, causative serotypes, antimicrobial-resistance patterns, and mortalities of pneumococcal infection in HIV-positive patients are similar to those in HIV-negative patients. Severe infections, unusual extrapulmonary manifestations, and late relapses, however, are more common in these patients. Pneumococcal vaccine should be administered as soon as possible after the diagnosis of HIV infection[13]; despite the decreased efficacy of vaccine in patients with advanced AIDS, vaccination is a cost-effective preventive intervention at all stages of HIV infection.[14]

Other Pneumococcal Infections

Upper respiratory tract infections Pneumococci spread from the nasopharynx to the upper respiratory tract to produce acute otitis media, especially in children. Acute mastoiditis, once a frequent sequela of acute otitis media, is now unusual. Pneumococci are a cause of acute purulent sinusitis in all age groups [see 5 Bacterial Infections of the Upper Respiratory Tract].

Meningitis Pneumococci can reach the central nervous system either by bacteremic spread from a pulmonary focus or by direct extension from otitis or sinusitis. Patients with skull fractures and cerebrospinal fluid rhinorrhea or otorrhea are particularly prone to recurrent attacks of pneumococcal meningitis [see 13 Bacterial Infections of the Central Nervous System].

Septic arthritis and osteomyelitis Pneumococci are a relatively common cause of acute septic arthritis, which results from bacteremic seeding; prosthetic joints may be involved [see 11 Septic Arthritis]. Pneumococcal osteomyelitis is uncommon.

Cardiac infections Antibiotics have greatly reduced the incidence of pneumococcal pericarditis, which can result from direct extension from pneumonia or empyema or hematogenous seeding. Pneumococcal endocarditis has also become uncommon in the antibiotic era.[15]

Postsplenectomy infections Overwhelming postsplenectomy pneumococcal infection is an uncommon but important syndrome. Patients at risk include those with sickle cell disease or other hemoglobinopathies that produce functional asplenia, postsurgical splenectomy, and congenital asplenia. Patients often have acute onset of fever, hemorrhagic skin lesions suggestive of disseminated intravascular coagulation or purpura fulminans, and shock. Hypoglycemia may be present. If therapy is not administered, death often occurs in less than 24 hours. Even when patients receive penicillin and cardiovascular support, mortality exceeds 50%. A similar syndrome can occur in healthy adults but is rare.[16]

Other infections Primary pneumococcal peritonitis can occur in patients who have cirrhosis, nephrotic syndrome, systemic lupus erythematosus, or other host defects [see 8 Peritonitis and Intra-Abdominal Abscess]. In rare cases, pneumococci can infect the liver, gallbladder, or pelvic organs; soft tissue infections and cellulitis caused by *S. pneumoniae* are also unusual.

TREATMENT OF PNEUMOCOCCAL INFECTIONS

For many years, all isolates of *S. pneumoniae* were penicillin sensitive; until 1965, most isolates in the United States were sensitive to less than 0.04 μg/ml penicillin, and all had minimum inhibitory concentrations (MICs) of less than 0.1 μg/ml. Since then, however, resistance to penicillin has become progressively more prevalent. Although pneumococci do not display plasmid-mediated penicillinase production, they can develop chromosomal mutations that confer resistance to penicillin by altering the affinity of the penicillin-binding proteins present in their cell walls. Gradual remodeling of three or four of the penicillin-binding proteins in parallel produces a stepwise increase in the level of resistance. The DNA sequences responsible for resistance probably originated in other streptococcal species and were transferred to pneumococci by heterologous recombination.[16]

Pneumococci with penicillin MICs of less than 0.1 μg/ml are considered penicillin sensitive. Above this threshold, organisms are classified as nonsusceptible or resistant. Those with MICs of 0.1 to 1.0 μg/ml are considered intermediately resistant, and those with MICs of greater than 1.0 μg/ml are considered resistant. About 24% of pneumococcal organisms isolated in the United States are penicillin-nonsusceptible *S. pneumoniae* (PNSP), but in some areas, more than one third of isolated pneumococci are resistant to penicillin.[17] The prevalence of PNSP increases among patients who have been using antibiotics and is highest in children younger than 6 years and in adults older than 65 years. Resistant strains can be spread from person to person, especially in closed population groups, such as those in day care centers and nursing homes. Infection with PNSP is associated with an increased likelihood of an adverse outcome.[18]

Pneumococci that are resistant to penicillin are often resistant to other antimicrobial drugs.[17] First- and second-generation cephalosporins are generally ineffective against these organisms, but third-generation cephalosporins, particularly ceftriaxone and cefotaxime, and carbapenems are usually active. Erythromycin and the other macrolides are generally ineffective, as are clindamycin and trimethoprim-sulfamethoxazole (TMP-SMX); chloramphenicol has variable efficacy. Rifampin and vancomycin are active against virtually all isolates, but vancomycin tolerance has been identified and may become a concern in the future.[19] Whereas many pneumococci have become resistant to the older quinolones, such as ciprofloxacin,[20] the newer members of this group, such as levofloxacin, sparfloxacin, gatifloxacin, and moxifloxacin, are active against penicillin-resistant pneumococci. However, levofloxacin resistance has been documented, especially in elderly nursing home patients with chronic obstructive pulmonary disease (COPD) and prior exposure to fluoroquinolones.[20] Linizolide,[21] which received approval from the Food and Drug Administration in 2000, is active against nearly all pneumococci, as are quinupristin-dalfopristin and the still investigational antimicrobial ketolide.

Because of the increasing problem of PNSP, organisms isolated from clinical sources should be screened for penicillin resistance with a 1 µg oxacillin disk. Isolates with oxacillin zone sizes of less than 19 mm should be studied further to determine the MICs for penicillin and other antimicrobial agents that are likely to be used in treatment.

Guidelines for treatment of patients with PNSP are being formulated.[22] Ceftriaxone and cefotaxime are generally effective, but treatment failures in patients with meningitis have been reported. Until the results of susceptibility testing are available, it may be advisable to add vancomycin to the regimen of cefotaxime or ceftriaxone for patients with life-threatening pneumococcal infections such as meningitis. Vancomycin is an effective alternative for patients in whom treatment fails and for those who cannot tolerate cephalosporins; however, because of the limited CSF penetration of I.V. vancomycin in patients with pneumococcal meningitis, concurrent therapy with intrathecal vancomycin or I.V. rifampin may be advisable. Oral rifampin has been effective in eradicating PNSP from the nasopharynx of asymptomatic carriers. The role of imipenem or meropenem in treating patients with PNSP is being explored. The new fluoroquinolones (levofloxacin, sparfloxacin, gatifloxacin, and moxifloxacin) will probably prove extremely useful, as will linezolid. To limit the spread of PNSP, physicians should be advised against the inappropriate use of antibiotics and encouraged in the appropriate use of the pneumococcal vaccine.

Penicillin remains the drug of choice for susceptible pneumococci; cephalosporins are also active against such organisms but must be used with caution in patients allergic to penicillin. Other drugs that can be used to treat susceptible pneumococci include erythromycin and the new macrolides, clindamycin, vancomycin, and the newer quinolones. TMP-SMX is a particularly good choice for patients with sinusitis or otitis; chloramphenicol may be useful in treating meningitis caused by susceptible pneumococci in patients who cannot tolerate penicillin, third-generation cephalosporins, or meropenem. Patients with pneumococcal pneumonia can be switched from intravenous to oral antibiotics once they are clinically stable, even if bacteremia was present.[23]

PREVENTION OF PNEUMOCOCCAL INFECTIONS

A vaccine containing 50 mg of purified capsular polysaccharide from 14 pneumococcal types was approved by the FDA in 1977, and an expanded vaccine containing 25 µg of polysaccharide from 23 pneumococcal types was released in 1983. These 23 types account for the great majority of serious pneumococcal infections in the United States, including 88% of invasive infections with penicillin-resistant strains.[17] Because polysaccharide vaccines are not effective in children younger than 2 years, a protein-polysaccharide conjugate vaccine containing approximately 2 µg of polysaccharides from the seven most important strains was introduced for pediatric use in 2000.[24]

Pneumococcal vaccination produces serum antibody titers that are protective in healthy adults; although most elderly people mount an adequate serologic response, some produce low antibody titers or functionally deficient antibodies. Patients with Hodgkin disease respond better to vaccination before staging laparotomy and splenectomy; chemotherapy markedly impairs the response to vaccination and accelerates the decline in antibody titers. Dialysis and transplant patients[25] may respond to vaccination suboptimally, as do many patients with myeloma, lymphoma, leukemia, AIDS, and low serum vitamin B_{12} levels.

The pneumococcal vaccine is safe.[26] Mild erythema and pain at the injection site may occur in up to one third of vaccine recipients, but fever, severe local reactions, and other serious side effects occur in fewer than 1%.

Despite its immunogenicity and safety, the pneumococcal vaccine still remains controversial.

The reason for controversy is that the efficacy of the vaccine has been difficult to demonstrate in certain population groups. In general, the evidence for efficacy has been stronger for the prevention of invasive pneumococcal disease than for nonbacteremic pneumonias; the evidence is also stronger for the protection of low-risk persons than for the protection of elderly or debilitated patients.

Perhaps because of conflicting data, pneumococcal vaccine has not been well accepted, and only 35% of vaccine candidates have been immunized. Because of the expense of large-scale field trials, the controversy is unlikely to be resolved in the near future, and recommendations for vaccine use must be formulated from the current information. Because of its safety and modest cost, the pneumococcal vaccine is cost-effective, even in the elderly.[27] The vaccine is recommended for healthy adults older than 65 years and for patients with chronic cardiopulmonary disease, asplenia or splenic dysfunction, Hodgkin disease, multiple myeloma, cirrhosis, alcoholism, renal failure, CSF leaks, immunosuppression, or HIV infection. Members of certain vulnerable population groups, such as Native Americans, are also candidates for the vaccine, as are patients with functional or anatomic asplenia, sickle cell disease, nephrotic syndrome, CSF leaks, or immunosuppression. When possible, the vaccine should be administered 2 weeks before elective splenectomy or chemotherapy.

The pediatric conjugate vaccine is safe and effective[28] and is recommended for all infants as well as for children up to 60 months of age who are at increased risk for pneumococcal infection; vulnerable children older than 5 years should continue to receive the adult 23-valent vaccine.[22]

Although antibody titers wane,[29] routine revaccination is not recommended. Apart from local reactions, however, revaccination after 5 or more years is safe[30] and should be considered for adults who are at the highest risk for pneumococcal infection. The safety of the pneumococcal vaccine during pregnancy has not been evaluated; women who are at high risk for pneumococcal infection should be vaccinated before they become pregnant. The pneumococcal and influenza vaccines may be administered simultaneously at different sites when both are indicated.

Because of vaccine failures, additional strategies have been devised to protect vulnerable patients from pneumococcal infection. Long-term prophylaxis with orally administered low-dose penicillin protects children with sickle cell anemia from acquiring pneumococcal septicemia. It has also been recommended for young children with anatomic or functional asplenia. For asplenic adults, many physicians prefer vaccination with pneumococcal, meningococcal, and *Haemophilus influenzae* type b vaccines; these vaccines can be administered simultaneously. Vulnerable patients should be instructed to seek medical care at the first sign of infection and should be provided with ampicillin for self-administration if medical attention is not immediately available.

Additional work to enhance the efficacy of pneumococcal vaccines is needed. The development of a conjugated polysaccharide-protein vaccine for adults is particularly promising.

Streptococci

The streptococci, a large and diverse group of organisms widely distributed in nature, are part of the normal human flora. They vary in their pathogenic potential from many harmless species to a few very significant pathogens, such as *S. pneumoniae* and *S. pyogenes*.

Streptococci are gram-positive, round to ovoid cocci that can appear in pairs but more characteristically grow in chains of varying length. They are fastidious organisms requiring many nutrients. Although most are facultative anaerobes, some are obligate anaerobes. All species are nonmotile and nonsporulating and lack the enzyme catalase.

When grown on blood agar plates, most streptococci form small (1 to 2 mm), round, nonpigmented colonies. Streptococci are often characterized by changes in the appearance of the blood agar surrounding their colonies. Three types of reaction may occur: α-, β-, and γ-hemolysis. In α-hemolysis, green discoloration results from reduction of red blood cell hemoglobin and not from true hemolysis. In β-hemolysis, lysis of the red blood cells produces clearing of the blood agar, and in the γ reaction, there is no change in the agar. Hemolysis alone, however, cannot be used for classification, because biologically dissimilar species can cause identical hemolytic reactions.

A far superior classification is the serologic system. In 1933, Rebecca Lancefield demonstrated that an antigenic carbohydrate could be extracted from the cell wall of streptococci. On the basis of chemical composition and immunologic reactivity of this carbohydrate, streptococci can be divided into 18 groups (A through H and K through T). The species within each group tend to be biologically similar and to have a similar human pathogenic potential [*see Table 1*]. There are also

Table 1 Medically Important Streptococci and Enterococci

Streptococcus Group	*Representative Species*	*Hemolysis*	*Characteristics*	*Human Habitat*	*Human Diseases*
A	*S. pyogenes*	β (rarely γ)	Bacitracin sensitive; produces many extracellular enzymes and toxins	Nasopharynx Skin Rectum	Many diseases (*S. pyogenes* is the major human pathogen)
B	*S. agalactiae*	β (α, γ)	May be bacitracin sensitive; hydrolyzes sodium hippurate	Nasopharynx Genitourinary tract	Neonatal sepsis and meningitis Puerperal infections Urinary tract infections Endocarditis
C	*S. equi*	β (α, γ)	May be bacitracin sensitive; produces extracellular enzymes similar to those made by group A	Nasopharynx Genitourinary tract GI tract Skin	Skin and wound infections Bacteremias Endocarditis Pharyngitis
G	*S. canis*	β (α, γ)	Similar to group C	Similar to group C	Similar to group C
D	*S. bovis* *S. equinus*	β, γ (α)	Heat resistant; bile resistant; NaCl sensitive; penicillin sensitive	GI tract Genitourinary tract	Urinary tract infections Bacteremia Endocarditis
F	*S. anginosus*	β (α, γ)	Tiny colonies on blood agar; growth enhanced by 10% CO_2	Oropharynx GI tract Genitourinary tract	Sinusitis Meningitis Brain abscess Pneumonia Endocarditis
H	*S. sanguis*	α (β, γ)	Bile resistant	Oropharynx GI tract	
K	*S. salivarius*	γ (α)	Can grow at 45° C	Oropharynx	
Nongroupable	Viridans streptococci, including *S. mitis*, *S. mutans*, and others	α	No group-specific carbohydrate antigen yet recognized	Oropharynx	Endocarditis
Anaerobic streptococci	Many, including the peptostreptococci	γ (β, α)	Obligate anaerobes; tiny colonies on blood agar; no group-specific carbohydrate	Oropharynx GI tract Genitourinary tract	Sinusitis Pneumonia Lung abscess Empyema Brain abscess Soft tissue infections Bone and joint infections
Enterococci	*Enterococcus faecalis* *E. faecium*	β, γ (α)	Heat resistant; bile resistant; 6.5% NaCl resistant; penicillin resistant	GI tract Genitourinary tract	Endocarditis Peritonitis Urinary tract infections Wound infections

separately classified nongroupable and anaerobic streptococci.

GROUP A STREPTOCOCCI

The group A streptococcus, *S. pyogenes*, ranks as one of the most important human pathogens. This organism can be recognized in the laboratory by the generous zone of β-hemolysis produced by most isolates. Up to 4% of group A streptococci, however, may be nonhemolytic while still retaining their full pathogenic potential. Because many other streptococci can produce β-hemolysis, a confirmatory test is necessary to identify a β-hemolytic streptococcus as group A. The traditional screening test is the bacitracin test; almost all group A streptococci are inhibited by very low concentrations of bacitracin. Definitive speciation of group A streptococci can now be accomplished rapidly through identification of the group A carbohydrate by immunologic techniques.

The group A streptococcus is structurally complex. The capsule consists of hyaluronic acid, which is similar to the hyaluronic acid of human connective tissue and is therefore nonantigenic. The cell wall is composed of group-specific carbohydrates, structural proteins, and mucopeptide. The group-specific carbohydrate is responsible for the Lancefield serologic grouping, and in group A streptococci, it is a polymer of rhamnose and *N*-acetyl glucosamine. Three structural proteins are part of the cell wall. The most important is the M protein, which is a crucial marker of virulence because it impedes phagocytosis by polymorphonuclear leukocytes. Anti-M antibodies are protective because they opsonize the bacteria, thus promoting phagocytosis and killing. Among group A streptococci, there are more than 80 antigenically distinct M proteins and hence more than 80 M types. M types are important because immunity is type specific and only certain M types produce acute poststreptococcal glomerulonephritis.

The third component of the group A cell wall is a mucopeptide composed of repeating units of *N*-acetyl glucosamine and *N*-acetyl muramic acid. This element can produce carditis in laboratory rabbits, but its role in human rheumatic fever is unknown. The final structural element is the lipid-protein protoplast membrane. This membrane has certain antigens that cross-react with antigens in human cardiac muscle. The importance of this phenomenon in the pathogenesis of rheumatic fever is uncertain.

Epidemiology of Streptococcal Infections

The most important mode of spread of group A streptococci is by droplets, either from asymptomatic nasopharyngeal carriers or from patients with symptomatic pharyngitis.[31] Both the carrier rate and the incidence of pharyngitis are highest in late winter and early spring, in temperate climates, and in school-aged children. The epidemiology of streptococcal pyoderma is quite different. It is most common in young children and has its peak in late summer and early fall. Group A streptococci can colonize normal skin and spread from person to person by direct contact. Nosocomial transmission can occur, resulting most often in postoperative wound infections or postpartum sepsis. On occasion, streptococcal infections can occur in epidemic fashion as a result of contaminated foods.

Pathogenesis of Streptococcal Infections

Direct invasion is the most common way that group A streptococci cause disease. The organisms elaborate enzymes such as streptolysins O and S and nicotinamide adenine dinucleotide glycohydrolase (NADase), which can account for their characteristic ability to produce inflammation and tissue damage and to spread rapidly in tissues. Streptokinase catalyzes the conversion of plasminogen to plasmin and thus promotes fibrinolysis. Four distinct streptococcal deoxyribonuclease (DNase) enzymes have been identified; most streptococcal strains produce DNase B. Group A streptococci also produce hyaluronidase, known as spreading factor because of its ability to digest the hyaluronic acid of connective tissue. Except for streptolysin S, these enzymes are all antigenic. Although antibodies directed against these enzymes do not protect the patient against recurrent streptococcal infections, the tests for such antibodies can be used to obtain accurate serodiagnosis.

The second most common way in which group A streptococci cause disease is by elaboration of exotoxins that are responsible for scarlet fever and streptococcal toxic-shock syndrome (TSS). Three antigenically distinct erythrogenic toxins—types A, B, and C—have been recognized; type A toxin is more cytotoxic than types B and C. Elaboration of erythrogenic toxin depends on lysogeny of the streptococci by a bacteriophage; on occasion, certain group C or G streptococci or even staphylococci can produce an erythrogenic toxin. From the site of the streptococcal infection, which is usually in the pharynx, the toxin enters the circulation and damages small blood vessels, producing the characteristic rash of scarlet fever. In addition, these toxins function as superantigens, stimulating the production and release of cytokines by host cells; the cytokines, in turn, appear to play a role in the pathogenesis of shock and possibly rheumatic fever. Antibodies to the toxins prevent development of a rash but do not protect against the underlying infection.

Finally, group A streptococci can produce nonsuppurative, delayed postinfectious syndromes apparently caused by an immune response to the antecedent streptococcal infection. Acute rheumatic fever and acute glomerulonephritis begin 1 to 3 weeks after a group A streptococcal infection, usually when the infection is no longer active. Despite their common origins as poststreptococcal disorders, acute rheumatic fever and acute glomerulonephritis have important differences in their epidemiologic and pathogenetic features.

Diseases Caused by Direct Bacterial Invasion

Upper respiratory tract infection Group A streptococci are the most important cause of bacterial pharyngitis and tonsillitis.[32] They also cause sinusitis, otitis, mastoiditis, cervical lymphadenitis, peritonsillar abscesses, retropharyngeal abscesses, and Ludwig angina [see 5 Bacterial Infections of the Upper Respiratory Tract].

Pneumonia Streptococcal pneumonia is uncommon, accounting for less than 5% of all bacterial pneumonias. Although it is recognized most frequently as a sequela of influenza, it can occur as a primary infection and may even produce epidemics in closed groups. Streptococcal pneumonia presents acutely with fever, chills, and productive cough. The distinguishing feature of streptococcal pneumonia is the very high incidence of pleuritic chest pain; empyemas occur in approximately 60% of patients with streptococcal pneumonia.

Lymphadenitis Group A streptococci are frequently responsible for suppurative lymphadenitis, particularly in patients with streptococcal infections of the respiratory tract or skin.

Wound infections The characteristic features of group A streptococcal wound infections include an early onset, often within 24 hours after surgery or injury; an acute presentation with fever and systemic toxicity; and, frequently, a wound that appears relatively benign. A modest amount of thin serosanguineous fluid is often present in the wound. Gram stain of a smear of the fluid reveals gram-positive cocci in chains, and group A streptococci can be isolated from the wound culture.

Bone and joint infections Group A streptococci are relatively common causes of infections of bones and joints, usually from bacteremic seeding.

Postpartum infections The incidence of puerperal fever (childbed fever) has diminished markedly but has not been eliminated. The onset is abrupt, most often within 24 to 48 hours after delivery. Fever, chills, systemic toxicity, abdominal or pelvic pain, and a serosanguineous and odorless vaginal discharge are common; without treatment, endometritis may rapidly progress to pelvic peritonitis and bacteremia. Group A streptococci are the classic cause of puerperal fever, but other organisms, including group B and other streptococci and gram-negative bacilli, can cause infections with similar clinical features.

Bacteremia The incidence of group A streptococcal bacteremia appears to be rising. It often develops from a primary infection of skin, soft tissue, or a wound.[33] The respiratory tract is the second most common source, but bacteremia after uncomplicated streptococcal pharyngitis is uncommon. In 18% of cases, no primary focus of infection can be identified. About 80% of patients have underlying problems, ranging from diabetes or malignancies to drug abuse. Osteomyelitis, septic arthritis, meningitis, and endocarditis[34] are among the potential complications; overall mortality is 15%. Although meningitis can result from group A streptococcal bacteremia, this rare infection is more often a sequela of neurosurgical conditions.[35]

Skin and soft tissue infections Group A streptococci are important causes of cutaneous infections, ranging from very superficial infections of the epidermis (e.g., impetigo) to deep infections with systemic symptoms (e.g., erysipelas or cellulitis)[36] to life-threatening processes (e.g., necrotizing fasciitis or gangrenous myositis) that require surgery and antibiotic therapy[37].

Necrotizing fasciitis The widespread publicity that has been given to necrotizing fasciitis (previously known as streptococcal gangrene) has fueled popular concern about invasive group A streptococcal infections. An estimated 10,000 to 15,000 cases of invasive group A streptococcal infections occur each year in the United States; of these, necrotizing fasciitis occurs in 5% to 10%, with a case-fatality rate of about 30%. Most group A streptococci that cause invasive disease produce erythrogenic toxin, but the genetic heterogenicity of causative strains does not support a clonal basis for the resurgence of invasive streptococcal infections.

Group A streptococcal necrotizing fasciitis is usually community acquired,[37] but many patients have predisposing conditions that include varicella, trauma, diabetes, and immunosuppressive disorders.[38,39] Because the organisms reside deep within fascia and muscle, cutaneous changes are initially less prominent than pain, swelling, and systemic toxicity. Without aggressive therapy, however, the necrosis spreads to the skin and deep tissues. Computed tomography or magnetic resonance imaging can help define the depth and extent of necrosis. In addition to antibiotics and meticulous metabolic and circulatory support, prompt and aggressive surgical debridement is required; amputation may be necessary. Bacteremia and toxic streptococcal syndrome often complicate necrotizing fasciitis and are adverse prognostic features.

Diseases Caused by Toxin Production

Streptococcal toxic-shock syndrome Since the first description of streptococcal TSS in 1987, the incidence of this disorder has been increasing. Like staphylococcal TSS [*see* Staphylococci, *below*], streptococcal TSS appears to be mediated by a toxin, which in the case of the streptococcal form is usually type A toxin. The increase in the incidence of invasive streptococcal infections may be linked to the spread of toxigenic strains of streptococci, particularly M types 1 and 3. Like the staphylococcal toxin, the streptococcal toxin enters the circulation and functions as a superantigen, stimulating the release of host proteins that appear to mediate the shock syndrome.

Although persons of all ages are vulnerable to streptococcal TSS, it occurs most often in the very young and very old; about half the patients have underlying diseases. When a primary focus is identified, it is most often a soft tissue infection, with respiratory infections the next most common focus. Hypotension occurs in all patients and is often severe. Clinical features often include a generalized erythematous rash that may undergo desquamation; acute respiratory distress syndrome or soft tissue necrosis, such as necrotizing fasciitis or myositis, may be present. Laboratory evidence of multiorgan involvement typically can be found and characteristically includes evidence of renal impairment, hepatic abnormalities, and disseminated intravascular coagulation.[40] Even after aggressive treatment (high-dose I.V. penicillin, circulatory and respiratory support, and surgical debridement when necessary), mortality ranges from 30% to 58%. I.V. immunoglobulin has been advocated as an adjunct to therapy,[41] but clinical trials are required to determine its usefulness.

Scarlet fever The incidence of scarlet fever has declined sharply in the antibiotic era. The initial symptoms are fever and sore throat. Within 1 to 5 days, the characteristic fine, red, sandpaper-like eruption appears, often beginning on the chest and rapidly spreading to other parts of the body. Although the tongue and buccal mucosa are classically involved, the perioral area may be spared, thus accounting for the typical circumoral pallor. The rash is caused by hyperemia and capillary damage produced by erythrogenic toxin. In areas of trauma, such as the antecubital fossae, punctate hemorrhages (Pastia sign) may occur. Nausea and vomiting may be present, and fever and prostration may be severe. Desquamation of skin and mucous membranes is prominent during healing; one characteristic feature is the strawberry tongue. Therapy is the same as that for the underlying streptococcal infection.

Delayed Diseases Caused by the Host Immune Response

Group A streptococci can produce disease by a mechanism that is rarely a feature of other infections—a host immune response that subsequently produces tissue damage. Acute rheumatic fever (ARF) and acute glomerulonephritis (AGN) are the major syndromes produced in this fashion; both are characterized by a latent period between the streptococcal infection and its inflammatory consequences. Erythema nodosum is a third poststreptococcal syndrome, but it is less specific and less serious than ARF and AGN.

Acute rheumatic fever ARF is strictly a sequela of streptococcal pharyngitis. Although many strains of group A streptococci can provoke ARF, it most often follows pharyngeal infection by certain M types (especially M5, M18, and M3) that are heavily encapsulated, mucoid organisms. In about half the cases, the antecedent pharyngitis is clinically silent, but all patients with ARF have serologic evidence of a recent group A streptococcal infection. The risk of ARF after untreated streptococcal pharyngitis is less than 3%; the latent period between the pharyngitis and the onset of ARF averages 18 days.

Although common in developing nations, ARF is now quite uncommon in industrialized nations. However, the occurrence of several outbreaks in the United States in the 1980s demonstrates that ARF can still be an important problem in affluent societies. The disease occurs most often in children between 5 and 15 years of age; adults may present with atypical features, including synovitis without carditis.

Despite intensive study, the pathogenesis of ARF is unclear. The most widely held theory proposes that a genetically susceptible host develops an autoimmune response to epitopes in the organism that are cross-reactive with epitopes in tissues of the heart, joints, skin, or CNS.[42] Alternatively, streptococcal toxins or immune complexes may create alterations in tissue antigens that in turn provoke an autoimmune response that damages host tissues.

There are five major clinical manifestations of ARF. (1) Carditis develops in about 60% of patients; it involves the endocardium, myocardium, and pericardium. The typical manifestations of rheumatic carditis are sinus tachycardia (sometimes with first-degree heart block), mitral regurgitation, a pericardial friction rub, and cardiomegaly; congestive heart failure indicates severe carditis. Although most cases of carditis resolve within 3 months, patients with moderate to severe carditis or recurrent ARF are at risk for the late manifestation of mitral or aortic valve scarring. (2) Polyarthritis develops in about 70% of patients with ARF. It is characteristically a migratory arthritis involving the large joints of the extremities; it resolves without sequelae in days to weeks.[43] On rare occasions, adults may develop a persistent arthropathy of the hands and feet. (3) Chorea, (4) subcutaneous nodules, and (5) erythema marginatum are all self-limited; each occurs in fewer than 10% of children with ARF and only very rarely in adults.

The minor manifestations of ARF are fever, arthralgias, and inflammation, as demonstrated by elevated erythrocyte sedimentation rates and C-reactive protein levels.

The diagnosis of ARF is made on the basis of clinical features. The classic Jones criteria include the presence of either two major manifestations or one major and two minor manifestations and laboratory evidence of a recent streptococcal infection (e.g., a positive throat culture or rising antistreptococcal antibody levels).

Patients with ARF should receive treatment to eradicate streptococcal pharyngitis and to reduce inflammation. Most clinicians recommend a course of penicillin or, as an alternative, other antistreptococcal antibiotics, even if the throat culture is negative at the time ARF is diagnosed. Anti-inflammatory therapy includes aspirin and bed rest until inflammatory symptoms resolve; corticosteroids may have a role in patients with severe carditis.

ARF can be prevented by adequate treatment of streptococcal pharyngitis, even if antibiotics are delayed for up to 9 days after the onset of pharyngitis. Patients with a history of ARF are particularly vulnerable to recurrent attacks. Consequently, they should receive continuous prophylaxis for at least 5 years with daily oral penicillin (250 mg twice a day) or monthly injections of 1.2 million units of benzathine penicillin G. Oral sulfadiazine or erythromycin may be administered to patients allergic to penicillin. Prophylaxis can be discontinued when young patients who are at low risk for recurrence reach adulthood.

Acute glomerulonephritis Acute poststreptococcal glomerulonephritis appears to result from the deposition of circulating antigen-antibody complexes and complement in renal glomeruli. Only group A streptococci of certain M protein types can produce glomerulonephritis; it is unknown why only approximately 15 of the more than 80 M types are nephritogenic. Acute glomerulonephritis can follow either streptococcal pharyngitis or pyoderma but is more common after skin infections.

The incidence of acute glomerulonephritis after infection with nephritogenic streptococci varies but may reach 10% to 15% in certain epidemic situations. The prognosis is generally good, especially in children, and recurrences are uncommon; therefore, penicillin prophylaxis is not indicated. In fact, it is not certain that penicillin therapy for streptococcal pharyngitis or pyoderma affects the incidence of subsequent acute glomerulonephritis.

Erythema nodosum Erythema nodosum is another nonsuppurative sequela of streptococcal infection. It can develop after streptococcal infections of the skin, pharynx, or other sites. However, these painful pretibial nodules may be associated with other infectious processes, such as tuberculosis or systemic mycoses, and with noninfectious processes, such as inflammatory bowel disease or hypersensitivity reactions.

Diagnosis and Treatment of Streptococcal Infections

The diagnosis of group A streptococcal infections depends on recognizing the clinical syndromes and culturing the bacterium from appropriate specimens. Streptococcal pharyngitis can be diagnosed rapidly by detecting streptococcal antigens on throat swab specimens [see 5 Bacterial Infections of the Upper Respiratory Tract]. Serologic tests may be extremely useful, albeit retrospectively, in documenting recent streptococcal infection. Many of the enzymes and toxins produced by group A streptococci are antigenic, and a variety of antibody tests are available. The most widely used is the anti–streptolysin O titer, which is elevated after most respiratory tract infections; anti-DNase B titers are also elevated after most group A streptococcal infections.

Despite the widespread use of penicillin, group A streptococci continue to be uniformly sensitive to this agent, which remains the drug of choice. The dose schedule and duration vary enormously. The standard therapy for pharyngitis is 10 days of low-dose oral penicillin (or a single I.M. dose of benzathine penicillin G), but a recent trial suggests that 5 days of therapy with various β-lactams or macrolides may be as effective.[44] Similarly, although oral penicillin is usually administered four times a day, a recent meta-analysis found that twice-daily dosing is as effective for children.[45] In contrast, more invasive streptococcal infections require much more intensive treatment, such as prolonged high-dose I.V. therapy for osteomyelitis or endocarditis. In patients who are allergic to penicillins, cephalosporins are effective but must be used with caution because of the risk of allergic cross-reactivity. Erythromycin, vancomycin, and clindamycin are generally excellent alternatives, although occasionally, clinical isolates are resistant to these agents. Erythromycin-resistant strains have become prevalent, especially in Japan and Finland; reducing the use of macrolide antibiotics can control this problem. Many strains of group A streptococci are now resistant to tetracyclines and TMP-SMX. The new fluoroquinolones levofloxacin, sparfloxacin, gatifloxacin, and moxifloxacin are active against group A streptococci.

INFECTIONS CAUSED BY NON–GROUP A STREPTOCOCCI

Streptococci belonging to all the Lancefield groups can cause disease ranging in severity from urinary tract infections to meningitis, bacteremia, and endocarditis [*see Table 1*]. None of the non–group A organisms, however, has been implicated in rheumatic fever.

Groups C and G Streptococci

Groups C and G streptococci have many similarities to group A streptococci, although they are much less commonly implicated as pathogens. Most strains of groups C and G are β-hemolytic, and some are bacitracin sensitive. Bacteria in both groups can produce many of the same enzymes and toxins produced by group A streptococci, including streptolysin O, streptokinase, NADase, DNase, hyaluronidase, and erythrogenic toxin. The group-specific carbohydrate of group C is similar to that of group A, and groups A, C, and G all have cross-reacting cell membrane antigens.

First recognized as animal pathogens, groups C and G streptococci may be part of the resident flora of the pharynx, skin, genitourinary tract, and gastrointestinal tract.[46] Group C streptococci can cause pharyngitis in adults. Groups C and G streptococci can cause skin and wound infections, puerperal sepsis, bacteremia, endocarditis, pericarditis, septic arthritis, meningitis, scarlatiniform eruptions, myositis, and toxic-shock syndrome.[47] In rare instances, groups C and G streptococci cause poststreptococcal glomerulonephritis. Groups C and G streptococci are sensitive to penicillin, which is the drug of choice, and to erythromycin, vancomycin, and other antibiotics.

Group B Streptococci

Group B streptococci are important human pathogens.[48] Most group B streptococci are β-hemolytic; up to 20% are sensitive to low-dose bacitracin. They can be presumptively separated from group A streptococci on the basis of their ability to hydrolyze sodium hippurate, but definitive identification depends on immunologic identification of the group B carbohydrate.

Group B streptococcal infections are the leading cause of bacterial disease and death in newborns; maternal infections can also occur in the peripartum period.[48] The organisms reside in the vagina and infect neonates during passage through the birth canal; premature labor, prolonged membrane rupture, and intrapartum fever are risk factors for neonatal infection. The intrapartum administration of antibiotics to women at high risk can prevent neonatal infection; screening and treatment have substantially reduced the incidence of perinatal and peripartum group B streptococcal infections.[49]

Group B streptococci can cause a broad range of infections in nonpregnant adults. Persons of any age can be affected, but elderly patients are most vulnerable.[50] Other risk factors include genitourinary disorders, diabetes, cancer, HIV infection, and other debilitating conditions. In addition to bacteremia, infections caused by group B streptococci include urinary tract infections, septic arthritis, endocarditis, meningitis, pulmonary infections, and infections of the skin, soft tissue, and wounds. Necrotizing fasciitis and streptococcal TSS[51] have also been reported.

Although group B streptococci are sensitive to clinically achievable levels of penicillin, the MICs are somewhat higher than those for group A streptococci. The great majority of group B streptococci are sensitive to cephalosporins, vancomycin, erythromycin, and clindamycin but are resistant to tetracycline. Penicillin-gentamicin synergism is evident in some strains; although clinical trials are lacking, synergistic therapy for serious group B streptococcal infections may merit consideration.

Group D Streptococci

Group D streptococci (*S. bovis* and *S. equinus*) can be identified in the laboratory by their ability to resist heat and bile but not 6.5% NaCl. Both species reside in the human GI and genitourinary tracts.

S. equinus rarely causes human disease, but *S. bovis* is a relatively common cause of endocarditis, which may be more severe than the subacute bacterial endocarditis caused by viridans streptococci.[52] *S. bovis* bacteremia is significantly linked to carcinoma of the colon; therefore, the GI tract of any patient with this infection should be aggressively evaluated. *S. bovis* is sensitive to penicillin and other antibiotics and responds well to therapy with penicillin alone.

Nongroupable Streptococci

Up to 30% of streptococcal isolates are not groupable under the currently available Lancefield antisera classification. These organisms are capable of producing a great variety of pyogenic infections, among which subacute bacterial endocarditis stands out as the most important. Nongroupable streptococci can also cause bacteremia and pneumonia, especially in immunosuppressed patients[53]; meningitis is rare.[54] Members of the *S. milleri* group have a propensity to produce abscesses, particularly in the brain or liver.[55]

Classically, subacute endocarditis is caused by viridans streptococci-nongroupable, α-hemolytic bacteria that are part of the normal flora of the oropharynx [see 7 Infective Endocarditis]. Many species of viridans streptococci can cause endocarditis; *S. sanguis*, *S. mutans*, *S. mitis*, and *S. milleri* group are commonly responsible. Infections caused by members of the *S. milleri* group may be more destructive than those caused by the other species. About 10% of viridans streptococci are nutritionally variant, requiring supplementary pyridoxal to grow on agar plates. Up to one third of these organisms require serum penicillin levels of greater than 0.1 μg/ml to inhibit growth. Although this level is higher than the levels that kill most other streptococci, this concentration can be easily achieved clinically. Synergistic penicillin-aminoglycoside therapy has been recommended for endocarditis caused by these organisms. Penicillin-tolerant and penicillin-resistant strains of viridans streptococci have been increasingly recognized; vancomycin or penicillin-aminoglycoside therapy has been recommended for endocarditis caused by penicillin-resistant streptococci.

Anaerobic Streptococci

Various anaerobic and microaerophilic streptococci reside in the oropharynx, GI tract, and genitourinary tract. These organisms cause a great variety of infections, including aspiration pneumonia, lung abscess, empyema, sinusitis, brain abscess, bone and joint infections, and skin and wound infections. Anaerobic streptococci often participate in these processes along with other anaerobic or aerobic bacteria. Foul-smelling pus is characteristic of these infections, and gas may be present in soft tissues. The anaerobic streptococci are penicillin sensitive.

Enterococci

Although they were long considered to be streptococci, the enterococci have been reclassified into the genus *Enterococcus*. Of the infections caused by enterococci, 80% to 85% are caused by *E. faecalis* and most of the others are caused by *E. faecium*, but *E. durans*, *E. avium*, and other species can also cause disease in humans. Morphologically indistinguishable from streptococci and immunologically similar to members of group D streptococci, the enterococci are metabolically unique in their ability to resist heat, bile, and 6.5% NaCl. Unlike streptococci, enterococci are uniformly penicillin resistant. Both major enterococcal species reside in the GI and genitourinary tracts, and both can cause urinary, abdominal, and disseminated infections, which are often marked by tissue invasion and destruction.

PATHOGENESIS OF ENTEROCOCCAL INFECTIONS

The primary reason enterococci have emerged as major human pathogens is that these organisms are resistant to many antibiotics. Enterococci are intrinsically resistant to penicillin because they have unique penicillin-binding proteins that permit cell wall synthesis to proceed even in the presence of β-lactam antibiotics. In addition, enterococci that produce β-lactamase have been recognized; although these strains are still relatively uncommon, they may pose problems in the future. Enterococci can also demonstrate low-level resistance to aminoglycosides, but synergistic therapy with a penicillin and an aminoglycoside has been successful against most species. However, high-level resistance to the aminoglycosides streptomycin and gentamicin has emerged during the past 20 years. More recently, vancomycin-resistant enterococci (VRE) have been recognized as nosocomial pathogens.[56] VRE colonization of the GI tract and skin often precedes overt infections. Colonization and infection are usually hospital acquired and are most common in patients who have prolonged hospitalizations, have serious underlying diseases, or have had previous therapy with multiple antibiotics; antibiotics that are active against anaerobes are particularly likely to promote intestinal colonization.[57] VRE are often carried by medical personnel and can spread from patient to patient. Because they often occur in very ill patients and are so difficult to treat, VRE infections pose a major threat. The mortality associated with VRE bacteremia approaches 45%.[55]

CLINICAL ENTEROCOCCAL INFECTIONS

Enterococci, alone or with other enteric organisms, are relatively common causes of urinary tract infections, wound infections, and peritonitis and intra-abdominal abscesses. Enterococci have become an increasingly prominent cause of bacteremia,[58] which usually originates from a focus in the urinary tract or abdomen; the incidence of nosocomial bacteremias caused by these organisms is also increasing, particularly in patients who have received cephalosporins or other broad-spectrum antibiotics. Enterococcal endocarditis may affect normal, diseased, or prosthetic valves and may pursue an acute destructive course. Enterococcal meningitis is much less common but may be very difficult to treat. Enterococcal infections are most common in persons with underlying genitourinary or GI disease, in the elderly, and in debilitated persons. Enterococci have become an important cause of disease in hospitalized patients; they are now the second most common nosocomial pathogen in the United States, occurring less commonly than *Escherichia coli* but more commonly than *Pseudomonas aeruginosa* and *Staphylococcus aureus*.

TREATMENT OF ENTEROCOCCAL INFECTIONS

Changing resistance patterns will necessitate changes in antibiotic therapy for patients with enterococcal infections. Traditionally, ampicillin has been the drug of choice for enterococcal urinary tract infections. In penicillin-allergic patients, nitrofurantoin, a fluoroquinolone, or TMP-SMX may be effective for the treatment of simple urinary tract infections; however, because in vitro susceptibility testing of enterococci is often misleading and because resistance to these agents may rapidly emerge, patients should be continually evaluated through assessment of their clinical response and by use of follow-up cultures.

Deep tissue and bloodstream infections have traditionally been treated with ampicillin and gentamicin, with vancomycin, or with vancomycin and gentamicin. Although these agents are still appropriate for most enterococcal infections, all clinically significant isolates should be subjected to testing for β-lactamase production, high-level aminoglycoside resistance, and vancomycin resistance to determine whether an alternative therapy is necessary. Infections caused by enterococci that produce β-lactamase can be treated with an antimicrobial agent that combines a penicillin with a β-lactamase inhibitor. Infections caused by strains that are highly resistant to aminoglycosides can be treated with vancomycin. Infections caused by vancomycin-resistant strains are the most difficult to treat; linezolid has been particularly helpful, and quinupristin-dalfopristin is also effective.[59] Doxycycline, chloramphenicol, and, for urinary tract infections, nitrofurantoin have also been used. In all cases, removal of infected indwelling catheters and foreign bodies and drainage of septic foci are essential. It is also essential to limit the spread of VRE by intensive surveillance, infection-control measures,[60] and prudent use of vancomycin and other antibiotics.

Staphylococci

Staphylococci are nonsporulating, nonmotile gram-positive cocci that have an average diameter of 1 μm. Microscopically, staphylococci tend to be larger and rounder than streptococci. Because cell division occurs on three planes, these organisms are typically found in grapelike clusters and tetrads as well as in pairs and sometimes short chains. When grown on blood agar, staphylococci form small (1 to 2 mm), smooth, round colonies that are often pigmented and may be surrounded by a zone of β-hemolysis.

Staphylococci are very hardy organisms and can withstand much more physical and chemical stress than pneumococci and streptococci. For example, staphylococci resist drying, withstand 10% NaCl, and will survive and even replicate at temperatures between 10° and 45° C. Because staphylococci are facultative anaerobes, they will grow in the presence or absence of oxygen. Staphylococci are catalase positive.

Of the species of staphylococci, *S. aureus* is by far the most important human pathogen. *S. aureus* can be tentatively identified in the laboratory on the basis of its production of a golden-yellow pigment. Because some strains are nonpigmented, definitive identification of *S. aureus* depends on its ability to produce the enzyme coagulase and to ferment mannitol.

The most important coagulase-negative organism is *S. epidermidis*, which is universally present as part of the normal skin flora but can produce disease in certain circumstances, such as infection of an indwelling prosthesis. Another important coagulase-negative species is *S. saprophyticus*, which causes urinary tract infections.

STAPHYLOCOCCUS AUREUS

The cellular structure of *S. aureus* is complex.[61] Most strains have polysaccharide microcapsules. The cell wall of *S. aureus* is structurally similar to that of group A streptococci: both have a carbohydrate antigen, a protein component, and a mucopeptide. The carbohydrate antigen is a teichoic acid, which in *S. aureus* is a polymer of *N*-acetylglucosamine and polyribitol phosphate. Antibodies to teichoic acid can be detected in normal human serum, and elevated antibody titers are present in patients with deep-seated staphylococcal infections. Teichoic acid has no established role in virulence, and antibodies to this carbohydrate are not protective. The protein component of the cell wall includes protein A, which reacts with IgG of normal human serum. Protein A interacts with the Fc component rather than the Fab component of IgG and hence is not a true antigen. Protein A may be antiphagocytic, but its role in virulence has not been clearly established. The cell wall mucopeptide of staphylococci is structurally similar to the mucopeptide of other gram-positive bacteria.

Epidemiology of Staphylococcal Infections

S. aureus is an extremely widespread organism; it can be cultured from environmental surfaces, clothing, bedding, and the air, although transmission of staphylococci by airborne droplets or fomites does not appear to be a major route of infection. Humans—either asymptomatic carriers or persons with staphylococcal lesions—are the reservoir of infection. Nasal carriage is common; rates of nasal carriage range from 15% to more than 50% and are increased in hospitalized patients, dialysis patients, narcotics addicts, and insulin-injecting diabetic patients. Other relatively common sites of colonization include the rectum, the perineum, and the pharynx. *S. aureus* can often be cultured from normal skin, but skin colonization is probably brief, with repeated repopulation occurring from the nose. It is unclear why some persons are prolonged carriers, others are transient carriers, and others resist colonization and why some persons carry many organisms, whereas others have low colony counts. Person-to-person transmission is more likely from nasal carriers of large numbers of organisms and from persons with active staphylococcal infections of the skin or respiratory tract. Nasal carriage increases the risk of skin and wound infections and bacteremia[62]; upper respiratory tract viral infections appear to increase bacteria shedding by *S. aureus* nasal carriers. Periodic application of mupirocin ointment in nasal carriers reduces the rate of carriage and lowers the risk of skin infections.

Minor staphylococcal infections are extremely common. It is the rare person who has not at some time experienced a staphylococcal furuncle (boil), paronychia, or hordeolum (sty). Serious staphylococcal infections generally require a predisposing insult to host defenses. Most often, this takes the form of skin disease, trauma, or a viral infection of the respiratory tract, especially influenza or measles. Other predisposing factors include foreign bodies, liver disease, neoplasia, diabetes, renal failure, defects in leukocyte or immunoglobulin function, narcotics addiction, and broad-spectrum antibiotic therapy.

Unlike the incidence of other gram-positive cocci, the incidence of serious staphylococcal infection increased sharply after the introduction of antibiotics. Much of this increase can be attributed to the development of antibiotic resistance. When penicillin was first introduced, fewer than 10% of staphylococci were penicillin resistant; this percentage has increased steadily to include the great majority of staphylococci. During the late 1950s, staphylococcal infection reached epidemic proportions, and hospital-acquired infections were a particularly grave problem. With the introduction of methicillin in 1959 and other penicillinase-resistant antibiotics in the 1960s, the incidence of nosocomial staphylococcal infection temporarily declined. Unfortunately, however, methicillin-resistant staphylococci have emerged as major nosocomial pathogens, and vancomycin-resistant strains loom on the horizon.[63]

Pathogenesis of Staphylococcal Infections

The earliest tissue response in staphylococcal infection is acute inflammation with a vigorous exudation of polymorphonuclear leukocytes. Vascular thrombosis and tissue necrosis quickly lead to abscess formation. As a result of the development of a fibrin meshwork and, later, fibroblast proliferation, these abscesses become walled-off zones of loculated infection and tissue destruction, with dying leukocytes and viable bacteria at the center. Fibrosis and scarring are often prominent in healing.

Most strains of *S. aureus* produce a variety of extracellular products, including both enzymes and toxins, that may account for the tendency to produce burrowing, destructive, localized infections. The enzyme coagulase causes plasma to clot, thus promoting the fibrin meshwork that contributes to abscess formation. Staphylococci can also produce lipase, protease, hyaluronidase, and DNAse, which can add to tissue damage. Another important enzyme is penicillinase. Because penicillinase has no role in pathogenicity, staphylococci that produce penicillinase are no more virulent than non–penicillinase-producing strains. Nevertheless, this enzyme is clinically and epidemiologically important because it hydrolyzes the β-lactam ring of penicillin, thereby inactivating the molecule. The production of penicillinase is controlled by plasmids, or episomes, which are extrachromosomal DNA molecules that replicate during cell division. Unlike the R factors of gram-negative bacilli, however, the plasmids responsible for penicillinase production do not usually mediate resistance to multiple antibiotics.

Of even greater interest are the nonenzymatic toxins produced by *S. aureus*. α-Toxin is a cytotoxin that produces pores in cell membranes, thereby altering their permeability and resulting in cell damage or death. α-Toxin damages red and white blood cells and activates platelets. Injection of α-toxin into animals can produce dermal necrosis and contraction of vascular smooth muscle, leading to tissue ischemia. Another potential virulence factor is leukocidin, which consists of two leukotoxic proteins that are capable of disrupting lysosomal membranes. Occasionally, strains of staphylococci produce exfoliatin, which causes the epidermolysis of staphylococcal scalded skin syndrome (SSSS). Some strains of staphylococci can also produce one of four antigenically distinct enterotoxins that cause the vomiting and diarrhea characteristic of staphylococcal food poisoning. In rare instances, staphylococci produce an erythrogenic toxin that causes scarlet fever. Finally, a staphylococcal exotoxin, toxic-shock syndrome toxin–1 (TSST-1), appears to be responsible for staphylococcal TSS.

Host resistance and immunity to staphylococci are poorly understood. The importance of the granulocyte is supported by the susceptibility to staphylococcal infections seen in patients with neutropenia or various disorders of neutrophil function, such as chronic granulomatous disease, Chédiak-Higashi syndrome, and various disorders of chemotaxis. The most important factors predisposing to staphylococcal infections are not immunologic defects but mechanical defects. Minute skin abrasions, for example, probably provide the portal of entry in staphylococcal skin infections and in many cases of staphylococcal bacteremia. I.V. drug abuse accounts for many cases of staphylococcal bacteremia and endocarditis. Indwelling venous catheters are particularly important in nosocomial infections; plastic catheters become coated with fibrinogen and fibrin, which interact with adhesins on the bacterial cell surface and bind staphylococci to the catheter.

Clinical Staphylococcal Infections

Skin and soft tissue infections The most frequent manifestations of staphylococcal disease are skin and soft tissue infections. These range from processes that can cause great discomfort but are rarely hazardous, such as impetigo, folliculitis, furuncles, carbuncles, and paronychia, to much more serious deep tissue infections, such as cellulitis and wound sepsis.

Staphylococcal skin infections are epidemiologically significant in the transmission of serious staphylococcal disease. Even localized infections can give rise to bacteremia and endocarditis, and furuncles of the nose and face may occasionally produce CNS infection by spreading along venous channels.

Bone and joint infections Staphylococci are among the principal causes of septic arthritis and osteomyelitis [see 11 Septic Arthritis and 12 Osteomyelitis] of the long bones and of vertebral bodies and disk spaces. These infections may result from hematogenous or contiguous spread of infection; infections of orthopedic prostheses are particularly serious.[64] In addition to causing acute osteomyelitis, staphylococci have a propensity for causing chronic bone infections in which active localized infection can persist for many decades without undergoing dissemination. *S. aureus* is also the leading cause of septic bursitis.

Respiratory tract infections Although staphylococci reside in the nasopharynx, they do not cause pharyngitis and they are rarely involved in acute otitis, sinusitis, or mastoiditis, but they can participate in chronic infections of these regions [see 5 Bacterial Infections of the Upper Respiratory Tract].

S. aureus accounts for fewer than 10% of all bacterial pneumonias, but it is nevertheless an important pathogen of the lower respiratory tract. Staphylococcal pneumonia can occur either by spread from the upper airways or by hematogenous seeding. Except in infants, airborne staphylococcal pneumonia is rare as a primary infection. It usually occurs after viral respiratory tract infections, especially influenza. Thus, clinical illness often follows a biphasic course: viral symptoms lasting 4 or 5 days precede an abrupt deterioration. Staphylococcal pneumonia also occurs as a nosocomial infection, particularly in elderly, debilitated patients[65]; in such patients, mortality is 32%. *S. aureus* can cause pneumonia in HIV-infected persons; these infections are often community acquired and have a mortality of 38%, even with appropriate antibiotic therapy.

Patients with staphylococcal pneumonia are acutely ill; purulent sputum production is the rule, and polymorphonuclear leukocytes and staphylococci can be identified on Gram stain of the sputum. Radiographs show a characteristic patchy bronchopneumonic pattern, often with multiple areas of consolidation. Because these organisms tend to produce tissue necrosis, cavitation is relatively common, and lung abscesses and empyemas may develop; fibrosis and scarring often occur during healing. Hematogenous staphylococcal pneumonia is a complication of staphylococcal bacteremia, especially when endocarditis of the tricuspid valve leads to septic embolization. Sputum production tends to occur later and is less prominent than in airborne pneumonias. Typical radiographic features include multiple small areas of infiltration, which, although sometimes evanescent, often progress to cavitation. Staphylococcal pneumonia is a life-threatening disease requiring high-dose parenteral antibiotic therapy, often for 2 to 4 weeks. Patients with abscess formation and empyema generally require therapy for 3 to 4 weeks; empyemas must be drained.

Bloodstream infections Most patients with *S. aureus* bacteremia are acutely ill; more than 50% have temperatures in excess of 40° C (104° F), and most experience chills and exhibit systemic toxicity. Serious underlying diseases are present in 75% to 85% of patients. The overall mortality is about 23%.[66] Up to 80% of patients with staphylococcal bacteremia acquire the infection in the hospital, often from infected I.V. catheters, skin and wound infections, or pulmonary tract infections.[67] Drug addiction is responsible for more than 50% of the community-acquired cases. Patients with community-acquired bacteremias are more likely to have endocarditis and secondary metastatic infections than patients with nosocomial infections, who are more likely to have an evident portal of entry and severe underlying diseases. Bacteremic seeding can lead to secondary staphylococcal infection of the lungs, bones and joints, and genitourinary tract. Evidence of CNS involvement is suggestive of endocarditis and is an adverse prognostic sign.

Patients with staphylococcal bacteremia have generally been treated with parenteral antibiotics for 4 to 6 weeks. This recommendation has been made on the basis of the results of a study conducted from 1940 to 1954 in which endocarditis developed in 64% of 55 patients with staphylococcal bacteremia.[68] Subsequent investigations[69] suggested that patients with a removable or treatable primary focus of infection (most often, infected I.V. devices) and no clinical evidence of endocarditis can be treated safely with only 10 to 21 days of I.V. antibiotics. Other studies, however, have reported development of endocarditis in 22% to 38% of patients with a primary focus of bacteremia. Therefore, the possibility of endocarditis should not be ignored, even if a primary focus is present. Moreover, major complications, including shock, acute respiratory distress syndrome, and metastatic infection, can occur even in the absence of endocarditis.

Controlled trials are necessary to determine the safety and efficacy of short-term therapy for staphylococcal bacteremia. It may therefore be prudent to treat patients with staphylococcal bacteremia as though they have endocarditis, unless there is clear evidence of only a transient bacteremia or of a removable primary focus with a benign clinical course, rapid clearing of bacteremia, absence of echocardiographically demonstrable valvular abnormalities and metastatic infection, and intact host defenses. Negative titers of teichoic acid antibodies would bolster the decision to abbreviate I.V. therapy, which should, in any case, be continued for at least 10 to 15 days. A regimen of I.V. antibiotics followed by oral antibiotic therapy has been suggested, but more studies are needed before this regimen can be widely recommended. Clearly, the physician must individualize therapy by balancing the morbidity and expense of 4 to 6 weeks of antibiotic therapy against the risks of undertreating endocarditis, which is a life-threatening infection.[70] Transesophageal echocardiography can establish a diagnosis of *S. aureus* endocarditis [see 7 Infective Endocarditis].[71]

Because of the high mortality associated with staphylococcal bacteremia and endocarditis, combination therapies utilizing nafcillin or vancomycin with gentamicin or rifampin are being studied. Thus far, combination therapy appears to offer few advantages, although it may be useful in patients who fail to respond to conventional single-drug treatment. I.V. drug abusers with uncomplicated right-sided endocarditis may respond well to abbreviated therapy.

Because of the propensity of staphylococci to form abscesses, it is particularly important to evaluate bacteremic patients for a loculated infection that may require surgical drainage. Management of staphylococcal bacteremia in patients with Hickman catheters almost always requires catheter removal in addition to antibiotic therapy. Staphylococcal endocarditis appears to be increasing in frequency; its clinical features and therapy are reviewed elsewhere[72] [see 7 Infective Endocarditis].

CNS infection Staphylococcal infections of the CNS present most often as aseptic meningitis in the course of staphylococcal bacteremia, especially in patients with endocarditis; the CSF typically reveals modest pleocytosis, and cultures and Gram stains are negative. *S. aureus* is an uncommon cause of purulent meningitis. Direct extension of infection from traumatic or neurosurgical wounds or from osteomyelitis of the mastoids or other cranial bones is a more frequent cause of staphylococcal meningitis than hematogenous seeding. Nafcillin has been shown to penetrate the CSF and should be administered in dosages of approximately 2 g I.V. every 4 hours for the average-sized adult with normal renal function. When nafcillin cannot be used because of methicillin-resistant organisms[73] or penicillin-allergic patients, therapy must be individualized. Options such as high-dose I.V. vancomycin and rifampin should be considered. In patients who are not responding favorably, there may be a role for intrathecal vancomycin or bacitracin or for I.V. TMP-SMX or erythromycin and chloramphenicol.

Another uncommon infection of the CNS in which *S. aureus* is a major pathogen is spinal epidural abscess. Patients with this disease often have underlying vertebral osteomyelitis. These patients present with fever and back pain; radicular pain, weakness, and paralysis evolve as cord compression occurs. Immediate surgical decompression is mandatory.

GI tract infections Staphylococci can also affect the GI tract. Staphylococcal food poisoning occurs when food handlers who have contaminated superficial wounds or who are shedding infected nasal droplets inoculate foods with enterotoxin-producing strains of *S. aureus*. If the contaminated food is not refrigerated, the organisms produce enterotoxin within 4 to 6 hours. The symptoms begin abruptly within 1 to 6 hours after the ingestion of preformed enterotoxin. They consist of salivation, nausea, vomiting, abdominal pain, diarrhea, and prostration. The symptoms usually subside within 24 hours; there is no specific therapy other than fluid and electrolyte repletion, although I.V. hydration may be necessary in cases of severe disease.

Genitourinary infections *S. aureus* can occasionally produce genitourinary infections. Between 7% and 27% of patients with staphylococcal bacteremia have positive urine cultures. Most of these patients have no gross renal infection, but in some, hematogenous pyelonephritis, renal cortical abscesses, renal carbuncles, perinephric abscesses, or prostatic abscesses may develop. These processes should be considered in all patients with positive urine cultures and in patients with staphylococcal bacteremia and persistent fever, flank pain, or abnormal urine sediments. I.V. pyelography, nephrotomography, renal ultrasonography studies, and CT may be diagnostically helpful. Prostatic abscesses may require repeated rectal examination or ultrasound for diagnosis. *S. aureus*, either alone or with other genitourinary pathogens, can also cause nosocomial urinary tract infections in patients with indwelling catheters.

Other staphylococcal infections *S. aureus* can produce infection of sebaceous glands of the eyelid (sty), purulent conjunctivitis, and orbital cellulitis. It can cause parotitis, which occurs most often in patients who are elderly, debilitated, and dehydrated. Mastitis is most frequent in nursing mothers in the early postpartum period but may occur in neonates or in nonlactating women. Infection of muscle is rare in temperate climates but common in the tropics. Tropical pyomyositis presents with fever and multiple muscle abscesses. The diagnosis should be suspected in recent immigrants from tropical areas but should also be considered in patients who have not traveled and in patients with AIDS. CT may be helpful in detecting muscle abscesses. Purulent pericarditis can result either from direct extension of a pneumonia or empyema or from hematogenous seeding. Staphylococcal bacteremia can produce metastatic abscesses of any organ, including the liver and spleen. Patients who have metastatic abscesses may have persistent fever; in such cases, diagnosis may be difficult if localizing symptoms are absent. *S. aureus* can cause peritonitis in patients on continuous ambulatory peritoneal dialysis.

Treatment of Staphylococcal Infections

In addition to paronychia and sties, minor staphylococcal infections of the skin, such as folliculitis and furunculosis, generally respond well to the topical application of warm soaks. Larger focal infections such as carbuncles may have to be incised and drained. Antibiotics should be added when fever or systemic symptoms are present, when lesions are large or numerous, when lesions fail to respond to local therapy, when patients have underlying medical problems such as valvular heart disease or a cardiac prosthesis, or when the nose or face is involved. Cloxacillin or dicloxacillin in an oral dosage of 250 to 500 mg every 6 hours is generally sufficient. Cephalexin, erythromycin, or the newer macrolides are excellent alternatives, as is clindamycin in an oral dosage of 150 to 300 mg every 6 hours.

For serious staphylococcal infections, such as cellulitis, deep wound sepsis, pneumonia, septic arthritis, osteomyelitis, bacteremia, endocarditis, or meningitis, parenteral antibiotics are mandatory. Oxacillin or nafcillin in a dosage of 1 g every 4 hours may suffice for cellulitis or pneumonia [see 2 Chemotherapy of Infection], but a dosage of 2 g every 4 hours should be used for osteomyelitis, endocarditis, or CNS infections in the average-sized adult with normal renal function. Parenteral cephalosporins are excellent alternatives unless CNS infection is present. Whereas erythromycin and clindamycin have produced good results in penicillin-allergic patients with cellulitis, pneumonia, or osteomyelitis, vancomycin is preferred for the treatment of endocarditis in these patients because it is a bactericidal antibiotic.

Although only about 10% of all *S. aureus* strains are penicillin sensitive, penicillin G remains the drug of choice for sensitive organisms. Care must be taken in sensitivity testing, however, because penicillinase is an inducible enzyme. It is best to reserve penicillin G for staphylococci that are shown to be penicillinase negative or for staphylococci that have extremely large zones of inhibition by penicillin on Kirby-Bauer sensitivity testing. Methicillin resistance may also be overlooked occasionally on routine sensitivity testing because it is more readily expressed at lower temperatures (30° C), at higher salt concentrations, or after 48 hours of incubation.

Synergism between penicillins and aminoglycosides against *S. aureus* can be shown in vitro and in experimental staphylococcal infections. However, a clinical benefit of combination therapy for *S. aureus* endocarditis has not yet been demonstrated. Most staphylococci are extremely sensitive to rifampin, which may be combined with other antistaphylococcal drugs in certain difficult clinical situations. However, staphylococci rapidly develop resistance to rifampin when the drug is used alone, and resistance may even arise during combination therapy. The utility of ciprofloxacin is limited by the emergence of resistance. Only time will tell if the newer fluoroquinolones, such as levofloxacin and sparfloxacin, will be more successful; combinations of rifampin and a fluoroquinolone are being investigated.

Since its first appearance in 1970, methicillin-resistant *S. aureus* (MRSA) has constituted a growing problem. These organisms produce a cell wall penicillin-binding protein with a low affinity for β-lactam antibiotics. Initially, MRSA appeared as a nosocomial pathogen in university hospitals. Although hospitals are still the most common setting, these organisms have also become important problems in long-term care facilities and are increasingly being acquired in the community.[74] MRSA has proved to be difficult to control; infected patients should be subjected to strict barrier precautions.[75] Both patients and hospital personnel may become asymptomatic carriers. The carrier state is typically prolonged, often exceeding 3 years; antibiotics are usually ineffective. Topical mupirocin ointment can reduce the MRSA carrier rate,[76] but because recolonization is common, mupirocin is not recommended for extended use in long-term care facilities.

The virulence and clinical manifestations of MRSA are no different from those of methicillin-susceptible *S. aureus*.[77] Most MRSA strains are also resistant to penicillin, cephalosporins, erythromycin, and chloramphenicol; even if the organisms appear to be sensitive to cephalosporins in disk diffusion testing, one should not rely on these agents. Vancomycin is the drug of choice, with results comparable to those achieved with β-lactam antibiotic treatment of infections caused by methicillin-sensitive strains. Linezolid and quinupristin-dalfopristin are also active against MRSA; but until more experience is available, these new drugs should probably be reserved for infections in which vancomycin is ineffective or unsuitable.

With the increased use of vancomycin, strains of *S. aureus* with reduced susceptibility to vancomycin have begun to appear.[63] Although these organisms are still very uncommon in the United States, vigorous control measures are required to prevent them from joining VRE as major nosocomial pathogens.[78]

In addition to vigorous antibiotic therapy, other measures are often necessary to treat staphylococcal infections. In particular, it is important to remove indwelling venous catheters or other foreign bodies that may be a portal of entry for staphylococcal bacteremia as well as a nidus for persistent infection. Patients must be evaluated for the presence of staphylococcal abscesses, which often must be drained. Finally, endocarditis and metastatic infection are a concern in all patients with staphylococcal bacteremia.

Epidemiologic control of staphylococcal infection requires ongoing surveillance and reporting of infections. Contact precautions should be followed in the management of patients with active infections of the skin or wounds. Respiratory precautions may be useful in the management of patients with staphylococcal pneumonia, although droplet spread is much less important than transmission by direct contact. The treatment of nasal or rectal carriers can be frustrating, particularly if the carriers are hospital personnel or persons suffering from recurrent furunculosis. Topical treatment with germicidal soaps, povidone-iodine, or antibiotic ointments has been advocated, but long-term results have been disappointing. Orally administered antibiotics, including rifampin, TMP-SMX, and ciprofloxacin, have also failed to live up to initially promising findings. Bacterial interference, which attempts to replace epidemiologically virulent strains of staphylococci with strains that have been deliberately colonized and are less virulent, has generally been abandoned, in part because infection has been caused by these supposedly less virulent strains. Attempts to develop staphylococcal vaccines are continuing.[79]

Intranasal therapy with mupirocin ointment may help control the staphylococcal carrier state. A naturally occurring antibiotic produced by *P. fluorescens*, mupirocin, inhibits *S. aureus* (including penicillin- and methicillin-resistant strains) and other aerobic gram-positive cocci by binding reversibly to bacterial isoleucyl transfer RNA synthetase; no cross-resistance has been observed between mupirocin and other antibiotics. A placebo-controlled trial of mupirocin in 34 patients who were *S. aureus* carriers found that a monthly course of nasal mupirocin reduced the incidence of nasal colonization and skin infections for at least 1 year. Mupirocin was administered intranasally twice daily for 5 days; side effects were minimal. Additional studies have confirmed the benefits of mupirocin. However, because resistance to mupirocin[76] and recolonization after therapy can occur, indiscriminate use of mupirocin should be avoided. The Food and Drug Administration has approved mupirocin for the topical treatment of impetigo.

Staphylococcal Toxic-Shock Syndrome

Staphylococcal TSS was first reported in 1978; by 1990, more than 3,300 cases had been reported in the United States, 90% of which occurred during menstruation in women who were using tampons. The incidence of staphylococcal TSS declined precipitously after superabsorbable tampons were withdrawn from the market. Currently, fewer than 100 cases occur each year, and nonmenstrual cases occur more often than those associated with menstruation. Many cases are nosocomially acquired, often as a result of postoperative staphylococcal wound infections.

Diagnosis TSS is a multisystem disease with diverse clinical manifestations [*see Table 2*]. Leukocytosis and thrombocytopenia (< 100,000 platelets/mm^3) are common findings. Urinalysis may show mild pyuria and, occasionally, microscopic hematuria. Blood urea nitrogen and creatinine levels are elevated in more than 50% of patients. Serum bilirubin and hepatic enzyme levels are raised in about half of patients. Serum creatine kinase levels are high in more than one third of patients, and myoglobinuria has developed in some patients. Elevated serum amylase levels are also found but may be related to the azotemia rather than to clinically evident pancreatitis. Unexplained marked hypocalcemia is often observed. The drop in serum calcium level is out of proportion to the degree of hypoalbuminuria noted in some patients and may be caused by elevated serum calcitonin levels. Blood cultures show no growth in almost all cases. Group A streptococci can produce a severe form of TSS that resembles staphylococcal TSS, except for

Table 2 Clinical Manifestations of Staphylococcal Toxic-Shock Syndrome

High fever

Scarlatiniform eruption

Hypotension and shock

Desquamation, particularly of palms and soles, during convalescence

MANIFESTATIONS OF SPECIFIC ORGAN INVOLVEMENT

- Mucous membranes: hyperemia of conjunctivae, pharynx, and vagina
- Gastrointestinal tract: vomiting and diarrhea at onset
- Muscle: severe myalgias (elevated serum creatine kinase level; rhabdomyolysis in some patients)
- Central nervous system: toxic encephalopathy (disorientation, delirium, or obtundation in absence of high fever or shock)
- Kidney: azotemia; pyuria in absence of demonstrable urinary tract infection
- Liver: elevations of serum bilirubin and aspartate aminotransferase
- Blood: thrombocytopenia

the paucity of cutaneous manifestations [*see* Streptococcal Toxic-Shock Syndrome, *above*].

Treatment The management of staphylococcal TSS calls for immediate treatment of hypotension and shock with vigorous fluid replacement (and supplemental catecholamines if needed), attention to the site of *S. aureus* colonization or infection (removal of tampon and drainage of any abscess), and systemic antimicrobial therapy with an antistaphylococcal agent. A retrospective analysis of 45 patients suggested that glucocorticoids may assist in recovery, but more data are needed before glucocorticoids can be recommended for all patients with staphylococcal TSS. Most patients recover in 1 to 2 weeks; mortality is about 5%.

COAGULASE-NEGATIVE STAPHYLOCOCCI

S. epidermidis and other coagulase-negative staphylococcal species are organisms of low pathogenic potential that are universally present as part of the normal skin flora. Because of their ubiquity, coagulase-negative staphylococci are frequently isolated from clinical specimens, including blood cultures, but are most often skin contaminants rather than true pathogens; unfortunately, neither clonal variability[80] nor molecular typing[81] can reliably distinguish between contaminants and pathogens. In certain circumstances, however, these organisms can cause significant disease. In the great majority of cases, coagulase-negative staphylococci are opportunistic pathogens, producing infection only in patients with significant underlying medical problems.[82] They most often produce infections in patients with indwelling I.V. catheters or implanted prosthetic devices. Many strains produce an exopolysaccharide that functions as a capsule.[83] This slime layer is an adhesion that binds the organism to implanted devices; it also inhibits the action of antibiotics, further contributing to pathogenicity.

Coagulase-negative staphylococci are now the leading cause of nosocomial bacteremia, which most often result from the use of I.V. catheters, especially centrally placed catheters. Patients with this infection may have signs of phlebitis at the needle or catheter site and may present with persistent low-grade fevers or high-spiking temperature elevations. The I.V. needle or catheter should be removed and a course of parenteral antibiotics administered. Metastatic infection is uncommon but can be serious. These organisms can also be an important cause of bacteremia in immunosuppressed patients. The mortality of patients with coagulase-negative staphylococcal bacteremia approaches 40%, in part because the patients have such serious underlying diseases; mortality attributable to the infection itself is about 13%.

An even more serious problem occurs when *S. epidermidis* or other coagulase-negative staphylococci infect indwelling ventriculoatrial shunts. Patients with this condition may present with bacteremia, meningitis, or both. In addition to high-dose antibiotic therapy, management must often include shunt removal or revision. Vascular grafts and joint prostheses may also become infected. These infections are generally indolent and are more likely to produce pain and joint dysfunction than fever and local inflammatory signs. Diagnosis may be difficult because coagulase-negative staphylococci can be recovered from joint aspirates either as pathogens or contaminants. These organisms can sometimes cause indolent wound infections or osteomyelitis. Here, too, diagnosis may be difficult, but visualization of the staphylococci on Gram stain, their consistent isolation on culture, and the absence of other pathogens should suggest their etiologic role.

The most serious therapeutic problem caused by coagulase-negative staphylococci is prosthetic valve endocarditis. The disease typically has a subacute course, but eradication of the organisms is often very difficult because of antibiotic resistance. Medical therapy with high-dose antibiotics should be attempted, but valve replacement is necessary if infection persists or if significant valve dysfunction occurs. Mortality is high, approaching 50% with or without surgical therapy. Coagulase-negative staphylococci may also cause endocarditis on native valves.[82]

Antibiotic therapy for deep-seated coagulase-negative staphylococcal infections is difficult. Many strains are resistant to methicillin and other semisynthetic penicillins. Whereas most strains appear to be sensitive to cephalosporins on disk diffusion testing, these results correlate poorly with actual bactericidal activity. Vancomycin, gentamicin, and rifampin are bactericidal against most coagulase-negative staphylococci. Vancomycin or rifampin resistance is rare but may emerge during therapy. Vancomycin is generally the drug of choice, but for serious infections, the addition of rifampin or gentamicin should be strongly considered. Linezolid and quinupristin-dalfopristin have been effective, but experience with these new antimicrobials is limited.

S. saprophyticus is a coagulase-negative member of the normal skin flora that can be distinguished from *S. epidermidis* by its resistance to the antibiotic novobiocin. Previously dismissed as a nonpathogen, *S. saprophyticus* is now clearly recognized to be an important cause of urinary tract infections. *S. saprophyticus* is second only to *E. coli* as a cause of cystitis in sexually active young women, accounting for 11% of all bladder infections encountered in one university health service. *S. saprophyticus* is much less likely to produce infections in men; however, *S. saprophyticus* commonly infects elderly men who have undergone urinary tract instrumentation. The clinical features of *S. saprophyticus* infections resemble those of other urinary tract infections; bacteremia and systemic toxicity are rare even when upper urinary tract infection occurs. *S. saprophyticus* is sensitive to most antimicrobial agents that are used to treat urinary tract infections.

References

1. Gillespie SH, Balakrishnan I: Pathogenesis of pneumococcal infection. J Med Microbiol 49:1057, 2000

2. Obaro SK, Monteil MA, Henderson DC: The pneumococcal problem. BMJ 312:1521, 1996

3. Nuroti JP, Butler JC, Farley MM, et al: Cigarette smoking and invasive pneumococcal disease. N Engl J Med 342:681, 2000

4. Dean N: Pneumococcus is number one. Am J Med 106:486, 1999

5. Feikin DR, Schuchat A, Kolczak M, et al: Mortality from invasive pneumococcal pneumonia in the era of antibiotic resistance, 1995–1997. Am J Public Health 90:223, 2000

6. Mufson MA, Stanek RJ: Bacteremic pneumococcal pneumonia in one American city: a 20-year longitudinal study, 1978–1997. Am J Med 107(1A):34S, 1999

7. Fiore AE, Moroney JF, Farley MM, et al: Clinical outcomes of meningitis caused by *Streptococcus pneumoniae* in the era of antibiotic resistance. Clin Infect Dis 30:71, 2000

8. Rubins JB, Cheung S, Carson P, et al: Identification of clinical risk factors for nosocomial pneumococcal bacteremia. Clin Infect Dis 29:178, 1999

9. O'Brien KL, Walters MI, Sellman J, et al: Severe pneumococcal pneumonia in previously healthy children: the role of preceding influenza infection. Clin Infect Dis 30:784, 2000

10. Osler W: The Principles and Practice of Medicine: Designed for the Use of Practitioners and Students of Medicine. D Appleton & Co, New York, 1892, p 517

11. Dowell SF, Garman RL, Liu G, et al: Evaluation of binax NOW, an assay for the detection of pneumococcal antigen in urine samples, performed among pediatric patients. Clin Infect Dis 32:824, 2001

12. Harrison LH, Dwyer DM, Billmann L, et al: Invasive pneumococcal infection in Baltimore, MD: implications for immunization policy. Arch Intern Med 160:89, 2000

13. Dworkin MS, Ward JW, Hanson DL, et al: Pneumococcal disease among human immunodeficiency virus-infected persons: incidence, risk factors, and impact of vaccination. Clin Infect Dis 32:794, 2001

14. Breiman RF, Keller DW, Phelan MA, et al: Evaluation of effectiveness of the 23-valent pneumococcal capsular polysaccharide vaccine for HIV-infected patients. Arch Intern Med 160:2633, 2000

15. Siegel M, Timpone J: Penicillin-resistant *Streptococcus pneumoniae* endocarditis: a case report and review. Clin Infect Dis 32:972, 2001

16. Tomasz A: New faces of an old pathogen: emergence and spread of multidrug-resistant *Streptococcus pneumoniae*. Am J Med 107(1A):55S, 1999

17. Whitney CG, Farley M, Hadler J, et al: Increasing prevalence of multidrug-resistant *Streptococcus pneumoniae* in the United States. N Engl J Med 343:1917, 2000

18. Metlay JP, Hofmann J, Cetron MS, et al: Impact of penicillin susceptibility on medical outcomes for adult patients with bacteremic pneumococcal pneumonia. Clin Infect Dis 30:520, 2000

19. Normark BH, Novak R, Ortqvist A, et al: Clinical isolates of *Streptococcus pneumoniae* that exhibit tolerance of vancomycin. Clin Infect Dis 32:552, 2001

20. Ho PL, Tse WS, Tsang KWT, et al: Risk factors for acquisition of levofloxacin-resistant *Streptococcus pneumoniae*: a case-control study. Clin Infect Dis 32:701, 2001

21. Plouffe JF: Emerging therapies for serious gram-positive bacterial infections: a focus on linezolid. Clin Infect Dis 31(suppl 4):S144, 2000

22. Ball P: Therapy for pneumococcal infection at the millennium: doubts and certainties. Am J Med 107(1A):77S, 1999

23. Ramirez JA, Bordon J: Early switch from intravenous to oral antibiotics in hospitalized patients with bacteremic community-acquired *Streptococcus pneumoniae* pneumonia. Arch Intern Med 161:848, 2001

24. Recommendations of the Advisory Committee on Immunization Practices (ACIP): Preventing pneumococcal disease among infants and young children. MMWR Morb Mortal Wkly Rep 49:1, 2000

25. Blumberg EA, Brozena SC, Stutman P, et al: Immunogenicity of pneumococcal vaccine in heart transplant recipients. Clin Infect Dis 32: 307, 2001

26. Recommendations of the Advisory Committee on Immunization Practices (ACIP): Prevention of pneumococcal disease. MMWR Morb Mortal Wkly Rep 46:1, 1997

27. Ament A, Baltussen R, Duru G, et al: Cost-effectiveness of pneumococcal vaccination of older people: a study of 5 Western European countries. Clin Infect Dis 31:444, 2000

28. Eskola J, Kilpi T, Palmu A, et al: Efficacy of a pneumococcal conjugate vaccine against acute otitis media. N Engl J Med 344:403, 2001

29. Mufson MA: Antibody response of pneumococcal vaccine: need for booster dosing? Int J Antimicrob Agents 14:107, 2000

30. Jackson LA, Benson P, Sneller V-P, et al: Safety of revaccination with pneumococcal polysaccharide vaccine. JAMA 281:243, 1999

31. Carapetis JR, Currie BJ, Kaplan EL: Epidemiology and prevention of group A streptococcal infections: acute respiratory tract infections, skin infections, and their sequelae at the close of the twentieth century. Clin Infect Dis 28:205, 1999

32. Bisno AL, Gerber MA, Gwaltney JM, et al: Diagnosis and management of group A streptococcal pharyngitis: a practice guideline. Clin Infect Dis 25:574, 1997

33. De Quirós JCLB, Moreno S, Cercenado E, et al: Group A streptococcal bacteremia: a 10-year prospective study. Medicine (Baltimore) 76: 238, 1997

34. Baddour LM: Infective endocarditis caused by α-hemolytic streptococci. The Infectious Diseases Society of America's Emerging Infections Network. Clin Infect Dis 26:66, 1998

35. Sommer R, Rohner P, Garbino J, et al: Group A β-hemolytic streptococcus meningitis: clinical and microbiological features of nine cases. Clin Infect Dis 29:929, 1999

36. Dupuy A, Benchikhi H, Roujeau J-C, et al: Risk factors for erysipelas of the leg (cellulitis): case-control study. BMJ 318:1591, 1999

37. Bisno AL, Stevens DL: Streptococcal infections of skin and soft tissues. N Engl J Med 334:240, 1996

38. Kaul R, McGeer A, Low DE, et al: Population-based surveillance for group A streptococcal necrotizing fasciitis: clinical features, prognostic indicators, and microbiologic analysis of seventy-seven cases. Am J Med 103:18, 1997

39. Zurawski CA, Bardsley M, Beall B, et al: Invasive group A streptococcal disease in metropolitan Atlanta: a population-based assessment. Clin Infect Dis 27:150, 1998

40. Stevens DL: The flesh-eating bacterium: what's next? J Infect Dis 179(suppl 2):S366, 1999

41. Kaul R, McGeer A, Norrby-Teglund A, et al: Intravenous immunoglobulin therapy for streptococcal toxic shock syndrome—a comparative observational study. Clin Infect Dis 28:800, 1999

42. Stollerman GH: Rheumatic fever. Lancet 349:935, 1997

43. Williamson L, Bowness P, Mowat A, et al: Lesson of the week: difficulties in diagnosing acute rheumatic fever—arthritis may be short lived and carditis silent. BMJ 320:362, 2000

44. Adam D, Scholz H, Helmerking M: Short-course antibiotic treatment of 4782 culture-proven cases of group A streptococcal tonsillopharyngitis and incidence of poststreptococcal sequellae. J Infect Dis 182:509, 2000

45. Lan AJ, Colford JM Jr: The impact of dosing frequency on the efficacy of 10-day penicillin or amoxicillin therapy for streptococcal tonsillopharyngitis: meta-analysis. Pediatrics 105:E19, 2000

46. Eriksson BKG: Anal colonization of group G β-hemolytic streptococci in relapsing erysipelas of the lower extremity. Clin Infect Dis 29: 1319, 1999

47. Hirose Y, Yagi K, Honda H, et al: Toxic shock-like syndrome caused by non-group Xβ-hemolytic streptococci. Arch Intern Med 157: 1891, 1997

48. Krohn MA, Hillier SL, Baker CJ: Maternal peripartum complications associated with vaginal group B streptococci colonization. J Infect Dis 179:1410, 1999

49. Schrag SJ, Zywicki S, Farley MM, et al: Group B streptococcal disease in the era of intrapartum antibiotic prophylaxis. N Engl J Med 342: 15, 2000

50. Henning KJ, Hall EL, Dwyer DM, et al: Invasive group B streptococcal disease in Maryland nursing home residents. J Infect Dis 183: 1138, 2001

51. Gardam MA, Low DE, Saginur R, et al: Group B streptococcal necrotizing fasciitis and streptococcal toxic shock-like syndrome in adults. Arch Intern Med 158:1704, 1998

52. Kupferwasser I, Darius H, Muller AM, et al: Clinical and morphological characteristics in *Streptococcus bovis* endocarditis: a comparison with other causative microorganisms in 177 cases. Heart 80:276, 1998

53. Shenep JL: Viridans-group streptococcal infections in immunocompromised hosts. Int J Antimicrob Agents 14:129, 2000

54. Cabellos C, Viladrich PF, Corredoira J, et al: Steptococcal meningitis in adult patients: current epidemiology and clinical spectrum. Clin Infect Dis 28:1104, 1999

55. Bert F, Bariou-Lancelin M, Lambert-Zechovsky N: Clinical significance of bacteremia involving the "Streptococcus milleri" group: 51 cases and review. Clin Infect Dis 27:385, 1998

56. Murray BE: Vancomycin-resistant enterococcal infections. N Engl J Med 342:710, 2000

57. Donskey CJ, Chowdhry TK, Hecker MT, et al: Effect of antibiotic therapy on the density of vancomycin-resistant enterococci in the stool of colonized patients. N Engl J Med 343:1925, 2000

58. Caballero-Granado FJ, Becerril B, Cuberos L, et al: Attributable mortality rate and duration of hospital stay associated with enterococcal bacteremia. Clin Infect Dis 32:587, 2001

59. Winston DJ, Emmanouilides C, Kroeber A, et al: Quinupristin/dalfopristin therapy for infections due to vancomycin-resistant *Enterococcus faecium*. Clin Infect Dis 30:790, 2000

60. Tenorio AL, Badri SM, Sahgal NB, et al: Effectiveness of gloves in the prevention of hand carriage of vancomycin-resistant *Enterococcus* species by health care workers after patient care. Clin Infect Dis 32:826, 2001

61. Lowy FD: *Staphylococcus aureus* infections. N Engl J Med 339:520, 1998

62. von Eiff C, Becker K, Machka K, et al: Nasal carriage as a source of *Staphylococcus aureus* bacteremia. N Engl J Med 344:11, 2001

63. Fridkin SK: Vancomycin-intermediate and -resistant *Staphylococcus aureus*: what the infectious disease specialist needs to know. Clin Infect Dis 32:108, 2001

64. Murdoch DR, Roberts SA, Fowler VG Jr, et al: Infection of orthopedic prostheses after *Staphylococcus aureus* bacteremia. Clin Infect Dis 32: 647, 2001

65. Gonzalez C, Rubio M, Romero-Vivas J, et al: Bacteremic pneumonia due to *Staphylococcus aureus*: a comparison of disease caused by methicillin-resistant and methicillin-susceptible organisms. Clin Infect Dis 29:1171, 1999

66. Mylotte MJ, Tayara A: *Staphylococcus aureus* bacteremia: predictors of 30-day mortality in a large cohort. Clin Infect Dis 31:1170, 2000

67. Jensen AG, Wachmann CH, Poulsen KB, et al: Risk factors for hospital-acquired *Staphylococcus aureus* bacteremia. Arch Intern Med 159: 1437, 1999

68. Wilson R, Hamburger M: Fifteen years' experience with *Staphylococcus* septicemia in a large city hospital: analysis of fifty-five cases in the Cincinnati General Hospital, 1940 to 1954. Am J Med 22:437, 1957

69. Nolan CM, Beaty HN: *Staphylococcus aureus* bacteremia: current clinical patterns. Am J Med 60:495, 1976

70. Rader BL, Wandall DA, Frimodt-Moller N, et al: Clinical features of *Staphylococcus aureus* endocarditis: a 10-year experience in Denmark. Arch Intern Med 159:462, 1999

71. Fowler VG Jr, Sanders LL, Kong LK, et al: Infective endocarditis due to *Staphylococcus aureus*: 59 prospectively identified cases with follow-up. Clin Infect Dis 28:106, 1999

72. Tornos P, Almirante B, Mirabet S, et al: Infective endocarditis due to *Staphylococcus aureus*: deleterious effect of anticoagulant therapy. Arch Intern Med 159:473, 1999

73. Lu C-H, Chang W-N: Adults with meningitis caused by oxacillin-resistant *Staphylococcus aureus*. Clin Infect Dis 31:723, 2000

74. Gorak EJ, Yamada SM, Brown JD: Community-acquired methicillin-resistant *Staphylococcus aureus* in hospitalized adults and children without known risk factors. Clin Infect Dis 29:797, 1999

75. Kotilainen P, Routamaa M, Peltonen R, et al: Eradication of methicillin-resistant *Staphylococcus aureus* from a health center ward and associated nursing home. Arch Intern Med 161:859, 2001

76. Harbarth S, Liassine N, Dharan S, et al: Risk factors for persistent carriage of methicillin-resistant *Staphylococcus aureus*. Clin Infect Dis 31:1380, 2000

77. Soriano A, Martinez JA, Mensa J, et al: Pathogenic significance of methicillin resistance for patients with *Staphylococcus aureus* bacteremia. Clin Infect Dis 30:368, 2000

78. Wenzel RP, Edmond MB: Vancomycin-resistant *Staphylococcus aureus*: infection control considerations. Clin Infect Dis 27:245, 1998

79. McKenney D, Poullot KL, Wang Y, et al: Broadly protective vaccine for *Staphylococcus aureus* based on an in vivo-expressed antigen. Science 284:1523, 1999

80. Van Eldere J, Peetermans WE, Struelens M, et al: Polyclonal staphylococcal endocarditis caused by genetic variability. Clin Infect Dis 31:24, 2000

81. Seo SK, Venkataraman L, DeGirolami PC, et al: Molecular typing of coagulase-negative staphylococci from blood cultures does not correlate with clinical criteria for true bacteremia. Am J Med 109:697, 2000

82. Proctor RA: Editorial response: coagulase-negative staphylococcal infections: a diagnostic and therapeutic challenge. Clin Infect Dis 31:31, 2000

83. Fey PD, Ulphani JS, Gotz F, et al: Characterization of the relationship between polysaccharide intercellular adhesion and hemagglutination in *Staphylococcus epidermidis*. J Infect Dis 179:1561, 1999

16 Infections Due to Gram-Positive Bacilli

Frederick S. Southwick, M.D.

Diphtheria

Diphtheria derives its name from the Greek word *diphtheria*, meaning leather hide, which is the character of the pharyngeal membrane that is a hallmark of this disease. Once the cause of major epidemics in Europe and the United States, diphtheria was nearly eradicated by medical discoveries in the late 1800s and early 1900s. Conditions in both developing and developed countries have led to several recent outbreaks and have raised concerns that diphtheria may again become a serious public health problem.

MICROBIOLOGY

Diphtheria is caused by *Corynebacterium diphtheriae*, a gram-positive rod with club-shaped swellings at each end. It is nonmotile and is capable of growing on blood agar plates, causing a narrow band of hemolysis. Most strains produce a highly lethal exotoxin, whose production requires the presence of a bacteriophage that carries a specific determinant for toxin production. The organism produces characteristic metachromatic granules that stain bluish purple with methylene blue. Their snapping division results in angular and palisade arrangements of the cells on smear that frequently take on the appearance of Chinese lettering.[1]

ETIOLOGY AND EPIDEMIOLOGY

Humans are the only natural host for *C. diphtheriae*. The organism is most commonly spread by upper respiratory tract droplets. Persons incubating the disease, those convalescing from the infection, and healthy carriers can spread the disease to others through close contact. Spread is more common during the colder months of the year, when people tend to be crowded indoors.[2] Patients with *C. diphtheriae* skin lesions can also serve as reservoirs for the organism, and contamination of the environment tends to be greater from skin infection than from upper respiratory tract infection.[3] Because the organism can survive as long as 6 months in fomites and dust, these objects and particles can serve as vehicles for transmission.

Diphtheria toxoid immunization prevents the serious complications of diphtheria, alleviating the clinical manifestations of the disease by blocking the toxin's ability to enter cells. Immunization reduces local colonization of the nasopharynx with toxin-producing strains by reducing their survival advantage. In the United States, with the advent of widespread vaccine administration in the 1940s, the carrier state has dropped to very low levels, and the incidence of diphtheria has steadily declined. Before the initiation of the vaccination program, as many as 125,000 cases and 10,000 deaths were reported annually in the United States. Subsequently, the incidence declined to zero to five cases a year from 1980 to 1990. History indicates that diphtheria outbreaks occur in cycles that may include quiescent periods of up to 100 years. Therefore, the downturn in incidence may represent a normal cycle rather than herd immunity. Occasional outbreaks have been observed in Texas, Washington, and South Dakota.[4] Two outbreaks were associated with urban alcoholics who practiced poor hygiene and lived in crowded environments; a third occurred in a Native American community. Day care centers can also serve as a site for the spread of diphtheria. Outbreaks that recently occurred in Russia (15,211 cases) and the Ukraine (2,987 cases) are thought to have resulted from the decreased immunization of infants and children, as well as because of waning immunity to diphtheria in older people.[5] The resurgence of diphtheria in developed countries raises concern that reductions in the immunization of young children and the failure to revaccinate older adults could lead to a worldwide increase in the incidence of this very serious disease.

PATHOGENESIS

C. diphtheriae attaches to mucosal surfaces, particularly in the nasopharynx. Ocular and genital mucosae are less often infected. The skin has become an increasingly common site of infection, particularly in the United States. The diphtheria bacillus rarely invades living tissue but generally remains in superficial layers of the mucosa and skin. The major manifestations of this often serious disease result from production of a potent exotoxin. When iron concentrations are low, diphtheria bacilli possessing the corynebacteriophage containing the *tox* gene produce high concentrations of the toxin. This protein has a molecular weight of 62,000 and consists of two major fragments, designated A and B. Fragment B binds to a specific host cell membrane receptor, resulting in endocytosis of the entire molecule. Once the toxin is in the endosome, acidification alters the conformation of the B fragment, and the hydrophobic domain of the B fragment forms a membrane channel that allows passage of fragment A into the host cell cytoplasm.[6] Fragment A then blocks protein synthesis and causes cell death within hours [*see Figure 1*]. Antitoxin antibody can neutralize toxin adsorbed to cells or the extracellular fluid. However, once the toxin penetrates cells, its toxic effects are irreversible.

In the host, the cytotoxic effects of the toxin are most marked in regions where bacterial growth is heavy and toxin concentrations are highest. Tissue necrosis is associated with an inflammatory response, leading to the formation of an adherent membrane that is greenish-gray to black and consists of fibrin, necrotic tissue, lymphocytes, polymorphonuclear leukocytes, erythrocytes, and bacterial colonies. All cells are susceptible to the lethal effects of the toxin; however, the heart, kidneys, and nervous system are injured most often.

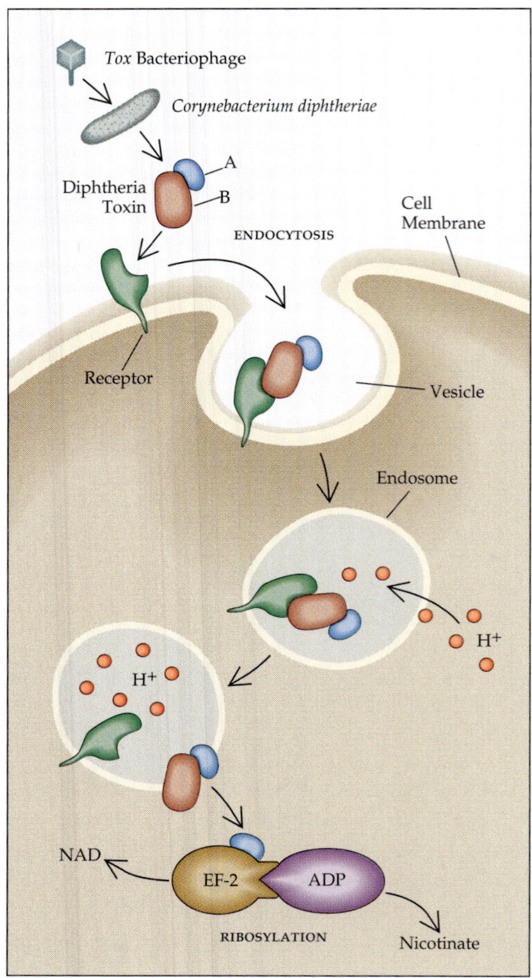

Figure 1 **Diphtheria toxin production is encoded by a bacteriophage carrying the *tox* gene that gains entry into *Corynebacterium diphtheriae*. The toxin consists of an A fragment and a B fragment. The B fragment binds to the receptor (heparin-binding epidermal growth factor precursor) on the cell surface, and the whole molecule is then taken into the cell by endocytosis. In the closed environment of the endosome, acidification occurs (H^+). The low pH level causes the B region to unfold and form a membrane channel, allowing the A domain to pass through the membrane into the cytoplasm. The disulfide bond linking the A and B regions is reduced, and the A subunit is then freed to bind with and to ADP-ribosylate elongation factor–2 (EF-2). Ribosylation interferes with the ability of EF-2 to add amino acids to a peptide chain, blocking protein synthesis and causing cell death. (A—A fragment; B—B fragment; NAD—nicotinamide adenine dinucleotide; ADP—adenosine diphosphate)**

CLINICAL MANIFESTATIONS

The incubation period for respiratory diphtheria is generally 2 to 4 days but can be as long as 7 days. Infection is usually associated with low-grade fever (approximately 38° C [100.4° F]), and systemic complaints early in the infection often are minimal. Symptoms depend on the location and duration of the infection before treatment. Concentrations of bacteria increase over time, resulting in the release of increasing amounts of the cytotoxic exotoxin. Early recognition and treatment are therefore critical for reducing the complications associated with toxin dissemination.

Respiratory Tract Infection

Pharyngeal infection, the most common form of diphtheria, presents as a sore throat and malaise. Symptoms may be mild in vaccinated patients, whereas unvaccinated patients tend to have more severe disease. Initially, diphtheria pharyngitis results in the development of a patchy white exudate that can be readily removed and is indistinguishable from group A streptococcal or viral pharyngitis. However, as the toxin begins to cause cell necrosis, a thin membrane begins to form that progressively thickens and spreads over the tonsils, posterior pharynx, and uvula [*see Figure 2*]. Initially, the membrane is white and smooth but later becomes gray, with patches of green and black necrosis. Particularly in children, the membrane can spread from the posterior wall up into the nose or down to the larynx or even the tracheobronchial tree. As the membrane spreads, it can interfere with normal airflow and lead to suffocation. Such extensive spread is generally associated with increased release of exotoxin, resulting in myocardial and neurologic complications and greatly increasing mortality. Laryngeal involvement results in hoarseness and may serve as a warning of impending respiratory compromise.[7] Less often, the membrane may be limited to the nasopharynx, causing a serosanguineous nasal discharge. Such limited involvement is less likely to be associated with generalized toxicity. Patients without the presence of the membrane, demonstrating only pharyngeal erythema, almost always have milder, uncomplicated disease. Other clinical manifestations include tachycardia, cervical adenopathy, leukocytosis, and proteinuria. Development of the classic bull neck, the result of massive adenopathy, is now uncommon.

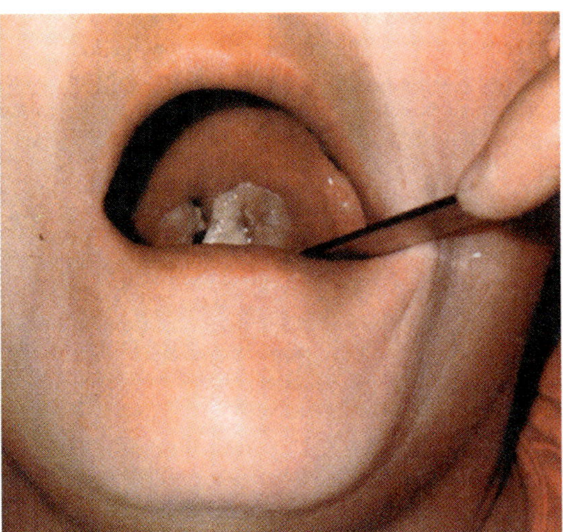

Figure 2 **Diphtheritic membrane extending across the uvula in a 47-year-old female. Neck edema also has developed.**[7]

Cutaneous Diphtheria

Although outbreaks of cutaneous diphtheria were originally described primarily in tropical areas, outbreaks over the past 3 decades have been reported in the Pacific Northwest, Midwest, and southern United States. Cutaneous infection may result in greater environmental contamination than respiratory diphtheria and may carry a greater risk of spread to others. Unlike pharyngeal diphtheria, which usually develops in the winter months, cutaneous infections tend to peak in the late summer and early fall. Most cases are reported among residents of Seattle's Skid Road district, who practice poor hygiene and often have preexisting sores.[8] Skin infections have also been described in young schoolchildren. The classic punched-out ulcerative lesion often found in the tropics is rare in temperate climates. When the lesion does develop, it generally begins as a pustule that progresses to an ulcer with a gray-brown membrane at its base. More commonly, diphtheria superinfects preexisting skin lesions, including traumatic breaks in the skin, insect bites, ecthyma, and impetigo. In association with *C. diphtheriae*, other skin pathogens, particularly *Staphylococcus* and *Streptococcus*, are found on culture. These infections tend to be indolent and are rarely associated with signs of intoxication, probably because cutaneous infections induce high levels of antitoxin antibody.

Other Sites of Infection

Less often, *C. diphtheriae* infects the conjunctiva, eye, ear, and vagina. In Seattle, ocular infections in Skid Road residents sometimes accompanied skin involvement.

Complications

Systemic complications are caused by release of the diphtheria exotoxin, which predominantly damages the heart and nervous system.

Myocarditis Subtle evidence of myocarditis is found in up to two thirds of patients with respiratory diphtheria.[9] Clinically significant cardiac dysfunction is observed in 10% to 20% of patients. The severity of cardiac compromise correlates with the extent and severity of respiratory tract involvement.

Cardiac toxicity generally occurs within 1 to 2 weeks after onset of the illness, often when pharyngeal symptoms are improving. The electrocardiogram generally reflects the severity of myocardial involvement and should be followed closely in all cases. ST segment and T wave changes and first-degree heart block are found in less severe disease, whereas left bundle branch block and AV block are associated with high mortality. In addition to causing damage to the Purkinje system, toxin causes necrosis of cardiac muscle cells that can result in acute congestive heart failure and circulatory collapse. A poor outcome is more likely in patients with extensive pharyngeal membrane and an aspartate aminotransferase level above 80 IU/L.[10] Recovery in more severe cases of myocarditis can result in normalization of the ECG; however, patients usually sustain permanent injury to the myocardium.

Neurologic toxicity Neurologic complications occur in approximately 10% of respiratory cases. As observed with myocardial involvement, the likelihood of neurologic involvement correlates with the severity of the respiratory infection. Symptoms develop 10 to 28 days after the onset of respiratory complaints. Two types of neuropathy are seen. The first, cranial nerve involvement, is generally limited to the ninth and 10th nerves, resulting in difficulty swallowing, aspiration, nasal regurgitation, and loss of the gag reflex. Less often, oculomotor and facial nerves become impaired. The second type of neuropathy tends to occur somewhat later in the course of the illness and resembles Guillain-Barré syndrome. Patients have quadriparesis associated with hyporeflexia. Degeneration of myelin sheaths and axon cylinders is observed in biopsy specimens. After treatment of the infection, slow but complete neurologic recovery ensues.[11]

DIAGNOSIS

Prompt recognition and treatment of respiratory diphtheria are critical for preventing complications and mortality. In the early stages, diphtheria pharyngitis mimics group A streptococcal pharyngitis and mononucleosis. As diphtheria progresses, unlike in pharyngitis and mononucleosis, the exudate changes, becoming darker and forming a membrane that cannot be removed without causing bleeding. Neurologic abnormalities, such as ninth and 10th nerve deficits or ECG changes, should also alert the clinician to the possibility of diphtheria. The microbiology laboratory staff must be notified of the possibility of *C. diphtheriae* because normal throat flora usually overgrow on blood agar plates. Nonnutritive, moist, reducing transport medium is helpful in preventing the overgrowth of competitors, and samples need to be inoculated on Löffler and tellurite media for proper identification. Assays for diphtheria toxin production also need to be performed.

TREATMENT

All patients in whom a clinical diagnosis of respiratory diphtheria is determined should be hospitalized and isolated because the course of illness is unpredictable. Rapid institution of antiserum is of primary importance. The sooner diphtheria antitoxin is administered, the more favorable the outcome. Antitoxin is most effective if given within 4 days after the onset of illness. The antibody blocks entry of toxin into cells and therefore is effective only in neutralizing toxin in the extracellular space before entry into the cytoplasm. Dosage of antitoxin is adjusted to the severity of disease. Patients with extensive involvement of the tonsils and pharynx or larynx who are expected to have higher concentrations of toxin should be given at least half the treatment dose of antitoxin by intravenous infusion over 60 minutes. If extensive disease has been present for 3 or more days or if a bull neck has developed, 80,000 to 120,000 U is recommended. For milder disease of shorter duration (48 hours or less), 20,000 to 40,000 U may be used. Antitoxin is given once; repeated doses provide no added benefit. Because antiserum is derived from horse serum, approximately 10% of patients have an allergic reaction. If skin or eye testing demonstrates hypersensitivity, desensitization should be attempted.

Antibiotic Treatment

Antibiotic therapy should be initiated as soon as possible and serves three purposes: (1) it shuts off toxin production; (2) it eradicates other potential pharyngeal pathogens, including group A streptococci; and (3) it eliminates the carrier state, preventing the spread of *C. diphtheriae* to other nonimmunized persons. Erythromycin (500 mg four times a day for 2 weeks) is considered the treatment of choice. Penicillin, given intramuscularly (600,000 U twice a day) until the patient is able to swallow, is also effective. The patient is then switched to penicillin V (250 mg p.o. four times a day) for the remainder of the 2-week therapy. A study of Vietnamese children found penicillin to be more efficacious than erythromycin.[12] *C. diphtheriae* is generally susceptible to clindamycin and rifampin. However, there has been less experience with the use of these antimicrobial agents.

Table 1 Clinical Syndromes Caused by Nondiphtheria *Corynebacterium* Species

Species	*Clinical Syndrome*	*Treatment of Choice*
C. ulcerans	Pharyngitis, skin ulcer, diphtheria	Erythromycin
C. pseudotuberculosis (C. ovis)	Suppurative lymphadenitis	Erythromycin or tetracycline
C. (Arcanobacterium) haemolyticum	Pharyngitis, scarlatiniform rash	Erythromycin, penicillin, clindamycin, or tetracycline
C. pseudodiphtheriticum (C. hofmannii)	Endocarditis, pneumonia, tracheobronchitis, lymphadenitis	Variable sensitivities
C. urealyticum (formerly group D2)	Alkaline-encrusted cystitis, urinary tract infections	Vancomycin
C. jeikeium (group JK)	Nosocomial septicemia, wound infection, endocarditis	Vancomycin
Rhodococcus equi (C. equi)	Necrotizing pneumonia in patients with acquired immunodeficiency syndrome	Erythromycin plus rifampin

Other Measures

Extensive pharyngeal and laryngeal membrane formation can lead to upper airway obstruction. Therefore, patients need to be closely monitored, and if signs of obstruction are detected, prompt intubation or tracheostomy must be performed. Sedatives may obscure the development of respiratory difficulties and should be avoided. Patients with myocarditis need cardiac monitoring and should initially be kept at bed rest. Treatment of congestive heart failure with digoxin may result in further impairment of electrical conduction and lead to heart block. Experience with cardiac pacemakers is limited, but pacemakers would be expected to reduce mortality from complete heart block.

Isolation and Treatment of the Carrier State

When diphtheria is suspected, the patient should be isolated until two cultures from the infected site are negative. Cultures should be obtained from all persons who have been in close contact with the patient to determine if they are pharyngeal carriers. All carriers need to be treated with erythromycin or penicillin for 14 days, and eradication of the carrier state must be documented by follow-up cultures.

PREVENTION

Active immunization using formalin-detoxified diphtheria toxin effectively prevents diphtheria. Preschool children (6 weeks to 7 years of age) should be immunized with three 0.5 ml intramuscular injections of diphtheria-pertussis-tetanus (DPT) vaccine spaced 4 to 8 weeks apart. A fourth dose should be given 6 to 12 months later. Immunity to the toxin is not lifelong, and if primary immunization was completed before 4 years of age, a booster is recommended at the time of school entry. Subsequently, booster injections need to be given every 10 years to maintain protective immunity. A single dose of vaccine is sufficient for most age groups, with the exception of persons 30 to 49 years of age, who may require three doses to generate protective antibody titers.[13] Surveys indicate that high percentages of adults in the United States and Europe fail to demonstrate a significant immune response to diphtheria toxoid. It has been estimated that epidemic diphtheria is favored when more than 70% of the population lacks protective immunity, a condition now present in many developed countries. A toxoid booster inoculation every 10 years is strongly recommended for all adults.

Nondiphtheria *Corynebacterium* and *Rhodococcus*

The genus *Corynebacterium*, in addition to diphtheria, contains a large number of organisms that for decades were considered to be culture contaminants and constituents of the normal human flora. These organisms were previously termed *diphtheroids*. As the number of immunocompromised hosts and persons with prosthetic devices has increased, the role of nondiphtheria corynebacteria as true pathogens has become evident[14] [*see Table 1*]. *C. urealyticum* and *C. jeikeium* are two nondiphtheria strains that are particularly important nosocomial pathogens.

C. UREALYTICUM

C. urealyticum, formerly a group D2 organism, is a slow-growing, urease-positive organism that is widely distributed on the skin of hospitalized patients. *C. urealyticum* is one cause of alkaline-encrusted cystitis, a urinary tract infection that is severe and difficult to treat.[15] The urea-splitting activity of the organism leads to an alkaline urine pH and the formation of struvite stones. Factors that predispose an individual to this infection include previous urinary tract infection urologic instrumentation, immunosuppression, underlying inflammation of the bladder, and bladder neoplasia. Less commonly, *C. urealyticum* can cause septicemia, endocarditis, osteomyelitis, and pneumonia. This organism is often resistant to most antibiotics; therefore, vancomycin is recommended for initial treatment pending sensitivity testing.

C. JEIKEIUM

C. jeikeium is a group JK organism that colonizes the skin of hospitalized patients. Patients at highest risk for colonization and subsequent infection with *C. jeikeium* include those receiving broad-spectrum antibiotics and those requiring prolonged hospitalization. In patients with neoplastic disease, other risk factors include prolonged neutropenia and breaks in the integument.[16] In most patients, infection presents as bacteremia. The incidence is highest in neutropenic patients and those who have undergone cardiac surgery.[14] Bacteremia is most often associated with an intravenous catheter. Prosthetic and native valve endocarditis have been reported, as have rare cases of extravascular infections, including cutaneous lesions, pneumonia, peritonitis, prosthetic knee infection, and ventriculostomy infection. Most isolates of this organism tend to be multiply resistant and frequently are sensitive only to vancomycin.[17] In patients with prosthetic valve infection, the foreign material often has to be removed to control the infection.

RHODOCOCCUS EQUI

Rhodococcus equi, also known as *C. equi*, primarily infects immunocompromised hosts with defects in cell-mediated immunity, particularly patients with AIDS[18] and those with solid organ transplants.[19] Cases in normal hosts have also been reported.[20] *R. equi* is found in the soil, and infection is generally acquired through the lungs. The primary manifestation in most cases is cavitary lung disease resembling tuberculosis, nocardiosis, or fungal infection. Lung consolidation without cavitation is also seen. Bronchoscopy, thoracentesis, or surgery may be required to make the diagnosis, although blood cultures are frequently positive.[18] The infection may be mistaken for contaminating diphtheroids or, because *R. equi* organisms are modified acid-fast positive, may be misdiagnosed as tuberculosis. Extrapulmonary infections may also occur. Erythromycin and rifampin act synergistically in combination, and this regimen is recommended. Short courses of therapy are associated with relapse; therefore, therapy needs to be continued for many weeks. The organism is also sensitive to vancomycin and aminoglycosides. Cephalosporins should be avoided because of the frequent development of resistance, and multidrug resistance is becoming more common.[21] Mortality in AIDS patients is approximately 15%; however, half of the patients are never completely cured of *R. equi* infection.[18]

Listeriosis

Listeria monocytogenes, a foodborne pathogen, is the cause of listeriosis, a serious and often fatal infection. Listeriosis varies in its clinical presentation; primary manifestations most often are sepsis, meningitis, or both.

MICROBIOLOGY

L. monocytogenes is an aerobic and facultatively anaerobic, non–spore-forming, gram-positive rod. As opposed to corynebacteria, this organism is motile, possessing one to five flagella. *Listeria* organisms grow at a wide range of temperatures (3° to 42° C), which explains its ability to contaminate refrigerated foods. This bacterium can also grow at acidic concentrations of pH 5 or higher and salt concentrations as high as 10% to 12%. *Listeria* organisms can be readily cultured on blood agar plates, where they cause slight zones of β-hemolysis. Gram stains of cerebrospinal fluid may be mistaken for diphtheroids or *Streptococcus pneumoniae* because *Listeria* organisms on occasion can appear somewhat coccoid. There are at least 11 serotypes of *L. monocytogenes*. Serotypes 1b and 4b are most commonly associated with listeriosis.

ETIOLOGY AND EPIDEMIOLOGY

L. monocytogenes is found in soil, dust fertilizer, sewage, stream water, plants, processed foods, and the intestinal tract of many mammals. Investigations of multiple outbreaks indicate that both sporadic and common source outbreaks of listeriosis are the result of food contamination.[7] Outbreaks have been linked to raw vegetables, Mexican-style cheese, milk, undercooked chicken, and foods purchased in delicatessens.[22] Prepared refrigerated foods stored for prolonged periods and requiring no further high-temperature heating are most likely to be contaminated because *Listeria* organisms can readily multiply on refrigerated foods.

The overall incidence of listeriosis is low: 0.7 cases per 100,000 population. This infection more often

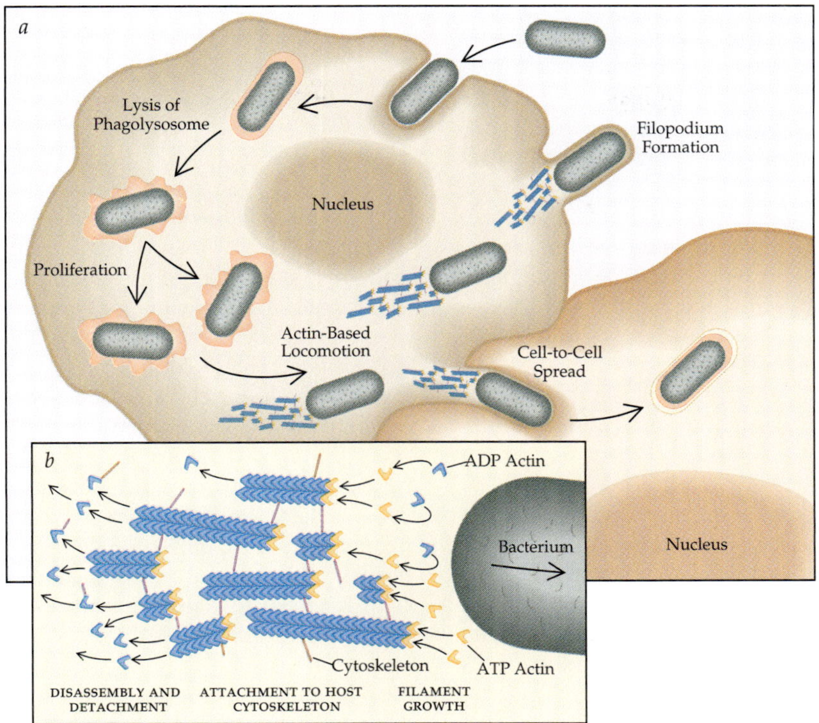

Figure 3 **(*a*) Life cycle of *Listeria monocytogenes* in host cells. (*b*) New actin filament assembly drives the bacterium through the cytoplasm. The *Listeria* surface protein ActA induces host cell actin to assemble into a rocket tail. The actin filament tail progressively lengthens, with new host cell actin monomers being added at the junction between the bacterium and the actin filament tail. The older regions of the actin tail attach to the host cell's cytoskeleton, providing a purchase so that the forces of actin filament lengthening can be applied to the bacterium to drive it through the cytoplasm. Bacteria are able to move at rapid speeds (0.02 to 1.4 μm/sec).[25]**

occurs in persons older than 70 years (2.1 cases per 100,000); pregnant women (12 cases per 100,000); patients with defects in cell-mediated immunity, including renal transplant patients; persons receiving high doses of corticosteroids; and patients with AIDS (100 cases per 100,000).[23] At a large referral hospital, *Listeria* organisms were the third most common cause of community-acquired bacterial meningitis in adults (11% of cases).[24] Despite its relatively low incidence, listeriosis concerns public health officials because this disease is associated with a high fatality rate (23%), unlike other foodborne pathogens, such as *Salmonella* organisms, which are rarely fatal. Given the increasing numbers of elderly and immunocompromised patients, the incidence of listeriosis is likely to increase.

PATHOGENESIS

L. monocytogenes has an unusual life cycle[25] [*see Figure 3, part a*]. Several proteins (internalins[26]) on the surface of the bacterium allow attachment and subsequent ingestion of *Listeria* organisms by host cells. On being internalized, the bacterium is surrounded by host cell membrane, forming a phagolysosome, a closed space that is generally toxic for pathogens. *Listeria* organisms escape by producing an exotoxin, listeriolysin O, that lyses the confining membranes. All pathogenic strains of *Listeria* organisms produce listeriolysin O, and their escape into cytoplasm of the host cell is required for pathogenesis. Once within the growth-permissive cytoplasm, the bacteria proliferate with doubling times of about 1 hour. The *Listeria* surface protein ActA possesses binding sequences to attract actin regulatory proteins that stimulate actin filament assembly.[25,27] About 2 hours after entry into the cytoplasm, actin filaments polarize at one end of the bacteria and provide the force for movement through the cytoplasm [*see Figure 3, part b*]. Many of the bacteria migrate to the periphery of the cytoplasm, where they push against the host cell's outer membrane to form elongated protrusions or filopods that can be ingested by adjacent cells. Once a bacterium enters the adjacent cell, the life cycle begins anew. *Listeria* organisms, therefore, can spread from cell to cell without directly contacting the extracellular environment. A number of other virulence factors, in addition to ActA and internalins, have been identified, and their contributions to *Listeria* pathogenesis are being defined.[28]

CLINICAL MANIFESTATIONS

The *Listeria* organism's intracellular lifestyle explains many of this pathogen's unique clinical characteristics.[25,29] Although the association between contaminated foods and the *Listeria* organism has been well documented, evidence of gastrointestinal disease has been absent in most cases. The *Listeria* organism's capacity to enter the gastrointestinal tract without causing erosive lesions is explained by the ability of this pathogen to stimulate phagocytosis by gastrointestinal cells and macrophages. Subsequently, the *Listeria* pathogen commandeers host cell actin regulatory proteins to spread from cell to cell and eventually enter the bloodstream either in monocytes or as free organisms after cell lysis.

The ability of the *Listeria* organism to avoid the extracellular environment also explains the increased incidence of listeriosis in immunocompromised patients, neonates, and pregnant women. Increased risk of listeriosis has not been associated with deficiencies of immunoglobulins or complement. However, clinical conditions and therapies (particularly corticosteroids) that lead to deficiencies in cell-mediated immunity, the primary defense for controlling intracellular pathogens, increase the risk for listeriosis. Treatment with fludarabine and prednisone, for example, in patients with chronic lymphocytic leukemia, markedly lowers their $CD4^+$ T cell counts and increases the incidence of listeriosis.[30] Patients with AIDS are most likely to contract *Listeria* infection when their $CD4^+$ T cell counts fall below 40/mm^3.[23]

Infection during Pregnancy

Nearly one third of individuals who contract listeriosis infection are pregnant women, with infection occurring most frequently in the third trimester. The symptoms tend to be relatively mild, mimicking a flulike illness, with chills, fever, and muscle aches. Back pain, a less frequent complaint, suggests a urinary tract infection; however, urinalysis and urine culture are normal. Blood cultures, although not always obtained, are positive. Symptoms usually resolve spontaneously without therapy.[31]

Neonatal Listeriosis

The *Listeria* organism can cross the placental barrier, probably as a result of cell-to-cell spread mediated by host cell actin. The organism may cause amnionitis as well as precipitate premature labor, leading to septic abortion. Transplacental transmission can also cause the unique clinical syndrome of granulomatosis infantiseptica. The organism can disseminate in utero, forming abscesses and granulomas involving the fetal liver, spleen, lungs, kidneys, brain, and skin.[32] Mortality is high, ranging from 35% to 55%. Chorioamnionitis is the most common early manifestation of perinatal *Listeria* infection. A Gram-stained smear of the meconium frequently reveals gram-positive bacilli, suggesting the diagnosis. Early antenatal treatment with ampicillin can markedly reduce mortality and result in the birth of healthy babies.[32] In addition to causing congenital infection, the *Listeria* pathogen can cause meningitis in neonates 7 to 28 days of age. Listerial meningitis is the third most common form of meningitis in neonates, accounting for 5% to 15% of cases.

Adult Meningitis and Meningoencephalitis

Meningitis is the most common manifestation of listeriosis. The *Listeria* pathogen has a predilection for the central nervous system, particularly the meninges. Although the clinical presentation of listerial meningitis is similar to that of other forms of bacterial meningitis (i.e., *Streptococcus pneumoniae, Haemophilus influenzae*, and *Neisseria meningitidis*), several characteristics distinguish *Listeria* infections. Meningeal signs develop less frequently in patients with listerial meningitis than in patients with other forms of bacterial meningitis.[33] However, tremor and grand mal or focal motor seizures are observed with a higher frequency, suggesting more extensive invasion of the nervous system.[25] The CSF response may reflect the intracellular nature of *Listeria* organisms. Compared with the CSF cell counts in other forms of bacterial meningitis, both the total number of white blood cells and the percentage of neutrophils tend to be reduced in patients with listerial meningitis. Because *Listeria* primarily grows within cells, it is less commonly found in Gram stains of CSF (positive in 5% to 33% of cultures versus 80% in other forms of bacterial meningitis).

Meningoencephalitis, a direct invasion of the cerebral cortex, can also result from *Listeria* infection, but it is not a recognized complication of other forms of bacterial meningitis. The ability of the *Listeria* pathogen to cross the meninges and blood-brain barrier is also likely to be the result of endothelial cell or macrophage phagocytosis of the organisms and utilization of the host cell contractile system to migrate to and grow within the brain. *Listeria* organisms most commonly invade the brain stem, causing a syndrome that has been called rhomboencephalitis.[34] The disease is usually biphasic; CNS manifestations are preceded by 7 to 10 days of malaise, fatigue, headache, nausea or vomiting, and fever. These symptoms are followed by the development of multiple cranial nerve deficits, particularly of the sixth and seventh nerves. Brain stem damage can also cause hemiparesis, ataxia, and respiratory dysfunction that is often followed by respiratory arrest.[35] In cases of meningoencephalitis, CSF monocyte counts may reach 80% to 90%.[35] In some cases, the CSF may contain no cells or only a few cells and have normal protein and glucose levels. Magnetic resonance imaging reveals areas of increased resonance and is the best way to visualize the brain stem. Computed tomography with contrast generally shows areas of increased uptake with or without ring enhancement.

The diagnosis of both listerial meningitis and meningoencephalitis frequently is delayed.[36] A monocytic response in the CSF and a negative CSF Gram stain can lead the clinician to confuse listerial meningitis and meningoencephalitis with herpes and other forms of viral encephalitis, viral meningitis, tuberculous meningitis, Lyme disease, syphilis, cryptococcal meningitis, Wegener granulomatosis, or CNS sarcoidosis. Particularly in the immunocompromised host, the possibility of *Listeria* infection must always be considered as a possible cause of CNS infection.

Bacteremia

Bacteremia without meningitis or focal infections occurs in 5% to 30% of adult cases. There are no distinctive clinical features except for peripheral monocytosis, which is present in a small percentage of patients. Diagnosis is based on blood culture findings.

Miscellaneous Infections

As observed with many pathogens that are able to enter the bloodstream, the *Listeria* organism can cause focal infections at many extravascular sites,[29] including bones, normal and prosthetic joints, eyes,[37] spinal cord, pleura, peritoneum, and liver.[38] Isolated brain abscesses have also been reported.[33] In rare cases, the *Listeria* organism may cause endocarditis, myocarditis, and mycotic aneurysms.

DIAGNOSIS

L. monocytogenes can be readily cultured. A diphtheroid-like organism discovered in blood or CSF cultures is frequently misinterpreted as a contaminant. In an immunocompromised host, treatment of listeriosis should be initiated pending the laboratory staff's final diagnosis. Diphtheroids can be rapidly differentiated from *Listeria* organisms by using a microscopic bacterial motility test. Decreasing motility is indicative of *Listeria* organisms. Gram stains of the cerebrospinal or meconium fluid showing gram-positive rods strongly suggest *Listeria* infection.

PREVENTION AND TREATMENT

It is not possible to eliminate the large reservoir of *Listeria* organisms found throughout our environment. Physicians can help prevent disease by instructing patients at risk on how to minimize the multiplication of *Listeria* organisms in foodstuffs and how to kill the organisms on potentially contaminated foods. Patients need to avoid unsterilized dairy products, undercooked meats, and prepared foods that have been refrigerated but not resterilized by high-temperature reheating. More detailed preventive instructions are provided by the Centers for Disease Control and Prevention [*see Table 2*].

Table 2 Dietary Recommendations for Preventing Food-Borne Listeriosis

General recommendations
- Thoroughly cook raw food from animal sources
- Wash raw vegetables thoroughly
- Keep uncooked meats separate from vegetables and cooked foods
- Avoid consumption of unpasteurized milk or foods made with raw milk
- Wash hands, knives, and cutting boards after handling uncooked foods

Additional recommendations for high-risk persons*
- Avoid soft cheeses (e.g., Mexican style, feta, Brie, Camembert, and blue veined); hard cheeses, cream cheese, cottage cheese, and yogurt can be eaten
- Leftovers or ready-to-eat foods (e.g., hot dogs) should be reheated until they are steaming hot
- Pregnant women and immunosuppressed persons should consider avoiding foods from delicatessen counters or thoroughly cooking cold cuts before eating

*High-risk persons include immunocompromised persons, pregnant women, neonates, and the elderly.

No clinical trials comparing various antibiotic regimens have been published. Bacteriostatic drugs, such as chloramphenicol and tetracycline, are associated with high failure rates in patients with listeriosis and cannot be recommended. Ampicillin or penicillin has generally been recommended as the treatment of choice, and the *Listeria* pathogen is generally sensitive to either agent.[39] These antibiotics should be given intravenously in high doses: ampicillin at a dosage of 200 mg/kg/day in six divided doses or penicillin at a dosage of 300,000 U/kg/day in six divided doses. In immunosuppressed patients, relapse has been reported after 2 weeks of penicillin therapy. The poor response to bacteriostatic drugs and the slow response to penicillin therapy are likely to result from the *Listeria* organism's ability to survive and grow within cells. The intracellular level of ampicillin or penicillin may not be sufficient for complete sterilization. Immunosuppression reduces the host's ability to clear infected cells, thereby allowing the *Listeria* organism to survive and spread for prolonged periods in a protected intracellular environment.

The exact duration of antibiotic treatment required to prevent relapse is not known; however, 3 to 6 weeks of therapy is probably prudent for immunosuppressed patients. Antibiotics that penetrate cells poorly, such as aminoglycosides, may be synergistic in vitro but are unlikely to prove efficacious in the living host. Although some experts have recommended that an aminoglycoside be added to ampicillin, the *Listeria* organism grows in cells in the presence of extracellular gentamicin concentrations of 10 to 20 μg/ml. Furthermore, addition of gentamicin to the ampicillin therapy has failed to improve outcome in a mouse infection model.[40] Therefore, aminoglycosides are unlikely to be efficacious in patients with listeriosis and certainly should be avoided in kidney transplant recipients and other patients with renal dysfunction. On the other hand, trimethoprim-sulfamethoxazole, a drug combination that readily enters cells and is bactericidal for *Listeria* organisms, may prove to be the most effective agent for treating *Listeria* infection. Trimethoprim-sulfamethoxazole has proved to be effective in patients with listeriosis and penicillin hypersensitivity.[34] The recommended dosage is 20 mg/kg/day of trimethoprim and 100 mg/kg/day of sulfamethoxazole, given in four divided doses. The *Listeria* pathogen is also sensitive to erythromycin, which is recommended at a dosage of 60 mg/kg/day intravenously in four divided doses. Tissue culture and animal studies suggest that levofloxacin may also be effective; however, treatment of human *Listeria* infection with this quinolone has not been reported.[41]

Listeria infection in the CNS is associated with a high mortality despite appropriate antibiotic treatment. In patients with meningoencephalitis, mortality ranges from 36% to 51%. Those who survive often have permanent neurologic sequelae. In patients with meningitis, mortality is somewhat lower (26%), but it is higher in patients with seizures and in those older than 65 years.[33] Early recognition and rapid institution of antibiotics are critical for improving outcome.[36]

Nocardiosis

MICROBIOLOGY

Nocardia species are thin, aerobic, gram-positive bacilli that form branching filaments that tend to fragment into coccobacilli. Gram stain is often taken up, variably resulting in an irregular, beaded appearance in exudates [*see Figure 4*]. *Nocardia asteroides* is the most common *Nocardia* species to cause human disease in the United States (80% to 90% of cases). *N. brasiliensis, N. otitidis-caviarum,* and *N. farcinica*[42] are rarer human pathogens. All four organisms are commonly found in soil. In addition to being gram positive, they are modified acid-fast positive. This characteristic helps differentiate *Nocardia* species from the *Actinomyces* organism, a gram-positive, anaerobic pathogen that also forms branching filaments. The *Nocardia* organism grows slowly on blood agar plates and Sabouraud dextrose agar. In sputum specimens, other organisms often overgrow, obscuring *Nocardia* colonies. Colonies

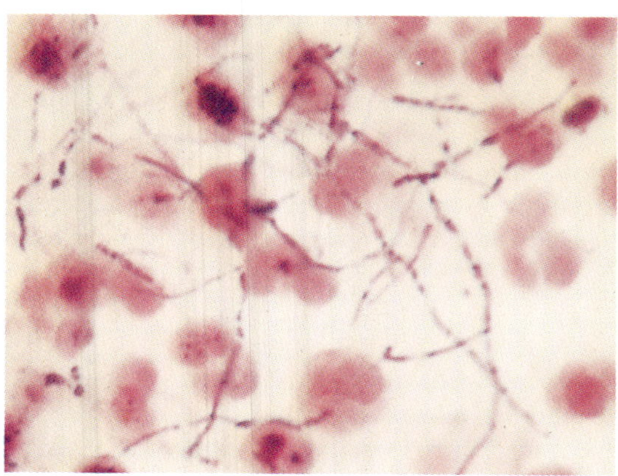

Figure 4 **Gram stain of joint fluid containing *Nocardia asteroides*.**

generally have an orange pigment and appear heaped up and folded. They can also be white or pink. Colony characteristics suggestive of the *Nocardia* organism may not develop for 2 to 4 weeks. Laboratory staff need to be alerted to incubate cultures for a prolonged period when a *Nocardia* species is suspected. Samples should be obtained when the patient is not taking antibiotics. Modified Thayer-Martin medium and buffered charcoal-yeast extract agar can be used to enhance recovery of *Nocardia* species.

ETIOLOGY AND EPIDEMIOLOGY

Nocardiosis is relatively rare, infecting approximately 1,000 people a year in the United States. Often found in soil, *Nocardia* organisms most often infect immunocompromised hosts and primarily cause pulmonary infections, brain abscesses, and skin infections. Nocardiosis has no pathognomonic characteristics, and delays in diagnosis are common. *Nocardia* organisms are slow growing and are difficult to identify on routine culture. When a potential case is encountered, it is important for the clinician to alert microbiology and pathology laboratory staffs that a *Nocardia* organism is a possibility.

PATHOGENESIS

In most cases, the *Nocardia* organism gains entry to the host through the respiratory tract. Inhaled bacteria elicit a neutrophil response that inhibits but does not kill the organism. *Nocardia* organisms are phagocytosed by neutrophils and incorporated into phagolysosomes. In this closed membrane space, the organism is able to survive for prolonged periods. Like *Mycobacterium tuberculosis*, pathogenic *Nocardia* species produce superoxide dismutase, a product that inactivates the toxic oxygen by-products of the neutrophils and macrophages. In addition, both *M. tuberculosis* and *Nocardia* species synthesize a second product: a mycolic acid that inhibits the fusion of lysosomes with the phagolysosomal compartment. This inhibitory activity prevents the release of toxic proteases and other antibacterial products from reaching the intracellular bacteria. The host defenses utilized to protect against nocardiosis are multifactorial and include neutrophils, macrophages, and cell-mediated and humoral immunity. Patients at risk for nocardiosis include those with chronic granulomatous disease (inability of neutrophils to produce toxic oxygen by-products) and those with dysgammaglobulinemia. The highest percentage of cases occur in patients with impaired cell-mediated immunity, including renal and cardiac transplant patients,[43] other patients on high-dose corticosteroids, patients with Cushing disease, and those with AIDS who have CD4$^+$ T cell counts below 250 cells/mm^3. Patients with chronic pulmonary disorders, particularly alveolar proteinosis, are also at increased risk. Approximately one third of those who acquire nocardiosis have no identifiable predisposing condition.

CLINICAL MANIFESTATIONS

Pulmonary Nocardiosis

Pulmonary infection is the most common manifestation of nocardiosis, occurring in approximately two thirds of cases. In most cases, pulmonary disease is subacute in onset, mimicking pulmonary tuberculosis. Patients complain of productive cough, pleuritic chest pain, dyspnea, fever, anorexia, and weight loss. Occasionally, hemoptysis develops, particularly in patients with large cavitary lung lesions. If left untreated, the disease tends to run a chronic waxing-and-waning course. Less often in the immunocompromised host, pneumonia is more acute in onset. Chest x-ray findings are variable and include the following, in order of most to least frequent: pulmonary nodules or mass lesions, areas of consolidation, cavitary lesions, interstitial infiltrates, and pleural effusions. In addition, CT may demonstrate areas of low attenuation within consolidations, multiple nodules, and chest wall extension of the infection. AIDS patients are more likely to have multiple pulmonary nodules, cavitary lung lesions, and upper lobe infiltrates.[44] On occasion, the infiltrate spontaneously resolves, particularly in patients with normal immune function. A brain abscess may develop later as a consequence of transient dissemination of the organism.

Central Nervous System Infection

In approximately one third of patients with nocardiosis, the CNS becomes infected. Brain abscess is the most common CNS infection. The lesions are often multilocular and can occur in any region of the brain.[45] CT or MRI with contrast demonstrates ring-enhancing lesions, as observed with other causes of pyogenic brain abscess. In AIDS patients, brain abscess is often accompanied by an abnormal chest x-ray, which suggests the diagnosis.[46] With other patients, abnormalities on chest x-ray are not always present. However, when detected, the combined findings of a lung nodule on chest x-ray and ring-enhancing CNS lesions are often mistaken for lung carcinoma with metastasis.[47] Patients undergoing surgical drainage of their abscesses have a higher survival rate. Nocardial meningitis is a less common CNS manifestation and is often associated with brain abscess (40% of meningitis cases). Patients typically have subacute to chronic meningitis characterized by fever, stiff neck, and headache. CSF analysis demonstrates a predominance of polymorphonuclear neutrophils, a low CSF glucose level, and an elevated protein level. CSF cultures are often negative, particularly in the first 3 days, and patients fail to fully respond to empirical antibiotic therapy. Appropriate treatment is often delayed, and mortality is high (50% to 60%).

Cutaneous Infection

Cutaneous involvement is uncommon and is generally caused by *N. brasiliensis*. A break in the skin caused by trauma, an insect bite, a thorn bush scratch,[48] and even a cat scratch can result in local invasion by *Nocardia* organisms. A pustule or a moderately erythematous, nonfluctuant nodule develops at the site of inoculation. Regional adenopathy is generally found. The presence of multiple subcutaneous nodules indicates dissemination of the organism and more often occurs in the immunocompromised patient. In the tropical regions of South and Central America, ulcerations and large tumorlike lesions called mycetomas occur on the lower legs and are caused by *N. asteroides*.

Other Infections

Dissemination occurs in approximately 40% of pulmonary *Nocardia* infections and can result in localized infection in any organ. Septic arthritis, osteomyelitis, endophthalmitis, sinusitis, peritonitis, and purulent pericarditis have all been reported.

DIAGNOSIS

Invasive procedures are generally required to obtain infected tissue samples. The histopathology of biopsy specimens usually reveals an acute inflammatory response with a predominance of neutrophils. Tissue necrosis with minimal fibrosis often results in the formation of multilocular abscesses with minimal capsular formation. Gram stain or Brown-Brenn stains often reveal gram-positive beaded branching forms. *Nocardia* species can also be visualized by using a modified acid-fast stain. The organism is not well seen after hematoxylineosin or periodic acid–Schiff stain. Obtaining a culture is the definitive way to prove the diagnosis. For sputum cultures, selective media may be required to prevent the overgrowth of more rapidly growing mouth flora. For the diagnosis of meningitis, large volumes of CSF should be obtained for culture. Clinical laboratory staff should be notified as to the possibility of *Nocardia* organisms so that cultures can be incubated for a longer period.

TREATMENT AND PROGNOSIS

Sulfonamides alone and trimethoprim-sulfamethoxazole remain the treatments of choice. High intravenous doses of these agents are required—sulfadiazine (1.5 to 2 g every 6 hours) or trimethoprim-sulfamethoxazole (20 mg/kg/day of trimethoprim and 100 mg/kg/day of sulfamethoxazole given in three divided doses) to maintain serum sulfonamide levels in the 12 to 15 mg/dl range. Once substantial improvement is documented, oral treatment can be substituted after 1 to 2 months of intravenous therapy. For sulfa-allergic patients, possible alternatives need to be determined on the basis of sensitivity testing. Minocycline, imipenem, amoxicillin–potassium clavulanate, and amikacin alone or in various combinations have been successful in individual patients.[49] Because of the intracellular nature of nocardiosis and the slow rates of bacterial growth, 12 months of antibiotic therapy is required to prevent relapse. In cases of abscess formation in the brain, subcutaneous tissue, or other organs (except the lung), surgical drainage is also required for cure.

The overall mortality from nocardiosis is approximately 25%. Otherwise healthy persons with pulmonary nocardiosis have a better prognosis (15% mortality). Fatality rates are higher in patients with bacteremia,[50] patients with acute infection (symptomatic for less than 3 weeks), patients receiving corticosteroids or cytotoxic agents, patients with disseminated disease involving two or more noncontiguous organs, and patients with meningitis.

Anthrax

Bacillus anthracis causes infections primarily in animals, particularly herbivores. However, contact with animals or animal products can produce infections in humans.[51] Although *B. anthracis* was once the cause of severe epidemics, our understanding of this pathogen's epidemiology and the vaccination of domestic animals have resulted in a marked reduction of anthrax in the United States. In developing countries and in one region of Russia, outbreaks continue to be reported. Cutaneous manifestations are most common (95% of cases in the United States); pulmonary disease is second in incidence (5%). Gastrointestinal disease, which has not been reported in the United States, is found primarily in Asia and Africa.

MICROBIOLOGY

B. anthracis is an aerobic, gram-positive rod that forms endospores. The spores are highly resistant to adverse conditions and are able to survive at extreme temperatures, at high pH and salinity levels, and in disinfectants. The organism can be readily cultured on standard blood and nutrient agar plates. For contaminated specimens (e.g., stool), selective media or decontamination methods can be used that take advantage of the spores' ability to resist heat, ethanol, and various antibiotics. The organism forms gray-white colonies and is nonhemolytic. A fluorescent antibody stain can be used to identify the organism.

ETIOLOGY AND EPIDEMIOLOGY

Anthrax is primarily a disease of herbivores (cattle, sheep, horses, goats, and swine). Humans become infected as a result of contact with infected animals (agricultural exposure) or through exposure of infected animal products (industrial exposure). Accidental laboratory-related infections have also been reported. *B. anthracis*, like all *Bacillus* species, is a saprophyte that grows in the soil, and animals generally contract the infection through contact with soil. Because domestic animals in the United States are vaccinated against anthrax, agricultural exposure is rare.

Most cases of anthrax in the United States occur as a result of contact with animal products imported from Asia, the Middle East, and Africa. Wool, goat hair, and animal hides are the most common sources of infection. Persons who work in the early stages of processing these materials are exposed to the highest inoculum of spores and are most likely to contract disease. Processed materials have also caused human disease. Cases have been traced to shaving-brush bristles, wool coats, yarn, goat-skin bongo drums, and heroin preparations.[52] The largest recent outbreak of anthrax occurred in Sverdlovsk (now Yekaterinburg), Russia, in 1979, resulting in approximately 96 inhalation cases and 64 deaths. The exact cause of the outbreak remains unclear. However, the explosion of a germ-warfare facility is suspected, and recent polymerase chain reaction analysis of tissue samples from 11 victims has identified multiple strains of *B. anthracis* in each sample, consistent with infection by a manufactured preparation of bacterial spores.[53] This incident underlines the potential risk of *B. anthracis* as a biologic weapon. False claims of contamination of letters and air ducts with anthrax in the United States emphasize the importance of training public health and law enforcement personnel on proper handling of potentially contaminated samples, decontamination, and prophylaxis.[54]

PATHOGENESIS

Spores gain entry into the epidermis through abrasions in the skin and can be inhaled into the lungs. Once in the host, the spores germinate, multiply, and produce toxins that cause tissue edema and necrosis. Later, bacilli in the skin or lung may gain entry into the lymphatic system, causing lymphangitis and lymphadenitis, and into the vascular system, causing bacteremia.

Three toxin components are synthesized on the bacterial surface and account for the major pathologic consequences of infection: protective antigen, lethal toxin, and edema toxin. Protective antigen binds host cell receptors and transports either lethal or edema toxin within the cells, which can cause cell swelling and death. Lethal toxin has a protease activity that cleaves specific kinases that in turn may induce cell lysis.[55]

CLINICAL MANIFESTATIONS

Skin Infection

Skin disease is the most common manifestation of anthrax. One to 7 days after spores are inoculated into the skin, a small papule develops that progresses to a vesicle over the ensuing few days. Erythema and nonpitting edema often surround the vesicle. Initially, the vesicular fluid is serous and contains large numbers of organisms. Once the vesicle ruptures, a black eschar becomes evident at the base of the ulcer [*see Figure 5*]. Despite the erythema and swelling, lesions are not painful but may be mildly pruritic. Lymphangitis, lymphadenopathy, fever, and malaise may accompany the skin infection. After 1 to 2 weeks, the skin lesion dries and a permanent scar is formed. Lesions occur primarily on exposed regions of the body. The arms are the most frequent site of infection; the face and neck are also commonly involved. A single lesion usually occurs, although multiple sites may occur as a result of simultaneous inoculations.[56]

Respiratory Infection (Woolsorters' Disease)

Inhalation anthrax is biphasic in its presentation.[57] From 1 to 5 days after inhalation of spores, the patient has symptoms suggestive of a viral syn-

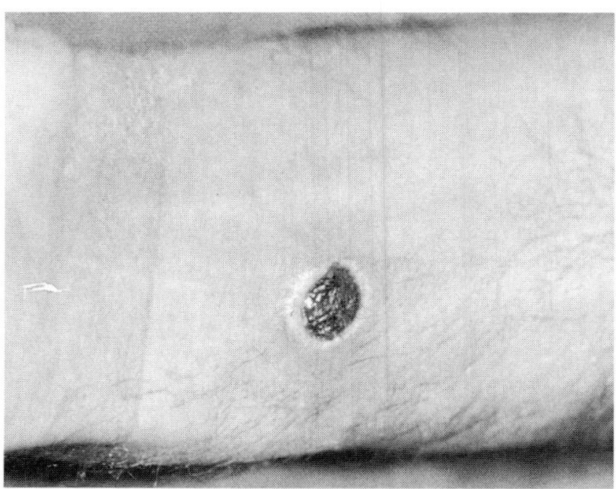

Figure 5 **Typical dark, necrotic, painless pruritic skin lesion of anthrax on the wrist of a shepherd from Morocco.**

drome: nonproductive cough, malaise, fatigue, myalgia, and mild fever. Occasionally, the sensation of chest heaviness is reported. Rhonchi may be heard on examination. Within 2 to 4 days, symptoms temporarily resolve but are rapidly followed by the second, more severe stage of the disease. This stage involves the sudden onset of severe respiratory distress with dyspnea, cyanosis, and diffuse diaphoresis, accompanied by fever, tachycardia, and tachypnea. On pulmonary auscultation, moist, crepitant rales are evident, and findings are consistent with pleural effusion. Chest x-ray demonstrates a widened mediastinum without a definite infiltrate. Death usually occurs within 24 hours and may be accompanied by septic shock. Autopsy usually reveals hemorrhagic necrosis of the thoracic lymph nodes, drainage from the lungs, and hemorrhagic mediastinitis. A high index of suspicion is critical because any delay in diagnosis and treatment greatly increases the likelihood of a fatal outcome.

Gastrointestinal Infection

Gastrointestinal infection has not been reported in the United States. It occurs primarily in developing countries, usually after ingestion of contaminated meat. The incubation period is usually 3 to 5 days. Patients initially have nausea, vomiting, anorexia, and fever. These symptoms are rapidly followed by acute abdominal pain, hematemesis, and bloody diarrhea. Findings on examination suggest an acute surgical abdomen, and there is moderate leukocytosis with immature band forms. Rapid progression to toxemia and shock leads to death within 2 to 5 days after the initial onset of symptoms. An oropharyngeal form of anthrax has also been described. Inflammatory lesions that resemble the cutaneous lesions develop on the posterior pharynx, hard palate, or tonsils. Tissue necrosis and edema are accompanied by sore throat, dysphagia, fever, regional lymphadenopathy, and toxemia.

Meningitis

Anthrax meningitis can result from bacteremia precipitated by cutaneous, respiratory, or gastrointestinal infection. This complication is relatively rare, occurring in fewer than 5% of patients. The onset of meningeal symptoms occurs simultaneously with the primary lesion or within several days after its onset. Meningitis is usually hemorrhagic and rapidly fatal (within 1 to 6 days).

DIAGNOSIS

A careful epidemiologic history is the single most important means of suggesting the diagnosis. A history of contact with herbivores or products from these animals, particularly if the products come from outside the United States, should raise the possibility of anthrax. The physical appearance of the skin lesions is characteristic, and Gram stains and cultures of the ulcer base are frequently positive. A history of exposure to dust from a contaminated animal product can usually be obtained in the prodromal phase of the respiratory illness, when symptoms are mild. In the absence of a thorough history, the disease is initially mistaken for a viral respiratory illness or bronchitis. Patients with gastrointestinal disease have a history of eating undercooked, often spoiled, meat. Enzyme-linked immunosorbent assays are available that measure antibody titers against lethal and edema toxin. A fourfold rise in titers over 4 weeks or a single titer of 1:32 is considered positive.

TREATMENT AND PROGNOSIS

Penicillin G is the treatment of choice; 4 million U administered parenterally every 4 to 6 hours is generally effective. Lesions usually become culture negative within hours of the initiation of therapy. However, treatment should be continued for 7 to 10 days. For penicillin-allergic patients, oral tetracycline (0.5 g every 6 hours) is effective for cutaneous disease. Erythromycin and chloramphenicol are also satisfactory alternatives. Excision of skin lesions is contraindicated because of the increased risk of precipitating bacteremia. However, after appropriate antibiotic therapy, excision and skin grafting may be necessary.[58]

Table 3 Clinical Syndromes Caused by *Bacillus* Species

Species	*Clinical Syndrome*	*Treatment*
B. alvei	Meningitis, pneumonia, empyema, bacteremia	Penicillin, cephalosporins, vancomycin
B. cereus	Ophthalmitis, bacteremia, pneumonia, osteomyelitis, endocarditis, soft tissue infection	Vancomycin, clindamycin, gentamicin, ciprofloxacin, imipenem
B. sphaericus	Peritonitis, pleuritis, lung infection, meningitis, bacteremia	Penicillin, cephalosporins, vancomycin
B. subtilis	Meningitis, otitis, mastoiditis, urinary tract infection, bacteremia, endocarditis, ventricular shunt infection	Penicillin, cephalosporins, vancomycin

Before antibiotics became available, cutaneous disease resulted in a mortality of 10% to 20%. With appropriate antibiotic treatment, fewer than 1% of patients die. Despite appropriate antibiotics and respiratory support, inhalation anthrax is almost always fatal. Gastrointestinal disease is also associated with high mortality (25% to 100%).

PREVENTION

A killed vaccine derived from a component of the exotoxin is available and is recommended for all industrial workers at risk for exposure to contaminated animal products. As a result of increased concerns about biologic warfare and bioterrorism, military personnel are now vaccinated. To date, surveillance studies have not detected any serious or unexpected adverse reactions.[59] In cases of suspected exposure to *B. anthracis*, antibiotic prophylaxis and vaccination are recommended. The regimens of choice are oral fluoroquinolones (ciprofloxacin, 500 mg b.i.d.; levofloxacin, 500 mg q.d.; or ofloxacin, 400 mg b.i.d.) or, if fluoroquinolones are contraindicated, doxycycline (100 mg b.i.d.). Prophylaxis should be continued until exposure is excluded. If exposure is confirmed, prophylaxis should be continued for 4 weeks and until three doses of vaccine have been administered. If vaccine is unavailable, prophylaxis should be continued for 8 weeks. Exposed skin should be washed extensively with soap and water, and personal items should be decontaminated with 0.5% hypochlorite (one part household bleach to 10 parts water).[54]

INFECTIONS AND DISORDERS DUE TO OTHER *BACILLUS* SPECIES

Bacillus organisms are found in soil, dust, decaying organic matter, and water. Some species are part of the normal flora, particularly in patients who have had prolonged hospitalizations. Despite their widespread distribution, these organisms rarely cause infection and are more often isolated as a contaminant. Risk factors associated with serious *Bacillus* infections include use of intravascular catheters; intravenous drug abuse; sickle cell disease; and immunosuppression caused by malignancy, neutropenia, corticosteroid therapy, or AIDS.[60] Because these organisms are frequently resistant to third-generation cephalosporins, prolonged antibiotic treatment regimens that include these agents may select out for *Bacillus* organisms.

B. cereus is the most frequent *Bacillus* species to cause invasive infection, followed by *B. subtilis* [*see Table 3*].

CLINICAL MANIFESTATIONS

With the exception of *B. cereus* eye infections, infections are rare and cannot be clinically distinguished from those caused by other pyogenic organisms. Pneumonia can develop in the compromised host, and necrotizing pneumonia caused by *B. cereus* has been reported in patients with acute leukemia and hepatic malignancy.

Bacterial endocarditis caused by *Bacillus* species is a well-recognized complication of intravenous drug abuse. The tricuspid valve is most often involved, and the course of illness tends to be indolent. The *Bacillus* species are among many pathogens that have infected the prosthetic valve.[61] Indwelling catheters may become colonized with *Bacillus* organisms, resulting in positive blood cultures.

High-grade bacteremia can be complicated by fatal meningoencephalitis in the immunocompromised host.[62] Necrotizing fasciitis can be caused by *B. cereus*.

In rare cases, bacterial meningitis may result from *Bacillus* species bacteremia, but more often, it has followed spinal anesthesia because of inadvertent inoculation of organisms into the CSF.[63] Because of their hardy growth characteristics, *Bacillus* species are common laboratory contaminants. Pseudobacteremia caused by contamination of alcohol swabs and rubber stoppers on blood culture bottles and pseudomeningitis caused by *Bacillus* contamination of commercial culture media have been reported.[64]

Motor vehicle accidents in which injuries result from direct contact with the road may result in *B. cereus* soft tissue and bone infections that necessitate extensive surgical debridement and amputation for cure. Close-range gunshot wounds have also been complicated by *B. cereus* infection.[65]

Ocular Infections

B. cereus is a primary pathogen for ocular infections. This species is one of the most common agents associated with posttraumatic endophthalmitis. When *B. cereus* is the causative agent, an intraocular foreign body is often present. Injuries caused by metal fragments and injuries associated with contamination by soil and dust increase the risk of infection by *B. cereus*. The onset of infection is rapid and leads to destruction of the vitreous and retinal tissue, causing loss of vision 12 to 48 hours after inoculation. Patients frequently become systemically ill, with fever and leukocytosis. Endophthalmitis and panophthalmitis can also be related to intravenous drug abuse. Early diagnosis and treatment are critical for preventing permanent structural changes and blindness.[66]

Food Poisoning

B. cereus produces two enterotoxins, diarrheal toxin and emetic toxin, that are responsible for two food poisoning syndromes. The emetic form is associated primarily with the ingestion of contaminated fried rice.[67] From 1 to 6 hours after ingestion, the individual experiences vomiting and symptoms identical to those of staphylococcal food poisoning. A case of fulminant fatal hepatic failure and rhabdomyolysis associated with ingestion of *B. cereus* emetic toxin has also been reported.[68] The diarrheal form has a longer incubation period (10 to 12 hours), and manifestations are related to lower rather than upper gastrointestinal symptoms. Symptoms include abdominal pain, profuse watery diarrhea, tenesmus, and nausea. This syndrome is usually self-limited and lasts 12 to 24 hours. Outbreaks are generally associated with ingestion of contaminated meat or vegetables.

TREATMENT

B. cereus is resistant to penicillin and other β-lactam antibiotics, including cephalosporins; it is sensitive to vancomycin, gentamicin, imipenem, and ciprofloxacin. Clindamycin, erythromycin, chloramphenicol, and tetracycline have also been shown to be active. Other *Bacillus* species are susceptible to penicillins and cephalosporins. Pending speciation and susceptibility testing, vancomycin or clindamycin with or without gentamicin is the empirical treatment of choice when infection with *Bacillus* species is suspected.

If *Bacillus* bacteremia develops in immunocompromised patients with long-term indwelling catheters, antibiotic therapy must be instituted and the catheter removed to prevent recurrence of the infection.[69] In addition to antibiotic treatment, the deep-seated soft tissue infection associated with necrotizing fasciitis requires aggressive surgical debridement.[70]

For intraocular infections, in addition to systemic therapy, intravitreous clindamycin and gentamicin are generally administered by an ophthalmologist. Intravitreous dexamethasone and early vitrectomy have been recommended for the management of sight-threatening endophthalmitis by *B. cereus*.[66]

For patients with food poisoning, antibiotics are not required because the disease is self-limited. Supportive care may include intravenous fluids if the patient becomes severely dehydrated.

Infections due to the *Erysipelothrix* Organism

Human infections by the *Erysipelothrix* organism are rare and are always caused by *Erysipelothrix rhusiopathiae* (formerly *E. insidiosa*). This aerobic gram-positive bacillus grows on routine nonselective media and is nonhemolytic, nonmotile, and catalase negative. Because of the cell wall's high lipid content (about 30%), *E. rhusiopathiae* is resistant to desiccation and may tolerate salting, pickling, and smoking. The organism is capable of growing over a broad temperature range (4° to 42° C) and is widespread in nature. *E. rhusiopathiae* can infect mammals, birds, fish, shellfish, and insects. Human infection results from handling dead infected animal parts. Infection can also result from cat bites.[71] Most cases of skin infection occur during the summer and early fall. Infection is almost always the result of occupational exposure of slaughterhouse workers, butchers, fishers, farmers, and veterinarians. The organism is usually traumatically inoculated. Bacilli remain extracellular and are often located deep in the skin near capillaries, where the organism can gain entry into the bloodstream.[72]

CLINICAL MANIFESTATIONS

Erysipeloid

Between 2 and 7 days after skin inoculation, a purplish-red, nonvesicular area arises with a sharply defined, raised, serpiginous border.

Lesions most often develop on the face and hands. Proximal regions of the hand and fingers are involved, whereas the distal phalanges are usually spared. Lesions spread peripherally at a slow pace (1 cm/day). Over time, the central part of the lesion begins to heal, resulting in a pale center surrounded by a fiery-red outer border. Lesions itch or burn and are rarely associated with lymphangitis or lymphadenitis. Fever and systemic complaints are rare.

Endocarditis

Endocarditis is rare but may occur on both deformed and normal heart valves. The onset is acute or subacute and most often involves the aortic valve. In approximately 40% of cases, a skin lesion is noted just before or at the time of diagnosis, suggesting the possibility of *E. rhusiopathiae*.[73] Often, the skin lesion has healed by the time endocarditis is apparent.

DIAGNOSIS

An appropriate epidemiologic history will suggest the diagnosis. Morphologically, the skin lesions resemble erysipelas (caused by group A streptococci). However, the rate of progression of *Erysipelothrix* infection is considerably slower, and unlike erysipelas, this skin lesion is not associated with tenderness or lymphadenopathy. Injection and culturing of nonbacteriostatic normal saline is rarely successful. Biopsy of a full-thickness skin specimen from the advancing border of the lesion and culturing in glucose-containing broth result in the highest yields. PCR assays for erysipelas have proved useful in swine and have recently been applied to humans.[72] Diagnosis of endocarditis depends on isolation of the organism from blood cultures.

TREATMENT

The treatment of choice for erysipeloid is penicillin; a single injection of 600,000 U of penicillin G benzathine generally is curative. For penicillin-allergic patients, oral erythromycin (0.25 to 0.50 g every 6 hours) is effective. This skin infection is usually self-limited and lasts about 3 weeks; however, antibiotic treatment hastens the healing. Bacterial endocarditis is best treated with intravenous penicillin G (12 to 20 million U/day in six divided doses for 4 to 6 weeks). For penicillin-allergic patients, intravenous cefazolin (4 to 6 g/day), in three divided doses, is recommended.[74] Most strains are resistant to vancomycin, which therefore should not be used for empirical therapy for endocarditis if *E. rhusiopathiae* is a possibility. Despite appropriate therapy, the mortality in patients with endocarditis is 30% to 40%.

Acknowledgments

Figure 1 R.J. Collier, M.D., Harvard Medical School. Adapted by Dimitry Schidlovsky.
Figure 3 Dimitry Schidlovsky.
Figure 4 Courtesy of Professor Jean Hilarie Saurat, Geneva University Hospital, Geneva, Switzerland.

References

1. Krech T, Hollis DG: *Corynebacterium* and related organisms. Manual of Clinical Microbiology, 5th ed. Balows A, Hausler WJ, Herrmann KL, et al, Eds. American Society for Microbiology, Washington, D.C., 1991, p 280

2. Bisgard KM, Hardy IR, Popovic T, et al: Respiratory diphtheria in the United States, 1980 through 1995. Am J Public Health 88:787, 1998

3. Koopman JS, Campbell J: The role of cutaneous diphtheria infections in a diphtheria epidemic. J Infect Dis 131:239, 1975

4. Golaz A, Lance-Parker S, Welty T, et al: Epidemiology of diphtheria in South Dakota. S D J Med 53:281, 2000

5. Control of epidemic diphtheria in the newly independent states of the former Soviet Union, 1990–1998. J Infect Dis 181(suppl 1):S1, 2000

6. Holmes RK: Biology and molecular epidemiology of diphtheria toxin and the *tox* gene. J Infect Dis 181(suppl 1):S156, 2000

7. Kadirova R, Kartoglu HU, Strebel PM: Clinical characteristics and management of 676 hospitalized diphtheria cases, Kyrgyz Republic, 1995. J Infect Dis 181(suppl 1):S110, 2000

8. Mofred A, Guérin JM, Falfoul-Borsali N, et al: Cutaneous diphtheria. Rev Med Interne 15:515, 1994

9. Loukoushkina EF, Boko PV, Kolbasova EV, et al: The clinical picture of diphtheritic carditis in children. Eur J Pediatr 157:528, 1998

10. Havaldar PV, Sankpal MN, Doddannavar RP: Diphtheritic myocarditis: clinical and laboratory parameters of prognosis and fatal outcome. Ann Trop Paediatr 20:209, 2000

11. Logina I, Donaghy M: Diphtheritic polyneuropathy: a clinical study and comparison with Guillain-Barré syndrome. J Neurol Neurosurg Psychiatry 67:433, 1999

12. Kneen R, Pham NG, Solomon T, et al: Penicillin vs. erythromycin in the treatment of diphtheria. Clin Infect Dis 27:845, 1998

13. Sutter RW, Hardy IR, Kozlova IA, et al: Immunogenicity of tetanus-diphtheria toxoids (Td) among Ukrainian adults: implications for diphtheria control in the newly independent states of the former Soviet Union. J Infect Dis 181(suppl 1):S197, 2000

14. Coyle MB, Lipsky BA: Coryneform bacteria in infectious diseases: clinical and laboratory aspects. Clin Microbiol Rev 3:227, 1990

15. Meria P, Desgrippes A, Arfi C, et al: Encrusted cystitis and pyelitis. J Urol 160:3, 1998

16. Zinner SH: Changing epidemiology of infections in patients with neutropenia and cancer: emphasis on gram-positive and resistant bacteria. Clin Infect Dis 29:490, 1999

17. Traub WH, Geipel U, Leonhard B, et al: Antibiotic susceptibility testing (agar disk diffusion and agar dilution) of clinical isolates of *Corynebacterium jeikeium*. Chemotherapy 44:230, 1998

18. Capdevila JA, Bujan S, Gavalda J, et al: *Rhodococcus equi* pneumonia in patients infected with the human immunodeficiency virus. Report of two cases and review of the literature. Scand J Infect Dis 29: 535, 1997

19. Munoz P, Burillo A, Palomo J, et al: *Rhodococcus equi* infection in transplant recipients: case report and review of the literature. Transplantation 65:449, 1998

20. Verville TD, Huycke MM, Greenfield RA, et al: *Rhodococcus equi* infections of humans: 12 cases and a review of the literature. Medicine (Baltimore) 73:119, 1994

21. Hsueh PR, Hung CC, Teng LJ, et al: Report of invasive *Rhodococcus equi* infections in Taiwan, with an emphasis on the emergence of multidrug-resistant strains. Clin Infect Dis 27:370, 1998

22. Schlech IIIWF: Foodborne listeriosis. Clin Infect Dis 31:770, 2000

23. Jurado RL, Farley MM, Pereira E, et al: Increased risk of meningitis and bacteremia due to *Listeria monocytogenes* in patients with human immunodeficiency virus infection. Clin Infect Dis 17:224, 1993

24. Durand ML, Calderwood SB, Weber DJ, et al: Acute bacterial meningitis in adults: a review of 493 episodes. N Engl J Med 328:21, 1993

25. Southwick FS, Purich DL: Intracellular pathogenesis of listeriosis. N Engl J Med 334:770, 1996

26. Braun L, Cossart P: Interactions between *Listeria monocytogenes* and host mammalian cells. Microbes Infect 2:803, 2000

27. Chakraborty T: Molecular and cell biological aspects of infection by *Listeria monocytogenes*. Immunobiology 201:155, 1999

28. Portnoy DA, Chakraborty T, Goebel W, et al: Molecular determinants of *Listeria monocytogenes* pathogenesis. Infect Immun 60:1263, 1992

29. Lorber B: Listeriosis. Clin Infect Dis 24:1, 1997

30. Anaissie E, Kontoyiannis DP, Kantarjian H, et al: Listeriosis in patients with chronic lymphocytic leukemia who were treated with fludarabine and prednisone. Ann Intern Med 117:466, 1992

31. Silver HM: Listeriosis during pregnancy. Obstet Gynecol Surv 53: 737, 1998

32. Nolla-Salas J, Bosch J, Gasser I, et al: Perinatal listeriosis: a population-based multicenter study in Barcelona, Spain (1990–1996). Am J Perinatol 15:461, 1998

33. Mylonakis E, Hohmann EL, Calderwood SB: Central nervous system infection with *Listeria monocytogenes*: 33 years' experience at a general hospital and review of 776 episodes from the literature. Medicine (Baltimore) 77:313, 1998

34. Armstrong RW, Fung PC: Brainstem encephalitis (rhombencephalitis) due to *Listeria monocytogenes*: case report and review. Clin Infect Dis 16:689, 1993

35. Uldry P-A, Kuntzer T, Bogousslavsky J, et al: Early symptoms and outcome of *Listeria monocytogenes* rhombencephalitis: 14 adult cases. J Neurol 240:235, 1993

36. Bartt R: *Listeria* and atypical presentations of *Listeria* in the central nervous. Semin Neurol 20:361, 2000

37. Lohmann CP, Gabel VP, Heep M, et al: *Listeria monocytogenes*-induced endogenous endophthalmitis in an otherwise healthy individual: rapid PCR-diagnosis as the basis for effective treatment. Eur J Ophthalmol 9:53, 1999

38. Vargas V, Aleman C, de Torres I, et al: *Listeria monocytogenes*–associated acute hepatitis in a liver transplant recipient. Liver 18:213, 1998

39. Temple ME, Nahata M C: Treatment of listeriosis. Ann Pharmacother 34:656, 2000

40. Hof H, Nichterlein T, Kretschmar M: Management of listeriosis. Clin Microbiol Rev 10:345, 1997

41. Nichterlein T, Bornitz F, Kretschmar M, et al: Successful treatment of murine listeriosis and salmonellosis with levofloxacin. J Chemother 10:313, 1998

42. Torres OH, Domingo P, Pericas R, et al: Infection caused by *Nocardia farcinica*: case report and review. Eur J Clin Microbiol Infect Dis 19: 205, 2000

43. Roberts SA, Franklin JC, Mijch A, et al: *Nocardia* infection in heart-lung transplant recipients at Alfred Hospital, Melbourne, Australia, 1989–1998. Clin Infect Dis 31:968, 2000

44. Javaly K, Horowitz HW, Wormser GP: Nocardiosis in patients with human immunodeficiency virus infection: report of two cases and review of the literature. Medicine (Baltimore) 71:128, 1992

45. Barnicoat MJ, Wierzbicki AS, Norman PM: Cerebral nocardiosis in immunosuppressed patients: five cases. Q J Med 72:689, 1989

46. LeBlang SD, Whiteman MLH, Post MJD, et al: CNS *Nocardia* in AIDS patients: CT and MRI with pathologic correlation. J Comput Assist Tomogr 19:15, 1995

47. Nenoff P, Kellermann S, Borte G, et al: Pulmonary nocardiosis with cutaneous involvement mimicking a metastasizing lung carcinoma in a patient with chronic myelogenous leukaemia. Eur J Dermatol 10:47, 2000

48. Angelika J, Hans-Jurgen G, Uwe-Frithjof H: Primary cutaneous nocardiosis in a husband and wife. J Am Acad Dermatol 41:338, 1999

49. Arduino RC, Johnson PC, Miranda AG: Nocardiosis in renal transplant recipients undergoing immunosuppression with cyclosporine. Clin Infect Dis 16:505, 1993

50. Kontoyiannis DP, Ruoff K, Hooper DC: *Nocardia bacteremia*. Report of four cases and review of the literature. Medicine (Baltimore) 77:255, 1998

51. Dixon T C, Meselson M, Guillemin J, et al: Anthrax (comments). N Engl J Med 341:815, 1999

52. Ringertz SH, Hoiby EA, Jensenius M, et al: Injectional anthrax in a heroin skin-popper (letter). Lancet 356:1574, 2000

53. Jackson PJ, Hugh-Jones ME, Adair DM, et al: PCR analysis of tissue samples from the 1979 Sverdlovsk anthrax victims: the presence of multiple *Bacillus anthracis* strains in different victims. Proc Natl Acad Sci U S A 95:1224, 1998

54. Bioterrorism alleging use of anthrax and interim guidelines for management: United States, 1998. MMWR Morb Mortal Wkly Rep 48: 69, 1999

55. Little SF, Ivins BE: Molecular pathogenesis of *Bacillus anthracis* infection. Microbes Infect 1:131, 1999

56. Smego RA Jr, Gebrian B, Desmangels G: Cutaneous manifestations of anthrax in rural Haiti. Clin Infect Dis 26:97, 1998

57. Shafazand S, Doyle R, Ruoss S, et al: Inhalational anthrax: epidemiology, diagnosis, and management. Chest 116:1369, 1999

58. Aslan G, Terzioglu A: Surgical management of cutaneous anthrax. Ann Plast Surg 41:468, 1998

59. Surveillance for adverse events associated with anthrax vaccination: U.S. Department of Defense, 1998-2000. MMWR Morb Mortal Wkly Rep 49:341, 2000

60. Sliman R, Rehm S, Shlaes DM: Serious infections caused by *Bacillus* species. Medicine (Baltimore) 66:218, 1987

61. Castedo E, Castro A, Martin P, et al: *Bacillus cereus* prosthetic valve endocarditis. Ann Thorac Surg 68:2351, 1999

62. Marley EF, Saini NK, Venkatraman C, et al: Fatal *Bacillus cereus* meningoencephalitis in an adult with acute myelogenous leukemia. South Med J 88:969, 1995

63. Barrie D, Wilson JA, Hoffman PN, et al: *Bacillus cereus* meningitis in two neurosurgical patients: an investigation into the source of the organism. J Infect 25:291, 1992

64. Loeb M, Wilcox L, Thornley D, et al: *Bacillus* species pseudobacteremia following hospital construction. Can J Infect Control 10:37, 1995

65. Krause A, Freeman R, Sisson PR, et al: Infection with *Bacillus cereus* after close-range gunshot injuries. J Trauma 41:546, 1996

66. Hemady R, Zaltas M, Paton B, et al: *Bacillus*-induced endophthalmitis: new series of 10 cases and review of the literature. Br J Ophthalmol 74:26, 1990

67. *Bacillus cereus* food poisoning associated with fried rice at two child day care centers: Virginia, 1993: Centers for Disease Control and Prevention. JAMA 271:1074, 1994

68. Mahler H, Pasi A, Kramer J M, et al: Fulminant liver failure in association with the emetic toxin of *Bacillus cereus* (comments). N Engl J Med 336:1142, 1997

69. Cotton DJ, Gill VJ, Marshall DJ, et al: Clinical features and therapeutic interventions in 17 cases of *Bacillus* bacteremia in an immunosuppressed patient population. J Clin Microbiol 25:672, 1987

70. Meredith FT, Fowler VG, Gautier M, et al: *Bacillus cereus* necrotizing cellulitis mimicking clostridial myonecrosis: case report and review of the literature. Scand J Infect Dis 29:528, 1997

71. Talan DA, Citron DM, Abrahamian FM, et al: Bacteriologic analysis of infected dog and cat bites. Emergency Medicine Animal Bite Infection Study Group. N Engl J Med 340:85, 1999

72. Brooke CJ, Riley TV: *Erysipelothrix rhusiopathiae*: bacteriology, epidemiology and clinical manifestations of an occupational pathogen. J Med Microbiol 48:789, 1999

73. Gorby GL, Peacock JE Jr: *Erysipelothrix rhusiopathiae* endocarditis: microbiologic, epidemiologic, and clinical features of an occupational disease. Rev Infect Dis 10:317, 1988

74. Venditti M, Gelfusa V, Tarasi A, et al: Antimicrobial susceptibilities of *Erysipelothrix rhusiopathiae*. Antimicrob Agents Chemother 34: 2038, 1990

17 Anaerobic Infections

Harvey B. Simon, M.D.

General Considerations

PATHOGENESIS OF ANAEROBIC INFECTIONS

Anaerobic bacteria dominate the microflora of healthy persons. Anaerobes outnumber aerobic and facultative bacteria in the colon by 1,000:1 and in the oral cavity and the female genital tract by 10:1. Even on the skin, where exposure to atmospheric oxygen might be expected to favor aerobes, anaerobic bacteria predominate in a ratio of about 10:1. Although more than 500 species of anaerobes have now been identified, only a small number of these organisms are clinically important.

The single property common to all anaerobes is oxygen intolerance; by definition, anaerobes are microorganisms that are unable to replicate in the presence of oxygen. Although Pasteur first recognized in 1863 that oxygen is toxic to certain bacteria, the mechanisms responsible for oxygen intolerance remain unclear. Moreover, anaerobic bacteria vary widely in their sensitivity to oxygen. Strict anaerobes grow best at an oxygen tension of less than 0.5%; some will be killed in 5 minutes by exposure to low concentrations of oxygen. This extreme oxygen sensitivity may partially be explained by the fact that many of these organisms lack the enzyme superoxide dismutase, which protects bacteria from the lethal effects of the superoxide radical. Many anaerobic bacteria that make up the normal flora of humans are strict anaerobes. However, most of the more pathogenic organisms are only moderate anaerobes; these bacteria grow best at an oxygen tension of less than 3%. Most of the moderate anaerobes contain at least small amounts of superoxide dismutase, and in some, such as *Bacteroides fragilis*, the enzyme is inducible by exposure to oxygen. Finally, some bacteria that are not strict anaerobes nevertheless grow much better anaerobically. These microaerophilic bacteria include a number of organisms capable of causing human disease, including certain *Clostridium, Streptococcus, Actinomyces,* and *Campylobacter* species.

The single most important requirement for virulence of anaerobes is a reduced environment. All anaerobes share this basic requirement, but their pathogenicity depends on diverse mechanisms.[1] Tissue invasion is one mechanism. Many anaerobes produce enzymes that can cause tissue damage; such enzymes include collagenase, hyaluronidase, and deoxyribonuclease. *Bacteroides* species appear to produce disease largely through direct tissue invasion. Many *Bacteroides* species make a heparinase that may account for their propensity to produce vascular thrombosis. In addition, these gram-negative bacilli contain endotoxins; the endotoxin of *Bacteroides* lacks a lipid A moiety, however, and is less potent than the endotoxins of aerobic and facultative gram-negative bacteria.[2] The virulence of *Clostridium* species depends on the production of various exotoxins. These toxins are so potent that life-threatening disease can result from mild or even inapparent local tetanus infection. *C. perfringens* produces toxins that may cause massive tissue necrosis in startlingly short periods. *Botulinum* toxin is the most potent of all exotoxins; ingestion of as little as 1 mg can induce lethal paralysis in a 70 kg man.

In addition to promoting the replication of anaerobes, a reduced environment impairs host defense mechanisms. Anaerobiosis impairs the bactericidal activity of polymorphonuclear leukocytes, probably by preventing the oxidative burst normally responsible for oxidant-mediated bactericidal activity. Hypoxia also impairs lymphocyte proliferation. Some anaerobic bacteria can directly impair host defenses by producing inhibitory products; *Bacteroides* species, for example, produce short-chain fatty acids that cause global impairment of the microbicidal activity of neutrophils.

Anaerobic infections frequently involve multiple bacterial species. In some infections, aerobic or facultative organisms are present together with anaerobes. Such infections are truly synergistic: the aerobic bacteria consume oxygen and thereby provide a reduced environment in which the anaerobes can thrive.

CLINICAL FEATURES OF ANAEROBIC INFECTIONS

Many anaerobic infections originate near a disrupted mucosal surface. Because anaerobes predominate in the indigenous microbiota of the oropharynx, colon, and female genital tract, most anaerobic infections are endogenous in origin. Thus, these infections depend on a primary insult to the patient's defense mechanisms rather than on transmission of a virulent agent from the outside environment.

Because of their intolerance for oxygen, anaerobes are often associated with ischemic, necrotic tissues; with the presence of foreign bodies; and with abscess formations. Anaerobic processes often begin as closed-space infections but frequently produce progressive necrosis and burrow through tissue planes. The presence of gas in tissues should raise the question of anaerobic or synergistic infection because many anaerobes are gas producers. Septic thrombophlebitis is a feature of anaerobic infections, especially those infections caused by *B. fragilis*.

A number of other clues should lead the clinician to suspect anaerobic infection. A foul smell is frequently associated with anaerobic infections, particularly when *Bacteroides* species are present. *Clostridium* species, however, do not share this tendency to cause putrid purulence. Because many anaerobes have characteristic morphologic properties, a Gram stain often provides the most rapid clue to the etiologic diagnosis. Negative aerobic cultures may indicate the presence of anaerobes, and although sterile pus can reflect the presence of mycobacteria or fungi, anaerobes are more often responsible. Finally, most antibiotics are less active at reduced oxygen tensions. If there is no response to therapy appropriate for aerobic or facultative organisms, the possibility of an anaerobic etiology should be considered.

Conditions that often result from polymicrobial or synergistic infection include aspiration pneumonias, lung abscesses, empyemas, intra-abdominal abscesses, pelvic infections, and certain necrotizing infections of skin and subcutaneous tissues.

PROCESSING OF SPECIMENS

Special processing of specimens is required of both the clinician and the laboratory if anaerobic infection is suspected. Because anaerobes constitute most of the normal flora of humans, specimens that have passed through the oropharynx, intestinal tract, or female genital tract inevitably become contaminated and are therefore useless. Thus, sputum, bronchoscopic washings, cervical or vaginal swabs, and stool specimens are unsuitable. The most useful specimens are blood, direct aspirates of abscesses or deep tissue infections, surgical specimens, or fluids that are normally sterile.

It is critical to get the specimen to the laboratory quickly and anaerobically. Aspirated fluids in sealed syringes are vastly preferable to swabs. When delay is unavoidable, special prereduced sterile anaerobic transport media should be used.

The microbiology laboratory faces a formidable task in the isolation and identification of anaerobes. A variety of techniques are available, and rapid progress in the development of new techniques continues. It has been estimated that in a microbiology laboratory that is equipped for the identification of anaerobes, approximately one third of all clinical specimens processed will grow one or more anaerobic bacteria and that another third of specimens will grow both anaerobes and aerobes. In such cases, the clinician must determine whether the identified organisms are pathogenic.

SPECIFIC ANAEROBIC INFECTIONS

Although anaerobic bacteria can cause various infections throughout the body, certain clinical syndromes typically involve anaerobes [*see Table 1*].

Clostridial Infections: Classification

Clostridia are gram-positive, spore-forming bacilli; all species are obligate anaerobes, but *C. perfringens* is relatively aerotolerant. There are three major groups of clostridia: histotoxic species (*C. perfringens*, *C. ramosum*, *C. novyi*, *C. septicum*, *C. bifermentans*, and *C. sordellii*), enterotoxigenic species (*C. perfringens* and *C. difficile*), and neurotoxic species (*C. tetani* and *C. botulinum*).

Diseases Due to Histotoxic Clostridia

Clostridia causing invasive infection are found in the lower gastrointestinal tract and in the soil. *C. perfringens* [*see Figure 1*] is the species most frequently responsible for human disease. Most invasive clostridial infections are of endogenous origin and are precipitated by trauma, underlying intestinal disorders, or lowered host resistance, all of which enable these organisms to enter sites outside

Table 1 Selected Antimicrobials for Anaerobic Infections*

Drug	*Representative Dose*†	*Interval*	*Typical Anaerobic Spectrum*	*Cost/Day ($)*	*Comments*
Penicillin G	1–4 million U	4–6 hr	Effective against peptostreptococci, oral *Bacteroides* species, *Veillonella* species, fusobacteria, peptococci, *Clostridium perfringens, Propionibacterium* species	10–20	Problems caused by these organisms include brain abscesses, subdural or extradural empyema, chronic sinusitis, lower respiratory tract infections, female genital tract infections, bone and joint infections, bacteremia, endocarditis, and intra-abdominal abscesses, as well as uncommon but severe skin and soft tissue infections such as myonecrosis, Meleney progressive synergistic gangrene, necrotizing fasciitis, and Fournier gangrene; in addition to antibiotics, most abscesses require percutaneous or surgical drainage. Necrotizing infections require surgical drainage and debridement.
Ampicillin-sulbactam	3 g	6 hr	Effective against peptostreptococci, *Bacteroides* species, fusobacteria, peptococci, many gram-negative bacilli	40–50	
Ticarcillin–clavulanic acid	3.1 g	4 hr	Effective against peptostreptococci, *Bacteroides* species, fusobacteria, peptococci	50–60	
Cefoxitin	2 g	8 hr	Effective against *Clostridium* species, microaerophilic streptococci, *Bacteroides* species	60–70	
Cefotetan	1–2 g	12 hr	Effective against *Clostridium* species, microaerophilic streptococci, *Bacteroides* species	20–30	
Ceftizoxime	2 g	8 hr	Effective against *Clostridium* species, microaerophilic streptococci, *Bacteroides* species	70–80	
Imipenem-cilastatin	500 mg	6 hr	Effective against *Clostridium* species, microaerophilic streptococci, *Bacteroides* species	100–150	
Meropenem	1 g	8 hr	Effective against *Clostridium* species, microaerophilic streptococci, *Bacteroides* species	150–200	
Clindamycin	600 mg	8 hr	Effective against *Clostridium* species, microaerophilic streptococci, *Bacteroides* species	30–40	
Metronidazole	500 mg	6 hr	Effective against most anaerobes, including *Clostridium* and *Bacteroides* species	100–150	

*See 2 Chemotherapy of Infection for details.
†Doses for major infections in adults with normal renal function.

their usual habitat. *C. septicum* infections are particularly likely to occur in patients with underlying malignancies.[3]

The spectrum of disease produced by *C. perfringens* is extensive [*see Table 2*]. Most often, isolation of *C. perfringens* represents simple contamination of a wound surface.

PATHOGENESIS

Even when severe wounds are contaminated with clostridia, gas gangrene develops in only a very small percentage of patients. For infection to occur, a lowered oxidation-reduction potential is needed, which allows spore germination and bacterial multiplication. Tissue necrosis, impaired blood supply, and introduction of foreign bodies provide the appropriate environment. Major determinants of pathogenicity for invasive clostridia are their potent exotoxins. The *C. perfringens* α-toxin, a lecithinase, is the most important, exhibiting hemolytic, necrotizing, and lethal properties. α-Toxin disrupts membranes containing phospholipid-lecithin complexes, including human cell and mitochondrial membranes, and has direct myocardial depressant properties. β-Toxin is a potent cytotoxin that has cytolytic activity, particularly against endothelial cells.[4] Once bacterial multiplication and toxin production occur at a site of injury, rapid invasion and destruction of healthy tissue ensue.[5] The paucity of leukocytes in the exudate of clostridial myonecrosis may reflect α-toxin and β-toxin cytotoxicities.

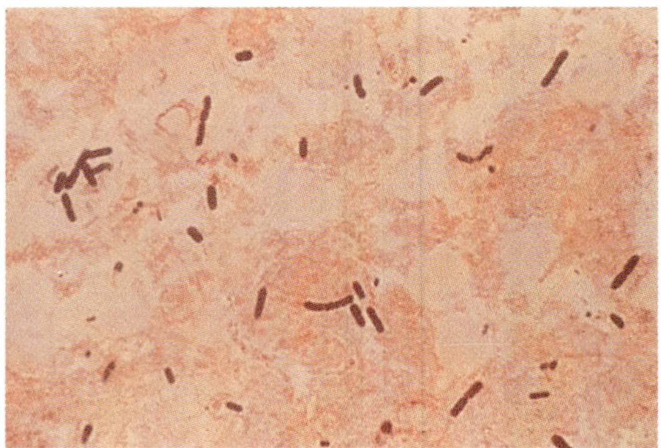

Figure 1 **Gram stain of *Clostridium perfringens* from a case of clostridial myonecrosis (magnification: ×1,000).**

SPECIFIC CLOSTRIDIAL INFECTIONS

C. perfringens and other histotoxic clostridia can cause a spectrum of disorders ranging in severity from relatively benign conditions (Welch abscess or anaerobic cellulitis) to infections associated with high mortality (clostridial myonecrosis or post-abortion uterine infection).

Table 2 Spectrum of Disease Produced by *Clostridium perfringens*

Traumatic Setting
Wound infection
Surface contamination
Localized Welch abscess (gas abscess)
Anaerobic cellulitis
Clostridial myonecrosis (gas gangrene)
Uterine infection (septic abortion; postpartum uterine infection)
Brain abscess secondary to penetrating foreign body
Burn wound sepsis
Mixed peritonitis secondary to penetrating trauma
Nontraumatic Setting
Postoperative gas gangrene (after cholecystectomy or bowel surgery)
Spontaneous gas gangrene (after bowel necrosis or infarction)
Postinjection gas gangrene
Isolated bacteremia (from decubitus ulcer, gangrene of extremity)
Septicemia (associated with leukemia or other malignant disease or with an intestinal lesion)
Miscellaneous infections (pneumonia, empyema, meningitis, cholecystitis, emphysematous cystitis, pyelonephritis)
Gastroenteritis
C. perfringens food poisoning
Enteritis necroticans

Welch Abscess

A Welch abscess is a localized collection of dark, foul fluid, sometimes mixed with gas, in a wound cavity. *C. perfringens* is isolated in pure culture. There is no invasion of surrounding tissues, and the process subsides after either spontaneous or surgical drainage.

Anaerobic (Clostridial) Cellulitis

Definition and etiology Anaerobic cellulitis is a moderately serious gas-forming infection of skin and subcutaneous tissues that does not invade muscle or produce the toxemic state seen with clostridial gas gangrene. It occurs in devitalized tissue in a dirty or inadequately debrided wound. Infection extends through tissue planes and is accompanied by the formation of large quantities of gas (more than is usually evident in cases of clostridial myonecrosis).

Clinical features and diagnosis The infection develops at a more gradual pace than gas gangrene. A thin, dark, gray-brown, foul exudate is produced. There is relatively little local pain or change in overlying skin. Radiographs of the involved area often show large gas bubbles that extend along fascial planes. Diagnosis is usually based on a Gram stain revealing plump, gram-positive bacilli (without spores) and variable numbers of polymorphonuclear leukocytes.

Differential diagnosis The presence of gas in subcutaneous tissue is not pathognomonic of clostridial infection [*see Table 3*]. Patients with diabetes mellitus are particularly prone to crepitant cellulitis caused by enteric bacteria or *Bacteroides* species. Perineal phlegmons, which result from extension of perirectal abscesses, may also be associated with subcutaneous gas formation; mixed infections with facultative organisms and with obligate anaerobes underlie such inflammations. Crepitus from trapped air [*see Table 3*] can usually be distinguished from crepitus caused by anaerobic cellulitis or myonecrosis by the fact that the former does not spread and by the patient's history. Surgery, with inspection of muscle for viability and the presence of clostridia, is necessary to distinguish anaerobic cellulitis from myonecrosis.[6]

Clostridial Myonecrosis

Definition and etiology Clostridial myonecrosis (gas gangrene, clostridial myositis) is an incredibly toxemic, rapidly progressive infection, usually caused by *C. perfringens*. It initially involves injured or devitalized muscle and then aggressively

Table 3 Causes of Gas in Soft Tissues

Bacterial Causes of Nonclostridial Crepitant Cellulitis
- *Escherichia coli*
- *Klebsiella* species
- *Peptostreptococcus* species
- *Bacteroides* and *Fusobacterium* species
- *Streptococcus pyogenes* (rare)
- Mixed cultures: facultative and anaerobic species, as seen in a perineal phlegmon

Sources of Crepitus after Trauma or after Manipulation
- Trapped air in open traumatic or surgical wounds
- Compressed air injection
- Gas released from H_2O_2 irrigations of a wound
- Air trapped around site of intravenous catheter placement

invades contiguous normal muscle.[6] Gas gangrene can occur after extensive injuries or penetrating war wounds; after surgery on the biliary tract or colon; in an infarcted bowel (incarcerated hernia); in arterial disease; or, very rarely, after an intramuscular injection, usually of epinephrine. Spontaneous, nontraumatic cases have also been reported. The incubation period is short, ranging from 8 to 72 hours.

Clinical features and diagnosis Onset is acute, and local pain is the earliest symptom, followed by pallor, apprehension, marked tachycardia, moderate fever, and lethargy. Hypotension, shock, and oliguria quickly supervene. Swelling of the involved area is marked. The overlying skin becomes dark yellow or bronze. In an involved extremity, the skin is pale and cold as a result of ischemia. Crepitus is present but not prominent. A thin, brownish discharge with a foul odor is evident; tense blebs containing dark, thin fluid often develop.

A presumptive diagnosis is based on a Gram stain of the wound drainage or of an aspirate from a bleb that reveals many clostridia but few leukocytes. Cultures ultimately reveal clostridia, often mixed with several other aerobic or anaerobic organisms. Bacteremia rarely complicates gas gangrene, and acute intravascular hemolysis is not usually a feature. The clinical setting, appearance of the involved area, and demonstration of large gram-positive rods in stained smears of the exudate provide support. It should be emphasized that *C. perfringens* does not form spores in tissues. Cultural confirmation of the presence of *C. perfringens* (or related histotoxic clostridia) takes several days and is not helpful in immediate management.

Differential diagnosis Definition of the specific clostridial syndrome requires surgical exploration and direct examination of healthy muscle for the presence of myonecrosis. In gas gangrene, involved muscle looks cooked and lacks contractility, whereas in cases of clostridial cellulitis, healthy muscle is not affected.

Uterine Infection

At least 5% of healthy women harbor *C. perfringens* in the genital tract. Almost all cases of clostridial uterine infection are caused by *C. perfringens*.

Etiology Infection occurs in the setting of an incomplete abortion, premature rupture of membranes, or operative termination of pregnancy. From the endometrium, the organisms may enter and remain confined to the myometrium, or instead, the infection may spread widely, as in the septicemic form of clostridial uterine infection.

Clinical features and diagnosis During an incubation period of 12 to 72 hours, vaginal bleeding, low-grade fever, and low abdominal pain occur. The onset of systemic symptoms, such as vomiting, diarrhea, marked tachycardia, high fever, and chills, is abrupt. A foul-smelling vaginal discharge is present, the uterus and adnexa are tender, and peritoneal signs may result from perforation of the uterus. The rapid development of jaundice and hemoglobinemia are the consequences of massive intravascular hemolysis secondary to intense bacteremia and toxemia. Hypotension, shock, and renal shutdown are common in such cases.

Other Clostridial Infections

Massive hemolysis can accompany intense *C. perfringens* bacteremia (originating from intestinal ulcerations) in patients with leukemia. Bacteremias caused by *C. septicum* and *C. perfringens* can occur without associated hemolysis in patients with leukemia and other neoplasms or in patients with bowel disease,[7] decubitus ulcers, or peripheral gangrene. *C. tertium* bacteremia is less common but can develop, especially in neutropenic patients.[8] Although rare, clostridial endocarditis can occur.[9]

Clostridia are occasionally found as part of a mixed flora that causes peritonitis or an intra-abdominal abscess after either a penetrating wound of the abdomen or perforation of a diseased colon. *C. perfringens* and *C. ramosum* are the most common clostridial species isolated in this setting. Clostridial brain abscesses can complicate penetrating head injuries; air-filled cavities have been observed in more than 50% of such injuries.

Clostridial infections of the respiratory and urinary tracts are rare, as is clostridial septic arthritis.[10]

TREATMENT OF INVASIVE CLOSTRIDIAL INFECTIONS

Surgery

Surgery should be performed immediately to define the nature and extent of the process and to eliminate all infected tissue. The procedure includes multiple incisions for drainage, fasciotomy for decompression of fascial compartments, and excision of involved muscle. Such surgery can control localized myositis. If the process is extensive and irreversible changes have occurred in an extremity, amputation becomes necessary. Widespread involvement of the abdomen makes extensive resection extremely difficult but not impossible. Such radical debridement is mutilating and presents problems of fluid loss. Plastic reconstruction is necessary after such surgery. Early use of hyperbaric oxygen therapy may limit the zone of frank muscle necrosis, reducing the extent of the surgical debridement.

Simple drainage, fasciotomy where indicated, and excision of necrotic tissue are usually sufficient for treating clostridial cellulitis.

Antibiotics

As an adjunct to surgical therapy, antibiotics are employed to eliminate organisms not removed by debridement and to control any bacteremia that may occur. Penicillin G (10 to 20 million U/day I.V. in divided doses for 2 weeks) is the drug of choice. When a Gram stain shows gram-negative bacilli, an aminoglycoside (e.g., gentamicin), a newer cephalosporin (e.g., ceftazidime), or a fluoroquinolone (e.g., levofloxacin) should be added initially. Clindamycin, metronidazole, and chloramphenicol are alternatives for patients who are highly allergic to penicillin.

Hyperbaric Oxygen

Hyperbaric oxygen therapy, consisting of the administration of 100% oxygen at 2 to 3 atm for approximately 2 hours, has been used as an adjunct to surgical debridement and antibiotics in the treatment of clostridial gas gangrene. Despite enthusiasm for hyperbaric oxygen therapy, there have been no controlled trials of its use in humans, and its precise role in the management of gas gangrene and other anaerobic infections remains to be defined.[11,12]

Other Measures

Transfusions, plasma infusions, and electrolyte replacement are required to treat anemia, hypovolemia, and shock. Polyvalent equine antitoxin was used in the treatment of clostridial myonecrosis, but its efficacy was not proved, and it is no longer available.

PROGNOSIS

The overall mortality in gas gangrene is 15% to 30%. Gas gangrene of the abdominal wall has a mortality of 50%. Mortality in postabortion uterine infection caused by *C. perfringens* with associated intravascular hemolysis is approximately 50%.

Diseases Due to Enterotoxigenic Clostridia

FOOD POISONING

Food poisoning caused by *C. perfringens* ranks second only to staphylococcal food poisoning in the annual number of outbreaks in the United States. Most strains of *C. perfringens* associated with food poisoning are heat-resistant type A organisms. The vehicle is usually a meat product that has been stewed or boiled and then left for a few hours before serving or rewarming. The initial cooking kills contaminating vegetative forms but not heat-resistant spores of *C. perfringens*. During cooling, the spores germinate and multiply in the anaerobic environment. Large numbers of viable organisms are then ingested. These organisms multiply and sporulate in the small intestine. Sporulation is associated with elaboration of an enterotoxin that produces ileal fluid accumulation and diarrhea.

Abdominal cramps and diarrhea develop about 8 to 12 hours after ingestion of contaminated food. Nausea occurs occasionally, but vomiting does not occur. Fever, headache, and systemic symptoms are absent. The illness is mild and runs its course in 24 hours.[13]

ENTERITIS NECROTICANS

In developing countries, intestinal infection with *C. perfringens* type C can cause a severe hemorrhagic, inflammatory, or ischemic necrosis of the jejunum known as enteritis necroticans or pigbel. Occasional cases have been reported in the United States, usually in chronically ill persons who consume pig intestines (chitterlings).[14]

COLITIS

Epidemiology

C. difficile is found in soil, in animals, and as part of the normal fecal flora in humans. Isolating *C. difficile* from stool is difficult but can be facilitated by the use of special selective media. The organism is acquired early in infancy, often in neonatal nurseries. Up to 78% of neonates harbor the organism, but the carrier rate declines to less than 50% in infants and older children.[15] Despite the high carrier rate, however, infants and young children are highly resistant to the clinical effects of *C. difficile*, possibly because the immature intestinal mucosa lacks receptors for the organism's toxins. The prevalence of positive cultures declines from a peak of about 78% in infants to about 5% in healthy adults.[16] The carrier rate is much higher in debilitated adults; the organism is usually acquired in a health care facility. Asymptomatic primary carriers have a lower risk of developing *C. difficile*-associated diarrhea (CDAD) than patients who acquire the organisms during a hospitalization,[17] possibly because of protection conferred by IgG antibody against *C. difficile* toxin A.[18]

Adult carriers may introduce *C. difficile* on admission to acute care or long-term care facilities.[19] In the hospital, the organism can spread from patient to patient; positive hand cultures suggest that medical personnel can transmit the infection.[20] About 20% of all patients acquire the organism during hospitalization, but two thirds remain asymptomatic. In rare instances, *C. difficile* causes colitis in patients who have not been hospitalized[21] or in those who have not previously been exposed to antibiotics; anticancer chemotherapy predisposes to *C. difficile* infection even in the absence of antibiotic therapy.

Etiology

CDAD occurs principally as a side effect of oral or parenterally administered antibiotic therapy. It accounts for about 25% of all cases of diarrhea in patients receiving antibiotics; CDAD may begin in the first few days of antibiotic therapy or as late as 6 weeks after antibiotics have been discontinued.[22] Antibiotics alter the normal fecal microflora and may allow *C. difficile* to proliferate and produce its two high-molecular-weight protein enterotoxins, toxin A (enterotoxin) and toxin B (cytotoxin), which cause CDAD. This syndrome was first observed in patients receiving clindamycin, but many other antibiotics may be responsible [see 2 Chemotherapy of Infection]. The risk is greatest from clindamycin, the cephalosporins, and ampicillin and is lowest from vancomycin, metronidazole, and the aminoglycosides.[23] Patients receiving tube feedings are at particular risk.[24]

Clinical Features and Diagnosis

At least 300,000 cases of CDAD occur in the United States every year.[22] The symptoms range from mild diarrhea to severe colitis with fever, leukocytosis, abdominal cramps, and bloody diarrhea[13,22,23]. Endoscopy reveals pseudomembrane formation in about half of the cases. Toxic megacolon may occur in severe cases, particularly in patients who have received antimotility agents. Intestinal perforation may occur in severe disease but is uncommon. Bacteremia and extracolonic infections with *C. difficile* are rare.[25]

The diagnosis of CDAD is most often established by demonstrating the toxins of *C. difficile* in stool specimens.[26] The original tissue culture cytotoxicity assay has been largely replaced by more rapid, less expensive immunoassays; enzyme-linked immunosorbent assays (ELISAs) are more reliable than latex agglutination tests, and a polymerase chain reaction assay is being studied. Perhaps 5% to 20% of patients require more than one stool assay to detect toxin; when ELISA results are negative but clinical suspicion is high, the tissue cytotoxicity assay will detect toxin in 5% to 10% of cases.[22]

Treatment

Patients with CDAD should be treated promptly. In nearly all cases, the offending antibiotic should be discontinued. Symptomatic patients should receive orally administered metronidazole or vancomycin. Administration of either agent at a dosage of 500 mg three times daily for 10 days produces a clinical cure in 94% of patients.[27] Metronidazole is considerably less expensive, but occasionally, *C. difficile* strains are resistant to the drug; because vancomycin is active against all isolates and is not absorbed in the upper gastrointestinal tract, it may be preferable for severely ill patients. For patients with CDAD who cannot tolerate oral therapy, intravenous therapy with vancomycin and metronidazole or with metronidazole alone has been recommended. Orally administered bacitracin is as effective in alleviating symptoms as either metronidazole or vancomycin but is less effective in eradicating *C. difficile* and its toxins from patients' stools.[15] Cholestyramine resin binds the toxin and may be useful for some patients.[15]

Regardless of which regimen is used, symptoms recur in about 20% of patients[28,29]; relapse is usually responsible but is less likely to occur in patients who mount a serum antibody response to toxin A during the initial episode.[30] In a few patients, reinfection with a new strain of *C. difficile* accounts for recurrent CDAD.[31] Patients whose symptoms recur should be treated again; various regimens, including a prolonged tapering course of vancomycin,[22] have been suggested, but none is ideal. Administration of the yeast *Saccharomyces boulardii* may improve the results of antibiotic therapy in some patients with relapses of *C. difficile* colitis[32]; lactobacillus is also being studied.[33]

Because *C. difficile* can be isolated from asymptomatic hospital personnel and from environmental surfaces,[20] enteric precautions are necessary when caring for patients with *C. difficile* colitis. Interpersonal spread of *C. difficile* colitis has been documented in hospitals and day care settings even in the absence of antibiotic use. Enteric precautions, hand washing, and restrictions on the use of antibiotics[31,34,35] and environmental disinfectants containing hypochlorite[36] can reduce the incidence of *C. difficile* acquisition and the subsequent development of disease. However, antibiotic therapy for asymptomatic carriers is not beneficial. In rare instances, *C. difficile* may cause extracolonic disease.[37–40]

Diseases Due to Neurotoxic Clostridia

TETANUS

Tetanus is a life-threatening acute disease caused by *C. tetani* in which all of the clinical features are produced by the effects of a potent neurotoxin, tetanospasmin. The disease is characterized by generalized rigidity and intermittent, intense muscle spasms.

Etiology

C. tetani is an anaerobic gram-positive bacillus commonly found in the soil, in the intestines of domestic animals, and occasionally in human feces. Spores are introduced into tissues after a penetrating injury. After the spores germinate, tetanus toxin is produced by replicating bacteria and is released by cell lysis. Tetanus and botulin toxins are of similar potency and are the most powerful bacterial toxins known. Only one antigenic type of tetanus toxin exists, making possible an effective toxoid for immunization.

Epidemiology

Tetanus is now rare in industrialized countries because of the widespread use of active immunization. In the United States, fewer than 50 cases are reported annually; at least 87% occur in inadequately immunized persons, and 35% occur in persons older than 60 years, which emphasizes the need to maintain immunity in older adults. Rural populations, immigrants, and abusers of I.V. narcotics are also at risk for tetanus and warrant special attention to ensure adequate immunization. In developing countries, tetanus is still a major problem, causing the deaths of an estimated one million persons annually, of which about half are newborns.

Pathogenesis

The organism is commonly introduced by a laceration or puncture wound that is usually sustained outdoors. Tetanus may also occur in association with pregnancy (postpartum and postabortion tetanus), surgery (postoperative tetanus), burns, vaccination, intramuscular injections, gangrene, chronic skin ulcers, dog bites, penetrating eye injuries, umbilical stump infection in newborns (neonatal tetanus), and narcotics addiction. In 10% to 20% of patients with tetanus, there is no history of injury or evidence of an infected lesion.

Tetanus toxin produced in a wound can spread centrally via intra-axonal transport along motor nerves to the spinal cord; it may also spread hematogenously. The toxin acts principally on the spinal cord, altering normal control of the reflex arc by suppressing the inhibition regularly mediated by the internuncial neurons. As a result of this suppression, for example, contraction of the biceps is accompanied by contraction of the antagonist muscle (the triceps), producing a spasm. When muscle spasms occur, the characteristic clinical features are determined by the relative strengths of the opposing muscles: the greater strength of the masseter over the opposing digastricus and mylohyoid results in trismus; the greater strength of the extensor groups over the flexors in the lower extremities produces characteristic extension at the hips and knees; and the greater strength of the biceps results in flexion of the forearms. This combination of flexion of the upper extremities and extension of the lower extremities is termed opisthotonos [*see Figure 2*].

The incubation period between injury and onset of symptoms ranges from 1 to 55 days. In more than 80% of patients, symptoms begin within 14 days. The length of the incubation period is a valuable prognostic sign in patients younger than 50 years: mortality is almost 100% when this period is only 1 or 2 days but 35% to 40% when it is more than 10 days.

Generalized tetanus Occasionally, local spasm at the wound site is the initial complaint. The usual presenting symptoms are restlessness; pain caused by muscle spasm; and stiffness of the back, neck, thighs, and abdomen. The patient notes difficulty in opening the mouth (trismus, or lockjaw), the hall-

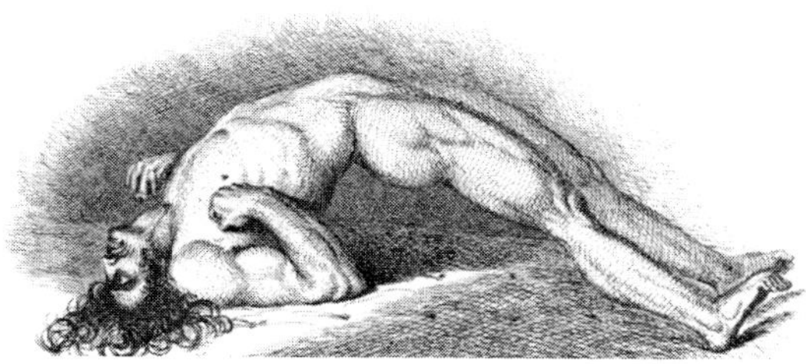

Figure 2 **Spasms in a wounded soldier with tetanus are illustrated in this drawing by Scottish surgeon and anatomist Sir Charles Bell in his book *The Anatomy and Philosophy of Expression*, published in 1832. The classic signs of tetanus—risus sardonicus, trismus, and opisthotonos—are shown.**

mark of tetanus; this is the first symptom in more than 50% of patients. Dysphagia, caused by spasm of pharyngeal muscles, may be an early symptom. Deep tendon reflexes are hyperactive, but the plantar responses are flexor. As the process progresses to generalized tetanus, violent spasms of the paraspinal, abdominal, and limb musculature occur, but the patient remains conscious. Trismus and stiffness of the facial muscles produce risus sardonicus, a characteristic sneering expression. Sudden stimuli (e.g., bright light or noise) can precipitate tonic seizure, accompanied by diaphragmatic, intercostal, glottal, or laryngeal spasm, and result in hypoxia and respiratory arrest. Fever (temperature of 38.3° to 38.9° C [100.9° to 102.0° F]) may be caused by the marked muscular rigidity and spasms alone.

Severe sympathetic hyperactivity has been associated with tetanus, which suggests that the toxin may directly affect the sympathetic portion of the CNS. Labile hypertension, tachycardia, arrhythmias, profuse sweating, marked intermittent vasoconstriction, tachypnea, and hypotension may occur singly or in varying combinations.

After the manifestations of tetanus have peaked, they persist at the same level for about a week and then gradually diminish over several weeks. Residual stiffness may persist for several more weeks. Among those patients who have survived moderate to severe tetanus, respiratory assistance was required for 2 to 4 weeks, and the average hospital stay was 5 to 8 weeks.

The major complications of tetanus are respiratory arrest secondary to tetanic spasms, pneumonia secondary to aspiration, pulmonary emboli, cardiac problems related to sympathetic overactivity or to cardiomyopathy, and fractures of thoracic vertebrae caused by violent spasms.

Cephalic tetanus Cephalic tetanus is a unique form of tetanus that results from the effects of toxin on the brain stem innervation of the jaw, ocular, facial, glossal, and pharyngeal musculature. It occurs when spores of *C. tetani* are introduced during trauma to the head or neck, into wounds of the eye, or during the course of chronic otitis media. Trismus is usually the first sign after a variable incubation period. A peripheral type of facial paralysis, ophthalmoplegias, and apparent palsies of cranial nerves IX, X, and XII are also evident. The apparent facial palsy is really a pseudoparalysis caused by hypertonia involving all of the muscles supplied by the facial nerve; voluntary movements are inhibited. If left untreated, most cases of cephalic tetanus progress to generalized tetanus.

Localized tetanus Localized tetanus is an unusual clinical form of the disorder characterized by intermittent painful spasms of muscles in a localized area, commonly a limb. Onset is usually preceded by a wound in the involved area. Stiffness of the involved muscles is the initial symptom, occurring days or several weeks after injury. The stiffness and spasms may persist for weeks in the local area and then gradually abate, or trismus and generalized tetanus may develop in a few days. Self-limited tetanus probably occurs only in persons with some degree of immunity or in persons whose wounds contain few *C. tetani* organisms.

Laboratory findings Blood counts, blood chemistries, and CSF values are normal. *C. tetani* is isolated from the wound in only 30% of cases, probably because of the fastidious anaerobic requirements of the organism.

Differential Diagnosis

The diagnosis of fully developed generalized tetanus presents little difficulty. Acute strychnine poisoning is the only disease that resembles tetanus. A greater problem in differential diagnosis occurs earlier in the course of the illness, when trismus is the principal manifestation. Trismus may also be present in patients with encephalitis, but in contrast to those with tetanus, these patients are not fully conscious. Trismus may occur in patients with intraoral disease, especially dental or jaw infections, and is rarely seen in those with trichinosis. Hepatic encephalopathy is sometimes associated with prominent muscular stiffness and rigidity. In this setting, trismus may also be present. The liver disease is usually obvious. A sudden stimulus, such as jarring a bed rail, is likely to cause spasms in a patient with tetanus but not in a patient with hepatic encephalopathy. Hysteria may mimic tetanus, particularly in the occurrence of trismus.

Trismus may also develop as an acute reaction, the so-called grimacing syndrome, to phenothiazine drugs. Unlike tetanus, the masseter spasm in this drug reaction is painful and intermittent and to some degree can be overcome voluntarily. The spasm in this drug-induced pseudotetanus may transiently pass from the masseter muscle to the pterygoid muscles; the jaw then opens wide for a short time, and the tongue protrudes. This drug reaction can be reversed promptly by administering diphenhydramine intravenously.

Treatment of Established Tetanus

General measures Treatment of tetanus is aimed at prevention of muscle spasms and respiratory complications, neutralization of circulating toxin, and elimination of the source of the toxin. Patients with tetanus should be placed in an intensive care unit, where they can be carefully monitored and receive constant nursing care. External stimuli (e.g., noise or bright lights) that may precipitate muscle spasms must be minimized. A urinary catheter is required.

Because of the danger of precipitating pharyngeal or laryngeal spasms by oral feedings, fluids and electrolytes are initially administered intravenously. Later, when the danger of aspiration is reduced, a nasojejunal tube may be used, provided that a cuffed endotracheal tube or tracheostomy tube is in place. Patients with severe and prolonged tetanus, who are in continued danger of aspiration, may require intravenous hyperalimentation or a feeding gastrostomy.[41]

Antitoxin Tetanus antitoxin does not appear to neutralize toxin already bound in the CNS, and its administration does not alter manifestations of tetanus already evident. Antitoxin does neutralize circulating toxin, however. Human tetanus immune globulin is given intramuscularly. A dose of 3,000 to 5,000 units was previously recommended, but 500 units is now considered sufficient.[41,42]

Control of muscular spasms and rigidity The use of muscle relaxants is essential. Their efficacy is enhanced by the use of sedatives to decrease responsiveness to sensory stimuli. Sedation requires careful titration to prevent respiratory depression, a complication that can best be minimized in the ICU setting.

Diazepam is the drug of choice and is widely used because it acts rapidly as a muscle relaxant and produces a sedative effect without inducing depression. The dosage (40 to more than 200 mg/day I.V.) is higher than that used for other conditions and is titrated to the patient's needs. If severe spasms cannot be controlled by diazepam, assisted ventilation and neuromuscular blockade may be required to produce paralysis.

Control of sympathetic overactivity Propranolol and labetalol are examples of beta-adrenergic blocking agents that have been used in patients with tetanus to treat marked sympathetic overactivity, including hypertension, tachycardia, and profuse sweating. In rare cases of extreme sympathetic overactivity, the addition of intravenous morphine to the therapeutic program (accompanied by controlled ventilation at all times) may be necessary to manage the autonomic dysfunction.

Antibiotic treatment The value of antimicrobial agents in the treatment of tetanus is doubtful. The only beneficial effect of antibiotics would be to eradicate from the wound vegetative cells of *C. tetani* that could produce additional toxin. Penicillin, administered intravenously for a week at intervals of 6 hours for a total daily dose of 10 to 15 million units, has been the traditional drug of choice, but metronidazole, in a 500 mg I.V. dose every 6 hours, is now preferred.[41,42]

Eradication of the infected site If feasible, wound debridement is carried out to eliminate the site of toxin elaboration. Wound material should be cultured aerobically and anaerobically at the time of surgery. Surgery should be performed only after the initial doses of tetanus immune globulin and antibiotics have been given and after muscle spasms have been controlled. The wound should be thoroughly irrigated and left open. Subsequent care of the wound should include irrigation with a 3% solution of hydrogen peroxide.

Tetanus toxoid Before discharge from the hospital, the patient should receive the first dose of adsorbed tetanus toxoid. Clinical tetanus does not establish natural immunity; thus, appropriate immunization to forestall a second episode of tetanus is mandatory; human tetanus immune globulin does not impede successful immunization.[41,42]

Prevention

The frequent exposure of children and adults to trauma and the ubiquity of *C. tetani* underscore the need for effective active immunization.

Immunization Infants should receive diphtheria-pertussis-tetanus (DPT) vaccine at 2 months of age. Two additional doses are given at 4 and 6 months of age. A booster injection of DPT is given at 18 months of age and again 4 years later. At 16 years of age, a booster dose of combined adult-type tetanus and diphtheria toxoids is administered. Thereafter, immunity is maintained by booster injections every decade. About 70% of Americans have protective levels of tetanus antibodies (> 0.15 IU/ml). Nearly 90% of children are protected, but the rate declines rapidly after 40 years of age, decreasing to less than 30% after 70 years of age.[43] Adults who have not been immunized should receive two doses of alum-precipitated tetanus toxoid intramuscularly, 1 month apart, followed by a booster dose after 1 year. Thereafter, immunity is maintained by booster injections every decade. In developing countries, immunization of pregnant women can prevent neonatal tetanus without teratogenicity.[44] Occasionally, persons who have received multiple booster injections experience hypersensitivity reactions such as local edema, erythema, pain, and fever. Because of these adverse reactions, the declining incidence of tetanus, and the expense of routine immunizations, British public health authorities no longer recommend boosters for persons who have had five doses of tetanus toxoid.[45]

Management of wounds About two thirds of cases of tetanus in the United States occur after puncture wounds, lacerations, and other penetrating trauma. Appropriate prophylaxis is directed against the development of trauma-induced tetanus; prompt and thorough debridement is of paramount importance. Prophylactic antibiotics do not reliably prevent subsequent tetanus. The United States Public Health Service has issued specific recommendations for tetanus prophylaxis [*see Table 4*].

BOTULISM

Like tetanus, botulism is a life-threatening disease caused by a potent clostridial neurotoxin; unlike tetanospasmin, which binds to inhibitory neurons and causes muscle spasms, *Botulinum* toxin targets peripheral cholinergic synapses and results in weakness that progresses to flaccid paralyses. About 100 cases of botulism are reported in the United States each year, but a surge in cases associated with black tar heroin[46] and the threat of international terrorism[47] have renewed interest in a disease that was first recognized in the early 17th century.

Table 4 Recommendations for Tetanus Prophylaxis in Routine Wound Management

History of Adsorbed Tetanus Toxoid	*Clean, Minor Wounds*		*All Other Wounds**	
	Td†	*TIG*	*Td†*	*TIG*
Unknown or fewer than three doses	Yes	No	Yes	Yes
Three or more doses‡	No§	No	No‖	No

*Such as, but not limited to, wounds contaminated with dirt, feces, soil, saliva, etc.; puncture wounds; avulsions; and wounds resulting from missiles, crushing, burns, and frostbite.
†For children younger than 7 yr, DTP (DT, if pertussis vaccine is contraindicated) is preferred to tetanus toxoid alone. For persons 7 yr of age or older, Td is preferred to tetanus toxoid alone.
‡If only three doses of fluid toxoid have been received, then a fourth dose of toxoid, preferably an adsorbed toxoid, should be given.
§Yes, if more than 10 yr since last dose.
‖Yes, if more than 5 yr since last dose.
DT—diphtheria and tetanus toxoids adsorbed (dose of diphtheria toxoid is higher than that in Td, dose of tetanus toxoid is the same)
DTP—diphtheria and tetanus toxoids and pertussis vaccine adsorbed Td—tetanus and diphtheria toxoids adsorbed TIG—tetanus immune globulin

Etiology

C. botulinum is an obligate, anaerobic spore-forming gram-positive bacillus. The organism is ubiquitous and has been isolated from soil everywhere in the world. The spores of *C. botulinum* are very hardy, resisting dryness and extremes of temperature that kill the bacteria themselves. Spores that are introduced into food, wounds, or the human intestinal tract can germinate and elaborate botulinum toxin, which is responsible for all manifestations of the disease. Although seven antigenically distinct forms of the toxin (termed A through G) have been identified, just three types (A, B, and E) account for nearly all human disease.

Epidemiology

Botulism occurs in three major forms: food-borne botulism, wound botulism, and infant botulism. From 1973 through 1996, a median of 24 cases of food-borne botulism, three cases of wound botulism, and 71 cases of infant botulism were reported annually in the United States.[48] Less often, botulism occurs in the absence of a predisposing cause; colonization of the adult intestinal tract may account for some of these cases.[49]

Food-borne botulism develops when spores of *C. botulinum* contaminate food. Because the spores can survive a temperature of 100° C at atmospheric pressure but not pressure-cooking, botulism is much more likely to result from home-processed foods than commercially prepared canned goods. Spores that survive processing will germinate if cooked food is not refrigerated properly. The vegetative organisms produce the toxin, which is heat labile and can be destroyed by boiling for 10 minutes or heating to 80° C for 30 minutes. However, if contaminated food is not heated sufficiently, the toxin resists gastric acid and intestinal trypsin and is absorbed from the intestinal tract. Food-borne botulism can occur sporadically or in outbreaks, which are often restaurant associated[48]; the largest outbreak in the United States since 1978 occurred in 1994, when 30 residents of El Paso, Texas, became ill after eating at a restaurant that served dips prepared from baked potatoes that had been wrapped in aluminum foil and kept at room temperature for several days.[50] Improperly prepared vegetables, meats, and seafood can all be vectors for botulism. About half the cases of food-borne botulism are caused by type A toxin; the rest are divided about evenly between types B and E.[48]

Wound botulism results when *C. botulinum* or its spores are inoculated into a wound or devitalized tissue. In an anaerobic milieu, the spores germinate and vegetative organisms produce the toxin, which enters the circulation. Severe trauma, such as a crush injury involving an extremity, is the classic cause of wound botulism. However, heroin use has become the leading predisposing factor in the United States; most cases have occurred in California after subcutaneous injection of black tar heroin from Mexico.[46] About 80% of wound botulism is caused by type A toxin; most of the rest is caused by type B toxin.[48]

Infant botulism is caused by ingestion of *C. botulinum* spores rather than preformed toxin. The spores then germinate, colonizing the intestinal tract with toxin-producing organisms. As such, infant botulism, like wound botulism, is an infection rather than an intoxication (e.g., food-borne botulism). Although the source of the spores eludes detection in most cases, honey has been implicated in about 15% of cases. Toxin types A and B each account for about half the cases of infant botulism.[48]

Pathogenesis

Despite structural and immunologic differences, all seven types of botulinum toxin act identically. A less potent protoxin is produced intracellularly; when it is released from the bacterial cell, this protoxin is enzymatically activated into the active toxin. Like tetanus toxin, botulinum toxin is composed of a heavy (100,000 kd) chain linked to a light (50,000 kd) chain by a disulfide bridge. Once absorbed in the bloodstream, the toxin binds irreversibly to presynaptic nerve endings of the cranial nerves and peripheral nervous system. Once bound, botulinum toxin prevents the release of the neurotransmitter acetylcholine, probably by blocking exocytosis, the process by which acetylcholine in synaptic vesicles is exported from nerve terminals. Because cholinergic fibers of motor neurons supply skeletal muscle, the toxin produces flaccid paralyses. Autonomic instability can also occur, but adrenergic fibers are spared.[48]

Small doses of purified botulinum toxin can be injected directly into muscles to reduce excessive muscle tone. The toxin is being used therapeutically to treat conditions such as anal fissures,[51] blepharospasm, strabismus, cervical dystonia (torticollis), laryngeal dystonia (spasmodic dysphasia), and achalasias,[52] as well as facial wrinkles.[53]

Diagnosis

Although food-borne botulism may be heralded by gastrointestinal symptoms such as nausea, vomiting, cramping abdominal distress, and diarrhea (earlier stage) or constipation (later stage), neurologic symptoms soon predominate. In wound botulism, gastrointestinal symptoms are absent and the wound may appear surprisingly benign, but the neurologic symptoms are identical to those of food-borne botulism. Cranial nerve symptoms are usually the earliest neurologic complaints; blurred vision, diplopia, dysphagia, dysarthria, and dry mouth are typical presenting features. Symmetrical motor paralysis ensues; it characteristically progresses in a descending fashion that begins with the arms and then involves the respiratory muscles and lower body. Autonomic dysfunction can produce constipation, urinary retention, and orthostatic hypotension. Sensory deficits are absent and mentation is normal; except in some cases of wound botulism, patients are afebrile. Physical findings reflect cranial nerve and motor neuron abnormalities.

The symptoms of botulism usually begin 18 to 36 hours after ingestion of the toxin; the incubation period for wound botulism is typically longer. Respiratory arrest occurs in severe cases; mechanical ventilation is needed to prevent death, and respiratory support may be required for weeks to months while cholinergic synapses recover function.

Infant botulism presents as lethargy, constipation, poor feeding, and floppiness, typically in the second month of life.

Because botulism is uncommon, the diagnosis may not be entertained despite characteristic clinical findings. Clustering of cases in a family or community and a history of eating home-canned or spoiled foods may be important clues.

Differential Diagnosis

The differential diagnosis of botulism includes the Guillain-Barré syndrome, the Eaton-Lambert syndrome, myasthenia gravis, cerebrovascular accidents, tick paralysis, and chemical intoxication. In patients with botulism, complete blood counts, blood chemistries, CNS imaging studies, and the CSF are all normal. Rapid repetitive electromyography, however, is highly suggestive of botulism if it demonstrates a pattern of facilitation. A positive diagnosis can be established by demonstrating botulinum toxin in serum or stool specimens; the toxin may also be detected in food samples.

Treatment

Enemas or cathartics may be useful in eliminating unabsorbed toxin in patients who are evaluated soon after they have ingested the toxin. Because antitoxin can only neutralize the toxin before it binds to cholinergic synapses, it should be administered promptly; the currently recommended dose is one vial of intravenous trivalent (types A, B, and E) antitoxin.[48] The only licensed antitoxin is of equine origin; hypersensitivity reactions occur in up to 7% of recipients and may be severe. A human botulism immune globulin is being developed for treatment of infant botulism. Botulism antitoxin is available from the Centers for Disease Control and Prevention (404-639-2206 during business hours; 404-639-2888 other times). Case reporting is extremely important to prevent outbreaks of food-borne botulism. Wound botulism should be managed with surgical debridement and intravenous penicillin. Patients with severe botulism require mechanical ventilation and metabolic support.[48]

Infections Due to *Bacteroides* Species

All members of the genus *Bacteroides* are thin, pleomorphic, gram-negative bacilli that are nonmotile and nonsporulating. All are obligate anaerobes, but the dominant pathogen, *B. fragilis* [*see Figure 3*], is relatively aerotolerant and can survive in the presence of oxygen for up to 8 hours. *Bacteroides* species are present in large numbers as part of the normal human flora, principally in the oropharynx and colon. Many *Bacteroides* species can be involved in mixed infections that arise from insults to mucosal integrity, and like other anaerobes, they can infect devitalized tissues, producing further necrosis, abscess formation, and gas.

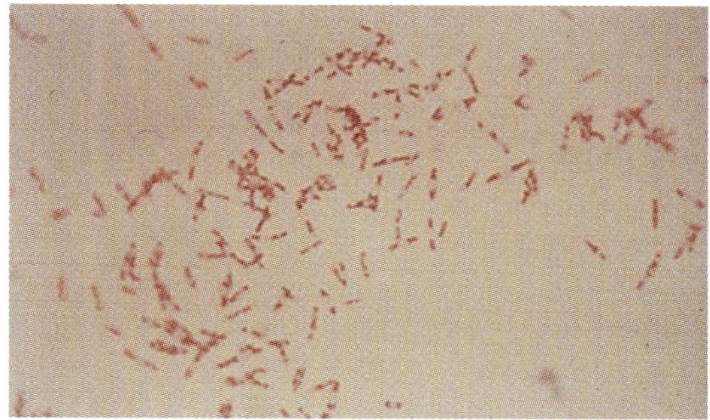

Figure 3 **Gram stain of *Bacteroides fragilis* from a pelvic abscess (magnification: ×1,000).**

Pathogenic *Bacteroides* species may be divided into two groups: the *B. fragilis* group, which dominates the colonic microflora, and the oral *Bacteroides* group, which resides in the oropharynx.

BACTEROIDES FRAGILIS GROUP

Of the nine species that constitute the *B. fragilis* group, *B. fragilis* is by far the most pathogenic. Although other members of the group, such as *B. ovatus*, *B. thetaiotaomicron*, *B. distasonis*, and *B. vulgatus*, are much more numerous in human feces, *B. fragilis* is far more likely to cause human disease. The virulence of *B. fragilis* is explained by several factors. Most important, it is the only species in the group that has a polysaccharide capsule; this capsule impairs phagocytosis and can itself cause inflammation and abscess formation. *B. fragilis* also produces the enzymes superoxide dismutase and catalase, which allow it to survive in the presence of oxygen. Other enzymes that contribute to its pathogenicity include bile salt–converting enzymes that may facilitate microbial survival in the gastrointestinal tract, a heparinase that may contribute to septic phlebitis, and proteases that may directly damage host tissues. As is the case with other *Bacteroides* species, however, the lipopolysaccharide component of the *B. fragilis* cell wall is only weakly active as an endotoxin. An enterotoxin produced by some strains has recently been associated with watery diarrhea in young children,[54] but the toxin is also present in the stools of healthy persons.[55] *B. fragilis* is a major contributor to intra-abdominal abscesses, pelvic infections, and peritonitis [see 8 Peritonitis and Intra-Abdominal Abscesses]. It is the most important cause of anaerobic bacteremia,[56,57] a life-threatening process[58] that occurs principally in debilitated patients who have intra-abdominal or pelvic disease.

All strains of *B. fragilis* produce β-lactamases and are resistant to penicillin, but extended-spectrum penicillins in combination with β-lactamase inhibitors (ampicillin-sulbactam, ticarcillin-clavulanate, and piperacillin-tazobactam) are active against most strains. Other β-lactam antibiotics that are active against most isolates are cefoxitin, cefotetan, ceftizoxime, imipenem, and meropenem. Metronidazole, clindamycin, and chloramphenicol all have excellent activity; metronidazole is the drug of choice for *B. fragilis* infection of the CNS, which occurs rarely. Because *B. fragilis* often is involved in polymicrobial infections, it may be necessary to select an antibiotic regimen that will eradicate other anaerobic or facultative organisms simultaneously. Patients with *B. fragilis* infections often require debridement of necrotic tissues and drainage of abscesses.

The antibiotic susceptibilities of the non-*fragilis* species of the *B. fragilis* group are more variable than those of *B. fragilis*. Only metronidazole, imipenem, and chloramphenicol are predictably active against nearly all isolates.

ORAL *BACTEROIDES* SPECIES

B. melaninogenicus, recognized in the laboratory by its production of a dark pigment, is the only encapsulated member of the group of oral *Bacteroides* species and is the most pathogenic. Other species in this group include *B. gingivalis*, *B. denticola*, and *B. intermedius*. All are natural inhabitants of the oropharynx, and all can be involved in aspiration pneumonias and putrid empyemas [see 6 Pulmonary Infections], head and neck infection [see 5 Bacterial Infections of the Upper Respiratory Tract], and brain abscesses [see 13 Bacterial Infections of the Central Nervous System]. Almost all organisms in this group are penicillin sensitive, but the minimum inhibitory concentration of penicillin for these organisms appears to be rising.

Infections Due to Actinomycosis

CLASSIFICATION AND MICROBIOLOGY

Actinomycetes are gram-positive bacteria that had been classified as fungi because of their filamentous, branching, hyphaelike appearance. Members of two genera of the family Actinomycetaceae, *Nocardia* and *Actinomyces*, may cause human disease. *Nocardia* species are aerobic [see 16 Infections Due to Gram-Positive Bacilli]; *Actinomyces* species are anaerobic or microaerophilic. One species, *A. israelii*, causes most cases of human actinomycosis. An obligate anaerobe, *A. israelii* is a normal resident of gingivodental crevices and tonsillar crypts. *A. naeslundii*, *A. eriksonii*, and *A. meyeri*[59] have been implicated in a few cases of actinomycosis. *A. bovis*, which causes lumpy jaw in cattle, rarely causes human disease.

SPECIFIC ACTINOMYCOTIC INFECTIONS

Actinomycosis is an uncommon but by no means rare infection.[60] Men are affected more often than women. Most patients have intact immune defenses. In many cases, actinomycosis follows an event that disrupts the integrity of a mucosal barrier. Like other anaerobic infections, actinomycosis thrives in the presence of necrotic tissues and foreign bodies and frequently is involved in polymicrobial infections. Many diverse clinical forms have been recognized, but the majority can be classified as cervicofacial (about 50% of all cases), pulmonary (20%), or gastrointestinal (20%). A fourth category is pelvic actinomycosis, which develops in women who use intrauterine devices (IUDs). Less often, actinomycosis affects the CNS, pericardium, endocardium, skin and soft tissue, bone, or intra-abdominal viscera. The disease may also present as widespread hematogenous dissemination to multiple organ systems.

Wherever the site of infection, actinomycosis characteristically produces chronic granulomatous inflammation that burrows deeply through contiguous tissues without respect to fascial planes. Consequently, draining sinus tracts are often present and may be purulent or sanguineous. If present, sulfur granules—small white-to-yellow aggregates of bacterial filaments—are an important clue to diagnosis. Actinomycosis usually pursues an indolent but progressive course. Typically, symptoms are present for 1 to 5 months before diagnosis; 90% of cases are diagnosed between 1 month and 2 years after the onset of symptoms. The most common clinical manifestations include a swollen mass, abscess, or draining sinus tract; pulmonary or abdominal complaints; fever; and weight loss.

Cervicofacial Infection

Cervicofacial actinomycosis often results from orofacial trauma, dental manipulation, or gingival infection in patients with poor oral hygiene. The initial symptom is often a firm, indurated swelling in the region of the mandible, and a tumor or cold abscess is often suspected clinically. On occasion, pain, inflammation, and fever are more prominent, and the disease may mimic a pyogenic infection. Sinus tracts may be involved in long-standing disease. Soft tissue infection is more common than bone involvement. Because actinomycosis spreads without regard for tissue planes, infection of regional nodes is not a characteristic feature, although it can occur. Extension of orofacial actinomycosis to the tongue, hypopharynx, larynx, orbit, or parotid or lacrimal glands is uncommon. As in other forms of actinomycosis, the cervicofacial infection is often clinically misdiagnosed as a tumor, tuberculosis, or mycotic or pyogenic infection. The diagnosis of actinomycosis can be established by biopsy or by smears and cultures of drainage from a sinus tract.

Pulmonary Infection

The aspiration of organisms from the oropharynx leads to pulmonary actinomycosis. A history of a discrete aspirational episode is unusual, however. The disease has an insidious onset and a subacute course. Typical symptoms include cough, hemoptysis, chest wall discomfort, fever, and weight loss. Pulmonary osteoarthropathy is less common. The radiographic findings are variable and include patchy infiltrates, mass lesions, or cavitary lesions. Often pleura based, the infection may extend directly into the pleural space, ribs, and chest wall to produce empyemas, osteomyelitis, and draining fistulous tracts. Less frequently, thoracic actinomycosis can extend to the mediastinum and present as pericarditis. The differential diagnosis includes carcinoma, tuberculosis, bacterial infections, nocardiosis, and systemic mycosis.

In the presence of pleural or chest wall involvement, the correct diagnosis of actinomycosis should not be problematic. Because *A. israelii* is part of the normal oral flora, culturing the organism from sputum or bronchoscopic washings is not diagnostic. Diagnosis often requires percutaneous needle aspiration, bronchoscopic biopsy, or open lung biopsy.

Gastrointestinal Infection

Gastrointestinal actinomycosis probably occurs when preexisting damage to the intestinal mucosa allows swallowed organisms access to vulnerable tissues. Any portion of the intestinal tract may be involved; ileocecal infection is most frequent. The disease can spread to the omentum, mesenteric lymph nodes, and intra-abdominal viscera and can produce fistulous invasions of the abdominal wall or perineum. Presenting symptoms include pain and fever; palpable mass lesions and draining sinus tracts are the most common physical findings. Carcinoma, tuberculosis, and Crohn disease are prominent considerations in the differential diagnosis. Unless draining sinus tracts are present, surgery is required for diagnosis. If the bladder is involved, sulfur granules may be present in the urine. A careful pathologic search may be needed to establish the diagnosis, even when excisional biopsy is performed. It is important to confirm the diagnosis because actinomycosis requires postsurgical administration of antibiotics to prevent recurrent disease.

Pelvic Infection

Once a rarity, pelvic actinomycosis has been recognized with greater frequency since its association with the use of IUDs was noted in 1974.[61] The pathogenesis of pelvic actinomycosis is not certain. The disease may originate from the upward spread of organisms that reach the perineum from the oropharynx via the intestinal tract. Although not generally considered a normal resident of the female genital tract, *A. israelii* may be a relatively frequent saprophyte in this region. Clinical disease may present as endometritis, salpingo-oophoritis, or tubo-ovarian abscess; bladder invasion or systemic infection arising from a vaginal focus is rare. Optimal management of *Actinomyces* colonization in asymptomatic women requires further study; removal of IUDs has been suggested. The role of antibiotics is uncertain. Pelvic inflammatory disease is the major consideration in differential diagnosis. Surgery is generally required to establish the diagnosis. Actinomycosis of the male genitourinary tract is rare, but prostate infection has been reported.

Disseminated Infection

Disseminated actinomycosis results most often from hematogenous spread from a pulmonary focus. These rare infections can involve soft tissues, bone, the brain, and viscera. Mass lesions, abscesses, and draining sinus tracts are prominent clinical features, as they are in the more common forms of actinomycosis.

DIAGNOSIS

The diagnosis of actinomycosis depends on identification of the organism by smear, culture, or both. Actinomycetes are slender, branching, gram-positive, filamentous organisms that can fragment into coccobacillary forms resembling diphtheroids. In these respects, actinomycetes are identical to *Nocardia* species [see 16 Infections Due to Gram-

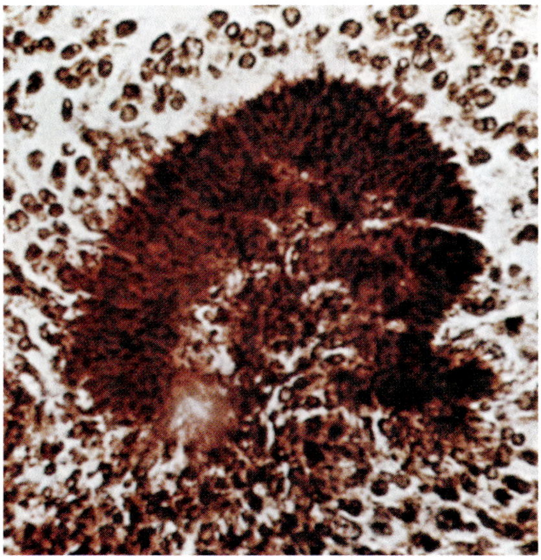

Figure 4 **Sulfur granules consist of masses of bacterial filaments that may be arranged in raylike projections. The finding of sulfur granules in visceral infections is specific for actinomycosis.**

Positive Bacilli]. Whereas it was traditionally believed that *Nocardia* and *Actinomyces* could be differentiated morphologically because only *Nocardia* is acid-fast, it was found that *A. israelii* can also be acid-fast when stained in tissue with modified acid-fast stains. The identification of sulfur granules in viscera establishes the diagnosis of actinomycosis; these structures are not present in nocardiosis. Sulfur granules may be identified grossly as small white-to-yellow particles and microscopically as masses of bacterial filaments that may be arranged in raylike projections [*see Figure 4*]. Tissue sections in actinomycosis may display tissue necrosis with polymorphonuclear infiltration, abscess formation, and prominent fibrosis with sinus tract formation and granulomatous inflammation.

Because *A. israelii* is a strict anaerobe, good anaerobic cultures are mandatory. The organisms will grow on ordinary bacteriologic media, but 3 to 7 days of incubation is often required before characteristic colonies become visible. A variety of anaerobic and aerobic bacteria may also be cultured from patients with actinomycosis, reflecting the polymicrobial nature of many anaerobic infections. Surgery is often required for the diagnosis of actinomycosis, and debridement may be helpful therapeutically. Wide surgical excision is not ordinarily required for treatment.

TREATMENT

Antibiotics are the mainstay of therapy for actinomycosis; penicillin is the drug of choice. Daily doses of 10 to 20 million units are usually administered intravenously for 2 to 4 weeks, followed by oral therapy for 3 to 6 months. These prolonged treatment schedules are designed to prevent recurrent infection. In penicillin-allergic patients, tetracycline is the preferred agent; clindamycin, ceftriaxone, and ciprofloxacin have also been used successfully in a few cases. With vigorous antibiotic treatment, the prognosis for patients with actinomycosis is excellent.

Miscellaneous Clinically Significant Anaerobes

Fusobacterium species, gram-negative bacilli that typically have pointed ends, reside in the oropharynx and, to a lesser extent, in the gastrointestinal tract. Six *Fusobacterium* species have been associated with human disease; of these, *F. nucleatum* is the most important. These bacteria can be involved in head and neck infections (including suppurative thrombophlebitis), pleuropulmonary infections, and, less often, bacteremias[62] or intra-abdominal abscesses. *Fusobacterium* species are penicillin sensitive.

Peptococci and peptostreptococci, small gram-positive cocci that are part of the normal oral, gastrointestinal, and genitourinary flora, can be involved in mixed infections arising in these regions. They are penicillin sensitive.

Veillonella species are anaerobic gram-negative cocci that are occasionally isolated from mixed infections, but their pathogenicity is uncertain. *P. acnes* is an anaerobic, gram-positive bacillus that is part of the normal skin flora and is occasionally isolated in blood cultures, almost always as a contaminant. Another anaerobic gram-positive bacillus with very low virulence is *Lactobacillus*, the dominant member of the normal vaginal flora. Despite their low virulence, *Lactobacillus* organisms occasionally cause serious infections.

References

1. Duerden BI: Virulence factors in anaerobes. Clin Infect Dis 18(suppl 4):S253, 1994

2. Botta GA, Arzese A, Minisini R, et al: Role of structural and extracellular virulence factors in gram-negative anaerobic bacteria. Clin Infect Dis 18(suppl 4):S260, 1994

3. Larson CM, Burbrick MP, Jacobs DM, et al: Malignancy, mortality, and medicosurgical management of *Clostridium septicum* infection. Surgery 118:592, 1995

4. Stevens DL, Bryant AE: Pathogenesis of *Clostridium perfringens* infection: mechanisms and mediators of shock. Clin Infect Dis 25(suppl 2): S160, 1997

5. Stevens DL: The pathogenesis of clostridial myonecrosis. Int J Med Microbiol 290:497, 2000

6. Nichols RL, Smith JW: Anaerobes from a surgical perspective. Clin Infect Dis 18(suppl 4):S280, 1994

7. Rechner PM, Agger WA, Mruz K, et al: Clinical features of clostridial bacteremia: a review from a rural area. Clin Infect Dis 33:349, 2001

8. Miller DL, Brazer S, Murdoch D, et al: Significance of *Clostridium tertium* bacteremia in neutropenic and nonneutropenic patients: review of 32 cases. Clin Infect Dis 32:975, 2001

9. Mendes CM, Oplustil CP, dos Santos TJL, et al: *Clostridium perfringens* as a cause of infectious endocarditis in a patient with a vascular prosthesis. Clin Infect Dis 22:866, 1996

10. Gredlein CM, Silverman ML, Downey MS: Polymicrobial septic arthritis due to *Clostridium* species: case report and review. Clin Infect Dis 30:590, 2000

11. Grim PS, Gottlieb LJ, Boddie A, et al: Hyperbaric oxygen therapy. JAMA 263:2216, 1990

12. Tibbles PM, Edelsberg JS: Hyperbaric-oxygen therapy. N Engl J Med 334:1642, 1996

13. Borriello SP: Clostridial disease of the gut. Clin Infect Dis 20(suppl 2):S242, 1995

14. Petrillo TM, Beck-Sague CM, Songer JG, et al: Enteritis necroticans (pigbel) in a diabetic child. N Engl J Med 342:1250, 2000

15. Yassin SF, Young-Fadok TM, Zein NN, et al: *Clostridium difficile*–associated diarrhea and colitis. Mayo Clin Proc 76:725, 2001

16. Barbut F, Corthier G, Charpak Y, et al: Prevalence and pathogenicity of *Clostridium difficile* in hospitalized patients: a French multicenter study. Arch Intern Med 156:1449, 1996

17. Shim JK, Johnson S, Samore MH, et al: Primary symptomless colonization by *Clostridium difficile* and decreased risk of subsequent diarrhoea. Lancet 351:633, 1998

18. Kyne L, Warney M, Qamar A, et al: Asymptomatic carriage of *Clostridium difficile* and serum levels of IgG antibody against toxin A. N Engl J Med 342:390, 2000

19. Samore MH, DeGirolami PC, Tlucko A, et al: *Clostridium difficile* colonization and diarrhea at a tertiary care hospital. Clin Infect Dis 18: 181, 1994

20. Samore MH, Venkataraman L, DeGirolami PC, et al: Clinical and molecular epidemiology of sporadic and clustered cases of nosocomial *Clostridium difficile* diarrhea. Am J Med 100:32, 1996

21. Kyne L, Merry C, O'Connell B, et al: Community-acquired *Clostridium difficile* infection. J Infect 36:287, 1998

22. Mylonakis E, Ryan ET, Calderwood SB: *Clostridium difficile*–associated diarrhea. Arch Intern Med 161:525, 2001

23. Johnson S, Gerding DN: *Clostridium difficile*-associated diarrhea. Clin Infect Dis 26:1027, 1998

24. Bliss DZ, Johnson S, Savik K, et al: Acquisition of *Clostridium difficile* and *Clostridium difficile*–associated diarrhea in hospitalized patients receiving tube feeding. Ann Intern Med 129:1012, 1998

25. Jacobs A, Barnard K, Fishel R, et al: Extracolonic manifestations of *Clostridium difficile* infections: presentation of 2 cases and review of the literature. Medicine (Baltimore) 80:88, 2001

26. Gerding DN: Diagnosis of *Clostridium difficile*–associated disease: patient selection and test perfection. Am J Med 100:485, 1996

27. Wenisch C, Parschalk B, Hasenhundl M, et al: Comparison of vancomycin, teicoplanin, metronidazole, and fusidic acid for the treatment of *Clostridium difficile*–associated diarrhea. Clin Infect Dis 22:813, 1996

28. Fekety R, McFarland LV, Surawicz CM, et al: Recurrent *Clostridium difficile* diarrhea: characteristics of and risk factors for patients enrolled in a prospective, randomized, double-blinded trial. Clin Infect Dis 24:324, 1997

29. Do AN, Fridkin SK, Yechouron A, et al: Risk factors for early recurrent *Clostridium difficile*–associated diarrhea. Clin Infect Dis 26:954, 1998

30. Kyne L, Warny M, Qamar A, et al: Association between antibody response to toxin A and protection against recurrent *Clostridium difficile* diarrhoea. Lancet 357:189, 2001

31. Jones EM, MacGowan AP: Back to basics in management of *Clostridium difficile* infections. Lancet 352:505, 1998

32. Surawicz CM, McFarland LV, Greenberg RN, et al: The search for a better treatment for recurrent *Clostridium difficile* disease: use of high-dose vancomycin combined with *Saccharomyces boulardii*. Clin Infect Dis 31:1012, 2000

33. Pochapin M: The effect of probiotics in *Clostridium difficile* diarrhea. Am J Gastroenterol 95(suppl):S11, 2000

34. Wilcox MH: Cleaning up *Clostridium difficile* infection. Lancet 348: 767, 1996

35. Climo MW, Israel DS, Wong ES, et al: Hospital-wide restriction of clindamycin: effect on the incidence of *Clostridium difficile*–associated diarrhea and cost. Ann Intern Med 128:989, 1998

36. Mayfield JL, Leet T, Miller J, et al: Environmental control to reduce transmission of *Clostridium difficile*. Clin Infect Dis 31:995, 2000

37. Feldman RJ, Kallich M, Weinstein MP: Bacteremia due to *Clostridium difficile*: case report and review of extraintestinal *C. difficile* infections. Clin Infect Dis 20:1560, 1995

38. Byl B, Jacobs F, Struelens MJ, et al: Extraintestinal *Clostridium difficile* infections. Clin Infect Dis 22:712, 1996

39. Wolf LE, Gorbach SL, Granowitz EV: Extraintestinal *Clostridium difficile*: 10 years' experience at a tertiary-care hospital. Mayo Clin Proc 73:943, 1998

40. Bhargava A, Sen P, Swaminathan A, et al: Rapidly progressive necrotizing fasciitis and gangrene due to *Clostridium difficile*: case report. Clin Infect Dis 30:954, 2000

41. Hsu SS, Groleau G: Tetanus in the emergency department: a current review. J Emerg Med 20:357, 2001

42. Sanford JP: Tetanus—forgotten but not gone (editorial). N Engl J Med 332:812, 1995

43. Gergen PJ, McQuillan GM, Kiely M, et al: A population-based serologic survey of immunity to tetanus in the United States. N Engl J Med 332:761, 1995

44. Silveira CM, Caceres VM, Dutra MG, et al: Safety of tetanus toxoid in pregnant women: a hospital-based case-control study of congenital anomalies. Bull World Health Organ 73:605, 1995

45. Bowie C: Tetanus toxoid for adults: too much of a good thing. Lancet 348:1185, 1996

46. Werner SB, Passaro D, McGee J, et al: Wound botulism in California, 1951–1998: recent epidemic in heroin injectors. Clin Infect Dis 31: 1018, 2000

47. Arnon SS, Schechter R, Inglesby TV, et al: Botulinum toxin as a biological weapon: medical and public health management. JAMA 285: 1059, 2001

48. Shapiro RL, Hatheway C, Swerdlow DL: Botulism in the United States: a clinical and epidemiologic review. Ann Intern Med 129:221, 1998

49. Fenicia L, Franciosa G, Pourshaban M, et al: Intestinal toxemia botulism in two young people, caused by *Clostridium butyricum* type E. Clin Infect Dis 29:1381, 1999

50. Angulo FJ, Getz J, Taylor JP, et al: A large outbreak of botulism: the hazardous baked potato. J Infect Dis 178:172, 1998

51. Brisinda G, Maria G, Bentivoglio AR, et al: A comparison of injections of botulinum toxin and topical nitroglycerin ointment for the treatment of chronic anal fissure. N Engl J Med 341:65, 1999

52. Münchau A, Bhatia KP: Uses of botulinum toxin injection in medicine today. BMJ 320:161, 2000

53. Hallett M: One man's poison: clinical applications of botulinum toxin. N Engl J Med 341:118, 1999

54. Sears CL, Myers LL, Lazenby A, et al: Enterotoxigenic *Bacteroides fragilis*. Clin Infect Dis 20(suppl 2):S142, 1995

55. Pantosti A, Menozzi MG, Frate A, et al: Detection of enterotoxigenic *Bacteroides fragilis* and its toxin in stool samples from adults and children in Italy. Clin Infect Dis 24:12, 1997

56. Goldstein EJ: Anaerobic bacteremia. Clin Infect Dis 23(suppl 1): S97, 1996

57. Salonen JH, Eerola E, Meurman O: Clinical significance and outcome of anaerobic bacteremia. Clin Infect Dis 26:1413, 1998

58. Redondo MC, Arbo MDJ, Grindlinger J, et al: Attributable mortality of bacteremia associated with the *Bacteroides fragilis* group. Clin Infect Dis 20:1492, 1995

59. Apotheloz C, Regamey C: Disseminated infection due to *Actinomyces meyeri*: case report and review. Clin Infect Dis 22:621, 1996

60. Smego RA Jr, Foglia G: Actinomycosis. Clin Infect Dis 26:1255, 1998

61. Fiorino SA: Intrauterine contraceptive device–associated actinomycotic abscess and *Actinomyces* detection on cervical smear. Obstet Gynecol 87:142, 1996

62. Bourgault AM, Lamothe F, Dolce P, et al: *Fusobacterium bacteremia*: clinical experience with 40 cases. Clin Infect Dis 25(suppl 2):S181, 1997

18 Infections Due to *Neisseria*

Jeanne M. Marrazzo, M.D., M.P.H.

Infections caused by *Neisseria* species are among the most frequently encountered and potentially dangerous diseases. The two major species of concern are *N. meningitidis* and *N. gonorrhoeae*. Both are gram-negative cocci that reside primarily in polymorphonuclear white blood cells and tend to cluster in pairs [*see Figure 1*]. No nonhuman reservoir exists for either organism. Although there is some overlap in the clinical syndromes these two species elicit, they are commonly known for distinctly different presentations.

Infections Caused by *Neisseria meningitidis*

The most clinically relevant classification scheme for *N. meningitidis* utilizes the organism's capsular polysaccharides and includes at least 13 serogroups. The most common of these are A, B, C, X, Y, L, and W135.[1] In addition to serogroup, the organism can be classified by class 1 outer-membrane proteins (OMP) (serosubtype), class 2 or 3 OMP (serotype), and lipo-oligosaccharide (immunotype).

Invasive disease caused by *N. meningitidis* is a significant source of morbidity and mortality worldwide. Important trends include increased recognition of the Y serogroup's role in outbreaks, consideration of college freshmen as candidates for vaccination, and the relative increase of *N. meningitidis* as a pathogen in children as the success of immunization against *Haemophilus influenzae* type b is increasingly realized.

EPIDEMIOLOGY AND TRANSMISSION

N. meningitidis is most commonly found in the setting of asymptomatic nasopharyngeal carriage. The prevalence of nasopharyngeal colonization in the United States is estimated at 5% to 10%.[2] Duration of colonization varies from transient (days) to as long as 2 years, with a median of 9 to 10 months. Development of humoral immunity to the colonizing strain of the organism is common and may last at least 4 to 6 months after exposure.

Transmission results from direct transfer of respiratory or oral secretions and requires prolonged intimate contact. Consequently, habitation in very close quarters (e.g., military barracks, correctional facilities, and college dormitories) can facilitate colonization, the prevalence of which can reach 20% to 40% during outbreaks.[3] Facilitation of transmission within close quarters is also reflected by seasonal patterns in invasive infection. Although disease occurs year-round, the incidence peaks in late winter and early spring. Transmission has also been documented through prolonged exposure to an infected person on an airplane and in laboratory technicians working with isolates on open laboratory benches.[4,5]

Despite longstanding availability of antibiotics and meningococcal vaccine, most areas of the world continue to have stable rates of endemic disease. After *Streptococcus pneumoniae*, *N. meningitidis* is the most common cause of bacterial meningitis worldwide, causing an estimated 25% of cases.[6] In

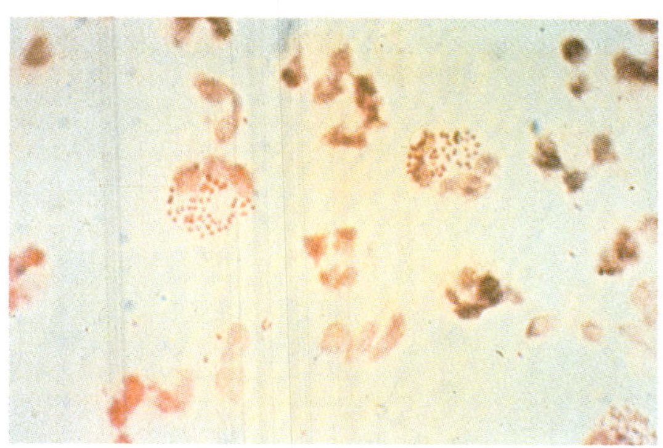

Figure 1 **Gram stain of urethral secretions showing abundant *N. gonorrhoeae* as gram-negative diplococci within polymorphonuclear cells.**

the United States, laboratory-based surveillance for invasive meningococcal disease from 1992 to 1996 revealed an average annual incidence of 1.1 cases per 100,000 population (approximately 2,454 cases a year).[2,6,7] Incidence was highest in infants younger than 1 year, with a rate of 15.9/100,000 for children 4 to 5 months of age. The serogroup associated with the most cases of invasive disease was serogroup C (35%); however, significant geographic variation was seen, and the incidence of disease from serogroup Y increased during the study period.[7] For reasons that are unclear, rates of invasive meningococcal disease in the United States are higher in blacks than in nonblacks.

The risk of invasive meningococcal infection in college students has been summarized by the Centers for Disease Control and Prevention (CDC),[8] which initiated surveillance in this group in 1998. Whereas the incidence in undergraduates overall was lower than that in persons 18 to 23 years of age who were not enrolled in college, rates were relatively high in the approximately 590,000 freshmen who lived in dormitories (4.6/100,000).

Sporadic outbreaks of invasive meningococcal disease also continue to occur in sub-Saharan Africa, in an area extending from Senegal in the west to Ethiopia in the east, known as the meningitis belt. Outbreaks caused primarily by serogroup A occur there during the dry season, from December to June. However, serogroups B and C have caused large epidemics elsewhere, including the United States.[7]

PATHOGENESIS AND IMMUNITY

The cascade of events from exposure to colonization and from invasion to specific manifestations of clinical disease is complex. Most persons who develop invasive meningococcal disease do so after recent colonization.[1] Concomitant upper respiratory viral infection, cigarette smoking, underlying chronic illness, and preceding *Mycoplasma* infection may facilitate meningococcal infection and colonization. Colonization requires attachment to nonciliated columnar mucosal cells of the nasopharynx. Meningococci secrete proteases that cleave IgA, which may disable a major mucosal defense mechanism; how this mechanism contributes to pathogenesis is unclear, however. Endocytosis and intracellular transport of meningococci-laden vacuoles mediate the organisms' passage to the submucosa.

Immunity to meningococcus involves interactions at the nasopharyngeal mucosa, innate immune mechanisms, and acquired antibody.[9,10] The importance of antibody is highlighted by several findings. Natural immunity is acquired after, and boosted by, meningococcal colonization of the nasopharynx. Immunity correlates with bactericidal antibody levels in serum, and the age-specific attack rate of meningococcal disease is reciprocally related to the presence of serogroup-specific antibodies.[9] Further, hypogammaglobulinemia is a risk factor for invasive disease. In military recruits, risk of disease is highest in the absence of bactericidal activity against the prevalent pathogenic strain.[11] Specific antibody directly binds the meningococcus and activates complement-mediated phagocytosis.

Both pathways of the complement system—classic and alternative—appear critical in controlling meningococcal infection.[9] Persons with deficiencies in the terminal complement system (C5, C6, C7, C8, or C9) develop antibody to meningococci, but the rates of meningococcal infection in these individuals are 1,400-fold to 10,000-fold higher than in the general population.[12] Approximately 50% of affected persons have at least one episode of meningococcal infection, and 20% to 25% have more than one episode. Of note, infections in persons with complement deficiency often involve unusual serogroups and are less severe. Persons with deficiencies of properdin (an alternative-pathway component) or factor D are also at increased risk for meningococcal disease, with a case-fatality rate of over 50%. Recurrent meningococcal disease should prompt screening for complement deficiencies,[13] which involves testing the serum for hemolytic whole-complement activity.

Coagulopathy and microvascular thrombosis are hallmarks of meningococcal sepsis. The most visible manifestation of these processes is purpura fulminans [*see Figure 2a and 2b*]. Dysfunction of the activation pathway of protein C appears to play a key role in these thrombotic events. When activated by its binding to thrombomodulin and the endothelial protein C receptor, protein C normally functions to keep thrombin's procoagulant properties in check. In children with purpuric lesions from meningococcal sepsis, endothelial protein C activation is impaired.[14]

CLINICAL PRESENTATIONS

Meningococcal Bacteremia

Meningococcal bacteremia occurs across a spectrum of clinical presentations, ranging from an acute fulminant disease that is fatal within hours to asymptomatic infection. The presence of *N. meningitidis* in the blood is usually associated with severe illness. However, bacteremia may occasionally be

a

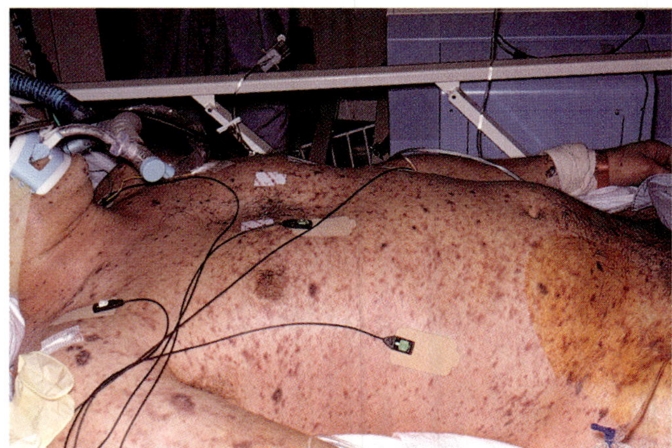

b

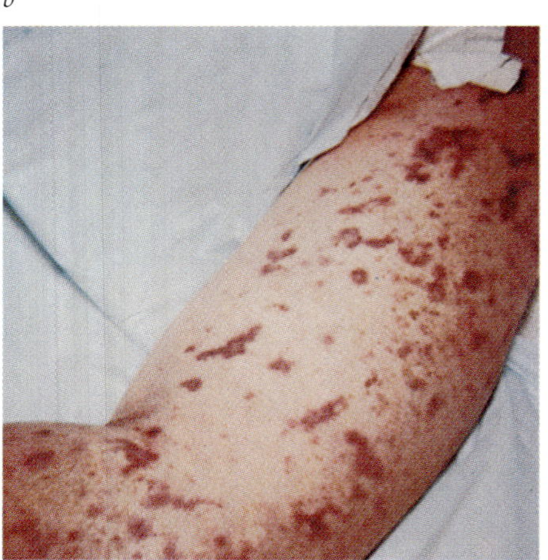

Figure 2 **(*a*) The rash of purpura fulminans, seen here with petechiae as well as larger, coalescent hemorrhagic lesions, in a patient with meningococcal sepsis and meningitis caused by serogroup B. (*b*) Closer view of petechiae, some of which have coalesced into purpuric and intracutaneous hemorrhagic lesions.**

found in persons who appear healthy or who have only mild systemic symptoms (usually fever and, sometimes, upper respiratory symptoms or rash resembling a viral exanthem).

Symptoms associated with so-called benign bacteremia usually resolve before the infection is identified by isolation of meningococcus from blood cultures. This syndrome differs from the so-called chronic meningococcemia associated with low-grade fever, rash, and polyarticular arthritis that can be confused with disseminated gonococcal infection (DGI).

The rash of chronic meningococcemia usually takes the form of a nonspecific maculopapular eruption, but it may be petechial. Unlike persons who experience recurrent meningococcal meningitis (see below), patients with chronic meningococcemia appear immunologically normal and are usually infected with typical serogroups. *N. meningitidis* should be considered in the evaluation of any patient with a chronic arthritis-dermatitis syndrome.

The most notorious presentations of meningococcal disease take two forms: meningococcemia and meningococcal sepsis. The two forms may occur simultaneously.

The term meningococcemia usually denotes bacteremia accompanied by signs of sepsis and frequently by the classic purpuric or petechial rash typical of this syndrome, which occurs in 75% of patients with this disease [*see Figure 2a and 2b*]. Although the rash of purpura fulminans is obvious, patients presenting early in the course of disease may have more subtle abnormalities of the skin and mucous membranes. These abnormalities include palpebral and conjunctival petechiae and lesions in areas subject to physical pressure, such as the waist and soles of the feet. Because these findings can herald the development of full-blown meningococcemia, they should be carefully sought in persons in whom this illness is a consideration; so that a thorough examination can be performed, the patient should be examined without clothes. Affected patients may also complain of intense, diffuse myalgias in the initial period of their illness. Evolution of individual petechiae to coalescence and eventual frank ecchymosis proceeds apace with the progression of the thrombocytopenia of disseminated intravascular coagulation (DIC).

Meningococcal sepsis is characterized by a rapid progression from general, nonspecific complaints that may resemble a viral illness to hypotension, multiorgan failure, and DIC. Despite the availability of antibiotics and advances in critical care, meningococcal sepsis still carries a mortality of up to 40%.[2] Concomitant adrenal hemorrhage, known as the Waterhouse-Friderichsen syndrome, may also occur. Myocarditis has been noted on histopathologic examination in more than 70% of patients with fatal meningococcemia.[15,16] Meningococcemia may also precipitate pericarditis, sometimes to the point of tamponade. The formation of arterial thrombi can result in peripheral gangrene.

Meningitis

Acute meningococcal meningitis results from hematogenous dissemination of the organism and is usually accompanied by classic signs of bacterial meningeal inflammation: fever, headache, and nuchal rigidity. Other findings typical of meningitis may occur, including photophobia, nausea, vomiting, focal neurologic signs, seizures, and progression to obtundation and coma.[17] From 50% to 75% of patients have a petechial rash suggestive of meningococcemia.[18] The cerebrospinal fluid is typically purulent, with numerous polymorphonuclear neutrophils (PMNs), low glucose (< 50 mg/dl, present in 75% of cases), and an elevated protein concentration. In contrast, the uncommon syndrome of recurrent meningococcal meningitis produces less severe clinical and CSF findings.

Bacteremic Pneumonia

Bacteremic pneumonia from *N. meningitidis* constituted 3% of cases of invasive meningococcal disease reported by Schuchat[6] in 1997 and may be more commonly associated with serogroup Y isolates. However, meningococcal pneumonia probably occurs more frequently than is indicated by detection through positive blood cultures, and this disease has occurred in outbreaks. In a well-described outbreak involving 68 military recruits, most of the individuals had fever, rales, and pharyngitis.[19] Although disease was multilobar in 40% of the patients, no deaths occurred. Diagnosis by sputum culture is problematic, given the potential confounding effect of upper airway colonization. Instead, most patients are diagnosed either at bronchoscopy or, if they have systemic infection, with positive cultures at nonpulmonary sites.

Other Meningococcal Infections

Uncommonly, *N. meningitidis* can cause syndromes for which *N. gonorrhoeae* is well known, including urethritis in men and cervicitis in women. One proposed mechanism of meningococcal genital infection is acquisition through orogenital sex, which may transmit nasopharyngeal colonizers to genital sites.[20] These syndromes respond well to the antibiotics typically used for gonococcal genital infections (see below).[21] Sex partners should be treated, but no further chemoprophylaxis (e.g., treatment of household contacts) is indicated.

Cases of *N. meningitidis* infecting numerous other body sites have been reported, including endocarditis, cellulitis, conjunctivitis, otitis media, epiglottitis, and arthritis.[2,22,23]

DIAGNOSIS

N. meningitidis is a fastidious aerobic organism that grows best on chocolate agar and is distinguished from *N. gonorrhoeae* by its ability to ferment both maltose and glucose. The bacteria can be isolated from blood in approximately 75% of persons with invasive meningococcal disease and from the CSF in approximately 46% to 94% of persons with meningitis.[17] Sepsis occurs in an estimated 5% to 20% of persons with positive blood cultures. Gram stain of CSF remains a very useful means of detecting the meningococcus; however, its sensitivity is probably no higher than 50% to 70% and, like that of culture, is reduced by recent antibiotic use. Detection assays for polysaccharide antigens using countercurrent immunoelectrophoresis or latex agglutination are frequently applied to CSF. Their advantages include rapid turnaround time, high specificity, and ability to individuate serogroups. Their major disadvantage is relatively low sensitivity (meaning that false negatives occur), particularly if serogroup B is responsible; in addition, they are not reliable when used to detect antigen in urine or serum. The polymerase chain reaction (PCR) has been successfully applied to the detection of *N. meningitidis*, especially in the United Kingdom, but is not commercially available in the United States.[24] Of note, the isolation of meningococci from upper respiratory secretions does not itself indicate meningococcal disease.

COMPLICATIONS AND PROGNOSIS

Meningococcal sepsis confers a mortality of up to 40%, and 11% to 19% of survivors suffer sequelae, including hearing loss, neurologic disability, and amputation because of peripheral gangrene.[25] The case-fatality rate for all invasive meningococcal disease is estimated to be 11%, and it is significantly higher in the presence of bacteremia (17%) than with meningitis alone (3%). Mortality from *N. meningitidis* is most profound in children: in developed countries, invasive meningococcal disease is the leading cause of death in this age group. Among 295 adolescents and young adults with invasive meningococcal disease in Maryland during the 1990s, 22.5% of those 15 through 24 years of age died.[26] Clearly, this disease continues to present a major challenge to physicians, communities, and the public health system.

DIFFERENTIAL DIAGNOSIS

In its earliest stage, the presentation of invasive meningococcal disease can be nonspecific, resembling a typical viral illness with fever and myalgias. Appearance of a rash should prompt consideration of common viral etiologies, including the enteroviruses. The presence of severe systemic illness should bring to mind Rocky Mountain spotted fever (RMSF), vasculitides (polyarteritis nodosa, Churg-Strauss syndrome, and anaphylactoid [Henoch-Schönlein] purpura), and toxic shock syndromes associated with staphylococcal, streptococcal, and, less commonly, clostridial infections. Less common infections that can present in similar fashion include epidemic typhus, infections caused by *Streptobacillus moniliformis* and *Spirillum minus* (rat-bite fever), gonococcemia, septicemia caused by *H. influenzae* type b, typhoid fever, and acute *S. aureus* endocarditis. Key pieces of information can help narrow the differential diagnosis. Tick-borne diseases such as RMSF usually occur within specific geographic confines and are generally associated with outdoor exposure to animal or insect vectors during the temperate months, principally in summer. Travel history is important in consideration of typhoid fever, as is information regarding the host's general immune status.

TREATMENT

Emergency Management

Infected patients should be isolated and droplet precautions observed until effective antimicrobial therapy has been given for at least 24 hours.[27] Antibiotic therapy should be started as soon as possible. Earlier initiation of antibiotics has been demonstrated to favorably affect outcome in some, though not all, studies,[28] but the disease is frequently so severe that reasonable measures to impact its early course should be undertaken.

Penicillin has constituted the mainstay of antibiotic therapy of meningococcal disease for several decades. Although β-lactamase–producing strains with high-level resistance (minimum inhibitory concentration [MIC] ≥ 250 μg/ml) exist, and strains with altered penicillin-binding proteins and intermediate resistance (MIC, 0.1 to 1.0 μg/ml) have been isolated clinically, treatment failures with penicillin have not been reported.[29] Similarly, isolates with high-level resistance to chloramphenicol have been reported outside the United States. Given these data, meningococcal isolates from blood and CSF should be routinely evaluated for penicillin susceptibility at a reference laboratory.

Antibiotic Therapy

Until the presence of meningococcus is confirmed, the patient should receive empirical treatment for bacterial meningitis [see 13 Bacterial Infections of the Central Nervous System]. Once *N. meningitidis* is identified in the CSF or blood, monotherapy with penicillin G (300,000 U/kg/day I.V., up to 24 million U/day) or ceftriaxone (50 mg/kg/day, up to 2 g) may be used. For persons who cannot tolerate penicillins or cephalosporins, chloramphenicol is an option; however, hematologic toxicity remains a concern. These antibiotics provide adequate CSF penetration, especially in the presence of meningeal inflammation. Treatment for 10 to 14 days is commonly recommended.[29] Although fluoroquinolones provide excellent activity against *N. meningitidis* and achieve very good CSF levels, their role in the treatment of invasive meningococcal disease requires further study.

Adjunctive Therapy

Adjunctive therapy of meningococcal infection with corticosteroids has been a subject of intense debate. Steroid therapy has not been shown to improve outcomes associated with meningococcal disease and is therefore not recommended. Another strategy under pursuit is repletion of activated protein C, which is severely depleted in severe meningococcemia.[30] One small open-label study showed that compared with predicted outcomes, there were reductions in morbidity and mortality from severe meningococcemia in patients treated with activated protein C.[31] In a large, randomized, placebo-controlled study of patients with sepsis, recombinant protein C reduced mortality but also increased bleeding events.[32] None of the patients in this study had sepsis from *N. meningitidis*. However, protein C depletion appears to be more severe in meningococcal disease than in related conditions that commonly cause sepsis, suggesting that further study is warranted. Recombinant protein C is commercially available, and its use in patients with sepsis from *N. meningitidis* should be considered.

PREVENTIVE THERAPY

Although outbreaks account for only 2% to 3% of all cases of meningococcal disease in the United States, prevention of the spread of disease carries a high priority. The risk of invasive disease in family members of persons with invasive meningococcal disease is increased by a factor of 400 to 800. Further, case clusters cause great alarm in the community. Consequently, assessment of the need for prophylaxis and coordination of its administration are critical steps in the management of invasive meningococcal disease. Assistance in carrying out

Table 1 Chemoprophylaxis for Meningococcal Disease[1]

Drug	*Dosage*	*Relative Efficacy*	*Comments*
Rifampin	Children < 1 mo: 5 mg/kg p.o., q. 12 hr for 2 days Children ≥ 1 mo: 10 mg/kg p.o., q. 12 hr for 2 days Adults: 600 mg q. 12 hr for 2 days	First choice	Not recommended for pregnant women, because it is teratogenic in animals; because reliability of oral contraceptives may be affected by rifampin, alternative contraceptive measures should be considered during its administration
Ciprofloxacin	Adults: 500 mg p.o. once	Alternative	Not generally recommended for persons < 18 yr or for pregnant and lactating women, because it causes cartilage damage in immature laboratory animals; however, ciprofloxacin has been used extensively in children with cystic fibrosis without reported adverse outcomes; CDC recommends it for chemoprophylaxis in children when no acceptable alternative is available.
Ceftriaxone	Children < 15 yr: 125 mg I.M. once Adults: 250 mg I.M. once	Alternative	Indicated for pregnant women

these steps can be provided by the public health agencies to which cases of meningococcal disease must be reported (see below).

Prophylaxis is recommended for close contacts of infected persons [*see Table 1*]. Close contacts are defined as household members, day care center contacts, and anyone directly exposed to the patient's oral secretions (e.g., by kissing, by mouth-to-mouth resuscitation, during endotracheal intubation, or during endotracheal tube management by health care workers not wearing masks).[33] The likelihood of contracting invasive disease from close contact is highest in the first few days after exposure; thus, prophylaxis should ideally be administered within 24 hours after identification of the index case and is unlikely to be of value if given beyond 14 days after onset of illness in the index case.[34]

IMMUNIZATION

Vaccine

A quadrivalent polysaccharide vaccine for protection against *N. meningitidis* serogroups A, C, Y, and W-135 (Menomune) is currently available.[35] It is administered subcutaneously as a single 0.5 ml dose, induces protective antibody within 7 to 10 days, and is generally well tolerated. No serious side effects have been reported. The vaccine may be administered to pregnant and lactating women, because no adverse events associated with immunization during pregnancy have been reported. An important consideration is that the vaccine does not provide protection against serogroup B infection, which causes over half of cases in infants younger than one year. Vaccine efficacy against serogroups A and C is estimated at 85% to 100% in older children and adults.[36] Although protective immunity to serogroup A can be conferred in infants older than 3 months, immunity to serogroup C is difficult to attain in children younger than 1 year. No data are available on efficacy of the Y and W-135 polysaccharides in older children and adults, but these polysaccharides are safe and immunogenic. For all serogroups, limited data suggest that the duration of immunoprotection is probably no more than 3 years. Given this, as well as the difficulty of inducing an adequate immune response in infants, routine vaccination of infants is not recommended.

Several new meningococcal conjugate vaccines are under study for serogroups A, C, Y, and W-135, and they are likely to become available in the United States in the next few years.[37] Unlike polysaccharide vaccines, they induce a stronger, longer-lasting immune response that can be boosted by subsequent doses. Serogroup C conjugate vaccines were introduced in the United Kingdom in 1999.

Recommendations for Vaccine Use

Vaccination is recommended for persons at increased risk, for prospective travelers, and for the control of outbreaks.

Persons at increased risk Persons at increased inherent risk include military recruits and persons with terminal complement pathway deficiencies or functional or anatomic asplenia. Persons exposed routinely to *N. meningitidis* through occupational exposure (e.g., clinical or research laboratory personnel) should also consider vaccination.

Prospective travelers Vaccination is recommended for travelers to areas endemic for invasive meningococcal disease, including parts of sub-Saharan Africa during peak periods of disease incidence (generally the dry season, from December to June). In addition, a large international outbreak in pilgrims to the Hajj in Saudi Arabia in 2001 prompted recommendations that travelers to this site also be immunized.[38] Updated recommendations for this and other travel-related immunizations can be obtained at www.cdc.gov/travel.

Control of outbreaks Vaccination may be considered as a means of controlling outbreaks caused by serogroups covered by the vaccine. The Advisory Committee on Immunization Practices (ACIP) recommends that mass vaccination of persons 2 years of age or older be considered when three cases of serogroup C meningococcal disease occur within a 3-month period in a community or organization (e.g., a school), with an incidence of 10 cases per 100,000 population or greater.[39]

Immunization of college freshmen, particularly those living in dormitories, deserves special mention. Although the rate of invasive infection in this group exceeds that of any age group other than children younger than 2 years, it is still below the threshold recommended for initiating meningococcal vaccination campaigns. Thus, ACIP recommends that health care providers and colleges inform students and their parents about the vaccine's availability and potential benefits.[8] Many colleges recommend meningococcal vaccination to incoming freshmen, and some offer the vaccine through their student health service.

Requirements for Reporting Meningococcal Disease

Infection with *N. meningitidis* is reportable by law to most local and state health departments. Public health agencies will assist clinicians in the identification and treatment of exposed contacts; in the case of outbreaks, these agencies may institute other control measures. Physicians should not assume that clinical laboratories will execute reporting. Contact information for reporting communicable diseases can be found through state health departments, Web sites for which can be found at http://www.cdc.gov/mmwr/international/relres.html.

Infections Caused by *Neisseria gonorrhoeae*

Known primarily as a cause of sexually transmitted infections, *N. gonorrhoeae* remains an important cause of cervicitis, urethritis, proctitis, and pelvic inflammatory disease (PID) [see 10 Sexually Transmitted Diseases]. No vaccine is available.

EPIDEMIOLOGY

An estimated 600,000 new cases of gonococcal infection occur in the United States each year.[40] These cases are a mix of symptomatic infections, which occur mostly in men, and asymptomatic infections detected through routine testing, largely in women.

The incidence of gonorrhea declined steadily in the United States from 1978 through 1997, but rates increased in 1998 and have not declined since then. In particular, the incidence in adolescents, especially those in large cities, remains high; in addition, sustained outbreaks have occurred recently in men who have sex with men. In the United States in 2000, the highest reported rates of gonorrhea were in women 15 to 19 years of age (715.6 per 100,000 population) and in men 20 to 24 years of age (589.7 per 100,000 population).[41] In 42 states, the incidence of gonorrhea in women remains above the objective of 19 new cases per 100,000 population from Healthy People 2010 (http://www.health.gov/healthypeople/document/html/objectives/25-02.htm), a set of health objectives for the United States developed through the Office of Disease Prevention and Health Promotion of the United States Department of Health and Human Services.

Rates of gonococcal infection have increased among men who report having sex with other men.[42] In a surveillance project at six sexually transmitted disease clinics in five U.S. cities, positivity of urethral gonorrhea in this population was 21% for those who were HIV positive and 12% for those who were HIV negative. These findings have spurred some government agencies to recommend routine screening at least annually for gonorrhea in this population.[43]

Typing methods for the gonococcus are generally less clinically useful than for meningococcus and are used primarily to study gonococcal epidemiology. Most widely used are auxotyping, which classifies the organism on the basis of nutritional requirements, and protein I-serotyping, which is based on the stable antigenic diversity of its largest surface protein and further classifiable into different serovars by coagglutination assays. These two methods are combined into auxotype/serovar (A/S) classes for nomenclature of many strains (e.g., AHA/IA-1 denotes a strain that requires arginine, hypoxanthine, and uracil for growth and exhibits protein IA with a type 1 coagglutination pattern).[21]

PATHOGENESIS

The pathogenesis of *N. gonorrhoeae* has been closely studied in an experimental model using male human volunteers.[44] Like *N. meningitidis*, the gonococcus possesses a protease that may be important in cleaving IgA at the mucosal surface. Columnar or cuboidal epithelium is the main target for attachment, which is mediated primarily by pili that protrude from the cell surface and by outer membrane proteins termed Opa proteins.[45] Because they require iron for growth, gonococci possess transferrin receptors; they also contain lipo-oligosaccharide (LOS). The toxicity of LOS may be especially important in incapacitating the ciliary function of cells lining the fallopian tubes.[45] Within 24 to 48 hours after attachment, the organism's penetration into submucosa elicits an intense neutrophilic inflammatory response. Submucosal microabscesses form, purulent exudate collects, and the affected epithelium sloughs, resulting in ready detection of intracellular gram-negative diplococci in neutrophils on Gram stain.

The role of systemic antibody in gonococcal infection is unclear, given that individuals may be infected multiple times. Gonococcal strains can differ in the clinical manifestations they induce. Some strains, such as AHU/IA-1, AHU/IA-2 and CU, have been associated with the uncommon finding of asymptomatic urethral infection in men and a higher incidence of DGI.[46]

CLINICAL PRESENTATIONS

N. gonorrhoeae is known primarily for its propensity to cause superficial mucosal infections that are transmitted through sexual contact. In men, these infections most commonly involve the urethra. After an incubation period of 1 to 14 days, 95% of men infected at this site experience dysuria and urethral discharge. The discharge is typically purulent but can be serous or seropurulent, especially early in the course of disease. Mild edema and erythema of the urethral meatus may be seen. If left untreated, infection usually resolves over the course of several weeks, and persistent asymptomatic carriage is thought to be unlikely. In some men with untreated urethral infection, infection may spread to cause epididymitis, prostatitis, seminal vesiculitis, and infections of the Cowper and Tyson glands.[21] The urethra may also be infected in women, but isolated urethral infection is unusual except in women who have undergone a hysterectomy. Urethral infection in women is less frequently symptomatic.

Endocervical Infection

In women, the most common site of infection is the endocervical canal, where *N. gonorrhoeae* may cause mucopurulent cervicitis (MPC). MPC presents as either mucopurulent endocervical discharge or easily induced endocervical bleeding. Cervical ectopy, if present, may appear edematous. However, at least half of women with gonococcal infection of the cervix have neither signs of MPC nor gonococci detected on Gram stain of endocervical secretions. If symptoms develop, they are nonspecific and typical of most lower genital tract infections: abnormal, increased, or malodorous vaginal discharge; bleeding between menses; menorrhagia; pelvic pain; or pain with intercourse. If cervical infection is left untreated, *N. gonorrhoeae* may ascend to infect the upper genital tract—including the endometrium, fallopian tubes, ovaries, or adnexa (PID)—or the perihepatic space (Fitz-Hugh-Curtis syndrome). PID is estimated to occur in 10% to 20% of infected women. Finally, abscesses of Bartholin glands are not uncommon.[47]

Infection at Other Mucosal Sites

Both men and women can be infected at common mucosal sites, including the rectum, pharynx, and conjunctiva. Approximately 35% to 50% of women with endocervical infection are also infected at the rectum, usually without local symptoms. Receptive anal sex is not a prerequisite for rectal infection in women; rather, these infections may result from perianal inoculation with infected cervicovaginal secretions. Men who practice receptive anal sex with other men are also at risk of rectal infection. The presentation of rectal gonococcal infection ranges from asymptomatic colonization detected at routine screening to overt proctitis. Even in symptomatic patients, the range of manifestations is wide, including mild perianal pruritus, painless mucopurulent rectal discharge, mild rectal bleeding, severe rectal pain, tenesmus, and constipation.

Gonococcal infection of the pharynx is rarely symptomatic. Acquired by receptive oral sex (by either fellatio or cunnilingus but more efficiently by fellatio), pharyngeal infection is usually detected through routine screening. In persons with gonococci detected at nonpharyngeal sites, the prevalence of pharyngeal infection ranges from

3% to 7% in heterosexual men, 10% to 20% in heterosexual women, and 10% to 25% in men who have sex with other men.[21]

Gonococcal conjunctivitis occurs uncommonly in adults. It usually results from autoinoculation, particularly in laboratory and medical personnel.

Disseminated Gonococcal Infection

The term disseminated gonococcal infection refers to gonococcal infections that have spread beyond the genitourinary tract. The most common presentation is the acute arthritis-dermatitis syndrome, which is estimated to occur in 0.5% to 3.0% of persons with untreated mucosal gonococcal infection.[48,49] This syndrome may comprise the triad of tenosynovitis, dermatitis, and polyarthralgias without purulent arthritis, or it may appear as purulent arthritis alone. DGI should be strongly considered in any young, sexually active person with acute, nontraumatic oligoarthritis or tenosynovitis.

The arthritis of DGI can affect joints of any size and is typically asymmetrical.[50] With tenosynovitis, major tendon sheaths and their insertions are often tender and inflamed; the clinician should palpate these sites if this diagnosis is at all entertained. The classic rash of DGI usually consists of relatively few (< 20) tender, necrotic pustules on an erythematous base that often resolve within several days if left untreated.

Diagnosis of DGI is made more often in women than in men. Predisposing factors include recent menstruation, recent pregnancy, and terminal complement deficiency. The gonococcal strains that cause DGI are often those associated with asymptomatic genital disease and with resistance to complement-mediated bactericidal activity of normal human serum. The organism is recovered by culture from normally sterile sites, including blood or joint fluid, in less than 50% of persons with DGI; however, it can be cultured from mucosal sites or from sexual partners in more than 80% of cases. Amplified nucleic acid assays, such as PCR, have increased the yield of *N. gonorrhoeae* detection in joint fluid, but a subset of those affected still have sterile joint fluid in the presence of urogenital gonococci, suggesting that immunomodulatory responses are important in the pathogenesis of DGI.[51,52]

More invasive infection with *N. gonorrhoeae* is uncommon. Endocarditis and meningitis have been reported, however.[53,54]

DIAGNOSIS

N. gonorrhoeae may be diagnosed presumptively by direct visualization on a Gram stain smear of secretions from a compatible clinical site and, specifically, by growth in culture or detection by antigen detection, nonamplified DNA probe, and a nucleic acid amplification test (NAAT). In men with urethral discharge from *N. gonorrhoeae*, the organism is seen on Gram stain in 95% [*see Figure 1*]. Although reasonably specific for detection of endocervical *N. gonorrhoeae* (> 95%), Gram stain is considerably less sensitive (50% to 70%) and thus not recommended as the sole means of diagnosis of endocervical infection. Gram stain of anoscopically obtained rectal secretions has a sensitivity of 70% to 80% and thus may assist in making a specific diagnosis of gonococcal proctitis.[21] Because nongonococcal *Neisseria* species colonize the pharynx, Gram stain of the pharynx is not specific to infection with *N. gonorrhoeae* and thus is not recommended.

Traditional bacterial culture remains the mainstay of microbiologic diagnosis for normally sterile specimens in which invasive disease is suspected, such as blood and joint fluid, and is commonly used for the diagnosis of cervical, urethral, pharyngeal, and rectal infections. Cultures are obtained from these sites with a sterile Dacron swab that is then swept across the surface of a plate containing chocolate agar supplemented with glucose, vancomycin, colistin, and nystatin (Thayer-Martin media) and held in an environment with a high level of CO_2. The organism grows best under aerobic conditions at 35° to 37° C; however, it can also grow under anaerobic conditions. Unlike *N. meningitidis*, it does not ferment lactose. Relative to an expanded diagnostic standard that incorporates results of NAAT, culture for *N. gonorrhoeae* has an estimated sensitivity of 90% and specificity of greater than 99%.[55]

Other tests commonly used to diagnose gonococcal infection are a nonamplified DNA probe and several types of NAAT. The DNA probe is a nucleic acid hybridization test with a sensitivity of approximately 85% and specificity of 98%.[56] Available NAATs include PCR, ligase chain reaction (LCR), transcription-mediated assay (TMA), and hybrid capture tests. In general, the performance of these tests exceeds that of the nonamplification techniques, enhancing sensitivity while maintaining excellent specificity.[56] Further, NAATs have the major advantage of performing well on noninvasive specimens: urine in men and, in women, urine and vaginal swabs. Vaginal swabs may be collected either by patients or by clinicians, which provides opportunities for novel screening strategies. The NAATs in general have sensitivities for detection of *N. gonorrhoeae* of 95% to 99%, with a

Table 2 Treatment of Gonorrhea[1]

Disease	*Drug*	*Dosage*	*Relative Efficacy*	*Comments*
Uncomplicated infection of the cervix, urethra, or rectum*	Cefixime	400 mg p.o. once	First choice	Quinolones not recommended in areas where resistance is a concern; spectinomycin is used for patients intolerant of cephalosporins and quinolones, it is unreliable against pharyngeal infection, and posttreatment cultures are recommended
	Ciprofloxacin	500 mg p.o. once	Alternative first choice	
	Ofloxacin	400 mg p.o. once	Alternative first choice	
	Levofloxacin	250 mg p.o. once	Alternative first choice	
	Ceftriaxone	125 mg I.M. once	Second choice	
	Spectinomycin	2 g I.M. once	Second choice	
Conjunctivitis (not ophthalmia neonatorum)	Ceftriaxone	1 g I.M. once	—	—
Disseminated gonococcal infection (DGI)	*Parenteral*			Parenteral therapy is given for 24–48 hr after improvement, then followed by oral therapy for 1 wk total antibiotic therapy
	Ceftriaxone	1 g I.M. or I.V. q. 24 hr	First choice	
	Cefotaxime	1 g I.V. q. 8 hr	Alternative	
	Ceftizoxime	1 g I.V. q. 8 hr	Alternative	
	Ciprofloxacin	400 mg I.V. q. 12 hr	Alternative	
	Ofloxacin	400 mg I.V. q. 12 hr	Alternative	
	Levofloxacin	250 mg I.V. q.d.	Alternative	
	Spectinomycin	2 g I.M. q. 12 hr	Alternative	
	Oral			
	Cefixime	400 mg p.o., b.i.d.		
	Ciprofloxacin	500 mg p.o., b.i.d.		
	Ofloxacin	400 mg p.o., b.i.d.		
	Levofloxacin	500 mg p.o., q.d.		
Meningitis	Ceftriaxone	1–2 g I.V. q. 12 hr for 10–14 days	—	—
Endocarditis	Ceftriaxone	1–2 g I.V. q. 12 hr for ≥ 4 wk	—	—
Ophthalmia neonatorum	Ceftriaxone	25–50 mg/kg I.V. or I.M. in a single dose, not to exceed 125 mg	—	Topical antibiotic therapy alone is inadequate

*Treatment of gonorrhea in the adult should always be accompanied by treatment of chlamydial infection (azithromycin, 1 g orally in a single dose, or doxycycline, 100 mg orally b.i.d. for 7 days), and patients should abstain from sex during treatment. Test of cure is not routinely recommended.

specificity greater than 99% for cervical and urethral specimens. However, none is currently recommended for use on specimens other than urine, cervical, or urethral samples.[56]

TREATMENT

Recommended treatment of gonorrhea varies according to the site of infection and the likelihood of antibiotic resistance [*see Table 2*]. Currently recommended regimens for the treatment of gonorrhea are available online at www.cdc.gov/std/treatment.[43]

The gonococcus has multiple means of acquiring resistance to antibiotics. Plasmid-mediated mechanisms confer resistance to penicillin by encoding altered penicillin-binding proteins (PBPs). Resistance to tetracyclines is mediated by chromosomal mechanisms. Resistance to fluoroquinolones is conferred by production of an altered DNA gyrase to which these antibiotics are unable to bind and hence are rendered ineffectual. The Gonococcal Isolate Surveillance Project (GISP) annually updates important trends in gonococcal resistance patterns (http://www.cdc.gov/ncidod/dastlr/gcdir). Because these patterns can emerge and progress surprisingly rapidly, physicians should be aware of them. Although some problems begin in relative geographic isolation, they often mark the start of significant nationwide trends.[57–59] For example, recommendations for the empirical use of single-dose fluoroquinolone therapy were prominent in the CDC's 1998 Sexually Transmitted Disease Treatment Guidelines; the 2002 document emphasizes that because up to 14% of gonococcal isolates in Hawaii exhibit resistance to fluoroquinolones, these drugs should not be used in this area.[60,61] Patients in whom physicians should consider the possibility of quinolone-resistant *N. gonorrhoeae* (QRNG) include those who (1) have had failures with fluoroquinolone therapy, (2) have traveled to Hawaii or Southeast Asia (where resistance is endemic) or have sexual partners who may have acquired a gonococcal infection there, and (3) reside in California, where recent data indicate an increasing prevalence of QRNG. Because active surveillance is critical, physicians who encounter documented or suspected cases of QRNG should report this to their local health department. In 2000, 25% of GISP isolates were resistant to penicillin, tetracycline, or both. To date, no isolates resistant to cephalosporins have been detected in GISP. Because persons with gonococcal infection are at risk for other STDs, particularly chlamydial infection, the CDC recommends that treatment regimens for gonorrhea be partnered with an antibiotic effective against *C. trachomatis* as well. Although azithromycin is active against the gonococcus, a dose of 2 g orally is required to effect acceptable cure rates. This is double the dose required to treat chlamydial infection, and such a high dose frequently causes gastrointestinal side effects. Similarly, ciprofloxacin remains effective for gonococcal infections not caused by QRNG, but it is not effective against chlamydial infection. Both infections can be treated with a 1-week course of levofloxacin or ofloxacin, however.

COMPLICATIONS AND PROGNOSIS

The best-known complications of *N. gonorrhoeae* infection include PID and neonatal conjunctivitis (ophthalmia neonatorum). PID in which gonococci play an etiologic role may be more purulent and severe than PID caused by *C. trachomatis*. If left untreated, 10% to 40% of women with gonococcal cervical infection will develop PID.[62] Ophthalmia neonatorum caused by *N. gonorrhoeae* can be severe, resulting in perforation of the globe and blindness. Moreover, accruing evidence suggests that gonococcal infection may profoundly impact global morbidity through its role in facilitating transmission and acquisition of HIV. In men infected with HIV, the presence of gonococcal urethritis was shown to increase the quantity of HIV shed in semen by approximately eightfold.[63,64] Remarkably, treatment with routine antibiotics aimed at *N. gonorrhoeae* resulted in significant reduction of the associated HIV shedding.[64] Similarly, cervical inflammation in women, commonly caused by gonococcal infection, is associated with increased shedding of HIV; treatment of cervicitis reduces this shedding.[65,66] These observations suggest that the inflammation associated with gonococcal infection significantly increases the likelihood that HIV may be more efficiently transmitted through unprotected sex. In persons who are not infected with HIV, the same inflammatory cells elicited by gonococcal infection provide a ready target for HIV infection; thus, risk of HIV acquisition is very likely increased in this setting.[67]

MANAGEMENT OF SEXUAL PARTNERS AND CHEMOPROPHYLAXIS

Persons infected with *N. gonorrhoeae* should be interviewed and counseled about the importance of treatment for their sexual partners. The CDC recommends that sexual partners with whom patients have had sex within the past 60 days be tested and treated for both gonococcal infection and chlamydial infection.[43] If the patient's last sexual contact was more than 60 days before being interviewed, the last partner should be evaluated and treated. For infants, most states require by law that, at birth, an agent be administered to prevent gonococcal ophthalmia neonatorum. Options include single applications of one of several agents, including silver nitrate 1% aqueous solution, erythromycin 0.5% ophthalmic ointment, and tetracycline 1% ophthalmic ointment.

Other *Neisseria* Species

Several typically nonpathogenic *Neisseria* species are found as saprophytes in the upper respiratory tract: the nonchromogens *N. lactamica*, *N. mucosa*, and *N. sicca* and the chromogens *N. flavescens* and *N. subflava*. All of these species can occasionally cause disease.[68,69] Meningitis that is clinically indistinguishable from that caused by *N. meningitidis* has been attributed to each of these species, most frequently to *N. subflava* and *N. mucosa*. Endocarditis has also been attributed to nonpathogenic species, particularly *N. sicca*, *N. mucosa*, and *N. subflava*. Odontogenic infections or bite wounds may also harbor these species.[70] Infections with nonpathogenic *Neisseria* species can be treated effectively with penicillin, but occasionally, strains are resistant. The antimicrobial susceptibility of the strain causing the infection should be used to guide therapy.

References

1. Apicella MA: *Neisseria meningitidis*. Principles and Practice of Infectious Diseases, 5th ed. Mandell GL, Bennett JE, Dolin R, Eds. Churchill Livingstone, Philadelphia, 2000, p 2228

2. Rosenstein NE, Perkins BA, Stephens DS, et al: Meningococcal disease. N Engl J Med 344:1378, 2001

3. Tappero JW, Reporter R, Wenger JD, et al: Meningococcal disease in Los Angeles County, California, and among men in the county jails. N Engl J Med 335:833, 1996

4. Exposure to patients with meningococcal disease on aircrafts—United States, 1999–2001. MMWR Morb Mortal Wkly Rep 50:485, 2001

5. Laboratory-acquired meningococcal disease—United States, 2000. MMWR Morb Mortal Wkly Rep 51:141, 2002

6. Schuchat A, Robinson K, Wenger JD, et al: Bacterial meningitis in the United States in 1995. Active Surveillance Team. N Engl J Med 337: 970, 1997

7. Rosenstein NE, Perkins BA, Stephens DS, et al: The changing epidemiology of meningococcal disease in the United States, 1992–1996. J Infect Dis 180:1894, 1999

8. Meningococcal disease and college students. Recommendations of the Advisory Committee on Immunization Practices (ACIP). MMWR Recomm Rep 49:13, 2000

9. Pollard AJ, Frasch C: Development of natural immunity to *Neisseria meningitidis*. Vaccine 19:1327, 2001

10. Kolb-Maurer A, Unkmeir A, Kammerer U, et al: Interaction of *Neisseria meningitidis* with human dendritic cells. Infect Immun 69:6912, 2001

11. Goldschneider I, Gotschlich EC, Artenstein MS: Human immunity to the meningococcus: I. The role of humoral antibodies. J Exp Med 129: 1307, 1969

12. Figueroa JE, Densen P: Infectious diseases associated with complement deficiencies. Clin Microbiol Rev 4:359, 1991

13. Fijen CA, Kuijper EJ, te Bulte MT, et al: Assessment of complement deficiency in patients with meningococcal disease in The Netherlands. Clin Infect Dis 28:98, 1999

14. Faust SN, Levin M, Harrison OB, et al: Dysfunction of endothelial protein C activation in severe meningococcal sepsis. N Engl J Med 345: 408, 2001

15. Garcia NS, Castelo JS, Ramos V, et al: Frequency of myocarditis in cases of fatal meningococcal infection in children: observations on 31 cases studied at autopsy. Rev Soc Bras Med Trop 32:517, 1999

16. Hardman JM, Earle KM: Myocarditis in 200 fatal meningococcal infections. Arch Pathol 87:318, 1969

17. Kaplan SL: Clinical presentations, diagnosis, and prognostic factors of bacterial meningitis. Infect Dis Clin North Am 13:579, 1999

18. Acute meningococcal meningitis: analysis of features of the disease according to the age of 255 patients. Copenhagen Meningitis Study Group.J Infect 34:227, 1997

19. Koppes GM, Ellenbogen C, Gebhart RJ: Group Y meningococcal disease in United States Air Force recruits. Am J Med 62:661, 1977

20. Tayal SC, Rashid S, Muttu KM, et al: Meningococcal carriage: prevalence and sex-related risk factors. J Infect 34:101, 1997

21. Hook EW 3rd, Handsfield HH: Gonococcal infections in the adult. Sexually Transmitted Diseases, 3rd ed. Holmes KK, Mardh P-A, Lemon SM, et al, Eds. McGraw-Hill Book Co, New York, 1999, p 451

22. Joao I, Marques P, Namora J, et al: *Neisseria meningitidis* native valve endocarditis: a case report. Rev Port Cardiol 20:877, 2001

23. Lin VH, Parekh RS, McQuillan MA, et al: Meningococcal endocarditis presenting as cellulitis. Clin Infect Dis 21:1023, 1995

24. Taha MK: Molecular detection and characterization of *Neisseria meningitidis*. Expert Rev Mol Diagn 2:143, 2002

25. Kirsch EA, Barton RP, Kitchen L, et al: Pathophysiology, treatment and outcome of meningococcemia: a review and recent experience. Pediatr Infect Dis J 15:967, 1996

26. Harrison LH, Pass MA, Mendelsohn AB, et al: Invasive meningococcal disease in adolescents and young adults. JAMA 286:694, 2001

27. Guideline for isolation precautions in hospitals. Part II. Recommendations for isolation precautions in hospitals. Hospital Infection Control Practices Advisory Committee.Am J Infect Control 24:32, 1996

28. Strang JR, Pugh EJ: Meningococcal infections: reducing the case fatality rate by giving penicillin before admission to hospital. BMJ 305: 141, 1992

29. Quagliarello VJ, Scheld WM: Treatment of bacterial meningitis. N Engl J Med 336:708, 1997

30. Smith OP, White B, Vaughan D, et al: Use of protein-C concentrate, heparin, and haemodiafiltration in meningococcus-induced purpura fulminans. Lancet 350:1590, 1997

31. White B, Livingstone W, Murphy C, et al: An open-label study of the role of adjuvant hemostatic support with protein C replacement therapy in purpura fulminans–associated meningococcemia. Blood 96:3719, 2000

32. Bernard GR, Vincent JL, Laterre PF, et al: Efficacy and safety of recombinant human activated protein C for severe sepsis. N Engl J Med 344:699, 2001

33. Prevention and control of meningococcal disease. MMWR Morb Mortal Wkly Rep 49:1, 2000

34. Peltola H: Prophylaxis of bacterial meningitis. Infect Dis Clin North Am 13:685, 1999

35. Rosenstein NE, Fischer M, Tappero JW: Meningococcal vaccines. Infect Dis Clin North Am 15:155, 2001

36. Rosenstein N, Levine O, Taylor JP, et al: Efficacy of meningococcal vaccine and barriers to vaccination. JAMA 279:435, 1998

37. Jodar L, Feavers IM, Salisbury D, et al: Development of vaccines against meningococcal disease. Lancet 359:1499, 2002

38. Update: assessment of risk for meningococcal disease associated with the Hajj 2001. MMWR Morb Mortal Wkly Rep 50:221, 2001

39. Control and prevention of serogroup C meningococcal disease: evaluation and management of suspected outbreaks: recommendations of the Advisory Committee on Immunization Practices (ACIP). MMWR Recomm Rep 46:13, 1997

40. Fox KK, Whittington WL, Levine WC, et al: Gonorrhea in the United States, 1981–1996: demographic and geographic trends. Sex Transm Dis 25:386, 1998

41. Sexually Transmitted Disease Surveillance, 2000. Centers for Disease Control and Prevention, U.S. Department of Health and Human Services Atlanta, 2001

42. Fox KK, del Rio C, Holmes KK, et al: Gonorrhea in the HIV era: a reversal in trends among men who have sex with men. Am J Public Health 91:959, 2001

43. Sexually transmitted disease treatment guidelines. MMWR Morb Mortal Wkly Rep 51(RR-6):1, 2002

44. Cohen MS, Cannon JG: Human experimentation with *Neisseria gonorrhoeae*: progress and goals. J Infect Dis 179 (suppl 2):S375, 1999

45. Sparling PF: Biology of *Neisseria gonorrhoeae*. Sexually Transmitted Diseases, 3rd ed. Holmes KK, Mardh P-A, Lemon SM, et al, Eds. McGraw Hill Book Co, New York, 1999, p 433

46. Whittington WL, Holmes KK: Unique gonococcal phenotype associated with asymptomatic infection in men and with erroneous diagnosis of nongonococcal urethritis. J Infect Dis 181:1044, 2000

47. Hoosen AA, Nteta C, Moodley J, et al: Sexually transmitted diseases including HIV infection in women with Bartholin's gland abscesses. Genitourin Med 71:155, 1995

48. Rompalo AM, Hook EW 3rd, Roberts PL, et al: The acute arthritis-dermatitis syndrome: the changing importance of *Neisseria gonorrhoeae* and *Neisseria meningitidis*. Arch Intern Med 147:281, 1987

49. O'Brien JP, Goldenberg DL, Rice PA: Disseminated gonococcal infection: a prospective analysis of 49 patients and a review of pathophysiology and immune mechanisms. Medicine (Baltimore) 62:395, 1983

50. Rice PA, Handsfield HH: Arthritis associated with sexually transmitted diseases. Sexually Transmitted Diseases 3rd ed. Holmes KK, Mardh P-A, Lemon SM, et al, Eds. McGraw Hill Book Co, New York, 1999 p 921

51. Liebling MR, Arkfeld DG, Michelini GA, et al: Identification of *Neisseria gonorrhoeae* in synovial fluid using the polymerase chain reaction. Arthritis Rheum 37:702, 1994

52. Muralidhar B, Rumore PM, Steinman CR: Use of the polymerase chain reaction to study arthritis due to *Neisseria gonorrhoeae*. Arthritis Rheum 37:710, 1994

53. Lin MF, Lau YJ, Hu BS, et al: Gonococcal meningitis and intra-abdominal abscess in the presence of a ventriculoperitoneal shunt. Scand J Infect Dis 32:567, 2000

54. Mofredj A, Baraka D, Madec Y, et al: Disseminated gonococcal infection and meningitis. Am J Med 109:71, 2000

55. Black CM, Morse SA: The use of molecular techniques for the diagnosis and epidemiologic study of sexually transmitted infections. Curr Infect Dis Rep 2:31, 2000

56. Koumans EH, Johnson RE, Knapp JS, et al: Laboratory testing for *Neisseria gonorrhoeae* by recently introduced nonculture tests: a performance review with clinical and public health considerations. Clin Infect Dis 27:1171, 1998

57. Ehret JM, Judson FN: Quinolone-resistant *Neisseria gonorrhoeae*: the beginning of the end? Report of quinolone-resistant isolates and surveillance in the southwestern United States, 1989 to 1997. Sex Transm Dis 25:522, 1998

58. Bal C: Increasing antimicrobial resistance in STDs and the need for surveillance: *Neisseria gonorrhoeae* as a model. FEMS Immunol Med Microbiol 24:447, 1999

59. National sentinel surveillance of antimicrobial resistance in *Neisseria gonorrhoeae*. Commun Dis Rep CDR Wkly 10:195, 2000

60. Trees DL, Sandul AL, Neal SW, et al: Molecular epidemiology of *Neisseria gonorrhoeae* exhibiting decreased susceptibility and resistance to ciprofloxacin in Hawaii, 1991–1999. Sex Transm Dis 28:309, 2001

61. Fox KK, Knapp JS, Holmes KK, et al: Antimicrobial resistance in *Neisseria gonorrhoeae* in the United States, 1988–1994: the emergence of decreased susceptibility to the fluoroquinolones. J Infect Dis 175:1396, 1997

62. Platt R, Rice PA, McCormack WM: Risk of acquiring gonorrhea and prevalence of abnormal adnexal findings among women recently exposed to gonorrhea. JAMA 250:3205, 1983

63. Moss GB, Overbaugh J, Welch M, et al: Human immunodeficiency virus DNA in urethral secretions in men: association with gonococcal urethritis and CD4 cell depletion. J Infect Dis 172:1469, 1995

64. Cohen MS, Hoffman IF, Royce RA, et al: Reduction of concentration of HIV-1 in semen after treatment of urethritis: implications for prevention of sexual transmission of HIV- 1. AIDSCAP Malawi Research Group. Lancet 349:1868, 1997

65. Kreiss J, Willerford DM, Hensel M, et al: Association between cervical inflammation and cervical shedding of human immunodeficiency virus DNA. J Infect Dis 170:1597, 1994

66. McClelland RS, Wang CC, Mandaliya K, et al: Treatment of cervicitis is associated with decreased cervical shedding of HIV-1. AIDS 15: 105, 2001

67. Weir SS, Feldblum PJ, Roddy RE, et al: Gonorrhea as a risk factor for HIV acquisition. AIDS 8:1605, 1994

68. Tronel H, Chaudemanche H, Pechier N, et al: Endocarditis due to *Neisseria mucosa* after tongue piercing. Clin Microbiol Infect 7:275, 2001

69. Baraldes MA, Domingo P, Barrio JL, et al: Meningitis due to *Neisseria subflava*: case report and review. Clin Infect Dis 30:615, 2000

70. Capitini CM, Herrero IA, Patel R, et al: Wound infection with *Neisseria weaveri* and a novel subspecies of *Pasteurella multocida* in a child who sustained a tiger bite. Clin Infect Dis 34:E74, 2002

19 Infections Due to *Escherichia coli* and Other Enteric Gram-Negative Bacilli

Michael S. Donnenberg, M.D.

This chapter describes infections caused by *Escherichia coli* and related members of the family Enterobacteriaceae, excluding genera that principally cause enteric infections. Infections caused by *Salmonella, Shigella,* and *Yersinia* are described elsewhere [see 20 Infections Due to the Enteric Pathogens *Campylobacter, Salmonella, Shigella, Yersinia, Vibrio,* and *Helicobacter*]. The family Enterobacteriaceae comprises facultative anaerobic gram-negative bacilli that ferment sugars. These organisms are often motile because of the presence of peritrichous flagella (i.e., flagella that are distributed around the entire cell). Many Enterobacteriaceae species reside principally in the gastrointestinal tract of vertebrates, though some are found primarily in the environment. They are oxidase negative and catalase positive and are capable of reducing nitrate to nitrite. They cause a variety of diseases, including diarrhea, urinary tract infections (UTIs), and nosocomial infections.

Escherichia coli Infections

E. coli, the most common facultative anaerobe in the human intestine, is distinguished from other members of the family Enterobacteriaceae primarily on the basis of *E. coli*'s ability to ferment lactose and to produce indole and its inability to hydrolyze urea. Although the many different strains of *E. coli* can cause a diverse array of diseases, several virulence factors are shared by most members of the species; these include the ability to produce a highly reactive lipopolysaccharide in the cell wall, the ability to produce type 1 mannose-binding fimbriae, and, in many strains, the ability to produce an antiphagocytic capsule and to sequester iron.

E. coli and *Salmonella* diverged from a common ancestor about 100 million years ago.[1] Ample time for diversifying selection and a prodigious capacity for genetic exchange have fostered a tremendous degree of genetic diversity in *E. coli* strains. Thus, it is not surprising that this species has the ability to cause a diverse array of infectious diseases. In fact, the organisms that are commonly referred to as *Shigella* are in fact members of the species *E. coli*,[2] but because of historical and clinical considerations, they are often discussed separately [see 20 Infections Due to the Enteric Pathogens *Campylobacter, Salmonella, Shigella, Yersinia, Vibrio,* and *Helicobacter*]. The ability of *E. coli* to cause a variety of clinical syndromes by a plethora of mechanisms is entirely dependent upon unique virulence attributes that are encoded by distinct sets of virulence genes. Each group of *E. coli* that causes a particular clinical syndrome by a recognized pathogenic mechanism may be referred to as a pathotype [*see Table 1*]. However, the recent publication of the complete genome sequences of the nonpathogenic *E. coli* strain K-12 and of a highly pathogenic serotype O157:H7 strain provides a humbling reminder of our ignorance regarding pathogenic mechanisms.[3] These two strains, which are so alike in most characteristics that they could easily be regarded as identical in clinical microbiology laboratories, are remarkably different in genetic content. Although 3,574 genes are common to both organisms, the pathogenic strain contains 1,387 genes that are not present in the K-12 strain, and 528 genes have the opposite distribution. It is not known what roles the overwhelming majority of these genes play in the biology of the organism or in the pathogenesis of infections.

Because each pathotype of *E. coli* produces disease that has more or less distinct epidemiologic, pathogenetic, and clinical features, the discussion of specific pathotypes is organized on the basis of whether the infections caused by those pathotypes occur within or outside of the GI tract.

DIARRHEA

Six pathotypes of *E. coli* cause diarrhea[4] [*see Table 1*]. Of these, the epidemiologic, pathogenetic, and

Table 1 Clinical, Epidemiologic, Pathogenetic, and Therapeutic Aspects of Infection with Various Pathotypes of *E. coli*

Pathotype	*Clinical Features*	*Epidemiologic Features*	*Virulence Factors*	*Management*
Enterotoxigenic	Watery diarrhea	Childhood diarrhea in developing countries; traveler's diarrhea	Pili, heat-labile and heat-stable enterotoxins	Fluid replacement; ciprofloxacin + loperamide
Enteropathogenic	Watery diarrhea, vomiting	Infants in developing countries	Bundle-forming pilus, attaching and effacing effect	Fluid replacement
Enterohemorrhagic	Watery diarrhea, hemorrhagic colitis, hemolytic-uremic syndrome	Food-borne and waterborne outbreaks in developed countries	Shiga toxins, attaching and effacing effect	Fluid replacement, supportive care; antibiotics and antimotility agents are contraindicated
Enteroaggregative	Diarrhea with mucus	Childhood diarrhea	Pili, cytotoxins	Fluid replacement; antibiotic treatment for patients with AIDS?
Diffuse-adhering	Diarrhea	Older children?	Unknown	Fluid replacement
Extraintestinal	UTI, neonatal meningitis, nosocomial infections	Sexually active women, neonates, hospitalized patients	Fimbriae of types 1, P, and others; hemolysin; capsule; iron-acquisition systems	Antibiotics for symptomatic patients and in selected patients with asymptomatic UTI; antibiotic therapy guided by susceptibility testing for other infections

UTI—urinary tract infection

clinical features of enteroinvasive *E. coli* are the same as those of *Shigella*, and they are described elsewhere [see 20 Infections Due to the Enteric Pathogens *Campylobacter, Salmonella, Shigella, Yersinia, Vibrio,* and *Helicobacter*].

Diarrhea Due to Enterotoxigenic E. coli

Epidemiology Enterotoxigenic *E. coli* (ETEC) is a common cause of watery diarrhea in children in developing nations and in people of all ages who visit these countries. ETEC infections are spread through ingestion of contaminated food and water in regions where sanitation is inadequate. A relatively large inoculum is required to produce illness; therefore, person-to-person transmission is not significant for this organism.

Pathogenesis ETEC produces either a heat-labile toxin (LT), a heat-stable toxin (ST), or both. LT has the same three-dimensional structure, receptor, and mechanism of action as cholera toxin [see 20 Infections Due to the Enteric Pathogens *Campylobacter, Salmonella, Shigella, Yersinia, Vibrio,* and *Helicobacter*]. Like cholera toxin, LT toxin induces a chain of events that leads to an elevation in the intracellular concentration of cyclic adenosine monophosphate (cAMP) and the opening of the cystic fibrosis transmembrane conductance regulator [*see Figure 1*]. The efflux of chloride ions into the intestinal lumen is accompanied by sodium ions and water, and diarrhea ensues. ST is a small disulfide-rich peptide that resembles the endogenous hormone guanylin. Like its homologue, ST toxin causes increased cyclic guanosine monophosphate (cGMP) levels, which also lead to electrolyte efflux and fluid efflux through the cystic fibrosis transmembrane conductance regulator. For these toxins to reach their targets in sufficient quantity and for a sufficient duration to induce symptoms, the organisms must adhere to the intestinal mucosa.[5] This binding is accomplished through an antigenically and morphologically diverse array of pilus and nonpilus adhesins known as colonization factor antigens.[4]

Diagnosis After ingestion of food or water that is contaminated with large numbers of ETEC organisms, there is an incubation period of 0 to 2 days before the onset of symptoms. The disease begins abruptly with the onset of watery diarrhea without blood or mucus. Nausea, vomiting, abdominal cramps, and fever are rarely prominent. The disease is self-limited, lasting 3 to 5 days in travelers.[4] The endemic disease is sometimes more

reporting. Fortunately, unlike most strains of *E. coli*, O157:H7 ferments sorbitol slowly, enabling the identification of these organisms on specific indicator plates. However, not all microbiology laboratories offer this test, and many of those that perform it do so only on request. Therefore, the recognition of sporadic cases and outbreaks of EHEC infection depends largely on the acumen of the astute clinician, who must suspect the diagnosis and request the test.

The diagnosis of *E. coli* infection caused by Shiga toxin–producing organisms other than O157:H7 is more difficult, because these organisms do not have a distinguishing phenotype that can be assayed in most laboratories. Colonies cultured from the stool of patients with suspected non-O157:H7 Shiga toxin–producing *E. coli* infection should be sent to referral laboratories, state health laboratories, or the Centers for Disease Control and Prevention for assays to detect Shiga toxins or the genes that encode them.

Treatment The treatment of EHEC infection is supportive and includes oral rehydration, observation, and, if necessary, hospital admission for the management of complications. Many antibiotics induce the production of Shiga toxins. The bacteriophages that encode Shiga toxins in vitro and in animal models[26] have been associated with an increased risk of HUS in people[27]; therefore, antibiotics are contraindicated in patients with known or suspected EHEC infection. In some studies, antimotility agents were found to be associated with an increased risk of HUS.[24] In addition, the use of antimotility agents is associated with a theoretical risk of increasing the duration of toxin exposure. For these reasons, antimotility agents are also contraindicated in patients with EHEC infection. The risk of EHEC infection can be reduced by routine adherence to good hygienic practice in food preparation. Ground beef should always be cooked to an internal temperature of 68.3° C (well done or until the juices run clear).[14] A broad array of efforts to reduce EHEC infections is under development. These include measures to reduce colonization in cattle; vaccine development; and improved food-safety measures.

Diarrhea Due to Enteroaggregative E. coli *and Diffuse-Adhering* E. coli

Enteroaggregative *E. coli* (EAEC) and diffuse-adhering *E. coli* (DAEC) are distinguished by characteristic patterns of adherence to tissue culture cells on in vitro assays. It is likely that these pathotypes contain a heterogeneous mixture of strains that do not entirely share pathogenetic or clinical features.[4,28,29] Our understanding of the epidemiology, pathogenesis, and management of these infections is rudimentary, but several interesting features have been defined.

Epidemiology EAEC organisms are associated with acute and chronic diarrhea in children in developing countries[30]; they have also been identified in epidemiologic studies in Europe[31] and have been isolated from patients with AIDS.[32,33] Interestingly, carriage of EAEC, even in the absence of overt symptoms, is associated with evidence of growth retardation in children.[34] DAEC has been associated with diarrhea in older children in developing countries.[35,36]

Pathogenesis EAEC strains produce a variety of pili and toxins, but further study is needed to clarify the role that these factors play in causing disease. The pathogenetic mechanisms of DAEC remain obscure.

Diagnosis Diarrhea caused by EAEC may contain mucus or blood and may be accompanied by cramps. In some cases, particularly in patients with AIDS, the diarrhea can be protracted. The clinical features of DAEC infection have not been well described. The diagnosis of these infections requires tissue culture assays that are performed only in the research setting.

Treatment Case reports and studies in small series of patients have suggested that AIDS patients who are infected with EAEC may respond to antibiotic treatment.[37]

EXTRAINTESTINAL INFECTIONS

E. coli can infect a variety of extraintestinal sites, including the urinary tract, the meninges (in neonates), the lungs, the peritoneum, the gallbladder, and the biliary tree; *E. coli* infections can also occur in association with intravascular and prosthetic devices [*see Table 1*]. *E. coli* can be involved in polymicrobial infections such as intra-abdominal abscesses and skin and soft tissue infections. Bacteremia can complicate extraintestinal *E. coli* infections. Although the virulence factors responsible for all of these diseases have not been well studied, it is clear that the strains that cause extraintestinal infections are not a random sample of *E. coli* from the host intestine. On the other hand, these strains lack most of the virulence factors associated with those that cause diarrhea; rather, the strains that cause extraintestinal infections are more likely to possess the genes for hemolysin, iron-acquisition systems, capsule, and a variety of fimbriae than are strains isolated from the GI tract.

E. coli is by far the leading cause of UTIs in otherwise healthy persons, and it is an important cause of UTIs in those patients whose urinary tracts are compromised by anatomic abnormalities, foreign bodies, or host immune defects. The bacteria that cause UTIs are more likely than fecal *E. coli* isolates to possess the genes for a variety of factors under study as potential virulence determinants. Of these factors, P fimbriae and hemolysin are prominent.[38] Interestingly, however, the ubiquitous type 1 fimbriae that are produced by virtually all strains of *E. coli* and related organisms play a critical role in the pathogenesis of *E. coli*–associated UTI and are a promising target for the development of vaccine.[39] However, there is much more to the pathogenesis of UTI than the production of type 1 fimbriae, because the presence of these organelles does not distinguish uropathogenic *E. coli* from other strains. Genomic sampling of prototype strains confirms that these strains possess many genes that are absent from *E. coli* K-12.[40–43] More detailed information on the pathogenesis, clinical features, and treatment of UTI is presented elsewhere [see 9 Infections of the Urinary Tract]. The similarity in the repertoire of putative virulence factors in strains isolated from UTIs and other extraintestinal infections has led some investigators to propose that extraintestinal pathogenic *E. coli* (ExPEC) be considered a single pathotype.[44]

The diagnosis of these infections is confirmed by isolating the organism in culture from appropriate clinical specimens. Treatment is guided by susceptibility testing. The rising prevalence of resistance to trimethoprim-sulfamethoxazole in *E. coli* isolates from the community and the rising prevalence in nursing homes and hospitals of strains that produce extended-spectrum β-lactamases are causes for concern.[45,46]

Proteus Infections

Named after a character in Homer's *Odyssey* who could change shape, organisms belonging to the genus *Proteus* are noted for their ability to take two forms: typical bacillary swimmer cells, which express a variety of surface fimbriae as well as flagella, and highly elongated swarm cells, which express hundreds of flagella and few other surface structures. Swarm cells provide a challenge to the clinical microbiologist because the organisms frequently swarm over culture plates and interfere with the isolation of individual colonies. By far, the most commonly isolated *Proteus* species is *P. mirabilis*.

PATHOGENESIS

Proteus rapidly hydrolyzes urea to form carbon dioxide and ammonium hydroxide. In the urinary tract, this reaction results in an increase in pH. This reaction also alters the solubility of polyvalent ions and leads to the formation of struvite calculi. These stones can then obstruct urinary catheters, leading to bacterial persistence and urosepsis. In a murine model of ascending UTI, a urease-negative mutant of *P. mirabilis* was found to be severely limited in its ability to colonize the urinary tract, and this mutant strain failed to form stones.[47] Studies in animal models have confirmed the ability of *P. mirabilis* to produce several fimbriae.[48]

EPIDEMIOLOGY AND ETIOLOGY

Although *P. mirabilis* occasionally causes UTI in otherwise healthy persons, it is more commonly isolated from patients with abnormalities of the urinary tract, particularly those with indwelling urethral catheters and those with stones. Notably, *Proteus* has a predilection for causing upper urinary tract infections.[49] Whereas *P. mirabilis* rarely causes infections outside the urinary tract, other members of the genus and closely related organisms such as *Morganella morganii* may be isolated from skin infections and soft tissue infections, especially skin ulcers in patients with diabetes mellitus.

DIAGNOSIS

The diagnosis of a urinary tract infection caused by *Proteus* can be suspected in patients with compatible symptoms and signs who have complicated urinary tracts, including those patients with indwelling urinary catheters and functional or anatomic abnormalities. Evidence of upper urinary tract involvement (e.g., fever, flank pain, and sepsis), catheter obstruction, or known renal calculi strongly supports the diagnosis, which can be confirmed by culture.

TREATMENT

Most strains of *P. mirabilis* are susceptible to many antibiotics, but some *Proteus* species are highly resistant. In the treatment of UTIs caused by *Proteus* organisms, the underlying urinary abnormality and the clinical appearance of the patient must be taken into account. Treatment of asymptomatic bacteriuria in patients with urinary calculi or anatomic or functional abnormalities provides no long-term benefit to the patient and merely increases the potential for antimicrobial resistance [see 9 Infections of the Urinary Tract].

Klebsiella Infections

The genus *Klebsiella* includes five species, but *K. pneumoniae* and, to a lesser extent, *K. oxytoca* are responsible for the vast majority of human *Klebsiella* infections. These organisms are found in the environment and in the GI tract.

EPIDEMIOLOGY AND ETIOLOGY

Although *Klebsiella* species occasionally cause UTI in otherwise healthy persons, the majority of *Klebsiella* infections occur in compromised hosts. *K. pneumoniae* can cause community-acquired pneumonia, classically in patients with alcoholism with dramatic findings such as currant jelly sputum and a bulging fissure sign (Friedländer pneumonia). In practice, pulmonary infections caused by *Klebsiella* are difficult to distinguish from those caused by other organisms on clinical grounds.[50] Most *Klebsiella* infections occur in hospitals, where these bacteria cause UTI, pneumonia, wound infections, biliary infections, and primary bacteremia.[51] *Klebsiella* are often second only to *E. coli* as a cause of nosocomial gram-negative bacteremia.[51,52] These infections can occur as epidemics or sporadically.[53] Particularly problematic are outbreaks of nosocomial infections caused by strains of *Klebsiella* that produce extended-spectrum β-lactamases.[46] These organisms are frequently resistant to multiple antibiotics, owing to the presence of plasmids that encode multiple antibiotic-resistance genes.

PATHOGENESIS

The primary virulence factor for *Klebsiella* is a luxuriant polysaccharide capsule, which has antiphagocytic properties. *Klebsiella* organisms also make type 1 fimbriae; like ExPEC organisms, they also produce other fimbriae and have iron-acquisition systems and a reactive lipopolysaccharide.[54]

DIAGNOSIS

The clinical features of community-acquired pneumonia caused by *K. pneumoniae* are not sufficiently distinctive to differentiate patients with infections caused by this organism from those who have infections caused by other agents. Similarly, nosocomial infections and urinary tract infections caused by *Klebsiella* cannot be diagnosed on the basis of clinical features.

In the microbiology laboratory, a presumptive identification of *Klebsiella* infection is often made when a highly mucoid, lactose-fermenting, ampicillin-resistant, gram-negative bacillus is isolated and is confirmed by further testing.

TREATMENT

Treatment of *Klebsiella* infections requires consultation with a clinical microbiology laboratory or specialists in infectious diseases to ensure selection of an antibiotic to which the organism is susceptible. *Klebsiella* isolates that do not produce extended-spectrum β-lactamases are usually resistant to ampicillin but are sensitive to cephalosporins, trimethoprim-sulfamethoxazole, aminoglycosides, combinations of penicillins and β-lactamase inhibitors, and fluoroquinolones, any of which may be used to treat infections caused by susceptible organisms.

Enterobacter and *Serratia* Infections

EPIDEMIOLOGY AND ETIOLOGY

Enterobacter and *Serratia* are closely related to *Klebsiella;* like *Klebsiella,* they are principally opportunistic pathogens that cause a variety of nosocomial infections. In addition, *S. marcescens* has been frequently isolated from the blood or other clinical specimens of patients who use injection drugs.[55] Although several species of *Enterobacter*, including *E. cloacae, E. aerogenes,* and *E. agglomerans,* cause infections, *S. marcescens* is the only *Serratia* species that has been isolated from patients with appreciable frequency.

PATHOGENESIS

Enterobacter and *Serratia* organisms share with *Klebsiella* organisms the ability to produce antiphagocytic capsules. One important clinical difference is that *Enterobacter* species have an inducible chromosomal cephalosporinase. This enzyme renders the organisms resistant not only to first-generation cephalosporins but also to many second- and third-generation cephalosporins after high-level induction of *Enterobacter* in the presence of these antibiotics. Such resistance may not be detected in the microbiology laboratory on initial testing and may become apparent only in vitro when the organism is again isolated from patients who fail to respond to therapy.

DIAGNOSIS

As with infections caused by *Klebsiella*, infections caused by *Enterobacter* and *Serratia* do not have distinguishing clinical features and are diagnosed by culture of the organism from a normally sterile site or from a nonsterile site in a patient with associated signs or symptoms.

TREATMENT

Second- and third-generation cephalosporins should be used cautiously in patients with serious *Enterobacter* infections, even if the isolate appears to be susceptible on initial testing.[56] When the organism is susceptible to alternative agents such as extended-spectrum penicillins or fluoroquinolones, their use may be advisable.

Acknowledgment

Figures 1 through 3 Seward Hung.

References

1. Whittam TS: Genetic variation and evolutionary processes in natural populations of *Escherichia coli. Escherichia coli* and *Salmonella*. Cellular and Molecular Biology Neidhardt FC, Ed. ASM Press, Washington, DC, 1996, p 2708

2. Pupo GM, Karaolis DK, Lan R, et al: Evolutionary relationships among pathogenic and nonpathogenic *Escherichia coli* strains inferred from multilocus enzyme electrophoresis and *mdh* sequence studies. Infect Immun 65:2685, 1997

3. Perna NT, Plunkett G 3rd, Burland V, et al: Genome sequence of enterohaemorrhagic *Escherichia coli* O157:H7. Nature 409:529, 2001

4. Nataro JP, Kaper JB: Diarrheagenic *Escherichia coli*. Clin Microbiol Rev 11:142, 1998

5. Zafriri D, Oron Y, Eisenstein BI, et al: Growth advantage and enhanced toxicity of *Escherichia coli* adherent to tissue culture cells due to restricted diffusion of products secreted by the cells. J Clin Invest 79:1210, 1987

6. DuPont HL, Ericsson CD: Prevention and treatment of traveler's diarrhea. N Engl J Med 328:1821, 1993

7. Petruccelli BP, Murphy GS, Sanchez JL, et al: Treatment of traveler's diarrhea with ciprofloxacin and loperamide. J Infect Dis 165:557, 1992

8. Donnenberg MS, Whittam TS: Pathogenesis and evolution of virulence in enteropathogenic and enterohemorrhagic *Escherichia coli*. J Clin Invest 107:539, 2001

9. Schroeder SA, Caldwell JR, Vernon TM, et al: A waterborne outbreak of gastroenteritis in adults associated with *Escherichia coli*. Lancet 1:737, 1968

10. Viljanen MK, Peltola T, Junnila SY, et al: Outbreak of diarrhoea due to *Escherichia coli* O111:B4 in schoolchildren and adults: association of Vi antigen-like reactivity. Lancet 336:831, 1990

11. Donnenberg MS: Enteropathogenic *Escherichia coli*. Infections of the Gastrointestinal Tract. Blaser MJ, Smith PD, Ravdin JI, et al, Eds. Raven Press, New York, 1995, p 709

12. Tarr PI: *Escherichia coli* O157:H7: clinical, diagnostic, and epidemiological aspects of human infection. Clin Infect Dis 20:1, 1995

13. Michino H, Araki K, Minami S, et al: Massive outbreak of *Escherichia coli* O157:H7 infection in schoolchildren in Sakai City, Japan, associated with consumption of white radish sprouts. Am J Epidemiol 150:787, 1999

14. Bell BP, Goldoft M, Griffin PM, et al: A multistate outbreak of *Escherichia coli* O157:H7–associated bloody diarrhea and hemolytic uremic syndrome from hamburgers: the Washington experience. JAMA 272:1349, 1994

15. Foodborne Diseases Active Surveillance Network 1996. MMWR Morb Mortal Wkly Rep 46:258, 1997

16. Griffin PM, Tauxe RV: The epidemiology of infections caused by *Escherichia coli* O157:H7, other enterohemorrhagic *E. coli*, and the associated hemolytic uremic syndrome. Epidemiol Rev 13:60, 1991

17. Outbreaks of *Escherichia coli* O157:H7 infections among children associated with farm visits—Pennsylvania and Washington, 2000. MMWR Morb Mortal Wkly Rep 50:293, 2001

18. Hilborn ED, Mermin JH, Mshar PA, et al: A multistate outbreak of *Escherichia coli* O157:H7 infections associated with consumption of mesclun lettuce. Arch Intern Med 159:1758, 1999

19. Boyce TG, Swerdlow DL, Griffin PM: *Escherichia coli* O157:H7 and the hemolytic-uremic syndrome. N Engl J Med 333:364, 1995

20. Tzipori S, Gunzer F, Donnenberg MS, et al: The role of the *eaeA* gene in diarrhea and neurological complications in a gnotobiotic piglet model of enterohemorrhagic *Escherichia coli* infection. Infect Immun 63:3621, 1995

21. O'Brien AD, Newland JW, Miller SF, et al: Shiga-like toxin-converting phages from *Escherichia coli* strains that cause hemorrhagic colitis or infantile diarrhea. Science 226:694, 1984

22. Sears CL, Kaper JB: Enteric bacterial toxins: mechanisms of action and linkage to intestinal secretion. Microbiol Rev 60:167, 1996

23. Griffin PM, Ostroff SM, Tauxe RV, et al: Illnesses associated with *Escherichia coli* O157:H7 infections: a broad clinical spectrum. Ann Intern Med 109:705, 1988

24. Bell BP, Griffin PM, Lozano P, et al: Predictors of hemolytic uremic syndrome in children during a large outbreak of *Escherichia coli* O157:H7 infections. Pediatrics 100:E12, 1997

25. Siegler RL, Pavia AT, Christofferson RD, et al: A 20-year population-based study of postdiarrheal hemolytic uremic syndrome in Utah. Pediatrics 94:35, 1994

26. Zhang X, McDaniel AD, Wolf LE, et al: Quinolone antibiotics induce Shiga toxin–encoding bacteriophages, toxin production, and death in mice. J Infect Dis 181:664, 2000

27. Wong CS, Jelacic S, Habeeb RL, et al: The risk of the hemolytic-uremic syndrome after antibiotic treatment of *Escherichia coli* O157:H7 infections. N Engl J Med 342:1930, 2000

28. Okeke IN, Lamikanra A, Czeczulin J, et al: Heterogeneous virulence of enteroaggregative *Escherichia coli* strains isolated from children in Southwest Nigeria. J Infect Dis 181:252, 2000

29. Czeczulin JR, Whittam TS, Henderson IR, et al: Phylogenetic analysis of enteroaggregative and diffusely adherent *Escherichia coli*. Infect Immun 67:2692, 1999

30. Bhan MK, Raj P, Levine MM, et al: Enteroaggregative *Escherichia coli* associated with persistent diarrhea in a cohort of rural children in India. J Infect Dis 159:1061, 1989

31. Huppertz HI, Rutkowski S, Aleksic S, et al: Acute and chronic diarrhoea and abdominal colic associated with enteroaggregative *Escherichia coli* in young children living in western Europe. Lancet 349: 1660, 1997

32. Polotsky Y, Nataro JP, Kotler D, et al: HEp-2 cell adherence patterns, serotyping, and DNA analysis of *Escherichia coli* isolates from eight patients with AIDS and chronic diarrhea. J Clin Microbiol 35: 1952,1997

33. Wanke CA, Mayer H, Weber R, et al: Enteroaggregative *Escherichia coli* as a potential cause of diarrheal disease in adults infected with human immunodeficiency virus. J Infect Dis 178:185, 1998

34. Steiner TS, Lima AA, Nataro JP, et al: Enteroaggregative *Escherichia coli* produce intestinal inflammation and growth impairment and cause interleukin-8 release from intestinal epithelial cells. J Infect Dis 177:88, 1998

35. Giron JA, Jones T, Millan-Velasco F, et al: Diffuse-adhering *Escherichia coli* (DAEC) as a putative cause of diarrhea in Mayan children in Mexico. J Infect Dis 163:507, 1991

36. Gunzburg ST, Chang BJ, Elliott SJ, et al: Diffuse and enteroaggregative patterns of adherence of enteric *Escherichia coli* isolated from aboriginal children from the Kimberley region of Western Australia. J Infect Dis 167:755, 1993

37. Wanke CA, Gerrior J, Blais V, et al: Successful treatment of diarrheal disease associated with enteroaggregative *Escherichia coli* in adults infected with human immunodeficiency virus. J Infect Dis 178: 1369, 1998

38. Stamm WE, Hooton TM, Johnson JR, et al: Urinary tract infections: from pathogenesis to treatment. J Infect Dis 159:400, 1989

39. Langermann S, Mollby R, Burlein JE, et al: Vaccination with FimH adhesin protects cynomolgus monkeys from colonization and infection by uropathogenic *Escherichia coli*. J Infect Dis 181:774, 2000

40. Swenson DL, Bukanov NO, Berg DE, et al: Two pathogenicity islands in uropathogenic *Escherichia coli* J96: cosmid cloning and sample sequencing. Infect Immun 64:3736, 1996

41. Kao JS, Stucker DM, Warren JW, et al: Pathogenicity island sequences of pyelonephritogenic *Escherichia coli* CFT073 are associated with virulent uropathogenic strains. Infect Immun 65:2812, 1997

42. Bahrani-Mougeot FK, Pancholi S, Daoust M, et al: Identification of putative urovirulence genes by subtractive cloning. J Infect Dis 183(suppl 1):S21, 2001

43. Zhang L, Foxman B, Manning SD, et al: Molecular epidemiologic approaches to urinary tract infection gene discovery in uropathogenic *Escherichia coli*. Infect Immun 68:2009, 2000

44. Russo TA, Johnson JR: Proposal for a new inclusive designation for extraintestinal pathogenic isolates of *Escherichia coli*: ExPEC. J Infect Dis 181:1753, 2000

45. Talan DA, Stamm WE, Hooton TM, et al: Comparison of ciprofloxacin (7 days) and trimethoprim-sulfamethoxazole (14 days) for acute uncomplicated pyelonephritis in women: a randomized trial. JAMA 283:1583, 2000

46. Wiener J, Quinn JP, Bradford PA, et al: Multiple antibiotic-resistant *Klebsiella* and *Escherichia coli* in nursing homes. JAMA 281:517, 1999

47. Johnson DE, Russell RG, Lockatell CV, et al: Contribution of *Proteus mirabilis* urease to persistence, urolithiasis, and acute pyelonephritis in a mouse model of ascending urinary tract infection. Infect Immun 61: 2748, 1993

48. Mobley HLT: Virulence of *Proteus mirabilis*. Urinary Tract Infections: Molecular Pathogenesis and Clinical Management. Mobley HLT, Warren JW, Eds. ASM Press, Washington, DC, 1996, p 245

49. Fairley KF, Carson NE, Gutch RC, et al: Site of infection in acute urinary-tract infection in general practice. Lancet 2:615, 1971

50. Sahly H, Podschun R, Ullmann U: *Klebsiella* infections in the immunocompromised host. Adv Exp Med Biol 479:237, 2000

51. Carpenter JL: *Klebsiella* pulmonary infections: occurrence at one medical center and review. Rev Infect Dis 12:672, 1990

52. Garcia de la Torre M, Romero-Vivas J, Martinez-Beltran J, et al: *Klebsiella* bacteremia: an analysis of 100 episodes. Rev Infect Dis 7:143, 1985

53. Geerdes HF, Ziegler D, Lode H, et al: Septicemia in 980 patients at a university hospital in Berlin: prospective studies during 4 selected years between 1979 and 1989. Clin Infect Dis 15:991, 1992

54. Jarvis WR, Munn VP, Highsmith AK, et al: The epidemiology of nosocomial infections caused by *Klebsiella pneumoniae*. Infect Control 6: 68, 1985

55. Mills J, Drew D: *Serratia marcescens* endocarditis: a regional illness associated with intravenous drug abuse. Ann Intern Med 84:29, 1976

56. Chow JW, Fine MJ, Shlaes DM, et al: *Enterobacter* bacteremia: clinical features and emergence of antibiotic resistance during therapy. Ann Intern Med 115:585, 1991

57. Bieber D, Ramer SW, Wu CY, et al: Type IV pili, transient bacterial aggregates, and virulence of enteropathogenic *Escherichia coli*. Science 280:2114, 1998

20 Infections Due to the Enteric Pathogens *Campylobacter, Salmonella, Shigella, Yersinia, Vibrio,* and *Helicobacter*

Marcia B. Goldberg, M.D.

In the United States, diarrhea is the third most common medical complaint, with an annual incidence of 1.5 to 5.0 illnesses per person. Rates of occurrence are highest in children, followed by the elderly. Worldwide, diarrhea is the second most common cause of death for all age groups and the leading cause of death in children.

The most common bacterial causes of diarrhea in the United States are gram-negative bacteria. *Campylobacter* species are the most common infectious organisms (46%), followed by *Salmonella* (28%), *Shigella* (17%), and *Escherichia coli* O157 (5%) [*see Figure 1*].[1]

Campylobacter Infections

EPIDEMIOLOGY

Campylobacter organisms are the most common cause of bacterial gastroenteritis in the United States, with 2.1 to 2.4 million cases estimated to occur each year.[2] This disease is most common in children. The incidence of *Campylobacter* enteritis is as much as 39-fold higher in HIV-infected persons than in the general population[3]; recurrent infection and infection with antibiotic-resistant strains are also more common.[4,5]

Campylobacter infection is acquired by ingestion of contaminated foodstuffs in 80% of cases. Exposure to infected dogs, unpasteurized milk, contaminated unchlorinated water, and infected persons has also been reported to spread the organism. Improper handling of uncooked chicken and consumption of undercooked chicken are the most common food-related causes. The infectious inoculum is only approximately 800 organisms[6]; therefore, secondary infection occurs in as many as two thirds of household contacts. Neonates born to infected mothers are at extremely high risk for infection, which can be life threatening.

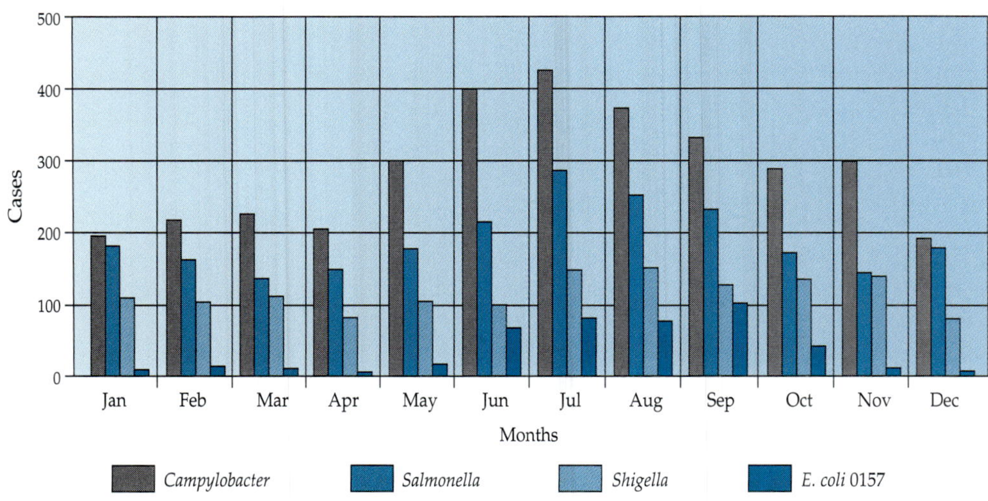

Figure 1 **Cases of gastroenteritis caused by *Campylobacter, Salmonella, Shigella,* and *E. coli* O157 reported to the Collaborating Sites Foodborne Disease Active Surveillance Network (CDC/USDA/FDA), 1996.**[1]

C. jejuni is the most common cause of *Campylobacter* enteritis. Other species of *Campylobacter*, particularly *C. coli* and *C. upsaliensis* (for which dogs are the normal host), are common causes of enteritis in AIDS patients. *C. fetus* is the predominant cause of systemic infection. Two thirds of patients with systemic *Campylobacter* infection are males. Many are in their middle 50s; more than 25% are farm workers, butchers, or abattoir workers; and most have a major underlying illness, such as alcoholism, cirrhosis, diabetes, lymphoproliferative disorder, or valvular or atherosclerotic heart disease.

PATHOGENESIS

Campylobacter enteritis is thought to involve bacterial invasion of intestinal epithelial cells,[7] as does *Salmonella* or *Shigella* enteritis. Intestinal lesions are similar to those of granulomatous or idiopathic ulcerative colitis. The pathogenesis of systemic *Campylobacter* infection is poorly understood. Genetic techniques have been developed that will allow molecular characterization of the pathogenesis of *Campylobacter* infection.[8,9]*C. jejuni* infection may be complicated by Guillain-Barré syndrome. In such cases, antibodies to ganglioside GM1 and other peripheral nerve gangliosides are frequently detected. The lipopolysaccharide from *C. jejuni* isolates displays molecular mimicry with several gangliosides, which suggests that the neurologic syndrome is caused by autoimmune recognition of gangliosides induced by exposure to the *C. jejuni* lipopolysaccharide.

DIAGNOSIS

Clinical Manifestations

The incubation period for *Campylobacter* enteritis is usually 2 to 4 days. Illness typically begins with crampy periumbilical pain and fever, which is followed by diarrhea with profuse, watery, foul-smelling stools. Abdominal pain can range from mild to severe, mimicking acute appendicitis, bowel perforation, or intussusception. Stool is grossly bloody or melanotic in 30% of patients and guaiac positive in 60%.

Patients with *Campylobacter* bacteremia present with symptoms common to many bacteremias: fever, malaise, headache, chills, night sweats, anorexia, and abdominal pain. Lethargy and confusion may occur without focal neurologic findings. A nonproductive cough may be present in the absence of focal pulmonary findings. Endocarditis may occur in 10% of patients. Meningitis is uncommon, although neonates are at extremely high risk.

Physical Examination

Physical findings in both *Campylobacter* enteritis and systemic *Campylobacter* infection are nonspecific.

Laboratory Tests

In *Campylobacter* enteritis, stool examination may reveal the diagnosis in as many as two thirds of cases. In fresh stool, *Campylobacter* organisms are small, motile, comma- or corkscrew-shaped; in Gram stains, they may be gull winged, curved, gram-negative organisms. Leukocytes are present in the stool in about 75% of cases.

Campylobacter organisms do not grow on standard media used in the detection of enteric pathogens but, rather, require specific media and specific environmental conditions.[10] If a stool sample cannot be delivered to a laboratory quickly, storage of the sample in an airtight container at 4° C or inoculation of transport medium (e.g., Cary-Blair) can improve the recovery of organisms.

Diagnosis of systemic *Campylobacter* infection is based on the isolation of the organism in blood cultures. *Campylobacter* organisms may grow slowly, so cultures should be incubated for 2 weeks or longer. In both systemic and intestinal infection, leukocytosis is common.

DIFFERENTIAL DIAGNOSIS

In the setting of acute onset of watery diarrhea, fever, and abdominal pain, *Campylobacter* infection should be considered. The differential diagnosis of diarrheal disease with polymorphonuclear leukocytes in the stool is enteritis caused by *Campylobacter, Salmonella, Shigella,* or *Yersinia enterocolitica* infection or by idiopathic ulcerative colitis. *Salmonella* and *Yersinia* infections are less likely when there is detectable blood in the stool. Systemic *Campylobacter* infection cannot be easily distinguished from other bacteremias.

TREATMENT

Campylobacter enteritis is usually self-limited, making specific therapy unnecessary. However, it may be prudent to administer antibiotics to patients with moderately severe disease (i.e., those with high fever, bloody diarrhea, or bacteremia or those who pass more than eight stools a day), immunosuppressed patients, pregnant women, or patients with symptoms that worsen or persist more than 7 days after diagnosis. Administration of antibiotics before laboratory confirmation of infection has been shown to reduce the median duration of symptoms from 10 days to 5 days.[11] However, empirical institution of antibiotics for diarrheal syndromes suggestive of enterohemorrhagic *E. coli* may increase the risk of hemolytic-uremic syndrome.[12]

Erythromycin is the treatment of choice for *Campylobacter* enteritis [*see Table 1*]. The newer macrolides, including azithromycin, and fluoroquinolones have also been used successfully [*see Table 1*]. However, resistance to fluoroquinolones is increasing rapidly worldwide; in 1998, approximately 10% of isolates in Minnesota were resistant to fluoroquinolones.[13] Moreover, strains resistant to both fluoroquinolones and macrolides have been isolated in Thailand. Fluid replacement should be administered as needed. On the basis of data for *Shigella* and *Salmonella* enteritis, antimotility agents such as Lomotil (diphenoxylate hydrochloride with atropine sulfate) should probably be avoided.

For systemic *Campylobacter* infection, imipenem or gentamicin, or a combination of the two, is the treatment of choice. Chloramphenicol, other aminoglycosides, and tetracyclines are also effective. Most isolates are resistant to penicillin, cephalosporins, vancomycin, and rifampin.

COMPLICATIONS

Postinfectious arthritis occurs in approximately 1% of patients, Guillain-Barré syndrome (or its variant, Miller Fisher syndrome) occurs in approximately 0.1%,[14] and hemolytic-uremic syndrome occurs rarely. Postinfectious arthritis presents as a sterile monoarticular or migratory polyarticular arthritis—particularly involving the knee—that begins 7 to 10 days after the onset of diarrhea and may persist for months or become chronic; 60% of patients carry the HLA-B27 haplotype, which is associated with an increased prevalence of ankylosing spondylitis and related spondyloarthropathies. In patients with Guillain-Barré syndrome, up to 40% have evidence of recent *Campylobacter* infection,[14] 20% are left with some long-term disability, and 5% die of the syndrome or its complications. Both postinfectious arthritis and Guillain-Barré syndrome are thought to be caused by autoimmune processes.

PROGNOSIS

Recurrence or relapse of *Campylobacter* infection may occur. Severe, persistent, or bacteremia-associated enteritis may occur in AIDS patients.

Salmonella Infections

EPIDEMIOLOGY

Disease caused by *Salmonella* organisms can be divided into two categories: typhoidal and nontyphoidal. *S. typhi* and *S. paratyphi* are the pathogens in typhoidal disease. Nontyphoidal disease results from all other serovars that infect humans. In the United States, nontyphoidal *Salmonella* organisms, most commonly *S. typhimurium* and *S. enteritidis*, are the second most frequently isolated cause of bacterial diarrhea (approximately 1.4 million cases annually).[15]

More than 95% of nontyphoidal *Salmonella* infections are food-borne; the remainder are nosocomial infections or are acquired from pets (reptiles and birds); from infected persons; or from contaminated water, drugs, or solutions. Outbreaks have been linked to eggs, cheese, fresh fruits and vegetables, juice, dry cereal, and ice cream premix.[16] *Salmonella* organisms can be passed transovarially from chicken to egg, and most *S. enteritidis* cases are traced to undercooked eggs.[16] *Salmonella* organisms are commonly carried by farm animals, and antibiotic resistance, particularly of *S. typhimurium*, has been linked to the use of antibiotics in animal feed.[17]

In the United States, *S. typhi* and *S. paratyphi* cause fewer than 1,000 cases of infection annually, more than 70% of which are acquired abroad.[15] Humans are the only host of these pathogens, and spread is person-to-person or via contaminated foodstuffs or water.

The inoculum for *Salmonella* infection is approximately 10^5 to 10^9 organisms but is lower in infants, in persons with pernicious anemia, and in persons taking antacids or H_2 receptor blockers. Additional risk factors are old age, alteration of the endogenous bowel flora (e.g., by recent antimicrobial therapy), HIV infection, therapeutic immunosuppression, alteration of the reticuloendothelial system (e.g., malaria or *Bartonella* infection), sickle-cell disease, splenectomy, diabetes, malignancy, and rheumatologic disorders, including lupus. HIV-infected persons have a 20- to 100-fold increased risk of *Salmonella* infection and a significantly increased risk of severe invasive disease.

Classification of *Salmonella* organisms is confusing because disease may be caused by more than 2,500 serovars, all of which belong to a single species, designated *S. enterica* and *S. choleraesuis*. However, in clinical settings, serovars are commonly referred to as species (e.g., *S. enterica* serovar *enteritidis* is called *S. enteritidis)*, as will be done herein.

PATHOGENESIS

Salmonella organisms are internalized by intestinal M cells, which are specialized epithelial cells that overlie Peyer patches and are enriched in the ileum. Organisms are transported to the lymphoid tissue of the Peyer patches, from which they may enter the systemic circulation. *Salmonella* organ-

Helicobacter	Proton-pump inhibitor (omeprazole [Prilosec] or lansoprazole [Prevacid]) *or* Ranitidine bismuth citrate (Tritec) *plus* Two of the following: Amoxicillin Clarithromycin (Biaxin) Metronidazole (Flagyl)	Omeprazole 20 mg or lansoprazole 30 mg p.o. twice a day for 14 days 400 mg p.o. twice a day for 14 days 1 g p.o. twice a day 500 mg p.o. twice a day 500 mg p.o. twice a day for 14 days	Suggested therapy	100.00–149.99/mo 90.00–99.99/mo 100.00–149.99/mo 0.25–0.49/day 7.00–7.99/day 0.50–0.74/day	Triple-therapy combination[50]; for resistant *H. pylori*, ranitidine bismuth citrate may be slightly better than proton-pump inhibitor; metronidazole may cause nausea, metallic taste, headaches, or disulfiram-like reaction (avoid alcohol)
	Proton-pump inhibitor (omeprazole [Prilosec] or lansoprazole [Prevacid]) *plus* Tetracycline *plus* Bismuth subsalicylate (Pepto-Bismol) *plus* Metronidazole (Flagyl)	Omeprazole 20 mg or lansoprazole 30 mg p.o. twice a day for 14 days 500 mg p.o. four times a day for 14 days 525 mg p.o. four times a day for 14 days 500 mg p.o. three times a day for 14 days	Suggested therapy	100.00–149.99/mo 90.00–99.99/mo 0.10–0.24/day 3.00–3.99/day 0.50–0.74/day	Quadruple-therapy combination[50]; metronidazole may cause nausea, metallic taste, headaches, or disulfiram-like reaction (avoid alcohol)
	Proton-pump inhibitor (omeprazole [Prilosec] or lansoprazole [Prevacid]) *plus* Tetracycline *plus* Bismuth subsalicylate (Pepto-Bismol) *plus* Furazolidone (Furoxone)	Omeprazole 20 mg or lansoprazole 30 mg p.o. twice a day for 14 days 500 mg p.o. four times a day for 14 days 525 mg p.o. four times a day for 14 days 500 mg p.o. three times a day for 14 days	For patients who have failed combination therapies listed above	100.00–149.99/mo 90.00–99.99/mo 0.10–0.24/day 3.00–3.99/day —	Quadruple-salvage-therapy combination[50]; furazolidone, a monoamine oxidase inhibitor, may cause nausea, vomiting, headache, tachycardia, and elevated blood pressure; must consider potential interactions with other medications and foods

isms have specialized mechanisms for survival inside of macrophages. Recruitment of inflammatory cells, including macrophages, into the Peyer patches may lead to their enlargement and necrosis after several weeks of infection. *Salmonella* organisms are also able to induce internalization into and transit across nonspecialized intestinal epithelial cells into deeper tissues.

Salmonella serovars vary in their pathogenesis. *S. anatum*, *S. derby*, and *S. newport* are usually limited to the intestine. *S. choleraesuis* rapidly enters the bloodstream and causes little damage in the intestine. *S. typhi* bacteremia often leads to seeding of the liver and biliary tree.

GASTROENTERITIS

Diagnosis

Clinical manifestations The incubation period for gastroenteritis caused by *Salmonella* organisms typically ranges from 6 to 72 hours. Symptoms of the disorder include nausea, vomiting, fever, diarrhea, and abdominal cramps. Stools are typically loose, of moderate volume, and do not contain blood. In rare cases, the presentation may mimic appendicitis or inflammatory bowel disease. Diarrhea is generally self-limited, lasting 3 to 7 days.

Physical examination Physical findings are nonspecific. Fever with temperatures to 39° C (102° F) for 1 to 2 days, mild abdominal tenderness, and hyperactive bowel sounds may be present. A more prolonged or more hectic fever pattern suggests bacteremia, metastatic foci, or both.

Laboratory tests Microscopic examination of stool reveals leukocytes and, rarely, red blood cells. *Salmonella* organisms are readily cultured from stool on selective media used routinely in clinical microbiology laboratories. Isolation of *Salmonella* organisms from otherwise sterile body fluids is also accomplished using routine media. The mean duration of fecal carriage after resolution of diarrhea for nontyphoidal *Salmonella* organisms is 1 month in adults and 7 weeks in young children.[18]

Differential Diagnosis

The presentation of *Salmonella* gastroenteritis is similar to that of other febrile diarrheal syndromes, including infection caused by *Campylobacter* organisms, infection caused by *Shigella* organisms, infection caused by *Y. enterocolitica*, and inflammatory bowel disease. Frankly bloody diarrhea is more suggestive of *Shigella* or enterohemorrhagic *E. coli* infection than of *Salmonella* infection.

Treatment

Antibiotics are not recommended for patients with uncomplicated gastroenteritis, because the illness is generally self-limited, and antibiotic therapy may prolong intestinal carriage.[19]

Antibiotics should be administered to patients who are severely ill or at risk for extraintestinal spread of infection, including infants; persons older than 50 years; and patients with cardiac valvular or mural abnormalities, patients with prosthetic vascular grafts, or patients who are receiving immunosuppressive therapy. Effective therapeutic agents include fluoroquinolones, trimethoprim-sulfamethoxazole, ampicillin, and third-generation cephalosporins. Because resistance to trimethoprim-sulfamethoxazole or ampicillin is common, treatment with a fluoroquinolone or a third-generation cephalosporin is appropriate when susceptibilities of the isolate are not known. Duration of therapy should be only 48 to 72 hours or until the patient becomes afebrile; longer therapy may increase the likelihood of long-term carriage.

Complications

Infants are at high risk for central nervous system infection. In some patients, *Salmonella* organisms invade the intestinal epithelium and enter the bloodstream, causing septicemia. Septicemia may in turn cause metastatic infection of other organs, including endovascular sites, the hepatobiliary tract, the spleen, bone, and, less commonly, the brain.

CARRIER STATE

The carrier state, defined as carriage of *Salmonella* organisms in the stool for more than 1 year after initial infection, occurs in 0.2% to 0.6% of persons infected with nontyphoidal *Salmonella* and 3% of persons infected with *S. typhi*.[20] The site of chronic infection is the biliary tree. The presence of stones or chronic scarring makes eradication more difficult. Long-term carriage may occur more rarely in the urinary tract, particularly in the setting of obstructive uropathy, tuberculosis, or schistosomiasis.

Diagnosis

Clinical manifestations The carrier state is generally asymptomatic. If the carrier state is accompanied by obstructive uropathy or gallstones, symptoms associated with that syndrome may be present.

Physical examination The physical examination of a patient in the carrier state is unremarkable.

Laboratory tests The carrier state is documented by culture of *Salmonella* organisms utilizing routine techniques.

Treatment

Ampicillin or amoxicillin [*see Table 1*] will eradicate the *Salmonella* organisms in 80% of persons in the carrier state. Alternative therapy is trimethoprim-sulfamethoxazole or ciprofloxacin [*see Table 1*]. Long-term gallbladder carriage can be effectively eliminated by cholecystectomy accompanied by 10 to 14 days of any of the regimens recommended for treatment of bacteremia. However, this approach should be reserved for individuals in whom eradication is required for public health reasons (e.g., food handlers and health care workers).

BACTEREMIA AND VASCULAR INFECTION

Nontyphoidal *Salmonella* organisms have a propensity to colonize sites of vascular abnormality, such as prosthetic vascular grafts, atherosclerotic plaques, and aneurysms.[21] The presence of high-grade bacteremia (more than 50% of three or more blood cultures are positive) is suggestive of endovascular infection.

Diagnosis

Clinical manifestations Patients with endovascular infection typically have high fevers that persist even after several days of therapy.

Physical examination The physical examination may reveal tenderness at the site of the infection, but it may also yield normal results.

Laboratory tests High-grade bacteremia (i.e., more than 50% of three or more blood cultures are positive) is suggestive of endovascular infection. Echocardiography and other imaging studies should be conducted to search for endovascular lesions.

Treatment

Life-threatening bacteremia, endovascular infection, or focal metastatic infection should be empirically treated with both a fluoroquinolone and a third-generation cephalosporin until antibiotic susceptibilities are known. For documented or suspected endovascular infection, 6 weeks of I.V. therapy with a β-lactam antibiotic, such as ampicillin or a cephalosporin, should be administered. For low-grade bacteremia, 7 to 14 days of I.V. therapy is adequate. Endovascular infection may require surgical intervention. However, in cases in which surgical resection of infected grafts is not feasible, lifelong oral suppressive therapy has been successful.[22]

In patients with AIDS, a first episode of *Salmonella* bacteremia should be treated with 7 to 14 days of I.V. antibiotics, followed by 4 weeks of an oral fluoroquinolone. AIDS patients who experience relapses of *Salmonella* bacteremia should be treated with an oral fluoroquinolone or trimethoprim-sulfamethoxazole for long-term suppression.

ENTERIC FEVER

Diagnosis

Clinical manifestations The incubation period for organisms that cause enteric fever ranges from 5 to 21 days. Initially, diarrhea or constipation may develop, followed by fever and then by headache, malaise, anorexia, myalgias, arthralgia, cough, and sore throat.[23] Approximately 1 week later, systemic toxemia, neuropsychiatric manifestations (psychosis and confusion), coryza, cough, sore throat, chest pain, and nausea and vomiting with or without abdominal pain may occur. Symptoms resolve spontaneously after 2 to 4 weeks.

Physical examination Results of the physical examination vary depending on the phase of the illness. During the toxemic phase of the illness, the patient's condition is acute. In 50% of patients, splenomegaly and hepatomegaly are present. In 30% of patients, rose spots (2 to 4 mm, slightly raised, discrete, irregular, blanching pink macules) appear on the anterior chest in crops of 5 to 15. The spots last 3 to 4 days and fade without a scar.

Laboratory tests The probability of culturing the organism from various sites varies during the course of illness [*see Table 2*].[24] Cultures of bone marrow and punch biopsies of rose spots may be positive when other cultures are negative, particularly during or after antibiotic therapy. Leukopenia, anemia, and moderately elevated liver function test results and muscle enzyme levels are common. Leukocytosis, transient thrombocytopenia, and clotting abnormalities are less common.

Differential Diagnosis

Enteric fever may be confused with other systemic febrile illnesses.

Treatment

Enteric fever can be successfully treated with ampicillin or amoxicillin, third-generation cephalosporins, fluoroquinolones, or trimethoprim-sul-

Table 2 Probability of Positive Cultures from Various Sites during Enteric Fever[24]

Phase of Illness (Time since Initial Exposure)	Disease Manifestations	Cultures				
		Blood	Stool	Urine	Bone Marrow	Rose Spots
Incubation period (0–1 wk)	Diarrhea in 10%–20%; constipation in some	Negative	Transiently positive	Negative	Negative	Negative
Active invasion (1–2 wk)	Fever, headache, malaise, anorexia, myalgia, arthralgia, cough, and sore throat	80%–90% positive	Negative	Negative	Negative	Negative
Established disease (2–4 wk)	Systemic toxemia, neuropsychiatric manifestations (psychosis and confusion), coryza, cough, sore throat, chest pain, nausea, vomiting, and abdominal pain	80%–90% positive	80% positive	25% positive	90% positive	60% positive
Convalescent period (4–5 wk)	—	Negative, except with ongoing disease or relapse	50% positive	10% positive	Decreasingly positive	Decreasingly positive
Late focal complications (> 5 wk)	Cholecystitis, osteomyelitis, soft tissue abscess	Negative, except with ongoing disease or relapse	Decreasingly positive	Decreasingly positive	—	—

famethoxazole [*see Table 1*]. However, given the prevalence of organisms resistant to ampicillin and third-generation cephalosporins among isolates from the Indian subcontinent, Southeast Asia, and Africa, therapy should consist of a fluoroquinolone or trimethoprim-sulfamethoxazole until antibiotic susceptibilities are known.[25] In cases of severe disease (associated shock, coma, stupor, obtundation, or delirium), dexamethasone [*see Table 1*] has been shown to improve survival,[26] although continuation of steroids beyond 48 hours may increase the rate of relapse.[27]

Several enteric fever vaccines are available [*see Table 3*]. Vaccination is recommended for individuals traveling to developing countries who will have prolonged exposure to contaminated food

Table 3 Vaccination for Enteric Fever

Vaccine	Dose	Relative Efficacy	Cost ($)	Comment
Ty21a (Vivotif Berna)	One enteric-coated capsule 1 hr before a meal every day for 4 days	43%–96%; not effective if administered with concomitant antimicrobial or antimalarial therapy	18.92	Live-attenuated vaccine; not recommended for immunosuppressed or children younger than 6 yr; boost every 5 yr; few side effects
Vi capsular polysaccharide [ViCPS] (Typhim Vi)	25 μg in 0.5 ml I.M. once	55% in one study[51]	30.21	Side effects: fever (1%), headache (1.5%–3%), local erythema or induration (7%); not recommended for children younger than 2 yr; boost every 2 yr
Heat-killed whole organism *Salmonella typhi*	0.5 ml I.M. for 2 doses administered more than 4 wk apart	51%–77%	9.39	Side effects: fever (17%–29%), severe headache (10%), pain at injection site (35%–60%), rare severe reactions; boost (0.1 ml) every 3 yr; dose for children 6 mo to 10 yr of age is 0.25 ml

and drink. Vaccination is an adjunct and not a replacement for careful eating and drinking.

Complications

Nonmetastatic complications, which include pneumonia (5% of cases), intestinal hemorrhage (3% to 20% of cases), intestinal perforation (2% to 3% of cases), acute cholecystitis (2% of cases), and myocarditis (1% to 2% of cases), often occur 2 to 4 weeks after the initial onset of symptoms. Less commonly, endocarditis, pericarditis, orchitis, and splenic or liver abscesses may occur. In the setting of intestinal perforation, repeat blood cultures should be drawn, and antibiotics should be broadened to cover anaerobic and aerobic bowel flora.

Shigella Infections

EPIDEMIOLOGY

Shigella organisms are estimated to cause 450,000 cases of diarrhea annually in the United States,[15] and they are an important cause of diarrhea and death worldwide.[28] *Shigella* includes four species: *S. dysenteriae, S. sonnei, S. boydii,* and *S. flexneri.* In industrialized countries, *S. sonnei* is currently most common, and *S. flexneri* accounts for essentially all other cases. In developing countries, *S. dysenteriae* is also common. Humans are the only natural host of *Shigella* organisms, and they are spread by fecal-oral contact or, in 20% of cases, through contaminated food or water.

The infectious inoculum is as few as 10 to 100 organisms.[29] Consequently, outbreaks spread readily and recurrences are common in day care centers, mental institutions, and other crowded settings. Disease is most common among young children, and secondary infection rates in families are as high as 20%.

PATHOGENESIS

Initially, *Shigella* organisms colonize the proximal small bowel, where secretion of an enterotoxin probably causes the initial symptoms. The organisms then pass into the colon, where they invade and spread through the epithelial layer. *Shigella* organisms induce the release of proinflammatory cytokines. Bacterial spread, in conjunction with the intense acute inflammatory response, leads to the formation of ulcerations and microabscesses in the colonic epithelium. *Shigella* organisms rarely gain access to the bloodstream or infect deeper tissues. The toxin Stx (formerly called Shiga toxin) is present only in *S. dysenteriae* and contributes to the more severe diarrhea that can accompany *S. dysenteriae* infection. Related enterotoxins are produced by members of all *Shigella* species.

DIAGNOSIS

Clinical Manifestations

The incubation period for *Shigella* organisms is typically 3 days, with a range of 1 to 7 days. Initial symptoms usually include fever, abdominal cramps, and watery diarrhea, which are followed by abdominal cramps, tenesmus, rectal urgency, and small-volume diarrhea. Diarrhea during this later stage is frequent (eight to 10 episodes a day), and stools may be bloody with mucus. If left untreated, disease is generally self-limited, lasting 7 days or less.

Physical Examination

Physical findings are nonspecific. Patients may appear toxic and have a high temperature (up to 41° C [106° F]). Abdominal tenderness, particularly in the left lower quadrant, and hyperactive bowel sounds are common.

Laboratory Tests

Stool cultures are usually positive during the acute illness. Later, *Shigella* organisms may be isolated by direct culture of material from rectal ulcerations. Direct microscopic examination of stool stained with methylene blue (or another stain) is extremely important because the presence of abundant leukocytes in the proper clinical setting is strongly suggestive of shigellosis. In *Salmonella* enteritis, *Campylobacter* enteritis, and idiopathic ulcerative colitis, leukocytes may also be present in the stool. The white blood cell count may be elevated with an increase in the percentage of immature forms, and metabolic abnormalities may be present.

DIFFERENTIAL DIAGNOSIS

In the setting of high fever, tenesmus, rectal urgency, and diarrhea with blood- and mucus-containing stools, *Shigella* infection should be suspected. However, *Shigella* infection can resemble any febrile diarrheal syndrome, including those caused by *Campylobacter, Y. enterocolitica,* and *Salmonella* organisms and by inflammatory bowel disease.

TREATMENT

For patients with significant dehydration, particularly young children and the elderly, oral and, if necessary, intravenous rehydration should be administered. Antibiotics are not essential, but administration of an antibiotic to which the organism is susceptible has been shown to shorten the course of clinical illness and the period of fecal excretion.[30,31] Given the ease of person-to-person *Shigella* transmission, many experts recommend that all individuals with documented infection be treated for public health reasons. For *Shigella* infection acquired in the United States with an unknown antibiotic susceptibility pattern, the treatment of choice is trimethoprim-sulfamethoxazole [*see Table 1*] because ampicillin resistance is common. The alternative therapy or therapy for trimethoprim-resistant isolates is norfloxacin, ciprofloxacin, or ofloxacin [*see Table 1*]. For *Shigella* acquired in Southeast Asia, Africa, the Middle East, Japan, South America, Spain, or Canada, the treatment of choice is a fluoroquinolone, because resistance to trimethoprim-sulfamethoxazole is common [*see Table 1*]. Azithromycin has also been used successfully. Cephalosporins have limited efficacy.

COMPLICATIONS

Complications are generally rare but include intestinal obstruction in the setting of severe colonic disease (2.5% of cases), bacteremia (4% of cases), colonic perforation (1.7% of fatal cases), and toxic megacolon (3% of *S. dysenteriae* infections). Proctitis and rectal prolapse (in children) also occur as complications. Metabolic disturbances are relatively common, although severe dehydration is uncommon because stool volume is generally low. Seizures occur in approximately 5% of infected children, generally in the setting of high fever and metabolic abnormalities.[32]

Reactive arthritis may occur 1 to 2 weeks after diarrhea, either alone or accompanied by conjunctivitis and urethritis (Reiter syndrome); 70% of these patients have the HLA-B27 haplotype. Although most commonly caused by enterohemorrhagic *E. coli* infection, hemolytic-uremic syndrome may occur after *Shigella* infection. Hemolytic-uremic syndrome is associated with infection caused by *S. dysenteriae* and is thought to be mediated by Stx.

PROGNOSIS

Prognosis is generally excellent. Settings that predispose to recurrence of disease are those with suboptimal hygiene, such as day care centers or crowded living conditions.

Yersinia Infections

EPIDEMIOLOGY

All three *Yersinia* species, *Y. enterocolitica, Y. pseudotuberculosis,* and *Y. pestis,* are pathogenic for humans. *Y. enterocolitica* and *Y. pseudotuberculosis* are widely distributed in nature and cause a variety of zoonoses. In the United States, *Y. enterocolitica* is estimated to cause approximately 100,000 cases of diarrhea annually,[15] predominantly in children. *Y. pseudotuberculosis* is a sporadic cause of purulent mesenteric adenitis.

Transmission of *Y. enterocolitica* is usually by ingestion of contaminated foodstuffs, including meat, milk and other dairy products, mussels, tofu, and oysters. Person-to-person transmission has also been reported, with a significant rate of secondary cases within families.[33] Transfusion of *Y. enterocolitica*-contaminated red blood cells has been a cause of severe transfusion reactions with high mortality.[34] Among the approximately 60 serogroups of *Y. enterocolitica,* three (O:3, O:8, and O:9) cause most human disease. Individuals with underlying cirrhosis or hemochromatosis, particularly if being treated with desferrioxamine, are at increased risk for bacteremia and metastatic disease.

PATHOGENESIS

Y. enterocolitica and *Y. pseudotuberculosis* transit the stomach, invade the mucosa of the terminal ileum at Peyer patches, and colonize mesenteric lymph nodes. *Yersinia* organisms are able to both replicate intracellularly and bind to macrophages and inhibit phagocytosis. The inflammatory response that ensues in the terminal ileum may be clinically mistaken for appendicitis or Crohn ileitis.

DIAGNOSIS

Clinical Manifestations

In older children and adults, *Y. enterocolitica* causes a febrile diarrheal syndrome in which the prominent symptom is colicky abdominal pain, predominantly localized to the right lower quadrant. In younger children, the illness may include vomiting and bloody diarrhea. Exudative pharyngitis has also been reported.[35] Septicemia, which occurs in individuals with iron overload or other chronic diseases, is often complicated by metastatic abscesses formation. *Y. pseudotuberculosis* causes mesenteric adenitis, which mimics acute appendicitis, with fever and right lower quadrant pain.

Physical Examination

On physical examination, patients with *Yersinia* infection are typically found to have fever and right lower quadrant tenderness.

Laboratory Tests

Leukocytosis is common. Microscopic examination of the stool will reveal fecal leukocytes.

Whereas isolation of *Yersinia* organisms from normally sterile body fluids is straightforward, isolation from stool is difficult because the organisms appear similar to and grow more slowly than other Enterobacteriaceae organisms; selective media for *Yersinia* organisms have not been developed. *Yersinia* serology, which turns positive 1 to 2 weeks after infection, may be useful in the setting of one of the autoimmune syndromes that may complicate infection. *Y. enterocolitica* is carried in the stool for an average of 1 month after the resolution of symptoms.

DIFFERENTIAL DIAGNOSIS

The differential diagnosis of diarrheal disease with polymorphonuclear leukocytes in the stool is enteritis caused by infection with *Campylobacter, Salmonella, Shigella,* or *Y. enterocolitica* or caused by idiopathic ulcerative colitis. Mesenteric adenitis caused by *Yersinia* infection may mimic appendicitis.

TREATMENT

Enteritis and mesenteric adenitis caused by *Y. enterocolitica* or *Y. pseudotuberculosis* are generally self-limited, and no clear role for antibiotic therapy has been established. Although direct proof is lacking, in principle, antiperistaltic agents should be avoided.

Septicemia caused by either *Y. enterocolitica* or *Y. pseudotuberculosis* should be aggressively treated with antibiotics because mortality is high. The suggested agents for treatment of *Y. enterocolitica* septicemia are gentamicin, doxycycline, trimethoprim-sulfamethoxazole, or a fluoroquinolone, alone or in combination [*see Table 1*].[36] *Y. enterocolitica* organisms produce a β-lactamase and are therefore resistant to penicillins and cephalosporins. The suggested agents for treatment of *Y. pseudotuberculosis* septicemia are ampicillin, streptomycin, and tetracycline [*see Table 1*]. For either *Y. enterocolitica* or *Y. pseudotuberculosis*, enteric precautions should be adopted.

COMPLICATIONS

Either reactive polyarthritis or erythema nodosum complicates 1% to 5% of *Y. enterocolitica* infections in adults in the United States and 10% to 30% of such infections in Scandinavia. On occasion, *Y. pseudotuberculosis* infections in adults are also complicated by reactive polyarthritis or erythema nodosum. These disorders may be the presenting complaint. Therefore, in individuals with such complaints, *Yersinia* infection should be considered and serology and cultures should be performed. These complications of *Yersinia* infections rarely occur in young children.

Reactive polyarthritis develops 2 days to 1 month after the onset of gastrointestinal symptoms. It persists for more than a month in two thirds of patients and for more than 4 months in one third of patients. Knees, ankles, toes, fingers, and wrists may be involved. Synovial fluid usually contains fewer than 25,000 white blood cells/ml, with a preponderance of polymorphonuclear leukocytes and negative cultures. The disorder may be particularly severe in individuals with the HLA-B27 haplotype, presenting as full-blown ankylosing spondylitis or as Reiter syndrome.

Erythema nodosum develops 2 to 20 days after the onset of gastrointestinal symptoms. It typically resolves spontaneously within a month and is twice as common in women than in men. Skin lesions are usually on the legs and trunk.

PROGNOSIS

The prognosis for *Y. enterocolitica* enteritis is excellent. In contrast, *Y. enterocolitica* septicemia is fatal in 50% of cases and *Y. pseudotuberculosis* septicemia is fatal in 75% of cases, despite appropriate antimicrobial therapy.

Vibrio Infections

CHOLERA

Epidemiology

The natural reservoir of *V. cholerae* is aquatic invertebrates in brackish or marine environments. Certain strains have become pathogenic for humans and have caused seven pandemics throughout history, the most recent of which began in Asia in 1961. There are 139 serotypes of *V. cholerae,* defined by the O surface antigen. Initially, the seventh pandemic was caused by an O1 strain of biotype El Tor, but in 1992, a new strain emerged from the pandemic strain that carried a new O antigen, which was designated O139. The emergence of the new strain was concurrent with rapid spread of cholera through Latin America and Africa. Currently, the continuing pandemic is caused by two strains, O139 and an O1 strain that differs from the initial O1 strain and likely emerged from the O139 strain.[37]

Spread of cholera is primarily through ingestion of fecally contaminated water and food, especially, but not exclusively, seafood. Only about 50 cases of cholera are estimated to occur in the United States annually,[15] predominantly in persons who acquire it while traveling in endemic areas. The rate of secondary infection in households is very high, suggesting that person-to-person transmission is occurring. Because *V. cholerae* is sensitive to gastric acid, the infectious inoculum in normal hosts is 10^{10} organisms, but in persons taking antacids or who have achlorhydria, the inoculum may be 10^6 organisms or fewer. Natural immunity to cholera is long lasting, with specificity to the O1 antigen. Thus, in endemic areas, disease is most common in children, but nonimmune adults traveling in the region are susceptible. Furthermore, alteration of the O antigen, as seen with the shift from O1 to O139 in 1992, leads to widespread susceptibility in adults.

Pathogenesis

V. cholerae colonize the proximal small intestine and secrete one major and at least two minor enterotoxins. The major toxin, cholera toxin (CTX), binds the ganglioside GM1 on the intestinal epithelium and activates adenylate cyclase, which in turn leads to the accumulation of cyclic adenosine monophosphate (cAMP). Increased levels of cAMP cause chloride secretion and inhibit sodium absorption, resulting in the characteristic profuse isotonic watery diarrhea.

V. cholerae does not invade intestinal tissue, and there is no tissue inflammatory response. Absorptive processes unaffected by cAMP, including glucose-facilitated salt and water absorption, are unaltered, allowing oral rehydration with glucose-electrolyte solutions.

Diagnosis

Clinical manifestations The hallmark of cholera is massive watery diarrhea consisting of thin, gray-brown, mucus-containing fluid (so-called rice-water stools). The diarrhea begins a few days after initial exposure to *V. cholerae* and is soon followed by copious vomiting without retching. Notably absent are fever (which occurs in only 5% of cases), abdominal pain, tenesmus, and strain. Muscle cramps may occur as a result of electrolyte shifts. Dehydration ranges from mild to severe. A rare variant in the presentation is so-called cholera sicca, in which abdominal ileus and distention occur, and diarrhea is absent. If left untreated, symptoms of cholera resolve in 1 to 7 days.

Physical examination Patients appear anxious and restless, with sunken eyes, dry mucous membranes, poor skin turgor, hyperactive bowel sounds, hypotension, and tachycardia. Obtundation may occur with severe dehydration. As much as 1 L/hr of fluid may be excreted in stools.

Laboratory tests Microscopic examination of Gram stains of stool reveals the small (1 to 3 µm long), comma-shaped, gram-negative organisms. *V. cholerae* grow well on a variety of selective media; TCBS (thiosulfate-citrate-bile salt-sucrose) agar is commonly used.

In patients with moderate-to-severe dehydration, packed cell volume, serum specific gravity, and total protein levels are elevated. In patients with severe disease, prerenal azotemia, metabolic acidosis with an elevated anion gap, normal to low serum potassium levels, normal to slightly low serum sodium and chloride levels, and leukocytosis are seen.

Differential Diagnosis

In patients with severe dehydration, cholera resembles little else. In patients with mild to moderate dehydration, the presentation is similar to that of enterotoxigenic *E. coli* (ETEC) or rotavirus.

Treatment

The cornerstone of management is prompt replacement of lost fluid and electrolytes. Replacement fluid and electrolytes should be administered intravenously for patients with severe dehydration, patients with moderate dehydration who do not tolerate oral intake, and patients who are purging large amounts of fluid (10 to 20 ml/kg/hr). Initially, replacement fluid should consist of lactated Ringer solution or a solution containing 5 g NaCl, 4 g $NaHCO_3$, and 1 g KCl for each liter of sterile distilled water. The goal is to return the patient to normal hydration status within 4 hours, which, in severely dehydrated persons, may require administration of fluids at 50 to 100 ml/kg/hr. Once rehydration has been accomplished, as determined by hemodynamic status and urine production, normal hydration status should be maintained by replacement of continuing losses of fluid. For those patients with mild disease, rehydration can be accomplished by oral administration of a glucose-electrolyte solution that consists of 20 g glucose, 3.5 g NaCl, 2.5 g $NaHCO_3$, and 1.5 g KCl for each liter of water.

Antibiotics are an adjunct to rehydration therapy; they can reduce the duration of symptoms and infection, as well as the overall fluid requirements. Tetracycline is the drug of choice [*see Table 1*]. Tetracycline-resistant isolates have been identified in Latin America, Bangladesh, and Tanzania; appropriate therapy for these isolates is ciprofloxacin, erythromycin, or trimethoprim-sulfamethoxazole. The only cholera vaccine (Wyeth Laboratories) commercially available in the United States provides protection in only 30% to 50% of cases and has a high rate of side effects.[38] In general, the vaccine should be administered only if required for entry into a foreign country.

Complications and Prognosis

Acute renal failure has complicated cholera in patients with severe dehydration who did not receive proper rehydration. In patients with severe dehydration who receive no treatment, mortality is about 50%.

OTHER INFECTIONS CAUSED BY *VIBRIO* SPECIES

In the United States, other *Vibrio* species are estimated to cause approximately 8,000 cases of disease annually.[15] These species include *V. parahaemolyticus, V. vulnificus,* and nontoxigenic strains of *V. cholerae.*

V. parahaemolyticus

V. parahaemolyticus is a common cause of diarrhea in the Chesapeake Bay area, the Gulf Coast region, and the Pacific Northwest. The organism is ubiquitous in coastal waters and is typically acquired by ingestion of raw or undercooked shellfish. Clinical illness most commonly consists of explosive watery diarrhea, crampy abdominal pain, and low-grade fever. Wound infections and septicemia also occur. The organism can be cultured from stool on selective media such as TCBS and from sterile body fluids in routine blood culture media or on blood agar plates. The illness is self-limited, lasting less than 7 days. Antibiotic treatment has not been shown to shorten the course of the illness, although if administered, tetracycline is probably the best choice because of its documented efficacy against *V. cholerae.*

V. vulnificus

V. vulnificus, an important cause of serious disease, can be isolated from waters of the eastern and western coasts of the United States, as far north as Cape Cod and the northern Pacific coast,[39] particularly during the summer months. In compromised persons, particularly those with chronic liver disease or iron-overload states but also other immunosuppressed persons, *V. vulnificus* can cause an overwhelming sepsis, accompanied by metastatic cutaneous lesions in the form of hemorrhagic bullae or vesicles that evolve into necrotic ulcers. This syndrome with bacteremia is fatal in over 50% of cases. More than 90% of patients have consumed raw oysters within a week of the onset of illness. Therapy consists of adequate debridement and parenteral antibiotics. Tetracycline is probably the drug of choice; either cefotaxime or ciprofloxacin is an alternative. Animal studies suggest that the combination of tetracycline and cefotaxime may be better than either drug alone.[40]

In both immunocompromised and healthy hosts, *V. vulnificus* can cause a second syndrome—a rapidly progressive cellulitis, fasciitis, or myositis that follows infection of a superficial wound, typically after cleaning shellfish. In addition to antimicrobials, incision and drainage with debridement are often necessary.

Non-O1 V. cholerae

Strains of *V. cholerae* (non-O1 *V. cholerae*) that do not produce cholera toxin can cause an acute febrile gastroenteritis. Non-O1 *V. cholerae* are distributed worldwide in saltwater and freshwater. Exposure is generally by ingestion of raw shellfish, particularly oysters. Diarrhea can range from mild to severe. Usually, no treatment is necessary, but in severe disease, rehydration and tetracycline are recommended.

Helicobacter Infections

EPIDEMIOLOGY

Helicobacter pylori is directly linked to the development of duodenal ulcer, gastric ulcer disease, and gastritis and to the long-term complications of gastric adenocarcinoma and gastric mucosa–associated lymphoid tissue (MALT) lymphoma. The organism is believed to be the cause of peptic ulcer disease in 90% of individuals with duodenal ulcers and in 70% to 90% of individuals with gastric ulcers. Cure of the infection significantly decreases the risk of long-term malignant complications.[41] Whether *H. pylori* also plays a role in peptic ulcer disease in the setting of nonsteroidal anti-inflammatory drug usage is less clear.

H. pylori infection is the most common long-term bacterial infection worldwide, with higher prevalence in developing countries than in industrialized countries. In the United States, the prevalence is 10% for persons 18 to 30 years of age, 30% to 45% for persons 30 to 60 years of age, and 50% for persons older than 60 years.[42,43] The prevalence is severalfold higher in African Americans and Hispanics than in non-Hispanic whites,[44] which is likely a reflection of the impact of socioeconomic status and living conditions on transmission as

Table 4 Sensitivity and Specificity of Tests for *Helicobacter pylori* Infection[52,53]

Test	Sensitivity (%)		Specificity (%)	
	Before Treatment*	After Treatment†	Before Treatment*	After Treatment†
UBT	95.3	88.5	97.7	99.4
HpSA	94.3	92.3	91.8	96.2
ELISA	> 90	Not useful	> 90	Not useful

*N = 501.
†N = 133.
ELISA—enzyme-linked immunosorbent assay HpSA—*H. pylori* stool antigen UBT—13C-urea breath test

well as possibly an indication of a minor role of hereditary susceptibility.

Evidence suggests that transmission occurs from person to person by the fecal-oral or oral-oral route.[45] Humans appear to be the major reservoir, although the organism has also been isolated from other primates and domestic cats. A second *Helicobacter species, H. heilmanii,* has been observed in the stomachs of humans,[46] but whether it has a role in the pathogenesis of gastric disease is unknown.

PATHOGENESIS

H. pylori organisms colonize the gastric mucus and adhere to gastric epithelial cells. They survive the acidic environment of the stomach by surrounding themselves with pH-buffering ammonia that is produced from hydrolysis of urea by a bacterial urease. *H. pylori* induces autocrine stimulation and proinflammatory cytokine release, causing alterations in acid secretion and acute and chronic inflammation that, in turn, potentiate the disease process and contribute to the development of the malignant complications of infection. The exact mechanisms are not fully understood, although a cluster of genes known as the *cag* pathogenicity island appears to be involved.

DIAGNOSIS

Clinical Manifestations

Acute *H. pylori* infection produces symptoms of gastroenteritis in up to 60% of patients, including nausea, vomiting, epigastric pain, and fever. Symptoms last 3 to 14 days. A period of hypochlorhydria begins a few weeks after clinical symptoms resolve and lasts 2 to 8 months. Hypochlorhydria is associated with gastritis, which causes the symptoms that frequently bring patients to medical attention.

Physical Examination

During the acute gastroenteritis syndrome, physical findings are nonspecific. Epigastric tenderness and fever may be present. Long-term findings are those of gastritis or peptic ulcer disease.

Laboratory Tests

Three of the more useful diagnostic tests in the initial diagnosis of *H. pylori* infection are (1) the carbon-13 (^{13}C) urea breath test (UBT), (2) the stool antigen test (HpSA), and (3) the enzyme-linked immunosorbent assay (ELISA) serology test [*see Table 4*]. The UBT and HpSA are noninvasive. The UBT does not pose a significant radiation exposure risk and is therefore safe for pregnant women and children. Because proton-pump inhibitors reduce the load of *H. pylori,* they should be stopped 2 weeks before either the UBT or the HpSA is performed.

DIFFERENTIAL DIAGNOSIS

The differential diagnosis of the acute gastroenteritis syndrome caused by *H. pylori* includes other causes of acute small intestinal infection, including toxin-induced gastroenteritis caused by *Clostridium perfringens, Bacillus cereus, Staphylococcus aureus,* ETEC, giardiasis, and viral gastroenteritis.

TREATMENT

Given the potential serious long-term complications of *H. pylori* infection, any individual who has documented infection should be treated. Recommended treatment regimens all consist of combinations of antibiotics and antisecretory agents or a bismuth formulation [*see Table 1*]. For duodenal ulcer disease caused by antibiotic-susceptible *H. pylori,* success rates range from 95% to 99%. Success rates may be lower in patients without duodenal ulcer disease. Success rates have been shown to be reduced by treatment with two agents rather than three or four; shortening of the course of therapy from 14 days to 10 or 7 days; or lowering of the dose of metronidazole from 500 mg to 250 mg. The combination of clarithromycin and metronidazole may be more successful than the combination of clarithromycin and ampicillin, although rigorous comparisons have not yet been performed.

Cure should be confirmed in all treated patients. The optimal tests for confirmation are the UBT and the HpSA [*see Table 4*] because serum antibody levels will remain elevated for at least 9 months. To ensure that any residual organisms have had the chance to multiply to detectable levels, UBT or HpSA should be delayed until at least 4 weeks after the course of therapy is completed, and proton-pump inhibitors should be stopped 2 weeks before the test. H_2 receptor antagonists can be continued until the day of testing because they have no effect on *H. pylori*.

Resistance to clarithromycin currently occurs in 11% of isolates in the United States and is an increasing problem. Resistance to metronidazole has also been reported; however, the combination of 500 mg of metronidazole with ampicillin or clarithromycin and a proton-pump inhibitor is effective even in the setting of metronidazole resistance.

Although information about the antibiotic susceptibility of the infecting strain is always useful, isolation of *H. pylori* is not trivial, requiring endoscopy and biopsy. Therefore, it is reasonable to treat suspected *H. pylori* infection empirically and obtain antibiotic susceptibility tests only if the initial therapy fails. In general, if a 14-day course of combination therapy fails, the possibility of resistance should be considered. Moreover, if the failed course of therapy included metronidazole and clarithromycin, antibiotic susceptibilities should be determined. Particular antibiotic combinations should not be repeated unless in vitro susceptibility is demonstrated.

COMPLICATIONS

H. pylori infection is probably the cause of the majority of MALT lymphomas. More than 90% of individuals with MALT lymphoma have evidence of *H. pylori* infection, and eradication of the infection during the premalignant phase leads to cure of the lymphomatous process.[47,48]

H. pylori gastritis can progress to chronic atrophic gastritis, which is thought to be a precursor for gastric adenocarcinoma. A prospective study of 1,526 patients in Japan who had duodenal ulcers, gastric ulcers, gastric hyperplasia, or nonulcer dyspepsia showed that gastric cancer developed in patients infected with *H. pylori*, but not in uninfected patients.[49] Treatment of *H. pylori* infection may reduce the risk of adenocarcinoma. However, gastric adenocarcinoma will develop in only a minority of patients with *H. pylori* gastritis, and some gastric adenocarcinomas occur in patients without evidence of prior *H. pylori* infection.

PROGNOSIS

In follow-up to a course of combination therapy, infection is again detected in a small but significant percentage of cases. Presence of *H. pylori* organisms usually represents recurrence rather than reinfection because most isolates are identical to the original isolate. If standard combination therapies fail, antibiotic susceptibility testing of the isolate and salvage therapy should be considered [*see Table 1*].

References

1. Altekruse SF, Stern NJ, Fields PI, et al: *Campylobacter jejuni*—an emerging foodborne pathogen. Emerging Infect Dis 5:28, 1999
2. Tauxe RV: Epidemiology of *Campylobacter jejuni* infections in the United States and other industrialized nations. Campylobacter, 2nd ed. Nachamkin I, Blaser MJ, Eds. American Society for Microbiology, Washington, DC, 2000, p 9
3. Sorvillo FJ, Lieb LE, Waterman SH: Incidence of campylobacteriosis among patients with AIDS in Los Angeles County. J Acquir Immune Defic Syndr 4:598, 1991
4. Perlman DM, Ampel NM, Schifman RB, et al: Persistent *Campylobacter jejuni* infections in patients infected with the human immunodeficiency virus (HIV). Ann Intern Med 108:540, 1988
5. Angulo FJ, Swerdlow DL: Bacterial enteric infections in persons infected with human immunodeficiency virus. Clin Infect Dis 21(suppl 1):S84, 1995
6. Black RE, Levine MM, Clements ML, et al: Experimental *Campylobacter jejuni* infection in humans. J Infect Dis 157:472, 1988
7. Rivera-Amill V, Kim BJ, Seshu J, et al: Secretion of the virulence-associated *Campylobacter* invasion antigens from *Campylobacter jejuni* requires a stimulatory signal. J Infect Dis 183:1607, 2001
8. Hendrixson DR, Akerley BJ, DiRita VJ: Transposon mutagenesis of *Campylobacter jejuni* identifies a bipartite energy taxis system required for motility. Mol Microbiol 40:214, 2001
9. Colegio OR, Griffin TJ 4th, Grindley ND, et al: In vitro transposition system for efficient generation of random mutants of *Campylobacter jejuni*. J Bacteriol 183:2384, 2001
10. Allos BM: *Campylobacter jejuni* infections: update on emerging issues and trends. Clin Infect Dis 32:1201, 2001
11. Salazar-Lindo E, Sack RB, Chea-Woo E, et al: Early treatment with erythromycin of *Campylobacter jejuni*–associated dysentery in children. J Pediatr 109:355, 1986
12. Wong C, Jelacic S, Habeeb R, et al: The risk of the hemolytic-uremic syndrome after antibiotic treatment of *Escherichia coli* O157:H7 infections. N Engl J Med 342:1930, 2000
13. Smith KE, Besser JM, Hedberg CW, et al: Quinolone-resistant *Campylobacter jejuni* infections in Minnesota, 1992–1998. N Engl J Med 340: 1525, 1999
14. Allos BM: Association between *Campylobacter* infection and Guillain-Barre syndrome. J Infect Dis 176:S125, 1997
15. Mead PS, Slutsker L, Dietz V, et al: Food-related illness and death in the United States. Emerging Infect Dis 5:607, 1999
16. Hohmann EL: Nontyphoidal salmonellosis. Clin Infect Dis 32:263, 2001
17. Rabsch W, Tschape H, Baumler AJ: Non-typhoidal salmonellosis: emerging problems. Microbes Infect 3:237, 2001
18. Buchwald D, Blaser M: A review of human salmonellosis: II. Duration of excretion following infection with non-typhi *Salmonella*. Rev Infect Dis 6:345, 1984
19. Neill MA, Opal SM, Heelan J, et al: Failure of ciprofloxacin to eradicate convalescent fecal excretion after acute salmonellosis: experience during an outbreak in health care workers. Ann Intern Med 114: 195, 1991

20. Pegues DA, Hohmann EL, Miller SI: *Salmonella* including *S. typhi*. Infections of the Gastrointestinal Tract. Blaser MJ, Smith PD, Ravdin JI, et al, Eds. Raven Press, New York, 1995, p 785

21. Benenson S, Raveh D, Schlesinger Y, et al: The risk of vascular infection in adult patients with nontyphi *Salmonella* bacteremia. Am J Med 110:60, 2001

22. Donabedian H: *Salmonella* aortitis [letter]. Clin Infect Dis 22:739, 1996

23. Butler T, Islam A, Kabir I, et al: Patterns of morbidity and mortality in typhoid fever dependent on age and gender: review of 552 hospitalized patients with diarrhea. Rev Infect Dis 13:85, 1991

24. Goldberg MB, Rubin RH: The spectrum of *Salmonella* infection. Infect Dis Clin North Am 2:571, 1988

25. Rowe B, Ward LR, Threlfall EJ: Multidrug-resistant *Salmonella typhi*: a worldwide epidemic. Clin Infect Dis 24(suppl 1):S106, 1997

26. Punjabi NH, Pulungsih SP, Woodward TE: Treatment of severe typhoid fever in children with high dose dexamethasone. Pediatr Infect Dis J 7:598, 1988

27. Cooles P: Adjuvant steroids and relapse of typhoid fever. J Trop Med Hyg 89:229, 1986

28. Kotloff KL, Winickoff JP, Ivanoff B, et al: Global burden of *Shigella* infections: implications for vaccine development and implementation of control strategies. Bull WHO 77:651, 1999

29. DuPont HL, Levine MM, Hornick RB, et al: Inoculum size in shigellosis and implications for expected mode of transmission. J Infect Dis 159:1126, 1989

30. Islam MR, Alam AN, Hussain MS, et al: Effect of antimicrobial (nalidixic acid) therapy in shigellosis and predictive values of outcome variables in patients susceptible or resistant to it. Trop Med Hyg 98:212, 1995

31. Haltalin KC, Nelson JD, Ring R 3rd, et al: Double-blind treatment study of shigellosis comparing ampicillin, sulfadiazine, and placebo. J Pediatr 70:970, 1967

32. Khan WA, Dhar U, Salam MA, et al: Central nervous system manifestations of childhood shigellosis: prevalence, risk factors, and outcome. Pediatrics 103:488, 1999

33. Lee LA, Taylor J, Carter GP, et al: *Yersinia enterocolitica* O:3: an emerging cause of pediatric gastroenteritis in the United States. J Infect Dis 163:660, 1991

34. From the Centers for Disease Control and Prevention: Red blood cell transfusions contaminated with *Yersinia enterocolitica*—United States, 1991–1996, and initiation of a national study to detect bacteria-associated transfusion reactions. JAMA 278:196, 1997

35. Adamkiewicz TV, Berkovitch M, Krishnan C, et al: Infection due to *Yersinia enterocolitica* in a series of patients with β-thalassemia: incidence and predisposing factors. Clin Infect Dis 27:1362, 1998

36. Crowe M, Ashford K, Ispahani P: Clinical features and antibiotic treatment of septic arthritis and osteomyelitis due to *Yersinia enterocolitica*. J Med Microbiol 45:302, 1996

37. Reeves PR, Lan R: Cholera in the 1990s. Br Med Bull 54:611, 1998

38. Ryan ET, Calderwood SB: Cholera vaccines. Clin Infect Dis 31:561, 2000

39. Strom MS, Paranjpye RN: Epidemiology and pathogenesis of *Vibrio vulnificus*. Microb Infect 2:177, 2000

40. Chuang YC, Ko WC, Wang ST, et al: Minocycline and cefotaxime in the treatment of experimental murine *Vibrio vulnificus* infection. Antimicrob Agents Chemother 42:1319, 1998

41. Cohen H: Peptic ulcer and *Helicobacter pylori*. Gastroenterol Clin North Am 29:775, 2000

42. Pounder RE, Ng D: The prevalence of *Helicobacter pylori* infection in different countries. Aliment Pharmacol Ther 9(suppl 2):33, 1995

43. Dooley CP, Cohen H, Fitzgibbons PL, et al: Prevalence of *Helicobacter pylori* infection and histologic gastritis in asymptomatic persons. N Engl J Med 321:1562, 1989

44. Staat MA, Kruszon-Moran D, McQuillan GM, et al: A population-based serologic survey of *Helicobacter pylori* infection in children and adolescents in the United States. J Infect Dis 174:1120, 1996

45. Perez-Perez GI, Taylor DN, Bodhidatta L, et al: Seroprevalence of *Helicobacter pylori* infections in Thailand. J Infect Dis 161:1237, 1990

46. Svec A, Kordas P, Pavlis Z, et al: High prevalence of *Helicobacter heilmannii*–associated gastritis in a small, predominantly rural area: further evidence in support of a zoonosis? Scand J Gastroenterol 35:925, 2000

47. Wotherspoon AC, Doglioni C, Diss TC, et al: Regression of primary low-grade B-cell gastric lymphoma of mucosa-associated lymphoid tissue type after eradication of *Helicobacter pylori*. Lancet 342:575, 1993

48. Roggero E, Zucca E, Pinotti G, et al: Eradicaton of *Helicobacter pylori* infection in primary low-grade gastric lymphoma of mucosa-associated lymphoid tissue. Ann Intern Med 122:767, 1995

49. Uemura N, Okamoto S, Yamamoto S, et al: *Helicobacter pylor* infection and the development of gastric cancer. N Engl J Med 345:784, 2001

50. Shiotani A, Nurgalieva ZZ, Yamaoka Y, et al: *Helicobacter pylori*. Med Clin North Am 84:1125, 2000

51. Klugman KP, Koornhof HJ, Robbins JB, et al: Immunogenicity, efficacy, and serological correlate of protection of *Salmonella typhi* Vi capsular polysaccharide vaccine three years after immunization. Vaccine 14: 435, 1996

52. Vaira D, Malfertheiner P, Megraud F, et al: Diagnosis of *Helicobacter pylori* infection using a novel, noninvasive antigen based assay in a European multicentre study. Lancet 354:30, 1999

53. Vaira D, Malfertheiner P, Megraud F, et al: Noninvasive antigen-based assay for assessing *Helicobacter pylori* eradication: a European multicenter study. The European *Helicobacter pylori* HpSA Study Group. Am J Gastroenterol 95:925, 2000

21 Infections Due to *Haemophilus, Moraxella, Legionella, Bordetella,* and *Pseudomonas*

Shawn J. Skerrett, M.D.

Haemophilus, Moraxella, Legionella, Bordetella, and *Pseudomonas* are gram-negative bacteria that are important respiratory pathogens. All can also cause other types of infections. Vaccines have markedly reduced the incidence of disease from *Haemophilus* and *Bordetella,* but these organisms remain sources of morbidity and potentially life-threatening infection.

Haemophilus influenzae Infections

In 1892, the German bacteriologist Richard Pfeiffer made the sensational claim that he had identified the etiologic agent of influenza.[1] He had repeatedly observed a bacillus in purulent sputum obtained from influenza victims and found that this organism could be cultured on media supplemented with blood. Pfeiffer's blood-loving bacillus was named *Haemophilus influenzae*.[1] Although the causative link with influenza proved false, *H. influenzae* was subsequently recognized as the leading cause of meningitis in young children and an important agent of respiratory infections.

H. influenzae occurs in encapsulated and unencapsulated forms.[2] Encapsulated strains express one of six antigenically distinct capsular polysaccharides, designated *a* through *f*. The type b strain was responsible for most invasive *Haemophilus* infections before the widespread use of conjugate vaccines began in the 1980s. The other capsular groups are rarely implicated as pathogens. Unencapsulated strains do not react with antisera directed at the polysaccharide antigens and thus are nontypeable. These strains are common commensals but can cause mucosal and invasive infections.

EPIDEMIOLOGY

H. influenzae is strictly a human parasite: no nonhuman host is known, and *H. influenzae* is not found free in nature. Essentially all persons are colonized by one or more strains of *Haemophilus* by 1 year of age.[2] The primary reservoir for *H. influenzae* is the human upper respiratory tract, although the organism can also be carried on the conjunctivae and in the genital tract. Population studies have found that 40% to 80% of persons harbor unencapsulated strains of *H. influenzae* in the nasopharynx.[2,3] Type b strains were recovered from nasopharyngeal swabs of 2% to 4% of children before the widespread use of the conjugate vaccines, but now such strains are found in less than 1% of children in vaccinated populations. The specific strains colonizing a person's pharynx change over time, and multiple strains can be found concurrently.[2,3] Colonization of the normally sterile tracheobronchial tree with nontypeable strains of *H. influenzae* occurs commonly in people with chronic airway disease, such as cystic fibrosis, bronchiectasis, and chronic obstructive pulmonary disease (COPD), and in asymptomatic smokers.[2,4] In very young infants, nasopharyngeal colonization with *H. influenzae* is associated with an increased risk of otitis media.[2] Persistent colonization of the lower respiratory tract with *H. influenzae* is associated with increased airway inflammation[5] and may contribute to the progression of COPD.[4]

H. influenzae can be transmitted from person to person, leading to secondary cases of infection in households, day care centers, and institutions.[2] The risk of invasive *H. influenzae* infection is age related. The incidence is highest in children younger than 5 years, with a second peak late in life.[6] The distribution and burden of invasive *H. influenzae* infection have been dramatically altered by the use of conjugate vaccines directed against the type b capsular polysaccharide.[7] In unvaccinated populations, the incidence of infection peaks between 6 and 18 months of age, but in vaccinated populations, the risk is highest in the first 6 months of life, before the primary immunization series is completed. In the prevaccine era, there were approximately 20,000 cases a year of invasive *H. influenzae* infection in children younger than 5 years in the United States. Meningitis accounted for 60% of these cases, and 95% of the infections were caused by type b strains.[7] Now, fewer than 300 cases of invasive *H. influenzae* infection in children younger than 5 years are reported to the Centers for Disease Control and Prevention (CDC) each year, and less than a third of these are type b infections.[6] Conjugate vaccine usage has also reduced the overall incidence of invasive *H. influenzae* infection in older children and adults, although an increase in non–serotype b infections has been observed.[8] Most cases of invasive *H. influenzae* in the United States now occur in adults, with pneumonia being the most common type of infection.[6] Certain population groups remain at increased risk, including Native Americans, Alaskan Natives, and African Americans.[7] An increased risk of invasive *H. influenzae* type b infection is also observed in association with complement deficiencies, hypogammaglobulinemia, and splenic dysfunction. The incidence of *H. influenzae* pneumonia is increased in the settings of recent influenza, HIV infection, alcoholism, advanced age, and underlying COPD.

PATHOGENESIS AND IMMUNITY

All *Haemophilus* organisms are small, pleomorphic, nonmotile, gram-negative coccobacilli. They are facultative anaerobes with fastidious nutritional requirements. Aerobic growth of *H. influenzae* requires X and V factors, both of which are contained in red blood cells. X factor (hematin) is not a single nutrient but, rather, refers to several diffusable pigments that supply protoporphyrins. V factor is nicotinamide adenine dinucleotide, a coenzyme that is released by lysis of red cells. All species of *Haemophilus* grow well on chocolate agar, which contains red cells that have been disrupted by heating.

Unencapsulated strains of *H. influenzae* selectively colonize and locally invade the respiratory tract. *H. influenzae* binds to airway mucins but evades mechanical clearance by inhibiting ciliary beat frequency and damaging ciliated epithelium. The ciliotoxic properties of *H. influenzae* have been attributed to the lipid A, peptidoglycan, and lipoprotein components of the bacterial cell wall. Most strains of *H. influenzae* also produce a protease that cleaves both serum and secretory IgA, thus inactivating a major component of mucosal host defense.[2,3] *H. influenzae* attaches to respiratory epithelial cells with the aid of several adhesins, including pili, high-molecular-weight hemagglutinins, and other surface proteins.[3] *H. influenzae* preferentially binds to nonciliated cells and to epithelium damaged by recent viral infection or exposure to toxins such as cigarette smoke.[2,3] *H. influenzae* not only can attach to the surface of respiratory epithelium but can enter and survive in epithelial cells and mucosal macrophages and penetrate intercellular junctions to invade the submucosal interstitium.[4]

H. influenzae type b is less efficient at colonization than unencapsulated strains, but it has a much greater capacity to invade and survive within the bloodstream.

The magnitude and duration of bacteremia is a critical determinant in the development of *H. influenzae* meningitis, which results mainly from hematogenous seeding rather than direct spread from contiguous infection.[2] The type b capsule facilitates invasion by shielding the organism from complement- and antibody-mediated phagocytosis.[2] The lipo-oligosaccharide in the *H. influenzae* outer membrane is another important factor in the pathophysiology of invasive *H. influenzae* infection: its lipid A component has typical endotoxin activity and contributes to local and systemic inflammatory manifestations of infection, including septic shock.[3]

Antibodies constitute the principal defense against *H. influenzae* type b. These antibodies are directed against the bacteria's capsule, which is composed of repeating units of polyribosyl ribitol phosphate (PRP). Anticapsular antibodies facilitate ingestion of *H. influenzae* by phagocytes and mediate the complement-dependent bactericidal activity of immune serum. Antibodies specific for the PRP component of *H. influenzae* appear by 4 years of age and coincide with the age-related decline in susceptibility to invasive disease.[2] Host resistance to nontypeable strains of *H. influenzae* is less well understood but also involves humoral immunity.[2,3]

CLINICAL SYNDROMES

In the prevaccine era, *H. influenzae* type b was responsible for nearly all invasive *H. influenzae* infections in young children and approximately 50% of invasive infections in adults.[9–11] Meningitis accounted for more than half of the childhood cases of invasive *H. influenzae* type b infection, followed by pneumonia, epiglottitis, primary bacteremia, cellulitis, and musculoskeletal infections.[12] In adults, pneumonia has been the most common manifestation of invasive *H. influenzae* infection, followed by primary bacteremia, epiglottitis, meningitis, obstetric infections, and septic arthritis.[9–11] Widespread use of conjugate vaccines has dramatically reduced the overall incidence of invasive type b infections, but infections caused by nontypeable *H. influenzae* remain important in both children and adults. Unencapsulated strains of *H. influenzae* are principally associated with otitis media, sinusitis, bronchitis, and pneumonia but also can infect other sites.

Meningitis

H. influenzae type b is the leading cause of meningitis in children younger than 5 years in unvaccinated populations but has become rare in immunized communities.[7,12] In adults, *H. influenzae* (predominantly type b) accounts for approximately 4% of cases of community-acquired and nosocomial meningitis.[9,13,14] Adult cases often are associated with contiguous infection of the paranasal sinuses, mastoids, or middle ear or with antecedent head trauma.[13–15] Childhood cases, in contrast, result from bacteremic seeding and often follow an upper respiratory infection.

The clinical manifestations of *H. influenzae* meningitis in both children and adults are typical of acute bacterial meningitis.[9,15] Most patients present with fever, headache, and lethargy. The cerebrospinal fluid is usually cloudy, with a neutrophilic pleocytosis, increased protein concentration, and reduced glucose levels. The diagnosis is made by detecting *H. influenzae* in blood or CSF (see below). The clinical course may be fulminant, leading to death within 24 hours. The overall mortality of *H. influenzae* meningitis in young children is approximately 5%, but 20% to 30% of survivors suffer residual neurologic sequelae. Morbidity is reduced in children treated with dexamethasone.[16] The mortality in adult cases is 10% to 30%.

Epiglottitis

Epiglottitis is a life-threatening infection that is most prevalent in children 2 to 7 years of age but also occurs in older children and adults. *H. influenzae* type b is the most common cause of epiglottitis in all age groups, and the incidence of epiglottitis has declined since the availability of conjugate vaccines.[2,17]

The usual presenting symptoms of epiglottitis are sore throat, odynophagia, dyspnea, and fever; respiratory symptoms are more common in children than adults.[17] The onset of epiglottitis often is abrupt, and the progression can be very rapid. On examination, patients are anxious and may assume an airway-protective posture, sitting erect with the neck extended and the chin protruding forward. Drooling and a muffled voice are useful clues. Stridor, tachypnea, and use of accessory muscles to breathe are common findings in children. The diagnosis can be confirmed by laryngoscopy, with visualization of the cherry-red swollen epiglottis in children or the diffuse supraglottic edema more typical of adult cases. Laryngoscopy must be undertaken with care because the procedure may precipitate acute airway obstruction. A lateral neck x-ray also can be diagnostic, but the supine position should be avoided and patients with suspected epiglottitis should not travel to the radiology suite unless accompanied by a physician prepared to secure an airway. Blood cultures are positive in many cases.

An artificial airway (endotracheal intubation or tracheostomy) should be established emergently in all children with epiglottitis and in adults with evidence of airway compromise. All patients with epiglottitis should be admitted to the hospital for observation and treatment with parenteral antibiotics. Death can result from acute airway obstruction or from septic shock. The mortality is less than 5%.

Pneumonia

H. influenzae is the second or third most common cause of community-acquired pneumonia in adults, identified in 1% to 12% of hospitalized cases.[18] Most of the isolates in these cases are nontypeable strains.[19] In contrast, community-acquired *H. influenzae* pneumonia in children is caused mainly by type b and now is rare in vaccinated populations.[12]

In adults, the risk factors for *H. influenzae* pneumonia include COPD, advanced age, alcoholism, and HIV infection.[9,19,20] *H. influenzae* has also been identified as an important cause of nosocomial pneumonia in the first 5 days of hospitalization, before the indigenous flora of the upper respiratory tract have been replaced.[21]

H. influenzae pneumonia presents as a typical acute pneumonia, with fever, cough productive of purulent sputum, chest pain, and dyspnea.[9,19] Crackles and diminished breath sounds usually are evident on lung auscultation. The chest x-ray may reveal a bronchopneumonic pattern or focal consolidation, often multilobar. Pleural effusions are common. The diagnosis of *H. influenzae* pneumonia is made most often from the sputum Gram stain and culture, although the organism is frequently missed on sputum smears.[18] Blood cultures are positive in 20% to 30% of cases. Complications of *H. influenzae* pneumonia include empyema, purulent pericarditis, and metastatic infection. The reported mortality of *H. influenzae* pneumonia is 5% to 20%, but it is higher in patients with bacteremia or suppurative complications.

Tracheobronchitis

H. influenzae can cause tracheobronchitis in patients with underlying COPD and, more rarely, in immunocompromised patients.[4,19] The airways of patients with chronic lung disease are often colonized with nontypeable strains of *H. influenzae*, and infection with these organisms contributes to acute exacerbations of chronic bronchitis.[4] The clinical presentation is characterized by an increase in cough, purulent sputum production, and dyspnea. Fever and leukocytosis also may be present, but the chest film is clear. The sputum Gram stain shows abundant leukocytes, with a predominance of gram-negative coccobacilli.

Otitis Media and Sinusitis

Nontypeable strains of *H. influenzae* are isolated from 15% to 30% of purulent middle-ear effusions in both children and adults and are second in frequency to *Streptococcus pneumoniae* strains.[22] As with all cases of otitis media, infants typically present with fever and irritability and older children and adults complain primarily of ear pain. The clinical diagnosis is made by otoscopy. A bacteriologic diagnosis requires tympanocentesis; however, that is rarely indicated, because antibiotic therapy can be directed empirically at the common pathogens.

Nontypeable strains of *H. influenzae* can also be isolated from maxillary aspirates in approximately 25% of children and adults with acute sinusitis.[23] In addition to experiencing common cold symptoms such as rhinorrhea and cough, patients with sinusitis often have unilateral pain, purulent nasal discharge, and reduced transillumination. Confirmatory sinus x-rays and diagnostic aspiration are usually unnecessary.[23] Empirical management includes topical or systemic decongestants, or both, and antibiotics that are effective against *S. pneumoniae, H. influenzae,* and *Moraxella (Branhamella) catarrhalis.*

Extrapulmonary Infections

Cellulitis *H. influenzae* type b is an important cause of cellulitis in unvaccinated children younger than 5 years and is rarely implicated in skin infections of older persons.[9,12,24] The face is the most common site in young children. A raised, warm, tender area of erythema on the cheek or periorbital area is typical, sometimes with a distinctive bluish hue. Underlying sinusitis is common with periorbital and orbital infection. Blood cultures are often positive.

Bone and joint infections In the prevaccine era, *H. influenzae* type b caused approximately 10% of cases of septic arthritis and hematogenous osteomyelitis in infants and young children, but this is now uncommon.[25] Most cases of *H. influenzae* septic arthritis in children are monoarticular, involving large weight-bearing joints. A respiratory source of infection is usually evident. The diagnosis is established by arthrocentesis.

Rare cases of *H. influenzae* pyarthrosis have been described in adults.[9,26] About half of these cases are polyarticular, and most are in patients with alcoholism, immunodeficiency, joint disease, or trauma. Extra-articular sites of infection are apparent in 50% of patients. As in children, most adult cases of *H. influenzae* septic arthritis are caused by type b strains and accompanied by bacteremia.

Conjunctivitis Nontypeable strains of *H. influenzae* have long been appreciated as common causes of purulent conjunctivitis. These infections are contagious, and outbreaks can occur, particularly in day care centers.[2] *H. influenzae* conjunctivitis is easily diagnosed from stains and cultures of conjunctival swabs.

Robert Koch was the first to identify small gram-negative rods in conjunctival exudates collected in Egypt in 1883.[1] This organism was successfully cultured 3 years later by John Weeks, an American ophthalmologist. The Koch-Weeks bacillus, formerly named *Haemophilus aegyptius*, is now known to be a variant of *H. influenzae.* A particularly virulent strain of this organism has been responsible for outbreaks and sporadic cases of Brazilian purpuric fever in young children. This is a fulminant illness in which resolution of an episode of purulent conjunctivitis is followed by high fever, vomiting, abdominal pain, petechiae, purpura, peripheral necrosis, and vascular collapse.[2]

Bacteremia *H. influenzae* b bacteremia without localizing infection can occur in children younger than 5 years and in older persons with defective humoral immunity.[9,12] These patients can deteriorate rapidly, and in rare cases, the bacteremia resembles meningococcemia with purpura fulminans or the Waterhouse-Friderichsen syndrome.[24] Nontypeable strains of *H. influenzae* have also been implicated in neonatal and puerperal sepsis.[9,10,24]

Other infections *H. influenzae* is a rare cause of genitourinary infections, including salpingitis, endometritis, chorioamnionitis, epididymitis, and prostatitis.[10,24] Other rare manifestations of *H. influenzae* infection include appendicitis, cholecystitis, peritonitis, and endocarditis.[9,24]

MICROBIOLOGIC DIAGNOSIS

The diagnosis of invasive *H. influenzae* infection is generally made from positive cultures of blood, CSF, joint fluid, or other normally sterile sites. CSF and joint fluid Gram stains reveal bacteria in 70% to 80% of cases of meningitis and septic arthritis, respectively. However, the morphology of the organisms is often misleading: plump gram-negative rods, filamentous organisms, gram-negative diplococci, and underdecolorized gram-positive cocci have been described.[9,15,26] Similarly, sputum Gram stains of patients with tracheobronchitis or pneumonia usually show abundant leukocytes and the characteristic gram-negative coccobacilli, but misinterpretations are common.[18] The small gram-negative rods can be overlooked in the pink background on the slide or misinterpreted as gram-positive cocci if the specimen is poorly decolorized.

Type b capsular antigen can be detected by latex agglutination or enzyme-linked immunosorbent assay (ELISA) in CSF, serum, or concentrated urine in up to 90% of invasive infections. Antigen detection is particularly attractive in patients who have already received antibiotic therapy at the time of presentation, but the results rarely influence outcome, because cultures or Gram stains are diagnostic in nearly all antigen-positive cases.[27]

ANTIBIOTIC TREATMENT

The initial antibiotic of choice for meningitis and other invasive *H. influenzae* infections is a third-generation cephalosporin such as ceftriaxone or cefotaxime. These agents are highly active against all isolates of *H. influenzae*, penetrate the CSF, and eradicate nasopharyngeal carriage of *H. influenzae* type b. The pediatric dose of ceftriaxone is 50 mg/kg every 12 hours and that for cefotaxime is 50 mg/kg every 6 hours. For adults, the maximum dose of ceftriaxone is 2 g every 12 hours and that for cefotaxime is 2 g every 6 hours. The preferred alternative treatment for *H. influenzae* meningitis is chloramphenicol (75 to 100 mg/kg/day in six divided doses). Children with *H. influenzae* meningitis also should receive dexamethasone (0.6 mg/kg/day in four divided doses). Other antibiotics that are highly active against nearly all strains of *H. influenzae* include carbapenems, aztreonam, β-lactam/β-lactamase inhibitor combinations, fluoroquinolones, azithromycin, and tetracycline[28,29] [*see* Table 1].

Table 1 Antibiotics Effective against *Haemophilus influenzae* and *Moraxella catarrhalis*[50,51]

Antibiotic	H. influenzae *Susceptible (%)*	M. catarrhalis *Susceptible (%)*
Cefepime	100	100
Ceftriaxone	100	100
Cefotaxime	100	100
Cefixime	100	100
Cefpodoxime	100	99
Cefuroxime	95–99	99
Cefaclor	80–90	99
Ampicillin	60–65	< 10
Ampicillin-clavulanate	> 99	100
Fluoroquinolones	> 99	100
Azithromycin	> 99	100
Clarithromycin	60–90	100
Tetracycline	> 98	100
Chloramphenicol	> 99	100
Trimethoprim-sulfamethoxazole	77–88	> 99

Ampicillin is highly effective against sensitive strains, but 35% to 40% of North American isolates of *H. influenzae* are resistant to ampicillin. Most ampicillin resistance is mediated by β-lactamase production, but conventional susceptibility testing is recommended for invasive isolates to detect all resistant strains. Intravenous antibiotic therapy is recommended for meningitis and endocarditis and for the initial treatment of other invasive infections. Less severe *H. influenzae* infections can be managed with oral antibiotics. Most *H. influenzae* infections can be cured with 7 to 10 days of therapy, but treatment should continue for 3 to 6 weeks in cases of osteomyelitis or endocarditis.

PREVENTION

Immunization

The introduction of conjugate vaccines in the late 1980s has resulted in a greater than 97% reduction in the incidence of invasive *H. influenzae* type b infections in children younger than 5 years.[7,12] Currently, four conjugate vaccines are licensed in the United States.[30] All are composed of the PRP component of the *H. influenzae* type b capsule in covalent linkage with a carrier protein and elicit protective antibodies directed at PRP. Conjugate vaccines have succeeded the polysaccharide vaccines introduced in the 1970s; those earlier polysaccharide vaccines did not contain a carrier protein and were less effective.[12]

The vaccines are given in a primary series starting at 2 months of age, with the schedule depending on the product. A booster dose is given at 12 to 15 months of age. Immunocompromised children may require additional boosters.[30] Local reactions are experienced by about 25% of persons, but systemic reactions are rare. All of the vaccines are effective, but the PRP-OMP vaccine, which uses the outer membrane protein of *Neisseria meningitidis* as the carrier protein, elicits a stronger first-dose response and is recommended for immunization of high-risk infants such as Native Americans and Alaskan Natives.[30] Adults at high risk for invasive *H. influenzae* infection as a result of sickle cell disease, splenectomy, immunoglobulin or complement deficiency, B cell malignancy, or HIV infection should be considered for vaccination, but specific guidelines have not been developed.

Secondary Prevention

Chemoprophylaxis with rifampin (20 mg/kg/day; maximum, 600 mg a day for 4 days) is more than 95% effective in eliminating nasopharyngeal carriage of *H. influenzae* and is recommended to prevent secondary cases of invasive infection in children at risk. Rifampin prophylaxis should be administered to all adults and children in households with at least one member (other than the index case) who is younger than 4 years and is unimmunized or incompletely immunized.[30] Treatment should also be given to all contacts in households with at least one member younger than 1 year who has completed the primary series but has not yet received a booster dose. Chemoprophylaxis of children and supervisory adults in child care and nursery school settings is recommended if at least two cases of invasive disease have occurred in the attendees within 60 days and if incompletely immunized children are in attendance. Finally, rifampin should be given to victims of invasive disease if they were treated with ampicillin or chloramphenicol, which do not eradicate the carrier state.

Other *Haemophilus* Infections

There are now 15 recognized species of the genus *Haemophilus. H. parainfluenzae, H. aphrophilus*, and *H. paraphrophilus* can be found among the flora of the oral cavity and upper respiratory tract. These organisms are primarily commensals, but in rare cases, they cause endocarditis and respiratory tract infection. Endocarditis caused by *Haemophilus* species usually develops on a diseased valve, is typically subacute in onset, and is often complicated by major systemic emboli. Combination antibiotic therapy is generally curative, but valve replacement is frequently necessary. Non-*influenzae* species of *Haemophilus* have antimicrobial susceptibilities that are similar to *H. influenzae*, but they are less likely to be ampicillin resistant.[31]

Moraxella (*Branhamella*) *catarrhalis* Infections

M. catarrhalis was first described by the German microbiologist Seifert in 1882. Originally called *Micrococcus catarrhalis*, the organism was renamed *Neisseria catarrhalis* in 1920, then assigned to the new genus *Branhamella* in 1970, and subsequently reclassified as *Moraxella (Branhamella) catarrhalis*. Although recognized as a cause of tracheobronchitis and pneumonia by early investigators, *M. catarrhalis* was dismissed as a harmless commensal for much of the 20th century, until regaining stature as a potential pathogen over the past 25 years.[32]

EPIDEMIOLOGY

The distribution of *M. catarrhalis* is limited to the human respiratory tract, except for occasional isolates from the conjunctiva and genital tract. Nearly 80% of children harbor *M. catarrhalis* in the nasopharynx by 2 years of age, but colonization declines with age. Fewer than 6% of healthy adults carry *M. catarrhalis*, although the organism can be isolated from the sputum of 10% to 28% of patients with chronic bronchitis or bronchiectasis. Colonization is a dynamic process, with individual strains persisting for only a few months. Carriage of *M. catarrhalis* also exhibits seasonal variation, with colonization and infection being more prevalent in the winter months.[33]

M. catarrhalis is the third most common cause of otitis media, sinusitis, and acute exacerbations of chronic bronchitis, after *H. influenzae* and *S. pneumoniae*.[23,33] The majority of lower respiratory tract infections attributed to *M. catarrhalis* in adults occur in patients with underlying COPD.[33]

PATHOGENESIS

M. catarrhalis is a nonmotile, gram-negative diplococcus that is morphologically indistinguishable from *Neisseria* species. *M. catarrhalis* grows well aerobically on blood agar and chocolate agar. The characteristic convex, opaque colonies can be pushed across the agar surface in the manner of a hockey puck. Other species of *Moraxella* are predominantly gram-negative coccobacilli that can be found among the normal flora of humans and other mammals, but they rarely cause disease.

The virulence of *M. catarrhalis* is related to its capacity to colonize the respiratory mucosa. *M. catarrhalis* expresses a number of potential adhesins, but the mechanisms underlying the respiratory tropism of this organism are poorly understood.[33] Similarly, the factors that influence the transition from asymptomatic colonization to infection have not been deciphered. In the case of otitis media and sinusitis, it is likely that nasopharyngeal bacteria will gain access to adjacent spaces after mucosal injury. The expression of particular virulence factors also may be important in pathogenesis. For example, strains of *M. catarrhalis* isolated from symptomatic persons are more likely to exhibit resistance to the bactericidal activity of serum complement than strains harbored by asymptomatic carriers. Recovery from *M. catarrhalis* infection is accompanied by strain-specific antibody responses,[33] but the key elements of host defense against this organism are unknown.

CLINICAL SYNDROMES

Tracheobronchitis

Acute exacerbations of chronic bronchitis are the most common manifestations of *M. catarrhalis* infection in adults.[33,34] As with exacerbations caused by other organisms, dyspnea and cough productive of purulent sputum are the cardinal symptoms; fever also may be present. *M. catarrhalis* can be implicated by the predominance of gram-negative diplococci on Gram stains of purulent sputum, with isolation of *M. catarrhalis* in culture. In approximately 30% of cases involving *M. catarrhalis*, additional pathogens are present in the sputum.

Pneumonia

Most cases of pneumonia caused by *M. catarrhalis* occur in the elderly, particularly those with underlying COPD.[34,35] The clinical features are those of a mild, acute pneumonia: fever, cough productive of purulent sputum, dyspnea, and chest pain are the common symptoms. Focal evidence of consolidation may be evident on physical examination. The chest x-ray usually reveals patchy alveolar or interstitial opacities that are often multilobar.[35] Pleural effusions are uncommon. The diagnosis is usually made from the sputum Gram stain and culture. Bacteremia, empyema, and other suppurative complications are rare.

Otitis Media and Sinusitis

M. catarrhalis can be isolated from middle-ear effusions in approximately 15% of cases of acute otitis media in children, usually in pure culture.[33] Polymerase chain reaction detects *M. catarrhalis* DNA in an even higher proportion of middle-ear exudates. Similarly, maxillary aspirates yield *M. catarrhalis* in about 20% of children with acute sinusitis.[23] However, only 2% of episodes of acute sinusitis in adults can be attributed to *M. catarrhalis*.[23]

Other Infections

Nosocomial outbreaks of *M. catarrhalis* infection, predominantly involving the respiratory tract and occurring mainly in patients with underlying cardiopulmonary disease, have been reported in children and adults.[34] The mode of transmission has not been clear. *M. catarrhalis* has also been reported as a rare cause of invasive infections, including meningitis, endocarditis, septic arthritis, and bacteremia.[33] Underlying lung disease and neutropenia have been identified as risk factors for *M. catarrhalis* bacteremia, but invasive infections originating in the upper respiratory tract have occurred in previously healthy individuals. *M. catarrhalis* can also cause conjunctivitis and rare urogenital infections.[33]

ANTIBIOTIC TREATMENT

More than 90% of clinical isolates of *M. catarrhalis* produce β-lactamases that render ampicillin and amoxicillin ineffective.[28,29] Penicillin–β-lactamase–inhibitor combinations, second- and third-generation cephalosporins, fluoroquinolones, macrolides, and tetracyclines are active against nearly all strains of *M. catarrhalis* [*see Table 1*].

Legionellosis

In the summer of 1976, a mysterious outbreak of pneumonia occurred among participants in the American Legion's bicentennial convention in Philadelphia, killing 34 of the 221 people afflicted.[36] The disorder became known as Legionnaires disease. Its cause remained obscure until Joseph McDade and his colleagues at the CDC isolated a novel bacterium from the spleens of guinea pigs that had been injected with lung tissue harvested from victims of the epidemic.[37] The new agent was named *Legionella pneumophila*. Studies with stored sera identified this organism as the cause of Pontiac fever—so named after an outbreak of a nonpneumonic, influenzalike illness that occurred in Pontiac, Michigan, in 1968—as well as other cases of epidemic and sporadic respiratory disease dating back to 1943.[38] *L. pneumophila* was the first of several previously unknown agents to emerge as important human pathogens in the late 20th century. In the years since the Philadelphia outbreak of legionellosis, many other *Legionella* species have been identified and implicated in a growing spectrum of human disease.

The family Legionellaceae now includes more than 40 species of the genus *Legionella,* with over 60 distinct serotypes.[39] Almost all of these organisms have been isolated from the environment, and approximately half of them have been associated with human disease. *L. pneumophila* remains the most important human pathogen in this family, accounting for more than 80% of legionellosis cases diagnosed in the United States.[39,40] Other species of *Legionella* produce a similar spectrum of disease and may be underappreciated as causes of human infection.[41]

EPIDEMIOLOGY

The Legionellaceae are widely distributed in freshwater habitats throughout the world.[38,42] They thrive in warm water enriched with iron, often in biofilms with other organisms that supply essential nutrients, such as blue-green algae or macrophytes. Legionellae can also replicate in free-living protozoa, and amebae may be their natural hosts. Man-made aquatic environments that often harbor legionellae include hot-water systems, cooling towers, air conditioners, industrial coolants, whirlpool baths, and humidifiers. The factors that promote the growth of legionellae in water tanks and potable water supplies include a temperature between 30° and 60° C, stagnation, decayed or rusted pipes and fixtures, and infrequent or ineffective decontamination. Water systems harboring legionellae can be disinfected by superheating (> 70° C) and flushing, hyperchlorination, or metallic ionization.[40,42]

Legionellosis is acquired mainly by the inhalation of aerosolized bacteria from an environmental source,[38,40] typically a man-made device. Examples of proven disseminators include showerheads, water faucets, cooling towers, evaporative condensers, respiratory therapy equipment, produce misters, whirlpool baths, and decorative fountains. Only a few cases of legionellosis have been linked to natural aquatic sources such as hot springs. Potting soil also has been identified as a source of infection. Transient contamination of the oropharynx followed by microaspiration may occur occasionally, particularly in patients with nasogastric tubes; stable colonization of the upper respiratory tract by legionellae has not been described. Wounds can be infected by direct inoculation with contaminated water, and oral ingestion has been postulated as a potential source of rare intestinal infections. There is no evidence for person-to-person transmission.

The epidemiologic patterns of legionellosis include common-source epidemics, sporadic cases, and endemic disease in institutions with contaminated water supplies. The infection is more common in the summer months, when seasonal conditions promote the growth of legionellae in the environment, and the use of air conditioners and other cooling devices facilitates the dissemination of airborne bacteria.

Legionella species have been reported to cause from 1% to 15% of community-acquired pneumonias leading to hospitalization,[18] but they consistently rank among the leading causes of severe community-acquired pneumonia leading to respiratory failure.[43] In hospitals with contaminated water supplies, legionellae are important agents of nosocomial pneumonias.

The risk factors for *Legionella* pneumonia include cigarette smoking; alcoholism; recent travel; chronic lung, heart, or kidney disease; diabetes mellitus; cancer; and the use of immunosuppressive medications (especially corticosteroids).[40] Transplant recipients are at particularly high risk and have been the sentinel victims in several nosocomial outbreaks. *Legionella* infections are uncommon but unusually severe in HIV-infected patients.

The epidemiologic features of pneumonic and nonpneumonic legionellosis differ in several respects.[38,44] During epidemics, the attack rate of *Legionella* pneumonia varies from 0.2% to 7%, whereas nonpneumonic legionellosis afflicts over 65% of the people exposed. The incubation period of Legionnaires disease varies from 2 to 12 days, but Pontiac fever usually strikes within 48 hours of exposure. One or more risk factors can be identified in most victims of *Legionella* pneumonia. In contrast, nonpneumonic legionellosis readily affects the normal host. Common sources have resulted in cases of both Legionnaires disease and Pontiac fever, suggesting that bacterial inoculum and host factors are important in determining the clinical course of infection. It is possible that Pontiac fever results primarily from the inhalation of bacterial endotoxin.[44]

PATHOGENESIS AND PATHOLOGY

The Legionellaceae are small, pleomorphic, flagellated gram-negative bacilli that often appear coccobacillary in tissue.[38] They are enveloped by a laminated outer membrane with a unique lipid structure that differs from the lipopolysaccharide of other gram-negative bacteria. Legionellae are facultative intracellular parasites: they can replicate independently or in other cells. They are strictly aerobic but grow best in a reduced-oxygen environment. Buffered charcoal–yeast extract agar supplemented with L-cysteine, ferric iron, and α-ketoglutarate is the most suitable artificial medium.

After inhalation into the lungs, *L. pneumophila* enters alveolar macrophages via coiling or conventional phagocytosis and replicates in a specialized vacuole.[45] The formation of this protected intracellular compartment is directed by the *dot* (defective organelle trafficking) and *icm* (intracellular multiplication) genes of *L. pneumophila*. These genes encode for a type IV secretion system that modifies the endocytic pathway of the host cell and delays fusion of the phagosome with lysosomes. As nutrients become scarce, the production of cytotoxins by the stressed bacteria leads to rupture of the macrophage, and the cycle begins anew. The secretion of proteases by *L. pneumophila* contributes to tissue injury.[45,46] Spreading infection leads to the recruitment of blood-borne phagocytes, but *L. pneumophila* is relatively resistant to killing by neutrophils and multiplies within monocytes. Humoral immunity appears to play little role in host defense against this infection, because *L. pneumophila* is resistant to the lytic effects of antibody and complement, and opsonization by specific antibody promotes uptake of the organism by phagocytic cells without stimulating bacterial killing. Ultimately, the infection is probably contained by suppression of intracellular replication by interferon-gamma–mediated activation of macrophages and the destruction of infected cells by cytotoxic lymphocytes.[47]

Impairments in specific host defenses underlie the increased risk of legionellosis in certain groups. For example, the alveolar macrophages of smokers are greater in number and more susceptible to parasitism by *L. pneumophila* than the macrophages of nonsmokers.[48] Smokers' macrophages exhibit greater expression of the CD11b/CD18 integrin complex that mediates uptake of *L. pneumophila*, and they also contain more iron, an essential bacterial nutrient, than the alveolar macrophages of nonsmokers. Conditions associated with impaired cellular immunity, such as T cell malignancies, HIV infection, and the use of immunosuppressive medications, result in deficient macrophage activation and failure to contain intracellular infection.

Pathologically, pneumonic legionellosis is characterized by confluent multilobular or lobar consolidation, with no predilection for particular segments.[49] Involvement is bilateral in approximately half the cases. Small pleural effusions are common, but empyema is unusual. The most common histologic pattern is an acute fibrinopurulent alveolitis, with little or no involvement of the conducting airways. There is a dense intra-alveolar infiltrate of macrophages and polymorphonuclear leukocytes, accompanied by an abundant fibrinous exudate and proteinaceous debris. The alveolar septae are congested, and there may be a minor vasculitic component. The bacteria are found in the alveolar exudate and are located mainly within macrophages.

A second histologic pattern of Legionnaires disease is diffuse alveolar damage. This is characterized by an intra-alveolar, fibrinoserous exudate with hyaline membrane formation and evidence of epithelial injury. Few organisms can be identified in this setting, but bacterial invasion of the interstitium may be observed. These features may coexist with the fibrinopurulent pattern and are predominantly found in immunocompromised patients. Fibrosis may occur with resolution of the infection. Bronchiolitis obliterans organizing pneumonia is an unusual complication.

CLINICAL SYNDROMES

Two distinct clinical syndromes of legionellosis have been recognized: the pneumonic form known as Legionnaires disease, and the nonpneumonic, self-limited syndrome called Pontiac fever. The spectrum of infection also includes asymptomatic seroconversion and rare focal infections of extrapulmonary organs.

Legionnaires Disease

The classic picture of Legionnaires disease is that of a chronically ill, middle-aged smoker with rapidly progressive pneumonia associated with nonpurulent sputum, diarrhea, confusion, hyponatremia, and abnormal liver function tests. The clinical features of Legionnaires disease are protean, however, so the disorder cannot reliably be distinguished from other pneumonias on clinical grounds alone[38,50,51] [*see Table* 2].

Legionnaires disease typically begins with a brief prodrome of profound weakness, malaise, myalgias, and headache. High fever and shaking chills accompany the development of a cough that is productive in approximately half the cases. Sputum is generally nonpurulent. Chest pain is common, and progressive dyspnea is the rule. Watery diarrhea, nausea, and vomiting are often reported.

Physical examination usually reveals a distressed, tachypneic patient. High fever is a hallmark of legionellosis, and temperatures exceeding 39° C (102.2° F) are found in most patients, even those who are immunosuppressed.[50] Relative bradycardia

Table 2 Manifestations of Legionnaires Disease[83–86]

Manifestations	*Percentage of Cases*
Symptoms and signs	
Fever	67–100
Chills	42–77
Cough	65–92
Sputum production	41–75
Hemoptysis	0–41
Chest pain	14–52
Dyspnea	14–59
Headache	17–56
Myalgias	20–43
Altered mental status	21–43
Diarrhea	21–47
Nausea, vomiting	9–37
Abdominal pain	5–20
Laboratory abnormalities	
Leukocytosis	53–78
Hyponatremia	17–55
Elevated liver enzymes	14–88
Hypophosphatemia	25–51
Azotemia	15–60
Proteinuria	25–56
Hematuria	0–50

(a heart rate less than 100 beats a minute despite a temperature of 40° C [104° F] or higher) may be present. Evidence of consolidation is typically evident on lung auscultation. An encephalopathy ranging from mild confusion to obtundation is common, and focal neurologic deficits have been described.

Routine laboratory tests also typically show an array of abnormalities[38,50,51] [*see Table 2*]. The complete blood count typically demonstrates leukocytosis with a left shift, although a white blood cell count above 15,000/mm^3 is unusual. Hyponatremia and abnormal liver enzymes are reported in approximately half the cases. Hypophosphatemia, azotemia, an elevated creatine kinase level, and an increased serum amylase level may also be found. Urinalysis often reveals proteinuria, hematuria, or both.

The chest x-ray in *Legionella* pneumonia may demonstrate poorly marginated, rounded nodules; patchy alveolar infiltrates; or consolidation in a segmental or lobar distribution.[50,52] The infiltrates are unilobar at presentation in most cases, but radiologic progression to multilobar disease is common. Small pleural effusions are frequently evident, but empyema is unusual. Cavitation is an uncommon finding that is most often seen in immunocompromised patients.

Extrapulmonary manifestations of Legionnaires disease can be striking and may reflect the effects of bacterial toxins, host-derived mediators, or metastatic infection.[40] Neurologic deficits are usually metabolic in origin, but focal bacterial encephalitis has been described. The pathogenesis of the watery diarrhea that often accompanies *Legionella* pneumonia is obscure, but intestinal abscesses and peritonitis have been reported. Acute renal failure may complicate legionellosis, as a result of acute tubular necrosis, rhabdomyolysis, or glomerulonephritis. Pyelonephritis is rare. Overt dissemination of *Legionella* infection from the lungs to other organs occurs most commonly in immunocompromised persons.

Unusual sites of *Legionella* infection include the skin (cellulitis and wound infection), the heart (myocarditis, pericarditis, and prosthetic valve endocarditis), and the abdomen (pancreatitis, colitis, and appendicitis).[40] Infections at these sites have been reported in the absence of pneumonia. In some instances, the infection appears to have resulted from direct inoculation of tissue or a prosthetic device with contaminated water. Other cases may result from bacteremic seeding from the lungs.

Pontiac Fever

The most common nonpneumonic form of legionellosis is Pontiac fever.[38] This syndrome is characterized by a prodrome of malaise, diffuse myalgias, and headache, followed hours later by fever and chills. A mild, nonproductive cough and sore throat may develop, but respiratory tract symptoms are not prominent. Nausea, vomiting, and diarrhea are common, as are neurologic disturbances such as dizziness, neck pain or stiffness, confusion, irritability, nightmares, and ataxia. The physical examination is unremarkable except for the presence of fever, and laboratory tests reveal only leukocytosis. The chest film is clear. The diagnosis is primarily made serologically and supported by the isolation of *Legionella* from an environmental source. Evidence of infection can be detected by PCR or, in some cases, urinary antigen testing. The acute illness resolves spontaneously in 2 to 5 days, but full recovery may take weeks.

MICROBIOLOGIC DIAGNOSIS

The diagnosis of legionellosis requires the isolation of the organism in culture, detection of microbial antigens or nucleic acids in body fluids, or demonstration of serologic evidence of infection [*see Table 3*]. However, an early clue to the diagnosis of Legionnaires disease can be obtained from nonspecific stains of sputum, bronchoalveolar lavage fluid, or lung tissue.[18] Although legionellae are poorly seen on routine Gram stain, visualization of these small, pleomorphic gram-negative bacilli is improved if basic fuchsin is used as the counter-

Table 3 Diagnostic Tests for Legionellosis[30]

Test	*Specimen*	*Sensitivity (%)*	*Specificity (%)*	*Comment*
Culture	Sputum, BALF	11–80	100	All species; requires selective media
Direct fluorescent antibody	Sputum, BALF	22–75	> 90	*Legionella pneumophila* only
Urinary antigen	Urine	55–90	> 95	*L. pneumophila* serogroup 1 only
Serology				
Fourfold change*	Blood	60–80	> 90	*L. pneumophila* only
Single titer		10–27	> 85	
PCR	Throat swab, sputum, BALF	83–100	> 95	All species; not widely available

*Between acute and convalescent samples.
BALF—bronchoalveolar lavage fluid PCR—polymerase chain reaction

stain in place of safranin O. The intracellular organisms can also be seen on Gimenez, Dieterle, or Wright-Giemsa stains. *L. micdadei* is unique among the Legionellaceae in appearing acid fast in clinical specimens.

Culture of sputum, bronchoalveolar lavage fluid, or lung tissue is the preferred means of confirming the diagnosis.[18,40] Specialized media are required for the isolation of *Legionella* (see above), so cultures for these pathogens must be specifically requested of the laboratory. All *Legionella* species can be isolated after 3 to 5 days of incubation, and the recovery of organisms from any body fluid or tissue is diagnostic of infection. Sputum submitted from patients with suspected legionellosis should not be discarded even if epithelial cell contamination occurs, because poor-quality specimens may still yield the organism. Experienced microbiology laboratories can recover legionellae from pretreatment sputum in most cases of legionellosis, but not all laboratories are skilled in this regard, and many patients do not produce sputum.

Antigen detection provides an opportunity for more rapid diagnosis.[18,53] The direct fluorescent antibody (DFA) test can identify organisms in sputum, bronchoalveolar lavage fluid, or lung tissue, even after a few days of antibiotic therapy. However, the interpretation of DFA preparations requires considerable expertise, and the sensitivity of this test is limited to specific antigens. The most commonly used monoclonal antibody preparation detects only *L. pneumophila* serogroups 1 through 12, and commercially available pooled antisera are limited to a few species. Urinary antigen detection is currently the most helpful test for rapid diagnosis of legionellosis. Antigens appear in the urine within 3 days of the onset of illness and may persist for months, although most patients stop excreting antigen within 6 weeks. The major limitation of this approach is that currently available tests reliably detect only *L. pneumophila* serogroup 1.

DNA amplification techniques are very promising for the rapid diagnosis of legionellosis.[18,53] Preliminary experience suggests that PCR can detect any species of *Legionella* in sputum, throat swabs, and bronchoalveolar lavage fluid with high sensitivity and specificity. *Legionella* DNA has also been detected in the urine and blood of patients with legionellosis. These tests hold great promise but require additional evaluation and refinement to establish their role in clinical practice.

Serologic evidence of infection can be obtained by indirect immunofluorescence, microagglutination, or ELISA.[18] A fourfold increase in titer between acute and convalescent samples is very specific for infection with *L. pneumophila* serogroup 1, but tests for other serogroups and species are more subject to cross-reactivity and have not been standardized. Approximately half of patients with Legionnaires disease will seroconvert within 4 weeks from the onset of illness, and 75% will do so within 9 weeks. A small number of patients take as long as 14 weeks to demonstrate an antibody response, and no serologic response will be detected in up to 25% of cases. The major limitation of seroconversion is the delay in diagnostic information. A single titer of 1:256 or higher suggests acute infection with *L. pneumophila* but is found in less than 30% of patients during the acute phase of illness.

TREATMENT AND PROGNOSIS

There are no controlled trials to guide the treatment of legionellosis, but retrospective observations, anecdotal experience, animal studies, and in vitro testing support the efficacy of fluoroquinolones, macrolides, tetracyclines, and rifampin in the treatment of Legionnaires disease [*see Table 4*].[40,54] Fluoroquinolones may be preferred in immunocompromised patients because they are bactericidal, in contrast to macrolides and tetracyclines, and exhibit the most activity in experimental models.[54] All of the fluoroquinolones appear to be effective, but cipro-

Table 4 Treatment of Legionellosis

Antibiotic Class	*Drug*	*Dosage*	*Cost*	*Comment*
Fluoroquinolones	Levofloxacin	500 mg p.o. or I.V. q. 24 hr for 10 days	500 mg p.o., $11.40	May be preferred in immunocompromised patients because the agents are bactericidal
	Gatifloxacin	400 mg p.o. or I.V. q. 24 hr for 10 days	400 mg p.o., $9.30	
	Moxifloxacin	400 mg p.o. q. 24 hr for 10 days	400 mg p.o., $9.30	
	Ofloxacin	400 mg p.o. or I.V. q. 24 hr for 10 days	400 mg p.o., $7–7.99; 400 mg I.V., $20–29.99	
Macrolides	Azithromycin	500 mg p.o. or I.V. q. 24 hr for 5–10 days	500 mg p.o., $10–19.99	Most active of its class against *Legionella*
	Clarithromycin	500 mg p.o. or I.V. q. 24 hr for 10 days	500 mg p.o., $7–7.99	—
	Erythromycin	500 mg p.o. or 1 g I.V. q. 6 hr for 10–14 days	p.o.: $2–2.99/day I.V.: $3–3.99/day	Less well tolerated than other macrolides
Tetracyclines	Doxycycline	100 mg p.o. or I.V. q. 12 hr for 10–14 days	p.o.: $0.20–0.49/day	May be less effective than fluoroquinolones or macrolides

floxacin is less active than other agents in this class. Azithromycin is the most active macrolide against *Legionella*. Both azithromycin and clarithromycin are more effective and better tolerated than erythromycin. Rifampin is highly active against *Legionella*, and anecdotal evidence supports its use in combination with erythromycin in severely ill or immunocompromised patients. Of the tetracyclines, doxycycline and minocycline are the most active agents, but these drugs appear to be less effective than fluoroquinolones or macrolides. Trimethoprim-sulfamethoxazole also may be effective, but clinical experience is limited. All of these agents share the ability to penetrate the intracellular environment of macrophages, where legionellae replicate. β-Lactam antibiotics and aminoglycosides generally are ineffective in legionellosis.

The optimum duration of therapy is unknown. Immunocompromised persons and patients with unusually severe disease may warrant treatment for 2 to 3 weeks, but experience with newer macrolides and fluoroquinolones suggests that shorter courses are adequate.[40,54]

The prognosis of *Legionella* pneumonia is influenced by the status of host defenses and the timely initiation of effective antibiotic treatment.[40,55] With appropriate treatment, the mortality of Legionnaires disease varies from approximately 5% in healthy persons to 25% in immunocompromised patients.

Pertussis (Whooping Cough)

Whooping cough was first described in 16th-century France.[56] The name pertussis was coined by the English physician Thomas Sydenham in 1679, in reference to the intensive cough that is the hallmark of this disease. *Bordetella pertussis*, the causative agent, was first isolated by Bordet and Gengou in 1906. Other members of the genus include *B. parapertussis, B. bronchiseptica, B. avium, B. hinzii, B. holmesii,* and *B. trematum. B. parapertussis* lacks pertussis toxin but causes a mild form of whooping cough in humans and also infects pigs. Other species of *Bordetella* rarely cause human disease.

EPIDEMIOLOGY

B. pertussis is exclusively a human pathogen: no carrier state, animal host, or natural reservoir is known. The infection is transmitted from person to person by aerosol droplets and is very contagious, spreading quickly among close contacts. Pertussis is endemic year-round, but epidemics occur at intervals of 2 to 5 years.[57,58] The attack rate is highest in infants younger than 1 year and is higher in females than males.[58] In the prevaccine era, pertussis was the leading cause of death in children younger than 14 years in the United States. The introduction of the killed whole cell vaccine in the 1940s led to a marked reduction in the prevalence of pertussis, which fell steadily until reaching its nadir in 1981. Since 1982, there has been a resurgence of reported cases of pertussis in the United States. During this time, the incidence in children younger than 5 years has remained relatively constant, but an increasing proportion of cases has been recognized in adolescents and young adults.[59] More than half of the 7,288 cases of pertussis reported to the CDC in 1999 occurred in persons older than 10 years.[6] Most early childhood cases of pertussis now occur in children who either are too young to have received vaccine or have been inadequately vaccinated.[59,60] Cases in adolescents and adults probably reflect the waning of immunity 5 to 10 years after vaccination. It is likely that pertussis is markedly underreported in older children and adults because the characteristic whooping cough is usually absent in these age groups. Mildly ill or asymptomatic adults with unrecognized pertussis serve as important reservoirs for the infection of more susceptible children.

Although effective vaccines have dramatically reduced the importance of pertussis in developed countries, the disease remains a leading cause of morbidity and mortality in unvaccinated populations. An estimated 50 million cases of pertussis occur worldwide each year, leading to 350,000 deaths.[61]

PATHOGENESIS

Bordetellae are small, aerobic, gram-negative coccobacilli. They have fastidious growth requirements (see below). Pertussis is primarily a disease of the conducting airways, characterized histologically by generalized inflammation of the bronchi and bronchioles with a mucopurulent luminal exudate.[56] The bacilli grow on the surface of ciliated epithelium, where they thrive through the expression of surface components and secreted toxins that suppress mechanical and cellular host defenses [*see Table 5*].

Pertussis toxin is the most intriguing factor produced by *B. pertussis.* This heterodimeric protein catalyzes adenosine diphosphate (ADP)–ribosylation of guanine nucleotide–binding (G) proteins, thereby inhibiting signal transduction through G-coupled transmembrane receptors.[61] How this action is linked to the pathophysiology of pertussis is not well understood. Pertussis toxin causes lymphocytosis, hyperinsulinemia, and possibly encephalopathy, but its role in the respiratory manifestations of whooping cough remains enigmatic.[61] Antibodies directed against pertussis toxin are protective against disease, yet *B. parapertussis,* which does not produce the toxin, can cause a similar (albeit milder) respiratory illness.

Relatively little is known of the essential elements of host defense against pertussis, but cellular and humoral immunity are both involved.[61,62] Protective maternal antibodies are not transferred across the placenta, contributing to the susceptibility of infants. The resolution of whooping cough is accompanied by the disappearance of *B. pertussis* from the airway epithelium.

Table 5 Virulence Factors of *Bordetella pertussis*[61,62]

Virulence Factor	*Effects*
Filamentous hemagglutinin	Attachment to ciliated epithelium; uptake by leukocytes via complement receptor 3
Agglutinogens, fimbriae	Attachment to epithelium
Lipopolysaccharide	Endotoxin activity
Tracheal cytotoxin	Ciliostasis, epithelial injury
Adenylate cyclase toxin	Induces increased cyclic adenosine monophosphate; impairs leukocyte function
Dermonecrotic toxin	Vascular smooth muscle contraction, ischemic necrosis
Pertussis toxin	Inhibits G protein-coupled signaling; lymphocytosis, hyperinsulinemia, encephalopathy
Type III secretion system	Delivers proteins into cytoplasm of target cells

CLINICAL MANIFESTATIONS

Classic pertussis is a three-stage illness lasting 4 to 8 weeks.[56,58,61] After an incubation period of 6 to 20 days, the clinical manifestations begin with the catarrhal stage. This phase lasts 1 to 2 weeks and resembles the common cold, with rhinorrhea, conjunctivitis, lacrimation, low-grade fever, and mild nonproductive cough. The distinctive paroxysmal stage follows for 2 to 4 weeks and is characterized by violent spasms of coughing. In a typical episode, a single expiration is punctuated by five to 20 explosive coughs in rapid succession, followed by a gasping, forceful inhalation through a narrowed glottis that produces the characteristic whoop. Paroxysms often are accompanied by cyanosis and followed by emesis. Infants have less pronounced whoops but may become apneic during coughing fits. The violent coughing can result in epistaxis, conjunctival hemorrhage, petechiae, rib fractures, pneumothorax, incontinence, hernias, and rectal prolapse. Paroxysms occur 10 to 30 times a day, often begin without warning, and can be triggered by activities such as eating, drinking, sneezing, yawning, or exposure to airborne irritants. The paroxysms are exhausting, and patients avoid oral intake, leading to dehydration and weight loss.

Physical examination during the spasmodic stage often is unremarkable. Eyelid edema may be present, and auscultation of the chest may reveal coarse rales and rhonchi. Fever is unusual in the absence of complications. The blood count at this time is characterized by marked lymphocytosis: the total WBC count often exceeds 30,000/mm^3, of which more than 60% are lymphocytes. Hypoglycemia is occasionally observed. Chest radiographs are usually normal but may demonstrate hyperinflation, atelectasis, or perihilar infiltrates.[56,63] Complications that can develop during the paroxysmal phase include pneumonia, otitis media, seizures, and encephalopathy. Pneumonia, caused either by *B. pertussis* or by a secondary invader, develops in 10% to 15% of young children and is responsible for most deaths.[59] The convalescent third stage of pertussis, during which the frequency and severity of the cough gradually diminish, usually lasts 1 to 3 weeks but may extend for months.

Adults and adolescents with partial immunity have a less severe illness and typically present with a persistent cough of several weeks' duration. The cough is paroxysmal and often productive of purulent or nonpurulent sputum, but whoops are unusual. As in children, violent coughing in adults with pertussis may result in posttussive vomiting, syncope, urinary incontinence, and rib fractures. About half of adult patients report a preceding catarrhal illness. Lymphocytosis is usually absent. Numerous recent studies suggest that 10% to 32% of adolescents and adults with cough lasting longer than 1 to 2 weeks have serologic evidence of pertussis.[57,64] Annual serologic screening programs have found that undiagnosed pertussis is common in adolescents and adults.

A presumptive diagnosis of pertussis can be made in susceptible children with the characteristic whooping cough and lymphocytosis. However, the typical whoop is not uniformly present, and similar illnesses can be caused by *B. parapertussis*, respiratory viruses (particularly adenovirus, parainfluenza, and respiratory syncytial virus), *Mycoplasma pneumoniae*, and *Chlamydia pneumoniae*.[62]

MICROBIOLOGIC DIAGNOSIS

Microbiologic confirmation of pertussis is best made during the catarrhal or early paroxysmal stages, when *B. pertussis* can be detected in the nasopharynx by culture, immunofluorescence, or PCR.[61,62,65] Cultures of nasopharyngeal aspirates have higher yields than those of nasopharyngeal swabs; if the latter are used, calcium alginate or Dacron are the preferred materials. Throat specimens are unsatisfactory because the oropharynx lacks the ciliated epithelium to which *B. pertussis* adheres. The nasopharyngeal sample should be directly streaked on suitably enriched media, such as charcoal-blood agar or Bordet-Gengou agar. If a delay in plating is anticipated, a charcoal-containing transport medium (e.g., Regan-Lowe) should be used.[65] Typical colonies of tiny gram-negative bacilli appear after 3 to 7 days of culture, and identification can be confirmed by agglutination or immunofluorescence. Culture yield is reduced by antibiotic therapy or prior immunization and falls with the duration of illness. Cultures are usually negative during the paroxysmal phase and in adults with persistent cough.

B. pertussis can also be detected in respiratory secretions by DFA staining in 30% to 65% of cases during the catarrhal stage.[61,65] Polyclonal antibody preparations have been plagued by variable sensitivity and poor specificity, but a monoclonal reagent has been found to be more satisfactory.[65] Nonetheless, immunofluorescence is mainly used as a screening test for outbreak investigation.

PCR testing of nasopharyngeal specimens has been found to be more sensitive than culture or immunofluorescence for the diagnosis of pertussis, with specificity greater than 85%.[61,62] This very promising technique has become increasingly available, but the methods and reagents for the diagnosis of pertussis by PCR have not yet been standardized.

Detection of serum antibody responses to *B. pertussis* by ELISA remains an important if imperfect diagnostic tool. Serologic tests are most useful for the diagnosis of pertussis in unvaccinated children, in whom the sensitivity of paired specimens or a single elevated titer more than 5 weeks after the onset of symptoms is 50% to 90%.[62,65] Multiple antigens are often used in antibody assays to enhance sensitivity, but pertussis toxin is the only antigen unique to *B. pertussis*.[62,65] The interpretation of serologic results in vaccinated persons is more difficult. The meaning of a single elevated antibody titer should be defined in relation to age-matched, population-specific controls.[62,64,65] Paired specimens have limited utility because the anamnestic response to infection is usually so rapid that no significant rise in antibody concentrations occurs between acute and convalescent sera.[64,65]

TREATMENT

Antibiotic therapy with erythromycin speeds elimination of *B. pertussis* from the nasopharynx and reduces transmission of infection.[61,62] Antibiotic treatment may also ameliorate the severity of disease, even if it is started in the paroxysmal phase, but this is less clear. The estolate form of erythromycin, 40 mg/kg/day (maximum, 2 g/

day) divided in two to four doses, is preferred and should be administered for 7 to 14 days.[62] There is limited evidence that the newer macrolides, clarithromycin and azithromycin, also are effective.[62] Alternative agents that speed elimination of *B. pertussis* include trimethoprim-sulfamethoxazole, tetracycline, and chloramphenicol.[61] Fluoroquinolones are active against *B. pertussis* in vitro, but their efficacy in the treatment of pertussis has not been demonstrated.

The value of antibiotic therapy in adults with persistent cough and suspected pertussis is unknown.

Infants with pertussis should be hospitalized for monitoring, airway suctioning, oxygen supplementation, hydration, and nutritional support. Treatment of severe cases with pertussis immune globulin has shown promise in animal studies and human trials.[66] Systemic corticosteroids may be helpful in infants with life-threatening disease.[61] Inhaled corticosteroids and bronchodilators are of uncertain value in ameliorating symptoms.

PREVENTION

Pertussis can be prevented by quarantine of infected individuals, prophylactic antibiotic treatment of exposed infants, and vaccination. Patients with active pertussis in the catarrhal and early paroxysmal stages should be isolated for 5 to 7 days after starting antibiotics. Prophylactic treatment of household contacts with a full course of erythromycin can reduce the spread of disease and is recommended for young children who have not completed primary immunization. In neonates, however, erythromycin prophylaxis is associated with an increased risk of hypertrophic pyloric stenosis.[67]

Immunization with inactivated whole cell vaccine was introduced in 1948, and acellular vaccines composed of inactivated pertussis toxin and one or more additional components were licensed in 1991. Current recommendations call for primary immunization with an acellular vaccine, which is combined with diphtheria and tetanus toxoids (DTaP), at ages 2, 4, and 6 months, with boosters at 15 to 18 months and at 4 to 6 years.[68] Pertussis vaccines provide approximately 80% protection from clinical pertussis, and immunized persons who become ill after exposure experience less severe disease.[62,68] Protection declines with time and is largely lost by 12 years after the last dose.[62] Historically, boosters have not been given to older children and adults because of the unacceptable toxicity of the whole cell vaccine. The acellular vaccine is immunogenic and well tolerated by adolescents and adults, but recommendations for boosters in these age groups have not been established. Reactions to whole cell pertussis vaccine (DTP) in children include local pain and swelling, fever, anorexia, irritability, vomiting, hypotonic hyporesponsiveness, seizures, and anaphylaxis. All of these reactions are much less common with the acellular vaccines.[62,68]

Pseudomonas aeruginosa Infections

P. aeruginosa is an important opportunistic pathogen, with a prominent role in cystic fibrosis. The organism was first isolated from a surgical wound in 1882 by the French pharmacist Carle Gessard.[69] The species designations in both the original name for the organism, *Bacillus pyocyaneus,* and its modern name, *P. aeruginosa,* refer to the blue-green pigments produced by these bacteria, which may serve as clinical markers for infection.[70] More than a dozen species of *Pseudomonas* are now recognized, but only *P. aeruginosa* is an important human pathogen.

EPIDEMIOLOGY

P. aeruginosa is widely distributed in nature, particularly in water, soil, and vegetation. Nutritional versatility, suppression of competitors, and resistance to antibiotics contribute to the diverse habitat of this organism.[70] *P. aeruginosa* is not part of the normal flora of most humans, but it can be cultured from the stool, throat, nose, or moist areas of the skin of up to 20% of healthy persons.[69,70]

P. aeruginosa is mainly an opportunistic and nosocomial pathogen. It has a marked predilection for colonizing damaged epithelium, such as burned skin, bronchiectatic airways, and sites of indwelling appliances such as tracheostomy tubes, endotracheal tubes, urinary catheters, intravascular devices, and peritoneal dialysis catheters.[69] Patients with cystic fibrosis are especially prone to airway colonization. The risk of colonization at any site increases with exposure to broad-spectrum antibiotics and duration of hospitalization.[70] Colonization is an important antecedent to invasive infection, particularly in neutropenic patients.[69,70] Additional risk factors for invasive disease include cytotoxic chemotherapy, treatment with corticosteroids, and HIV infection.[69,71] Persons with diabetes mellitus are at risk for invasive external otitis.

Outbreaks of *P. aeruginosa* infection can result from common-source exposures. Community outbreaks of folliculitis have been associated with swimming pools, whirlpool baths, and hot tubs. Ocular infections have resulted from contaminated cosmetics and contact lens solution.[69] In hospitals, epidemics of *P. aeruginosa* infection have been linked to contaminated sinks, mops, cleaning solutions, therapy pools, respiratory therapy equipment, endoscopic devices, flowers, vegetables, and water pitchers.[69]

PATHOGENESIS

P. aeruginosa is a motile gram-negative bacillus that is typically thin and either straight or slightly curved. It does not ferment sugars and grows strictly aerobically. *P. aeruginosa* has simple nutritional requirements and tolerates a wide range of environmental conditions. It grows well on most laboratory media and emits a sweet, grapelike odor. Most strains produce one or more diffusable pigments, including pyocyanin, pyoverdin, pyorubin, and pyomelanin.[69]

P. aeruginosa is a formidable pathogen that is well equipped to colonize and invade epithelial surfaces, undermine host defenses, and induce systemic toxicity. *P. aeruginosa* attaches to tracheobronchial mucus and replicates in a biofilm on the mucosal surface.[72] Although *P. aeruginosa* adheres poorly to normal epithelium, it readily attaches to damaged epithelial cells via pili and other adhesins.[71,72] The persistence of some strains of *P. aeruginosa* on epithelial surfaces is aided by the abundant secretion of tenacious mucopolysaccharide, which facilitates adherence to host cells, inhibits ciliary activity, and blocks ingestion by phagocytes. Mucociliary clearance is further impaired by the production of bacterial toxins that reduce ciliary beat frequency and directly injure cilia.[72] Invasion across epithelial surfaces by *P. aeruginosa* is made possible by proteolytic enzymes that damage epithelial cells, loosen tight junctions, and digest extracellular matrix.[71] These enzymes also interfere with host defenses by cleaving immunoglobulins, complement, and cytokines. Exotoxin A, leukocidin, and other products exert cytotoxic effects on macrophages, neutrophils, and lymphocytes. Vascular injury by exotoxin A can result in local or distant hemorrhagic necrosis. Damage to epithelial and endothelial barriers permits the entry of bacteria, bacterial products, and endogenous proinflammatory mediators into the systemic circulation, leading to systemic toxicity and shock.[73]

The striking association of *P. aeruginosa* with cystic fibrosis (CF) is an area of special interest.[74] Most patients with CF are initially colonized with an environmental, nonmucoid strain of *P. aeruginosa*. These bacteria eventually undergo a phenotypic shift in the CF airway to express an unusual lipopolysaccharide structure and hypersecrete mucoid exopolysaccharide (alginate).[74] The factors controlling these adaptations and the mechanisms underlying the persistence of *P. aeruginosa* in the CF airway remain incompletely understood. *P. aeruginosa* binds somewhat more avidly to CF epithelium than to normal epithelial cells.[72,74] However, the uptake of *P. aeruginosa* by epithelial cells is defective in CF. The cystic fibrosis transmembrane conductance regulator (CFTR) may serve as a receptor for the internalization of surface bacteria, and shedding of these infected cells may be a normal defense mechanism against *P. aeruginosa* that is defective in CF.[72,74] Also, human β defensin 1, an antibacterial peptide secreted by airway epithelial cells, is inactive in the high salt concentrations that some investigators have found in CF airways.[72,74] Chronic inflammation precipitated by *P. aeruginosa* infection contributes to the airway injury and progressive loss of pulmonary function that characterize CF.

CLINICAL SYNDROMES

Pneumonia

Nosocomial pneumonia *P. aeruginosa* is one of the most common causes of hospital-acquired pneumonia and is implicated in 20% to 50% of cases complicating mechanical ventilation.[75–77] Risks for nosocomial *P. aeruginosa* pneumonia include prolonged hospitalization, mechanical ventilation for 7 days or longer, and exposure to broad-spectrum antibiotics.[75,76,78] Tracheal colonization with *P. aeruginosa* usually precedes infection.[78]

The clinical features of ventilator-associated pneumonia are nonspecific: fever, purulent tracheal secretions, leukocytosis, and new or changing infiltrates on chest films.[75,76] The radiographic abnormalities are multifocal and bilateral in most cases of *P. aeruginosa* pneumonia, and are more severe than those observed with other nosocomial pathogens.[76] Cavitation is evident on plain films or chest tomography in about 25%.[79]

The diagnosis of hospital-acquired pneumonia in critically ill patients is challenging because tracheal colonization with potential pathogens cannot be distinguished easily from infection on clinical grounds.[80] The diagnosis of *P. aeruginosa* pneumonia, particularly in intubated patients, is most accurately made from quantitative cultures of bronchoscopic specimens.[77] Yields of 1,000 colony-forming units per milliliter from a protected specimen brush or 10,000 colony-forming units per milliliter from a bronchoalveolar lavage are indicative of infection. Blood cultures are positive in less than 10% of cases.

Hospital-acquired pneumonia caused by *P. aeruginosa* is associated with a worse outcome than infections caused by other pathogens. In well-documented cases of *P. aeruginosa* ventilator-associated pneumonia, the crude mortality is 45% to 85% and the attributable mortality is about 40%.[75,80,81] In fatal cases, death usually results from septic shock or multiple-organ failure.[75] Relapses are relatively common after successful treatment.[75,82]

Community-acquired pneumonia *P. aeruginosa* is a rare cause of community-acquired pneumonia but is disproportionately represented among the most severe cases, accounting for approximately 2% of community-acquired pneumonias that result in admission to critical care units.[43] Most patients with *P. aeruginosa* pneumonia have underlying conditions that place them at particular risk for colonization of the lower airways with *P. aeruginosa* (e.g., cystic fibrosis, bronchiectasis, or tracheostomy), or they have important defects in host defenses caused by malignancy, aplastic anemia, cytotoxic chemotherapy, or advanced HIV infection.[83] The few cases of *P. aeruginosa* pneumonia that have been reported in healthy persons have occurred predominantly in smokers.[83]

Community-acquired *P. aeruginosa* pneumonia is typically acute in onset and rapidly progressive.[70,83] Fever, cough, chest pain, and progressive dyspnea are the usual symptoms. The cough is generally productive of purulent sputum that may be streaked with blood. On examination, patients are apprehensive, often confused, and acutely ill, with fever, tachypnea, tachycardia, hypotension, and cyanosis. The chest x-ray typically reveals multifocal, nodular alveolar infiltrates, often bilateral. Small areas of parenchymal cavitation may be evident, but large effusions and empyema are unusual. Routine laboratory findings are nonspecific and may include leukocytosis or leukopenia, elevated transaminase levels, and azotemia. Sputum Gram stains demonstrate gram-negative bacilli in nearly all cases, and sputum cultures grow *P. aeruginosa* in greater than 80%.[70,83] Blood cultures often are positive. The clinical course is usually rapidly progressive despite therapy, with most patients experiencing respiratory failure. Mortality exceeds 30%.[83]

Pneumonia in HIV disease *P. aeruginosa* infections of the lower respiratory tract are unusually common in patients with advanced HIV disease, and the incidence may be increasing.[71,84] These infections occur in the setting of very low $CD4^+$ T cell counts (median, < 25 cells/mm^3). Additional risk factors in some cases include neutropenia, recent antibiotic therapy, and treatment with corticosteroids. Most infections are community acquired. The clinical course can be fulminant, but a subacute presentation also has been described, characterized by productive cough, fever, and dyspnea for days to weeks. The radiographic features are similar to those of other cases of community-acquired *P. aeruginosa* pneumonia. *P. aeruginosa* is readily identified in purulent sputum in the majority of cases; blood cultures are positive in 10% to 30%.

Most patients with *P. aeruginosa* pneumonia complicating HIV infection respond to antibiotic treatment, but relapses are common.

Cystic Fibrosis

More than 80% of patients with CF develop chronic airway infection with mucoid strains of *P. aeruginosa*. This infection is associated with chronic airway inflammation, progressive loss of pulmonary function, and eventual death from respiratory failure.[71,74] Intensive and prolonged treatment of initial infection with aerosolized tobramycin or colistin may delay chronic infection and preserve pulmonary function.[85] Once chronic infection with mucoid *P. aeruginosa* is established, it is virtually impossible to eradicate.

Patients with CF experience pulmonary exacerbations that are associated with an increased density of *P. aeruginosa* in sputum. These episodes are characterized symptomatically by increased coughing, more purulent or bloody sputum, chest congestion, and dyspnea. Physical signs include tachypnea, use of accessory muscles for breathing, fever, and weight loss. A decline in airflow is evident on pulmonary function testing, and the chest x-ray may demonstrate new or changing infiltrates.[86]

Treatment of pulmonary exacerbations in CF includes chest physiotherapy, bronchodilators, and combination antibiotic therapy guided by in vitro susceptibility testing of sputum isolates.[86] Intermittent maintenance therapy with inhaled tobramycin (300 mg twice daily during alternate months) can suppress *P. aeruginosa*, improve airflow, and reduce the need for hospitalization.[87]

Bacteremia

P. aeruginosa bacteremia occurs predominantly in hospitalized patients with severe underlying disease.[71,88,89] The most common sources of infection are the lower respiratory tract, the urinary tract, and the skin; intravascular catheters are implicated in 7% to 16% of cases. No primary source of infection can be identified in up to one third of episodes. The overall mortality of *P. aeruginosa* bacteremia is approximately 20%. An increased risk of death is observed in patients with pneumonia, severe sepsis, and fatal underlying disease.

Endocarditis

P. aeruginosa is a rare cause of infective endocarditis. The majority of reported cases have occurred in injection drug users, particularly those from the Detroit area.[71,90] Occasional episodes have complicated cardiac surgery or involved seeding of a prosthetic device. Most cases have been localized to the right side of the heart and have developed on normal valves.

Patients with right-sided infection often present with a prolonged febrile illness and may complain of cough or chest pain associated with radiographic evidence of septic pulmonary emboli.[90] Patients with aortic or mitral valve involvement follow a more acute clinical course that may include evidence of congestive heart failure, myocardial abscess, or systemic embolization.[90] The diagnosis of *P. aeruginosa* endocarditis is made from blood cultures, cardiac auscultation, and echocardiography.

Most right-sided infections can be cured by 6 weeks of high-dose parenteral treatment with an extended-spectrum penicillin and an aminoglycoside.[71] Left-sided infections usually require valve replacement surgery in conjunction with medical therapy.[71,90] The overall survival in left-sided infections is approximately 50%.

Urinary Tract Infections

P. aeruginosa is a common cause of urinary tract infection in hospitals and chronic care facilities. These infections usually follow instrumentation, surgery, or catheterization of the urinary tract, often in patients recently treated with antibiotics.[70,71] Symptomatic infections can be treated with single-agent antibiotic therapy, including oral indanyl carbenicillin or a fluoroquinolone. Catheter-associated infections are unlikely to be eradicated unless the catheter is removed.

Gastrointestinal Infections

P. aeruginosa can cause outbreaks of enteritis and enteric fever in young children exposed to contaminated water.[70,71] Infants with *P. aeruginosa* enteritis present with symptoms ranging from mild irritability, diarrhea, and abdominal distention to severe dehydration and vascular collapse. *P. aeruginosa* has also been linked with a typhoidlike illness called Shanghai fever. This syndrome consists of fever, diarrhea or constipation, and spotted skin rash and lasts for 1 to 2 weeks. The diagnosis of enteric infection is supported by culturing *P. aeruginosa* from stool or blood. Mild cases are self-limited, but severe disease should be treated with antibiotics. Surgical intervention may be required in necrotizing infections complicated by bowel perforation or abscess formation.

P. aeruginosa is also associated with necrotizing enterocolitis, typhlitis, and perirectal abscesses in patients with neutropenia resulting from chemotherapy or hematologic malignancy.[70,71] These infections typically follow colonization of the gut after displacement of the normal flora by broad-spectrum antibiotic therapy. Necrotizing enterocolitis can involve any portion of the alimentary tract, but it most often affects the distal ileum, cecum, and colon. Typhlitis refers to localized gangrenous necrosis of the cecum, which often leads to perforation and peritonitis. Patients with necrotizing enteric infections present with fever, abdominal pain, distention, and tenderness. In typhlitis, pain and tenderness are localized to the right lower quadrant. Computed tomography and ultrasonography can reveal evidence of focal bowel edema. Blood or stool cultures may be positive. Antibiotics and intravenous fluids are the mainstays of therapy, but surgical intervention may be necessary. *P. aeruginosa* is also one of many organisms that can cause perirectal abscess formation in neutropenic patients. Surgical drainage is required.

Ear Infections

Swimmer's ear *P. aeruginosa* is commonly isolated from cases of acute diffuse external otitis (swimmer's ear), which is associated with freshwater swimming in warm, humid climates.[71] This condition is characterized by an inflamed, draining, pruritic, and sometimes painful external auditory canal. Local cleansing followed by topical treatment with an otic solution containing 2% acetic acid or an antibiotic in combination with corticosteroids speeds recovery. Recurrences are common.

Malignant otitis externa *P. aeruginosa* is the pathogen in nearly all cases of malignant external otitis, a chronic, invasive infection of the external auditory canal that predominantly afflicts elderly persons with diabetes mellitus.[71,91] The infection spreads to the temporal bone and mastoid, often involving the adjacent cranial nerves as they exit the skull. Severe otalgia is the presenting symptom, and most patients have purulent otorrhea. Facial nerve paresis is evident in 30% to 40% of cases; other cranial neuropathies are less common. Fever and other systemic signs of infection are usually absent. CT and magnetic resonance imaging are useful for defining the extent of disease, with MRI being more sensitive for delineating the soft tissue component.[71,91] The diagnosis can be made from the clinical presentation, imaging studies, and cultures of diseased bone or granulation tissue in the external canal.

Local debridement and antibiotic therapy for 4 to 8 weeks are successful in most cases. An oral fluoroquinolone may be sufficient in mild infections without cranial nerve involvement or osteomyelitis, but parenteral combination therapy with an antipseudomonal β-lactam and an aminoglycoside is recommended for more extensive disease.[71] The mortality ranges from 10% to 20%.

Eye Infections

P. aeruginosa is an important cause of keratitis, particularly in contact lens wearers.[92] This infection develops as a complication of corneal injury, which permits bacterial attachment to the damaged epithelium and subsequent invasion.

The clinical manifestations begin with a small, painful ulcer that spreads with gray discoloration and edema of the cornea, anterior chamber reaction, and mucopurulent exudate. The microbiologic diagnosis can be made by Gram stain and culture of purulent material in the base of the ulcer.

Emergent treatment is with frequent (every 15 to 30 minutes) topical applications of an ophthalmic solution containing high concentrations of an aminoglycoside or fluoroquinolone. *P. aeruginosa* is also occasionally implicated in posttraumatic endophthalmitis and nosocomial conjunctivitis.

Central Nervous System Infections

Meningitis caused by *P. aeruginosa* occurs most often as a complication of neurosurgery.[71] Rare cases result from *P. aeruginosa* bacteremia, particularly in debilitated patients with cancer or severe burns.

Fever and depressed consciousness are the cardinal manifestations. The onset often is insidious in postoperative cases. The diagnosis is made from culture and Gram stain of the cerebrospinal fluid.

Ceftazidime is the preferred treatment, often given in combination with an intravenous aminoglycoside. Alternative agents that achieve adequate levels in the cerebrospinal fluid include meropenem, aztreonam, and ciprofloxacin. Intrathecal therapy with aminoglycosides may be required for refractory cases or highly resistant organisms.[71]

Bone and Joint Infections

P. aeruginosa is associated with a distinctive spectrum of acute and chronic osteochondral infections that result from hematogenous seeding, direct inoculation, or contiguous spread from adjacent tissues.[71] Hematogenous infections are most commonly seen in injection drug users and typically involve the sternoclavicular joints, symphysis pubis, sacroiliac joints, or cervical vertebrae. Lumbosacral vertebral osteomyelitis may complicate instrumentation of the urinary tract via contamination of the venous plexus shared by the pelvis and the spine. *P. aeruginosa* is also the most common cause of osteochondritis after puncture wounds of the foot. This syndrome is most often seen in children and results from direct inoculation of bacteria colonizing the moist insoles of their sneakers. Chronic osteomyelitis caused by *P. aeruginosa* can develop as a complication of orthopedic surgery, sternotomy, or contiguous infection of pressure sores or ischemic skin ulcers.

The cardinal symptom of acute osteochondral *P. aeruginosa* infection is pain lasting days to weeks. Examination is notable for local tenderness and diminished mobility, frequently with warmth and erythema. Fever and leukocytosis are often present, and the erythrocyte sedimentation rate is almost always elevated. The clinical presentation of chronic osteomyelitis is subtler than that of acute infection. Pain, nonunion, and draining ulcers are common, often without systemic manifestations.

Imaging studies are important in the evaluation of *P. aeruginosa* bone and joint infections.[93] Plain x-rays or CT scans can reveal evidence of bony destruction or periosteal reaction but may be negative early in the clinical course. MRI is more sensitive than radiography, particularly for nonosseous changes. Technetium-99m bone scans are invariably positive in osteomyelitis but may be normal when the infection is confined to the joint. Confirmation of *P. aeruginosa* as the pathogen is made from joint aspiration or bone biopsy. Blood cultures are negative in most cases.

Treatment of *P. aeruginosa* osteochondral infections usually requires 4 to 6 weeks of antibiotic therapy. An antipseudomonal β-lactam in combination with an aminoglycoside is generally recommended, but single-agent therapy, particularly with a fluoroquinolone, may be effective.[71,93] Surgical debridement is necessary when bone necrosis is evident, but most infections confined to a joint can be treated with antibiotics alone. In the case of *P. aeruginosa* osteochondritis of the foot in children, 1 week of antibiotic therapy after debridement is sufficient for cure. Chronic infections are difficult to eradicate, and suppressive therapy may be required.

Skin Infections

P. aeruginosa causes a variety of cutaneous infections that can affect normal skin after submersion in contaminated water.

Folliculitis Outbreaks of folliculitis, or swimmer's itch, have been associated with the use of hot tubs, whirlpools, therapy baths, and swimming pools.[71] The presenting feature is a diffuse, pruritic eruption that may be follicular, maculopapular, vesicular, or pustular. The rash develops 8 hours to 5 days after exposure and usually involves skin that had been covered by a swimsuit. Mild headache and other complaints may be present, but fever is unusual. *P. aeruginosa* can be identified from stains and cultures of pustular lesions. Topical drying agents may ease symptoms, but the rash resolves within 7 days without specific therapy.

Hot-foot syndrome Another waterborne infection is the recently described *Pseudomonas* hot-foot syndrome, which is characterized by the development of tender, warm, erythematous 1 to 2 cm nodules on a background of plantar or palmar erythema.[94] These lesions appeared in children 10 to 40 hours after being in a contaminated wading pool and resolved without antibiotic treatment within 7 to 14 days.

Green-nail syndrome This syndrome results from discoloration of the nail plate by pyocyanin and occurs in persons who frequently submerge their hands. Local cleansing and debridement, including draining of any associated paronychia, are generally successful.[71,95]

Toe web infection *P. aeruginosa* is a frequent cause of toe web infections. These occur most often in tropical climates and may complicate minor trauma or tinea pedis. The affected toe webs are macerated, thickened, and painfully fissured; a purulent exudate is often present. Examination under a Wood lamp can reveal green-white fluorescence from the elaboration of pyoverdin. Toe web infections often can be managed with local measures, but systemic antibiotics may be needed in severe cases.[71,95]

Burn wound sepsis In years past, *P. aeruginosa* was the most common agent of burn wound sepsis, which was the leading cause of death after thermal injury. With the development of effective topical antimicrobials, wound excision, and other advances in burn wound care, burn sepsis has become far less common. Fungi are now the dominant pathogens, but *P. aeruginosa* remains an important consideration. Suspicion of wound sepsis should be aroused by the appearance of dark-brown, black, or violaceous discoloration of the wound. Hemorrhage, purulent drainage, or green pigment also may be present. Blood cultures may be positive, but the diagnosis of invasive infection is made from wound biopsies demonstrating microbial invasion of normal tissue. Treatment of *P. aeruginosa* infection is with systemic antibiotics, topical mafenide acetate cream, and surgical debridement.[96] *P. aeruginosa* can also cause post-traumatic cellulitis, deep abscesses, necrotizing fasciitis, and other locally invasive pyodermas, particularly in immunocompromised persons.[71]

Ecthyma gangrenosum Ecthyma gangrenosum is a distinctive skin infection that results in most cases from *P. aeruginosa* bacteremia, usually in the setting of neutropenia, cancer, burns, AIDS, or other severely debilitating conditions.[71,95] The lesions may be discrete or multiple and begin as painless macules or nodules that may become vesicular or bullous. The lesions undergo central hemorrhagic necrosis and ulceration over a period of 12 to 24 hours, with a surrounding rim of tender erythema. Ecthyma gangrenosum is characterized histologically by bacterial invasion of dermal veins. Blood cultures are usually positive, and *P. aeruginosa* can be demonstrated in biopsies or scrapings from the base of the ulcer. Treatment requires prompt administration of intravenous antibiotics and management of the underlying condition.

ANTIBIOTIC TREATMENT

The treatment of *P. aeruginosa* infections is particularly challenging because of the remarkable resistance of this organism to most antibiotics and its propensity to develop further resistance during the course of therapy. The intrinsic antimicrobial insensitivity of *P. aeruginosa* arises from several complementary mechanisms.[97] First, a relatively impermeable outer membrane limits the access of antibiotics to their binding sites. Second, an active efflux pump can expel agents that penetrate the outer barrier. Third, expression of a chromosomally encoded β-lactamase is induced on exposure to β-lactam antibiotics. Furthermore, mutations in *P. aeruginosa* can result in the rapid selection of resistant organisms during the course of treatment. This is particularly evident with carbapenem monotherapy, during which resistance can emerge in 30% to 50% of episodes, often within 1 week after starting treatment.[75,97] Finally, *P. aeruginosa* can acquire plasmids bearing additional resistance genes, such as those encoding for extended-spectrum β-lactamases, carbapenemases, and enzymes that inactivate aminoglycosides.[97,98]

Antimicrobial agents that are effective against most strains of *P. aeruginosa* include β-lactams, fluoroquinolones, and aminoglycosides [see 2 Chemotherapy of Infection]. In the United States, the β-lactam showing the greatest activity against *P. aeruginosa* is meropenem; the most active aminoglycoside is amikacin. Local resistance patterns vary, however, so it is important to determine the antibiotic susceptibilities of individual strains by in vitro testing. Hospital isolates exhibit greater resistance than outpatient isolates, and organisms cultured in intensive care units are the most resistant. Multidrug-resistant strains may be susceptible to antibiotic combinations or polymyxins.[98]

Treatment of suspected *P. aeruginosa* infection should begin with high doses of an antipseudomonal β-lactam in combination with an aminoglycoside or fluoroquinolone. The use of two agents increases the likelihood of effective initial therapy, which is associated with reduced mortality.[88] Whether combination therapy should be continued after sensitivities are known is unclear. On the one hand, the combination of an aminoglycoside with a β-lactam antibiotic results in synergistic killing of *P. aeruginosa* and improves outcome in some animal models of infection.[83,99] Prospective observational studies have found combination therapy with β-lactams and aminoglycosides to be associated with improved survival in neutropenic or bacteremic patients with *P. aeruginosa* infections.[99,100] On the other hand, aminoglycosides are relatively toxic, and other antibiotic combinations are less predictably synergistic against *P. aeruginosa*.[83] Recent retrospective clinical studies have not identified any survival advantage of dual-drug therapy over treatment with a single effective agent.[75,88,89] Combination therapy also has not been shown to suppress the emergence of resistant strains. Despite this uncertainty, it may be prudent to use combination therapy whenever possible because of the high mortality and refractory nature of *P. aeruginosa* infections. An exception is urinary tract infection, which can be treated effectively with a single agent. Most *P. aeruginosa* infections can be cured with 2 to 3 weeks of antibiotic therapy, but longer courses are required for endocarditis and osteomyelitis.

References

1. Turk DC, May JR: *Haemophilus influenzae*: its clinical importance. English Universities Press, London, 1967

2. Moxon ER, Murphy TF: *Haemophilus influenzae*. Principles and Practice of Infectious Diseases 5th ed. Mandell GL, Bennett JE, Dolin R, Eds. Churchill Livingstone, Philadelphia, 2000, p 2369

3. Rao VK, Krasan GP, Hendrixson DR, et al: Molecular determinants of the pathogenesis of disease due to nontypable *Haemophilus influenzae*. FEMS Microbiol Rev 23:99, 1999

4. Murphy TF: *Haemophilus influenzae* in chronic bronchitis. Semin Respir Infect 15:41, 2000

5. Bresser P, Out TA, van Alphen L, et al: Airway inflammation in nonobstructive and obstructive chronic bronchitis with chronic *Haemophilus influenzae* airway infection: comparison with noninfected patients with chronic obstructive pulmonary disease. Am J Respir Crit Care Med 162:947, 2000

6. Summary of notifiable diseases, United States—1999. MMWR Morb Mortal Wkly Rep 48:1, 2001

7. Bisgard KM, Kao A, Leake J, et al: *Haemophilus influenzae* invasive disease in the United States, 1994–1995: near disappearance of a vaccine-preventable childhood disease. Emerg Infect Dis 4:229, 1998

8. Perdue DG, Bulkow LR, Gellin BG, et al: Invasive *Haemophilus influenzae* disease in Alaskan residents aged 10 years and older before and after infant vaccination programs. JAMA 283:3089, 2000

9. Hirschmann JV, Everett ED: *Haemophilus influenzae* infections in adults: report of nine cases and a review of the literature. Medicine (Baltimore) 58:80, 1979

10. Invasive *Haemophilus influenzae* disease in adults: a prospective, population-based surveillance. CDC Meningitis Surveillance Group. Ann Intern Med 116:806, 1992

11. Sarangi J, Cartwright K, Stuart J, et al: Invasive *Haemophilus influenzae* disease in adults. Epidemiol Infect 124:441, 2000

12. Peltola H: Worldwide *Haemophilus influenzae* type b disease at the beginning of the 21st century: global analysis of the disease burden 25 years after the use of the polysaccharide vaccine and a decade after the advent of conjugates. Clin Microbiol Rev 13:302, 2000

13. Durand ML, Calderwood SB, Weber DJ, et al: Acute bacterial meningitis in adults: a review of 493 episodes. N Engl J Med 328:21, 1993

14. Hussein AS, Shafran SD: Acute bacterial meningitis in adults: a 12-year review. Medicine (Baltimore) 79:360, 2000

15. Spagnuolo PJ, Ellner JJ, Lerner PI, et al: *Haemophilus influenzae* meningitis: the spectrum of disease in adults. Medicine (Baltimore) 61:74, 1982

16. Quagliarello VJ, Scheld WM: Treatment of bacterial meningitis. N Engl J Med 336:708, 1982

17. Kucera CM, Silverstein MD, Jacobson RM, et al: Epiglottitis in adults and children in Olmsted County, Minnesota, 1976 through 1990. Mayo Clin Proc 71:1155, 1996

18. Skerrett SJ: Diagnostic testing for community-acquired pneumonia. Clin Chest Med 20:531, 1999

19. Musher DM, Kubitschek KR, Crennan J, et al: Pneumonia and acute febrile tracheobronchitis due to *Haemophilus influenzae*. Ann Intern Med 99:444, 1983

20. *Haemophilus influenzae* pneumonia in human immunodefiency virus–infected patients. Grupo Andaluz para el Estudio de las Enfermedades Infecciosas. Clin Infect Dis 30:461, 2000

21. Hospital-acquired pneumonia in adults: diagnosis, assessment of severity, initial antimicrobial therapy, and preventive strategies. A consensus statement, American Thoracic Society, November 1995. Am J Respir Crit Care Med 153:1711, 1996

22. Klein JO: Otitis media. Clin Infect Dis 19:823, 1994

23. Gwaltney JM Jr: Acute community-acquired sinusitis. Clin Infect Dis 23:1209, 1996

24. Kostman JR, Sherry BL, Fligner CL, et al: Invasive *Haemophilus influenzae* infections in older children and adults in Seattle. Clin Infect Dis 17:389, 1993

25. Sonnen GM, Henry NK: Pediatric bone and joint infections: Diagnosis and antimicrobial management. Pediatr Clin North Am 43:933, 1996

26. Borenstein DG, Simon GL: *Hemophilus influenzae* septic arthritis in adults: a report of four cases and a review of the literature. Medicine (Baltimore) 65:191, 1986

27. Perkins MD, Mirrett S, Reller LB: Rapid bacterial antigen detection is not clinically useful. J Clin Microbiol 33:1486, 1995

28. Thornsberry C, Ogilvie PT, Holley HP Jr, et al: Survey of susceptibilities of *Streptococcus pneumoniae, Haemophilus influenzae,* and *Moraxella catarrhalis* isolates to 26 antimicrobial agents: a prospective U.S. study. Antimicrob Agents Chemother 43:2612, 1999

29. Doern GV, Jones RN, Pfaller MA, et al: *Haemophilus influenzae* and *Moraxella catarrhalis* from patients with community-acquired respiratory tract infections: antimicrobial susceptibility patterns from the SENTRY antimicrobial Surveillance Program (United States and Canada, 1997). Antimicrob Agents Chemother 43:385, 1999

30. *Haemophilus influenzae* Infection. 2000 Red Book: Report of the Committee on Infectious Diseases, 25th ed. Pickering LK, Ed. American Academy of Pediatrics, Elk Grove Village, Illinois, 2000, p 262

31. *Haemophilus* endocarditis: report of 42 cases in adults and review. Haemophilus Endocarditis Study Group. Clin Infect Dis 24:1087, 1997

32. Berk SL: From *Micrococcus* to *Moraxella*: The reemergence of *Branhamella catarrhalis*. Arch Intern Med 150:2254, 1990

33. Murphy TF: *Branhamella catarrhalis*: epidemiology, surface antigenic structure, and immune response. Microbiol Rev 60:267, 1990

34. Murphy TF: Lung infections. 2. *Branhamella catarrhalis*: epidemiological and clinical aspects of a human respiratory tract pathogen. Thorax 53:124, 1998

35. Wright PW, Wallace RJ Jr, Shepherd JR: A descriptive study of 42 cases of *Branhamella catarrhalis* pneumonia. Am J Med 88:2S, 1990

36. Fraser DW, Tsai TR, Orenstein W, et al: Legionnaires' disease: description of an epidemic of pneumonia. N Engl J Med 297:1189, 1977

37. McDade JE, Shepard CC, Fraser DW, et al: Legionnaires' disease: isolation of a bacterium and demonstration of its role in other respiratory disease. N Engl J Med 297:1197, 1977

38. Winn WC Jr: Legionnaires disease: historical perspective. Clin Microbiol Rev 1:60, 1988

39. Benson RF, Fields BS: Classification of the genus *Legionella*. Semin Respir Infect 13:90, 1998

40. Stout JE, Yu VL: Legionellosis. N Engl J Med 337:682, 1997

41. McNally C, Hackman B, Fields BS, et al: Potential importance of *Legionella* species as etiologies in community acquired pneumonia (CAP). Diagn Microbiol Infect Dis 38:79, 2000

42. Atlas RM: *Legionella*: from environmental habitats to disease pathology, detection and control. Environ Microbiol 1:283, 1999

43. So HY: Severe community-acquired pneumonia. Anaesth Intensive Care 25:222, 1997

44. Fields BS, Haupt T, Davis JP, et al: Pontiac fever due to *Legionella micdadei* from a whirlpool spa: possible role of bacterial endotoxin. J Infect Dis 184:1289, 2001

45. Swanson MS, Hammer BK: *Legionella pneumophila* pathogenesis: a fateful journey from amoebae to macrophages. Annu Rev Microbiol 54: 567, 2000

46. Dowling JN, Saha AK, Glew RH: Virulence factors of the family Legionellaceae. Microbiol Rev 56:32, 1992

47. Friedman H, Yamamoto Y, Newton C, et al: Immunologic response and pathophysiology of *Legionella* infection. Semin Respir Infect 13:100, 1998

48. Skerrett SJ: Host defenses against respiratory infection. Med Clin North Am 78:941, 1994

49. Winn WC, Myerowitz RL: The pathology of the legionella pneumonias: a review of 74 cases and the literature. Hum Pathol 12:401, 1981

50. Kirby BD, Snyder KM, Meyer RD, et al: Legionnaires' disease: report of sixty-five nosocomially acquired cases of review of the literature. Medicine (Baltimore) 59:188, 1980

51. Sopena N, Sabria-Leal M, Pedro-Botet ML, et al: Comparative study of the clinical presentation of *Legionella* pneumonia and other community-acquired pneumonias. Chest 113:1195, 1998

52. The radiologic manifestations of Legionnaire's disease. The Ohio Community-Based Pneumonia Incidence Study Group. Chest 117:398, 2000

53. Waterer GW, Baselski VS, Wunderink RG: *Legionella* and community-acquired pneumonia: a review of current diagnostic tests from a clinician's viewpoint. Am J Med 110:41, 2001

54. Edelstein PH: Antimicrobial chemotherapy for Legionnaires disease: time for a change. Ann Intern Med 129:328, 1998

55. el-Ebiary M, Sarmiento X, Torres A, et al: Prognostic factors of severe *Legionella* pneumonia requiring admission to ICU. Am J Respir Crit Care Med 156:1467, 1997

56. Lapin JH: Whooping cough. Charles C. Thomas, Springfield, Illinois, 1943

57. Cherry JD: Epidemiological, clinical, and laboratory aspects of pertussis in adults. Clin Infect Dis 28 (suppl 2):S112, 1999

58. Cherry JD: Pertussis in the preantibiotic and prevaccine era, with emphasis on adult pertussis. Clin Infect Dis 28 (suppl 2):S107, 1999

59. Guris D, Strebel PM, Bardenheier B, et al: Changing epidemiology of pertussis in the United States: increasing reported incidence among adolescents and adults, 1990-1996. Clin Infect Dis 28:1230,1999

60. Halperin SA, Wang EE, Law B, et al: Epidemiological features of pertussis in hospitalized patients in Canada, 1991–1997: report of the Immunization Monitoring Program—Active (IMPACT). Clin Infect Dis 28:1238, 1999

61. Kerr JR, Matthews RC: *Bordetella pertussis* infection: pathogenesis, diagnosis, management, and the role of protective immunity. Eur J Clin Microbiol Infect Dis 19:77, 2000

62. Heininger U: Recent progress in clinical and basic pertussis research. Eur J Pediatr 160:203, 2001

63. Gordon M, Davies HD, Gold R: Clinical and microbiologic features of children presenting with pertussis to a Canadian pediatric hospital during an eleven-year period. Pediatr Infect Dis J 13:617, 1994

64. Senzilet LD, Halperin SA, Spika JS, et al: Pertussis is a frequent cause of prolonged cough illness in adults and adolescents. Clin Infect Dis 32:1691, 2001

65. Muller FM, Hoppe JE, Wirsing von Konig CH: Laboratory diagnosis of pertussis: state of the art in 1997. J Clin Microbiol 35:2435, 1997

66. Bruss JB, Malley R, Halperin S, et al: Treatment of severe pertussis: a study of the safety and pharmacology of intravenous pertussis immunoglobulin. Pediatr Infect Dis J 18:505, 1999

67. Honein MA, Paulozzi LJ, Himelright IM, et al: Infantile hypertrophic pyloric stenosis after pertussis prophylaxis with erythromycin: a case review and cohort study. Lancet 354:2101, 1999

68. Pertussis vaccination: use of acellular pertussis vaccines among infants and young children. Recommendations of the Advisory Committee on Immunization Practices (ACIP). MMWR Morb Mortal Wkly Rep 46(RR-7):1, 1997

69. Morrison AJ Jr, Wenzel RP: Epidemiology of infections due to *Pseudomonas aeruginosa.* Rev Infect Dis 6 (suppl 3):S627, 1984

70. Bodey GP, Bolivar R, Fainstein V, et al: Infections caused by *Pseudomonas aeruginosa*. Rev Infect Dis 5:279, 1983

71. Pollack M: *Pseudomonas aeruginosa*. Principles and Practice of Infectious Diseases, 5th ed. Mandell GL, Bennett JE, Dolin R, Eds. Churchill Livingstone, Philadelphia, 2000, p 2310

72. Wilson R, Dowling RB: Lung infections: 3. *Pseudomonas aeruginosa* and other related species. Thorax 53:213, 1998

73. Kurahashi K, Kajikawa O, Sawa T, et al: Pathogenesis of septic shock in *Pseudomonas aeruginosa* pneumonia. J Clin Invest 104:743, 1999

74. Pier GB: Role of the cystic fibrosis transmembrane conductance regulator in innate immunity to *Pseudomonas aeruginosa* infections. Proc Natl Acad Sci USA 97:8822, 2000

75. Crouch Brewer S, Wunderink RG, Jones CB, et al: Ventilator-associated pneumonia due to *Pseudomonas aeruginosa*. Chest 109:1019, 1996

76. Trouillet JL, Chastre J, Vuagnat A, et al: Ventilator-associated pneumonia caused by potentially drug-resistant bacteria. Am J Respir Crit Care Med 157:531, 1998

77. Fagon JY, Chastre J, Wolff M, et al: Invasive and noninvasive strategies for management of suspected ventilator-associated pneumonia: a randomized trial. Ann Intern Med 132:621, 2000

78. Bonten MJ, Bergmans DC, Ambergen AW, et al: Risk factors for pneumonia, and colonization of respiratory tract and stomach in mechanically ventilated ICU patients. Am J Respir Crit Care Med 154: 1339, 1996

79. Winer-Muram HT, Jennings SG, Wunderink RG, et al: Ventilator-associated *Pseudomonas aeruginosa* pneumonia: radiographic findings. Radiology 195:247, 1995

80. Fagon JY, Chastre J, Domart Y, et al: Mortality due to ventilator-associated pneumonia or colonization with *Pseudomonas* or *Acinetobacter* species: assessment by quantitative culture of samples obtained by a protected specimen brush. Clin Infect Dis 23:538, 1996

81. Papazian L, Bregeon F, Thirion X, et al: Effect of ventilator-associated pneumonia on mortality and morbidity. Am J Respir Crit Care Med 154:91, 1996

82. Rello J, Mariscal D, March F, et al: Recurrent *Pseudomonas aeruginosa* pneumonia in ventilated patients: relapse or reinfection? Am J Respir Crit Care Med 157:912, 1998

83. Hatchette TF, Gupta R, Marrie TJ: *Pseudomonas aeruginosa* community-acquired pneumonia in previously healthy adults: case report and review of the literature. Clin Infect Dis 31:1349, 2000

84. Afessa B, Green B: Bacterial pneumonia in hospitalized patients with HIV infection: the Pulmonary Complications, ICU Support, and Prognostic Factors of Hospitalized Patients with HIV (PIP) Study. Chest 117:1017, 2000

85. Ratjen F, Doring G, Nikolaizik WH: Effect of inhaled tobramycin on early *Pseudomonas aeruginosa* colonisation in patients with cystic fibrosis. Lancet 358:983, 2001

86. Ramsey BW: Management of pulmonary disease in patients with cystic fibrosis. N Engl J Med 335:179, 1996

87. Intermittent administration of inhaled tobramycin in patients with cystic fibrosis. Cystic Fibrosis Inhaled Tobramycin Study Group. N Engl J Med 340:23, 1999

88. Vidal F, Mensa J, Almela M, et al: Epidemiology and outcome of *Pseudomonas aeruginosa* bacteremia, with special emphasis on the influence of antibiotic treatment: analysis of 189 episodes. Arch Intern Med 156:2121, 1996

89. Chatzinikolaou I, Abi-Said D, Bodey GP, et al: Recent experience with *Pseudomonas aeruginosa* bacteremia in patients with cancer: retrospective analysis of 245 episodes. Arch Intern Med 160:501, 2000

90. Komshian SV, Tablan OC, Palutke W, et al: Characteristics of left-sided endocarditis due to *Pseudomonas aeruginosa* in the Detroit Medical Center. Rev Infect Dis 12:693, 1990

91. Rubin J, Yu VL: Malignant external otitis: insights into pathogenesis, clinical manifestations, diagnosis, and therapy. Am J Med 85:391, 1988

92. O'Brien T: Keratitis. Principles and Practice of Infectious Diseases, 5th ed., Mandell GL, Bennett JE, Dolin R, Eds. Churchill Livingstone, Philadelphia, 2000, p 1257

93. Lew DP, Waldvogel FA: Osteomyelitis. N Engl J Med 336:999, 1997

94. Fiorillo L, Zucker M, Sawyer D, et al: The pseudomonas hot-foot syndrome. N Engl J Med 345:335, 2001

95. Agger WA, Mardan A: *Pseudomonas aeruginosa* infections of intact skin. Clin Infect Dis 20:302, 1995

96. Pruitt BA Jr, McManus AT, Kim SH, et al: Burn wound infections: current status. World J Surg 22:135, 1998

97. Hancock RE: Resistance mechanisms in *Pseudomonas aeruginosa* and other nonfermentative gram-negative bacteria. Clin Infect Dis 27 (suppl 1):S93, 1998

98. Gales AC, Jones RN, Turnidge J, et al: Characterization of *Pseudomonas aeruginosa* isolates: occurrence rates, antimicrobial susceptibility patterns, and molecular typing in the global SENTRY Antimicrobial Surveillance Program, 1997-1999. Clin Infect Dis 32(suppl 2): S146, 2001

99. Hilf M, Yu VL, Sharp J, et al: Antibiotic therapy for *Pseudomonas aeruginosa* bacteremia: outcome correlations in a prospective study of 200 patients. Am J Med 87:540, 1989

100. Leibovici L, Paul M, Poznanski O, et al: Monotherapy versus beta-lactam-aminoglycoside combination treatment for gram-negative bacteremia: a prospective, observational study. Antimicrob Agents Chemother 41:1127, 1997

22 Infections Due to *Brucella, Francisella, Yersinia pestis,* and *Bartonella*

W. Conrad Liles, M.D., Ph.D.

Brucellosis, tularemia, (bubonic) plague, and bartonellosis are zoonoses (i.e., infectious diseases that can be transmitted from animals to humans) caused by gram-negative bacilli. The causative agents of these diseases are *Brucella* species, *Francisella tularensis, Yersinia pestis,* and *Bartonella* species, respectively. Infected arthropods, such as ticks or fleas, can serve as vectors for the transmission of tularemia, plague, and bartonellosis. In general, the diagnosis of these zoonoses requires the physician to consider the clinical presentation (which is not always distinctive) in light of the epidemiology of these diseases [*see Table 1*]. Treatment is principally with appropriate empirical antimicrobials [*see Table 2*].

Brucellosis

Brucellosis continues to be a major zoonosis worldwide.[1] The animal reservoirs for the disease include a variety of domesticated animals: cattle, goats, sheep, pigs, and dogs. Human brucellosis (variously known as undulant fever, Malta fever, and Mediterranean fever) is rare in the United States but remains a significant health problem in developing countries. In humans, brucellosis is a disease of protean manifestations, ranging from an indolent febrile syndrome to fulminant endocarditis. Like plague and tularemia, brucellosis is recognized as a potential agent of biological terrorism.[2]

EPIDEMIOLOGY

Virtually all cases of brucellosis arise from direct or indirect exposure to animals.[1,3–5] In animals, brucellosis is a chronic disease that persists lifelong and causes infectious abortion and sterility. *B. abortus* infects predominantly cattle; *B. melitensis,* goats and sheep; and *B. suis,* domestic and wild swine. *B. canis,* the least common cause of human brucellosis, is mostly found in kennel-raised dogs. Infected animals shed large numbers of *Brucella* organisms in their milk, urine, and afterbirth. Hence, brucellosis is considered an occupational hazard for farmers, ranchers, veterinarians, abattoir workers, and laboratory personnel.[3,4,6]

Brucellosis is distributed worldwide, but its incidence varies markedly, depending largely on the degree of its control in domestic animals and the pasteurization of milk. The disease is relatively common in southern Europe, the Middle East, the Indian subcontinent, parts of Africa, Mexico, and Central and South America.[1,3–5]

In the United States, the incidence of brucellosis has declined to less than 100 cases annually, coincident with public health programs and the virtual elimination of *B. abortus* infection in cattle. Currently, most cases of brucellosis acquired in the United States are caused by *B. melitensis* and can be linked to ingestion of unpasteurized goat-milk products from foreign countries, such as Mexico, and exposure to *Brucella* cultures in microbiology laboratory personnel.[4,6–8] Transmission of brucellosis by bone marrow transplantation was recently reported.[9]

ETIOLOGY

Brucellosis is transmitted to humans by direct contact with infected animals or their body fluids (inoculation occurs through cuts or abraded skin); via inhalation of aerosolized organisms; or by ingestion of unpasteurized dairy products. Because of the low density of organisms in muscle, consumption of meat products has rarely been implicated in infection.[1,3–5]

PATHOGENESIS

Brucella organisms are small, nonmotile, non–spore-forming, gram-negative coccobacilli. The organisms are relatively hardy and can survive in dairy products or refrigerated meats for weeks to months. Although they grow aerobically, some species require supplemental carbon dioxide for

Table 1 Diagnosis of Diseases Caused by *Brucella, Francisella, Yersinia,* and *Bartonella* Species

	Brucella *(Brucellosis)*	Francisella tularensis *(Tularemia)*	Yersinia pestis *(Plague)*	Bartonella *(Oroya Fever, Bacteremia, Cat-Scratch Disease)*
Animal reservoir	Cattle, goats, sheep, swine, dogs	Widespread: mammals, birds, fish, amphibians, arthropods	Rodents (rats, ground squirrels, prairie dogs); other animals possible	Cats, phlebotomine sandflies (Andes Mts.)
Transmission	Direct contact through skin lesions, airborne, ingestion of contaminated dairy products	Direct contact, airborne, arthropod bites	Flea bites, animal bites or scratches, airborne	Oroya fever: sandfly bites Bacteremia: body lice Cat-scratch disease: cat bites or scratches; possibly, cat flea bites
Incubation period (range)	10–14 days (5 days to several months)	3–7 days (1–21 days)	Bubonic: 2–7 days Pneumonic: 2–3 days (1–14 days)	Oroya fever: 3–12 wk Bacteremia: days to months Cat-scratch disease: 3–10 days
Clinical manifestations	Protean: fever and tachycardia, flulike syndrome, liver or spleen enlargement, lymphadenopathy, rashes or skin lesions	Flulike illness, ulcer at site of skin inoculation, regional lymphadenopathy, rash, GI symptoms	Flulike illness, buboes (inguinal/axillary lymphadenopathy) Septicemic: GI symptoms	Oroya fever: flulike illness, lymphadenopathy, hemolytic anemia, thrombocytopenia Bacteremia: fever, malaise, anemia, thrombocytopenia, splenomegaly, cardiac murmur, bacillary angiomatosis (in HIV) Cat-scratch disease: inoculation-site lesion, regional lymphadenopathy, low-grade fever
Laboratory tests	WBCs normal or decreased; RBCs and platelets typically decreased; ESR variable; culture of body fluid and tissue; serology	Screening tests often unremarkable; mild to moderate elevation of AST and ALT; serology (late)	WBCs 15,000–25,000/µl, left shift; fibrin split products ↑; DIC possible; AST, ALT, and bilirubin elevated; culture of body fluid and tissue; direct immunofluorescence	Oroya fever: blood culture Bacteremia: blood culture Cat-scratch disease: diagnosis usually clinical

ALT—alanine aminotransferase AST—aspartate aminotransferase ESR—erythrocyte sedimentation rate RBC—red blood cell WBC—white blood cell

primary isolation. In culture, *Brucella* strains are relatively slow growing; isolation from clinical specimens can require incubation for 30 days or more.[1,4]

Infection can occur via the gastrointestinal tract, broken skin, oral mucosa, conjunctiva, or respiratory tract. Once inoculated, bacteria travel to regional lymph nodes and multiply. They then enter the bloodstream and localize in cells of the reticuloendothelial system (particularly the liver, spleen, bone marrow, and lymph nodes) and kidney. At tissue sites of infection, noncaseating granulomas characteristically develop. Bacteremia can lead to metastatic infection at various sites, including bone, joints, meninges, and cardiac valves.[1,3–5]

DIAGNOSIS

Clinical Manifestations

The incubation period for brucellosis is usually 10 to 14 days, but it ranges from 5 days to several months. Onset of illness can be abrupt or insidious. The presentation is nonspecific; fever, chills, headache, myalgias, anorexia, malaise, and fatigue are common. Fever and tachycardia are present in approximately 90% of cases, hepatomegaly in 25% to 30%, splenomegaly in about 40%, and lymphadenopathy (most commonly cervical) in 10% to 40%. Cutaneous manifestations, which occur in approximately 5% of patients, include a variety of nonspecific maculopapular rashes, erythema nodosum,

Table 2 Treatment of Diseases Caused by *Brucella, Francisella, Yersinia,* and *Bartonella* Species

Infection	*Drug*	*Dosage*	*Relative Efficacy*	*Cost*	*Comments*
Brucella (*Brucellosis*)	Doxycycline *plus* Gentamicin *or* Streptomycin	100 mg p.o., b.i.d., for 6 wk; 3–5 mg/kg/day I.V. in divided doses for 2–3 wk; 1 g I.M. q.d. for 2–3 wk	First choice	$0.05–0.12/day; 120 mg I.V. q. 8 hr: $5.00–5.99/day; 500 mg I.M. b.i.d.: $3.00–3.99/day	Relapse rate ~ 6%
	Doxycycline *plus* Rifampin	100 mg p.o., b.i.d., for 6 wk; 600–900 mg p.o., b.i.d., for 6 wk	Alternative choice	$0.05–0.12/day; 600 mg p.o. once daily: $60.00–69.99/mo.	Relapse rate ~ 15%
	Ciprofloxacin	500 mg p.o., b.i.d., for 30 days, with rifampin (see above)	Adjunctive therapy	—	Adjunctive therapy
Francisella tularensis (*Tularemia*)	Streptomycin	500 mg–1 g I.M. q. 12 hr for 7–14 days	First choice	500 mg I.M. b.i.d.: $3.00–3.99/day	—
	Gentamicin	3–5 mg/kg/day I.V. in divided doses q. 8 hr for 7–14 days	Equally effective	120 mg I.V. q. 8 hr: $5.00–5.99/day	—
	Tetracycline	500 mg p.o., q.i.d., for 21–28 days	Alternative choice	500 mg p.o., q.i.d.: $0.10–0.24/day	Relapse can occur if therapy < 21 days
	Doxycycline	100 mg p.o., b.i.d., for 21–28 days	Alternative choice	—	Relapse can occur if therapy < 21 days
	Chloramphenicol	1 g I.V., p.o.* q. 6 hr for 21–28 days	Alternative choice	1 g I.V. q. 6 hr: $150.00–199.99/day	Relapse can occur if therapy < 21 days; consider for treatment if signs or symptoms of meningitis are present
	Ciprofloxacin	500 mg p.o., b.i.d., for 14–21 days	Alternative choice	500 mg p.o., b.i.d.: $7.00–7.99/day	Limited data
Yersinia pestis (*Bubonic Plague*)	Streptomycin	30 mg/kg/day I.M. in divided doses q.12 hr, for 10 days or at least 3 days after clinical recovery; or for 5 days, followed by gentamicin for 5–10 days (see below)	First choice	500 mg I.M. b.i.d.: $3.00–3.99/day	Continue antibiotic therapy for 10 days, or at least 3 days after clinical recovery
	Gentamicin	2 mg/kg I.V. loading dose, then 1.7 mg/kg I.V. q. 8 hr	Equally effective	120 mg I.V. q. 8 hr: $5.00–5.99/day	Continue antibiotic therapy for 10 days, or at least 3 days after clinical recovery
	Tetracycline	500 mg I.V./p.o., q.i.d.	Alternative choice	500 mg p.o., q.i.d.: $0.10–0.24/day	Continue antibiotic therapy for 10 days, or at least 3 days after clinical recovery
	Doxycycline	100 mg I.V./p.o., b.i.d.	Alternative choice	100 mg p.o., b.i.d.: $0.05–0.12/day	Continue antibiotic therapy for 10 days, or at least 3 days after clinical recovery
	Chloramphenicol	500 mg–1 g I.V./p.o.* q.i.d.	Alternative choice	1 g I.V. q. 6 hr: $150.00–199.99/day	Continue antibiotic therapy for 10 days, or at least 3 days after clinical recovery
	Tetracycline	500 mg p.o., q.i.d.	Chemoprophylaxis	$0.10–0.24/day	Chemoprophylaxis for contacts of patients with pneumonic plague

Table 2 (continued)

Infection	*Drug*	*Dosage*	*Relative Efficacy*	*Cost*	*Comments*
Yersinia pestis *(Bubonic Plague) (continued)*	Doxycycline	100 mg p.o., b.i.d.	Chemoprophylaxis	$0.05–0.12/day	Chemoprophylaxis for contacts of patients with pneumonic plague
	Streptomycin	20 mg/kg/day I.M. in two divided doses	Chemoprophylaxis	500 mg I.M., b.i.d.: $3.00–3.99/day	Chemoprophylaxis for contacts younger than 8 yr of age of patients with pneumonic plague
	Trimethoprim-sulfamethoxazole	40 mg/kg p.o., b.i.d.	Chemoprophylaxis	800/160 mg p.o., b.i.d.: $0.10–0.24/day	Chemoprophylaxis for contacts younger than 8 yr of age of patients with pneumonic plague
Bartonella *(Bartonellosis)*	OROYA FEVER				
	Chloramphenicol	500 mg p.o.*/I.V. q.i.d. for ≥ 1 wk	First choice	1 g I.V. q. 6 hr: $150.00–199.99/day	—
	Tetracycline	500 mg p.o./I.V. q.i.d. for ≥ 2 wk	Alternative choice	$0.10–0.24/day	—
	Doxycycline	100 mg p.o./I.V. q.i.d. for ≥ 2 wk	Alternative choice	$0.05–0.12/day	—
	Ampicillin	500 mg p.o./I.V. q.i.d. for ≥ 2 wk	Alternative choice	500 mg p.o., q.i.d.: $0.75–0.99/day	—
	URBAN TRENCH FEVER WITH BACTEREMIA				
	Erythromycin	500 mg p.o., q.i.d., for 14 days	—	—	Azithromycin and clarithromycin are probably equally effective
	Doxycycline	100 mg p.o., b.i.d., for 14 days	—	$0.05–0.12/day	—
	URBAN TRENCH FEVER WITH ENDOCARDITIS				
	Gentamicin	2 mg/kg I.V. loading dose, then 1.7 mg/kg I.V. q. 8 hr	—	120 mg I.V. q. 8 hr: $5.00–5.99/day	In conjunction with valve replacement
	Ciprofloxacin *plus* Rifampin	Ciprofloxacin, 500 mg p.o., b.i.d., plus rifampin, 600 mg p.o., q.d., for ≥ 4–6 mo	—	—	Limited data; monitor for surgical valve replacement; levofloxacin can be substituted for ciprofloxacin
	Ciprofloxacin *plus* a macrolide	Ciprofloxacin, 500 mg p.o., b.i.d., plus an oral macrolide (erythromycin, clarithromycin, or azithromycin) for ≥ 4–6 mo	—	—	Limited data; monitor for surgical valve replacement; levofloxacin can be substituted for ciprofloxacin
	CAT-SCRATCH DISEASE				
	Azithromycin	500 mg p.o. once, then 250 mg p.o., q.d., for 4 days	—	250 mg p.o., q.d.: $6.00–6.99/day	Azithromycin is only agent shown to be effective in placebo-controlled, double-blind clinical trial; alternative choices include rifampin, gentamicin, trimethoprim-sulfamethoxazole, doxycycline, ciprofloxacin, and levofloxacin
	BACILLARY ANGIOMATOSIS				
	Erythromycin	500 mg p.o., q.i.d., for 2 mo (4 mo for osteomyelitis or peliosis hepatis)	First choice	250 mg (base) p.o., q.i.d.: $1.00–1.49/day	—

(continued)

Table 2 (continued)

Infection	Drug	Dosage	Relative Efficacy	Cost	Comments
Bartonella (*Bartonellosis*) (*continued*)	Doxycycline	100 mg p.o., b.i.d., for 2 mo (4 mo for osteomyelitis or peliosis hepatis)	First choice	$0.05–0.12/day	—
	Clarithromycin	500 mg p.o., b.i.d., for 2 mo (4 mo for osteomyelitis or peliosis hepatis)	Alternative choice	500 mg p.o., b.i.d.: $7.00–7.99/day	—
	Azithromycin	250 mg p.o., q.d., for 2 mo (4 mo for osteomyelitis or peliosis hepatis)	Alternative choice	250 mg p.o., q.d.: $6.00–6.99/day	—
	Ciprofloxacin	500–750 mg p.o., b.i.d., for 2 mo (4 mo for osteomyelitis or peliosis hepatis)	Alternative choice	500 mg p.o., b.i.d.: $7.00–7.99/day	—
	Doxycycline *plus* Rifampin	Doxycycline: 100 mg I.V./po., b.i.d., plus rifampin, 300 mg p.o., b.i.d., for 2 mo (4 mo for osteomyelitis or peliosis hepatis)	Alternative choice	$0.05–0.12/day	For severe or relapsed cases

*Note: Chloramphenicol is not distributed as an oral drug in the United States.

petechiae, and purpura. Other symptoms and signs will depend on specific organ involvement in individual cases.

Brucellosis can follow an acute, subacute, or chronic course. Untreated disease may persist for months to years and may cause a syndrome of relapsing fevers. Because the symptoms and signs of brucellosis may be nonspecific, it is important to obtain a detailed history that includes occupation, travel, exposure to animals, or ingestion of high-risk foods, such as unpasteurized dairy products[1,3–5] [*see Table 1*].

Laboratory Tests

The leukocyte count is typically normal or decreased. Anemia and thrombocytopenia are relatively common. The erythrocyte sedimentation rate is variable and rarely helpful.

Definitive diagnosis of brucellosis depends on isolation of the organism from blood, bone marrow, urine, cerebrospinal fluid, or other body fluids or tissues. The sensitivity of a single blood culture ranges from 15% to 70%, depending on the method used and the length of incubation. Because *Brucella* organisms grow slowly, cultures should be maintained for at least 4 weeks to increase recovery. The use of lysis centrifugation culture systems has been reported to hasten recovery. Culture of bone marrow is reportedly more sensitive than conventional blood culture.

Presumptive diagnosis of brucellosis can be made by serologic studies showing specific brucella IgG antibodies or the presence of IgM antibody to *Brucella*. [3–5,10] It should be noted that the standard brucella serum agglutination test does not detect antibodies to *B. canis*. In suspected *B. canis* infection, serologic tests specific for that species should be ordered. Molecular diagnosis using polymerase chain reaction has been developed but is currently not available for routine clinical use.[11]

DIFFERENTIAL DIAGNOSIS

The differential diagnosis of brucellosis includes enteric fever, malaria, infectious mononucleosis (Epstein-Barr virus [EBV] infection), atypical mononucleosis (cytomegalovirus infection), Q fever, miliary tuberculosis, subacute bacterial endocarditis, HIV infection, and visceral leishmaniasis (kala-azar).[4]

TREATMENT

Brucellosis requires prolonged treatment with a tetracycline, typically supplemented with a second antibiotic: an aminoglycoside, rifampin, or perhaps a fluoroquinolone[1,3–5] [*see Table 2*]. Significant resistance to trimethoprim-sulfamethoxazole has limited the use of this agent.[5] Recent studies from Spain and the Middle East suggest that the best initial regimen is doxycycline (100 mg p.o., b.i.d.) for 6 weeks, plus either gentamicin (3 to 5 mg/kg a day I.V. in divided doses) or streptomycin (1 g/day I.M.) for the first 2 to 3 weeks. Relapse occurs in approximately 6% of patients treated with this regimen.[12] Doxycycline can also be combined with 6 weeks of rifampin (600 to 900 mg p.o., b.i.d.), although relapse has been reported in approximately 15% of patients treated with this regimen.[13] Fluoroquinolones have demonstrated good activity against *Brucella* in vitro, but clinical results have been disappointing; therefore, those agents should be regarded as adjunctive rather than primary therapy.[13] Although corticosteroid therapy has been recommended for management of brucellosis involving the central nervous system, no controlled studies have demonstrated its efficacy. No satisfactory vaccines for human brucellosis are currently available.[1]

COMPLICATIONS

Brucellosis can cause complications in almost any organ system. Endocarditis occurs in less than 2% of cases but accounts for the majority of brucellosis-related deaths. Infected aneurysms of the brain, aorta, and other vessels can occur. Direct invasion of the central nervous system occurs in only about 5% of cases. Meningitis is the most frequent CNS complication. Bone and joint involvement is relatively common, with a reported occurrence of 20% to 60%. Sacroiliitis and spondylitis are the most common musculoskeletal complications.[14] The GI tract is involved in as many as 70% of patients. Inflammation of Peyer patches can cause ileitis or colitis. Brucellosis can cause granulomatous hepatitis, pyogenic hepatic abscesses, or cholecystitis. Although renal involvement in brucellosis is unusual, orchitis has been reported in 20% of men with brucellosis. Respiratory tract involvement in brucellosis ranges from flulike symptoms to pneumonia with or without pleural effusions. A variety of ocular complications have been reported, including uveitis and endophthalmitis.

PROGNOSIS

A relapse rate of 5% to 25% can be expected in patients treated for brucellosis, depending on the antibiotic regimen employed (see above). Relapse is especially common in spondylitis.[14] Mortality is highest in cases of endocarditis. Cardiac valve replacement surgery, in addition to prolonged antimicrobial therapy, is often required for successful resolution of endocarditis.[15]

Tularemia

Infection by *Francisella tularensis* causes clinical tularemia. This disease is a zoonosis of substantial complexity whose natural hosts or vectors include more than 100 species of wild mammals; several species of birds, fish, and amphibians; and more than 50 species of blood-sucking arthropods (including ticks, fleas, and deerflies). Tularemia has been recognized widely throughout the Northern Hemisphere, where it was formerly known by a variety of names, such as rabbit fever, deerfly fever, market men's disease, wild-hare disease, Ohara disease (Japan), and water-rat trappers' disease (Russia). *F. tularensis* could potentially be used in biological warfare or terrorism.[16]

EPIDEMIOLOGY

Tularemia is most commonly found in the temperate zones of the Northern Hemisphere. Five subspecies of *F. tularensis* have been recognized on the basis of biologic properties and geographic location. Type A biovar (*F. tularensis* biovar *tularensis*), the most virulent, is found only in North America, where it causes 70% to 90% of all cases of tularemia. This biovar is transmitted by infected rabbits and ticks, and untreated infection can be fatal. The less virulent type B biovar (*F. tularensis* biovar *palearctica*) is present in temperate zones worldwide. It is transmitted by rodents or aquatic animals and can cause mild or subclinical disease. *F. tularensis* biovar *palearctica mediasiatica* and *F. tularensis* biovar *palearctica japonica* are found in central Asia and Japan, respectively. *F. tularensis* biovar *novicida* rarely causes disease in humans or animals.

In the United States, human tularemia has been reported from every state except Hawaii.[17,18] In 1993, the last year in which tularemia was designated a notifiable disease by the Centers for Disease Control and Prevention (CDC), 132 cases were reported in the United States[19] [*see Figure 1*]. The disease clusters in the lower midwestern states, especially Arkansas, Oklahoma, and Missouri.[17,20]

The most important reservoirs of *F. tularensis* are rabbits, hares, and hard ticks.[18] The three major North American tick vectors of tularemia are *Dermacentor variabilis* (dog tick), which is widely distributed throughout North America; *Amblyomma americanum* (Lone star tick) in the southeastern and south central United States; and *D. andersoni* in the western United States. Infected *Ixodes* ticks can also transmit tularemia.[18,21,22] Aside from hard ticks, other reported arthropod vectors for transmission of tularemia to humans include deerflies, horseflies, and mosquitoes.[17,20,21]

Hunters, trappers, game wardens, veterinarians, meat handlers, laboratory workers, and pet owners are considered populations at increased risk for tularemia. However, as many as 40% of patients with tularemia relate no history of contact with a potential animal reservoir or arthropod vector.

ETIOLOGY

Humans generally acquire tularemia by direct contact with infected wild mammals or via bites

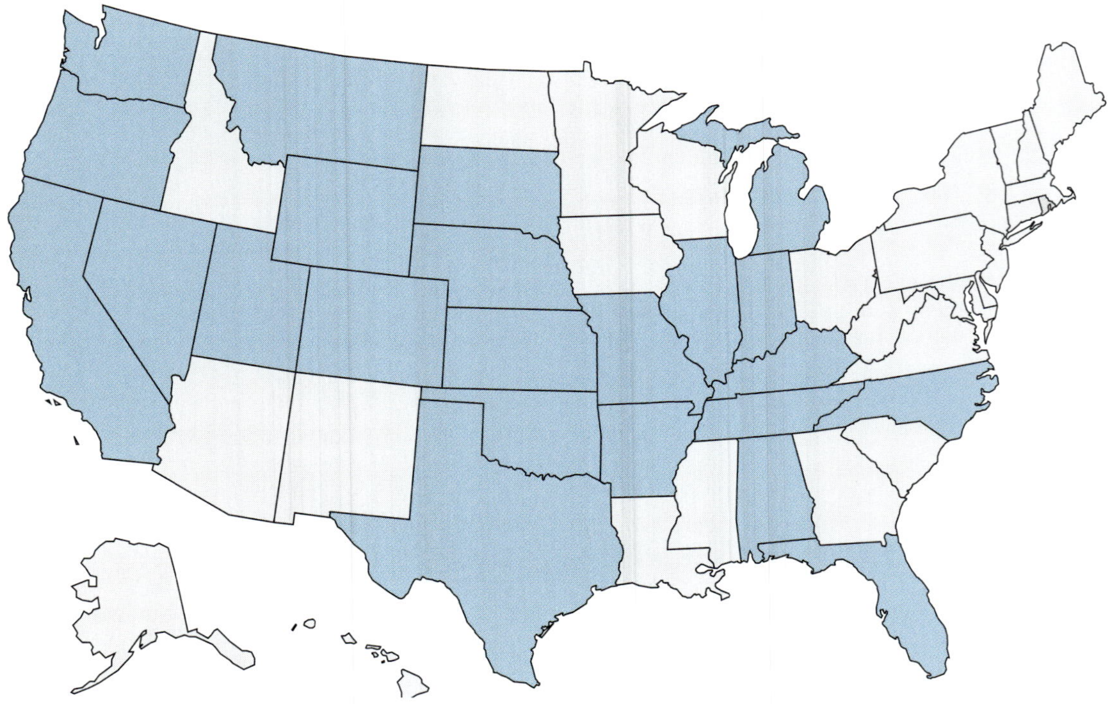

Figure 1 **States in blue are those reporting cases of tularemia in 1993.**

from infected arthropods. Domestic animals, such as pet cats and dogs that have preyed on infected wild animals, can serve as sources of tularemia transmission to humans via bites, scratches, or licks.[23,24] Transmission has also resulted from inhalation of aerosolized organisms or ingestion of contaminated meat or water.[17,18,25] No documented human-to-human transmission of tularemia has been reported.[17,18,25,26]

The etiology of human tularemia shows some seasonal variation. During the summer, most cases occur as a result of arthropod bites. During the fall and winter, hunters and trappers may acquire tularemia while skinning and dressing wild game.

PATHOGENESIS

F. tularensis is a small, pleomorphic, nonmotile, intracellular, gram-negative coccobacillus that grows fastidiously as an obligate aerobe. In culture, it requires cysteine-enriched blood agar for growth. In the environment, it can remain viable at low temperatures for 3 to 4 months in mud, water, or decayed animal carcasses.

F. tularensis is highly infectious. As few as 10 to 50 organisms can cause clinical tularemia after inhalation or intradermal injection, and 10^8 organisms can cause disease if ingested. The skin and mucous membranes are the most common portals of entry for *F. tularensis*. After inoculation, the organism multiplies locally to produce an erythematous, tender papule within 2 to 5 days, which subsequently becomes an ulcer with a black base (chancriform lesion). Bacteria then usually spread to regional lymph nodes, causing lymphadenopathy. Sepsis syndrome can occur with bacteremia or in cases of widely disseminated disease.

Histopathologically, tularemia is characteristically associated with mononuclear cell infiltration and granuloma formation. Those features can resemble the pathology of tuberculosis.

DIAGNOSIS

Clinical Manifestations

The usual incubation period of tularemia is 3 to 7 days (range, 1 to 21 days). Classically, tularemia presents as a severe illness with a sudden onset of fever, chills, headache, malaise, fatigue, and generalized myalgias and arthralgias. However, the severity of illness, especially in tick-borne disease, is highly variable, ranging from mild, afebrile, self-limited disease to rare cases of septic shock. Typically, an ulcer with surrounding inflammation develops at the site of inoculation. The inoculation ulcer may persist for weeks to months in untreated cases.

Most patients (70% to 90%) acquire infection by inoculation of the skin. Regional lymphadenopathy often develops in the inguinal/femoral nodes in adults and the cervical nodes in children. A generalized rash, usually maculopapular but occasionally pustular, is seen in approximately 20% of patients. Erythema nodosum has been reported infrequently.

The clinical manifestations of tularemia have been categorized into six recognized syndromes: (1) ulceroglandular, (2) glandular, (3) oculoglandular, (4) oropharyngeal, (5) pleuropulmonary, and (6) typhoidal.

Ulceroglandular tularemia and glandular tularemia are the most common forms of clinical tularemia, accounting for 75% to 85% of cases. Both result from inoculation of the skin. Ulceroglandular disease is characterized by an ulcerated lesion at the site of inoculation and regional lymphadenopathy. The glandular and ulceroglandular syndromes are similar except that the skin lesion is absent in glandular tularemia.

Oculoglandular tularemia is caused by accidental inoculation of the eye with contaminated fingers. Conjunctival inflammation is extremely painful, and numerous ulcers and a yellow exudate are often apparent. Conjunctival involvement is typically associated with preauricular lymphadenopathy (Parinaud complex).

Oropharyngeal tularemia can follow oral inoculation. This syndrome is characterized by an exudative or membranous pharyngitis and cervical lymphadenopathy. A subcategory of oropharyngeal tularemia that can develop after massive ingestion of *F. tularensis* is gastrointestinal tularemia. It is characterized by fever, intestinal ulceration, mesenteric lymphadenopathy, diarrhea, abdominal pain, nausea, vomiting, and gastrointestinal bleeding.

Pleuropulmonary tularemia can be a primary infection, following inhalation of aerosolized organisms, or a secondary manifestation resulting from hematogenous spread of infection to the lungs. The latter occurs in about 10% to 15% of cases of ulceroglandular tularemia. Mediastinal lymphadenopathy may evolve during the course of pleuropulmonary tularemia.

Typhoidal tularemia is the most difficult presentation to diagnose and is associated with the highest mortality.[17,18,25–27] Neither skin lesions nor lymphadenopathy are present; fever and malaise may be the only clinical manifestations. Secondary pleuropulmonary involvement occurs in approximately 50% of cases of typhoidal tularemia.

Laboratory Tests

Laboratory screening tests are often unremarkable in cases of tularemia. The leukocyte count may be slightly elevated or normal. Serum levels of hepatic aminotransferases tend to be mildly to moderately elevated. With pleuropulmonary involvement, chest films show parenchymal infiltrates (typically patchy, in one or multiple lobes), and pleural effusions are common.[17,18,25,26]

Definitive laboratory diagnosis of tularemia is generally based on detection of antibodies to *F. tularensis*. Serum agglutinins are usually detectable by day 10 to 14 of illness and peak approximately 2 to 6 weeks later. Early, appropriate antimicrobial therapy may blunt the rise in antibody titer. A fourfold increase in titer between acute-phase and convalescent-phase specimens is considered diagnostic, but a single specimen with a titer of 1:160 or greater is highly suggestive. A specific enzyme-linked immunosorbent assay (ELISA) for *F. tularensis* antibodies is now available and may eventually replace the serum agglutinins assay. PCR technology has been employed for molecular diagnosis but is not widely available for clinical use.[28–30]

Airborne transmission of *F. tularensis* is possible, so attempts to isolate and culture the organism should be avoided in most clinical laboratories. Biosafety level 2 is recommended for clinical laboratory work with material where contamination with *F. tularensis* is suspected. Biosafety level 3 is required for culture of the organism in large quantities.[31]

DIFFERENTIAL DIAGNOSIS

The skin lesion of ulceroglandular tularemia may resemble that seen in sporotrichosis, ecthyma from *Staphylococcus aureus* or *Streptococcus pyogenes*, skin infection with atypical mycobacteria (e.g., *Mycobacterium marinum*), syphilis, anthrax, rat-bite fever, or rickettsial disease. The lymphadenopathy of tularemia may be similar to that of plague, lymphogranuloma venereum, cat-scratch disease, or necrotizing lymphadenitis. Oropharyngeal tularemia can mimic the exudative pharyngitis caused by *S. pyogenes, Arcanobacterium haemolyticus, Corynebacterium diphtheriae,* and EBV. Pleuropulmonary tularemia is often similar to any of the atypical pneumonias, including those caused by respiratory viruses, *Mycoplasma pneumoniae, Legionella pneumophila, Chlamydia pneumoniae, C. psittaci, Coxiella burnetii, Histoplasma capsulatum,* and *Coccidioides immitis*.[26] Typhoidal tularemia may be confused with enteric fever (typhoid or paratyphoid fever), rickettsial infections, brucellosis, EBV, primary toxoplasmosis, miliary tuberculosis, sarcoidosis, or lymphoma.

TREATMENT

Because of the lack of rapid diagnostic laboratory tests for tularemia, initial treatment is often empirical and based on clinical suspicion. Although streptomycin (500 mg to 1 g I.M. every 12 hours) is the conventional drug of choice, evidence indicates that gentamicin (3 to 5 mg/kg daily I.V. in divided doses every 8 hours) is equally effective. With either agent, treatment should be given for 10 to 14 days in cases of severe clinical illness.[32] Tetracycline (or chloramphenicol) can be used, but relapse may occur if the duration of therapy is less than 21 days.[33] Ciprofloxacin was recently reported to be effective for treatment, but clinical experience is limited.[34–36]

Only partial immunity develops after infection with *F. tularensis*, and cases of reinfection have been documented. Chemoprophylaxis is not recommended for persons potentially exposed to tularemia. A live attenuated tularemia vaccine has been developed. It may be useful for the partial protection of laboratory workers but is not commerciallyavailable.[37,38]

COMPLICATIONS

Tularemia can be complicated by bacteremia, meningitis (usually marked by a lymphocytic pleocytosis in the CSF), rhabdomyolysis, acute renal failure, endocarditis, osteomyelitis, pericarditis, and septic shock.

PROGNOSIS

Typhoidal and ulceroglandular tularemia have the worst prognosis, with approximately 5% mortality reported in untreated cases. Prognosis is excellent for patients treated with appropriate antibiotics, with significant clinical improvement generally occurring within 48 hours of starting therapy.[17,18,25]

Plague

Yersinia infections primarily affect rodents, pigs, and birds; humans are accidental hosts. Nevertheless, *Yersinia pestis* (formerly *Pasteurella pestis*) has made its mark in human history as the causative agent of plague—also known as bubonic plague, black plague, and the Black Death. Plague was initially described in biblical times; in the Middle Ages, epidemic bubonic plague killed an estimated one fourth of Europe's population.[39] This disease of antiquity has persisted to the present. Although human plague is now relatively infrequent worldwide, aerosolized *Y. pestis* is well recognized for its potential use as a biological weapon.[40]

EPIDEMIOLOGY

Plague currently exists in widely scattered foci in Asia, Africa, and the Americas. In the 1990s, countries with the greatest number of cases included Tanzania, Madagascar, Democratic Republic of Congo, Vietnam, Peru, India, Myanmar, Zimbabwe, Mozambique, Uganda, and China [*see Figure 2*]. In the United States, about 10 cases of plague are reported annually, primarily from the Four Corners area, where Utah, Colorado, New Mexico, and Arizona meet. In that region, plague is endemic in prairie dog colonies.[41,42]

ETIOLOGY

Plague is a zoonotic infection that affects predominately urban and sylvatic rodents (e.g., rats and ground squirrels, respectively). It is transmitted to its natural animal reservoirs by flea bites or ingestion of contaminated animal tissues. Humans represent accidental hosts who usually acquire infection via bites from infected fleas.[39] Bites or scratches from an infected animal can also transmit plague to humans. In endemic areas, risk factors for acquiring plague include direct contact with rodents or carnivores that prey on them (e.g., cats, dogs), the presence of wild rodents near the place of residence, and pet dogs or cats with fleas.[43]

Plague may also result from inhalation of aerosolized bacilli. Airborne transmission can occur via the cough of an infected patient with pulmonary involvement or from close contact with an infected animal or cadaver.

PATHOGENESIS

Y. pestis is a pleomorphic, non–spore-forming, gram-negative, bipolar-staining coccobacillary member of the family Enterobacteriaceae. It is a nonmotile, facultative anaerobe that is able to grow aerobically on routine microbiologic media. The organism can survive at room temperature in dried blood or the environment for weeks to months.

Y. pestis is one of the most virulent bacteria known. It is usually inoculated through the skin or mucous membranes, where it invades cutaneous lymphatics. Monocytes and macrophages, which can phagocytize *Y. pestis* without killing it, may play a role in spread of infection from the inocula-

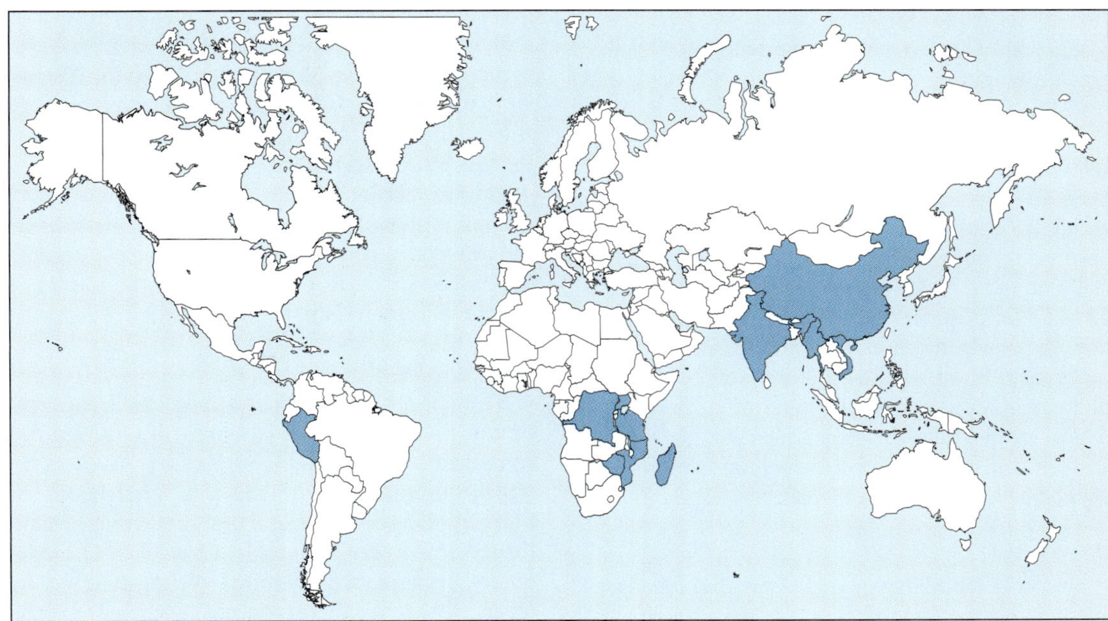

Figure 2 **Shaded countries reported more than 100 cases of plague from 1990–1995.**

tion site. Plague can involve almost any tissue or organ and cause massive destruction if left untreated. Initially, infected lymph nodes are tender and edematous. Later, hemorrhagic necrosis develops in affected nodes, and bacteria enter the bloodstream, where they disseminate to other sites (e.g., liver, spleen, lungs, and central nervous system). Infarcts and hemorrhagic, necrotic nodules are characteristic histopathologic findings at affected tissue sites.[39]

DIAGNOSIS

Clinical Manifestations

The usual incubation periods for bubonic plague and pneumonic plague are 2 to 7 days and 2 to 3 days, respectively (range, 1 to 14 days). Plague generally presents as an acute illness characterized by the abrupt onset of fever, chills, headache, gastrointestinal symptoms, and local pain, followed within hours by the development of a painful, swollen mass of lymph nodes (buboes) in the groin or axilla. Skin overlying buboes is usually red-purple in color. Buboes are initially tense and hard but rapidly become fluctuant. Spontaneous rupture and drainage can occur. Buboes do not develop in patients with septicemic plague; instead, these patients have gastrointestinal signs and symptoms: nausea, vomiting, diarrhea, and abdominal pain. Severe pharyngitis, severe diarrhea, and cough with or without hemoptysis may also be early clinical manifestations of plague[39,44] [*see Table 1*].

Laboratory Tests

The leukocyte count is typically elevated in the range of 15,000 to 25,000 cells/µl, with a shift to the left; leukemoid reactions (> 50,000 cells/µl) can occur. The platelet count may be normal or mildly depressed or may be very low if disseminated intravascular coagulation (DIC) is present. The level of fibrin split products is frequently elevated, even in patients without frank DIC. Serum levels of hepatic aminotransferases and bilirubin are often increased.

Definitive diagnosis of plague is usually based on isolation of *Y. pestis* from cultures of blood, other body fluids, or tissues. Aspiration of buboes may readily yield material for diagnosis. The organism can be easily grown on blood and MacConkey agar, as well as in infusion broth. A direct immunofluorescence test has been developed for rapid identification of *Y. pestis* in clinical specimens, and a passive hemagglutination test is available for presumptive diagnosis based on serology. Both of those tests are available from the CDC Division of Vector-Borne Infectious Diseases, Fort Collins, Colorado (970-221-6400).

DIFFERENTIAL DIAGNOSIS

Clinical suspicion based on knowledge of plague epidemiology is essential for timely diagnosis and institution of appropriate antimicrobial therapy. Plague should be suspected in febrile individuals who have been exposed to rodents or other mammals in regions of the world where plague is endemic. Illness may resemble that caused by a number of other serious infectious diseases, especially tularemia. Other causes of acute, painful lymphadenitis include staphylococcal, streptococcal, and *Pasteurella* infection. Plague pneumonia can be confused with other causes of atypical pneumonia or the hantavirus pulmonary syndrome. The combination of plague-associated abdominal symptoms and DIC can resemble an acute surgical abdomen or *Capnocytophaga canimorsus* sepsis.[44]

TREATMENT

Streptomycin (30 mg/kg I.M. in divided doses every 12 hours) remains the drug of choice for the treatment of plague. Timely administration of streptomycin reduces mortality to approximately 5%. Gentamicin, which is more widely available than streptomycin, also appears to be effective. To prevent relapses, antibiotic treatment should be continued for 10 days or for at least 3 days after defervescence and clinical recovery. Most patients improve rapidly and defervesce within 72 hours of initiation of antimicrobial therapy, although buboes can persist for weeks. Some authorities advocate switching from streptomycin to a different antibiotic for completion of therapy after 5 days of treatment in order to minimize the risk of ototoxicity and nephrotoxicity.

Tetracycline or doxycycline can also be used for plague. Chloramphenicol is the preferred agent for the treatment of plague meningitis, pleuritis, endophthalmitis, and myocarditis because of superior penetration into those tissues. Penicillins, cephalosporins, and macrolides are suboptimal agents for treatment of plague. Trimethoprim-sulfamethoxazole and fluoroquinolones appear to be active against plague in vitro and in animal models, but clinical experience with these agents for the treatment of plague is limited[39,44,45] [*see Table 2*].

All cases of suspected or documented plague should be reported to the state and city or county health departments, the CDC, and the World Health Organization. Plague patients with cough or other signs or symptoms of pneumonia should be placed in strict respiratory isolation for at least 48 hours after initiation of appropriate antibiotic therapy.

Contacts of patients with pneumonic plague or suspected septicemic plague with pulmonary involvement should receive chemoprophylaxis with either tetracycline (500 mg p.o., q.i.d.) or doxycycline (100 mg p.o., b.i.d.). Streptomycin (20 mg/kg/day I.M. in two divided doses) or trimethoprim-sulfamethoxazole (40 mg/kg p.o., b.i.d.) can be used for children younger than 8 years.

Plague vaccine (Cutter Laboratories) is a killed, formalin/phenol-fixed whole-bacteria vaccine that provides only partial protection against infection. Vaccinated individuals who are exposed to plague should still receive chemoprophylaxis.[46]

COMPLICATIONS

Septic shock, DIC, acute respiratory distress syndrome (ARDS), and meningitis are recognized complications of plague, especially in cases in which antimicrobial therapy is inadequate or delayed. Plague meningitis, a rare complication that typically occurs more than 1 week after inadequate antimicrobial therapy, is characterized by fever, headache, meningismus, and neutrophilic pleocytosis of the cerebrospinal fluid.

PROGNOSIS

Reported mortality of untreated plague ranges from 40% to 90%. Mortality is greatest in pneumonic plague. The overall mortality for cases of plague in the United States during the past 20 years has been approximately 15%.[42]

Bartonella Infections

Bartonella (formerly *Rochalimaea*) organisms are small, gram-negative bacilli that are extremely fastidious. They require specialized culture methods for isolation and specific staining techniques for detection in clinical specimens.[47–49] Infections by these organisms can occur in both immunocompromised and immunocompetent individuals.[47,49] Four *Bartonella* species have been documented to be pathogenic in humans: *B. bacilliformis, B. quintana, B. henselae,* and *B. elizabethae.*[47,49] The spectrum of diseases caused by *Bartonella* can be divided into five categories: (1) Oroya fever (classic bartonellosis), (2) trench fever, (3) bacteremia and endocarditis, (4) cat-scratch disease, and (5) bacillary angiomatosis.

OROYA FEVER (CLASSIC BARTONELLOSIS)

Oroya fever (chronic bartonellosis; Carrión disease) is caused by infection with *B. bacilliformis* transmitted to humans by the bite of infected phlebotomine sandflies. The disease is geographically restricted to valleys of the Andes Mountains at elevations between 800 m (2,624 ft) and 2,500 m (8,200 ft) above sea level, which are found in Peru, Ecuador, and Colombia.

Diagnosis

Oroya fever, caused by primary bacteremia, develops 3 to 12 weeks after inoculation. The onset of illness can be either insidious or abrupt. Clinical manifestations include fever, chills, headache, myalgias and arthralgias, abdominal pain, generalized lymphadenopathy, progressive hemolytic anemia, and thrombocytopenia.[47,49,50]

Definitive diagnosis of acute bartonellosis is based on the isolation of *B. bacilliformis* from blood cultures. The organism can be grown on Colombia agar with 5% defibrinated human blood or semisolid nutrient agar with 10% rabbit hemoglobin aerobically at 28° C. Colonies usually appear in 7 to 10 days. The presence of intraerythrocytic bacilli in a Giemsa-stained thin blood smear provides rapid confirmation of acute bartonellosis. Serologic tests have been developed in research laboratories but are not widely available.[47,49]

Treatment

Standard treatment consists of chloramphenicol (2 g/day p.o. or I.V.) for at least 1 week. Alternative agents include tetracycline (or doxycycline) or ampicillin.[51] Without treatment, mortality is high. Survivors are temporarily at risk for secondary salmonellosis or toxoplasmosis. Asymptomatic bacteremia is estimated to persist in approximately 15% of survivors.

In untreated cases, resolution of primary infection may be followed weeks to months later by the onset of verruca peruana. This manifestation of chronic bartonellosis consists of recurrent crops of nodular skin lesions, which may ulcerate and bleed. Mucosal and visceral lesions may also occur. Histopathologic examination of active lesions demonstrates neovascular proliferation and occasional bacilli in the interstitium.[47,49]

TRENCH FEVER

Trench fever is caused by infection with *B. quintana,* which is transmitted to humans via feces of infected human body lice (*Pediculus humanus*).[52] Epidemics of the disease occurred in troops engaged in trench warfare in World War I and in World War II troops deployed in crowded and unsanitary conditions.

Diagnosis

The incubation period of classic trench fever was 3 to 38 days, and illness was typically characterized by the abrupt onset of fever, associated with headache, dizziness, conjunctival injection, myalgias, arthralgias, hepatosplenomegaly, a transient maculopapular rash, leukocytosis, and albuminuria. The duration of acute illness was generally 3 to 5 days, and relapses were not uncommon. Less commonly, unremitting fever would persist for 2 to 6 weeks.[47,49]

Treatment

Much of the clinical experience with trench fever predates the antibiotic era. It is not known whether one regimen is superior to another.

BACTEREMIA AND ENDOCARDITIS

Recently, a syndrome termed urban trench fever was recognized in urban homeless persons (usually with a history of alcoholism and malnutrition) and in HIV-infected individuals.[47,49,53,54] In the urban homeless population, the syndrome is caused by *B. quintana* bacteremia and is often associated with apparently culture-negative endocarditis.[47,49,53–56] In the HIV-infected population, the bacteremia can be caused by either *B. quintana* or *B. henselae,* and concomitant bacillary angiomatosis (see below) is often present.[47,49,57,58] As with classic trench fever, the human body louse is the vector for transmission of *B. quintana* (the animal reservoir remains unknown); cats transmit *B. henselae.* Clinical manifestations of urban trench fever include fever, malaise, anemia, thrombocytopenia, splenomegaly, and cardiac murmurs.[47,49,53–56]

Diagnosis

Diagnosis is based on the isolation of *B. henselae* or *B. quintana* from blood, which is best accomplished using lysis-centrifugation blood culture. Growth of those organisms is slow, and incubation for more than 30 days may be required. Acridine orange staining can be used to enhance detection of *Bartonella* organisms in culture. An antibody titer of 1:1,600 or higher against either *B. henselae* or *B. quintana* also strongly suggests bartonellosis as the cause of endocarditis in a patient with valvular vegetations.[47,49]

Treatment

For bacteremia without endocarditis, a 14-day regimen of either a macrolide or a tetracycline (e.g., doxycycline, 100 mg p.o., b.i.d.) is recommended. No definitive treatment regimen has been established for endocarditis. Surgical valve replacement plus aminoglycoside therapy has been used. An alternative approach has been to give prolonged (4 to 6 months or more) combination therapy with a fluoroquinolone plus either rifampin or a macrolide. Patients treated with that regimen should be followed carefully for clinical deterioration that would necessitate valve replacement[47,49,54–56] [*see Table 2*].

CAT-SCRATCH DISEASE

Although *Afipia felis* was first identified as the causative agent of cat-scratch disease, it is now clear that *B. henselae* causes the overwhelming majority of cases.[47,49,59] The domestic cat serves as the major reservoir of *B. henselae*, which is transmitted to humans by a scratch or bite—usually from a kitten or feral cat—or possibly via infected cat fleas.[47,49] The incubation period is generally 3 to 10 days.

Typically, a primary cutaneous papule or pustule develops at the site of inoculation. Regional lymphadenopathy follows in approximately 90% of cases and persists for 10 to 120 days. Lymphadenopathy is most common at axillary, cervical, and submandibular sites. Less commonly, epitrochlear, inguinal, femoral, or supraclavicular nodes may be involved. Approximately 10% of involved nodes suppurate spontaneously. Low-grade fever occurs in approximately 50% of patients and lasts for several days. Less frequent symptoms and signs include malaise, fatigue, headache, and rash.[47,49]

Relatively common presentations of atypical cat-scratch disease are Parinaud oculoglandular syndrome—a self-limited syndrome of granulomatous conjunctivitis and preauricular lymphadenitis—and encephalitis, which occurs primarily in children.[47,49,60,61] About one half of patients with cat-scratch disease encephalitis experience seizures. Although full recovery from cat-scratch disease encephalitis may require weeks to months, the overall prognosis is good, with few patients experiencing permanent neurologic sequelae.[47,49,61] Other atypical manifestations of cat-scratch disease include self-limited granulomatous hepatitis or splenitis, atypical pneumonitis, osteitis, and neuroretinitis.[47,49,62–66]

Most cases of cat-scratch disease are diagnosed presumptively, on the basis of the clinical presentation and a history of exposure to cats. The differential diagnosis of typical cat-scratch disease includes tularemia, mycobacterial infection, plague, brucellosis, mononucleosis, syphilis, lymphogranuloma venereum, sporotrichosis, histoplasmosis, toxoplasmosis, and lymphoma.

Serologic confirmation of cat-scratch disease is usually not required. When clinically warranted, either immunofluorescence antibody testing or ELISA, available through commercial clinical diagnostic laboratories, can be used to detect antibodies against *B. henselae*. Those serologic studies have essentially supplanted the cat-scratch disease skin test in clinical practice. In biopsy specimens obtained from lymph nodes, skin, or conjunctiva, cat-scratch disease can be confirmed by the detection of small, pleomorphic bacilli in sections prepared with a Warthin-Starry or Brown-Hopps stain.[47–49] PCR technology has been used to detect *B. henselae* in clinical specimens but is currently not widely available for routine clinical diagnosis.[47–49,67]

In immunocompetent patients, both typical and atypical CSD generally resolve spontaneously without antimicrobial therapy. Most *B. henselae* isolates are susceptible in vitro to a wide variety of antimicrobials, including β-lactams, tetracyclines, macrolides, aminoglycosides, fluoroquinolones, vancomycin, and rifampin. However, clinical response does not correlate well with susceptibility testing for *B. henselae*.[47,49,68] Although a variety of agents have been reported to be effective in anecdotal reports and case series (including rifampin, gentamicin, trimethoprim-sulfamethoxazole, doxycycline, ciprofloxacin, and ofloxacin), only azithromycin (500 mg p.o. for 1 day, then 250 mg p.o. daily for 4 days) has been shown to accelerate resolution of typical cat-scratch disease lymphadenopathy in a placebo-controlled, double-blind clinical trial.[69]

BACILLARY ANGIOMATOSIS

Bacillary angiomatosis (epithelioid angiomatosis, bacillary epithelioid angiomatosis) is a form of neovascular proliferation associated with infection by either *B. henselae* or *B. quintana*. It was first described as a disease of the skin and regional lymph nodes of HIV-infected persons. Subsequently, bacillary angiomatosis was documented in a large variety of tissues, including liver, spleen, bone, brain, respiratory tract, gastrointestinal tract, and uterine cervix. It has also been found, albeit rarely, in other immunocompromised hosts and in apparently immunocompetent patients. In HIV-infected persons, it is a relatively late opportunistic infection, usually occurring after the $CD4^+$ lymphocyte count has declined to less than 100 cells/μl.[47,49,57,58]

Cutaneous disease is the most frequently recognized manifestation of bacillary angiomatosis. Lesions generally appear in crops and can have verrucous, papular, or pedunculated features. They often have an erythematous base and vascular appearance but may occasionally be dry, scaly, hyperkeratotic, or plaquelike. Painful subcutaneous nodules and osseous lesions can develop. Regional lymphadenopathy is common, but involved nodes rarely suppurate or drain.[47,49]

Peliosis hepatis, consisting of venous lakes in the hepatic parenchyma, is a relatively common manifestation of bacillary angiomatosis. Splenitis can also occur. Hepatosplenomegaly is often present, and an increased serum alkaline phosphatase level is a common laboratory finding. Peliotic spaces in the liver and spleen appear as hypodense lesions on abdominal computed tomography. Thrombocytopenia and pancytopenia may develop, as well as concomitant bacteremia or endocarditis, in patients with bacillary peliosis.[47,49,57,58]

The lesions of bacillary angiomatosis may be indistinguishable clinically from Kaposi sarcoma, and biopsy is usually necessary to distinguish between the two disorders and guide management. Both hematoxylin-eosin staining, which differentiates bacillary angiomatosis from Kaposi sarcoma, and Warthin-Starry staining, which detects *Bartonella* bacilli, should be performed on biopsy specimens. Lesions of bacillary angiomatosis are characterized by lobular proliferation of endothelial-lined capillaries; the endothelial cells are protuberant, unlike the spindle-shaped endothelial cells in Kaposi sarcoma. Recovery of *Bartonella* organisms by culture from lesions of bacillary angiomatosis is difficult.[47–49]

The recommended first-line therapy for bacillary angiomatosis in HIV-infected patients is either erythromycin (500 mg p.o., q.i.d.) or doxycycline (100 mg p.o., b.i.d.). Alternative agents include clarithromycin (500 mg p.o., b.i.d.), azithromycin (250 mg p.o. daily), and ciprofloxacin (500 to 750 mg p.o., b.i.d.). For severe cases, consideration should be given to combination therapy with doxycycline (100 mg p.o. or I.V., b.i.d.) plus rifampin (300 mg p.o., b.i.d.). Bacillary angiomatosis usually responds rapidly to either erythromycin or doxycycline therapy. A Jarisch-Herxheimer reaction may occur with the initiation of antimicrobial therapy. Patients who have only cutaneous lesions should receive at least 2 months of treatment; in those with osteomyelitis or peliosis hepatis, therapy should be continued for a minimum of 4 months. Relapses can occur after discontinuance of therapy. HIV-infected patients who experience relapses should be treated lifelong with either a tetracycline or a macrolide.[47,49]

References

1. Corbel MJ: Brucellosis: an overview. Emerg Infect Dis 3:213, 1997

2. Leggiadro RJ: The threat of biological terrorism: a public health and infection control reality. Infect Control Hosp Epidemiol 21:53, 2000

3. Solera J, Martinez-Alfaro E, Espinosa A: Recognition and optimum treatment of brucellosis. Drugs 53:245, 1997

4. Sanford JP: *Brucella* pneumonia. Semin Respir Infect 12:24, 1997

5. Memish Z, Mah MW, Al Mahmoud S, et al: *Brucella* bacteraemia: clinical and laboratory observations in 160 patients. J Infect 40:59, 2000

6. Fiori PL, Mastrandrea S, Rappelli P, et al: *Brucella abortus* infection acquired in microbiology laboratories. J Clin Microbiol 38:2005, 2000

7. Summary of notifiable diseases, United States—1999. MMWR Morb Mortal Wkly Rep 48:1, 2001

8. Doyle TJ, Bryan RT: Infectious disease morbidity in the US region bordering Mexico, 1990–1998. J Infect Dis 182:1502, 2000

9. Ertem M, Kurekci AE, Aysev D, et al: Brucellosis transmitted by bone marrow transplantation. Bone Marrow Transplant 26:225, 2000

10. Gad El-Rab MO, Kambal AM: Evaluation of a *Brucella* enzyme immunoassay test (ELISA) in comparison with bacteriological culture and agglutination. J Infect 36:197, 1998

11. Morata P, Queipo-Ortuno MI, Reguera JM, et al: Posttreatment follow-up of brucellosis by PCR assay. J Clin Microbiol 37:4163, 1999

12. Solera J, Espinosa A, Martinez-Alfaro E, et al: Treatment of human brucellosis with doxycycline and gentamicin. Antimicrob Agents Chemother 41:80, 1997

13. Agalar C, Usubuntun S, Turkyilmaz R: Ciprofloxacin and rifampicin versus doxycycline and rifampicin in the treatment of brucellosis. Eur J Clin Microbiol Infect Dis 18:535, 1999

14. Solera J, Lozano E, Martinez-Alfaro E, et al: Brucellar spondylitis: review of 35 cases and literature survey. Clin Infect Dis 29:1440, 1999

15. Uddin MJ, Sanyal SC, Mustafa AS, et al: The role of aggressive medical therapy along with early surgical intervention in the cure of *Brucella* endocarditis. Ann Thorac Cardiovasc Surg 4:209, 1998

16. Franz DR, Jahrling PB, Friedlander AM, et al: Clinical recognition and management of patients exposed to biological warfare agents. JAMA 278:399, 1997

17. Boyce JM: Recent trends in the epidemiology of tularemia in the United States. J Infect Dis 131:197, 1975

18. Spach DH, Liles WC, Campbell GL, et al: Tick-borne diseases in the United States. N Engl J Med 329:936, 1993

19. Summary of notifiable diseases, United States, 1993. MMWR Morb Mortal Wkly Rep 42:i, 1, 1994

20. Taylor JP, Istre GR, McChesney TC, et al: Epidemiologic characteristics of human tularemia in the southwest-central states, 1981–1987. Am J Epidemiol 133:1032, 1991

21. Guerrant RL, Humphries MK Jr, Butler JE, et al: Tickborne oculoglandular tularemia: case report and review of seasonal and vectorial associations in 106 cases. Arch Intern Med 136:811, 1976

22. Markowitz LE, Hynes NA, de la Cruz P, et al: Tick-borne tularemia: an outbreak of lymphadenopathy in children. JAMA 254:2922, 1985

23. Liles WC, Burger RJ: Tularemia from domestic cats. West J Med 158:619, 1993

24. Capellan J, Fong IW: Tularemia from a cat bite: case report and review of feline-associated tularemia. Clin Infect Dis 16:472, 1993

25. Evans ME, Gregory DW, Schaffner W, et al: Tularemia: a 30-year experience with 88 cases. Medicine (Baltimore) 64:251, 1985

26. Gill V, Cunha BA: Tularemia pneumonia. Semin Respir Infect 12: 61, 1997

27. Penn RL, Kinasewitz GT: Factors associated with a poor outcome in tularemia. Arch Intern Med 147:265, 1987

28. Fulop M, Leslie D, Titball R: A rapid, highly sensitive method for the detection of *Francisella tularensis* in clinical samples using the polymerase chain reaction. Am J Trop Med Hyg 54:364, 1996

29. Johansson A, Berglund L, Eriksson U, et al: Comparative analysis of PCR versus culture for diagnosis of ulceroglandular tularemia. J Clin Microbiol 38:22, 2000

30. Junhui Z, Ruifu Y, Jianchun L, et al: Detection of Francisella tularensis by the polymerase chain reaction. J Med Microbiol 45:477, 1996

31. Pike RM: Laboratory-associated infections: summary and analysis of 3921 cases. Health Lab Sci 13:105, 1976

32. Mason WL, Eigelsbach HT, Little SF, et al: Treatment of tularemia, including pulmonary tularemia, with gentamicin. Am Rev Respir Dis 121:39, 1980

33. Risi GF, Pombo DJ: Relapse of tularemia after aminoglycoside therapy: case report and discussion of therapeutic options. Clin Infect Dis 20:174, 1995

34. Limaye AP, Hooper CJ: Treatment of tularemia with fluoroquinolones: two cases and review. Clin Infect Dis 29:922, 1999

35. Johansson A, Berglund L, Gothefors L, et al: Ciprofloxacin for treatment of tularemia in children. Pediatr Infect Dis J 19:449, 2000

36. Ikaheimo I, Syrjala H, Karhukorpi J, et al: In vitro antibiotic susceptibility of *Francisella tularensis* isolated from humans and animals. J Antimicrob Chemother 46:287, 2000

37. Burke DS: Immunization against tularemia: analysis of the effectiveness of live *Francisella tularensis* vaccine in prevention of laboratory-acquired tularemia. J Infect Dis 135:55, 1977

38. Waag DM, Sandstrom G, England MJ, et al: Immunogenicity of a new lot of *Francisella tularensis* live vaccine strain in human volunteers. FEMS Immunol Med Microbiol 13:205, 1996

39. Perry RD, Fetherston JD: *Yersinia pestis*—etiologic agent of plague. Clin Microbiol Rev 10:35, 1997

40. Inglesby TV, Dennis DT, Henderson DA, et al: Plague as a biological weapon: medical and public health management. Working Group on Civilian Biodefense. JAMA 283:2281, 2000

41. Fatal human plague—Arizona and Colorado, 1996. MMWR Morb Mortal Wkly Rep 46:617, 1997

42. Summary of notifiable diseases, United States—1999. MMWR Morb Mortal Wkly Rep 48:1, 2001

43. Gage KL, Dennis DT, Orloski KA, et al: Cases of cat-associated human plague in the Western US, 1997–1998. Clin Infect Dis 30:893, 2000

44. Cleri DJ, Vernaleo JR, Lombardi LJ, et al: Plague pneumonia disease caused by *Yersinia pestis*. Semin Respir Infect 12:12, 1997

45. Wong JD, Barash JR, Sandfort RF, et al: Susceptibilities of *Yersinia pestis* strains to 12 antimicrobial agents. Antimicrob Agents Chemother 44:1995, 2000

46. Prevention of plague: recommendations of the Advisory Committee on Immunization Practices (ACIP). MMWR Morb Mortal Wkly Rep 45:1, 1996

47. Spach DH, Koehler JE: *Bartonella*-associated infections. Infect Dis Clin North Am 12:137, 1998

48. Doern GV: Detection of selected fastidious bacteria. Clin Infect Dis 30:166, 2000

49. Maguina C, Gotuzzo E: Bartonellosis: new and old. Infect Dis Clin North Am 14:1, 2000

50. Kosek M, Lavarello R, Gilman RH, et al: Natural history of infection with *Bartonella bacilliformis* in a nonendemic population. J Infect Dis 182:865, 2000

51. Sobraques M, Maurin M, Birtles RJ, et al: In vitro susceptibilities of four *Bartonella bacilliformis* strains to 30 antibiotic compounds. Antimicrob Agents Chemother 43:2090, 1999

52. Raoult D, Roux V: The body louse as a vector of reemerging human diseases. Clin Infect Dis 29:888, 1999

53. Brouqui P, Lascola B, Roux V, et al: Chronic *Bartonella quintana* bacteremia in homeless patients. N Engl J Med 340:184, 1999

54. Ohl ME, Spach DH: *Bartonella quintana* and urban trench fever. Clin Infect Dis 31:131, 2000

55. Baorto E, Payne RM, Slater LN, et al: Culture-negative endocarditis caused by *Bartonella henselae*. J Pediatr 132:1051, 1998

56. Brouqui P, Raoult D: Endocarditis due to rare and fastidious bacteria. Clin Microbiol Rev 14:177, 2001

57. Koehler JE, Sanchez MA, Garrido CS, et al: Molecular epidemiology of bartonella infections in patients with bacillary angiomatosis-peliosis. N Engl J Med 337:1876, 1997

58. Gasquet S, Maurin M, Brouqui P, et al: Bacillary angiomatosis in immunocompromised patients. AIDS 12:1793, 1998

59. Giladi M, Avidor B, Kletter Y, et al: Cat scratch disease: the rare role of *Afipia felis*. J Clin Microbiol 36:2499, 1998

60. Grando D, Sullivan LJ, Flexman JP, et al: *Bartonella henselae* associated with Parinaud's oculoglandular syndrome. Clin Infect Dis 28:1156, 1999

61. Armengol CE, Hendley JO: Cat-scratch disease encephalopathy: a cause of status epilepticus in school-age children. J Pediatr 134:635, 1999

62. Jacobs RF, Schutze GE: *Bartonella henselae* as a cause of prolonged fever and fever of unknown origin in children. Clin Infect Dis 26:80, 1998

63. Ormerod LD, Skolnick KA, Menosky MM, et al: Retinal and choroidal manifestations of cat-scratch disease. Ophthalmology 105: 1024,1998

64. Ormerod LD, Dailey JP: Ocular manifestations of cat-scratch disease. Curr Opin Ophthalmol 10:209, 1999

65. Reed JB, Scales DK, Wong MT, et al: *Bartonella henselae* neuroretinitis in cat scratch disease: diagnosis, management, and sequelae. Ophthalmology 105:459, 1998

66. Solley WA, Martin DF, Newman NJ, et al: Cat scratch disease: posterior segment manifestations. Ophthalmology 106:1546, 1999

67. Jensen WA, Fall MZ, Rooney J, et al: Rapid identification and differentiation of *Bartonella* species using a single-step PCR assay. J Clin Microbiol 38:1717, 2000

68. Rolain JM, Maurin M, Raoult D: Bactericidal effect of antibiotics on *Bartonella* and *Brucella* spp.: clinical implications. J Antimicrob Chemother 46:811, 2000

69. Bass JW, Freitas BC, Freitas AD, et al: Prospective randomized double blind placebo-controlled evaluation of azithromycin for treatment of cat-scratch disease. Pediatr Infect Dis J 17:447, 1998

23 Infections Due to Mycobacteria

Harvey B. Simon, M.D.

Mycobacteria are a large, diverse, and widely distributed group of aerobic, nonsporulating, nonmotile bacilli that have a high cell-wall lipid content and a slow growth rate. Members of the genus *Mycobacterium* vary tremendously in virulence—from many harmless organisms to a few significant pathogens, such as *M. tuberculosis*. Mycobacterial species are differentiated by their growth rate, pigment production, animal virulence, and biochemical reactivity [*see Table 1*].

Tuberculosis

EPIDEMIOLOGY

Tuberculosis is the second leading infectious cause of death in the world. It is estimated that about two billion people, or one third of the world's population, are infected with *M. tuberculosis*, with more than eight million new cases and nearly three million deaths occurring each year. Tuberculosis is directly responsible for 7% of all deaths worldwide, and the global epidemic is likely to worsen as a result of the spread of drug-resistant organisms and the ongoing HIV epidemic.

In the United States and other developed countries, the incidence of tuberculosis began to decline in about 1900 because of improved living conditions. In addition, the introduction of chemotherapy has greatly enhanced control of the disease. Except for the period from 1979 to 1981, when the influx of refugees from Indochina produced a slight increase, and from 1985 to 1992, when HIV and homelessness fueled a 20% rise, tuberculosis in the United States has decreased by about 6% a year since 1953. In 2000, 16,372 cases were reported—an all-time low.[1] About 80% of these cases were pulmonary tuberculosis; the remainder were a variety of extrapulmonary infections. Nearly two thirds of new cases occur in nonwhites, and 42% occur in foreign-born persons. Among immigrants, the risk is highest in males between the ages of 25 and 44 who had been in the United States for less than 5 years.[2] Among minorities, tuberculosis is a disease of the young, with a median age at onset of 39 years. Among whites, tuberculosis is a disease of the elderly, with a median age at onset of 62 years. In about 90% of older patients with active tuberculosis, clinical illness is a result of reactivation of previous disease; of this group, at least 7% have a history of clinical tuberculosis that was inadequately treated. In younger, urban members of minorities, however, more than one third of cases reflect recently acquired tuberculosis; poverty and HIV infection increase the likelihood of infection.[3]

The disease is most common among men, the economically disadvantaged, and inner-city residents.[4] Tuberculosis is 200 times more likely to occur in persons who are HIV positive than in persons who are HIV negative; all patients with tuberculosis should be tested for HIV infection.[5] Other population groups with a disproportionately high incidence of tuberculosis include Hispanics, African Americans, immigrants, alcoholics, drug-dependent persons, homeless persons,[6] nursing home residents, prison inmates, and patients with gastrectomies, neoplasia, renal transplants, uremia, or other debilitating conditions. People who travel to countries where tuberculosis is endemic are also at risk.[7]

Hospital employees, including physicians, are also at increased risk for tuberculous infections. Although airborne transmission resulting from inadequate ventilation is usually responsible for transmission in hospitals,[8] medical wastes may occasionally be the source of infection.[9] High-quality masks, augmented ventilation, improved air filters, and ultraviolet germicidal irradiation are recommended for prevention of the nosocomial transmission of tuberculosis. Because of atypical presentations, the diagnosis of pulmonary tuberculosis is often delayed in hospitalized patients[10]; early

Table 1 Classification of Mycobacteria

	Organism or Group	Skin Test	Growth Rate (Days)	Pigment	Niacin	Comment
Common or Medically Important Species	*M. tuberculosis*	PPD-S	15–40	None (buff)	+	Guinea pig virulent
	M. bovis	PPD-S	25–40	None	–	Rabbit and guinea pig virulent Drug sensitive
	Bacillus Calmette-Guérin (BCG vaccine)	PPD-S	25–40	None	–	Drug sensitive Urease positive Nonvirulent for normal humans
	M. leprae	Lepromin				Never grown in vitro Cause of leprosy (Hansen disease)
Atypical Mycobacteria	Group I Photochromogens (pigment is light dependent)	PPD-Y	7–21	Yellow	–	Often drug sensitive Representative species: *M. kansasii* (pulmonary disease; grows at 37° C), *M. marinum* (swimming pool granuloma; grows at 30° to 33° C)
	Group II Scotochromogens (pigment is not light dependent)	PPD-G	7–21	Yellow-orange	–	Drug resistant Representative species: *M. scrofulaceum* (cervical lymphadenitis, or scrofula, in children)
	Group III Nonchromogens (no pigment)	PPD-B PPD-A	7–21	None	–	Drug resistant Representative species: *M. avium* complex (pulmonary disease, disseminated infection in AIDS)
	Group IV Rapid growers	PPD-F	3–7	None	–	Drug resistant Representative species: *M. fortuitum* (grows on MacConkey agar)

Note: Nonmycobacteria that may be acid-fast include members of the order Actinomycetales. Unlike mycobacteria, these organisms stain gram-positive and typically grow in branching chains that may morphologically resemble fungal hyphae but are actually composed of individual bacterial cells. They are more weakly acid-fast than mycobacteria and sometimes retain carbolfuchsin only when decolorized with dilute sulfuric acid rather than acid alcohol (modified acid-fast stain). Representative organisms include *Nocardia asteroides* (aerobic) and *Actinomyces israelii* (anaerobic). Acid-fast organisms belonging to the rhodochrous taxon have now been identified as opportunistic human pathogens; these organisms are gram-positive and aerobic and have similarities to rapidly growing mycobacteria and to *Nocardia* species.

diagnosis and appropriate use of control measures can effectively prevent nosocomial tuberculosis.

ETIOLOGY

Although clinical tuberculosis is relatively uncommon in the United States, an estimated 7% of the population (approximately 17.5 million people) have positive tuberculin skin tests indicating previous infection by the organism. Unless they have received chemotherapy, these persons harbor small numbers of dormant but viable tubercle bacilli, which may reactivate, causing clinical disease. Because *M. tuberculosis* is highly adapted to humans and has no reservoir in nature, this population group is the reservoir for human tuberculosis.

With the virtual elimination of bovine tuberculosis in the United States, almost all cases of tuberculosis are acquired through person-to-person transmission via the aerosol route. Genetic factors account for the greater infectivity of certain strains of *M. tuberculosis* and for the greater susceptibility of certain human population groups.[11] Patients with active pulmonary infection shed infected airborne droplets into the environment.[12] Because most infectious patients discharge relatively few organisms, most secondary cases occur among household members or other close contacts of the index case. Infectivity is greatest from patients whose sputum smears test positive,[13] as well as from those with cavitary disease, tuberculosis of the larynx, or thin, watery sputum. Shedding is further enhanced by coughing. Once infected particles become airborne, they can remain aloft for many hours; hence, adequate ventilation is of prime importance for control of tuberculosis, particularly in the hospital setting. After the droplets have settled on environmental surfaces, however, they are essentially noninfectious, although they may still contain viable bacilli. High-quality masks are important for the protection of persons in contact with patients with pulmonary tuberculosis; gowns, gloves, and room disinfection are unnecessary.

MICROBIOLOGY AND PATHOGENESIS

M. tuberculosis is a 0.2 × 5.0 μm bacillus that has several clinically important biologic properties. First, it is an obligate aerobe. Consequently, it grows most successfully in those human tissues having the highest oxygen tension (Po_2), such as the lung apexes. Second, it is a slow-growing organism with a generation time estimated to be 12 to 18 hours. As a result, tuberculous lesions in humans typically evolve in a subacute to long-term course, and laboratory isolation of the organism requires 1 to 2 weeks or more. Third, it has a high cell-wall lipid content; because of the presence of various complex mycosides, the organisms are impermeable to the usual bacteriologic stains, such as Gram stain. Finally, although tubercle bacilli require special enriched media to grow in the laboratory, these organisms are extremely resistant to physical stress. Specimens from patients suspected of having tuberculosis can survive concentration and digestion procedures that would kill ordinary bacteria.

The pathogenesis of tuberculosis is unique among infectious diseases because of the highly variable but often extremely long latency period between infection and clinical illness. Although a single tubercle bacillus theoretically can cause infection, it must first bypass the upper airway defense mechanisms and lodge in the pulmonary alveoli; airborne particles 5 to 10 μm in diameter are thus most likely to transmit infection. Initial infection usually occurs in the lower lung fields because of gravity and the greater ventilation of the lung bases. Once in the alveoli, tubercle bacilli multiply slowly and, because they do not secrete any enzymes or toxins, provoke little initial inflammatory reaction in the nonimmune host. In about 3 weeks, a single organism can potentially give rise to more than a million progeny, and these bacilli will have invaded the lymphatics and will have spread to the draining regional nodes. With further multiplication, bacilli invade the bloodstream and can spread hematogenously to any organ. Even at this stage, the great majority of patients are completely asymptomatic; hence, hematogenous infection is truly a silent bacillemia.

Whereas any tissue can be hematogenously seeded, organs with high blood flow tend to receive the most bacilli, and tissues with the highest Po_2 provide the most favorable environment for multiplication. Hence, the lung apexes are by far the most common repositories. Other frequently infected areas include the renal cortex, the vertebral column, and the metaphyseal ends of long bones. After 6 to 8 weeks, cell-mediated immunity is well established, and results of tuberculin skin testing become positive. In addition, granulomatous inflammation develops in infected tissues in the lung and in the regions of metastatic spread. Granuloma formation in tuberculosis results from the interaction of specifically sensitized T cells with tubercle bacilli. The antigenically stimulated lymphocytes in turn activate macrophages, whose metabolic, phagocytic, and bactericidal potentials are then enhanced. Tubercle bacilli are engulfed by macrophages, and the great majority of the bacteria are killed. As a result, most patients experience complete healing of these initial tuberculous lesions, but if immunity is incomplete, progressive primary tuberculosis or even disseminated disease may develop.

In patients whose primary lesions heal, the chest x-ray may be normal, or it may show focal calcifications. The primary lower lobe lesion and its draining node may be recognized radiologically as the Ghon complex; apical calcifications (Simon foci) may be present. Although inactive, these lesions contain small numbers of dormant but viable tubercle bacilli, which can break down and lead to reactivation infection; histologically normal lung tissue may also harbor dormant bacilli.[14] Reactivation occurs in about 5% of patients within 2 years of the initial infection[15]; reactivation is also likely to occur at times of lowered host resistance, as in adolescence or in the postpartum period. Reactivation disease can occur many decades after initial infection and, in fact, is now most common in the elderly. At times, a discrete insult to host defenses (e.g., HIV infection, steroid therapy, malnutrition, and neoplastic disease) can be implicated, but more often, the reason for reactivation is impossible to identify. Reactivation tuberculosis has been estimated to occur in up to 10% of all infected persons,[15] the remainder having positive results on tuberculin skin testing but no clinical illness. Such previously infected persons appear resistant to exogenous reinfection from inhaled bacilli; in these patients, accelerated granuloma formation occurs, killing organisms that are newly lodged in the alveoli. However, in debilitated patients and in regions where there is a high prevalence of tuberculosis, exogenous reinfection can occur.

DIAGNOSIS

Tuberculin Test

The tuberculin test is an important tool in both diagnosis and prevention of tuberculosis; it is far more sensitive than the chest x-ray in identifying *M. tuberculosis* infection.[16] The Mantoux test, using the intradermal injection of Tween 80 (polysorbate 80–coated nanoparticles) stabilized purified protein derivative (PPD), is more reliable than multiple-puncture tests, such as the tine test. The standard test material is intermediate-strength (5 tuberculin units) PPD; the two commercially available preparations, Aplisol and Tubersol, are equally potent.[17] Tuberculosis testing should be used for persons at high risk for the disease (targeted tuberculin testing) rather than for persons at low risk (tuberculin screening).[18]

The tuberculin skin test should be evaluated 48 to 72 hours after administration. The diameter of induration rather than that of erythema determines the interpretation. Until recently, a single standard was used to interpret the tuberculin skin test in all patients, but the American Thoracic Society and the Centers for Disease Control and Prevention (CDC) now propose that different criteria be applied to different population groups[18]: (1) 5 mm of induration should be considered positive for patients with HIV infection or other major defects in cell-mediated immunity and for persons who are very likely to have tuberculosis, such as those in close contact with patients known to have tuberculosis and in patients with fibrosis or calcification on chest x-ray that is consistent with previous tuberculosis; (2) 10 mm of induration should still be used as the criterion for a positive reaction in members of population groups with a high prevalence of tuberculosis infection, including immigrants from endemic areas, prisoners, the homeless, I.V. drug abusers, nursing home residents, and other chronically ill patients; and (3) 15 mm of induration should be the criterion for a positive reaction in persons with no identifiable risk factors.

Among hospital workers or other groups in which repeated testing may be necessary, a booster reaction may be mistaken for conversion. This effect can be avoided by administering a second test 1 week later to anyone whose primary reaction is negative or whose test result is in doubt. Any increase in the diameter of induration after this second test may be attributed to the booster effect. However, if the size of the induration on retesting 1 year later has increased by 6 mm or more, a new tuberculous infection can be presumed. The booster reaction is most likely to occur in persons who have been vaccinated for bacillus Calmette-Guérin (BCG)[19] or who have had a prior infection with *M. tuberculosis* or other mycobacteria.[20,21]

Except in patients who have received chemotherapy, a positive skin test implies the presence of a few dormant but viable tubercle bacilli that have the potential for reactivation; obviously, however, a positive tuberculin test does not prove active disease. Conversely, negative reactions have been documented in about 20% of HIV-negative patients and 40% of HIV-positive patients with tuberculosis, particularly those persons with overwhelming or advanced disease, malnutrition, and debility. Viral infections, including measles and rubella, can depress tuberculin reactivity, but this effect is transient.

Because of the limited sensitivity and specificity of the tuberculin skin test, new methods for diagnosing infections by *M. tuberculosis* are being developed. A sandwich-capture, enzyme-linked immunosorbent assay that identifies circulating T cells that react with ESAT-6, a secreted antigen specific to *M. tuberculosis*, is particularly promising.[22]

Microbiology Studies

The Ziehl-Neelsen stain is the traditional method for visualizing mycobacteria in clinical specimens. Although the acid-fast stain remains useful, reference laboratories are turning increasingly to fluorescent staining methods. Unfortunately, the sensitivity of direct microscopy is only about 50%, and it cannot distinguish *M. tuberculosis* from other mycobacteria. New nucleic acid amplification (NAA) techniques can be used to identify mycobacterial DNA or RNA in clinical specimens. The tests are rapid, requiring less than 6 hours, but they are expensive. In sputum specimens that are smear positive, NAA tests have sensitivities and specificities greater than 95%; in smear-negative specimens, specificity remains above 95%, but sensitivity is only 40% to 77%.[23] In a clinical trial, NAA testing had better positive and negative predictive values than direct microscopy.[24] The Food and Drug Administration has approved NAA tests in conjunction with cultures of respiratory specimens from patients who have not been treated for tuberculosis[25]; with additional refinements and experience, NAA testing is likely to prove useful for other types of specimens, such as CSF, pleural fluid, blood, and tissue.[26]

Culture methods have also improved; the BACTEC radiometric system has greatly facilitated the isolation of mycobacteria. Clinical specimens are inoculated in bottles containing broth that has a carbon-14 (^{14}C) substrate specific for mycobacterial growth and antibiotics for the suppression of ordinary bacteria. If mycobacteria are present, their growth releases $^{14}CO_2$ into the atmosphere above the medium; an automated system can detect growth in as little as 7 to 10 days. Susceptibility testing can be performed by adding antituberculous drugs to the medium. Because *M. tuberculosis* is the only mycobacterial species that produces a significant amount of niacin, a positive niacin test confirms the identification. A DNA probe can be used to rapidly identify colonies of *M. tuberculosis* complex (*M. tuberculosis, M. bovis, M. africanum,* and *M. microti*); it has replaced the niacin test in many laboratories.

CLINICAL PRESENTATIONS OF TUBERCULOSIS

Pulmonary Tuberculosis

Primary infection More than 90% of patients are entirely asymptomatic at the time of primary infection and can be identified only through conversion of the tuberculin skin test from negative to positive. Most of these patients have normal chest x-rays, but in some patients, fibrocalcific residua of infection are radiographically demonstrable. In the past, primary tuberculosis was a pediatric disease, but as childhood infection has declined, primary infection has increased in adults. Adults who are debilitated, immunosuppressed, or HIV positive are particularly vulnerable to the tubercle bacillus and are at increased risk for symptomatic primary tuberculosis.

Among symptomatic patients, four broad syndromes can be identified. The most common is similar to atypical pneumonia, with fever and nonproductive cough. Chest x-rays may show unilateral, lower lobe, patchy parenchymal infiltrates; paratracheal or hilar adenopathy; or both. Although these patients should receive full antituberculous chemotherapy when diagnosed, the symptoms resolve even without therapy in the great majority.

The same prognosis applies to patients who present with the second syndrome, tuberculous pleuritis with effusion. These patients often have high fever, cough, and pleuritic chest pain; occasionally, they also have dyspnea. Chest x-rays reveal unilateral pleural effusions, often without identifiable parenchymal lesions; in immunocompetent persons, the tuberculin skin test is almost always strongly positive. Because cultures of sputum or gastric washings, or both, are positive in only about 30% of patients with tuberculous pleuritis, diagnosis depends on examination of the pleural fluid, which characteristically contains high levels of protein and lactic dehydrogenase (LDH) and low levels of glucose. Pleural fluid white cell counts typically range from 1,000 to 6,000/mm^3. Neutrophils may be predominant early, but lymphocytes eventually predominate in most cases. Whereas acid-fast smears and cultures of pleural fluid are positive in only about one third of patients, percutaneous needle biopsy of the pleura will reveal caseating granulomas in about two thirds of patients with tuberculous pleuritis. Primary tuberculous pleuritis will usually resolve spontaneously; however, without therapy, reactivation tuberculosis develops in up to 60% of patients. Combined chemotherapy is therefore indicated in all patients. Corticosteroids hasten symptomatic improvement but do not improve long-term results. Complications are rare, and surgery is almost never required to manage tuberculous pleuritis.

The third major syndrome of primary tuberculosis is direct progression to upper lobe disease. The fourth syndrome is manifested when patients experience extrapulmonary tuberculosis as a progression of primary infection. In the past, this pattern was most common in young children, who presented with cervical adenitis, miliary tuberculosis, or tuberculous meningitis; it is now most often observed in persons infected with HIV. Besides these major manifestations, erythema nodosum and other hypersensitivity reactions may develop in patients with primary tuberculosis.

Reactivation (postprimary) tuberculosis Reactivation tuberculosis is the most common clinical form of tuberculosis. It is seen most often in innercity residents, elderly persons, or debilitated patients; HIV infection greatly increases risk. Symptoms usually begin insidiously and progress over a period of many weeks or months before diagnosis. Systemic symptoms are often prominent. They include anorexia, weight loss, and night sweats. Most patients have low-grade fevers, but high temperatures and even chills may be seen if the disease progresses relatively rapidly. In addition, most patients present with pulmonary symptoms, including cough and sputum production; dyspnea is relatively uncommon in the absence of underlying chronic lung disease. A frequent complaint is hemoptysis, which is caused by bronchial irritation and is often in the form of bright-red streaks of blood. However, these classic symptoms are now often absent in patients with pulmonary tuberculosis,[27] thus making diagnosis more difficult. In addition, the diagnosis of pulmonary tuberculosis may be delayed in patients with advanced disease who present with respiratory failure, which may suggest a diagnosis of nontuberculous pneumonia.

Chest x-rays are highly suggestive of the diagnosis. Typical features include unilateral or bilateral infiltration in the posterior apical pulmonary segments that progresses to frank cavitation; chest tomography may be helpful in identifying cavitary lesions. In some patients with postprimary tuberculosis—particularly those infected with HIV—the lower lung fields may be involved. In some instances, the chest x-ray may appear normal; computed tomography scans, however, may show nodular or branching linear centrilobular lesions in very early disease.

The tuberculin skin test is positive in about 80% of immunocompetent patients with reactivation tuberculosis; patients with advanced disease are often malnourished and may be anergic, as are many patients with HIV infection or other immunosuppressive disorders. The diagnosis of pulmonary tuberculosis can be confirmed in many persons by examination of the sputum. Sputum specimens should be examined microscopically by using either the acid-fast stain or fluorescent stain; selected specimens[25] should also be tested with NAA techniques, which can identify an acid-fast bacillus as *M. tuberculosis* rather than as an atypical mycobacterium. Specimens should always be cultured; the sensitivity and specificity of smears are 53.1% and 99.8%, respectively, and the sensitivity and specificity of cultures are 81.5% and 98.4%, respectively. If patients are unable to produce sputum spontaneously, attempts should be made to induce sputum with the aid of pulmonary physiotherapy, intermittent positive-pressure breathing, and mucolytic agents. Bronchoscopy and bronchoalveolar lavage may be necessary to obtain appropriate specimens; care must be taken to avoid cross-infection from contaminated bronchoscopes. In one trial, induced sputum and bronchoscopic specimens were equally useful for diagnosing tuberculosis.[28] Blood cultures that use the BACTEC system may also help establish the diagnosis of pulmonary tuberculosis, especially in HIV-infected persons, who are often bacillemic.

Tuberculosis in HIV-infected persons *M. tuberculosis* is an important opportunistic pathogen in patients with AIDS. Tuberculosis in AIDS usually reflects reactivation of previously acquired latent infection; hence, tuberculosis occurs most commonly in HIV-infected patients with a high prevalence of tuberculous infection, such as I.V. drug abusers, Haitian-Americans, and inner-city residents. Because *M. tuberculosis* is more virulent than other latent intracellular pathogens, tuberculosis tends to occur early in the course of HIV infection, preceding other manifestations of AIDS in more than half the cases. Tuberculosis may have an adverse effect on the course of HIV infections[5]; antiretroviral therapy may produce a paradoxical worsening of tuberculosis,[29] but the effect is temporary and is caused by the restoration of immunologic competence.

When tuberculosis occurs early in the course of HIV infection before severe immunosuppression has occurred, the clinical and radiographic features resemble tuberculosis in patients who are HIV negative. In patients with $CD4^+$ T cell counts below $200/mm^3$, however, *M. tuberculosis* tends to produce infections that are more widespread, severe, and unusual than conventional tuberculosis. For example, when tuberculosis develops in patients with $CD4^+$ T cell counts greater than $200/mm^3$, the presentation is typically pulmonary; in patients who have symptomatic AIDS before the diagnosis of tuberculosis, up to 70% have tuberculous involvement of one or more extrapulmonary sites.

Although the tuberculin skin test is often negative in HIV-infected patients with tuberculosis, the diagnosis of tuberculosis can be established by identifying *M. tuberculosis* from sputum or from extrapulmonary sites; blood culture may be positive. However, radiographic features may be confusing. Chest x-rays are normal in 10% to 15% of HIV-positive patients with tuberculosis, and patients with low $CD4^+$ T cell counts often have intrathoracic adenopathy without parenchymal infiltrate. When infiltrates occur, lower lobe consolidation or diffuse infiltrates are much more common than upper lobe abnormalities, and cavitation is very uncommon. Pneumocystis and other opportunistic pathogens may produce radiographic abnormalities indistinguishable from tuberculosis in patients with AIDS, but the presence of intrathoracic adenopathy, pleural effusions, miliary infiltrates, or cavities is an important clue to tuberculosis.

With combination chemotherapy, the prognosis of pulmonary tuberculosis is good; HIV-positive patients respond well to treatment, except when they have multidrug-resistant tuberculosis. Without therapy, devastating complications, such as massive hemoptysis, may ensue. Another complication is bronchogenic spread of infection to other pulmonary segments. In extreme cases, such spread can result in massive tuberculous pneumonia with hypoxia and an acute lethal course despite chemotherapy. The infection can also spread to the pleural space, which results in a bronchopleural fistula or tuberculous empyema, or to the upper airway, which results in tuberculous laryngitis. Tuberculous pericarditis may result from direct extension of an adjacent pulmonary focus. Bronchial obstruction may also result from extrinsic compression caused by tuberculous lymphadenitis or by endobronchial granulomas; secondary bacterial pneumonias may develop in patients with bronchial obstruction. Swallowed organisms can produce tuberculous enteritis. Still another complication of pulmonary tuberculosis is hematogenous dissemination with simultaneous extrapulmonary disease. The syndrome of inappropriate antidiuretic hormone (SIADH) may develop as a metabolic complication of pulmonary tuberculosis. Hypercalcemia may complicate active infection. Anemia is common in patients with advanced or chronic disease. Polyclonal hyperglobulinemia, hypoalbuminemia, and elevated erythrocyte sedimentation rates are also common but nonspecific. Liver function tests are often elevated, possibly reflecting extrapulmonary dissemination.

Extrapulmonary Tuberculosis

Although the lungs are the portal of entry and bear the major clinical brunt of tuberculosis, the disease is actually a disseminated infection. Even before HIV became a widespread problem, about 15% of all newly recognized cases of tuberculosis in the United States were extrapulmonary. In recent years, an increasing number of tuberculosis patients have presented with extrapulmonary infection, largely because it occurs in 24% to 45% of patients with early HIV infection and in more than 70% of patients with advanced AIDS. In such patients, tuberculosis may affect multiple extrapulmonary sites and may be unusually severe or atypical in its clinical features.

Medical history is not a reliable guide to the diagnosis of extrapulmonary tuberculosis. Only 25% of patients have a history of tuberculosis, but virtually all of them have been inadequately treated. Except in children and in HIV-infected adults, there is typically a long latency period between the initial infection and the extrapulmonary presentation. Approximately 50% of patients with extrapulmonary tuberculosis have entirely normal chest x-rays; most of the others have stigmata of old, inactive pulmonary disease, and a minority have coexisting active pulmonary infection. All organ systems can be involved, either singly or in various combinations; the most commonly involved areas are the genitourinary tract, the musculoskeletal system, and the lymph nodes. Abdominal tuberculosis, with infection of lymph nodes and spleen, is common in patients infected with HIV.

Although generalizations about extrapulmonary tuberculosis are subject to many exceptions, it is clinically useful to divide the disorder into three large categories. The first is subacute, progressive, life-threatening disease. Patients in this category are generally febrile and have prominent systemic symptoms suggestive of infection. The tuberculin skin test may be negative in up to 20% of patients because of the overwhelming nature of the infection. Without therapy, these patients experience a progressive downhill course and an extremely high mortality; death often occurs in a matter of weeks. Important examples of this fulminating type are miliary tuberculosis, tuberculous meningitis, and tuberculosis of the pericardium and great vessels.

The second type is tuberculosis of the large serosal surfaces, such as tuberculous pleuritis and peritonitis. Patients in this category also have prominent systemic symptoms, including fever in almost all cases. However, the tuberculin skin test is positive more often, the clinical course is longer, and the prognosis, with or without therapy, is better than in subacute disease.

The third, and most common, type is infection of individual organ systems. Patients in this category are most often afebrile and can be entirely free of systemic complaints. The illness typically pursues a very indolent course characterized by local organ dysfunction and, eventually, destruction rather than by progressive general decline. In fact, the differential diagnosis suggests neoplastic disease more often than infection. Except in patients with HIV infection or other immunosuppressive disorders, the tuberculin skin test is almost always positive. Clinical syndromes of this type of extrapulmonary tuberculosis include genitourinary tuberculosis, tuberculous arthritis and osteomyelitis, and tuberculous lymphadenitis.

Miliary tuberculosis No other form of tuberculosis has had its epidemiology change more dramatically than miliary tuberculosis—first with the advent of chemotherapy and then with the onset of the HIV epidemic. In HIV-negative patients, miliary tuberculosis once occurred most commonly in children, but now it occurs principally in the elderly; more than half the patients are older than 60 years, and one third have an underlying debilitating illness. In contrast, HIV-positive patients with miliary tuberculosis are predominantly young adults.

The onset of miliary tuberculosis is usually subacute. Symptoms progress over a period of 1 to 4 months before diagnosis. Fever is present in at least 85% of patients, and anorexia, weight loss, and weakness are only slightly less common. Cough and dyspnea occur in up to 60% of patients, but hemoptysis is rare. Many other symptoms may appear; headache is particularly important because it may reflect coexisting tuberculous meningitis. Variant presentations include cryptic miliary tuberculosis, in which patients have normal chest x-rays and exhibit problems typical of fever of undetermined origin [see 1 Hyperthermia, Fever, and Fever of Undetermined Origin]; such cases account for approximately 10% of all cases of miliary tuberculosis. A rare occurrence is fulminating pulmonary disease, in which respiratory insufficiency and, often, disseminated intravascular coagulation are present. The physical examination in patients with miliary tuberculosis is usually nonspecific, disclosing various pulmonary findings in up to 50%, hepatomegaly in 30%, and splenomegaly or lymphadenopathy in 15% of observed cases. Choroidal tubercles are less common, but they are diagnostically more helpful.

Laboratory findings are often nonspecific. The complete blood count may be normal, but dramatic abnormalities, ranging from pancytopenia to leukemoid reactions, are well documented. Abnormal liver function test results, especially with the alkaline phosphatase test, occur in 30% of observed cases. Hyponatremia is less common but, if present, should raise the possibility of SIADH or adrenal insufficiency. The tuberculin skin test is initially positive in only 75% of HIV-negative patients with miliary tuberculosis. Whereas chest x-rays may be normal early in the course of disease, typical interstitial miliary lesions eventually develop in 90% of patients. Sputum smears are positive, however, in only 30% of patients. Fiberoptic bronchoscopy, bronchial brushings, and transbronchial biopsy specimens can establish the diagnosis in more than 70% of patients who have abnormal chest x-rays but negative sputum smears. Liver biopsy is especially helpful, revealing granulomas in about 60% of patients. These granulomas, however, are often noncaseating and are etiologically nonspecific. Bone marrow biopsy is positive in about one third of all patients with miliary tuberculosis and has an even higher yield in those with hematologic abnormalities.

About 40% of AIDS patients with extrapulmonary tuberculosis experience disseminated tuberculosis. They tend to be in generally poorer health than other patients with miliary tuberculosis, and only 32% demonstrate typical miliary infiltrates on chest radiographs. Sputum smears are positive in 25%, sputum cultures in 71%, and blood cultures in 56% of cases. A so-called nonreactive histologic pattern, characterized by acute inflammation, tissue necrosis, and many bacilli but no granulomas, is often seen in AIDS patients with disseminated tuberculosis but is otherwise rare.[30]

Miliary tuberculosis is uniformly fatal without chemotherapy; even with combined chemotherapy, mortality is 5% to 35%. Adverse prognostic features include the presence of meningitis, extremes of age (i.e., old age and early childhood), and underlying diseases. Clinical improvement with treatment is often very slow: fever can persist for 1 to 3 weeks. The major differential diagnosis includes histoplasmosis and other mycotic infections, sarcoidosis, and malignant disorders.

Tuberculous meningitis In HIV-negative patients, tuberculous meningitis has also markedly decreased in incidence, shifting from a disease of childhood to a disease of old age. Although tuberculous meningitis is much more likely to develop in HIV-positive patients than in HIV-negative patients, its clinical and laboratory manifestations, as well as its prognosis, are similar in the two groups.[31] Tuberculous meningitis may result from hematogenous seeding of the meninges, or it can be caused by breakdown of an old parameningeal granuloma, with rupture into the subarachnoid space. The intense inflammatory reaction is most prominent at the base of the brain and can have three effects: direct compression of neural tissues, especially cranial nerves; vasculitis leading to areas of infarction; and obstruction of the free flow of CSF, leading to cerebral edema, hydrocephalus, or subarachnoid block. CT scanning may show basal meningeal enhancement and hydrocephalus; angiography may show arteritis.

Clinically, tuberculous meningitis is the most rapidly progressive form of tuberculosis; 50% of patients are ill for less than 2 weeks before diagnosis. Without therapy, the illness progresses from headache, fever, and meningismus to cranial nerve palsies or other focal deficits, alterations of sensorium, seizures, coma, and eventually death.

Except in the relatively uncommon patient with coexisting active pulmonary or miliary tuberculosis, examination of the CSF is the only way to make the diagnosis. CSF pressure may be normal or elevated. The CSF glucose level is depressed in almost all patients. The CSF protein level is usually moderately elevated to between 50 and 200 mg/dl, but it may occasionally be very high, suggesting the presence of CSF block. A modest pleocytosis occurs in virtually all patients, typically ranging from 100 to 1,000 white cells/mm^3, at least 70% of which are lymphocytes. Acid-fast smears of CSF are positive in only about 25% of patients, but CSF cultures are eventually positive in up to 75%.

The major differential diagnosis includes cryptococcal and other less common forms of fungal meningitis, carcinomatous meningitis, and, if antibiotics have been given, partially treated bacterial meningitis [see 13 Bacterial Infections of the Central Nervous System]. Hence, if fungal stains, serologies, and CSF cytologies are negative, antituberculous therapy should be initiated immediately. Isoniazid, rifampin, and ethambutol are the preferred drugs because they all penetrate the CSF; patients infected with multidrug-resistant organisms may benefit from intrathecal therapy.[32] Corticosteroids are useful only for patients with cerebral edema or subarachnoid block. Ventricular shunting may be helpful in patients with hydrocephalus who fail to respond to antituberculous and pressure-reducing agents. With therapy, improvement is slow, mortality remains about 20%, and some survivors have neurologic residua.

Less common forms of CNS tuberculosis include radiculomyelitis and other infections of the spinal cord or epidural space[33] and cerebral tuberculomas,[34] which typically present as slowly enlarging mass lesions and are generally diagnosed as brain tumors before surgical exploration.

Tuberculous pericarditis Although infrequent, tuberculous pericarditis occurs most often in young to middle-aged adults. Tuberculous pericarditis is relatively uncommon in HIV-infected persons, but it may be the first manifestation of AIDS. Infection of the pericardium can result either from hematogenous dissemination of bacilli or from contiguous spread from lung or mediastinal nodes. Pathologically, the disease progresses from inflammation to effusion and eventually to fibrous organization. The earliest stages include insidious onset of fever and weight loss. Pericardial pain occurs in only about half of patients and is usually considerably milder than it is in viral or idiopathic pericarditis. Cough, dyspnea, orthopnea, and edema are present in more than half of patients with tuberculous pericarditis. Physical examination will disclose a pericardial rub in only about one third of patients; cardiomegaly and signs of pericardial tamponade are more common. Echocardiography reveals the presence of pericarditis but is etiologically nonspecific. In immunologically competent patients, the tuberculin skin test is almost always positive, but unless pulmonary tuberculosis is also present, the diagnosis of tuberculous pericarditis depends on direct examination of pericardial fluid or tissue. The pericardial fluid is turbid or hemorrhagic, with white cell counts that typically range from 5,000 to 10,000/mm^3. Lymphocytes are predominant. High protein levels and low glucose levels are typical. Acid-fast smears or cultures of pericardial fluid are positive in about half of cases, but pericardial biopsy has a higher yield. The major differential diagnosis includes idiopathic or viral pericarditis and tumor.

If left untreated, tuberculous pericarditis has a mortality of more than 80%, and constriction eventually occurs in many survivors. Surgery is needed if clinical tamponade progresses or recurs despite repeated pericardiocentesis. However, in the absence of this complication, medical therapy is generally preferred. Corticosteroids have been useful in reducing the need for surgery, the incidence of late constriction, and the overall mortality. In the absence of specific contraindications, antituberculous chemotherapy should be supplemented initially by corticosteroids for the treatment of tuberculous pericarditis; corticosteroids should be tapered over a 2- to 3-month period.

Tuberculous aortitis A rare disorder, tuberculous aortitis can result from hematogenous infection of the vasa vasorum or from contiguous spread from the lung or nodes. Most patients also have active pulmonary or miliary tuberculosis and present with chest pain and fever. Both surgical intervention and chemotherapy are necessary, but mortality is high.

Tuberculous pleuritis A relatively common condition, tuberculous pleuritis often occurs in HIV-infected persons. The clinical features are outlined in the discussion of primary tuberculosis. Acid-fast smears are positive in 69% of HIV-positive patients but in only 21% of HIV-negative patients, in whom pleural biopsies are often necessary for diagnosis. Corticosteroids do not improve the results of chemotherapy, which is usually effective.

Tuberculous peritonitis Resulting either from hematogenous seeding or from extension of tuberculous salpingitis, enteritis, or adenitis, tuberculous peritonitis is most common in women because of the contribution of salpingitis. Although rare, the disease has been reported in patients on continuous ambulatory peritoneal dialysis.[35] Clinically, the onset is insidious, and fever, weight loss, weakness, abdominal pain, and increasing girth are typically present for months before diagnosis. Tuberculous peritonitis progresses from an early wet (exudative) phase with free abdominal fluid on physical examination to a late dry (plastic) phase with fibrosis, adhesions, and a doughy abdomen on physical examination, often with palpable masses caused by matted bowel and omentum. The tuberculin skin test is almost always positive. CT scanning may reveal peritoneal and mesenteric nodularity, complex ascites, lymphadenopathy, and tubo-ovarian abscess. The peritoneal fluid typically has 100 to 3,000 white cells/mm^3, at least 75% of which are lymphocytes, and high protein levels. Acid-fast smears and cultures of peritoneal fluid are generally negative unless extremely large volumes of fluid are examined. Peritoneal biopsy has a much higher diagnostic yield; percutaneous or laparoscopic needle biopsy is preferable to open biopsy unless adhesions that increase the risk of perforation are present. Differential diagnosis includes carcinomatosis, lymphoma, and cirrhosis. When tuberculous peritonitis is untreated, mortality nears 50%, with bowel obstruction common in survivors; with therapy, the prognosis is excellent. Corticosteroids may reduce the risk of complications.[36]

Intra-abdominal tuberculosis Like tuberculous peritonitis, intra-abdominal tuberculosis is more common in HIV-positive patients than in patients who are HIV negative. Tuberculous enteritis often involves the ileocecal region and may mimic Crohn disease or cancer. CT scanning and barium examinations are helpful, but colonoscopy and biopsy are usually required for diagnosis.

Renal tuberculosis Renal infection, the most common form of extrathoracic tuberculosis, occurs in 3% to 4% of all patients with tuberculosis; the incidence is highest among young to middle-aged adults. Renal tuberculosis is relatively uncommon in patients with AIDS, but it has been reported in renal transplant recipients.[37] Because the disease arises from hematogenous seeding, bilateral cortical granulomas are demonstrable pathologically in most patients. Clinically, however, the disease is often unilateral. Renal tuberculosis is an insidious process that may produce progressive renal destruction over a period of many years before diagnosis. About 70% of affected patients present with urinary tract symptoms, including flank pain, hematuria, dysuria, and pyuria in various combinations, but 20% are asymptomatic and are diagnosed because of abnormal urine sediments. Fever and systemic complaints are uncommon, occurring in fewer than 10% of patients. The tuberculin skin test is almost always positive. The urine sediment is abnormal in about 95% of patients, revealing pyuria, hematuria, or both. Intravenous pyelography (IVP) shows abnormalities in 60% to 90% of patients; calcification, cavitation, and ureteral strictures and fibrosis suggest tuberculosis, but calyceal dilatation, cortical scarring, and papillary necrosis are nonspecific. CT scanning is as useful as IVP for visualizing advanced urinary tract tuberculosis, but ultrasonographic studies are less accurate. Because of the presence of nonpathogenic mycobacteria, acid-fast smears of urine are often misleading and should not be performed. The key to diagnosis is urine cultures; if three first-morning urine specimens are submitted, positive cultures will be obtained in at least 90% of patients with renal tuberculosis. NAA testing is also very useful and is much faster than urine culture tests.[38] The differential diagnosis includes nephrolithiasis, tumor, and bacterial urinary tract infection. Prognosis is excellent with chemotherapy; because ureteral strictures can progress during chemotherapy, serial IVP is important in patients with ureteral defects.

Male genital tuberculosis Male genital tuberculosis can result from hematogenous seeding or can spread from infected urine; about 50% of patients also have renal tuberculosis. Patients present with slowly enlarging mass lesions of the epididymis, prostate, or seminal vesicles. Because the most common clinical diagnoses are tumors or pyogenic infections, tuberculosis is usually discovered only during biopsy.

Female genital tuberculosis Hematogenous spread to the fallopian tubes causes female genital tuberculosis; coexisting renal tuberculosis is uncommon. Presenting complaints include infertility, abnormal menstrual bleeding, or pelvic pain. The physical examination may be normal, or it may reveal an adnexal mass. Endometrial curettage produces greater diagnostic yields than endometrial biopsy or culture of menstrual blood. Surgery is often needed for diagnosis of tubo-ovarian abscesses or pelvic peritonitis. Chemotherapy controls infection, but infertility persists despite treatment.

Musculoskeletal tuberculosis Once a childhood disease, musculoskeletal tuberculosis now presents most commonly in persons between 40 and 50 years of age. This variety of tuberculosis rivals genitourinary infection in frequency, but both are relatively uncommon in patients with AIDS. Because of high blood flow, bacilli frequently disseminate hematogenously to the anterior aspects of the vertebral bodies and to the metaphyses of long bones. It can erode through the epiphyseal plates, involve the joint space by causing progressive destruction and fibrous ankylosis, and spread to soft tissues, sometimes producing so-called cold abscesses. Spinal involvement (Pott disease) occurs in about half of patients. Vertebral disease may lead to diskitis, paraspinous abscesses, gibbus formation, and vertebral collapse with paraplegia. The hips and knees are the next most common sites of infection. Infection progresses very slowly, often over a period of many years, and usually produces pain and impaired mobility. Tuberculosis of bone appears radiographically as an array of destructive osteolytic lesions, with relatively little reactive bone formation. Definitive diagnosis often requires biopsy.

Tuberculous arthritis is characteristically a chronic, slowly progressive, destructive monoarticular process. The synovial fluid has a high protein level, a low glucose level, and a poor mucin clot. The white cell count is variable but is typically in the range of 10,000 to 20,000/mm^3; neutrophils often predominate. Acid-fast smears of synovial fluid are positive in only 20% of patients, but cultures are positive in 80%, and synovial biopsies are positive in 90%. In rare instances, tuberculous rheumatism, which is an acute polyarthritis that results from a hypersensitivity reaction rather than direct synovial infection, develops in patients. Prosthetic joint tuberculosis and tenosynovitis are uncommon.

Most patients with musculoskeletal and synovial tuberculosis have positive tuberculin skin tests. Tumor is the major differential diagnosis, and fungal and pyogenic infections are additional presenting considerations. Results of chemotherapy are excellent; nevertheless, orthopedic surgery may be required to provide spinal fixation or to fuse destroyed joints.

Tuberculous lymphadenitis Almost all forms of tuberculosis involve regional lymphatics and nodes. Aside from intrathoracic nodes, which may be infected even without parenchymal lesions, the cervical nodes are most commonly affected. HIV-negative patients are usually afebrile and present with slowly enlarging, painless mass lesions. Patients with AIDS are particularly vulnerable to tuberculous lymphadenitis and are usually febrile. Tuberculous nodes can become fluctuant and drain through skin or to contiguous tissues. Additional symptoms can be produced as a result of compression of adjacent structures. The tuberculin skin test is usually positive in HIV-negative patients who have tuberculous lymphadenitis but is often negative in patients with AIDS. Diagnosis depends either on fine-needle aspiration and culture or on biopsy and culture. Differential diagnosis includes lymphoma and other tumors, fungal disease, sarcoidosis, and, in children with cervical adenopathy, atypical mycobacterial infection. The last condition is important because excisional surgery is sufficient treatment for atypical infection, but chemotherapy is required for lymphadenitis caused by *M. tuberculosis*.

Other forms of tuberculosis Other, less common forms of extrapulmonary tuberculosis include infection of the eye, skin, upper respiratory tract, and many other organs. Adrenal infection is particularly important to consider because it is clinically silent unless Addison disease results. Adrenal insufficiency can occur even after successful chemotherapy; it is usually insidious but can be acute, and it should be considered in all patients with active or remote tuberculosis who are doing poorly, particularly if hypotension, hyponatremia, or hyperkalemia is present.

PREVENTION OF TUBERCULOSIS

Case Finding

All patients with tuberculosis should be reported to public health authorities so that case finding can be undertaken; in urban settings, the average patient has about six close contacts, two of whom will be tuberculin positive.[39]

Treatment of Latent Tuberculous Infection

HIV-positive persons All HIV-infected persons should receive the PPD tuberculin skin test; testing for anergy with two additional skin tests, such as the mumps-skin-test antigen and the *Candida* antigen, may be helpful. The prevalence of anergy correlates with the stage of HIV infection and is highest in patients with CD4$^+$ T cell counts below 200/mm³. Unless there are contraindications, all those in whom 5 mm of induration develops on the PPD test should receive isoniazid chemoprophylaxis daily for 9 months. When daily isoniazid administration is not feasible, twice weekly directly observed administration of isoniazid in a dose of 10 to 15 mg/kg (with a maximum of 900 mg) for 9 months appears beneficial. When isoniazid is contraindicated, latent tuberculosis can be treated with daily administration of pyrazinamide and rifampin for 2 months or with rifampin daily for 4 months.[40] Rifampin is contraindicated in patients taking protease inhibitors or nonnucleoside reverse transcriptase inhibitors (NNRTIs) [see 14 HIV and AIDS],[41] but rifabutin may be substituted in some circumstances.[41]

Tuberculin-negative HIV-infected persons who are anergic and are at low risk for tuberculosis do not need routine prophylaxis.[41] Prophylaxis may be considered on an individual basis for anergic HIV-positive patients if their risk of tuberculous infection is estimated to be 10% or greater; HIV-positive persons who are often at increased risk for tuberculosis include immigrants from countries with a high prevalence of tuberculosis, prisoners, homeless people, and I.V. drug abusers.[42]

HIV-negative persons Guidelines for the treatment of latent tuberculosis in HIV-negative adults depend on patient age, the strength of the tuberculin reaction, and the presence or absence of risk factors.[18] Persons who have recently been exposed to active pulmonary tuberculosis or who have evidence of old tuberculosis on chest radiography are also at high risk for tuberculosis. If such patients have a PPD skin reaction of 5 mm or more, they are candidates for preventive therapy regardless of age. Patients who have important but somewhat less potent risk factors, such as I.V. drug abuse and immunosuppression, are candidates for chemoprophylaxis if their PPD skin test is 10 mm or more, regardless of age. Patients younger than 35 years who have had a recent tuberculin conversion should be considered for chemoprophylaxis if their PPD skin test has increased by 10 mm, whereas patients older than 35 years who have had a recent tuberculin conversion are candidates if their PPD skin test has increased by 15 mm.

Patients who have no risk factors but who belong to high-incidence population groups, such as immigrants, low-income patients with inadequate medical care, prison inmates, and residents of long-term care facilities, should be considered for isoniazid chemoprophylaxis if their PPD skin test is 10 mm or more and they are younger than 35 years. Patients who have no risk factors and who belong to low-incidence population groups should be considered for isoniazid chemoprophylaxis if their PPD skin test is 15 mm or more and they are younger than 35 years.

The role of isoniazid prophylaxis in older patients is being reevaluated.[43,44] In a study of 1,935 nursing home residents (mean age, 79.4 years), isoniazid prophylaxis had a favorable risk-to-benefit ratio in persons with documented tuberculin conversions but was less helpful in those who had long-standing positive skin tests. Isoniazid hepatitis developed in 4.4% of patients, and other forms of drug intolerance developed in 6%; however, drug therapy did not contribute to any fatalities.[45]

When isoniazid is used for treatment of latent tuberculosis in HIV-negative adults, it should be administered daily for 9 months. Except in patients with fibrotic changes on chest radiographs, 6 months of daily therapy is also acceptable. When prophylaxis is given to tuberculin-negative persons because of a heavy exposure to tuberculosis, it can be discontinued at 3 months if the tuberculin skin test remains negative.[46] In noncompliant patients who require prophylaxis, isoniazid can be administered twice weekly for 9 months under direct observation in a dose of 15 mg/kg (maximum, 900 mg).[18] Isoniazid is less likely to be beneficial in regions with a high prevalence of isoniazid-resistant organisms. Alternative regimens include 2 months of daily rifampin and pyrazinamide and 4 months of daily rifampin alone[18]; the 2-month rifampin-pyrazinamide combination may allow prison inmates to complete their therapy before they are released.[47] For persons who are likely to be infected with multidrug-resistant tuberculosis and who are at high risk for tuberculosis, pyrazinamide plus ethambutol or a fluoroquinolone (ofloxacin or levofloxacin) for 6 to 12 months is recommended.[18]

Isoniazid prophylaxis is contraindicated in patients with active tuberculous infection, active acute liver disease, alcohol abuse, and isoniazid intolerance. The presence of chronic liver disease, poor patient understanding or compliance, or the requirement for multiple medications constitutes relative contraindications; chronic hepatitis B carriage, however, is not a contraindication to isoniazid prophylaxis. Isoniazid prophylaxis should be deferred in pregnant women until after delivery. Hepatitis is the major toxicity associated with isoniazid therapy[48]; severe or fatal hepatitis has also been reported with rifampin and pyrazinamide prophylaxis,[49] underscoring the need for clinical monitoring for adverse reactions in all patients receiving treatment for latent tuberculosis.

Vaccines BCG is a live attenuated strain of *M. bovis* that has been used for the prevention of tuberculosis since 1921. Although BCG has been administered to more people than any other vaccine, a wide variation in efficacy has been reported, ranging from 0% to above 80%. The best results have been reported in trials conducted at latitudes far from the equator; ironically, the results have been worst in tropical countries, where the vaccine is used most widely. Even in the tropics, however, administration of BCG has been associated with a decreased risk of leprosy.[50] Despite the heterogeneity of results, a meta-analysis of vaccine trials concluded that on average, BCG vaccination reduces the risk of tuberculosis by 50%.[51]

BCG is not recommended for routine use in the United States.[52] The vaccine produces a positive tuberculin test in recipients, and because of the low incidence of new tuberculous infections in the United States (estimated at 0.03%), case finding and treatment of latent tuberculous infection are considered more efficient. However, BCG may be useful for tuberculin-negative infants and children (1) who are unable to receive isoniazid but who are continuously exposed to active tuberculosis, (2) who are continuously exposed to isoniazid- and rifampin-resistant bacilli, or (3) who are members of groups with rates of new infection that exceed 1% a year. Because of the increase in drug-resistant tuberculosis, BCG may also have a use in adults who are at high risk for tuberculosis, such as homeless persons,[52] and possibly in health care providers and correctional officers. However, BCG is contraindicated in immunosuppressed persons, including those with HIV infection[53]; adverse reaction may occur up to 12 years after BCG administration in HIV-infected persons.[54]

BCG is now being used clinically for the intravesical therapy of superficial bladder cancer[55] and experimentally as an immunologic adjuvant in other cancer patients. Although most patients tolerate intravesical BCG without complications, adverse side effects may occur. Such side effects include prolonged episodes of fever with abnormal liver function tests, pulmonary granulomas (which can mimic metastatic disease), pneumonitis, osteomyelitis, brain abscess, and disseminated infection.[56] Antituberculous therapy is indicated for severe reactions. New vaccines for tuberculosis are being developed.[57]

ANTITUBERCULOUS CHEMOTHERAPY

General Principles

The chemotherapy for tuberculosis differs from other antimicrobial approaches.[58,59] The therapies for pulmonary and extrapulmonary tuberculosis are similar and should proceed according to six basic principles. (1) Cultures and drug-sensitivity testing are mandatory. In most cases, testing can be accomplished within a week by use of the BACTEC system; faster molecular methods of screening for drug susceptibility are currently under study.[60] (2) Multiple drugs should be used. The most important reason for using two or more agents simultaneously is to prevent the emergence of drug-resistant organisms. (3) Drugs should be changed in combination, rather than singly, in treatment failures. The reason is that the patient who is responding poorly to therapy may harbor drug-resistant organisms; therefore, the introduction of a single new drug may permit the selection of organisms resistant to that drug as well. (4) Single daily doses of drugs are preferred. Single-dose therapy is as effective as divided-dose therapy, perhaps because of the very slow generation time of the tubercle bacillus, and achieves greater patient acceptance and compliance. (5) Prolonged chemotherapy is necessary. Previous regimens employed multiple drugs for periods of 18 to 24 months, but with combinations of newer agents, shorter regimens of 6 months have been found to be equally effective. (6) No matter what regimen is chosen, it is important to follow patients closely to ensure compliance and to monitor drug efficacy and toxicity. The regimens are so effective, however, that relapse is unlikely and prolonged surveillance is not needed [*see Table 2*].

Hospitalization Most patients should be hospitalized initially. Patients with pulmonary tuberculosis who have positive sputum smears should be treated in isolation rooms until they show clinical improvement and until three consecutive sputum specimens, collected on separate days, test negative. As little as 2 weeks of combined therapy greatly decreases the infectiousness of pulmonary tuberculosis, although a few mycobacteria may persist in sputum smears or cultures. Hence, short-term isolation in general hospitals is preferred, with early home care for clinically stable patients who will follow their treatment regimens, even if they do not meet the standard of three negative sputum smears.[61] Patients with extrapulmonary

Table 2 Selected Drugs for Mycobacterial Infections*

Drugs	*Usual Daily Dose for Adults*	*Major Properties*	*Major Toxicities*
Drugs for tuberculosis			
Isoniazid	300 mg p.o. (may be given I.M.)	Bactericidal Active against *M. tuberculosis, M. bovis*, and *M. kansasii* Emerging resistance	Hepatotoxicity Hypersensitivity Neuropathy Drug interactions
Rifampin	600 mg p.o. (may be given I.V.)	Bactericidal Active against *M. tuberculosis* and many other species	Hepatotoxicity Hypersensitivity Hematologic Drug interactions
Pyrazinamide	15–30 mg/kg p.o. (maximum, 2 g)	Bactericidal	Hepatotoxicity Hypersensitivity Gout
Ethambutol	25 mg/kg p.o. initially, then 15 mg/kg p.o. (maximum, 2.5 g)	Bacteriostatic Active against many strains of *M. avium* complex	Optic neuritis Hypersensitivity Gastrointestinal
Streptomycin	15 mg/kg (maximum, 1 g) I.M.; reduce to twice weekly after 2–8 wk	Bactericidal	Ototoxicity
Ciprofloxacin	1.0–1.5 g in two divided doses	New use; not licensed for antituberculous therapy Bactericidal Use when major drugs are ineffective Active against some strains of *M. avium* complex	Gastrointestinal
Ofloxacin	600–800 mg in two divided doses	New use; not licensed for antituberculous therapy Bactericidal Use when major drugs are ineffective Active against some strains of *M. avium* complex	Gastrointestinal
Drugs for *M. avium* complex			
Rifabutin	300 mg	Licensed for use in patients with CD4+ cell counts ≤ 100/mm^3 Also useful for tuberculosis	Hepatotoxicity Hypersensitivity
Clarithromycin	1 g in two divided doses	New use in combination with other drugs for *M. avium* complex	Gastrointestinal
Azithromycin	250 mg	New use in combination with other drugs for *M. avium* complex	Gastrointestinal

*Other antituberculous drugs include rifapentine, ethionamide, cycloserine, kanamycin, amikacin, capreomycin, and aminosalicylic acid. Other drugs for *M. avium* complex include clofazimine and amikacin.

tuberculosis are much less infectious and can sometimes be managed entirely as outpatients.

Initial drug treatment In response to increasing drug resistance, the United States Public Health Service issued revised guidelines for the initial treatment of tuberculosis.[62] Until drug susceptibility data are available, patients with active tuberculosis should be treated with daily administration of isoniazid, rifampin, pyrazinamide, and either ethambutol or streptomycin; in communities with documented isoniazid resistance rates below 4%, only isoniazid, rifampin, and pyrazinamide are required. After 2 months of such therapy, the regimen for patients with drug-sensitive organisms should be changed to isoniazid and rifampin administered daily or two or three times weekly for an additional 4 months or until sputum cultures are negative for 3 months. Alternative regimens are recommended for patients who require directly observed therapy to ensure compliance [*see* Directly Observed Therapy, *below*].

Treatment of HIV-infected persons HIV-infected individuals who do not require antiretroviral therapy can receive standard antituberculous regimens. Directly observed therapy and other strategies that promote compliance should always be employed. The results are generally excellent.[63,64]

Although patients coinfected with HIV and drug-susceptible strains of *M. tuberculosis* respond well to antituberculous therapy, treatment is complicated by drug interactions.[41,65,66] Because rifamycins induce the hepatic cytochrome CYP450 enzyme system, they reduce blood levels and antiretroviral activities of protease inhibitors and NNRTIs [see 14 HIV and AIDS]. Rifampin is the most potent CYP450 inducer, followed by rifapentine and rifabutin. Conversely, the protease inhibitors are CYP450 inhibitors that raise rifamycin levels to potentially toxic concentrations; ritonavir has the greatest effect, and saquinavir has the smallest.

Because rifampin is contraindicated in patients receiving protease inhibitors or NNRTIs, antituberculous regimens must be modified in the presence of antiretroviral therapy. Two options are available. In one, rifabutin, isoniazid, pyrazinamide, and ethambutol are administered daily for either 2 weeks or 8 weeks to complete the induction phase; in either case, therapy is completed by administering rifabutin and isoniazid daily or twice a week for 4 months. The usual rifabutin dose of 300 mg should be reduced to 150 mg during daily rifabutin therapy in patients concurrently receiving indinavir, nelfinavir, or amprenavir; no reduction is necessary during twice-weekly rifabutin therapy. The other option is reserved for patients who cannot receive rifabutin. It consists of isoniazid, streptomycin, pyrazinamide, and ethambutol administered daily for either 2 weeks or 8 weeks and then twice a week for 6 weeks to complete the induction phase; in either case, therapy is completed by administering isoniazid, streptomycin, and pyrazinamide two or three times a week for 7 months.

Major Antituberculous Agents

Isoniazid Introduced into clinical use in the early 1950s, isoniazid remains the single most important antituberculous drug. It is bactericidal but is active against only dividing organisms. Its mechanism of action is not fully understood but probably involves impairment of cell-wall mycolic acid synthesis and possibly mycobacterial DNA synthesis.

Most strains of *M. tuberculosis* are inhibited by approximately 0.05 µg/ml of isoniazid. After a standard dose of the drug, peak serum levels reach 3 to 5 µg/ml at 2 hours, thus providing an excellent ratio of serum levels to inhibitory concentrations. Food greatly decreases the absorption of isoniazid.[67] Of great importance is the excellent tissue penetration of this small, water-soluble molecule. The distribution of isoniazid includes the CNS, tuberculous abscesses, and intracellular sites. The major metabolism of the drug is hepatic acetylation; the metabolites are then excreted by the kidneys. The rate of hepatic acetylation is a genetically determined trait, the half-life of isoniazid averaging approximately 80 minutes in patients in whom acetylation occurs rapidly and 180 minutes in those in whom acetylation occurs slowly. Peripheral neuropathy may be somewhat more common with slow acetylation. Because the metabolite acetylhydrazine may be responsible for isoniazid hepatotoxicity, hepatitis may be more common with rapid acetylation. Although metabolites are excreted by the kidneys, it is not necessary to modify doses except in advanced renal failure. Isoniazid resistance occurs naturally in about 1 per 10^5 mycobacteria.

Isoniazid is an inexpensive drug. It is available in both oral and intramuscular preparations. The parenteral preparation is temporarily unavailable commercially but can be obtained from the CDC Drug Service (404-639-3670). The usual dose is 5 mg/kg body weight, which averages 300 mg/day for adults. In initial therapy for life-threatening disease, dosages of 10 to 15 mg/kg/day may be used. For patients receiving isoniazid, pyridoxine in a daily dose of 50 mg is also recommended. The major toxicities associated with isoniazid administration include the following:

1. Neurologic toxicity, ranging from peripheral neuropathy (which is prevented by daily administration of 50 mg of pyridoxine) to much less common manifestations, such as encephalopathies, seizures, optic neuritis, and personality changes.
2. Hypersensitivity reactions, including fever, rash, and rheumatic syndromes with or without positive antinuclear antibodies and lupus erythematosus cell preparations.
3. Serious clinical hepatitis, which appears in fewer than 2% of patients receiving isoniazid. There is a transient, clinically insignificant rise in aspartate aminotransferase (AST) levels in 10% to 20% of patients. In the asymptomatic patient, mild transient AST elevations do not necessitate drug withdrawal, but close follow-up is mandatory. Isoniazid must be stopped if mild AST elevations persist, if even a single level is substantially elevated, or if signs or symptoms of hepatitis are present.

Isoniazid interacts with a variety of drugs[67]; results of these interactions include increases in serum levels of phenytoin, carbamazepine, primidone, and barbiturates and decreases in serum levels of ketoconazole. Prednisolone decreases the serum levels of isoniazid.

Rifampin Rifampin is the newest of the major antituberculous drugs, rivaling isoniazid in its efficacy. Rifampin is bactericidal for mycobacteria; it acts by inhibiting DNA-dependent RNA polymerase. Most mycobacteria are inhibited by 0.5 μg/ml, a concentration much lower than the average serum peak levels of 8 to 24 μg/ml. Rifampin is a large, fat-soluble molecule that achieves excellent penetration of tissues, including CNS tissues. The drug is excreted by the liver; modification of dosage is not required in renal failure but may be necessary in patients with hepatic insufficiency. Rifampin is usually given orally, ideally on an empty stomach.[68] In addition, an intravenous preparation has been available for use in the United States since 1989.

Unlike isoniazid and ethambutol, rifampin is a broad-spectrum antimicrobial agent that acts against some atypical mycobacteria, *M. leprae*, many bacteria (including staphylococci, meningococci, and various gram-negative bacilli), *Chlamydia trachomatis*, and some viruses. The average dosage for adults is 600 mg/day, given in a single dose. Patients should be cautioned to expect orange discoloration of urine, sweat, tears, and saliva. This manifestation has no clinical significance, although damage to contact lenses may occur. Toxicities include hypersensitivity reactions such as fever, rash, and eosinophilia; hematologic effects such as thrombocytopenia, leukopenia, and hemolytic anemia; and hepatitis accompanied by an elevated AST level in up to 10% of patients with toxic reactions.

Because rifampin is a potent inducer of the hepatic CYP450 oxidative enzymes, it accelerates the metabolism of many drugs, including warfarin, oral contraceptives, cyclosporine, glucocorticoids, itraconazole, ketoconazole, theophylline, quinidine, digitoxin, verapamil, nifedipine, and methadone. Rifampin increases thyroxine clearance and can induce hypothyroidism in patients receiving thyroid replacement. Rifampin is contraindicated in patients receiving antiretroviral therapy. Additional caution should be exercised if rifampin is given in intermittent chemotherapy. Low dosages (600 mg twice weekly) are well tolerated, but higher dosages (900 to 1,200 mg twice weekly) have produced hypersensitivity reactions, including hemolysis, thrombocytopenia, and renal failure.

Other Rifamycins

Rifabutin Rifabutin is structurally and pharmacologically similar to rifampin. Rifabutin is active against the same strains of *M. tuberculosis* and *M. leprae* as rifampin. Unlike rifampin, however, rifabutin demonstrates in vitro activity against most strains of *M. avium* complex.[69] Because it is a much less potent inducer of hepatic cytochrome CYP450, rifabutin should be substituted for rifampin in the antituberculous therapy of HIV-infected patients who are receiving antiretroviral therapy.

Rifapentine Rifapentine[70] is a long-acting analogue of rifampin that was approved for use in the United States in 1998, making it the first new antituberculous drug to be licensed in 25 years. Its spectrum of activity and potential toxicities resemble those of rifampin. Because of its longer half-life, however, rifapentine may be administered twice a week during the induction phase of chemotherapy and once a week during the continuation phase, always in conjunction with other antituberculous drugs. Despite this advantage, rifampin is preferred until data demonstrate that rifapentine is equally effective.

Pyrazinamide First introduced in 1952, pyrazinamide, a derivative of nicotinic acid, was relegated to secondary status for years but has regained its prominence because its bactericidal activity is important in short-course antituberculous regimens. Pyrazinamide is well absorbed from the gastrointestinal tract, achieving peak blood levels of 20 to 60 μg/ml, higher than the 12.5 μg/ml required to inhibit most mycobacteria. The drug is widely distributed in body tissues and fluids, including the CSF. Although its mechanism of action has not been fully elucidated, pyrazinamide is bactericidal and is particularly active against dormant bacilli at an acid pH in the intracellular milieu. Pyrazinamide seems to be excreted by both hepatic and renal mechanisms. The major toxicities of the drug include hepatic dysfunction, hyperuricemia, and hypersensitivity. Pyrazinamide is usually administered in a single daily dose of 15 to 30 mg/kg (maximum dose is 2 g).

Ethambutol Introduced clinically in the United States in 1967, ethambutol represented a major advance in antituberculous chemotherapy. Ethambutol is bacteriostatic, probably acting by impairing incorporation of mycolic acids into the cell wall. Most organisms are inhibited by 0.05 to 2.0 μg/ml, but serum peak levels (2 to 5 μg/ml) do not greatly exceed this concentration. Ethambutol penetrates tissues well, including those of the CNS when the meninges are inflamed. It is excreted by the kidneys; drug dosage must be modified in patients with renal failure. Serum ethambutol levels (available through the manufacturer) should be monitored in patients with renal failure who require the drug. Ethambutol is available only as an oral preparation; it is best administered on an empty stomach.[71] Many authorities recommend initial therapy with 25 mg/kg/day (maximum, 2.5 g) for the first 6 to 8 weeks of therapy, followed by dosages of 15 mg/kg/day for the remainder of the course. Although good results have also been obtained with use of the lower dosage throughout therapy, the relatively narrow ratio of serum levels to inhibitory concentrations makes the initial high-dosage regimen seem more attractive for severe cases. The major toxicities of ethambutol include hypersensitivity reactions, such as fever and rash, and optic neuritis. The optic neuritis is dose related and usually first manifested by a loss of color vision. Less common side effects include neuritis, gastrointestinal intolerance, headache, and hyperuricemia.

Streptomycin The first effective antituberculous drug, streptomycin remains therapeutically useful. It is bactericidal and acts by inhibiting protein synthesis. Most strains of *M. tuberculosis* are sensitive to levels of streptomycin ranging from 0.5 to 5.0 µg/ml, and peak serum levels exceed this greatly, averaging 30 to 45 µg/ml. Like other aminoglycosides, streptomycin has only fair tissue distribution; it is inactive at an acid pH or in an anaerobic milieu, and it penetrates the CSF very poorly. Because streptomycin is excreted via the kidneys, dosage must be reduced in patients with renal failure. Streptomycin must be given parenterally. The average adult dosage is 15 mg/kg (maximum, 1 g) daily for the first 2 to 8 weeks of therapy, followed by the same dosage twice a week; the total cumulative dose should not exceed 120 g. Major toxicities include hypersensitivity reactions and eighth nerve toxicity, especially to the vestibular division, with consequent vertigo. Streptomycin is not currently available commercially, but it can be obtained directly from the manufacturer (Pfizer, 800-254-4445).

Fluoroquinolones The fluoroquinolones are the most promising new antituberculous agents[72]; ofloxacin, levofloxacin, ciprofloxacin, and sparfloxacin are bactericidal against most strains of *M. tuberculosis* and many atypical mycobacteria, but resistance develops rapidly if they are used for monotherapy. Although clinical experience with these drugs is limited,[73] oral fluoroquinolone therapy (ciprofloxacin at a dosage of 750 mg twice daily, ofloxacin at a dosage of 400 mg twice daily, sparfloxacin at a dosage of 200 mg twice daily, or levofloxacin at dosage of 500 mg once or twice daily) is effective as part of multidrug regimens. The new quinolones are well tolerated for prolonged periods but are active against only 30% to 38% of *M. avium* complex strains.

Other Drugs

In addition to the major drugs, several other agents are available in the United States for the treatment of tuberculosis. Three of these are administered orally: aminosalicylic acid (PAS), ethionamide, and cycloserine. Two other drugs, kanamycin and capreomycin, are available for parenteral administration; these agents are pharmacologically similar to streptomycin. They tend to be less effective and more toxic than the standard agents, but occasionally, they are critically important for treating patients with drug-resistant tuberculosis or atypical mycobacterial infections and for treating patients who cannot tolerate the standard drugs.

Fixed-Dose Combinations

Although fixed-dose combination antimicrobial agents are generally considered less desirable than single-agent preparations for the treatment of infectious diseases, fixed-dose combinations of antituberculous drugs may be helpful for patients who are poorly compliant with multidrug regimens. Combinations of isoniazid and rifampin and of isoniazid, rifampin, and pyrazinamide are now available in the United States and have long been recommended by the World Health Organization and the International Union against Tuberculosis and Lung Disease.

DRUG RESISTANCE

Drug resistance has long been a problem in the management of tuberculosis, but in the 1990s, the problem developed new and worrisome features. Drug resistance seems to fall into two distinct categories. The older category includes organisms that typically have been resistant to isoniazid and streptomycin but remained susceptible to other standard antituberculous drugs. A new category comprises tubercle bacilli that have become resistant to multiple drugs, including most of the standard agents. In the United States as a whole, 8.4% of the tubercle bacilli isolated from patients between 1993 and 1996 were resistant to isoniazid; 6.2% were resistant to streptomycin; 3.0% were resistant to rifampin; and 2.2% were resistant to ethambutol. However, only 2.2% of isolates were classified as multidrug resistant because of resistance to both isoniazid and rifampin.[74] In urban areas, however, the rate of resistance is often much higher. Fortunately, measures to prevent and control tuberculosis have helped contain multidrug-resistant organisms; in New York City, the prevalence of such organisms decreased from 19% to 13% between 1991 and 1994.[75]

Three factors increase the likelihood of the older type of resistance: (1) the patient's country of origin is in Latin America or Southeast Asia, where these organisms are much more prevalent; (2) the patient has been residing in the United States a relatively short time (people who have lived less than 10 years in the United States are more likely to harbor resistant mycobacteria); and (3) the patient has undergone previous antituberculous therapy. Primary resistance is much more likely for older antituberculous drugs, such as isoniazid and streptomycin, than for newer agents, such as rifampin and ethambutol.

The newer and more dangerous type of multidrug resistance has developed in the AIDS era. Between 1990 and 1992, seven outbreaks of multidrug-resistant tuberculosis were reported to the CDC; about 90% of the patients were HIV positive, and many had advanced AIDS at the time of diagnosis. Nosocomial transmission of multidrug-resistant organisms was demonstrated in these outbreaks. The mortality in these original outbreaks was exceedingly high, ranging from 70% to 90%, but early diagnosis and aggressive multidrug therapy has produced some improvement.[75,76] Even with this progress, however, prevention is of greatest importance; the need is particularly acute in areas of the world with a high prevalence of resistant organisms.[77]

The management of multidrug-resistant tuberculosis is exceedingly difficult, and early diagnosis and individualized therapy are critical. To prevent the transmission of multidrug-resistant tuberculosis, stringent isolation procedures are mandatory. Aggressive chemotherapy with a combination of drugs is essential.[41] The choice of agents should depend on the results of susceptibility testing, but before the results are received, the drugs administered and most likely to be effective include pyrazinamide, streptomycin, ciprofloxacin, ofloxacin, levofloxacin, cycloserine, capreomycin, and ethambutol. Pulmonary resection may be warranted as an adjunct to medical therapy in some cases.[78]

The management of persons exposed to multidrug-resistant tuberculosis is also difficult. Such persons should be evaluated for the closeness of their contact with infected persons and their immune status. Persons at high risk are candidates for chemoprophylaxis. Possible regimens include pyrazinamide plus ethambutol in standard doses and pyrazinamide in standard doses plus ciprofloxacin (750 mg twice daily) or ofloxacin (400 mg twice daily).

Directly Observed Therapy

There are three major reasons for the failure of antituberculous therapy: the selection of resistant mutants, the persistence of dormant organisms, and poor patient compliance. The first two problems have been approached by using multiple drugs simultaneously and by continuing therapy for prolonged periods; the third problem can be corrected by directly observed therapy.

Directly observed therapy is helpful for patients who cannot be relied upon to comply with their treatment regimens and who therefore require supervised outpatient administration of their drugs. One option is to initiate therapy with daily doses of isoniazid, rifampin, pyrazinamide, and either ethambutol or streptomycin for 2 weeks, followed by twice-weekly administration of the same drugs for 6 weeks, followed by twice-weekly administration of isoniazid and rifampin. Another option is to treat with isoniazid, rifampin, pyrazinamide, and either ethambutol or streptomycin three times a week for 6 months. The rifampin dosage is not increased during twice- or thrice-weekly therapy, but the isoniazid dosage is increased to 15 mg/kg (maximum, 900 mg), the pyrazinamide dosage to 50 to 70 mg/kg (maximum, 4 g twice a week or 3 g three times a week), the ethambutol dosage to 50 mg/kg twice a week (maximum, 2.5 g) or 25 to 30 mg/kg three times a week (maximum, 2.5 g), and the streptomycin dosage to 25 to 30 mg/kg (maximum, 1.5 g twice a week or 1.0 g three times a week). Directly observed therapy reduces the frequency of drug resistance and relapse and is cost-effective.[79]

Other Considerations

Isoniazid, ethambutol, and rifampin appear to be safe in pregnant women who have tuberculosis; pyrazinamide also appears safe, but experience is limited.[80] Children with tuberculosis should be treated in the same manner as adults, except that ethambutol is generally avoided in children younger than 5 years. Treatment of extrapulmonary tuberculosis is the same as that of pulmonary tuberculosis. The availability of excellent chemotherapeutic agents has greatly reduced the role of surgery in the treatment of tuberculosis, but surgery occasionally may be helpful in treating complications, in repairing or removing damaged tissue, or in attempting to extirpate drug-resistant organisms. Corticosteroids are useful only in tuberculous meningitis complicated by hydrocephalus and by CSF block, in tuberculous pericarditis, and possibly in tuberculous peritonitis.[36,81] Elaborate programs of rest and diet are ineffective.

Nontuberculous Mycobacterial Diseases

Although *M. tuberculosis* is by far the most important human pathogen, numerous other species of mycobacteria can cause disease in humans [*see Table 1*]. Of these pathogens, *M. bovis* is the most closely related to *M. tuberculosis*. At one time, 5% of cattle in the United States harbored *M. bovis*, and the organism often caused disease in humans, particularly lymphadenitis, enteritis, pulmonary infection, and osteomyelitis, which are all clinically indistinguishable from disease caused by *M. tuberculosis*. However, as a result of the slaughter of tuberculin-positive herds and the pasteurization of milk, *M. bovis* rarely causes disease in the United States. However, immigrants from Mexico and other countries that have not controlled *M. bovis* in cattle may bring the organism into the United States, and *M. bovis* still causes outbreaks in other parts of the world.[82] *M. bovis* is usually sensitive to isoniazid and other chemotherapeutic agents.

Many mycobacterial species in addition to *M. tuberculosis* have been recognized in the laboratory for many years, but their potential as human pathogens was not demonstrated until 1951. A great problem in understanding this heterogeneous group of organisms was the lack of a workable classification system, which led to the designations of anonymous, unclassified, and atypical mycobacteria. In terms of their high lipid content, acid-fast properties, aerobic metabolism, and lack of motility and spore formation, these organisms are in fact typical mycobacteria. They differ from *M. tuberculosis*, however, in terms of their rate of growth, colonial morphology, pigment production, biochemical reactivity, and pathogenicity. It is therefore best to refer to them as nontuberculous, or atypical, mycobacteria. The understanding of these organisms was greatly enhanced in 1959 by Runyon's development of an excellent system that classifies these organisms (groups I to IV) by their rate of growth and pigment production [*see Table 1*].

Table 3 Relative Virulence of Mycobacteria Encountered in Clinical Situations

	Organism	*Runyon Group*
Pathogenic	*M. tuberculosis* *M. bovis* *M. leprae* *M. ulcerans*	—
Usually pathogenic	*M. marinum (M. balnei)* *M. kansasii* *M. avium* complex	I I III
Sometimes pathogenic	*M. scrofulaceum* *M. szulgai* *M. fortuitum* *M. chelonei* *M. xenopi*	II II IV IV —
Usually nonpathogenic	*M. gordonae* *M. smegmatis*	III IV
Nonpathogenic	*M. gastri* *M. terrae*	III III

Unlike *M. tuberculosis*, which is highly adapted to humans, the nontuberculous mycobacteria are widely distributed in the animal kingdom and in nature. The epidemiology of these organisms is not well understood, but person-to-person transmission has never been demonstrated; human infection probably results from inhalation or ingestion of bacilli from the environment. Some so-called atypical mycobacteria are concentrated in specific geographic regions, such as *M. kansasii* in the urban Midwest. Other atypical species, such as *M. scrofulaceum* and *M. marinum*, are more widespread. Infections caused by nontuberculous mycobacteria appear to be increasing, largely, but not exclusively, because of those produced by *M. avium* complex in AIDS patients.

On the basis of skin-test data, it is estimated that 40 million Americans have been infected with nontuberculous mycobacteria. Despite the fact that nearly three times more people have been infected with these atypical organisms than with *M. tuberculosis*, no more than 1% to 5% of all clinical mycobacterial infections are caused by nontuberculous mycobacteria because of their much lower virulence. In fact, the most common problem is determining whether the laboratory isolation of an atypical mycobacterium is of clinical significance. One clue may be the species of *Mycobacterium* isolated. Many of these organisms can cause human disease, but others are nonpathogens and may even be laboratory contaminants [*see Table 3*].

Criteria for the diagnosis of infection by an atypical *Mycobacterium* include repeated isolation of a potentially pathogenic species, the absence of other pathogens, and a compatible clinical, radiologic, or pathologic picture. Patients with nontuberculous mycobacterioses often exhibit a stronger cutaneous reactivity to antigens extracted from the atypical organism than to standard PPD. Unfortunately, these antigens are not generally available; however, patients infected with atypical mycobacteria often have a positive reaction to a second-strength PPD skin test, although their reaction to intermediate-strength PPD is weak or negative.

MYCOBACTERIUM AVIUM COMPLEX INFECTION IN AIDS

M. avium complex is the most frequent opportunistic bacterial infection in patients with AIDS; it typically occurs late in the course of AIDS, when other opportunistic infections and neoplasia have already occurred; almost all patients have $CD4^+$ T cell counts lower than $100/mm^3$. The mode of acquisition of *M. avium* complex in patients with AIDS is not clear. The genetic diversity of *M. avium* complex isolates from patients with AIDS implies that the organisms may be acquired from multiple environmental sources.

Diagnosis

M. avium complex produces widely disseminated infection in patients with AIDS.[83] Systemic symptoms predominate, including fever, chills, night sweats, and profound weight loss. Gastrointestinal symptoms, such as diarrhea and malabsorption, are often prominent. Pulmonary involvement is often present, but symptoms are difficult to interpret because other opportunistic pathogens, such as cytomegalovirus and *Pneumocystis*, are often present as well; pulmonary findings are absent in about 20% of patients.

Disseminated *M. avium* complex infection can be readily documented by mycobacterial smears and cultures in AIDS patients. Organisms are frequently present in the lungs, liver, spleen, bone marrow, and lymph nodes. Despite the presence of many mycobacteria in macrophages, well-formed granulomas are typically absent; this so-called lepromatous histology reflects the profound impairment of cell-mediated immunity in these patients and explains their inability to contain the infection. Intestinal infection can often be proved by culture of stool or of colonic biopsy specimens; *M. avium* complex may contribute to diarrhea in these patients. Intestinal or pulmonary infection may precede *M. avium* complex bacteremia, but smears and cultures of these sites are not sensitive enough to be used as screening tests for early infection. When the newer blood culture techniques are used, a high-grade *M. avium* complex bacteremia can be shown in almost all AIDS patients with such disseminated infection; the bacteremia may, however, be intermittent.

Treatment

The management of *M. avium* complex has improved greatly. Effective antiretroviral therapy can control the infection even without antibiotics,[84] although a severe inflammatory reaction may occur as immune competence is restored[85] and the infection can recur if $CD4^+$ T cell counts drop.[86] In addition, antimicrobials are effective for chemoprophylaxis. Patients with $CD4^+$ T cell counts of $50/mm^3$ or lower should receive azithromycin (1,200 mg weekly) or clarithromycin (500 mg twice daily). The drugs are equally efficacious, but azithromycin is often preferred for its greater convenience. Rifabutin is an alternative prophylactic agent for patients who cannot tolerate a macrolide.[87] Prophylaxis may be discontinued when the $CD4^+$ T cell counts exceed $100/mm^3$.[88] The treatment of disseminated infection has also improved. Although an optimal regimen has not been established, most patients should receive clarithromycin (or azithromycin) plus ethambutol and possibly rifabutin.[89,90] The dosage of clarithromycin should not exceed the recommended 500 mg twice a day. The azithromycin dosage is 600 mg a day.[91] Ethambutol is often given at a dosage of 15 mg/kg/day and rifabutin at a dosage of 300 mg/day. Other drugs that may be useful for individual patients include rifampin, clofazimine, amikacin, and the fluoroquinolones ciprofloxacin, ofloxacin, and sparfloxacin.[92]

OTHER NONTUBERCULOUS MYCOBACTERIAL INFECTIONS

A variety of syndromes can be caused by nontuberculous mycobacteria. Lymphadenitis in children may be caused by *M. scrofulaceum* or, less often, by *M. avium* complex, *M. kansasii*, or other species. These patients usually present with a single, slowly enlarging, painless submandibular node.[93] The clinical picture of scrofula caused by nontuberculous mycobacteria is identical to that of tuberculous lymphadenitis, and diagnosis depends on culture. Surgical excision is sufficient therapy for lymphadenitis caused by atypical organisms; in contrast, chemotherapy is needed for lymphadenitis caused by *M. tuberculosis*.

Pulmonary Infections

Pulmonary infection is most frequently caused by *M. kansasii*[94] or *M. avium* complex and can mimic tuberculosis. *M. kansasii* infections are most common in middle-aged men with chronic lung disease and are radiologically and clinically similar to reactivation tuberculosis; in some patients, however, chest radiographs reveal patchy nodular infiltrates without upper lobe predominance or cavitation. Spread of infection to the pleura or to extrapulmonary sites may occur in immunocompromised hosts.[95] Regimens containing rifampin, ethambutol, and isoniazid are recommended therapy. The newer macrolides and fluoroquinolones are active against most isolates; clarithromycin should be included in multidrug regimens used to treat rifampin-resistant strains. However, the patient's underlying disease is the most potent prognostic indicator.

M. avium complex is encountered most often as an opportunistic pathogen in immunosuppressed patients, especially in those with AIDS. When isolated from immunologically intact patients or those with cystic fibrosis,[96] *M. avium* complex may be a simple contaminant or a true pathogen. *M. avium* complex can cause cavitary disease in patients with chronic obstructive pulmonary disease or multiple small, slowly progressing lung nodules in patients with bronchiectasis.[97] Most patients respond to regimens that include clarithromycin or azithromycin.[98]

M. chelonei and other rapidly growing mycobacteria can also cause progressive pulmonary infections in immunocompetent hosts; patients with esophageal disorders are particularly vulnerable.[99]

Cutaneous Infections

Cutaneous infection can result from direct inoculation of organisms into the skin. The most common syndrome is the swimming-pool granuloma, caused by *M. marinum*, an organism common in pools and aquariums. After an incubation period of 5 to 270 days,[100] lesions develop on the extremities and present as slowly enlarging papules or verrucae, which may ulcerate. The granulomas usually heal spontaneously, but this process may take months to years, and the use of surgery or chemotherapy has been advocated. Both *M. fortuitum* and *M. chelonei* may cause localized abscesses; *M. chelonei* can cause disseminated skin and soft tissue infections in immunosuppressed patients. *M. ulcerans*, which is confined to parts of Africa, Asia, Australia, and Mexico, causes a progressively destructive process called Buruli ulcer.[101]

Rare Types of Nontuberculous Infection

On rare occasions, nontuberculous mycobacteria cause bacteremia and endocarditis.[102] Atypical mycobacteria can also cause nosocomial infections, such as wound infections, otitis media, abscesses,[103] osteomyelitis,[104] and peritonitis in dialysis patients.[105] *M. fortuitum* and *M. chelonei* can cause catheter-related infections.

Atypical mycobacteria can occasionally spread via the bloodstream to cause localized disease (e.g., arthritis, tenosynovitis, prostatitis, or meningitis) or systemic dissemination similar to miliary tuberculosis. These uncommon syndromes are most likely to occur in immunosuppressed patients; *M. avium* complex, *M. kansasii, M. fortuitum,* and *M. chelonei* are most often implicated.

Treatment

The treatment of nontuberculous mycobacterioses can be extremely difficult because the majority of these organisms are highly resistant to standard antituberculous regimens. Important exceptions are *M. kansasii, M. marinum,* and *M. xenopi,* which are often drug sensitive and respond to combined antituberculous therapy. *M. fortuitum* is often susceptible to amikacin, cefoxitin, clarithromycin, imipenem, sulfonamides, and the quinolones ciprofloxacin and ofloxacin. Many strains of *M. chelonei* are also susceptible to these agents, with the exception of the sulfonamides and the quinolones, and some strains are susceptible to doxycycline or erythromycin. Clarithromycin appears to be particularly valuable for the treatment of *M. kansasii, M. chelonei,* and many other nontuberculous mycobacteria, including *M. avium* complex. With all species, detailed sensitivity testing is mandatory, but surgery may be the only therapeutic modality available for localized disease. The prognosis for patients who have disseminated nontuberculous mycobacteriosis is poor.

Leprosy

A classic scourge of medieval Europe, leprosy (Hansen disease) is a mycobacterial disease that still afflicts a significant number of people; there are about one million persons with active disease and about 685,000 new cases annually throughout the world.[106] In the United States, however, fewer than 200 new cases appear each year, and most of these cases occur in immigrants from endemic areas.[107] Secondary transmission from imported cases has not been recognized.

PATHOGENESIS

The agent of leprosy, *M. leprae,* is an acid-fast bacillus, which, because it is easily decolorized, can best be visualized with the Fite-Faraco or other special stain. The organism has two unique properties: it is thermolabile, growing best at 27° to 30° C, and it divides very slowly—the generation time is 12 to 14 days. Consequently, leprosy in humans typically evolves very slowly and primarily affects the cooler peripheral tissues. The principal lesions are in the skin and peripheral nerves. Because of the long and variable incubation period of the disease, its epidemiology is incompletely understood. Prolonged intimate contact appears to be necessary for transmission by cutaneous inoculation; isolation of patients is not necessary.

DIAGNOSIS

The characteristic mutilation is caused by sensory loss in which the victim has no sensation of pain; infection of motor neurons causes paralysis. Early leprosy and indeterminate leprosy present as isolated nondescript skin lesions. Skin biopsy is required to make a diagnosis. Although many patients with indeterminate leprosy heal spontaneously, all such patients should receive chemotherapy.

More advanced infection can be divided into two polar forms: tuberculoid leprosy and lepromatous leprosy. The cell-mediated immunity of patients with tuberculoid leprosy is intact. Patients who have lepromatous leprosy are anergic and show severely impaired cell-mediated immunity.

Tuberculoid Leprosy

Skin lesions of patients with tuberculoid leprosy contain predominantly helper T cells, well-formed granulomas, and few organisms, whereas the lesions of lepromatous leprosy are practically devoid of granulomas and helper T cells, containing instead suppressor T cells and numerous bacilli. The major defect in lepromatous leprosy appears to be a specific inability of T cells to respond to *M. leprae*; as a result, they are unable to generate the lymphokines that normally activate macrophages and thereby enhance their ability to kill the organisms.

The presence of a few large, asymmetrical, well-defined skin lesions characterizes tuberculoid leprosy. The skin is rough, anhidrotic, and hypesthetic; central healing may occur. Neurologic involvement is limited to a few peripheral nerves. Although the damage to these nerves can be severe, the overall prognosis is good. A biopsy that shows well-formed granulomas but only very few organisms establishes the diagnosis.

Lepromatous Leprosy

A patient with lepromatous leprosy can serve as the host for an enormous bacterial burden because organisms multiply unchecked. The numerous symmetrical skin lesions are small and ill defined. At times, the entire skin surface can be involved, yielding a diffuse, waxy appearance. The loss of eyebrows and hypertrophy of earlobes produce the characteristic leonine facies. Neurologic involvement is widespread. A symmetrical peripheral neuropathy progresses proximally; sensory loss precedes paralysis. Other cool tissues, such as the anterior chamber of the eye, the upper airway, and the testes, are often involved; sustained bacillemia with multisystem infection can occur. A biopsy specimen showing many organisms and foam cells but no granulomas clinches the diagnosis, as does the finding of numerous acid-fast bacilli in smears of skin-slit preparations. If untreated, lepromatous leprosy is relentlessly progressive.

Borderline Leprosy

Many patients have a type of leprosy that falls between the tuberculoid and lepromatous forms and are classified as having borderline, or dimorphous, leprosy. In addition, the otherwise chronic course of leprosy can be punctuated by acute inflammatory reactions called erythema nodosum leprosum and the lepra reaction.

TREATMENT

Patients should be treated by physicians experienced in the management of this disease. Sulfones have been the mainstay of chemotherapy, but primary dapsone resistance has led to recommendation for combined chemotherapy with rifampin and clofazimine. Clofazimine, an oral phenazine dye that has been approved by the FDA for the treatment of leprosy, also exhibits activity against *M. avium* complex and is used experimentally in AIDS patients.

The enormous progress in chemotherapy, which has reduced the number of leprosy cases by nearly 90% over the past 10 years, makes the worldwide elimination of leprosy a realistic goal.

The fluoroquinolones discussed in this chapter have not been approved by the FDA for use in Mycobacteria *infections.*

References

1. US Department of Health and Human Services: World TB Day—March 24, 2001. MMWR Morb Mortal Wkly Rep 50:201, 2001

2. Talbot EA, Moore M, McCray E, et al: Tuberculosis among foreign-born persons in the United States, 1993–1998. JAMA 284:2894, 2000

3. Bishai WR, Graham NMH, Harrington S, et al: Molecular and geographic patterns of tuberculosis transmission after 15 years of directly observed therapy. JAMA 280:1679, 1998

4. Sotir MJ, Parrott P, Metchock B, et al: Tuberculosis in the inner city: impact of a continuing epidemic in the 1990s. Clin Infect Dis 29:1138, 1999

5. Havlir DV, Barnes PF: Tuberculosis in patients with human immunodeficiency virus infection. N Engl J Med 340:367, 1999

6. Moss AR, Hahn JA, Tulsky JP, et al: Tuberculosis in the homeless: a prospective study. Am J Respir Crit Care Med 162:460, 2000

7. Cobelens FGJ, van Deutekom H, Draayer-Jansen IWE, et al: Risk of infection with *Mycobacterium tuberculosis* in travelers to areas of high tuberculosis endemicity. Lancet 356:461, 2000

8. Menzies D, Fanning A, Yuan L, et al: Hospital ventilation and risk for tuberculosis infection in Canadian health care workers. Ann Intern Med 133:779, 2000

9. Johnson KR, Braden CR, Cairns KL, et al: Transmission of *Mycobacterium tuberculosis* from medical waste. JAMA 284:1683, 2000

10. Rao VK, Iademarco EP, Fraser VJ, et al: Delays in the suspicion and treatment of tuberculosis among hospitalized patients. Ann Intern Med 130:404, 1999

11. Bloom BR, Small PM: The evolving relation between humans and *Mycobacterium tuberculosis*. N Engl J Med 338:677, 1998

12. Behr MA, Warren SA, Salamon H, et al: Transmission of *Mycobacterium tuberculosis* from patients smear-negative for acid-fast bacilli (editorial). Lancet 353:444, 1999

13. Fine PEM, Small PM: Exogenous reinfection in tuberculosis. N Engl J Med 341:1220, 1999

14. Hernandez-Pando R, Jeyanathan M, Mengistu G, et al: Persistence of DNA from *Mycobacterium tuberculosis* in superficially normal lung tissue during latent infection. Lancet 356:2133, 2000

15. Small PM, Fujiwara PI: Management of tuberculosis in the United States. N Engl J Med 345:189, 2001

16. Diagnostic standards and classification of tuberculosis in adults and children (pt 1). Am J Respir Crit Care Med 161:1376, 2000

17. Villarino ME, Burman W, Wang Y-C, et al: Comparable specificity of 2 commercial tuberculin reagents in persons at low risk for tuberculous infection. JAMA 281:169, 1999

18. US Department of Health and Human Services: Targeted tuberculin testing and treatment of latent tuberculosis infection. MMWR Morb Mortal Wkly Rep 49:(RR-6), 2000

19. Moreno S, Blázquez R, Novoa A, et al: The effect of BCG vaccination on tuberculin reactivity and the booster effect among hospital employees. Arch Intern Med 161:1760, 2001

20. Menzies D: Interpretation of repeated tuberculin tests: boosting, conversion, and reversion. Am J Respir Crit Care Med 159:15, 1999

21. Warren DK, Foley KM, Polish LB, et al: Tuberculin skin testing of physicians at a Midwestern teaching hospital: a 6-year prospective study. Clin Infect Dis 32:1331, 2001

22. Lalvani A, Pathan AA, Durkan H, et al: Enhanced contact tracing and spatial tracking of *Mycobacterium tuberculosis* infection by enumeration of antigen-specific T cells. Lancet 357:2017, 2001

23. Pfyffer GE: Nucleic acid amplification for mycobacterial diagnosis. J Infect 39:21, 1999

24. Catanzaro A, Perry S, Clarridge S, et al: The role of clinical suspicion in evaluating a new diagnostic test of active tuberculosis: results of a multicenter prospective trial. JAMA 283:639, 2000

25. US Department of Health and Human Services: Update: nucleic acid amplification tests for tuberculosis. MMWR Morb Mortal Wkly Rep 49:593, 2000

26. Shah S, Miller A, Mastellone A, et al: Rapid diagnosis of tuberculosis in various biopsy and body fluid specimens by the AMPLICOR *Mycobacterium tuberculosis* polymerase chain reaction test. Chest 113: 1190, 1998

27. Miller LG, Asch SM, Yu EI, et al: A population-based survey of tuberculosis symptoms: how atypical are atypical presentations? Clin Infect Dis 30:293, 2000

28. Conde MB, Soares SLM, Mello FCQ, et al: Comparison of sputum induction with fiberoptic bronchoscopy in the diagnosis of tuberculosis: experience at an acquired immune deficiency syndrome reference center in Rio de Janeiro, Brazil. Am J Crit Care Med 162:2238, 2000

29. Narita M, Ashkin D, Hollender ES, et al: Paradoxical worsening of tuberculosis following antiretroviral therapy in patients with AIDS. Am J Respir Crit Care Med 158:157, 1998

30. Daikos GL, Uttamchandani RB, Tuda C, et al: Disseminated miliary tuberculosis of the skin in patients with AIDS: report of four cases. Clin Infect Dis 27:205, 1998

31. Verdon R, Chevret S, Laissy JP, et al: Tuberculous meningitis in adults: review of 48 cases. Clin Infect Dis 22:982, 1996

32. Berning SE, Cherry TA, Iseman MD: Novel treatment of meningitis caused by multidrug-resistant *Mycobacterium tuberculosis* with intrathecal levofloxacin and amikacin: case report. Clin Infect Dis 32:643, 2001

33. Hernandez-Albujar S, Arribas JR, Royo A, et al: Tuberculosis radiculomyelitis complicating tuberculosis meningitis: case report and review. Clin Infect Dis 30:915, 2000

34. Farrar DJ, Flanigan TP, Gordon NM, et al: Tuberculous brain abscess in a patient with HIV infection: case report and review. Am J Med 102:297, 1997

35. Talwani R, Horvath JA: Tuberculosis peritonitis in patients undergoing continuous ambulatory peritoneal dialysis: case report and review. Clin Infect Dis 31:70, 2000

36. Alrajhi AA, Halim MA, Al-Hokail A, et al: Corticosteroid treatment of peritoneal tuberculosis. Clin Infect Dis 27:52, 1998

37. Dowdy L, Ramgopal M, Hoffman T, et al: Genitourinary tuberculosis after renal transplantation: report of 3 cases and review. Clin Infect Dis 32:662, 2001

38. Moussa OM, Eraky I, El-Far MA, et al: Rapid diagnosis of genitourinary tuberculosis by polymerase chain reaction and non-radioactive DNA hybridization. J Urol 164:584, 2000

39. Marks SM, Taylor Z, Qualls NL, et al: Outcomes of contact investigations of infectious tuberculosis patients. Am J Respir Crit Care Med 162:2033, 2000

40. Gordin F, Chaissson RE, Matts JP, et al: Rifampin and pyrazinamide vs isoniazid for prevention of tuberculosis in HIV-infected persons: an international randomized trial. JAMA 283:1445, 2000

41. US Department of Health and Human Services: Prevention and treatment of tuberculosis among patients infected with human immunodeficiency virus: principles of therapy and revised recommendations. MMWR Morb Mortal Wkly Rep 47(RR-20):1, 1998

42. Gordin FM, Matts JP, Miller C, et al: A controlled trial of isoniazid in persons with anergy and human immunodeficiency virus infection who are at high risk for tuberculosis. N Engl J Med 337:315, 1997

43. Salpeter SR, Sanders GD, Salpeter EE, et al: Monitored isoniazid prophylaxis for low-risk tuberculin reactors older than 35 years of age: a risk-benefit and cost-effectiveness analysis. Ann Intern Med 127:1051, 1997

44. Gilroy SA, Rogers MAM, Blair DC: Treatment of latent tuberculosis infection in patients aged >35 years. Clin Infect Dis 31:826, 2000

45. Stead WW, To T, Harrison RW, et al: Benefit-risk considerations in preventive treatment for tuberculosis in elderly persons. Ann Intern Med 107:843, 1987

46. Nolan CM, Goldberg SV, Buskin SE: Hepatotoxicity associated with isoniazid preventive therapy: a 7-year survey from a public health tuberculosis clinic. JAMA 281:1014, 1999

47. Bock NN, Rogers T, Tapia JR, et al: Acceptability of short-course rifampin and pyrazinamide treatment of latent tuberculosis infection among jail inmates. Chest 119:833, 2001

48. Stead WW: Management of health care workers after inadvertent exposure to tuberculosis: a guide for the use of preventive therapy. Ann Intern Med 122:906, 1995

49. US Department of Health and Human Services: Fatal and severe hepatitis associated with rifampin and pyrazinamide for the treatment of latent tuberculosis infection—New York and Georgia, 2000. MMWR Morb Mortal Wkly Rep 50:289, 2001

50. Randomized controlled trial of single BCG, repeated BCG, or combined BCG and killed *Mycobacterium leprae* vaccine for prevention of leprosy and tuberculosis in Malawi. Karonga Prevention Trial Group. Lancet 348:17, 1996

51. Brewer TF: Preventing tuberculosis with bacillus Calmette-Guérin vaccine: a meta-analysis of the literature. Clin Infect Dis 31(suppl 3): S64, 2000

52. US Department of Health and Human Services: The role of BCG vaccine in the prevention and control of tuberculosis in the United States: a joint statement by the Advisory Council for the Elimination of Tuberculosis and the Advisory Committee on Immunization Practices. MMWR Morb Mortal Wkly Rep 45:1, 1996

53. Talbot EA, Perkins MD, Fagundes S, et al: Disseminated bacille Calmette-Guérin disease after vaccination: case report and review. Clin Infect Dis 24:1139, 1997

54. van Deutekom H, Smuldersy M, Roozendaal KJ, et al: Bacille Calmette-Guérin (BCG) meningitis in an AIDS patient 12 years after vaccination with BCG. Clin Infect Dis 22:870, 1996

55. Viallard J-F, Denis D, Texier-Maugein J-T, et al: Disseminated infection after bacille Calmette-Gúerin instillation for treatment of bladder carcinoma. Clin Infect Dis 29:451, 1999

56. US Department of Health and Human Services: Development of new vaccines for tuberculosis. Recommendations of the Advisory Council for the Elimination of Tuberculosis (ACET). MMWR Morb Mortal Wkly Rep 47(RR-13):1, 1998

57. Alexandroff AB, Jackson AM, O'Donnell MA, et al: BCG immunotherapy of bladder cancer: 20 years on. Lancet 353:1689, 1999

58. Horsburgh CR Jr, Feldman S, Ridzon R: Practice guidelines for the treatment of tuberculosis. Clin Infect Dis 31:633, 2000

59. Van Scoy RE, Wilkowske CJ: Antimycobacterial therapy. Mayo Clin Proc 74:1038, 1999

60. Woods GL: Susceptibility testing for mycobacteria. Clin Infect Dis 31:1209, 2000

61. Iseman MD: Editorial response: an unholy trinity-three negative sputum smears and release from tuberculosis isolation. Clin Infect Dis 25:671, 1997

62. US Department of Health and Human Services: Initial therapy for tuberculosis in the era of multidrug resistance: recommendations of the Advisory Council for the Elimination of Tuberculosis. MMWR Morb Mortal Wkly Rep 42(RR-7):1, 1993

63. Narita M, Hisada M, Thimmappa B, et al: Tuberculosis recurrence: multivariate analysis of serum levels of tuberculosis drugs, human immunodeficiency virus status, and other risk factors. Clin Infect Dis 32:515, 2001

64. El-Sadr WM, Perlman DC, Denning E, et al: A review of efficacy studies of 6-month short-course therapy for tuberculosis among patients infected with human immunodeficiency virus: differences in study outcomes. Clin Infect Dis 32:623, 2001

65. Burman WJ, Gallicano K, Peloquin C: Therapeutic implications of drug interactions in the treatment of human immunodeficiency virus–related tuberculosis. Clin Infect Dis 28:419, 1999

66. US Department of Health and Human Services: Updated guidelines of the use of rifabutin or rifampin for the treatment and prevention of tuberculosis among HIV-infected patients taking protease inhibitors or nonnucleoside reverse transcriptase inhibitors. MMWR Morb Mortal Wkly Rep 40:185, 2000

67. Self TH, Chrisman CR, Baciewicz AM, et al: Isoniazid drug and food interactions. Am J Med Sci 317:304, 1999

68. Peloquin CA, Namdar R, Singleton MD, et al: Pharmacokinetics of rifampin under fasting conditions, with food, and with antacids. Chest 115:12, 1999

69. Watt B: In-vitro sensitivities and treatment of less common mycobacteria. J Antimicrob Chemother 39:567, 1997

70. Rifapentine: a long-acting rifamycin for tuberculosis. Med Lett 41: 21, 1999

71. Peloquin CA, Bulpitt AE, Jaresko GS, et al: Pharmacokinetics of ethambutol under fasting conditions, with food, and with antacids. Antimicrob Agents Chemother 43:568, 1999

72. Alangaden GJ, Lerner SA: The clinical use of fluoroquinolones for the treatment of mycobacterial diseases. Clin Infect Dis 25:1213, 1997

73. Yew WW, Chan CK, Chau CH, et al: Outcomes of patients with multidrug-resistant pulmonary tuberculosis treated with ofloxacin/levofloxacin-containing regimens. Chest 117:744, 2000

74. Moore M, Onorato IM, McCray E, et al: Trends in drug-resistant tuberculosis in the United States, 1993–1996. JAMA 278:833, 1997

75. Fujiwara PI, Cook SV, Rutherford CM, et al: A continuing survey of drug-resistant tuberculosis, New York City, April 1994. Arch Intern Med 157:531, 1997

76. Franzetti F, Gori A, Iemoli E, et al: Outcome of multidrug-resistant tuberculosis in human immunodeficiency virus-infected patients. Clin Infect Dis 29:553, 1999

77. Espinal MA, Laszlo A, Simonsen L, et al: Global trends in resistance to antituberculosis drugs. N Engl J Med 344:1294, 2001

78. Pomerantz BJ, Cleveland JC Jr, Olson HK, et al: Pulmonary resection for multi-drug resistant tuberculosis. J Thorac Cardiovasc Surg 121:448, 2001

79. Directly observed therapy for treatment completion of pulmonary tuberculosis: Consensus Statement of the Public Health Tuberculosis Guidelines Panel. JAMA 279:943, 1998

80. Davidson PT: Managing tuberculosis during pregnancy. Lancet 346: 199, 1995

81. Dooley DP, Carpenter JL, Rademacher S: Adjunctive corticosteroid therapy for tuberculosis: a critical reappraisal of the literature. Clin Infect Dis 25:872, 1997

82. Rivero A, Marquez M, Santos J, et al: High rate of tuberculosis reinfection during a nosocomial outbreak of multidrug-resistant tuberculosis caused by *Mycobacterium bovis* strain B. Clin Infect Dis 32:159, 2001

83. Horsburgh CR Jr: The pathophysiology of disseminated *Mycobacterium avium* complex disease in AIDS. J Infect Dis 179(suppl 3):S461, 1999

84. Hadad DJ, Lewi DS, Pignatari ACC, et al: Resolution of *Mycobacterium avium* complex bacteremia following highly active antiretroviral therapy. Clin Infect Dis 26:758, 1998

85. Race EM, Adelson-Mitty J, Kriegel GR, et al: Focal mycobacterial lymphadenitis following initiation of protease-inhibitor therapy in patients with advanced HIV-1 disease. Lancet 351:252, 1998

86. Cinti SK, Kaul DR, Sax PE, et al: Recurrence of *Mycobacterium avium* infection in patients receiving highly active antiretroviral therapy and antimycobacterial agents. Clin Infect Dis 30:511, 2000

87. Benson CA, Williams PL, Cohn DL, et al: Clarithromycin or rifabutin alone or in combination for primary prophylaxis of *Mycobacterium avium* complex disease in patients with AIDS: a randomized, double-blind, placebo-controlled trial. J Infect Dis 181:1289, 2000

88. El-Sadr WM, Burman WJ, Bjorling L, et al: Discontinuation of prophylaxis against *Mycobacterium avium* complex disease in HIV-infected patients who have a response to antiretroviral therapy. N Engl J Med 342:1085, 2000

89. Ward TT, Rimland D, Kauffman C, et al: Randomized open-label trial of azithromycin plus ethambutol vs. clarithromycin plus ethambutol as therapy for *Mycobacterium avium* complex bacteremia in patients with human immunodeficiency virus infection. Clin Infect Dis 27:1278, 1998

90. Gordin FM, Sullam PM, Shafran SD, et al: A randomized, placebo-controlled study of rifabutin added to a regimen of clarithromycin and ethambutol for treatment of disseminated infection with *Mycobacterium avium* complex. Clin Infect Dis 28:1080, 1999

91. Dunne M, Fessel J, Kumar P, et al: A randomized, double-blind trial comparing azithromycin and clarithromycin in the treatment of disseminated *Mycobacterium avium* infection in patients with human immunodeficiency virus. Clin Infect Dis 31:1245, 2000

92. Koletar SL: Treatment of *Mycobacterium avium* in human immunodeficiency virus–infected individuals. Am J Med 102(5C):16, 1997

93. Hazra R, Robson CD, Perez-Atayde AR, et al: Lymphadenitis due to nontuberculous mycobacteria in children: presentation and response to therapy. Clin Infect Dis 28:123, 1999

94. Bloch KC, Zwerling L, Pletcher MJ, et al: Incidence and clinical implications of isolation of *Mycobacterium kansasii*: results of a 5-year, population-based study. Ann Intern Med 129:698, 1998

95. Jacobson KL, Teira R, Libshitz HI, et al: *Mycobacterium kansasii* infections in patients with cancer. Clin Infect Dis 30:965, 2000

96. Oliver A, Maiz L, Canton R, et al: Nontuberculous mycobacteria in patients with cystic fibrosis. Clin Infect Dis 32:1298, 2001

97. Griffith DE, Wallace RJ Jr: Treatment of pulmonary *Mycobacterium avium* complex lung disease in non-acquired immunodeficiency syndrome (AIDS) patients in the era of the newer macrolides and rifabutin. Am J Med 102(5C):22, 1997

98. Griffith DE, Brown BA, Murphy DT, et al: Initial (6-month) results of three-times-weekly azithromycin in treatment regimens for *Mycobacterium avium* complex lung disease in human immunodeficiency virus–negative patients. J Infect Dis 178:121, 1998

99. Hadjiliadis D, Adlakha A, Prakash BS: Rapidly growing mycobacterial lung infection in association with esophageal disorders. Mayo Clin Proc 74:45, 1999

100. Jernigan JA, Farr BM: Incubation period and sources of exposure for cutaneous *Mycobacterium marinum* infection: case report and review of the literature. Clin Infect Dis 31:439, 2000

101. van der Werf TS, van der Graaf WTA, Tappero JW, et al: *Mycobacterium ulcerans* infection. Lancet 354:1013, 1999

102. Spell DW, Szurgot JG, Greer RW, et al: Native valve endocarditis due to *Mycobacterium fortuitum* biovar *fortuitum*: case report and review. Clin Infect Dis 30:605, 2000

103. Villanueva A, Calderon RV, Vargas BA, et al: Report on an outbreak of postinjection abscesses due to *Mycobacterium abscessus*, including management with surgery and clarithromycin therapy and comparison of strains by random amplified polymorphic DNA polymerase chain reaction. Clin Infect Dis 24:1147, 1997

104. Sarria JC, Chutkan NB, Figueroa JE, et al: Atypical mycobacterial vertebral osteomyelitis: case report and review. Clin Infect Dis 26:503, 1998

105. Harro C, Braden GL, Morris AB, et al: Failure to cure *Mycobacterium gordonae* peritonitis associated with continuous ambulatory peritoneal dialysis. Clin Infect Dis 24:955, 1997

106. Jacobson RR, Krahenbuhl JL: Leprosy. Lancet 353:655, 1999

107. Ooi WW, Moschella SL: Update on leprosy in immigrants in the United States: status in the year 2000. Clin Infect Dis 32:930, 2001

24 Syphilis and the Nonvenereal Treponematoses

Michael Augenbraun, M.D.

Syphilis

Syphilis is an infectious disease with complex acute and chronic manifestations that is transmitted primarily through sexual contact. The disease has been recognized for many centuries, although its origin remains unknown.

EPIDEMIOLOGY

Transmissible syphilis in the United States has become increasingly concentrated in a few geographic areas, particularly in the southeastern part of the country [*see Figure 1*]. It disproportionately affects minority populations and occurs more frequently in men than in women. Recent outbreaks have been reported in homosexual men. Sexual transmission rates from infected to uninfected persons may range from 30% to 60%.[1-3]

The incidence of syphilis was declining from the 1940s through the 1980s, but a sharp and surprising increase occurred in the late 1980s. By 1990, the Centers for Disease Control and Prevention (CDC) reported the largest number of primary and secondary cases of syphilis in 40 years.[4] This increase was strongly linked to the epidemic use of crack cocaine. With the increased incidence of primary syphilis came an increase in the numbers of cases of congenital syphilis.[5]

Just as surprising as the increase in the number of syphilis cases in the late 1980s has been the rapid decline in the number of syphilis cases in the latter half of the 1990s.[6] The reasons for this decline are unclear, but by 1999 there had been an 87% decline from the peak number of cases in 1990. This was the lowest reported rate since the collection of reliable statistics began [*see Figure 2*].

As a result of the low incidence rates of primary and secondary syphilis, its geographic confinement to a limited number of areas, the continued efficacy of penicillin therapy, and the reliability of serologic diagnostic tests, the CDC has initiated a program intended to eliminate syphilis in the United States.[7] The stated goal is to reduce primary and secondary cases to 1,000 or fewer in a given year and to increase the number of syphilis-free counties to 90% by the year 2005. The CDC hopes to achieve this goal through the use of enhanced surveillance, greater cooperation with community groups in the remaining areas of high morbidity, and rapid outbreak response.

ETIOLOGY

Syphilis is transmitted primarily through sexual contact between infected and uninfected partners. Passage through the placenta in an infected pregnant woman may result in congenital disease. Although the disease can also be transmitted through nonsexual contact with infectious lesions, laboratory accidents, and the administration of contaminated blood products, these methods of transmission are relatively rare. Humans are the only known host of *Treponema pallidum*.

PATHOGENESIS AND DISEASE COURSE

T. pallidum is a bacterium belonging to the order Spirochaetales. This order also includes similar familiar bacteria genera, such as *Leptospira* and *Borrelia*. All of these organisms are slender, helically coiled, gram-negative bacteria. Treponemal species other than *T. pallidum* may live as commensals in the oral cavity or the genital tract (e.g., *T. denticola* and *T. oralis*).

T. pallidum probably gains entry to the subcutaneous tissues through small abrasions in overlying skin and mucous membranes. The organism does not possess well-recognized virulence factors, such as lipopolysaccharide. Once penetration of the epithelium occurs, organisms replicate locally at the site of inoculation and spread to regional lymph nodes. Depending on factors such as inoculation load and history of previous syphilis infection, the incubation period from exposure to clinical disease can range from 3 weeks to 3 months.

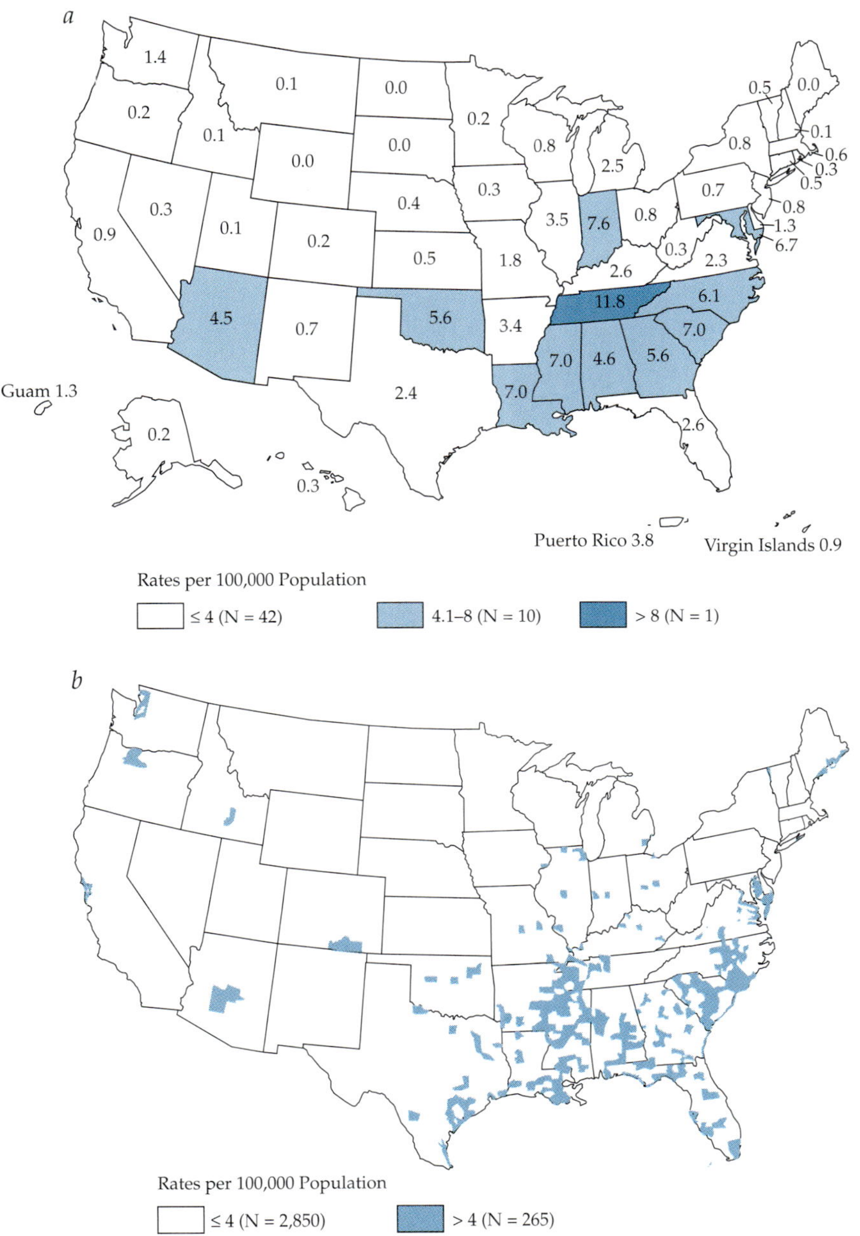

Figure 1 **Rates of primary and secondary syphilis by (*a*) state and (*b*) county.**

The characteristic first lesion of primary syphilis [*see Table 1*] is the chancre [*see Figure 3*]. It is a typically indurated and nontender ulcerative lesion, often accompanied by a nontender, nonsuppurative regional lymphadenopathy. In some patients, the chancre is inconspicuous, and in others it can be more than 1 to 2 cm in diameter. Although not common, multiple chancres may occur, particularly in HIV-infected persons. In the absence of effective therapy, the chancre resolves within 2 to 8 weeks. Healing may take longer in immunocompromised persons.

Spirochetemia develops soon after the appearance of the primary chancre, but clinical evidence of dissemination is rarely seen at the same time. Signs and symptoms of dissemination and secondary syphilis include fever, malaise, diffuse lymphadenopathy, patchy alopecia, headache, and

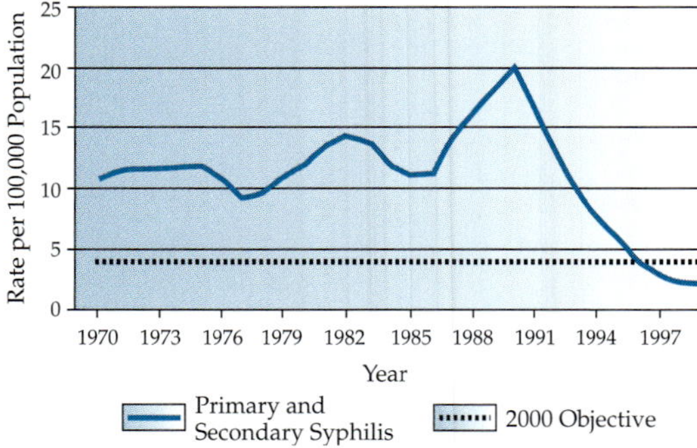

Figure 2 **Reported rates of primary syphilis in the United States over 3 decades. The highest rate occurred in the late 1980s and early 1990s, after which there has been a steep decline in the number of syphilis cases.**

classic hyperpigmented macular-papular rash on the palms and soles [*see Figure 4*]. Condylomata lata and mucous patches may appear in a variety of locations, such as the genitals and the gluteal and nasolabial folds [*see Figure 5*]. Other anatomic sites, such as the eyes, gastrointestinal mucosa, liver, and bones, may also be involved.

The clinical manifestations of secondary syphilis [*see Table 1*] resolve after weeks to months even without therapy, and the disease enters the latent stage. During the early latency period, the signs and symptoms of secondary syphilis may recrudesce. This period generally lasts 1 year after infection but can extend to 4 or 5 years.[8]

Latent syphilis is, by definition, recognized only by the presence of a reactive serologic test. During this period, the organisms evade any meaningful host immunologic responses. Although infected persons mount both significant cell-mediated and humoral responses to infection, neither response is adequate for control. Many reasons have been postulated for this phenomenon, including the lack of immunogenic proteins and polysaccharides in the outer membrane of *T. pallidum,* as well as the organism's ability to cloak itself with host proteins.[9]

Once syphilis enters the latent phase, the course of disease is variable.

Although the majority of infected persons will never suffer undue consequences, data from the Oslo[8] study suggests that years later, tertiary disease [*see Table 1*] will develop in approximately one third of these individuals, manifesting as neurosyphilis, cardiovascular syphilis, or gummatous (benign) syphilis. The pathology associated with tertiary syphilis is quite varied, and there is substantial overlap between clinical entities. Chronologically, meningeal and meningovascular symptoms (i.e., stroke) may be the earliest manifestations of symptomatic neurosyphilis. In later stages, parenchymatous disease with associated cognitive and long-tract signs becomes prominent. As in cardiovascular and gummatous syphilis, the lesion in CNS syphilis is endarteritis.

DIAGNOSIS

Depending on the stage of disease, the diagnosis of syphilis may be made by visualizing the organisms, by serologic studies, by pathology, or by clinical presentation. None of these methods is entirely sensitive or specific.

Clinical Manifestations

Primary syphilis In primary syphilis, the chancre [*see* Pathogenesis, *above*] typically occurs at the site of inoculation and thus may be seen any-

Table 1 Clinical Manifestations of Syphilis in Adults

Stage	*Manifestations*
Primary	Chancre and inguinal lymphadenopathy
Secondary	Rash, diffuse lymphadenopathy, fever, alopecia, condyloma latum, and mucous patches
Early latent	None (secondary syphilis may recur)
Late latent or latent syphilis of unknown duration	None
Tertiary	
Neurosyphilis	
Asymptomatic	None
Meningitis	Headache, cranial nerve palsies, delirium, seizures, and findings of raised intracranial pressure
Meningovascular	Hemiparesis, hemiplegia, aphasia, and seizures
Parenchymatous	
General paresis	Memory loss, personality changes, cognitive dysfunction, confusion, and seizures
Tabes dorsalis	Lightning pains, ataxia, pupillary abnormalities, and impaired proprioception
Cardiovascular	Aortic aneurysm, aortic regurgitation, chest wall mass, and hoarseness
Gummatous	Chronic inflammation with focal destructive lesions in nearly any tissue or organ of the body

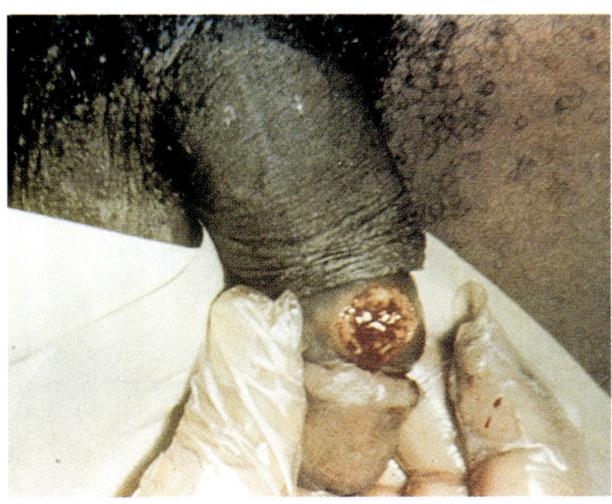

Figure 3 **Indurated, nontender ulcerative chancres are the first lesions of early syphilis.**

where in the genital region (i.e., penis, scrotum, inner thigh, buttocks, vaginal labia, cervix, or anus). Lesions may be single or multiple. Often, they occur where tissue proximates infected sites—so-called kissing lesions.

Typically, the chancre is indurated with a raised but clean margin. It is nontender. It may have a gray-white exudative covering, particularly if the lesion is secondarily infected. More commonly, it is clean without bleeding. There is associated nontender and nonsuppurative regional lymphadenopathy. Cervical or rectal chancres may result in deep pelvic noninguinal adenopathy.

Secondary syphilis The widely varied clinical manifestations of secondary syphilis reflect the capacity of *T. pallidum* to disseminate virtually anywhere in the body within weeks of the appearance (and resolution) of the primary chancre. With spirochetemia, which develops after the first chancre [*see* Pathogenesis, *above*], comes a host of systemic symptoms that are relatively nonspecific, including headache, malaise, fatigue, arthralgias, myalgias, and diffuse painless lymphadenopathy. The finding of enlarged epitrochlear lymph nodes in the absence of any upper extremity pathology is considered to be highly suspicious for secondary syphilis.

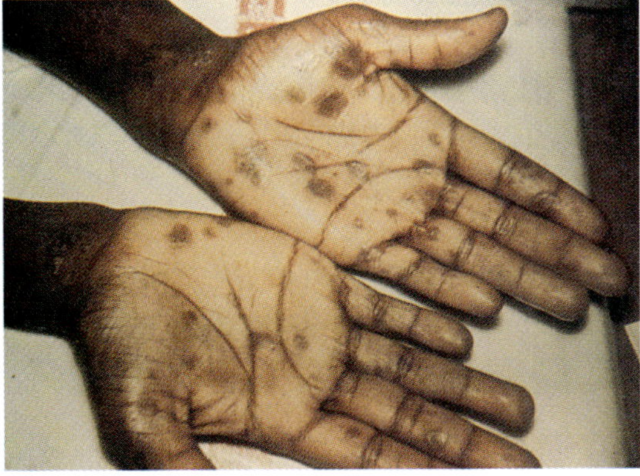

Figure 4 **A hyperpigmented maculopapular rash on the palms and soles is a classic sign of spirochetemia.**

The rash of secondary syphilis is one of the most common signs of the disease. The classic finding is maculopapular hyperpigmented lesions 3 to 10 mm in diameter, often with fine peripheral scaling on the palms and soles. There are so few clinical entities that cause these lesions that the presence of the lesions is nearly pathognomonic. Rash will be seen in 75% to 100% of patients at some point in the course of infection. However, the rash of secondary syphilis does not always fit this classic pattern. It may present in any of a variety of ways—macular, maculopapular, papular, pustular, or plaques of varying size—on virtually any site of the body. Raised, moist, nontender plaques known as condylomata lata may form in intertriginous areas, such as in the gluteal fold, under the breasts, and in the inguinal area. Similar mucous patches may form on mucosal surfaces, such as the nares, mouth, vagina, and anus. These lesions can be confused with chancres but are not, strictly speaking, ulcers. They teem with spirochetes and are highly infectious. Secondary syphilis can also involve hair follicles, leading to patchy alopecia of scalp hair, as well as thinning of the eyebrows, eyelashes, and beard.

Skeletal manifestations of secondary syphilis can include osteitis, arthritis, and bursitis.[10] Syphilitic hepatitis with hepatomegaly and an elevated alkaline phosphatase level may occur.[11] Various forms of nephropathy, including glomerulonephritis and nephrotic syndrome, have also been noted in secondary syphilis.[12] Gastritis with attendant abdominal pain, nausea, and vomiting can result from infiltration of the gastric mucosa by spirochetes.[13] Both anterior and posterior uveitis can occur and may be either asymptomatic or associated with altered vision.[14,15] Some of these cases come to light after failure to respond or after worsening of symptoms with steroids.

Involvement of the CNS occurs early in syphilis.[16] At least 40% of lumbar puncture samples from patients with secondary disease (more in some series) have been found to have CSF abnormalities. *T. pallidum* may actually be recovered from up to 30% of these samples. Whereas symptomatic parenchymatous neurosyphilis is often associated with

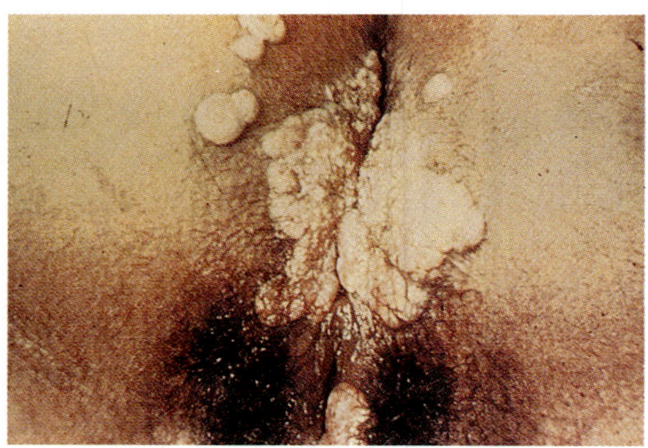

Figure 5 **Highly infectious condylomata lata appear on genitalia and gluteal folds.**

late-stage syphilis, meningeal involvement may be seen during or shortly after the nonneurologic symptoms of secondary syphilis. This condition is characterized by findings typical of a bacterial meningitis, including headache, stiff neck, photophobia, nausea, and vomiting. Cranial neuropathies associated with ocular and otic deficits, as well as facial nerve palsies, can occur. In some instances, papilledema associated with hydrocephalus has been reported, as have delirium, seizures, aphasia, and hemiplegia. Most patients no longer demonstrate the rash of secondary syphilis at the time these symptoms develop.

Latent syphilis By definition, latent syphilis is not associated with any clinical finding. Early latency delineates that period after the resolution of secondary disease during which the signs and symptoms of secondary disease may recur. Although this latency period may last as long as 5 years, the majority of cases of latent syphilis occur within the first to second year, followed by tertiary syphilis.

Neurosyphilis It is presumed that in the majority of patients with primary or secondary syphilis who experience invasion of the CNS by spirochetes, resolution of this aspect of infection occurs with or without the administration of systemic antibiotics. A small number of these patients have continuing CNS involvement with asymptomatic CSF changes and are at high risk for progressive symptomatic neurologic disease for a period of years. It is difficult to ascertain which individuals may be at risk, and anyone with presumably latent syphilis may harbor CSF changes suggesting continued neurosyphilis.

Late symptomatic neurosyphilis may present as one of several clinical syndromes that occur within the following conditions (the syndromes often overlap):

1. Meningovascular neurosyphilis. *T. pallidum* tends to cause endarteritis, which can compromise vascular supply to portions of the CNS and cause infarctions that clinically resemble any other cerebrovascular accident. These events can occur anywhere along the neuroaxis, including the cerebrum, the cerebellum, the brain stem, and the spinal cord. Signs and symptoms therefore correspond to the portion of the CNS involved. The time elapsed from primary syphilis to meningovascular syphilis is usually 5 to 12 years but may be as long as several decades.
2. Parenchymatous neurosyphilis. Direct involvement of the CNS parenchyma results in a wide range of clinical syndromes characterized pathologically by fibrosis and atrophy. General paresis is a meningoencephalitic syndrome that may be similar in presentation to many psychiatric and neurologic disorders. Patients exhibit emotional lability, delusions, paranoia, and memory loss and may progress to dementia, delirium, and seizures. They may have difficulty with speech, and their pupils may become constricted and unresponsive to light and painful stimuli (Argyll Robertson pupil). They may lose the capacity for facial expressions and are noted to have trembling of the lips and tongue. In tabes dorsalis, there is a pronounced involvement of the dorsal roots and the posterior columns of the spinal cord. Patients complain of shooting pains in the back and lower extremities, where they also notice paresthesias. These paroxysms of pain can be referred to other locations, including the abdomen and the throat. Patients lose proprioception and vibratory sense and develop a wide-based gait. Optic atrophy may occur. Knee and ankle reflexes are diminished or lost entirely, plantar responses are flexor, and ataxia is usually present. Symptomatic parenchymatous disease develops 15 to 25 years after primary infection. The long-term outlook in general paresis without treatment is grim. Death may occur within months or, more likely, 4 to 5 years after the onset of symptoms. Untreated tabes dorsalis leads to eventual incapacitation, although it has been known to remit spontaneously.

Cardiovascular syphilis After the introduction of antibiotics, cardiovascular syphilis became extremely rare. *T. pallidum* can cause endarteritis of the aortic vasa vasorum, leading to progressive medial necrosis and loss of elastic tissue, dilatation, and, eventually, aneurysm. The proximal thoracic aorta and the aortic arch are most commonly involved, whereas involvement of the abdominal aorta is extremely rare. Symptoms usually develop when the aneurysm begins to encroach upon or erode adjacent structures, such as the chest wall, the superior vena cava, the recurrent laryngeal nerve, the trachea, and the mainstem bronchi. These aneurysms rarely dissect. In 30% of cases, aortic root dilatation leads to aortic regurgitation in which there is no evidence of aortic stenosis. Uncommonly, the coronary artery ostia may be involved, causing ischemic heart disease. Cardiovascular syphilis is usually preceded by a latent period of 15 to 30 years.

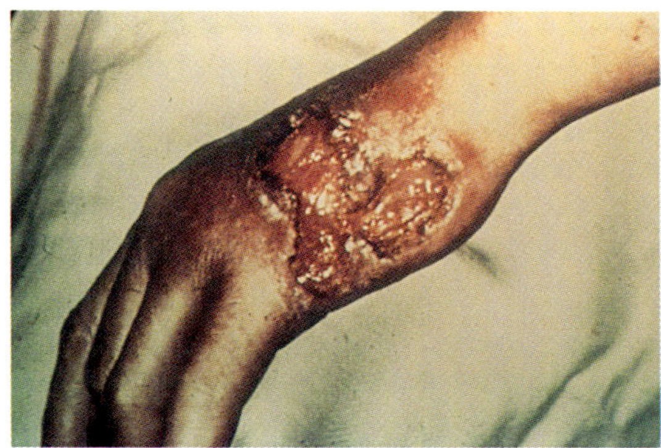

Figure 6 **Granulomatous lesions called gummas are particularly destructive to soft tissue and bone.**

Gummatous (benign) syphilis As with neurosyphilis and cardiovascular syphilis, the incidence of late gummatous syphilis has declined dramatically since the introduction of effective antimicrobial agents. The hallmark of this disease are gummas, which are indolent, destructive granulomatous lesions of soft tissue and bone [*see Figure 6*]. They can lead to dramatic scarring and disfigurement. They are primarily immunologically mediated responses. Although almost any part of the body may be involved, gummas most frequently occur in soft tissue and skeletal structures. Gummas do not develop until decades after infection. They appear slowly, often as a nodule with minimal attendant inflammation. Central coagulative necrosis develops, with softening and involution of the lesion. Eventually, fibrosis occurs, with deep scarring. Involvement of the nasal septum can lead to collapse of the nasal structures. Perforation of the hard palate may occur. Skeletal lesions can lead to fractures.

Laboratory Tests

Primary syphilis Clinical appearance of a genital ulcer is not adequate to establish its etiology. Dark-field microscopy of lesion exudate is a reliable diagnostic method. Incident light through a microscope fitted with polarizing lenses allows the viewer to identify the corkscrew morphology of treponemes as white against a black background [*see Figure 7*]. Exudate for dark-field microscopy can be collected from the base of a chancre that has been cleaned with saline and to which gentle pressure has been applied. Examination must be performed promptly because any drying of the specimen reduces the sensitivity of the test. Therapy, intentional or not, with antibiotics active against *T. pallidum* will rapidly reduce the yield of a dark-field specimen. Nonpathogenic treponemes in the oral cavity reduce the specificity of dark-field microscopy on lesions from this area. A direct fluorescent antibody test (DFA-TP) can also be performed on lesion exudate when the immediate collection of a specimen is not possible. Nucleic acid amplification tests have been developed for *T. pallidum,* but these tests should be considered research tools.

Besides dark-field microscopy, the most commonly used tests for primary syphilis are serologic tests. Syphilis serology testing requires the use of two tests performed in sequence—one for screening and the other for confirmation. Screening tests are characterized by high sensitivity but variable specificity. They make use of standardized amounts of cardiolipin, cholesterol, and lecithin, to which *T. pallidum*–directed immunoglobulins (IgG or IgM) have an affinity. These tests include the Venereal

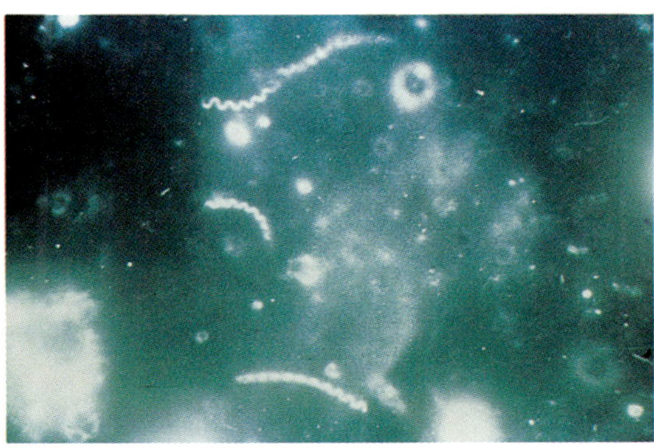

Figure 7 **In dark-field microscopy, treponemes appear white against a black background.**

Disease Research Laboratory (VDRL) test, rapid plasma reagin (RPR) test, unheated serum reagin (USR) test, and toluidine red unheated serum test (TRUST). All are flocculation tests in which visible (macroscopic, microscopic, or both) clumping occurs when test reagents are added to serum from a patient with syphilis. Results may be reported qualitatively or quantitatively. For quantitative results, testing is performed on sequentially diluted serum. The final dilution in which a reaction occurs is reported. In primary syphilis, the sensitivity of any of these nontreponemal serologic tests (NTSTs) ranges only from 78% to 86%. They may also be erroneously reactive in association with a number of other clinical factors, including older age, pregnancy, a history of intravenous drug use, and collagen vascular diseases.[17]

Treponemal-specific tests such as the fluorescent treponemal antibody absorption (FTA-ABS) and the *T. pallidum* particle agglutination (TP-PA) tests use fluorescent antibody and hemagglutinating antibody, respectively, to detect patients' antibodies to *T. pallidum*. In these cases, a suspension of *T. pallidum* serves as the antigenic target. These tests are not routinely quantified. Depending on the strength of the reaction, they may be reported as reactive, nonreactive, or inconclusive. In primary syphilis, these tests can become reactive before the NTSTs. False positive results occur in a small percentage of those tested, so these tests should not by themselves be used for screening. They are best used to confirm a reactive NTST.

Secondary syphilis Dark-field microscopy may be useful for examining exudate from condylomata lata and mucous patches, but ordinarily, this test has limited utility in the diagnosis of secondary syphilis. Serologic tests remain the standard for diagnosing syphilis at this stage. Because these tests quantitatively reflect the degree of immune response associated with infection, the highest NTST titers are generally seen during secondary syphilis. The likelihood of a false negative test in secondary syphilis is remote. An exception to this occurs in the event of the so-called prozone phenomenon, in which extremely high concentrations of reaginic antibodies block the flocculation process. This effect may be expected in no more than 2% of cases and can be overcome by performing repeated tests on diluted samples.

CSF findings in meningitis associated with secondary syphilis are nonspecific, except with use of the CSF-VDRL. A positive finding is invariably indicative of neurosyphilis unless there has been significant contamination of the CSF with blood. Sensitivity of the CSF-VDRL ranges only from 30% to 70%, so a negative test does not rule out neurosyphilis.[18] Other abnormalities of the CSF that may occur with or without a reactive CSF-VDRL include a mononuclear pleocytosis with counts of 10 to 500 cells/mm^3 and an elevated protein level of 46 to 200 mg/dl.

Latent syphilis As disease activity wanes and immunologic mechanisms exert some control, the height of titer in the NTST declines. Titers of between 1:1 and 1:16 are not uncommon. Higher titers suggest but do not confirm the presence of disease activity. The treponemal serologic tests are also reactive.

Neurosyphilis The laboratory diagnosis of neurosyphilis depends on the analysis of serologic tests and the CSF examination. The treponemal serologic test is almost always positive in neurosyphilis but it is not a specific marker for disease, because it is generally reactive for the life of the infected individual, whether treated or not. The NTSTs, generally regarded as sensitive but nonspecific in the evaluation of primary syphilis, are nonreactive in 25% to 30% of cases of neurosyphilis.[19]

CSF evaluation remains the gold standard by which neurosyphilis is diagnosed. Because lumbar puncture is associated with some morbidity, efforts have been made to define subgroups of patients with latent syphilis (i.e., asymptomatic with serologic evidence of disease) who may be at risk for asymptomatic neurosyphilis and therefore at a higher risk for progression to symptomatic late neurosyphilis. Current guidelines suggest that patients with latent syphilis in the setting of HIV and patients with latent syphilis whose titers rise or fail to decline after 2 to 3 years of therapy are at risk.[20] Some experts recommend CSF evaluation in latent syphilis if the serologic titer is at least 1:32.

CSF analysis is warranted in any patient with serologic evidence of syphilis and neurologic, ophthalmologic, otic, or psychiatric disease. Tests conducted on the CSF should include a quantitative CSF-VDRL, a cell count with differential, and a protein assay. The VDRL is the only nontreponemal test that is standardized for CSF. In 25% to 30% of neurosyphilis cases, this test may be nonreactive. It is otherwise extremely specific and by itself may be diagnostic of neurosyphilis. The CSF cell count can range from 5 to 200 cells/mm^3, with a lymphocytic predominance. The CSF protein concentration is also usually increased, although levels should not exceed 200 g/dl. Lymphocytic pleocytosis and increased CSF protein concentrations are nonspecific for neurosyphilis and may be seen in a wide range of pathologic processes. The diagnosis of neurosyphilis in which the results of only these tests are abnormal rests on these findings and clinical suspicion. In some instances when tabes dorsalis has run its course, the CSF is completely normal.

Cardiovascular syphilis As with other forms of tertiary syphilis, the nontreponemal serologic test for late cardiovascular syphilis may be nonreactive, whereas the treponemal-specific test is almost always reactive. Although a chest x-ray may be normal, it can also show a mediastinal mass consistent with the thoracic aortic aneurysm. Calcification of the aneurysm is often seen on radiograph but is not specific for syphilis.

Gummatous syphilis Clinical suspicion is the most important tool in the diagnosis of late gummatous syphilis. Nontreponemal serologic tests are nonreactive in a sizable number of cases. The treponemal serologic tests should always be reactive. Interestingly, spirochetes are not often demonstrated in biopsied tissue. Dark-field microscopy is of little use. More sensitive tests based on nucleic acid amplification may detect treponemal DNA in these lesions.[21]

DIFFERENTIAL DIAGNOSIS

Primary Syphilis

Any clinical condition likely to cause a genital ulcer should be considered in the differential diagnosis when primary syphilis is suspected. The most common cause of genital ulcer disease in the United States is herpes simplex virus type 2 (HSV-2). The ulcers of HSV-2 are usually preceded by prodromal symptoms of burning and tingling, and they pass through a series of predictable stages, including papules, vesicles, pustules, and ulcers, before healing. The ulcers are tender and shallow, with an erythematous base. Lesions are often multiple and can coalesce to form large irregularly shaped ulcers. The course of illness varies, depending on whether it is a primary infection or a recurrence of established infection. The former may last as long as 3 weeks, whereas the latter usually resolves after 10 days. Diagnosis may be made on clinical grounds or with viral culture. Regional lymphadenopathy is common. Worldwide, the other common infectious cause of genital ulcer is chancroid, caused by *Haemophilus ducreyi* [see 10 Sexually Transmitted Diseases]. Chancroid is seen sporadically in the United States, usually in conjunction with focal urban outbreaks, but is a common cause of genital ulcer disease in developing countries. Chancroid lesions are painful and indurated, with ragged margins. Gram stain of exudate may reveal gram-variable rods that characteristically line up together in patterns referred to as a school of fish or railroad tracks. Special nutrient media with antibiotic supplements should be used for isolation of *H. ducreyi.*

Secondary Syphilis

It would be nearly impossible to list all the conditions to which secondary syphilis bears some resemblance. A rash of any description, whose etiology may be construed as allergic, infectious, or immune mediated may potentially be syphilitic. Thus, syphilis testing for any patient with a rash of unknown etiology is warranted. The finding of a palmar rash or a rash on the soles of the feet—classic for syphilis—may be seen in a limited number of conditions, including Rocky Mountain spotted fever, atypical measles, and meningococcemia. A rash accompanying any of these alternative diagnoses would ordinarily be associated with more severe systemic illness than is seen with secondary syphilis. Syphilis needs to be considered in the differential diagnosis for aseptic meningitis. More typical causes for this problem may include enteroviruses, HSV-1, and medication-associated aseptic meningitis.

Latent Syphilis

In 1% to 2% of the general population, nontreponemal serologic tests such as the RPR, VDRL, and USR may be falsely reactive. In these circumstances, the treponemal serologic tests, such as the FTA-ABS and TP-PA, are nonreactive. An increased risk of this finding is commonly associated with older age, pregnancy, collagen vascular disease, and intravenous drug use.

Neurosyphilis

Although the pattern of classic meningovascular or parenchymatous neurosyphilis may be recognizable, the clinically varied manifestations of CNS syphilis require the clinician to consider it with nearly any presentation. A wide array of stroke syndromes caused by thrombotic or hemorrhagic mechanisms should be included in the differential diagnosis. Neurosyphilis should be considered in a relatively young person with a history of sexually transmitted diseases who otherwise has no risk factors for a cerebrovascular accident (e.g., atherosclerosis or hypertension) and suffers a stroke. Diabetic neuropathy has been said to mimic tabes dorsalis. Neurosyphilis should be considered in the differential diagnosis of any patient presenting with a dementia.

Cardiovascular Syphilis

Cardiovascular pathology leading to ischemia is more likely to result from atherosclerotic disease than from syphilis. Likewise, aortic aneurysm formation secondary to long-standing hypertension would be more common than syphilitic aneurysms. Aortic regurgitation often follows aortic stenosis. Besides syphilitic aortitis, pure valvular regurgitation without stenosis may be seen in patients with congenital valvular disease (e.g., Marfan syndrome), healed infective endocarditis, or other cardiac trauma.

Gummatous Syphilis

The lesions of late benign syphilis may be easily confused with other granulomatous processes, such as tuberculosis, sarcoid, fungal infection, and, occasionally, neoplastic disease.

TREATMENT

Penicillin remains the antimicrobial agent of choice in all stages of syphilis [*see Table 2*]. The studies that established this therapeutic standard were conducted decades ago. They used varying formulations of penicillin not currently available and would not meet present standards for randomization, blinding, sample size, and other aspects of good study design. These studies provide a weak basis for conclusions about optimal management today.

Primary and Secondary Syphilis

Therapy for primary syphilis should serve two overlapping goals: (1) to reduce and eliminate the capacity of the infected person to transmit disease and (2) to achieve the microbiologic eradication of *T. pallidum* from the host to resolve clinical manifestations and avoid long-term sequelae.

Sexual transmission of syphilis occurs almost exclusively during the early stages of disease, when contact with infectious lesions is most common. Penicillin eliminates infectivity relatively easily. Early studies of penicillin demonstrated the ability of the drug to rapidly convert dark-field–positive lesions to dark-field–negative lesions and hasten their resolution.

All the clinical manifestations of primary and secondary syphilis will resolve without therapy. However, the resolution of clinical manifestations does not ensure the eradication of *T. pallidum*. In such circumstances, patients are assumed to remain infected and to have entered the latent stage of disease. Studies of therapeutic efficacy rely on changes in serologic markers that may or may not reflect microbiologic activity of disease. There is general agreement today that a fourfold (two dilution) decrease in the NTST titer should occur as early as 3 months and as late as 12 or even 24 months after successful therapy. This notion is based on clinical experience and data from a study and subsequent reanalysis of the data.[22,23] The criteria for failure and the need for retreatment in both of these studies were poorly defined. Although it has thus been easy to create general categories for the patterns of response expected after therapy, few studies since the introduction of penicillin have followed patients long enough to establish the risk of disease progression.

Penicillin therapy For the past 3 decades, benzathine penicillin G (2.4 million units given once I.M.) has been the standard regimen for the treatment of primary syphilis and is currently recommended by both the CDC and the World Health Organization (WHO).[20,24] Studies have demonstrated the efficacy of benzathine penicillin but have also suggested a 3% to 10% failure rate by the serologic criteria mentioned above.[22] Where comparative data exist, this single injection appears to be nearly as effective, if not as effective, as a variety of more complicated regimens.[25] The ease and cost-effectiveness of a single injection clearly favors its use over multiple-injection–based therapies or therapies requiring hospitalization for intravenous treatment.

Nonpenicillin therapy It is advantageous to have alternative therapies to penicillin not only for the possibility of resistant *T. pallidum* but also to treat patients who are allergic to penicillin [*see* Complications, *below*]. There have been few comparative trials that have examined the role of nonpenicillin therapies. Tetracyclines have been used for decades as an alternative to penicillin, and the CDC currently recommends doxycycline (100 mg orally twice a day for 14 days) as second-line therapy in primary syphilis.[17] Retreatment rates after tetracycline therapy are higher than those after penicillin therapy.[22] Clinical experience supports the use of tetracyclines as alternatives to penicillin for cases of early stage syphilis in which penicillin cannot be used.

Table 2 Treatment of Syphilis

Stage	*Drug*	*Dose*	*Relative Efficacy*	*Cost/Day ($)*	*Comment*
Primary, secondary, and early latent syphilis	Benzathine penicillin G	2.4 million U I.M. once	Drug of choice	0.75–0.99	—
	Doxycycline	100 mg p.o. twice a day for 14 days	—	0.05–0.12	Therapy for nonpregnant patients who are allergic to penicillin
	Tetracycline	500 mg p.o. four times a day for 14 days	—	0.10–0.24	
	Ceftriaxone	1 g I.M. or I.V. daily for 8–10 days	—	60.00–69.99	Optimal dose has not been defined
	Azithromycin	2 g p.o. once	—	10.00–19.99	—
Late latent or latent syphilis of unknown duration	Benzathine penicillin G	2.4 million U I.M. once a wk for 3 wk (total 7.2 million U)	Drug of choice	0.75–0.99	May be associated with gastrointestinal upset
	Doxycycline	100 mg p.o. twice a day for 28 days	—	0.05–0.12	Therapy for nonpregnant patients who are allergic to penicillin
	Tetracycline	500 mg p.o. four times a day for 28 days	—	0.10–0.24	
Tertiary syphilis (gummatous and cardiovascular)	Benzathine penicillin G	2.4 million U I.M. once a wk for 3 wk	Drug of choice	0.75–0.99	—
	Doxycycline	100 mg p.o. twice a day for 28 days	—	0.05–0.12	Therapy for nonpregnant patients who are allergic to penicillin
	Tetracycline	500 mg p.o. four times a day for 28 days	—	0.10–0.24	—
Neurosyphilis	Aqueous crystalline penicillin G	18–24 million U/day, given as 3–4 million U I.V. every 4 hr for 10–14 days	—	10.00–19.99	—
	Procaine penicillin G and probenecid	Penicillin, 2–4 million U/day I.M. for 10–14 days; plus probenecid, 500 mg p.o. four times a day for 10–14 days	—	Penicillin, 2.00–2.99; probenecid, 10.00–19.99*	Can be used if compliance is good
	Ceftriaxone	2 g I.M. or I.V. daily for 10–14 days	—	60.00–69.99	Limited supporting data
Congenital syphilis	Aqueous crystalline penicillin G	100,000–150,000 U/kg/day, given as 50,000 U/kg/dose I.V. every 12 hr during the first 7 days of life and every 8 hr thereafter for a total of 10 days	—	10.00–19.99	—
	Procaine penicillin G	50,000 U/kg/day I.M. once a day for 10 days	—	2.00–2.99	—
Nonvenereal treponematoses (yaws, endemic syphilis, and pinta)	Benzathine penicillin G	Adults, 1.2 million U I.M. once; children, 600,000 U I.M. once	—	0.75–0.99	—
	Doxycycline	100 mg p.o. twice a day for 14 days	—	0.05–0.12	—
	Tetracycline	500 mg p.o. four times a day for 14 days	—	0.10–0.24	—

*Monthly cost.

Erythromycin congeners, primarily the potentially hepatotoxic estolate form, have also been studied and appear to be as effective as tetracyclines in the treatment of early stage syphilis.[22] However, oral absorption of erythromycin is erratic, and the difficulty of achieving adequate serum levels with the widely used base form makes this an unreliable choice for primary syphilis treatment. Questions regarding erythromycin resistance have also been raised. A high-dose amoxicillin-probenecid combination is another possible alternative, although compliance with such a complex oral regimen makes it difficult to recommend.

The role of first-generation cephalosporins for the treatment of primary syphilis has also been examined.[26,27] Some efficacy was demonstrated for these agents, but at least one study suggested an unacceptably high failure rate.[28] Given the unclear role of these agents in the treatment of penicillin-allergic patients, interest in them waned. The third-generation cephalosporin ceftriaxone is a suitable alternative agent for syphilis treatment. In vitro and animal-model data suggest that ceftriaxone has good antitreponemal activity.[29–31] Favorable pharmacokinetics and ceftriaxone's ability to penetrate the blood-brain barrier also make it an attractive choice for therapy. In small groups of patients with primary syphilis, ceftriaxone appeared to be effective.[32,33] Despite its perceived efficacy, ceftriaxone probably should not be given as a single dose for the treatment of primary syphilis, because it would not remain at treponemicidal levels for an acceptable period of time. The proper dosage and duration of therapy are matters of conjecture.

The azalide antibiotic azithromycin has many properties that suggest its usefulness as therapy for primary syphilis. It is active against *T. pallidum* in vitro and has been effective in experimental models of syphilis.[34,35] Although plasma concentration of azithromycin may be nearly unmeasurable, high levels are achievable in tissue.[36] Its extremely long half-life makes it ideal therapy for *T. pallidum*, an organism with a prolonged doubling time. In a number of small studies, azithromycin in varying doses appeared effective for incubating, primary, and secondary syphilis.[37,38]

Latent Syphilis

The successful treatment of latent syphilis is made problematic by a lack of clear and readily measurable clinical end points. By definition, there is no chancre or rash, the resolution of which would suggest response. The objective of therapy is the prevention of long-term sequelae. Except for waiting perhaps decades to see if late-stage disease develops, changes in serologic titers are the only indication of efficacy. Unfortunately, by its very nature, late latent syphilis elicits little in the way of an inflammatory response. Thus, nontreponemal serologic test results are often very low, and their decline after therapy may be proportionately slow. Seroreversal may never be achieved.

Because early latent syphilis occurs shortly after secondary syphilis appears to resolve, it should respond appropriately to similar single-dose and multiple-dose regimens. In most clinical settings, patients with latent-stage disease are unable to reliably give any history suggestive of recent primary disease and are usually treated as having late latent-stage disease.

Studies have suggested that penicillin, which is effective in primary disease, would be effective for latent disease as well. A variety of penicillin regimens were compared and patients followed over a wide range of periods,[39] and benzathine penicillin G provided equivalent duration of in vivo drug levels with fewer injections. Although there are no data directly supporting the current recommendation of three weekly injections of 2.4 million units of benzathine penicillin G (total, 7.2 million units), this therapy appears reasonable on the basis of theoretical assumptions regarding the slow doubling time of *T. pallidum* and the need for extended duration of therapy. The recommended regimen has been used effectively for decades and only rarely results in progression of disease.

There are virtually no useful data on the treatment of latent syphilis with nonpenicillin therapies. Recommendations of 28 days of tetracycline, chloramphenicol, or erythromycin are largely without clinical data to support their effectiveness.

Late Symptomatic Syphilis (Excluding Neurosyphilis)

Incidences of gummatous syphilis and cardiovascular syphilis have declined so dramatically in the penicillin era that it has been difficult to collect enough cases to conduct a study of newer therapeutic modalities. A few studies conducted on small groups of patients soon after the introduction of penicillin demonstrated that penicillin therapy probably halts the progression of gummatous disease, although existing damage to skin, mucous membranes, soft tissue, and skeletal structures is likely irreparable. The therapeutic efficacy of penicillin for cardiovascular syphilis has never been clearly established[40] because of the difficulty of establishing a diagnosis and determining the efficacy of therapy in individuals with already advanced disease (i.e., cardiac structural damage). Despite suggestions that penicillin appeared to have some efficacy in preventing the progression of otherwise uncomplicated aortitis, carefully controlled studies comparing various therapies have never been conducted. In over 4 decades, there have been no studies examining the newer, long-acting preparations of penicillin, nor have there been studies of alternatives to penicillin.

Given the relative safety and ease of use of penicillin therapy for the treatment of cardiovascular syphilis, the WHO and the CDC recommendations appear reasonable, provided that patients are adequately evaluated for other complications of syphilis, such as neurosyphilis, and that adequate clinical and serologic follow-up can be performed.

Neurosyphilis

Frank symptomatic neurosyphilis, like cardiovascular syphilis and gummatous syphilis, has to a certain extent disappeared from clinicians' experience because of the success of therapies for primary and latent-stage disease. Although there is a significant body of work describing and essentially confirming the efficacy of penicillin in the treatment of neurosyphilis, this literature, like much of the syphilis-treatment literature, is compromised by poor post-treatment follow-up and poorly defined outcomes. Nonetheless, penicillin appears to be effective against neurosyphilis, in many instances improving or halting the inexorable progression of neurologic symptoms.

In the 1970s, the CDC recommended either 7.2 million units of benzathine penicillin G I.M. over 3 weeks or 9 million units of aqueous procaine penicillin G over 15 days as therapy for neurosyphilis. The former regimen was also recommended as treatment for late latent syphilis and probably offered some assurance that adequate therapy would be provided for patients with unappreciated asymptomatic neurosyphilis. Serious questions about the efficacy of these regimens, particularly of 7.2 million units of benzathine penicillin G for neurosyphilis, emerged almost simultaneously with their recommendation. Reports detailed the inability of the regimen to achieve acceptable spirocheticidal levels in CSF,[41–45] as well as treatment failures.[46–48] The response of patients with reported treatment failures to increased doses of penicillin has led the CDC to recommend prolonged courses of aqueous or procaine penicillin G for the treatment of neurosyphilis.

Despite the new CDC recommendations for therapy, there are no data from randomized, controlled trials that demonstrate superior efficacy of the new recommendations over previous recommendations. Some experts still contend, also in the absence of supporting data, that lower-dose regimens may be appropriate for asymptomatic neurosyphilis.

The efficacy of high-dose intravenous therapy for neurosyphilis in certain circumstances is also questionable. It is probable that advanced parenchymal disease (e.g., paresis or tabes dorsalis) will not improve after even the most aggressive therapy and may in fact progress. In patients with neurosyphilis and concomitant HIV infection, disease progression may be seen after therapy.[49] Controversy also exists regarding the efficacy of procaine penicillin G.[49]

Ceftriaxone is an attractive alternative to penicillin in the treatment of neurosyphilis.[32,33,50] It has a long half-life, penetrates the CNS well, and has been shown in vivo and in vitro to have activity against *T. pallidum*. Although there are few well-designed trials supporting the clinical efficacy of ceftriaxone for the treatment of neurosyphilis, infectious disease specialists in the United States commonly use it as an alternative to penicillin.[51]

High-dose amoxicillin (2 g orally three times a day) combined with probenecid has been proposed as an alternative outpatient regimen for neurosyphilis because it has been documented to achieve treponemicidal levels of β-lactam antibiotic in the CSF.[52–54] No randomized, controlled studies have been done to evaluate this regimen for this purpose.

Both chloramphenicol and doxycycline have been examined in individual cases and in small groups of patients with neurosyphilis.[55,56] Limited data suggest that these drugs may have efficacy in the treatment of neurosyphilis, but there is not enough evidence to make final recommendations.

Oral steroids are a frequent adjunct in the therapy of sensorineural deafness complicating neurosyphilis,[57,58] but no controlled trials have been properly conducted to evaluate this practice.

Serologic Follow-up

In the treatment of syphilis, the lack of a microbe that can be cultured, the problem of latency, and the uncertainty of therapeutic efficacy combine to foster a unique clinical reliance on quantitative changes in serologic markers to determine response to and adequacy of therapy. Few, if any, infectious diseases require similar follow-up after treatment.

Current standards of care require patients with primary syphilis to return for clinical and serologic evaluation at 3, 6, and 12 months after therapy.[20] Patients with latent syphilis are followed less frequently, perhaps at 6-month intervals for up to 24 months. HIV-coinfected patients are followed more regularly. Recurrence of disease or lack of resolution of signs or symptoms of disease after treatment may be considered evidence of treatment failure. As a measure of disease activity, a two-tube, or fourfold, dilution increase in the NTST during follow-up is also widely accepted as a marker of treatment failure. In all of these instances, distinguishing treatment failure from reinfection may be difficult. At the opposite end of the therapeutic spectrum, cure may reasonably be assumed to have occurred if the NTST becomes nonreactive after therapy. Unfortunately, this development may occur slowly if at all.

A two-tube, or fourfold, dilution decrease in the NTST after treatment has become accepted as the measure of success. This finding will occur more rapidly after treatment for primary syphilis. Cumulative data and clinical experience over several decades indicate that in immunocompetent patients treated with standard regimens of benzathine penicillin G or tetracycline, the NTST should decline by two or three dilutions within 6 and 12 months of treatment, respectively. The proportion of patients expected to be seronegative within 12 to 24 months is less certain, but the weight of evidence suggests that at least 90% of patients with primary or secondary syphilis should serorevert within 1 or 2 years, respectively.

The treponemal-specific serologic tests revert to negative within 3 years in up to 25% of successfully treated patients with first-episode primary syphilis, so that a negative treponemal antibody test result does not always exclude a past history of syphilis.[20,59] However, seroreversal of the treponemal antibody test results occurs rarely, if ever, after treatment of syphilis at the secondary stage or beyond or after treatment of a second episode of primary syphilis. Some data suggest a higher prevalence of nonreactive treponemal antibody tests in HIV-infected patients after treatment of syphilis.[60] It is possible that HIV-infected persons serorevert more often than non–HIV-infected persons, but the issue is unresolved.

Serologic response after treatment in latent disease may be even more problematic than in primary disease. Long-term studies are not available. Another confounding issue is variation in the definition of late syphilis, which determines the dose or duration of therapy of latent infection. Most early writers defined late infection as syphilis of 4 years' duration, on the basis of observations that relapses of secondary syphilis in untreated individuals ceased after this interval. The usual cutoff in the United States, by contrast, is 1 year, after which sexual transmission is rare and classic tertiary syphilis begins to appear.[61] In 1986, the WHO defined late latent syphilis as infection of 2 years' duration.[24] All these definitions are arbitrary, and there are insufficient data for choosing among them on the basis of documented differences in the clinical or serologic response to various treatment regimens. Moreover, the duration of infection cannot be determined accurately in most asymptomatic seropositive patients, further confounding interpretation of the serologic response to treatment in most published studies.

Older data and the accumulated experience of recent years indicate that NTST results decline more slowly after treatment of late syphilis than after treatment of early syphilis and that these tests often remain reactive indefinitely, usually at low titer. Serologic titers in late latent syphilis and in tertiary syphilis decline slowly after treatment, and nonreactive tests will develop in only a minority of patients after upwards of 5 years.[25] The serologic response to the treatment of symptomatic late-stage syphilis may also result in only gradual declines in the NTST. Whether this reflects failure to achieve biologic cure or is merely a serologic phenomenon (so-called immunologic memory) is unresolved. For clinical application, a reasonable guideline is that failure of the NTST to decline by two or more dilutions within 12 months of treatment of late syphilis and any subsequent rise in titer are indications for comprehensive reevaluation and retreatment.

CSF abnormalities in neurosyphilis are also slow to respond after therapy. When reactive, the CSF-VDRL may remain so for years. Other parameters of inflammation, such as cell count and protein level, should resolve more rapidly. It appears to be a reasonable and acceptable practice to repeat CSF examination in patients treated for neurosyphilis at 3-month to 6-month intervals after therapy to ensure an appropriate response. Although the CDC suggests retreatment if CSF abnormalities persist after 2 years, there is no evidence that this condition is clearly indicative of treatment failure or that retreatment will result in an improved response. It is unclear whether serologic response can be expected to differ in all clinical settings, and it would be prudent to consider more frequent serologic follow-up for the HIV-infected patient treated for any stage of syphilis.

Despite considerable effort to develop guidelines for expected serologic response after treatment, it must be remembered that microbiologic response and serologic response are not synonymous. *T. pallidum* has been isolated by rabbit inoculation of lymph nodes of both patients and rabbits and has been identified histologically or immunochemically in aqueous humor after penicillin therapy that resulted in clinical and serologic resolution. Relapse (especially of neurosyphilis) has been reported after apparently adequate penicillin treatment of HIV-infected patients with primary syphilis.

Management of Sexual Partners and Incubating Syphilis

Syphilis treatment is not complete until treatment of sexual partners of the index case has been considered. The CDC recommends that sexual contacts exposed to an index case of primary, secondary, or early latent syphilis receive presumptive therapy within 90 days regardless of the serologic test results. For persons exposed more than 90 days before, therapy should be based on the serologic test results. The need for therapy for contacts of patients with latent or late-stage syphilis should be based on clinical evaluation.

High-risk sexual activity (as indicated by the recent acquisition of such sexually transmitted organisms as *Chlamydia trachomatis* and *Neisseria gonorrhoeae*) carries with it the risk of simultaneous acquisition of syphilis. Because the incubation period of syphilis may be much longer than that of diseases caused by these other organisms, neither clinical nor serologic evidence of syphilis may be present at the time of presentation for clinical care. It would therefore be advantageous for therapies directed toward *C. trachomatis* or *N. gonorrhoeae* to also adequately treat syphilis. Treatment with standard doses of ceftriaxone for gonorrhea will probably abort incubating syphilis. The same cannot be said for single-dose therapy with quinolone antibiotics that do not have activity against *T. pallidum*. Activity of single-dose cefixime against *T. pallidum* is uncertain. Spectinomycin is not active in this instance.[62] Although data are lacking to support a 7-day course of doxycycline, this therapy may in fact be effective. Single-dose azithromycin may also be useful for this purpose.[38]

COMPLICATIONS

Jarisch-Herxheimer Reaction

The Jarisch-Herxheimer reaction is an acute systemic syndrome characterized by fever, chills, headaches, myalgias, tachycardia, tachypnea, and nausea that occurs within the first few hours after the treatment of syphilis—usually secondary syphilis. It may result from the release of pyrogenic endotoxins from treponemes adversely affected by therapy. Treatment with anti-inflammatory agents during the first 24 to 48 hours is warranted. Some clinicians advocate the use of preemptive steroid therapy to mitigate any reaction in which additional end-organ damage (e.g., ocular or cardiovascular) may be problematic, but this practice is not supported by available data. In pregnancy, a Jarisch-Herxheimer reaction may precipitate premature labor or fetal distress.[63] Pregnant women should be advised to seek obstetric evaluation if they note contractions or decreased fetal movements after syphilis treatment.

Penicillin Allergy and Desensitization

In the United States, 5% to 10% of the population may have a history of penicillin allergy, and life-threatening complications may result in 2% to 13% of related allergic events.[64] Despite the relatively high risk of adverse events, there are certain clinical situations in which nonpenicillin therapies for syphilis are not acceptable and penicillin must be used (i.e., congenital syphilis, syphilis in pregnancy, and neurosyphilis).

Even where a history of penicillin allergy exists, the drug may not necessarily be contraindicated. A history of allergy may be inaccurate. Additionally, with the passage of time after an allergic event, many patients may stop expressing penicillin-specific IgE. Penicillin skin testing is a well-established means of securing the patient's true allergy status. The penicilloyl hapten moiety that is the largest product of penicillin metabolism is referred to as the major determinant and, conjugated to polylysine, is commercially available for skin testing. The remaining metabolites are referred to as the minor determinants and are available only at certain academic centers. Even in this setting, the quality criteria for their production have not been standardized. Major determinant skin testing, along with that for benzathine penicillin G (considered a minor determinant), should identify 90% to 97% of patients with penicillin allergy. Nearly all allergic patients will be identified if the other minor determinants are also used.[65] Patients who have a positive response to any of the major or minor determinants should undergo either oral or intravenous desensitization.[66]

Desensitization is usually performed only in a hospital setting. Syphilis treatment regimens may be initiated immediately after the successful completion of desensitization. Unless penicillin therapy is continued indefinitely after desensitization, patients should be considered potentially allergic.

SPECIAL SITUATIONS

Syphilis in Pregnancy

Routine screening and confirmatory serologic tests should reveal syphilis in pregnant women. In pregnancy, quantitative nontreponemal tests reflective of previously treated syphilis may not be specifically indicative of syphilis. An increase in titer in this setting should be considered nonspecific.

The treatment of syphilis in pregnancy must not only cure disease in the adult and prevent sexual transmission but also prevent fetal infection via transplacental passage of *T. pallidum* [*see* Congenital Syphilis, *below*]. These goals can be achieved with therapeutic regimens recommended for the nonpregnant individual. Studies have been conducted in small groups of pregnant women with syphilis using 2.4 to 4.8 million units of various forms of penicillin, often over the course of at least 1 week.[67–73] In each case, the incidence of congenital syphilis was exceedingly low. It was observed that where failures occurred, mothers had been treated late in pregnancy. More studies support the contention that treatment late in pregnancy carries a greater risk for congenital disease than treatment earlier in pregnancy.[74,75] No other factors appear to conclusively increase the risk of congenital syphilis after appropriate therapy of the mother, provided that currently recommended doses are used and that the serologic and clinical markers of disease do not suggest relapse or reinfection. Follow-up in this manner is no more difficult than would be expected after the treatment of the nonpregnant patient with syphilis.

Congenital Syphilis

Diagnosis The CDC recommends that, in screening for congenital syphilis, the mother's serum be tested rather than cord blood. Reactive standard serologic tests in the infant may reflect passive transfer of antibody. Although there is interest in the use of tests for IgM antibodies in the infant, such tests may be insensitive, and nonreactive tests should be interpreted with caution. Demonstration of the presence of *T. pallidum* by direct microscopic examination in the umbilical cord, placenta, nasal discharge, or skin lesions is considered definitive for diagnosis.

Any rise in the incidence of secondary syphilis is invariably accompanied by a rise in the incidence of congenital syphilis. In most cases, the newborn is asymptomatic. Symptomatic disease may occur early or later after birth. In the perinatal period, involvement of the mucocutaneous tissues may be seen, characterized by rhinitis and a desquamative, vesicular, or bullous rash of the skin, particularly on the palms and on the soles of the feet. Hepatic disease can also occur and may result in significant morbidity and mortality. Hepatomegaly, splenomegaly, and hematologic abnormalities occur in this setting. Osteochondritis and perichondritis lead to the classic findings of the so-called saddle-nose deformity and saber shins. After 6 to 12 months, the child enters a latent phase of disease not unlike that seen in adults. Late-stage disease in children may manifest as interstitial keratitis, eighth-nerve deafness, arthropathy, and dental malformations.

Treatment Except where adequate treatment and follow-up of the mother with syphilis can be documented more than 1 month before delivery, some therapeutic intervention will be necessary for the infant. No well-controlled study has determined the appropriate dose of penicillin for the infant suspected of having congenital syphilis, but for those with symptomatic disease at birth, 50,000 U/kg of I.V. aqueous crystalline penicillin G every 12 hours for 10 days or 50,000 U/kg of I.M. procaine penicillin G every day for 10 days appears to be satisfactory. These doses are somewhat arbitrary but are based on doses that may be used to treat bacterial meningitis and would also safely provide at least the standard spirocheticidal levels in the CSF. Because of the difficulty of ruling out active disease in the newborn, many experts recommend the same course of treatment for infants whose mothers' treatment histories are negative or unclear or who received nonpenicillin therapy during pregnancy or within 4 weeks of delivery.

For many years, a single dose of benzathine penicillin for the newborn was considered adequate therapy for congenital syphilis once neurosyphilis had been ruled out. However, reports of treatment failures have cast doubt on this assumption.[76] Benzathine penicillin continues to be recommended as an option in a variety of settings, particularly when the infant is asymptomatic and neurosyphilis has been excluded, but questions exist about the adequacy of maternal therapy and whether follow-up of the child can be assured.[20,77] There are no data to support the contention, largely based on clinical experience, that in low-risk situations these therapies result in nearly universal prevention of congenital syphilis. It is doubtful that most infants receiving this therapy have syphilis at all.

There are no clinical trials examining the role of other antibiotics for the treatment of congenital syphilis. Nonpenicillin therapies recommended for syphilis in adults cannot automatically be recommended for syphilis in infants. Tetracyclines are contraindicated in pregnancy and in infants because of their toxicity to deciduous teeth and long bones and because of concern that they may cause maternal hepatotoxicity, particularly when there is preexisting renal dysfunction.[78] Case reports of symptomatic congenital syphilis in instances in which women received erythromycin during pregnancy as therapy for syphilis suggest that this drug is not a suitable alternative to penicillin.[79–81] These clinical observations are supported by studies demonstrating that placental transfer of erythromycin may not be consistent.[82,83] Issues of compliance and gastrointestinal disturbance in pregnant women treated with erythromycin, although not studied, raise additional questions about this drug's role in pregnancy.

As in adults, serologic follow-up after treatment in infants is essential to ensure the adequacy of response. The ideal frequency of such follow-up is poorly defined, and recommendations range from every month to every 3 months during the first 6 months, with continued follow-up through 12 to 24 months, depending on response.

Syphilis in Children

Penicillin therapy Children with primary, secondary, or early latent syphilis should be treated with benzathine penicillin G (50,000 U/kg I.M., to 2.4 million units in a single dose). Children with late latent syphilis or syphilis of unknown duration should also receive benzathine penicillin G (50,000 U/kg I.M., to 2.4 million units administered as three doses at 1-week intervals). In both cases, a CSF examination should be performed to rule out neurosyphilis.

Alternative therapy The American Academy of Pediatrics recommends that tetracyclines be considered as an alternative to penicillin for both primary and latent disease after 9 years of age.[84] Erythromycin may be considered in early acquired syphilis even in children younger than 9 years (500 mg orally four times a day for 14 days). Follow-up must be ensured. Newer therapies, such as ceftriaxone and azithromycin, may also be effective. There are no studies to support any of these recommendations. Early interest in chloramphenicol as therapy for syphilis has waned because of the drug's well-known side effects.

Syphilis and HIV

Risk behaviors that contribute to the transmission of syphilis are often the same as those that contribute to the transmission of HIV, and therefore, coinfection is common. Each infection has been demonstrated to have some effect on the other. Substantial evidence suggests that early stage syphilis enhances the transmission of HIV.[85,86] Presumably, the inflammatory milieu of syphilitic lesions can serve either as a portal of entry of HIV or as the route through which HIV may be transmitted to an uninfected partner.

In coinfected persons, the deleterious effect of HIV on the immune system can alter the natural history, diagnosis, and management of syphilis. Since the earliest years of the HIV epidemic, case studies have reported on individuals who failed to respond to conventional doses of penicillin therapy and who often progressed rapidly from primary syphilis to neurosyphilis.[87,88] Other important findings have included seronegative secondary syphilis,[89] a likelihood of higher-titer NTSTs by stage,[90] and an increased incidence of biologic false positive NTSTs.[21,91]

A study prospectively followed both HIV-seronegative and HIV-seropositive patients with primary syphilis who received either conventional penicillin therapy or an enhanced regimen of high-dose amoxicillin and probenecid. No neurologic complications and no differences in response to therapy were noted between the groups.[52,92] Except for a tendency for HIV-infected persons to present with multiple chancres, as opposed to a single chancre in non–HIV-infected individuals, no significant differences were noted in presentation or rapidity to resolution of primary syphilis findings. In another study, the CSF white blood cell count, protein, and VDRL were slower to resolve after therapy in HIV-infected individuals than in non–HIV-infected individuals.[93] Clinical failures were not noted.

The propensity for *T. pallidum* to invade the CNS early during infection and the likely importance of immune mechanisms for its control suggest possible mechanisms for the risk of neurosyphilis in coinfected persons. This issue is further complicated by the likelihood for HIV-infected persons to have CSF abnormalities even in the absence of discernible CNS pathology.[94] Many experts recommend that HIV-infected persons with latent syphilis or primary syphilis undergo a CSF evaluation and that those with CSF abnormalities be treated accordingly.

Nonvenereal Treponematoses

The nonvenereal treponematoses—yaws, endemic syphilis, and pinta—are a group of infections distributed throughout tropical and semitropical areas of the world. They are primarily noted to cause a variety of skin and skeletal lesions. There is little biologic difference between the treponemes that cause these conditions.[95] Their distinguishing nomenclature is based primarily on the clinical disease that characterizes each. Each is linked to poor hygiene and person-to-person transmission and disproportionately affects children. As a result of mass treatment programs conducted in the 1950s and the 1960s, initiated primarily by the WHO in conjunction with local authorities, the incidences of all of the nonvenereal treponematoses are today quite low.

YAWS

Epidemiology

Yaws is a disease primarily affecting individuals who live in rural areas of the tropics. It is seen in parts of South America, Africa, Southeast Asia, and Oceania. In the Western Hemisphere, yaws occurs sporadically in small regions of Colombia, Haiti, Suriname, and Guyana. Propagation depends on a hot, humid climate. Persons younger than 15 years appear to be most at risk for acquisition of this infection. It is known by a number of names in different parts of the world, including frambesia, pian, bouba, and parangi.

Pathogenesis

T. pallidum subspecies *pertenue* is associated with yaws. Transmission occurs through skin-to-skin contact, where abrasions or other defects allow spirochetes to enter and cause infection. The incubation period of yaws is like that of syphilis. Within 9 days to 3 months, a granulomatous papule forms in the area of inoculation. This papule gradually enlarges and becomes either hyperkeratotic or frankly ulcerative, often with the development of an overlying amber crust of bacterial superinfection. As with syphilis, even in the absence of specific treatment, these primary lesions resolve.

Diagnosis

The diagnosis of yaws should be suspected in anyone with skin or bone lesions who has spent time in a tropical region.

Clinical manifestations Systemic symptoms of fever, arthralgias, and regional lymphadenopathy occur in conjunction with the development of a diffuse rash similar in appearance to the primary lesion. Osteitis and periosteitis can occur involving the fingers (polydactylitis), tibia (saber shin), and the paranasal maxillae. Secondary lesions may resolve and then relapse over the course of many years. Gummatous lesions with significant dermal scarring and destruction of underlying bone occur years after infection. Whether CNS involvement occurs is debatable.

Laboratory tests Dark-field microscopy of both primary and secondary lesions may yield spirochetes. Nonspecific treponemal serologic tests (e.g., VDRL or RPR) and treponemal-specific serologic tests (e.g., FTA-ABS or TP-PA) should be reactive in cases of yaws, but these tests cannot distinguish between yaws and other treponematoses.

Differential Diagnosis

The differential diagnosis includes syphilis, eczema, psoriasis, scabies, pyoderma, tuberculosis, leprosy, and ecthyma, as well as other processes.

Treatment

Penicillin remains the treatment of choice. For primary disease, doses of benzathine penicillin, 1.2 million units I.M. once in adults and 600,000 units I.M. once in children, should be adequate. Tetracyclines and chloramphenicol are acceptable alternatives. Close contacts of the patient should also be treated.

ENDEMIC SYPHILIS

Epidemiology

Unlike yaws, endemic syphilis, or bejel, is epidemiologically restricted to the arid regions of the Middle East and North Africa. Like the other treponematoses, endemic syphilis is transmitted by close personal contact and affects primarily children living in rural areas.

Pathogenesis

Endemic syphilis is caused by the spirochete *T. pallidum* subspecies *endemicum*. The primary lesion of endemic syphilis usually occurs at a site of inoculation on the oral mucosa and is often unappreciated. This has led to the suspicion that contaminated utensils and drinking vessels may be involved in the spread of the disease.

As in the case of yaws, gummatous late-stage lesions result in destruction and deformation of the mucosa and bony structures, particularly of the mouth and nasal structures. Long bones are sometimes involved. Hyperkeratosis of the soles of the feet occurs. CNS disease is uncommon.

Diagnosis

The diagnosis of endemic syphilis should be considered in any person from an endemic area who has skin or bone disease.

Clinical manifestations Secondary lesions, which may be the first manifestation of infection to be noticed, occur on and around the oral mucosa as well as on other moist, nonkeratinized epithelium and in the intertriginous areas. In rare cases, lesions are disseminated across the surface of the body. Diffuse lymphadenopathy and osteitis are also seen in this circumstance.

Laboratory tests Dark-field microscopy of primary and secondary lesions will be positive for spirochetes, and serologic testing will also be reactive.

Differential Diagnosis

The differential diagnosis of endemic syphilis includes many of the conditions considered in the differential diagnosis of yaws.

Treatment

As in the case of yaws, a single I.M. injection of 1.2 million units of benzathine penicillin is effective to eradicate disease.

PINTA

Epidemiology

Pinta (Spanish for blemish) occurs only in the Western Hemisphere and only in rural areas of southern Mexico and parts of Colombia. All age groups are susceptible to infection.

Pathogenesis

The organism that causes pinta, *T. carateum*, is transmitted through contact of broken skin with infectious lesions.

Within a few weeks of inoculation, a small papule develops at the infection site. The initial papule is followed rapidly by the appearance of other small, pruritic, erythematous papules around the site of the lesion.

Diagnosis

Pinta should be suspected in anyone with characteristic dermal lesions who has been in an endemic area.

Clinical manifestations Papules may coalesce to form squamous plaques. They may then persist for some time before resolving and leaving areas of hypopigmentation. Within 3 to 12 months, a disseminated form of skin lesion known as a pintid appears, which is similar to the initial lesion. These also may coalesce. Diffuse lymphadenopathy is common. Eventually, longstanding lesions leave atrophic and hypopigmented patches, particularly in the area of the wrists, elbows, and ankles.

Laboratory tests Except in the late stages of disease, lesions should yield dark-field microscopic results positive for spirochetes. Standard serologic tests for syphilis are usually reactive except during the earliest phases of disease.

Differential Diagnosis

Conditions with which pinta may be confused include tinea versicolor, vitiligo, and chloasma.

Treatment

The same penicillin doses used for yaws and endemic syphilis should be effective for pinta. Tetracyclines and chloramphenicol are acceptable alternatives. Lesions may be slow to heal. The hypopigmented, or achromic, lesions of late-stage pinta may never improve despite therapy.

References

1. Schroeter A, Turner RH, Lucas JB, et al: Therapy for incubating syphilis: effectiveness of gonorrhea treatment. JAMA 218:711, 1971
2. Schober P, Gabriel G, White P, et al: How infectious is syphilis? Br J Vener Dis 59:217, 1983
3. von Wessouwetz J: The incidence of infection in contacts of early syphilis. J Vener Dis Infect 28:132, 1948
4. Surveillence for primary and secondary syphilis. MMWR Morb Mortal Wkly Rep 42(SS3):13, 1993
5. Surveillence for geographic and secular trends in congenital syphilis. MMWR Morb Mortal Wkly Rep 42(SS6):59, 1993
6. Division of STD Prevention: Sexually Transmitted Disease Surveillence 1998. U.S. Department of Health and Human Services. Centers for Disease Control and Prevention, Atlanta, September 1999
7. The National Plan to Eliminate Syphilis from the United States. National Center for HIV, STD and TB Prevention. Division of STD Prevention. Centers for Disease Control and Prevention, Atlanta, October 1999
8. Clark E, Danbolt N: The Oslo Study of the natural course of untreated syphilis. Med Clin North Am 48:613, 1964
9. Musher D: The biology of *Treponema pallidum*. Sexually Transmitted Diseases. Homes K, Mardh P, Sparling P, et al, Eds. McGraw-Hill, New York, 1999
10. Tight R, Wagner J: Skeletal involvement in secondary syphilis detected by bone scanning. JAMA 235:2326, 1976

11. Campisi D, Whitcomb C: Liver disease in early syphilis. Arch Intern Med 139:365, 1978

12. Bhorade M, Carag HB, Lee HJ, et al: Nephropathy of secondary syphilis: a clinical and pathological spectrum. JAMA 216:1159, 1971

13. Winters H, Notar-Francesco V, Bromberg K, et al: Gastric syphilis: five recent cases and a review of the literature. Ann Intern Med 116:314, 1992

14. Tait I: Uveitis due to secondary syphilis. Br J Vener Dis 59:397, 1983

15. Ormerod LD, Puklin JE, Sobel JD: Syphilitic posterior uveitis: correlative findings and significance. Clin Infect Dis 32:1661, 2001

16. Lukehart S, Hook E, Baker-Zander S, et al: Invasion of the central nervous system by *Treponema pallidum*: implications for diagnosis and treatment. Ann Intern Med 109:855, 1988

17. Augenbraun M, Dehovitz J, Feldman J, et al: Biological false-positive syphilis test results for women infected with human immunodeficiency virus. Clin Infect Dis 19:1040, 1994

18. Hart G: Syphilis tests in diagnostic and therapeutic decision making. Ann Intern Med 104:368, 1986

19. Larsen S, Steiner B, Rudolph A: Laboratory diagnosis and interpretation of tests for syphilis. Clin Micro Rev 8:1, 1995

20. 1998 guidelines for treatment of sexually transmitted diseases. MMWR Morb Mortal Wkly Rep 47(RR-1):28, 1997

21. Horowitz H, Valsamis M, Wicher V, et al: Brief report: cerebral syphilitic gumma confirmed by polymerase chain reaction in a man with human immunodeficiency virus infection. N Engl J Med 331:1488, 1994

22. Schroeter A, Lucas J, Price E, et al: Treatment for early syphilis and reactivity of serologic tests. JAMA 221:471, 1972

23. Brown S, Zaidi A, Larsen S, et al: Serologic response to syphilis treatment: a new analysis of old data. JAMA 253:1296, 1985

24. Management of Patients with Sexually Transmitted Diseases. World Health Organization Technical Report Series. World Health Organization, Geneva, 1991, p 810

25. Idsoe O, Guthrie T, Wilcox W: Penicillin in the treatment of syphilis. Bull WHO 47(suppl):1, 1972

26. Duncan W, Knox J: Cephalexin therapy for infectious syphilis. Arch Dermatol 110:77, 1974

27. Nicolis G, Loucopoulos A: Cephalothin in the treatment of syphilis. Br J Vener Dis 50:270, 1974

28. Duncan W, Knox J: Cephalexin therapy for infectious syphilis. Arch Dermatol 110:77, 1974

29. Korting HC, Walther D, Riethmuller, et al: Comparative in vitro susceptibility of *Treponema pallidum* to ceftizoxime, ceftriaxone and penicillin G. Chemotherapy 32:352, 1986

30. Johnson R, Bey R, Wolgamot S: Comparison of the activities of ceftriaxone and penicillin G against experimentally induced syphilis in rabbits. Antimicrob Agents Chemother 21:984, 1982

31. Korting H, Walther D, Riethmuller U, et al: Ceftriaxone given repeatedly cures manifest syphilis in the rabbit. Chemotherapy 33:376, 1987

32. Hook EW 3rd, Rodd RE, Handsfield HH: Ceftriaxone therapy for incubating and early syphilis. J Infect Dis 158:881, 1988

33. Moorthy T, Lee C, Lim K, et al: Ceftriaxone for treatment of primary syphilis in men: a preliminary study. Sex Transm Dis 14:116, 1987

34. Stamm L, Parrish E: In-vitro activity of azithromycin and CP-63,956 against *Treponema pallidum*. J Antimicrob Chemother 25(suppl A):11, 1990

35. Lukehart S, Fohn M, Baker-Zander S: Efficacy of azithromycin for therapy of active syphilis in the rabbit model. J Antimicrob Chemother 25(suppl A):91, 1990

36. Drew R, Gallis H: Azithromycin-spectrum of activity, pharmacokinetics and clinical applications. Pharmacotherapy 12:161, 1992

37. Verdon MS, Handsfield H, Johnson R: Pilot study of azithromycin for treatment of primary and secondary syphilis. Clin Infect Dis 19:486, 1994

38. Hook E, Stephans J, Ennis D: Azithromycin compared with penicillin G benzathine for the treatment of incubating syphilis. Ann Intern Med 131:434, 1999

39. Hatos G: Evaluation of 460 cases of treated syphilis. Med J Aust 2: 415, 1972

40. St. John R: Treatment of cardiovascular syphilis. J Am Vener Dis Assoc 3:148, 1976

41. Yoder F: Penicillin treatment of neurosyphilis. JAMA 232:270, 1975

42. Mohr J, Griffiths W, Jackson R, et al: Neurosyphilis and penicillin levels in cerebrospinal fluid. JAMA 236:2208, 1976

43. Dunlop E, Al-Egaily S, Houang E: Penicillin levels in blood and CSF achieved by treatment of syphilis. JAMA 241:2538, 1979

44. Ducas J, Robson HG: Cerebrospinal fluid penicillin levels during therapy for latent syphilis. JAMA 246:2583, 1981

45. Goh B, Smith G, Smarasinghe L, et al: Penicillin concentrations in serum and cerebrospinal fluid after intramuscular injection of aqueous procaine penicillin 0.6 MU with and without probenecid. Br J Vener Dis 60:371, 1984

46. Hooshmand H, Escobar M, Kopf S: Neurosyphilis. JAMA 219:726, 1972

47. Greene B, Miller N, Bynum T: Failure of penicillin G benzathine in the treatment of neurosyphilis. Arch Intern Med 140:1117, 1980

48. Jorgenson J, Tikjob G, Weismann K: Neurosyphilis after treatment of latent syphilis with benzathine penicillin. Genitourin Med 62:129, 1986

49. Gordon S, Eaton M, George R, et al: The response of symptomatic neurosyphilis to high-dose intravenous penicillin G in patients with human immunodeficiency virus infection. N Engl J Med 331:1469, 1994

50. Marra CM, Boutin P, McArthur JC, et al: A pilot study evaluating ceftriaxone and penicillin G as treatment agents for neurosyphilis in human immunodeficiency virus-infected individuals. Clin Infect Dis 30:540, 2000

51. Augenbraun M, Workowski K: Ceftriaxone therapy for syphilis: report from the emerging infections network. Clin Infect Dis 29:1337, 1999

52. Rolfs R, Joesoef R, Hendershot EF, et al: A randomized trial of enhanced therapy for early syphilis in patients with and without human immunodeficiency virus infection. The Syphilis and HIV Study Group. N Engl J Med 337:307, 1997

53. Faber W, Bos J, Rietra P, et al: Treponemicidal levels of amoxicillin in cerebrospinal fluid after oral administration. Sex Transm Dis 10:148, 1983

54. Morrison R, Harrison S, Tramont E: Oral amoxycillin, an alternative treatment for neurosyphilis. Genitourin Med 61:359, 1985

55. Romanowski B, Starreveld E, Jarema A: Treatment of neurosyphilis with chloramphenicol: a case report. Br J Vener Dis 59:225, 1983

56. Yim C, Flynn N, Fitzgerald F: Penetration of oral doxycycline into the cerebrospinal fluid of patients with latent or neurosyphilis. Antimicrob Agents Chemother 28:347, 1985

57. Rothenberg R, Becker G, Wiet R: Syphilitic hearing loss [editorial]. South Med J 72:118, 1979

58. Steckelberg J, McDonald T: Otologic involvement in late syphilis. Laryngoscope 94:753, 1984

59. Romanowski B, Sutherland R, Fick G, et al: Serologic response to treatment of infectious syphilis. Ann Intern Med 114:1005, 1991

60. Haas J, Bolan G, Larsen S, et al: Sensitivity of treponemal tests for detecting prior treated syphilis during human immunodeficiency virus infection. J Infect Dis 162:862, 1990

61. Zenker P, Rolfs R: Treatment of syphilis, 1989. Rev Infect Dis 12 (suppl 6):S590, 1990

62. Peterman TA, Zaidi AA, Lieb S, et al: Incubating syphilis in patients treated for gonorrhea: a comparison of treatment regimens. J Infect Dis 170:689, 1994

63. Klein V, Cox S, Mitchell M, Wendel G: The Jarisch-Herxheimer reaction complicating syphilotherapy in pregnancy. Obstet Gynecol 75:375, 1990

64. Sullivan T, Yecies L, Shatz G, et al: Desensitization of patients allergic to penicillin using orally administered β-lactam antibiotics. J Allergy Clin Immunol 69:275, 1982

65. Lin R: A perspective on penicillin allergy. Arch Intern Med 152:930, 1992

66. Wendel G, Stark B, Jamison R, et al: Penicillin allergy and desensitization in serious infections during pregnancy. N Engl J Med 312:1229, 1985

67. Ingraham N: Prevention and treatment of prenatal syphilis. Am J Med 5:693, 1948

68. Cross J, McCain J, Heyman A: The use of crystalline penicillin G in the treatment of syphilis in pregnancy. Am J Obstet Gynecol 57:461, 1949

69. Bundeson H, Rodriques J, Aron H: Outcome of pregnancies of women treated with aqueous penicillin for early infectious syphilis. Arch Dermatol Syph 62:230, 1950

70. Wammock V, Carrozzino O, Ingraham N, et al: Penicillin therapy of the syphilitic pregnant woman. Am J Obstet Gynecol 59:806, 1950

71. Smith C, O'Brien J, Simpson W, et al: Treatment of early syphilis with N, N' Dibenzylenediamine penicillin G. Am J Syph 38:136, 1954

72. Nelson N, Struve V: Prevention of congenital syphilis by the treatment of syphilis in pregnancy. JAMA 161:869, 1956

73. Jackson F, Vanderstoep E, Knox J, et al: Use of aqueous benzathine penicillin G in the treatment of syphilis in pregnant women. Am J Obstet Gynecol 83:1389, 1962

74. Taber L, Huber T: Congenital syphilis. Prog Clin Biol Res 3:183, 1975

75. Mascola L, Pelosi R, Blount J, et al: Congenital syphilis: Why is it still occurring? JAMA 252:1719, 1984

76. Beck-Sague C, Alexander E: Failure of benzathine penicillin G treatment in early congenital syphilis. Pediatr Infect Dis 6:1061, 1987

77. Zenker P, Berman S: Congenital syphilis: trends and recommendations for evaluation and management. Pediatr Infect Dis J 110:516, 1991

78. Wendel G: Gestational and congenital syphilis. Clin Perinatol 15: 287, 1988

79. Hashiasaki P, Wertzberger G, Conrad G, et al: Erythromycin failure in the treatment of syphilis in a pregnant woman. Sex Transm Dis 10:36, 1983

80. Fenton L, Light I: Congenital syphilis after maternal therapy with erythromycin. Obstet Gynecol 47:492, 1976

81. Pavithran K: Failure of erythromycin to prevent prenatal syphilis and cure syphilis. Ind J Sex Transm Dis 7:30, 1986

82. Kiefer L, Rubin A, McCoy J, et al: The placental transfer of erythromycin. Am J Obstet Gynecol 69:174, 1955

83. Philipson A, Sabath L, Charles D: Transplacental passage of erythromycin and clindamycin. N Engl J Med 288:1219, 1973

84. American Academy of Pediatrics: Syphilis. Report of the Committee on Infectious Diseases. Red Book 25th ed. Pickering LK, Ed. American Academy of Pediatrics, Elk Grove, Illinois, 2000, p 547

85. Kreiss J, Coombs R, Plummer F, et al: Isolation of human immunodeficiency virus from genital ulcers in Nairobi prostitutes. J Infect Dis 160:380, 1989

86. Telzak E, Chaisson M, Bevie P, et al: HIV-1 seroconversion in patients with and without genital ulcer disease: a prospective study. Ann Intern Med 119:1181, 1993

87. Berry C, Hooten T, Collier A, et al: Neurologic relapse after benzathine penicillin therapy for secondary syphilis in a patient with HIV infection. N Engl J Med 316:1587, 1987

88. Johns D, Tierney M, Felsenstein D: Alteration in the natural history of neurosyphilis by concurrent infection with the human immunodeficiency virus. N Engl J Med 316:1569, 1987

89. Hicks C, Benson P, Lupton G: Seronegative secondary syphilis in a patient infected with human immunodeficiency virus with Kaposi's sarcoma. Ann Intern Med 107:492, 1987

90. Gourevitch M, Selwyn P, Davenny D, et al: Effects of HIV infection on the serologic manifestation and response to treatment of syphilis in intravenous drug users. Ann Intern Med 118:350, 1993

91. Rompalo A, Cannon R, Quinn T, et al: Association of biologic false positive reactions for syphilis with human immunodeficiency virus infection. J Infect Dis 165:1124, 1992

92. Rompalo AM, Joesoef MR, O'Donnell JA, et al: Clinical manifestations of early syphilis by HIV status and gender: results of the syphilis and HIV study. Sex Transm Dis 28:158, 2001

93. Marra C, Longstreith W, Maxwell C, et al: Resolution of serum and cerebrospinal fluid abnormalities after treatment of neurosyphilis. Sex Transm Dis 23:184, 1996

94. Hollander H: Cerebrospinal fluid normalities and abnormalities in individuals infected with human immunodeficiency virus. J Infect Dis 158:855, 1988

95. Noordhoek G, Hermans P, Paul A, et al: *Treponema pallidum* subspecies *pallidum* (Nichols) and *Treponema pallidum* subspecies *pertenue* (CDC 2575) differ in at least one nucleotide: comparison of two homologous antigens. Microb Pathogenesis 6:29, 1989

25 Leptospirosis, Relapsing Fever, Rat-Bite Fever, and Lyme Disease

David A. Relman, M.D.

Leptospirosis

Leptospirosis is an acute systemic disease caused by various serotypes of *Leptospira*, the smallest and most tightly coiled of the pathogenic spirochetes. Leptospirosis is endemic in animals; humans are only accidentally infected. There are more than 200 serotypes of *L. interrogans* that cause this disease.[1] For convenience in diagnosis, serotypes that have major antigens in common are combined into serogroups. Infection with any of a variety of serotypes can cause aseptic meningitis, Weil's disease, or fever of unknown origin. The *canicola* serogroup is the most common cause of leptospirosis in the United States.

EPIDEMIOLOGY

Leptospirosis occurs worldwide but is especially common in tropical regions. Cattle, swine, sheep, dogs, raccoons, and other animals serve as the disease reservoir. Infected animals may develop overt illness or become asymptomatic carriers, shedding leptospires in the urine for many months.

Leptospires may enter the human host directly through abraded skin, the conjunctivae, or oral mucous membranes.[2] Human disease often results from indirect contact with infected animals via contaminated water or soil; in nature, leptospires that are shed in neutral or alkaline urine can survive for several weeks in a warm, moist environment. Person-to-person transmission is very rare; however, breastfeeding has been associated with transmission of leptospirosis.

About 50 to 100 cases of leptospirosis were reported annually in the United States until 1995, when cases were no longer required to be reported. However, it is likely that many cases, including subclinical infections, go unrecognized.[2,3]

Leptospirosis occurs sporadically or as a common-source outbreak. It was once regarded primarily as an occupational disease, particularly among farmers, workers in rice paddies and sugarcane fields, veterinarians, sewer workers, and slaughterhouse workers. In the United States, however, leptospirosis is now most common among children, adolescents, and homemakers. It is contracted during recreational activities such as fishing, hunting, and swimming or wading in contaminated ponds, participating in other water sports, or exposure to rat urine in urban or rural settings.[3] Infections occur in most areas of the United States, but more cases have been reported in southern and western regions, usually during the summer and autumn months.

PATHOLOGY AND PATHOGENESIS

After the entry of leptospires through mucous membranes or abraded skin, the organisms are disseminated via the blood. Virulent *L. interrogans* serotypes have been shown to adhere to and penetrate cultured endothelial and kidney epithelial cells in vitro. The proximal renal tubules may be the natural habitat for these organisms.[1] The mechanisms by which leptospires cause multiorgan system dysfunction and, occasionally, diffuse vasculitis remain largely unknown. Direct spirochetal invasion of tissues may be one mechanism of cellular injury.

The major impact of severe infection is on the liver and kidneys. Aseptic meningitis is also common. Mild pulmonary symptoms may occur in 20% to 70% of patients with leptospirosis but are often overlooked.[4] Occasionally, myocarditis or hemorrhagic pneumonitis occurs. Histologic changes in the liver are not often striking, and such changes are not diagnostic. Jaundice is often observed without hepatocellular necrosis. The most common renal lesions in patients with leptospirosis are interstitial nephritis and tubular epithelial necrosis. The pathophysiology of these lesions may, in some cases, be a direct toxic effect by the leptospires as well as immune-mediated injury. The extent of renal damage generally correlates well with the degree of renal function impairment. Silver impregnation stains have shown leptospires to be present in renal tubules but only rarely in other organs. The pathologic changes that are observed in the kidney are reversible.

Typically, leptospirosis is a biphasic illness. In the initial febrile leptospiremic phase, organisms can be demonstrated in the blood and cerebrospinal fluid. The second febrile immune phase begins when IgM antibodies appear in the circulation. Renal involvement appears before the onset of the immune phase but may persist throughout much of it. Meningeal signs and CSF pleocytosis are common during the second phase.

CLINICAL FEATURES

General Manifestations

The incubation period usually lasts 7 to 12 days, with a range of 2 to 20 days. Most patients have an anicteric, self-limited illness clinically indistinguishable from viral or bacterial infections. Fever may be the only manifestation. The onset of acute disease is abrupt and is typically manifested by high fever, chills, headache, and prostration. Myalgias are prominent. The leptospiremic phase continues with spiking fevers and chills for 4 to 7 days, during which cough, chest pain, anorexia, nausea, and vomiting are common; abdominal pain and diarrhea are less common.[4]

The most prominent and frequent findings are relative bradycardia, muscle tenderness (particularly in the calves, thighs, and lumbar areas), and stiff neck. An important finding is a conjunctival suffusion (a dilatation of conjunctival vessels without purulent discharge), which occurs on the third or fourth day. Maculopapular, petechial, or purpuric rashes may appear, usually on the trunk. Splenomegaly, hepatomegaly, and lymphadenopathy are uncommon.

Coincident with the disappearance of leptospires from the circulation and CSF is an afebrile, almost symptom-free period, usually lasting from 1 to 3 days. Then a second phase is heralded by the return of fever and other earlier symptoms. Meningismus, photophobia, uveitis, and CSF pleocytosis are common. The second phase may last from a few days to as long as several weeks.

Specific Syndromes

Weil's disease, a severe form of leptospirosis, is characterized by fever, jaundice, cutaneous and visceral hemorrhages, anemia, azotemia, and altered state of consciousness. The syndrome develops in 5% to 10% of cases of leptospirosis. Initially, the illness resembles less severe forms of leptospirosis, but the second phase is characterized by higher fever and hepatic, renal, and encephalopathic manifestations. The liver is enlarged and tender. Serum aspartate aminotransferase (AST) and alanine aminotransferase (ALT) levels are only mildly elevated, even in the presence of marked direct hyperbilirubinemia. Rhabdomyolysis results in elevated serum creatine kinase (CK) levels in more than 50% of patients. Epistaxis, purpura, hemoptysis, and gastrointestinal bleeding can be marked and are believed to be the result of diffuse small vessel vasculitis.

Renal damage is manifested by proteinuria, hematuria, and increasing azotemia; peak renal damage is reached early in the second phase of illness. Oliguria may be so marked that dialysis is required. Although renal involvement is common, it is almost never fatal except in patients with the hepatorenal syndrome. In rare instances, myocarditis, congestive heart failure, and cardiac arrhythmias occur.[5]

Aseptic meningitis Many serotypes of *Leptospira* cause aseptic meningitis; the three most frequent are the *canicola*, *icterohaemorrhagiae*, and *pomona* serotypes. Leptospiral meningitis differs from viral meningitis in that there is no CSF pleocytosis during the first phase, although leptospires may be isolated from the CSF. Pleocytosis develops during the second phase; the cell count usually ranges from 20 to 1,000/mm^3, with a predominance of lymphocytes. In some patients, particularly those with higher cell counts, polymorphonuclear leukocytes predominate early. The CSF glucose level is usually normal. The CSF protein level is sometimes markedly elevated, above 100 mg/dl; such an elevation is unusual in the viral aseptic meningitides.

Pretibial fever The early manifestations of pretibial fever, also called Fort Bragg fever, resemble the initial phase of leptospirosis, but on the fourth or fifth day, slightly raised, erythematous, tender areas develop on both shins. Splenomegaly is common in pretibial fever but not in other forms of leptospirosis. The original outbreak, at Fort Bragg, North Carolina, was caused by the *autumnalis* serotype. Reports from England have described cases of leptospirosis with erythema nodosum; whether this syndrome and pretibial fever are the same is unclear.

LABORATORY FINDINGS

The leukocyte count may be normal, reduced, or elevated, with a prominent shift to the left. Thrombocytopenia is very common, particularly in severely ill patients. Proteinuria, hematuria, and azotemia occur during the initial phase in up to 70% of cases but disappear unless Weil's disease develops. Serum bilirubin, predominantly in conjugated form, is also elevated and may reach a concentration of 20 mg/dl or more in Weil's disease.

DIFFERENTIAL DIAGNOSIS

Leptospirosis initially resembles a viral infection. Definitive diagnosis requires a positive culture or a microscopic agglutination test result that shows a fourfold or greater rise in antibody titer. Serologic cross-reactions occur between various serotypes. Isolation of the organism is the only certain means of establishing the serotype.

Leptospires can be isolated from blood and CSF during the initial phase and from the urine during the second phase and for some months after recovery. Multiple blood cultures should be taken because the number of circulating organisms is low; cultures are incubated at 28° to 30° C in the dark for at least 5 to 6 weeks. Specimens may be sent to a reference laboratory for cultivation without compromising yield, because leptospires remain viable in non–citrate-treated anticoagulated blood for up to 11 days. Artifacts resembling leptospires in blood specimens and urine render dark-field microscopy unreliable. Use of the polymerase chain reaction for *Leptospira* detection in body fluids has proved useful in the early diagnosis of leptospirosis.[3]

TREATMENT

Although the efficacy of antimicrobial agents in the treatment of leptospirosis is controversial, data suggest that they shorten the duration of illness and reduce the likelihood of complications. Doxycycline, 0.1 g orally twice daily for 7 days, may favorably affect the course of leptospirosis when treatment is initiated within 2 to 4 days after the onset of symptoms. A prospective, randomized study has suggested that penicillin G, 6 million units I.V. daily for 7 days, has a beneficial effect on the course of late, severe leptospirosis,[6] but other studies have not confirmed this finding. A Jarisch-Herxheimer type of reaction may occur within a few hours after the initial dose of penicillin, indicating that the drug possesses some in vivo antileptospiral activity. Treatment of renal failure requires careful management of fluid and electrolyte balance. Because renal damage is often reversible, peritoneal dialysis or hemodialysis should be used in cases of renal failure.

PREVENTION

Prevention is difficult because of the large and diverse animal reservoir. Doxycycline, 0.2 g orally once a week, significantly reduces the attack rate of leptospirosis. *Leptospira* vaccines are available for dogs, but they have limited efficacy.

PROGNOSIS

The case-fatality rate is 3% to 6%. Mortality is highest (15% to 40%) in patients with jaundice and in the elderly. Dyspnea, oliguria, leukocytosis, and radiographic and electrocardiographic abnormalities have been associated with higher mortality.[7] Recovery is complete except for the rare occurrence of residual renal tubular dysfunction.

Relapsing Fever

Relapsing fever is an acute louse- or tick-borne infection caused by blood spirochetes of the genus *Borrelia*. It is characterized by recurrent febrile episodes separated by asymptomatic intervals. Unlike other spirochetes that cause human disease, the etiologic agent can be readily detected with Giemsa stain or Wright's stain. *B. recurrentis* is the cause of louse-borne relapsing fever. A variety of species produce the tick-borne disease; in the United States, the predominant species are *B. hermsii* and *B. turicatae*. These organisms cannot be cultivated on artificial media but can be grown in chick embryos.

EPIDEMIOLOGY

Louse-borne relapsing fever usually occurs in epidemics, often with epidemic typhus, in the wake of wars, famines, and natural disasters. It is not observed in the United States, but endemic foci persist in Ethiopia, South America, and the Far East. *B. recurrentis* is transmitted to humans by contamination of skin abrasions with crushed infected lice.

Tick-borne relapsing fever occurs sporadically during the summer in areas of the western United States where ticks of the genus *Ornithodoros* dwell. It also occurs in widely distributed areas of Africa, Asia, and South America. When ticks feed on infected rodents or other mammals, they ingest borrelias; borrelias can persist for years in a tick and can be passed transovarially, making the tick vector an efficient reservoir. Transmission to humans occurs through the tick feeding site. The number of reported cases of tick-borne relapsing fever is growing in some areas of the United States, perhaps because of improved disease awareness, improved diagnostic techniques, or increased tick-host contact.

PATHOGENESIS

After inoculation from an arthropod vector, borrelias produce a spirochetemia accompanied by an acute febrile illness. The most characteristic feature of the subsequent course is the phenomenon of relapse, which is caused by the ability of borrelias to undergo antigenic variation in an infected host. The mechanism of antigenic variation comprises recombination, deletion, and the transposition of silent gene copies that encode serotype-determining proteins to an active expression site.[8] By these processes, new antigenically distinct borrelias are created that can evade the host's immune response. After 3 to 6 days of overt illness, circulating antibodies appear, eliminating the original organisms from the bloodstream. Simultaneously, the fever resolves by crisis; however, during an afebrile interval of about 1 week, the new antigenic variant arises and multiplies. A second febrile illness, the initial relapse, results when large numbers of these variant borrelias reinvade the bloodstream. After several days, new antibodies to this variant are produced, followed by clearance of the organisms from the peripheral blood and a second defervescence. The cycle of new variant selection followed by specific antibody production may be repeated one or more times, producing the distinctive feature of relapsing fever.

CLINICAL FEATURES

Tick- and louse-borne relapsing fevers are clinically similar. The higher mortality seen in louse-borne disease may relate more to the host, who may have malnutrition or other illnesses, than to a difference in pathogenicity.

After a 7-day incubation period, symptoms begin abruptly, with high fever, shaking chills, and profound headache. Myalgias, prostration, nausea, vomiting, diarrhea, abdominal pain, and cough are early signs. The temperature remains elevated at 39.4° to 40.6° C (102.9° to 105.1° F) until defervescence by crisis. Tachycardia and tachypnea are present. The patient is somnolent and sometimes confused. Maculopapular or petechial rashes may appear. Splenomegaly is common.[9] Hepatomegaly, abdominal tenderness, and lymphadenopathy (particularly affecting cervical nodes) may develop. Jaundice caused by hepatocellular damage is uncommon in tick-borne disease but occurs in about one third of patients with louse-borne disease, usually late in the course. Epistaxis is common in louse-borne disease; in severe disease, extensive ecchymoses and mucosal bleeding may develop secondary to liver disease or disseminated intravascular coagulation. Neurologic complications occur in 10% to 30% of cases.[9] Iridocyclitis and myocarditis are uncommon complications; iridocyclitis occurs after several febrile cycles.

The initial febrile attack lasts 3 to 6 days, ending abruptly in another distinctive feature of this illness—the crisis. There is a sudden fall in temperature, accompanied by drenching sweats; hypotension and shock are rare. Spirochetes rapidly disappear from the peripheral blood at this time. After an afebrile period of 6 to 10 days, a febrile, symptomatic relapse occurs, but it is of shorter duration than the original episode. There is usually only a single relapse in louse-borne disease, but several additional relapses are common in tick-borne relapsing fever.[9] Each succeeding relapse is milder and of shorter duration, and each intervening afebrile period is longer than the previous period.

LABORATORY FINDINGS

The leukocyte count is usually normal. A mild normocytic anemia is common. The AST level may be elevated, and in severe cases, the serum bilirubin is markedly increased. Thrombocytopenia may be present, even without obvious disseminated intravascular coagulation. Serologic tests for syphilis are positive in about 5% of patients.

The most dramatic and diagnostically helpful laboratory observation is the finding of spirochetes on smears of peripheral blood obtained during febrile periods and stained with Wright's or Giemsa stain [*see Figure 1*]. Repeated examinations may be required to demonstrate the organisms, particularly during relapses. Organisms are not seen during afebrile intervals. Spirochetes may be seen on wet mounts examined with phase-contrast microscopy, but this method is unreliable in the hands of inexperienced observers because of the frequent occurrence of artifacts resembling spirochetes. When direct smears are negative for spirochetes, greater diagnostic sensitivity may be achieved by examination of smears of blood from mice that were previously inoculated with blood from a patient. The density of spirochetes in the blood may correlate with the likelihood of complications.

DIFFERENTIAL DIAGNOSIS

During the initial febrile episode, relapsing fever resembles many other acute infections, such as leptospirosis, salmonellosis, infectious mononucleosis, malaria, and a variety of bacteremias. Epidemiologic features can suggest the diagnosis, and careful examination of the blood smear can provide substantiation. Colorado tick fever is also endemic in

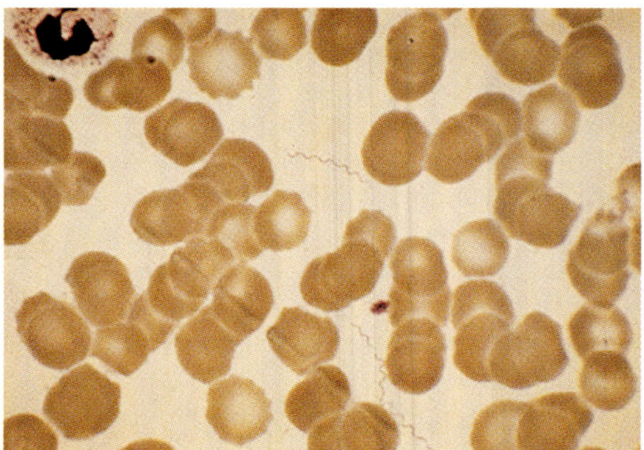

Figure 1 **In this thin Wright's stain of peripheral blood from a patient in the febrile stage of relapsing fever, several spirochetes can be seen.**

the western states and has a biphasic course; however, the febrile and afebrile periods are shorter in Colorado tick fever, and leukopenia is common. Rocky Mountain spotted fever may mimic relapsing fever in initial symptoms because of the presence of a rash and history of exposure to a tick vector. In Rocky Mountain spotted fever, however, the rash appears first on the extremities and is usually more extensive than in relapsing fever.

TREATMENT

For adults, the treatment of choice is tetracycline, 0.5 g orally four times daily for 10 days. Tetracycline rapidly eliminates organisms from the circulation and prevents relapses. A single 0.1 g dose of doxycycline has also been shown to be effective for the treatment of louse-borne disease in endemic areas; however, this regimen has not been studied in patients with tick-borne disease. Penicillin is also effective in the treatment of relapsing fever. Ceftriaxone may have a role in the treatment of relapsing fever with central nervous system involvement.

In most cases of louse-borne relapsing fever and, less often, in tick-borne relapsing fever, treatment is followed by a Jarisch-Herxheimer type of reaction. The reaction is characterized by rigors, high fever, headache, and tachycardia and is believed to be related to the destruction of spirochetes. Penicillin clears the blood of spirochetes more slowly than tetracycline and thus may prevent a severe reaction, but it may result in a more prolonged period of hypotension than occurs with tetracycline.

The mortality in untreated cases of louse-borne relapsing fever during epidemics has reached 40%. This high rate may in part be the result of concurrent typhus and salmonellosis epidemics. The mortality for either tick- or louse-borne relapsing fever with appropriate treatment is 2% to 5%.

Rat-Bite Fever

Rat-bite fever refers to infection caused by either *Streptobacillus moniliformis* or *Spirillum minus*. Although these two infections produce similar clinical syndromes, there are differences sufficient to warrant separate discussions. In the United States, *S. moniliformis* is the more common cause of rat-bite fever.

STREPTOBACILLUS MONILIFORMIS INFECTION

S. moniliformis is a highly pleomorphic, nonmotile, gram-negative, facultative anaerobe that has a remarkable capacity to produce stable L-forms during routine culture. Rapid bacteriologic diagnosis from blood cultures may be rendered difficult because prolonged incubation is needed for isolation and because the L-form predominates in cultures; thus, bacillary forms may not be revealed by Gram's stain of direct smears of initial cultures.

S. moniliformis has been found in the nasopharynx of up to 50% of rats, the apparent natural reservoir, and the organism is excreted in the urine. Rat-bite fever is uncommon, and most infections in humans result from bites or scratches by wild rats or other rodents. Worldwide, the illness occurs most often in crowded, urban, rodent-infested areas. Occasionally, epidemic *S. moniliformis* infection occurs as a result of contamination of food or water. Recent outbreaks of waterborne disease (Haverhill fever) have presented a diagnostic dilemma because there was no history of rodent bite.[10]

The incubation period is usually 2 to 10 days. The onset is abrupt, and the initial manifestations (fever, chills, headache, malaise, and myalgias) are nonspecific. The bite wound frequently has healed by the time symptoms appear. The clinical features of epidemic food-borne and waterborne disease are generally the same as those of rat bite–associated disease except that in the epidemic form no bite is present and upper respiratory tract symptoms are more common. A morbilliform or petechial rash, which is most marked on the extremities, particularly the hands and feet, develops in most patients shortly after the onset of fever. Arthralgias and polyarthritis in both large and small joints are characteristic features. The fever may recur. Abscesses sometimes complicate disseminated infection.[11] If untreated, the febrile illness and articular manifestations persist for several weeks. Prolongation of symptoms beyond several

Table 1 Characteristics of Rat-Bite Fever

	Streptobacillus moniliformis *Infection*	Spirillum minus *Infection*
Incubation period	Less than 10 days	1–4 wk
Bite site	Healed by the time symptoms appear	Inflammation at bite site; lymphangitis and regional lymphadenitis at onset of systemic symptoms
Onset	Chills, fever, joint symptoms	Fever without joint symptoms
Course	Relapsing course uncommon	Relapsing course common

weeks should raise suspicion of a complicating endocarditis.[12]

Diagnosis

The diagnosis is made by isolation of the organism from blood or, less commonly, from synovial fluid. The fever, rash, and articular manifestations of *S. moniliformis* infection may resemble those of meningococcemia, but meningitis is usually not a feature of streptobacillary infection. Rocky Mountain spotted fever, leptospirosis, and echovirus infection have similar presentations. Such epidemiologic factors as tick exposure, endemic areas, and season of the year should be considered. A history of recent rat bite should suggest possible infection by *S. moniliformis* or *S. minus* [*see Table 1*].

Treatment

Initial treatment is aqueous penicillin G, 600,000 to 1 million units parenterally every 4 hours. Patients with endocarditis should be treated with 10 to 20 million units of penicillin I.V. daily. It has been suggested that streptomycin, 15 mg/kg/day I.M. in two divided doses, be given in addition to penicillin for complicated cases, including those with endocarditis, to provide increased bactericidal activity and increased activity against L-forms. For patients with penicillin allergy, oral tetracycline, 0.5 g four times daily, is acceptable. When therapy is administered promptly, cure can be anticipated. Untreated disease results in mortality approaching 10%.

SPIRILLUM MINUS INFECTION

Acute infection by *S. minus* (sodoku) also results from the bite or scratch of a rat. This spirillary, gram-negative, motile organism is found in the blood and in the peritoneal and lacrimal fluids of infected rats. The organism cannot be grown on artificial media. Its isolation from humans requires inoculation of blood or fluid from the primary cutaneous lesion into disease-free mice or guinea pigs. A Giemsa-stained smear of blood or peritoneal fluid from these animals is subsequently examined by dark-field microscopy to demonstrate the presence of *S. minus*.

Several characteristics of rat-bite fever caused by *S. minus* distinguish it from *S. moniliformis* rat-bite fever: the incubation period is longer; the bite-site manifestations are decidedly pronounced, with swelling and pain returning at the onset of febrile illness; and the disease has a relapsing course of 3- to 4-day febrile periods with systemic symptoms followed by afebrile periods, a pattern that may continue for several months or longer if the patient goes untreated. Articular manifestations are uncommon. A macular rash may occur. Biologic false positive test results for syphilis are common.

Treatment is the same as for *S. moniliformis* rat-bite fever.

Lyme Disease

Lyme disease is a tick-borne illness caused by the spirochete *B. burgdorferi*. It is divided into early disease (stages 1 and 2) and late disease (stage 3). Stage 1 is characterized by the presence of a distinctive skin lesion, termed erythema migrans or erythema chronicum migrans. Stage 2 is a disseminated phase of the infection, with manifestations in the skin, CNS, musculoskeletal system, and heart. Late disease, or stage 3, reflects persistent infection that is clinically manifest for more than 1 year after the onset of disease.

Since 1982, when a surveillance system for Lyme disease was established in the United States, more than 100,000 cases have been reported, and the annual number of cases has increased about 20-fold.[13,14] Lyme disease is currently the most commonly reported vector-borne illness in the United States.[14] The protean manifestations of this illness probably account for many unrecognized cases in the United States and Europe.

EPIDEMIOLOGY

In 1975, a geographic clustering of arthritis cases in several rural communities in southeastern Connecticut, including the town of Lyme, led to the recognition of Lyme disease.[15] Erythema migrans, the unique dermatologic feature of Lyme disease,

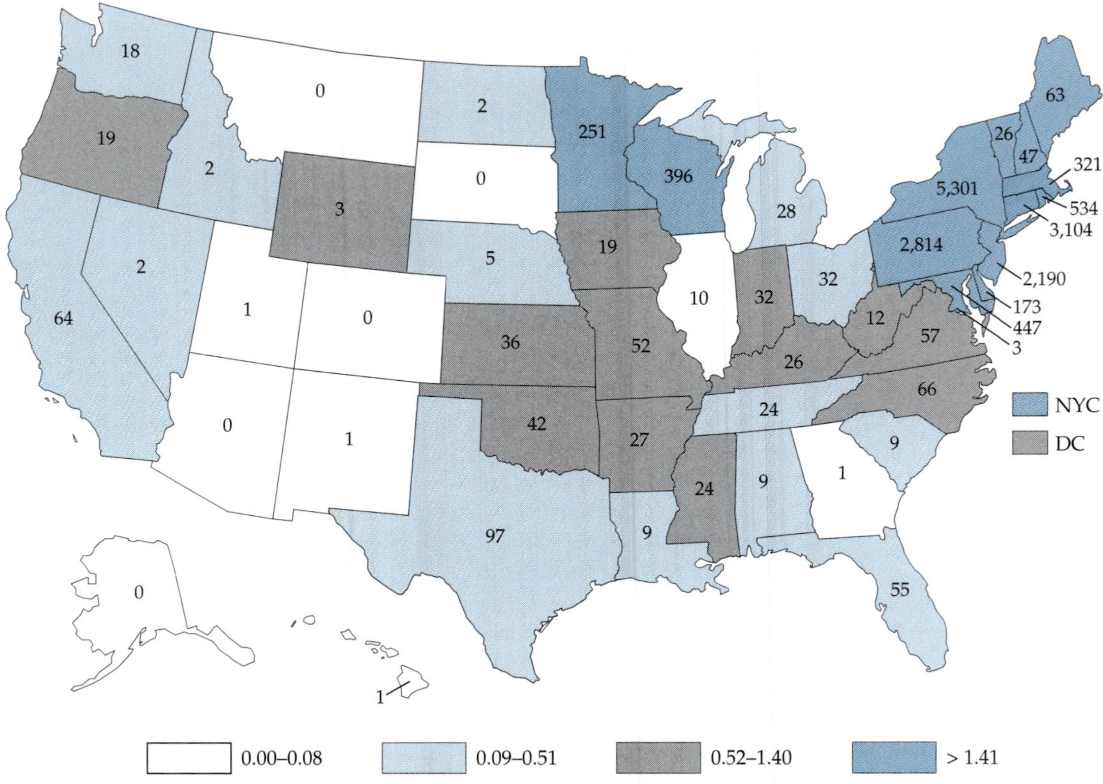

Figure 2 **This map shows the number of reported cases of Lyme disease for each state in 1996, as well as the number of reported cases per 100,000 population.[13] (NYC—New York City DC—District of Columbia)**

was observed in Europe in the early part of the 20th century, usually as the solitary manifestation of a disorder associated with tick bites. Other long-recognized clinical entities now included within the Lyme disease complex are acrodermatitis chronica atrophicans, a skin disorder seen particularly in Europe, and lymphocytic meningoradiculitis, which is also known as Bannwarth's syndrome.

There are three major endemic areas for Lyme disease in the United States: (1) coastal and wooded regions of southern New England, New York, and the Middle Atlantic states; (2) much of Wisconsin, Minnesota, and Michigan; and (3) coastal and wooded areas of California and Oregon [*see Figure 2*].[16] Despite reports of Lyme disease from nearly every state and of the gradual spread of the disease to new areas, enzootic foci have been identified in a limited number of states, and in 1996, eight states (Connecticut, Rhode Island, New York, New Jersey, Delaware, Pennsylvania, Maryland, and Wisconsin) accounted for 91% of all cases.[14] In any given state, Lyme disease is distinctly focal and may affect only certain counties and towns.[17]

Provisional data indicate just under 11,000 reported cases of Lyme disease in 1997, after a record number of cases (16,455) were reported the previous year [*see Figure 2*].[14] Increased awareness of Lyme disease, greater availability of diagnostic tests with varying reliability, and the spread of infected tick vector populations and animal reservoirs all contribute to its prevalence in the United States. Ten percent of asymptomatic persons in endemic loci have serologic evidence of exposure to the Lyme spirochete. Social factors play an important role in the epidemiology of Lyme disease; these factors include reforestation of agricultural land in the Northeast, which causes deer populations to expand, and human migration into these wooded areas.[17] Once established in a new locale, Lyme disease rapidly spreads to the local human population. Lyme disease occurs in widely distributed but focal areas throughout Europe, the former Soviet Union, South Africa, and Australia, as well as China, Japan, and other portions of the Far East.[17,18]

The chief vector of Lyme disease in the northeastern and upper midwestern regions of the United States is the tick *Ixodes dammini* (or *I. scapularis*); in the western United States, *I. pacificus*; in Europe, *I. ricinus*; and in Asia, *I. persulcatus*. In endemic areas of Connecticut and New York, as many as 50% to 70% of *I. dammini* ticks are infected with *B. burgdorferi*.[19] In contrast, only 1% to 6% of *I. pacificus* ticks are infected in endemic regions of California. This low infectivity rate is probably not sufficient to maintain *B. burgdorferi* in California; instead, a different tick, *I. neotomae*, may serve as the principal vector for enzootic cycles in that state.[20] Evidence to date does not suggest that insects other than ticks are important vectors of Lyme disease.

The reservoirs of the Lyme disease agent include a wide variety of wild and domestic animals and birds; the preferred hosts, however, are the white-tailed deer and the white-footed mouse. In the northeastern and north central United States, white-footed mice are the most important small mammal reservoir for *B. burgdorferi*. White-tailed deer are the preferred host for adult *I. dammini*, but deer are incompetent as reservoirs for *B. burgdorferi*. After a season of high acorn production, Lyme disease transmission risk may increase because tick density in oak forests is correlated with the abundance of this preferred mouse and deer food.[21] Migratory birds may disperse *I. dammini* infected with *B. burgdorferi* over wide regions of North America and northern Europe.[22] In the western United States, lizards serve as hosts for *I. pacificus*; however, lizards are resistant to *B. burgdorferi* infection and are not competent reservoirs. This contributes to the low rate of infection with *B. burgdorferi* in this tick species.

The likelihood of humans acquiring *B. burgdorferi* infection in Lyme disease–endemic areas depends on several factors. Tick exposure, both occupational and domestic, is a risk factor for Lyme disease seropositivity.[23] In addition, the risk of infection varies with the time of year. In the northeastern United States, the risk of spirochete transmission is greatest during May and June. In the northeastern and north central United States, Lyme disease occurs from May through August, peaking in July. In the western United States, disease most often occurs from January through May. Prospective studies with both mice and humans indicate that *B. burgdorferi* transmission is extremely unlikely with less than 48 to 72 hours of tick attachment (i.e., in the absence of engorgement).[24,25]

ETIOLOGY

B. burgdorferi, a spirochete that had been isolated from the *I. dammini* tick, was confirmed as the causative agent of Lyme disease in 1983.[26,27] The organism originally known as *B. burgdorferi* actually comprises at least three genomic groups, or genospecies, that are defined by chromosomal DNA relatedness and sequence analysis, protein polymorphisms, and differences in antigenicity.[16]

Nearly all strains of *B. burgdorferi* in the United States can be classified into the genomic group *B. burgdorferi sensu stricto*. Although some of these strains have also been found in Europe, the other important endemic region of the world, most European strains belong to the *B. burgdorferi* groups now known as *B. garinii* and *B. afzelii*. It was once believed that isolates from the United States were less diverse than those found in Europe; however, DNA sequence analysis reveals substantial and comparable genetic diversity among the former—especially among isolates from the Southeast and West, where tick vectors are more diverse as well.[28]

Unlike other bacterial genera, the genomic groups heretofore referred to as *B. burgdorferi* and, probably, the other *Borrelia* species have linear chromosomes and a mixture of linear and circular plasmids. Despite evidence of plasmid rearrangement and plasmid exchange in nature,[29] the overall population structure among *B. burgdorferi* isolates is clonal. Recently, the complete genome sequence of the original *B. burgdorferi* isolate (B31) was determined.[30] The genome sequence is notable for its paucity of genes that encode elements of biosynthetic pathways. Surprisingly, 6% of the linear chromosome is dedicated to motility and chemotaxis. The Lyme spirochete contains approximately 21 linear and circular plasmids, some of which can be viewed as minichromosomes. Many of the plasmid-encoded outer-surface lipoproteins (Osps) are immunodominant, and some, including the well-characterized OspA, OspB, and OspC, are protective antigens. The *B. burgdorferi* plasmids may provide genetic plasticity to this organism, as many of the genes show evidence of recombination and duplication. Depending on the strain and genospecies, each of these proteins can vary considerably.[31] The ability to recognize host environments and to regulate gene expression accordingly may be critical for virulence. These findings may have important implications for the reliability of some of the serologic tests currently available for Lyme disease and for the development of a vaccine.[32,33]

The *B. burgdorferi* complex is the cause of erythema migrans, acrodermatitis chronica atrophicans (ACA), Bannwarth's syndrome, and other disorders associated with Lyme disease in Europe. Each genospecies appears to have a propensity to cause different clinical manifestations.[34] In Europe, cutaneous disease, such as erythema migrans and ACA, is likely to be associated with *B. afzelii*, whereas extracutaneous disease, such as encephalomyelitis, is often associated with *B. garinii*. The early dissemination of infection and the arthritis that are more common in the United States than in Europe may reflect the particular properties of *B. burgdorferi sensu stricto*.

PATHOGENESIS

After inoculation in the skin of a human host, *B. burgdorferi* replicates and spreads within the dermis, resulting in erythema migrans. Studies suggest that the motility of this organism is adapted for viscous environments such as the extracellular matrix of the dermis. During this early phase of infection (stage 1), *B. burgdorferi* can be visualized in and grown from biopsy samples of most of these lesions.[35] The organism then disseminates to numerous organs by the hematogenous route. *B. burgdorferi* can be isolated from blood samples during this period.[36] Although there are rare reports of *B. burgdorferi* isolation from other human tissues, the organism exhibits particular tropism for the heart, CNS, and joints.

Direct tissue invasion and the resultant humoral and cellular immune responses all play a role in Lyme disease pathogenesis; however, their relative importance is unclear. *B. burgdorferi* DNA can often be detected with PCR early in the infectious process at many of the sites of disseminated disease. In addition, *B. burgdorferi* has been visualized in and grown from myocardium.[37] However, isolation of viable organisms from this and other sites of dissemination, including joints, occurs much less frequently than does detection of *B. burgdorferi* DNA. Positive test results are more likely to occur in patients who have relatively high fluid leukocyte counts and in those who remain untreated or are treated only for short periods. In addition, synovial fluid appears to contain greater numbers of plasmid DNA PCR targets (e.g., *ospA*) than chromosomal targets.[38] Thus, chronic Lyme arthritis may be caused by small numbers of persistent *B. burgdorferi* organisms that shed plasmid-containing, proinflammatory membrane blebs into the synovial fluid.

Similarly, cultures of CSF taken during the first 10 days of symptoms have yielded *B. burgdorferi* from approximately 10% of patients with neuroborreliosis[39]; however, results of PCR studies have shown that two thirds of patients with acute disseminated Lyme disease have *B. burgdorferi* DNA in the CSF.[40] This spirochete exhibits specific adherence to glial cells. The recently determined complete *B. burgdorferi* genome sequence should facilitate a more detailed understanding of pathogenic mechanisms.[30]

The host immune response within the CNS and other organs may be responsible for some of the resultant tissue damage. In particular, there are T cells and antibodies that recognize antigenic determinants shared by the *B. burgdorferi* 41 kd flagellar protein and human nerve cells. The role of immune autoreactivity in Lyme disease pathogenesis remains undetermined; however, certain human hosts may be predisposed toward this form of the disease. For example, patients with particular *HLA-DR4* and *HLA-DR2* alleles may be more susceptible to chronic Lyme arthritis.[41]

CLINICAL FEATURES

During stage 1, clinical manifestations of Lyme disease primarily involve the skin. During the disseminated and persistent stages of infection, the disease may affect, in decreasing likelihood, the skin, the musculoskeletal system, the CNS, and the heart.

Erythema Migrans

Three to 20 days after a tick bite (an incident recalled by 20% of patients with Lyme disease), a red macule or papule appears at the bite site in approximately 60% to 80% of cases.[42] It later expands to a large, annular, erythematous lesion that is 6 to 16 cm, and sometimes larger, in diameter. Occasionally, the lesion shows central clearing, and secondary concentric rings may develop within the original ring [*see Figure 3*]. Patients usually describe the lesion as burning. Multiple skin lesions develop in about half of patients during dissemination of the infection. There is no enanthema.

Most patients have a variety of symptoms that are associated with the onset of the skin lesion and that last for a few days. Such symptoms include malaise, fatigue, chills, fever, headache, stiff neck, and backache. Less often, diffuse myalgias, nausea, vomiting, and sore throat occur. On examination, the patient usually has a temperature of 38.0° to 39.5° C (100.4° to 103.1° F) and the distinctive erythema migrans skin lesion. Regional or generalized lymphadenopathy and splenomegaly are

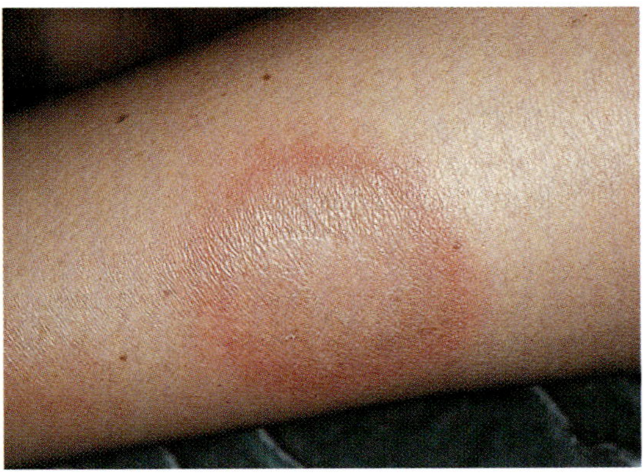

Figure 3 **An erythema migrans lesion has enlarged over several days and now has a red border with clearing in the center.**

occasionally present; several patients have had a malar rash.

In most patients, the erythema migrans skin lesion fades in 3 or 4 weeks, and recovery is complete. In some patients, disseminated and sometimes persistent disease develops in other organs: arthralgia or frank arthritis has been observed in up to 80% of patients, neurologic abnormalities in approximately 15%, and cardiac involvement in 4% to 8%.

Lyme Carditis

Cardiac conduction abnormalities may arise 4 to 80 days after the onset of erythema migrans. Such abnormalities usually consist of varying degrees of atrioventricular (AV) block. Skin lesions, which are frequently multiple, and fever are often still present at the time of cardiac involvement. Articular and neurologic manifestations are also present in many of these patients.

First-degree block, Wenckebach-type block, and complete heart block can all occur and may shift from one to another in the same patient. Complete heart block may be the sole clinical presentation of Lyme disease. Patients with high-degree AV block may have palpitations, dyspnea, substernal chest pain, dizziness, or syncope as the principal symptom of cardiac involvement. Physical examination may reveal tachycardia or bradycardia with irregularly occurring cannon A waves in the jugular vein pulse. Despite the risk of hemodynamic instability that accompanies this complication, the prognosis is favorable. Complete heart block rarely lasts longer than 1 week, and lesser degrees of heart block are usually reversible as well.[43] Myocardial disease with evidence of myopericarditis may develop and in some patients may lead to a chronic cardiomyopathy[37]; histologic examination reveals a lymphocytic infiltrate. Occasionally, a small pericardial effusion and an S_3 gallop develop. Valvular involvement does not occur during the active stage of carditis and does not develop after recovery from Lyme disease.

Neurologic Abnormalities

Lyme disease–related neurologic involvement occurs most often while the erythema migrans skin lesion is still present or within 6 weeks after its disappearance (during the disseminated stage of early disease), though some patients with neurologic abnormalities have no history of extraneural features.[44] Meningitis and cranial and peripheral neuropathies are probably the most common syndromes ascribed to Lyme neuroborreliosis. The most common neurologic symptoms of Lyme disease—headache, mild stiff neck, and photophobia—are also characteristic symptoms of viral meningitis, but in cases of Lyme disease, these symptoms may be accompanied by facial palsy or peripheral nerve paresthesias. CSF examination shows lymphocytic pleocytosis, with 25 to 450 leukocytes/mm^3; glucose and protein levels are normal. Other types of neurologic manifestations include the following:

1. Cranial nerve disorders—most commonly unilateral or bilateral facial palsy, which occurs in up to 50% of patients with neurologic manifestations and may be the sole neurologic manifestation of the disease. Cranial nerves III, V, and VIII are less often affected. These disorders usually resolve within 6 months.
2. Peripheral neuritis, most frequently a motor or sensory radiculoneuritis that involves the extremities or trunk. Usually, the neuritis subsides in a month or so. Mononeuritis multiplex and a Guillain-Barré–like syndrome have also been associated with Lyme disease. In some patients with the late stage of Lyme disease, intermittent paresthesias are reported, and there is neurophysiologic evidence of abnormal peripheral nerve function.[45]
3. Encephalitis, which is manifested by emotional lability, depression, poor memory and concentration, chorea in children, and cerebellar ataxia.
4. Cerebral vasculitis, which has been seen in a small number of patients with Lyme disease.
5. Chronic encephalopathy, which may occur during the late stage of Lyme disease. It is most often manifested by memory impairment,

mood changes, sleep disturbances, and difficulty with concentration.[46] The prevalence of this disorder is not known.

Many of these clinical disorders may be recurrent. Intrathecal production of antibodies against *B. burgdorferi* organisms may be useful as an indication of active Lyme neuroborreliosis.[47]

Lyme Arthritis

Articular manifestations develop in as many as 80% of patients with Lyme disease who do not receive antibiotic therapy. In approximately 20% of patients, only arthralgias occur, with onset between 1 day and 8 weeks after the appearance of erythema migrans. Frank arthritis is found in approximately 50% of patients 4 days to 2 years after disease onset. The most common clinical pattern is that of an asymmetrical monarthric or oligoarticular arthritis; polyarticular involvement is rare. Most patients have several recurrences of short duration, interspersed with longer periods of complete remission. Individual episodes may last from 3 days to 1 year. In children, the duration of episodes of arthritis and the frequency of recurrence may increase with age.[47] Approximately one third of children report arthralgias as long as 10 to 13 years after the initial onset of joint disease.

Large joints, especially the knees, are particularly affected. Chronic involvement, with pannus formation and cartilage erosion, of the knees or other large joints occurs in 10% of patients with Lyme arthritis. The knees in these patients are markedly swollen and demonstrate palpable synovial thickening. In several instances, popliteal cysts have formed and ruptured. The subsequent dissection of fluid into the calf produces a condition that simulates thrombophlebitis. The same phenomenon is sometimes observed in patients who have Reiter's syndrome.

Synovial fluid findings include a pleocytosis of 2,000 to 72,000 cells/mm^3, of which about 80% are granulocytes, and a protein concentration of 3 to 6 g/dl. Synovial biopsy shows synovial hypertrophy, vascular ingrowth, and marked infiltration by lymphocytes and plasma cells. *HLA-DR4* or *HLA-DR2* and antibodies to OspA or OspB may be associated with chronic arthritis that is relatively resistant to antimicrobial therapy.[48]

Other Clinical Manifestations

In a manner resembling that of *Treponema pallidum, B. burgdorferi* may cause disease in a variety of tissues. Ocular manifestations include conjunctivitis, keratitis, uveitis, retinitis, and optic neuritis.[49] Other manifestations are hepatitis, myositis, dermatomyositis, and acute respiratory distress syndrome. Some patients with Lyme disease develop signs and symptoms of fibromyalgia that antibiotic treatment fails to resolve.[50] Other forms of long-term morbidity are chronic or recurrent arthritis and arthralgias, memory and concentration deficits, and fatigue.[51] The relation between these clinical findings and *B. burgdorferi* infection is unclear. There is no clear evidence that Lyme disease has an adverse impact on pregnancy [*see* Prognosis and Treatment, *below*]. Recent reports suggest that concurrent infection with either *Babesia microti* or *Ehrlichia* species may modify the course of Lyme disease.[52] In particular, coexisting babesial infection increases the severity and duration of Lyme disease.[53]

LABORATORY FINDINGS

Routine hematologic test results are usually within normal limits. Most patients who have arthritis or show signs of involvement of other organs after an episode of erythema migrans have a mildly elevated erythrocyte sedimentation rate.

The human immune response to *B. burgdorferi* consists of an early T cell response, followed by a delayed B cell response and subsequent formation of antibodies. Specific IgM antibodies appear 3 to 4 weeks after onset of infection; specific IgG antibodies appear after 4 to 6 weeks. Disease activity correlates with levels of total serum IgM and circulating immune complexes. Serum IgG antibody levels peak months later and may persist for years, confusing the diagnosis of unrelated disorders in endemic areas.

Early humoral immune responses to *B. burgdorferi* are directed against both the 41 kd flagellar protein, with its mixture of broadly cross-reactive and highly specific epitopes, and OspC. Among the late humoral immune responses are those directed against OspA, OspB, and heat shock proteins. Serum antibodies may persist for years regardless of whether there is clinically apparent disease.[54] Specific antibodies are made, and can be detected, at sequestered sites of systemic infection. Prompt antibiotic treatment of erythema migrans may abrogate the humoral response to *B. burgdorferi.*

DIAGNOSIS

The diagnosis of Lyme disease can be made by noting the presence of the erythema migrans lesion and the subsequent development of neurologic, cardiac, or articular manifestations. In the absence of the telltale skin lesions, epidemiologic features

Table 2 Clinical Findings Suggestive of Lyme Disease* in the Absence of Erythema Migrans

Recurrent arthritis
Transient atrioventricular block
Myocarditis or myopericarditis
Facial palsy
Lymphocytic meningitis
Radiculoneuritis
Keratitis or choroiditis

*Multiple findings and positive serologic test results increase the likelihood of this diagnosis. Each finding alone is nonspecific.

such as location, time of year, and known tick exposure may suggest the diagnosis, as may certain clinical findings [*see Table* 2]. Specific laboratory tests play a role in the evaluation of atypical clinical presentations when Lyme disease is suspected; however, Lyme disease is diagnosed clinically early in the course of infection.[55]

Direct detection of *B. burgdorferi* by visualization in affected tissues or by growth in modified Kelly's medium is impractical for most clinical laboratories [*see Figure* 4]. Nevertheless, skin biopsy or cutaneous lavage of untreated erythema migrans for subsequent cultivation of *B. burgdorferi* in broth is a sensitive diagnostic method when performed by experienced personnel.[35,56] PCR-based techniques offer greatly improved sensitivity and specificity in detecting the organism[57,58]; however, they are neither widely available nor standardized. Consequently, serologic tests remain the basis for the laboratory diagnosis of Lyme disease.

Enzyme-linked immunosorbent assays (ELISAs) are the preferred method of detecting anti–*B. burgdorferi* antibodies. When class-specific antibody-capture ELISA methods are used, only about 60% of patients have detectable anti–*B. burgdorferi* IgM after 2 to 3 weeks of infection; therefore, a negative result early in the course of the disease does not exclude the diagnosis. In contrast, as many as 90% of patients have significant levels of IgM or IgG during the disseminated and persistent stages of infection. Immunoblotting provides more sensitive detection of early Lyme disease, but this technique should be reserved for diagnostic confirmation.[55,59,60] Despite the availability of more rapid, office-based tests, clinicians should reserve serologic testing for patients with risk factors and clinical findings suggestive of Lyme disease.

The overuse of serologic tests for Lyme disease has magnified the problem of false positive results and has led to unnecessary antibiotic treatment. Studies of patients who were referred to Lyme disease clinics found that only 23% of those in an endemic area[61] and 3% of those in a nonendemic area[62] had active disease. False positive results are seen in patients with other spirochetal infections, including syphilis, and with HIV infection [*see Table 3*]. The Venereal Disease Research Laboratory (VDRL) test can be used to discriminate between Lyme disease and syphilis. False negative serologic results may be caused by testing too early in the course of infection or by early antibiotic therapy. Well-documented and widespread intralaboratory and interlaboratory variations in test results with identical samples suggest that greater reliance be placed on clinical features when diagnosing Lyme disease.[63] In some cases, it may be appropriate to repeat the ELISA or perform a VDRL test, an HIV test, or Lyme disease immunoblotting tests. In all cases, paired serum samples, drawn at least 6 weeks apart, enhance the reliability of Lyme disease serologic testing.

DIFFERENTIAL DIAGNOSIS

The considerations in differential diagnosis depend on whether the manifestations of Lyme disease are primarily those of Lyme arthritis or those of carditis or neurologic dysfunction. Typical Lyme arthritis consists of brief episodes of synovitis, a feature that distinguishes it from most other rheumatoid diseases. A temporal relation between the

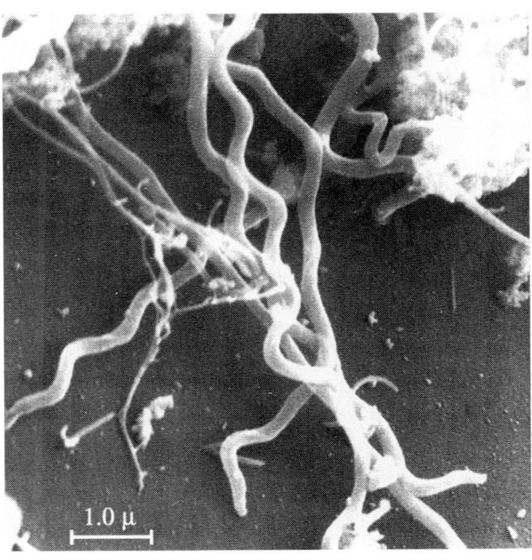

Figure 4 **Borrelia burgdorferi cultivated in Kelly's medium is shown in this scanning electron micrograph.**

Table 3 Causes of False Positive Serologic Results for Lyme Disease

Infectious Causes
- Syphilis and other treponemal infections
- Leptospirosis
- Relapsing fever
- HIV infection
- Infectious mononucleosis
- Rocky Mountain spotted fever

Other Causes
- Rheumatoid arthritis
- Systemic lupus erythematosus
- Inadequate laboratory proficiency and lack of test standardization

erythema migrans lesion and the arthritis strongly supports the diagnosis. The association of annular skin lesions with joint findings suggests the diagnosis of erythema marginatum and acute rheumatic fever. The lesions of erythema marginatum are smaller than erythema migrans lesions, however, and either migrate rapidly or come and go over the course of minutes to hours. The chronic form of Lyme arthritis in children may be differentiated from juvenile rheumatoid arthritis, which it resembles, by the absence of iridocyclitis and antinuclear antibodies. In adults, chronic Lyme arthritis may resemble the reactive arthritis that occurs in men after intestinal infections (caused by *Salmonella, Shigella,* or *Campylobacter* organisms) or chlamydial urethritis (Reiter's syndrome). Lyme arthritis, however, does not exhibit such characteristic features of Reiter's syndrome as conjunctivitis, mucocutaneous lesions, and urethritis. Adult rheumatoid arthritis can usually be distinguished from Lyme arthritis by the presence of morning stiffness, symmetrical polyarthritis, rheumatoid nodules, and rheumatoid factor in the blood.

The cardiac presentation of Lyme disease might suggest the diagnosis of acute rheumatic fever. Both diseases occur in children; however, Lyme disease is more common in adults, whereas acute rheumatic fever usually occurs in young children. Also, valvular involvement is common in acute rheumatic fever but does not occur in Lyme carditis. In contrast, complete heart block is rather common in Lyme carditis but rare in acute rheumatic fever.

The neurologic manifestations of Lyme disease are diverse and may suggest a variety of diagnoses, particularly viral meningitis, idiopathic Bell's palsy, encephalitis, peripheral neuritis, Behçet's syndrome, or leptospirosis. The presence of painless facial erythema and induration may distinguish Lyme facial palsy from Bell's palsy.[64] Measurement of intrathecal anti–*B. burgdorferi* antibodies should help determine whether certain etiologically obscure, self-limited neurologic illnesses are related to Lyme disease.

PROGNOSIS AND TREATMENT

Early studies indicated that oral tetracycline treatment of early localized Lyme disease reduces the likelihood of later neurologic, cardiac, and rheumatic complications. Doxycycline is currently the drug of choice for this early stage.[65]

Generally accepted regimens for early localized Lyme disease in adults include doxycycline, 0.1 g orally twice daily for 14 to 30 days, or amoxicillin, 0.5 g orally three to four times daily for 14 to 30 days. Cefuroxime axetil, 0.5 g orally twice daily for 14 to 30 days, is probably as effective.[65–67] Children younger than 8 years should receive amoxicillin, 20 mg/kg/day in divided doses, or cefuroxime axetil, 0.25 g twice daily, for 10 to 30 days. Ceftriaxone is no more effective than doxycycline in treating acute disseminated infection without meningitis.[68]

Treatment of the cardiac, neurologic, and rheumatologic manifestations of disseminated and persistent Lyme disease should include parenteral administration of ceftriaxone. For first-degree AV block, facial palsy without CSF abnormalities, or mild arthritis, one of the oral antibiotic regimens described above may be appropriate. In addition, many patients with Lyme arthritis may respond as well to a 3-week course of oral doxycycline as to a 2-week course of I.V. ceftriaxone.[66] However, treatment of chronic Lyme disease tends to be less successful than treatment of acute disease.[69]

Lyme neuroborreliosis may respond to penicillin G, 20 to 24 million units/day I.V. for 10 to 21 days,[65] though some studies suggest that ceftriaxone, 2 g I.V. once daily for 14 to 21 days, is more effective than penicillin G in these settings.[70] Symptomatic therapy for arthritis with nonsteroidal anti-inflammatory drugs is helpful. Synovectomy has been employed in some patients with chronic arthritis of the knee and marked functional impairment refractory to antibiotics.

Complete heart block is likely to develop in patients with Lyme carditis and a markedly prolonged PR interval or a high degree of AV block; thus, such patients should be hospitalized. Intravenous penicillin or ceftriaxone therapy is recommended in this setting, in the dosages given above, though this therapy has not received much clinical study. High-degree AV block is treated by insertion of a temporary pacemaker. Prednisone, 40 to 60 mg orally daily for 1 week, may be useful; the dosage can then be tapered rapidly. Reduction in the degree of block is commonly evident within 24 to 48 hours; return of normal conduction usually takes 1 to 2 weeks. Permanent pacemaker implantation is not necessary.[43]

Many patients with nonspecific, chronic clinical ailments, such as chronic fatigue and myalgia, who have positive results on serologic testing for Lyme disease receive I.V. antibiotics for presumed Lyme disease. However, because the incidence of false positive test results far exceeds the true incidence of Lyme disease, the costs and risks of such a practice far outweigh the benefits.[71,72]

Despite early clinical observations and theoretical concerns, there is no convincing evidence that Lyme disease has an adverse affect on the fetus during pregnancy.[73] A large prospective study found no association of maternal Lyme disease with fetal death, decreased birth weight, prematurity, or overall increase in the rate of fetal malformations.[74] The optimal treatment of pregnant women with Lyme disease is unclear. Many physicians prescribe a course of I.V. high-dose penicillin G or ceftriaxone.[73] Amoxicillin and cefuroxime axetil are reasonable alternatives for children and pregnant or lactating women. Penicillin and the macrolides are less effective. Cases of significant late complications have been reported, however, despite early antibiotic therapy.

PREVENTION

The most practical and least controversial means of preventing Lyme disease are to minimize exposure to ticks by wearing protective clothing and using acaricides and to remove ticks promptly. Several studies have examined the role of early antibiotic therapy for incubating infection after tick bites.[75,76] In one double-blind, placebo-controlled trial of amoxicillin conducted in southeastern Connecticut, where Lyme disease is endemic, only two of 387 persons who were bitten by deer ticks developed erythema migrans; both had received placebo.[76] At 1 year of follow-up, no one in either group had an asymptomatic seroconversion or developed late disease. The low rates of infection and late disease in untreated persons with recognized tick bites, the availability of effective treatment for early Lyme disease, and the potential toxicity of antibiotics suggest that routine antimicrobial prophylaxis of persons bitten by deer ticks is unwarranted.[65]

A vaccine derived from recombinant *B. burgdorferi* OspA (LYMErix) was approved by the Food and Drug Administration in 1998 for use in persons 15 to 70 years of age who were at high risk of acquiring infection. Studies showed the agent to be a protective, well-tolerated antigen,[77–80] but the vaccine was found cost effective only for individuals who live in areas where Lyme disease is endemic and who are frequently exposed to ticks.[81] Production of the vaccine was discontinued by the manufacturer in 2002 because of lack of demand.[82]

ADDITIONAL INFORMATION

The National Center for Infectious Diseases of the Centers for Disease Control and Prevention provides regularly updated information about Lyme disease on their Web site (www.cdc.gov/ncidod/index.htm).

Acknowledgments

Figure 2 John Blackford.
Figure 4 Micrograph courtesy of Dr. Willy Burgdorfer and S. F. Hayes, Rocky Mountain Laboratories, Hamilton, Montana.

References

1. Farr RW: Leptospirosis. Clin Infect Dis 21:1, 1995

2. Sasaki DM, Pang L, Minette HP, et al: Active surveillance and risk factors for leptospirosis in Hawaii. Am J Trop Med Hyg 48:35, 1993

3. Vinetz JM, Glass GE, Flexner CE, et al: Sporadic urban leptospirosis. Ann Intern Med 125:794, 1996

4. O'Neil KM, Rickman LS, Lazarus AA: Pulmonary manifestations of leptospirosis. Rev Infect Dis 13:705, 1991

5. Watt G, Padre LP, Tuazon ML, et al: Skeletal and cardiac muscle involvement in severe, late leptospirosis. J Infect Dis 162:266, 1990

6. Watt G, Padre LP, Tuazon ML, et al: Placebo-controlled trial of intravenous penicillin for severe and late leptospirosis. Lancet 1:433, 1988

7. Dupont H, Dupont-Perdrijet D, Perie LJ, et al: Leptospirosis: prognostic factors associated with mortality. Clin Infect Dis 25:720, 1997

8. Restrepo BI, Barbour AG: Antigen diversity in the bacterium *B. hermsii* through "somatic" mutations in rearranged *vmp* genes. Cell 78:867, 1994

9. Southern PM Jr, Sanford JP: Relapsing fever: a clinical and microbiological review. Medicine (Baltimore) 48:129, 1969

10. McEvoy MB, Noah ND, Pilsworth R: Outbreak of fever caused by *Streptobacillus moniliformis*. Lancet 2:1361, 1987

11. Pins MR, Holden JM, Yang JM, et al: Isolation of presumptive *Streptobacillus moniliformis* from abscesses associated with the female genital tract. Clin Infect Dis 22:471, 1996

12. Rupp ME: *Streptobacillus moniliformis* endocarditis: case report and review. Clin Infect Dis 14:769, 1992

13. Summary of notifiable diseases, United States, 1996. MMWR Morb Mortal Wkly Rep 45(53):1, 1997

14. Lyme disease—United States, 1996. MMWR Morb Mortal Wky Rep 46:531, 1997

15. Steere AC, Malawista SE, Snydman DR, et al: Lyme arthritis: an epidemic of oligoarticular arthritis in children and adults in three Connecticut communities. Arthritis Rheum 20:7, 1977

16. Steere AC: Lyme disease: a growing threat to urban populations. Proc Natl Acad Sci USA 91:2378, 1994

17. Barbour AG, Fish D: The biological and social phenomenon of Lyme disease. Science 260:1610, 1993

18. Barthold SW: Globalisation of Lyme borreliosis. Lancet 348:1603, 1996

19. Burgdorfer W, Barbour AG, Benach JL, et al: Lyme disease—a tick-borne spirochetosis? Science 216:1317, 1982

20. Brown RN, Lane RS: Lyme disease in California: a novel enzootic transmission cycle of *Borrelia burgdorferi*. Science 256:1439, 1992

21. Jones CG, Ostfeld RS, Richard MP, et al: Chain reactions linking acorns to gypsy moth outbreaks and Lyme disease risk. Science 279: 1023, 1998

22. Smith RP Jr, Rand PW, Lacomte EH, et al: Role of bird migration in the long-distance dispersal of *Ixodes dammini*, the vector of Lyme disease. J Infect Dis 174:221, 1996

23. Schwartz BS, Goldstein MD: Lyme disease in outdoor workers: risk factors, preventive measures, and tick removal methods. Am J Epidemiol 131:877, 1990

24. Sood SK, Salzman MB, Johnson BJB, et al: Duration of tick attachment as a predictor of the risk of Lyme disease in an area in which Lyme disease is endemic. J Infect Dis 175:996, 1997

25. Piesman J, Mather TN, Sinsky RJ, et al: Duration of tick attachment and *Borrelia burgdorferi* transmission. J Clin Microbiol 25:557, 1987

26. Steere AC, Grodzicki RL, Kornblatt AN, et al: The spirochetal etiology of Lyme disease. N Engl J Med 308:733, 1983

27. Benach JL, Bosler EM, Hanrahan JP, et al: Spirochetes isolated from the blood of two patients with Lyme disease. N Engl J Med 308:740, 1983

28. Mathiesen DA, Oliver JH Jr, Kolbert CP, et al: Genetic heterogeneity of *Borrelia burgdorferi* in the United States. J Infect Dis 175:98, 1997

29. Marconi RT, Samuels DS, Landry RK, et al: Analysis of the distribution and molecular heterogeneity of the *ospD* gene among the Lyme disease spirochetes: evidence for lateral gene exchange. J Bacteriol 176: 4572, 1994

30. Fraser CM, Casjens S, Huang WM, et al: Genomic sequence of a Lyme disease spirochaete, *Borrelia burgdorferi*. Nature 390:580, 1997

31. Zhang JR, Hardham JM, Barbour AG, et al: Antigenic variation in Lyme disease borreliae by promiscuous recombination of VMP-like sequence cassettes. Cell 89:275, 1997

32. de Silva AM, Fikrig E: Arthropod- and host-specific gene expression by *Borrelia burgdorferi*. J Clin Invest 99:377, 1997

33. Fikrig E, Tao H, Kantor FS, et al: Evasion of protective immunity by *Borrelia burgdorferi* by truncation of outer surface protein B. Proc Natl Acad Sci USA 90:4092, 1993

34. Van Dam AP, Kuiper H, Vos K, et al: Different genospecies of *Borrelia burgdorferi* are associated with distinct clinical manifestations of Lyme borreliosis. Clin Infect Dis 17:708, 1993

35. Berger BW, Johnson RC, Kodner C, et al: Cultivation of *Borrelia burgdorferi* from erythema migrans lesions and perilesional skin. J Clin Microbiol 30:359, 1992

36. Nadelman RB, Pavia CS: Isolation of *Borrelia burgdorferi* from the blood of seven patients with Lyme disease. Am J Med 88:21, 1990

37. Stanek G, Klein J, Bittner R, et al: Isolation of *Borrelia burgdorferi* from the myocardium of a patient with longstanding cardiomyopathy. N Engl J Med 322:249, 1990

38. Persing DH, Rutledge BJ, Rys PN, et al: Target imbalance: disparity of *Borrelia burgdorferi* genetic material in synovial fluid from Lyme arthritis patients. J Infect Dis 169:668, 1994

39. Karlsson M, Hovind-Hougen K, Svenungsson B, et al: Cultivation and characterization of spirochetes from cerebrospinal fluid of patients with Lyme borreliosis. J Clin Microbiol 28:473, 1990

40. Luft BJ, Steinman CR, Neimark HC, et al: Invasion of the central nervous system by *Borrelia burgdorferi* in acute disseminated infection. JAMA 267:1364, 1992

41. Steere AC, Dwyer E, Winchester R: Association of chronic Lyme arthritis with HLA-DR4 and HLA-DR2 alleles. N Engl J Med 323:219, 1990

42. Malane MS, Grant-Kels JM, Feder HM, et al: Diagnosis of Lyme disease based on dermatologic manifestations. Ann Intern Med 114:490, 1991

43. McAlister HF, Klementowicz PT, Andrews C, et al: Lyme carditis: an important cause of reversible heart block. Ann Intern Med 110:339, 1989

44. Reik L Jr, Burgdorfer W, Donaldson JO: Neurologic abnormalities in Lyme disease without erythema chronicum migrans. Am J Med 81: 73, 1986

45. Halperin JJ, Little BW, Coyle PK, et al: Lyme disease: cause of a treatable peripheral neuropathy. Neurology 37:1700, 1987

46. Logigian EL, Kaplan RF, Steere AC: Chronic neurologic manifestations of Lyme disease. N Engl J Med 323:1438, 1990

47. Szer IS, Taylor E, Steere AC: The long-term course of Lyme arthritis in children. N Engl J Med 325:159, 1991

48. Kalish RA, Leong JM, Steere AC: Association of treatment-resistant chronic Lyme arthritis with HLA-DR4 and antibody reactivity to OspA and OspB of *Borrelia burgdorferi*. Infect Immun 61:2774, 1993

49. Aaberg TM: The expanding ophthalmologic spectrum of Lyme disease. Am J Ophthalmol 107:77, 1989

50. Dinerman H, Steere AC: Lyme disease associated with fibromyalgia. Ann Intern Med 117:281, 1992

51. Shadick NA, Philips CB, Logigian EL, et al: The long-term clinical outcomes of Lyme disease: a population-based retrospective cohort study. Ann Intern Med 121:560, 1994

52. Persing DH: The cold zone: a curious convergence of tick-transmitted diseases. Clin Infect Dis 25(suppl 1):S35, 1997

53. Krause PJ, Telford SR III, Spielman A, et al: Concurrent Lyme disease and babesiosis: evidence for increased severity and duration of illness. JAMA 275:1657, 1996

54. Feder HM, Gerber MA, Luger SW, et al: Persistence of serum antibodies to *Borrelia burgdorferi* in patients treated for Lyme disease. Clin Infect Dis 15:788, 1992

55. Tugwell P, Dennis DJ, Weinstein A, et al: Laboratory evaluation in the diagnosis of Lyme disease. Ann Intern Med 127:1109, 1997

56. Nadelman RB, Nowakowski J, Forseter G, et al: Failure to isolate *Borrelia burgdorferi* after antimicrobial therapy in culture-documented Lyme borreliosis associated with erythema migrans: report of a prospective study. Am J Med 94:583, 1993

57. Persing DH, Telford SR III, Spielman A, et al: Detection of *Borrelia burgdorferi* infection in *Ixodes dammini* ticks with the polymerase chain reaction. J Clin Microbiol 28:566, 1990

58. Schmidt BL: PCR in laboratory diagnosis of human *Borrelia burgdorferi* infections. Clin Microbiol Rev 10:185, 1997

59. Recommendations for test performance and interpretation from the Second National Conference on Serologic Diagnosis of Lyme Disease. MMWR 44:590, 1995

60. Tilton RC, Sand MN, Manak M: The western immunoblot for Lyme disease: determination of sensitivity, specificity, and interpretive criteria with use of commercially available performance panels. Clin Infect Dis 25(suppl 1):S31, 1997

61. Steere AC, Taylor E, McHugh GL, et al: The overdiagnosis of Lyme disease. JAMA 269:1812, 1993

62. Burdge DR, O'Hanlon DP: Experience at a referral center for patients with suspected Lyme disease in an area of nonendemicity: first 65 patients. Clin Infect Dis 16:558, 1993

63. Bakken LL, Callister SM, Wand PJ, et al: Interlaboratory comparison of test results for detection of Lyme disease by 516 participants in the Wisconsin State Laboratory of Hygiene/College of American Pathologists Proficiency Testing Program. J Clin Microbiol 35:537, 1997

64. Markby DP: Lyme disease facial palsy: differentiation from Bell's palsy. BMJ 299:605, 1989

65. Treatment of Lyme disease. Med Lett Drugs Ther 39:47, 1997

66. Eckman MH, Steere AC, Kalish RA, et al: Cost effectiveness of oral as compared with intravenous antibiotic therapy for patients with early Lyme disease or Lyme arthritis. N Engl J Med 337:357, 1997

67. Nadelman RB, Luger SW, Frank E, et al: Comparison of cefuroxime axetil and doxycycline in the treatment of early Lyme disease. Ann Intern Med 117:273, 1992

68. Dattwyler RJ, Luft BJ, Kunkel MJ, et al: Ceftriaxone compared with doxycycline for the treatment of acute disseminated Lyme disease. N Engl J Med 337:289, 1997

69. Steere AC, Levin RE, Molloy PJ, et al: Treatment of Lyme arthritis. Arthritis Rheum 37:878, 1994

70. Dattwyler RJ, Halperin JJ, Pass H, et al: Ceftriaxone as effective therapy in refractory Lyme disease. J Infect Dis 155:1322, 1987

71. Lightfoot RW, Luft BJ, Rahn DW, et al: Empiric parenteral antibiotic treatment of patients with fibromyalgia and fatigue and a positive serologic result for Lyme disease: a cost-effectiveness analysis. Ann Intern Med 119:503, 1993

72. Appropriateness of parenteral antibiotic treatment for patients with presumed Lyme disease. American College of Rheumatology and the Council of the Infectious Diseases Society of America. Ann Intern Med 119:518, 1993

73. Silver HM: Lyme disease during pregnancy. Infect Dis Clin North Am 11:93, 1997

74. Strobino BA, Williams CL, Abid S, et al: Lyme disease and pregnancy outcome: a prospective study of two thousand prenatal patients. Am J Obstet Gynecol 169:367, 1993

75. Magid D, Schwartz B, Craft J, et al: Prevention of Lyme disease after tick bites: a cost-effectiveness analysis. N Engl J Med 327:534, 1992

76. Shapiro ED, Gerber MA, Holabird NB, et al: A controlled trial of antimicrobial prophylaxis for Lyme disease after deer-tick bites. N Engl J Med 327:1769, 1992

77. Keller D, Koster FT, Marks DH, et al: Safety and immunogenicity of a recombinant outer surface protein A Lyme vaccine. JAMA 271:1764, 1994

78. Meurice F, Parenti D, Fu D, et al: Specific issues in the design and implementation of an efficacy trial for a Lyme disease vaccine. Clin Infect Dis 25(suppl 1):S71, 1997

79. Sigal LH, Zahradnik JM, Lavin P, et al: A vaccine consisting of recombinant *Borrelia burgdorferi* outer-surface protein A to prevent Lyme disease. Recombinant Outer-Surface Protein A Lyme Disease Vaccine Study Consortium. N Engl J Med 339:216, 1998

80. Steere AC, Sikand VK, Meurice F, et al: Vaccination against Lyme disease with recombinant *Borrelia burgdorferi* outer-surface lipoprotein A with adjuvant. Lyme Disease Vaccine Study Group. N Engl J Med 339:209, 1998

81. Hsia EC, Chung JB, Schwartz JS, et al: Cost-effectiveness analysis of the Lyme disease vaccine. Arthritis Rheum 46:1439, 2002

82. Manufacturer discontinues only Lyme disease vaccine. FDA Consum 36:5, 2002

26 Rickettsial Diseases and Q Fever

David A. Relman, M.D.
Morton N. Swartz, M.D.

Pathogenesis, Pathophysiology, and Pathology of the Rickettsioses

The rickettsias are small coccobacillary obligate intracellular parasites. Almost all of the rickettsias that are pathogenic to humans have an arthropod–animal reservoir–arthropod cycle in nature; human infection is only an incidental phenomenon.[1] One exception is the agent of epidemic typhus, *Rickettsia prowazekii,* which is maintained in a human-louse cycle.

Four groups of rickettsial pathogens are now recognized: the spotted fever group, the typhus group, the *Ehrlichia* group, and the *Bartonella* (formerly *Rochalimaea*) group. *Bartonella* includes the causative agents of bacillary angiomatosis, cat-scratch disease, and trench fever [*see Table 1*]. All of these organisms belong to the α-proteobacteria group of bacteria, whose members often form close endosymbiotic relations with host cells [*see Figure 1*]. This feature explains why propagation of these organisms in the laboratory is difficult and why some were identified only recently by molecular methods. *Coxiella burnetii,* the causative agent of Q fever, is related to *Legionella pneumophila;* both are γ-proteobacteria and are only distantly related to the α-proteobacteria.

Rickettsias are often introduced into humans by an arthropod vector. *C. burnetii* is usually acquired by inhalation of infected dust. *B. henselae* is usually transmitted from cats to humans by direct inoculation [*see Table 1*]. Obvious lesions develop at the bite sites in rickettsialpox, Mediterranean spotted fever, scrub typhus, and cat-scratch disease, but not with other rickettsioses.

During the incubation period, rickettsias multiply locally and then invade the bloodstream. Most rickettsias infect endothelial cells throughout the microvasculature, but *Ehrlichia* organisms infect leukocytes. Rickettsemia recurs shortly after the onset of fever and overt systemic illness. Subsequent vascular lesions caused by rickettsia-induced damage to endothelial cells account for the pathologic changes that occur throughout the body, particularly in the skin, the heart, the brain, the lungs, and muscle. The vascular damage is most marked in Rocky Mountain spotted fever (RMSF), in which thromboses and microinfarcts are prominent features.

Vascular lesions in the meninges probably account for the severe headache characteristic of rickettsial diseases. In severe infections from the spotted fever or the typhus group, extensive loss of fluid from the intravascular compartment as a result of vascular injury can occur rapidly, resulting in shock and eventually death. Myocarditis and myocardial failure can develop in rickettsioses. Renal failure, marked hepatic dysfunction, and coma can occur in fulminant cases because of direct vascular damage to the kidneys, the liver, and the central nervous system and because of hypovolemia. Extensive hemorrhagic lesions indicate the development of disseminated intravascular coagulation (DIC).

Rocky Mountain Spotted Fever

RMSF is an acute tick-borne febrile illness caused by *R. rickettsii* and characterized by sudden onset, fever, headache, and a rash that begins on the extremities and spreads to the trunk.

ETIOLOGY AND EPIDEMIOLOGY

R. rickettsii (as well as other members of the spotted fever group) grows in the nucleus and in the cytoplasm of infected cells.[2] In the cell, *R. rickettsii* can induce formation of oxygen free radicals and depletion of intracellular antioxidants, leading ultimately to endothelial cell death.[3] At the same time, *R. rickettsii* may block programmed cell death, or apoptosis, thereby temporarily protecting its preferred site of growth.[4] Procoagulant materials from damaged endothelium can activate platelets and trigger both the coagulation and fibrinolytic pathways, resulting in thrombosis and DIC.

Table 1 Rickettsial Diseases

Group	Disease	Rickettsial Agent	Geographic Distribution	Means of Transmission to Humans	Rash: Type	Rash: Distribution	Preferred Laboratory Diagnostic Tests
Spotted Fever Group	Rocky Mountain spotted fever	*Rickettsia rickettsii*	Throughout the U.S., particularly in South Atlantic states and Oklahoma	Tick bite	Macular, maculopapular, petechial	Extremities to trunk; palms and soles	Immunofluorescent staining of skin biopsy specimen, IFA, IHA
Spotted Fever Group	Rickettsialpox	*R. akari*	U.S., former Soviet Union	Mite bite	Papulovesicular	Trunk, face, extremities	IFA
Typhus Group	Endemic (murine)	*R. typhi*	Worldwide; in southeastern and Gulf states in the U.S.	Inoculation of infected flea feces into abraded skin	Macular, maculopapular	Trunk to extremities	IFA, ?PCR
Typhus Group	Epidemic (louse-borne)	*R. prowazekii*	Worldwide	Inoculation of infected feces of body louse into abraded skin Contact with flying squirrels	Macular, maculopapular	Trunk to extremities	IFA
Ehrlichia *Group*	Human monocytic ehrlichiosis	*E. chaffeensis*	Southeastern, south central, and Middle Atlantic states	Tick bite	None	None	IFA, ?PCR
Ehrlichia *Group*	Human granulocytic ehrlichiosis	*Ehrlichia* species*	Northeastern, north central, and Pacific states	Tick bite	None	None	IFA, ?PCR
Bartonella *Group*	Bacillary angiomatosis	*B. henselae*, *B. quintana*	U.S., Europe	Inoculation by cat	Angiomatous papules	Widespread	Silver stain of biopsy, IFA, ?PCR
Bartonella *Group*	Trench fever	*B. quintana*	U.S., Europe, Russia, Mexico	Body louse	None	None	Blood culture, IFA
Bartonella *Group*	Cat-scratch disease	*B. henselae*	U.S. (especially the South), Europe	Inoculation by cat	Papule at inoculation site	Widespread	Silver stain of biopsy, IFA, ?PCR
Bartonella *Group*	Oroya fever, verruga peruana	*B. bacilliformis*	Andean region of South America	Sandfly bite	Angiomatous papules (verruga peruana)	Widespread	Blood culture
Other Rickettsia*-like Organisms*	Scrub typhus	*Orientia tsutsugamushi*	South and Southeast Asia, South Pacific	Mite bite	Eschar, then macular or maculopapular	Trunk to extremities	IFA
Other Rickettsia*-like Organisms*	Q fever	*Coxiella burnetii*	Worldwide	Inhalation of dried infected excreta from animals such as cattle and sheep Ingestion of raw milk	None	None	IFA, ELISA

*This organism is closely related to *E. phagocytophila* but has not yet been named.
ELISA—enzyme-linked immunosorbent assay IFA—indirect fluorescent antibody IHA—indirect hemagglutination antibody PCR—polymerase chain reaction

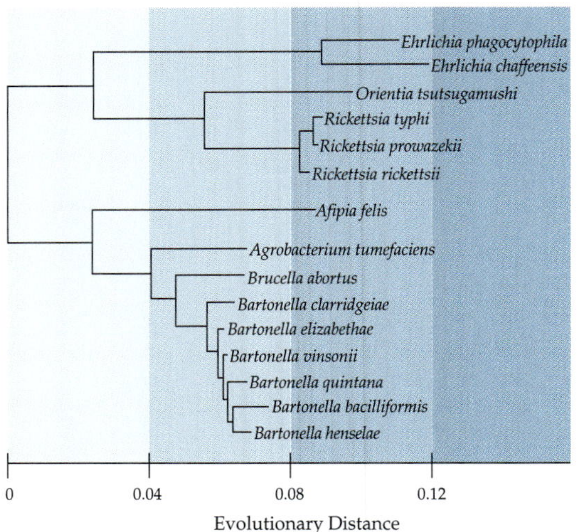

Figure 1 **This figure shows a phylogenetic tree of some α-proteobacteria. Most of the known rickettsias that are pathogenic for humans are classified within this group. Evolutionary distance is expressed in terms of point mutations per 16S ribosomal RNA sequence position. The evolutionary distance between any two organisms is proportional to the sum of the horizontal line segments that connect them. Branch points indicate putative common evolutionary ancestors.**

RMSF tick vectors include primarily the dog tick, *Dermacentor variabilis*, in the eastern United States and the wood tick, *D. andersoni*, in the West. Less frequently, the Lone Star tick, *Amblyomma americanum*, is a vector for RMSF in the South and Southeast. Ticks serve as a reservoir for *R. rickettsii* infection because they acquire nonlethal, lifelong infection either by feeding on infected animals or by maternal transovarial transmission. Infection usually requires the tick to remain attached for several hours. Infection may also be acquired through skin abrasions when ticks are being removed.

R. rickettsii, and hence RMSF, is found only in the Western Hemisphere. The incidence of RMSF in the United States is stable; approximately 600 cases of RMSF are reported each year.[5] A conspicuous characteristic of RMSF is its focal geographic distribution. The Rocky Mountain area, where the disease was originally discovered at the turn of the century, now accounts for fewer than 2% of cases. All states except Maine, Alaska, and Hawaii have reported cases, but approximately one third of the cases occur in Oklahoma and North Carolina [*see Table 1*]. Small, circumscribed regions account for a high percentage of the cases, including those in urban areas.

Ninety percent of cases of RMSF occur in the months of April through September, the period when ticks are active and people are often outdoors. Children are disproportionately affected: the incidence of this disease is highest in children 5 to 9 years of age. Because dogs can acquire RMSF, they may also serve as a means of transferring infected ticks from their natural reservoirs to the human environment. In rare cases, RMSF is acquired by transfusion or in the laboratory by inoculation or by aerosol inhalation.

CLINICAL FEATURES

After an incubation period of 3 to 12 days, illness usually begins abruptly, with severe headache, nausea, rigor and high fever, myalgias, and marked weakness. Abdominal pain, which may be pronounced, is caused by involvement of the abdominal musculature. Sometimes the onset is gradual, with nonspecific features such as anorexia, low-grade fever, and malaise. After 1 to 2 days, the fever rises rapidly up to 40.6° C (105.1° F) and then follows a spiking pattern. Intense headache remains a prominent symptom, and back stiffness may develop. In severe cases, mental confusion and obtundation may suggest encephalitis or aseptic meningitis, and the cerebrospinal fluid may show pleocytosis.[6]

The triad of fever, headache, and rash is reported in approximately 50% to 60% of confirmed RMSF cases.[6,7] The rash, which is the most valuable diagnostic sign, usually develops on the third through fifth days of illness but appears after the sixth day in 20% of cases. In 4% to 16% of patients, skin lesions are not observed; in others, the rash may be evanescent.[8] So-called spotless disease, which evinces no rash, may be more common in males, African Americans, and persons older than 25 years and is no less severe. Characteristically, when the rash appears, it begins as erythematous macules on the wrists and ankles; within 24 hours, it spreads up the extremities to the trunk and face. The lesions rapidly become maculopapular. If treatment is not instituted, the lesions become petechial after the fourth day of illness. There is no enanthema. The centripetal progression of the eruption and the presence of lesions on the palms and soles are the diagnostic features of the rash [*see Figure 2*]. Because of increased capillary fragility, lesions also appear after a tourniquet or blood pressure cuff is applied. In severe infections, particularly in patients with marked, persistent hypotension, large purpuric lesions may develop on the extremities and become necrotic.

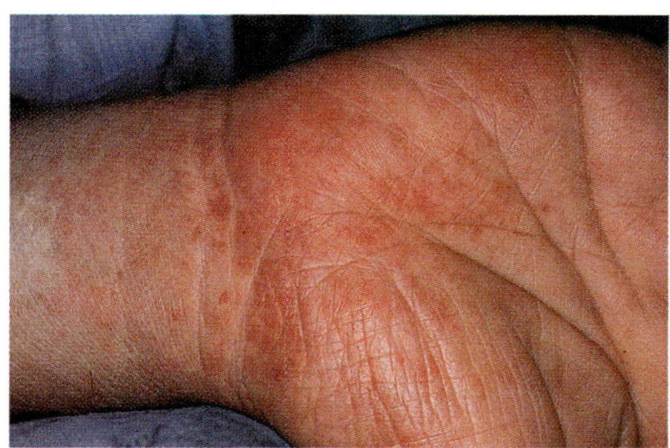

Figure 2 **Purpuric macules on the palm and wrist of a patient with Rocky Mountain spotted fever.**

Other features of RMSF are splenomegaly (seen in 25% of patients), muscle tenderness, nausea, vomiting, diarrhea, and abdominal pain. Nonproductive cough with radiologic findings of interstitial and alveolar infiltrates are common. Pulmonary edema secondary to capillary leakage is usually responsible for the impaired gas exchange.

Progressive hypotension secondary to peripheral circulatory changes in severe RMSF may be complicated by myocardial dysfunction. Acute renal insufficiency may occur as a result of inadequate renal perfusion. Advanced age and thrombocytopenia are both associated with an increased risk of developing renal failure.[9]

LABORATORY FINDINGS

The leukocyte count is usually slightly decreased or normal. Thrombocytopenia occurs in almost 50% of patients, and serial platelet counts may aid in early recognition of DIC. Laboratory abnormalities also include anemia, hyponatremia, elevated serum aminotransferase and bilirubin levels, and azotemia.

Laboratory diagnosis is usually established serologically, but none of the serologic tests are useful for early diagnosis. The most sensitive and specific test is the indirect fluorescent antibody (IFA) assay, followed by the indirect hemagglutination antibody (IHA) assay. Polymerase chain reaction technology is now being applied to the diagnosis of rickettsial diseases. A PCR-based assay permits early detection of *R. rickettsii* in patient serum.[10] An assay of this type is available from some state health departments or the Centers for Disease Control and Prevention (404-639-1075). The Weil-Felix reaction is now an outdated serologic test because it lacks sensitivity and specificity.

Between the third and eighth days of illness, it is possible with immunofluorescence or immunoperoxidase techniques to demonstrate rickettsias in biopsy specimens of macular skin lesions.[5,11] These techniques are currently the best means of making an early, specific diagnosis. Rickettsial isolation from blood in cell culture is possible but is rarely practical.

DIFFERENTIAL DIAGNOSIS

The preeruptive stage of RMSF is indistinguishable from a number of acute bacterial and viral infections, but the geographically focal and seasonal characteristics of the disease should suggest RMSF as a condition to be particularly considered in the differential diagnosis. A history of exposure to ticks is helpful but is lacking in 10% to 40% of cases. When rash is absent, RMSF is easily confused with ehrlichiosis because the two diseases occur in the same geographic regions and can be transmitted by the same tick species. Once skin lesions appear, RMSF is often mistaken for measles or meningococcemia. In measles, however, there is a distinctive enanthema (Koplik's spots), and the rash rapidly becomes confluent, whereas in RMSF, the lesions generally remain discrete. In fulminant meningococcemia, the macular lesions become petechial and purpuric, usually within 24 hours; in RMSF, the evolution is slower. In meningococcal meningitis, the CSF contains polymorphonuclear pleocytes. In RMSF, the CSF usually contains only 10 to 100 cells/µl; most are lymphocytes, with a smaller number of neutrophils.[5]

Other diseases that may be confused with RMSF are enterovirus infections (particularly those caused by echovirus 9), infectious mononucleosis, relapsing fever, leptospirosis, typhoid fever, and idiopathic thrombocytopenic purpura.

Rickettsialpox, the only other member of the spotted fever group occurring in the United States, is readily distinguished from RMSF by an eschar at the bite site, the papulovesicular nature of the eruption, and a mild clinical course. Murine (endemic) typhus, prevalent in the Gulf and southeastern states and in southern California, closely resembles RMSF; however, murine typhus is generally milder, and the rash is nonpurpuric and less extensive than that in RMSF. In epidemic typhus as well as endemic typhus, the rash begins on the trunk and spreads centrifugally to the extremities, but it usually spares the palms, the soles, and the face.

TREATMENT

Antimicrobial treatment is optimally effective when initiated early in the course of RMSF (i.e., before or at the appearance of the rash). In some patients, however, a rash appears late or does not develop. In the proper epidemiologic setting, treatment must therefore be considered even in the absence of rash. Doxycycline or tetracycline is the antibiotic of choice. Doxycycline is given orally in a dosage of 200 mg/day in divided doses every 12 hours. Tetracycline is administered orally in a dosage of 25 to 30 mg/kg/day in divided doses every 6 hours; there is no loading dose. Chloramphenicol is an effective alternative; it is given orally in a loading dose of 50 mg/kg, followed by 50 mg/kg/day in divided doses every 6 hours.

If the patient is critically ill or cannot take oral medication, antibiotics should be given intravenously. Doxycycline is given intravenously in a dosage of 4.4 mg/kg/day up to 200 mg/day in divided doses every 12 hours. Chloramphenicol is administered in a loading dose of 15 to 20 mg/kg I.V., followed by 30 to 50 mg/kg daily in divided doses every 6 hours. Medication is shifted to the oral route as soon as possible. Usually, symptoms lessen in severity within 24 hours and the fever subsides within 3 days. Antibiotic therapy can be discontinued after the patient has been afebrile for 2 or 3 days. Sulfonamides are not only ineffective but also potentially harmful; therefore, they should not be used.

In addition to the use of specific chemotherapy, treatment is aimed at correcting severe complications such as hypovolemia, congestive heart failure, electrolyte disturbances, azotemia, thrombocytopenia, and DIC. Intravenous glucocorticoids have been used as adjuvant therapy in severely ill patients, but there are no controlled studies to support this practice.

PREVENTION

Prevention entails minimizing contact with ticks; this can be accomplished by avoidance of tick-infested areas, wearing of protective clothing, application of insect repellents (e.g., dimethyl phthalate), and thorough inspection of the body several times daily (including at bedtime) and removal of attached ticks. The safest and most efficacious method of removing ticks is to grasp the tick's mouthparts with tweezers as close to the patient's skin as possible and to pull upward with a steady, even pressure. The use of a twisting movement is not recommended. Care should be taken not to crush the tick or to handle it with the bare hand. The bite area should be washed with soap and water or with an antiseptic to destroy any contaminating rickettsias. No vaccine against RMSF is available at present.

PROGNOSIS

The overall mortality for RMSF is approximately 4%. Treatment with appropriate antibiotics initiated before the sixth day of illness almost invariably cures the disease. Because rash is often absent in the first several days of illness, the differential diagnosis of fever and headache in a focal endemic area must include an early consideration of RMSF and must lead to consideration of early empirical therapy. If such steps are not taken, the consequences may be disastrous.[12] In addition to delay in diagnosis and treatment, features that are associated with increased mortality include patient age greater than 40 years, jaundice, and neurologic, cardiac, or renal complications.[7,9,13]

Rickettsialpox

Rickettsialpox is a mild, self-limited disease caused by *R. akari* and transmitted to humans by a mouse mite. The reservoir of infection is the house mouse, but because *R. akari* can be passed transovarially in mites, this arthropod vector is also a reservoir. Humans are infected primarily in urban settings when infected mites have been deprived of their preferred murine hosts by vigorous programs of rodent extermination. Cases are now seldom noted.

Seven to 14 days after the mite bite, a nonpainful primary papular lesion appears and enlarges to a diameter of about 1 cm. It then becomes vesicular, crusts over, and evolves into a blackish eschar, which persists for several weeks with associated regional lymphadenopathy.[14]

The onset of clinical illness occurs 4 to 7 days after the appearance of the initial lesion. The onset of illness is abrupt, with fever, sweats, headache, myalgias, and malaise. In untreated patients, daily temperature elevations to 39.4° C (102.9° F) continue for 7 to 10 days, but the systemic symptoms are generally mild. A maculopapular exanthema appears within the first 2 days of the illness and quickly becomes vesicular. The vesicles are small and are located on top of a papular base, which is sometimes surrounded by erythema. They may be numerous or few and may involve all parts of the body but usually spare the palms and soles. There is no clinical evidence of pulmonary or other visceral involvement.

The differential diagnosis includes chickenpox and other rickettsioses. Chickenpox, however, is

lated from blood, sputum, or urine by intraperitoneal inoculation in guinea pigs, inoculation into chick embryos, or inoculation of cultured human fetal diploid fibroblasts. Because this organism is so highly contagious in the laboratory, attempts at isolation should be made only in a special biologic containment facility. *C. burnetii* can be detected in human heart valve tissues by PCR.[36]

DIFFERENTIAL DIAGNOSIS

Early in its course, Q fever resembles a variety of acute febrile illnesses, including salmonellosis, infectious hepatitis, brucellosis, leptospirosis, and infectious mononucleosis. A history of contact with livestock is the only clue that can suggest the diagnosis at this point. When pulmonary involvement is apparent, illnesses considered in the differential diagnosis include *Mycoplasma pneumoniae* pneumonia, *Chlamydia pneumoniae* pneumonia, psittacosis, viral pneumonia, Legionnaires' disease, and pulmonary histoplasmosis. When hepatitis is present and noncaseating granulomas are found on liver biopsy, a host of causes of granulomatous hepatitis—such as tuberculosis, sarcoidosis, brucellosis, and histoplasmosis—must be considered. Q fever should always be considered in cases in which the clinical findings suggest endocarditis but the blood cultures are negative for routine bacterial pathogens.

TREATMENT AND PREVENTION

Tetracycline, 0.5 g orally every 6 hours, doxycycline, 0.1 g orally every 12 hours, or ciprofloxacin, 0.5 g orally every 12 hours, is effective in the treatment of acute Q fever. Most patients treated early in the course of the infection recover rapidly; however, acute Q fever is usually self-limited. In cases of Q fever endocarditis, prolonged antibiotic therapy seems to be necessary to effect a cure. Regimens employing different antimicrobial agents, either alone or in combination, have been tried with variable success.[33,36] Some experts recommend treatment with doxycycline plus rifampin or with doxycycline plus a fluoroquinolone for at least 3 years.[37] Chloroquine is being assessed as adjunctive therapy because of its ability to block intracellular vacuole acidification and, hence, growth of *C. burnetii*. Valve replacement may be required as well. If left untreated, this disease is usually fatal. Patients need not be isolated, because secondary cases do not occur.

Killed vaccines made from *C. burnetii* grown in chick embryo cultures are immunogenic and can provide protection for persons at high risk, such as dairy and slaughterhouse workers, woolsorters, tanners, and laboratory workers. However, vaccines against *C. burnetii* are not commercially available for human use in the United States.

Human Ehrlichiosis

Ehrlichia species are intraleukocytic parasites that are pathogenic for a wide variety of wild and domestic animals.[38,39] Their life cycle includes the formation of an intracellular vacuole, known as a morula, that contains multiple ehrlichiae. Until the mid-1980s, *E. sennetsu*, the cause of an infectious mononucleosis–like syndrome in the Far East, had been the only known human pathogen of the *Ehrlichia genus*. In 1986, however, the first documented case of human infection by an organism closely related to *E. canis* was reported. This organism caused an acute febrile illness after a tick bite that was similar to RMSF but without the rash. The diagnosis was based on the finding of characteristic intraleukocytic inclusion bodies and a serologic response to *E. canis* antigens. This agent of human (monocytic) ehrlichiosis, *E. chaffeensis*, has now been cultured and described and can be detected by PCR. In 1994, a second *Ehrlichia* species capable of causing disease in humans was identified in the United States.[40] This organism, which is closely related to *E. phagocytophila*, preferentially infects neutrophils—in contrast to *E. chaffeensis*, which prefers mononuclear leukocytes. The granulocytic and monocytic ehrlichiae are antigenically distinct, but the former has not yet been assigned a species name. Both forms of human ehrlichiosis are being recognized with increasing frequency.[41]

ETIOLOGY AND EPIDEMIOLOGY

More than 400 cases of human *E. chaffeensis*–associated, or monocytic, ehrlichiosis (HME) have been reported in more than 30 states since 1986, and more than 300 cases of human granulocytic ehrlichiosis (HGE) have been reported in the United States since 1994.[42] Undoubtedly, each figure is a gross underestimate of the true number of cases of human ehrlichiosis, because these diseases have protean manifestations and are difficult to recognize. For example, seroprevalence studies suggest that the incidence of human ehrlichiosis may be several times that of RMSF in some regions. A survey of persons in a retirement community in Tennessee found evidence of previous *E. chaffeensis* infection in 12.5% of residents; seropositivity was linked to tick exposure.[43]

The geographic and seasonal distributions of HME and HGE reflect the ecology and behavior of the relevant tick vectors. *A. americanum* transmits HME and is found throughout the southeastern and south central United States; *Dermacentor* species may transmit disease less frequently in other regions. *Ixodes* species serve as vectors for HGE as well as for Lyme disease [see 25 Leptospirosis, Relapsing Fever, Rat-Bite Fever, and Lyme Disease] and babesiosis and are active in the northeastern, upper midwestern, and Pacific regions of the United States. In Westchester County, New York, a hyperendemic region for Lyme disease, the HGE agent is found as often in *I. scapularis* ticks as is *B. burgdorferi*. Approximately 20% to 25% of adult ticks are infected with both[44]; in fact, simultaneous infection of humans with the two tick-borne agents has been well documented.[45] Transmission of ehrlichiosis to humans may require at least 24 to 48 hours of tick attachment.[46] The natural reservoirs for the HGE agent include the white-footed mouse and the white-tailed deer. HME occurs from April through September[47]; HGE occurs throughout the year, though most cases occur from midspring to the end of summer.[42,48] The median age of patients with HME is 44 years; that of patients with HGE is 60 years.[47,48] Perinatal transmission of the HGE agent has been reported.[49]

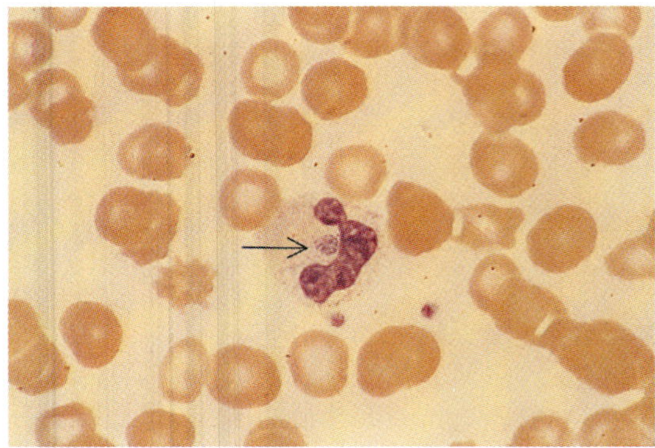

Figure 3 **In a peripheral blood smear from a patient with human granulocytic ehrlichiosis, a typical round ehrlichial morula is seen at the center of the neutrophil, adjacent to the nuclear lobes (arrow). Two platelets can be seen below and to the right of the neutrophil, for comparison. Wright-Giemsa stain was used; original magnification: × 370.**

CLINICAL FEATURES

A median of 8 or 9 days after tick exposure, patients with human ehrlichiosis experience the acute onset of fever, rigors, malaise, headache, and myalgias. Nausea, vomiting, and particularly rash occur less commonly in both forms of this disease than in RMSF; rash is reported in 36% of patients with HME and 2% of patients with HGE.[47,48] Cough occurs in 25% to 30% of patients, and pulmonary infiltrates are common. Like other rickettsial infections, human ehrlichiosis may be accompanied by aseptic meningitis; confusion is reported in 20% to 25% of all patients and may have a multifactorial etiology. Serious clinical complications, including renal insufficiency, DIC, and neurologic manifestations, develop in approximately 16% of patients with HME.[47] In earlier studies, 50% to 70% of patients with human ehrlichiosis, especially elderly patients, underwent hospitalization; however, most experts believe that many cases of mild or asymptomatic infection remain unidentified.[42,43] Although ehrlichiosis in humans may persist, as it often does in animals,[50] the median duration of gross clinical manifestations in HME is 23 days.[47] In a human host, coinfection with a combination of *Ehrlichia* species, *B. burgdorferi*, and *Babesia* species may modify the presentation and natural course of disease caused by each of these agents alone.[51]

LABORATORY FINDINGS

Human ehrlichiosis is accompanied by leukopenia, especially lymphopenia, in 50% to 75% of patients and by thrombocytopenia in 72% to 92% of patients. Nadirs in cell counts occur at the end of the first week of illness. Elevated serum aminotransferase levels occur in 85% to 90% of patients at some time during the clinical course. These findings help distinguish human ehrlichiosis from other diseases [*see* Differential Diagnosis, *below*]. Furthermore, in a study of 41 patients with HGE, 80% had visible morulae on acute-phase peripheral blood smears [*see Figure 3*]; these morulae are detected in 1% to 42% of neutrophils (median, 5%).[48] Other laboratory abnormalities, including anemia, are less specific and are not useful in making the diagnosis.

DIFFERENTIAL DIAGNOSIS

As acute febrile illnesses, HME and HGE resemble a number of other infectious diseases, including RMSF, typhus, Q fever, tularemia, early Lyme disease, viral hepatitis, influenza, and Colorado tick fever. Tick-borne transmission is common to several of these diseases. In addition to the detection of intraleukocytic morulae, the diagnosis of human ehrlichiosis is best made by use of serologic methods and paired acute and convalescent sera; however, this approach does not yield timely information. Because the causative agents of HME and HGE are antigenically distinct, separate IFA assays must be performed to detect antibody responses to *E. chaffeensis* and to the HGE agent. Both assays are available through state health departments. Both of the ehrlichial pathogens for humans in the United States can be cultivated[52]; however, the procedure is difficult and impractical for routine diagnostic purposes. PCR-based assays have also been developed for both agents and appear to be highly sensitive and specific, but again they are not yet routinely available.[41,53] The causative agents of human ehrlichiosis can be detected directly in tissue by an immunoperoxidase technique.[41]

TREATMENT

The drug of choice for both HME and HGE is doxycycline, 0.1 g orally twice daily; it may be given intravenously to patients who are unable to tolerate oral medications. Patients who receive doxycycline early in the course of disease have a more rapid recovery and lower mortality than do those who do not receive this drug.[47] The necessary duration of therapy is unclear. Most patients have a clinical response to doxycycline within several days, but some experts recommend 14 days of treatment, in part to treat coexistent Lyme disease.[48] The treatment of children is controversial: the same doses of chloramphenicol that are used for RMSF appear to be effective for human ehrlichiosis; however, observations of in vitro *E. chaffeensis* resistance to this drug and concerns about adverse effects have prompted physicians to reconsider administering doxycycline therapy to children. Brief treatment regimens with doxycycline may pose only a low risk of teeth discoloration, an adverse effect that once concerned many clinicians. A fatal outcome is associated with the delayed administration of effective therapy, advanced patient age, and higher percentages of infected peripheral leukocytes. Mortality ranges from 2% to 10% of all patients with human ehrlichiosis.[41]

Human Bartonellosis

Bartonella is a genus of fastidious bacilli that form complex relationships with cells of the endovascular compartment. Nine *Bartonella* species have been described; at least four of them cause disease in humans.[54,55] There are three principal clinical syndromes caused by *Bartonella*: persistent or relapsing bacteremia (trench fever, endocarditis, and Oroya fever), caused by *B. quintana*, *B. henselae*, *B. elizabethae*, and *B. bacilliformis*; vascular proliferative disease (bacillary angiomatosis-peliosis and verruga peruana), caused by *B. quintana*, *B. henselae*, and *B. bacilliformis*; and granulomatous disease (cat-scratch disease), caused by *B. henselae* and possibly *B. clarridgeiae*.

PERSISTENT OR RELAPSING BACTEREMIA

Trench fever, also called Wolhynia fever, is a louse-borne disease occurring in Mexico, North Africa, Poland, and the former Soviet Union. *B. quintana* is the causative agent. This disease is characterized by fever, headache, myalgias with pains in the shins, a macular rash, and splenomegaly. The fever tends to recur in cycles of 3 to 5 days for several weeks. The disease is generally mild and may occur in epidemics.

In 1993, a cluster of cases of *B. quintana* bacteremia (also known as urban trench fever), some of which were fatal, occurred in Seattle, Washington, in homeless persons who were chronic alcoholics.[56] These cases were identified, and the causative agent was isolated after special microbiologic methods were instituted at a large public hospital in that city. A follow-up study in a separate clinic found that 20% of the patients seen there in 1994 had significant serum levels of anti-*Bartonella* antibodies, in contrast to 2% of control subjects.[57] Similar findings have been reported in urban areas of western Europe. A minority of patients with urban trench fever also have endocarditis. *B. quintana*, *B. henselae*, and *B. elizabethae* can cause prolonged or recurrent bacteremia and endocarditis, without classic signs of endotoxemia.[58,59] Oroya fever, an acute, debilitating bacteremic illness associated with fever and hemolysis, is caused by *B. bacilliformis*, a sandfly-borne pathogen found in the Andean region of South America.

Bartonella bacteremic disease, including trench fever and endocarditis, can be diagnosed by cultivating these organisms from blood by use of lysis centrifugation procedures, special growth conditions, and incubation for 3 weeks (see below). Serologic methods may be more practical but still do not provide a timely diagnosis. *Bartonella* endocarditis should be treated either with erythromycin, 2 g/day in divided doses every 6 hours, plus rifampin or with doxycycline plus rifampin for at least 6 weeks. Most patients with endocarditis require valve replacement.

BACILLARY ANGIOMATOSIS-PELIOSIS

Bacillary angiomatosis is a vascular proliferative disorder that affects the skin and internal organs of primarily immunocompromised persons, especially

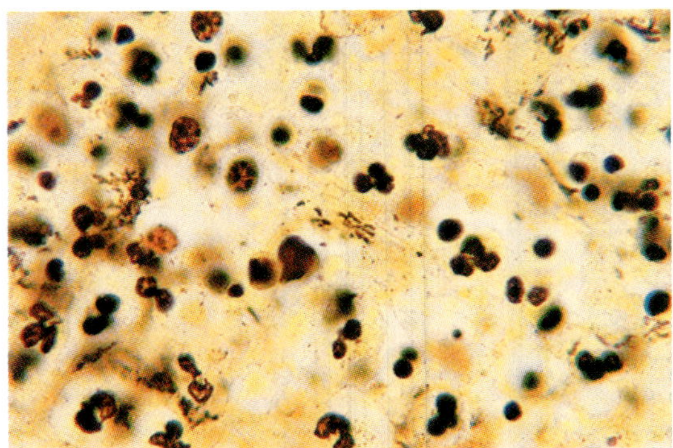

Figure 4 **Clumps of argyrophilic, pleomorphic bacilli are apparent after Warthin-Starry staining in a splenic nodule of a patient with bacillary angiomatosis.**

those infected with HIV. A similar form of pathology called verruga peruana occurs in patients with chronic *B. bacilliformis* infection. Bacteria-induced proliferation of atypical endothelial cells creates numerous poorly formed capillary channels. Adjacent to these channels are clumps of small argyrophilic bacilli [*see Figure 4*]. In 1990, these bacilli were identified as a novel α-proteobacterium, later named *B. henselae*, by means of a cultivation-independent, molecular approach[60] [*see Figure 1*]. Subsequent investigations have suggested that *B. quintana* causes an equal number of cases of bacillary angiomatosis.[61,62] However, the epidemiology of this disease differs according to causative species: *B. henselae*–associated cases are linked to exposure to cats and cat fleas, and *B. quintana*–associated cases are linked to louse exposure, poverty, and homelessness. *B. henselae* bacteremia has been documented in nearly 50% of all cats, suggesting that these animals serve as reservoirs for this organism.[63]

The most commonly recognized clinical manifestations of bacillary angiomatosis are angiomatous skin nodules or papules, whose gross appearance may be confused with that of the lesions of Kaposi's sarcoma [*see Figure 5*]. Bacillary angiomatosis disseminates in some patients and may affect the liver, the spleen, bone marrow, lymph nodes, the lungs, the brain, and other organ systems, with or without concurrent skin involvement. Infection with *B. quintana* tends to cause subcutaneous and underlying bone lesions; *B. henselae* is more often associated with lymph node and visceral disease, including bacillary peliosis in the liver and spleen.[62] If left untreated, visceral disease may be fatal.

Diagnosis of bacillary angiomatosis-peliosis is currently based on the characteristic microscopic histology, on demonstration of bacillary organisms with the Warthin-Starry silver stain [*see Figure 4*], on identification of *Bartonella* species by PCR or culture, or on serologic testing. Differentiation of this disease from Kaposi's sarcoma is important because the management of each varies considerably. *B. henselae* and *B. quintana* can be recovered from blood and tissue specimens by the use of centrifugation to process primary blood cultures after blood cell lysis or by cocultivation with endothelial cells.[61,64] Cultivation of *B. henselae* and *B. quintana* requires the use of blood agar, atmospheric conditions with elevated concentrations of carbon dioxide, and prolonged incubation times.[61] An indirect IFA serologic test for *B. henselae* and *B. quintana* has been developed, and a significant humoral response to these organisms has been measured in patients with associated disease (see below).

The treatment of choice for bacillary angiomatosis-peliosis is erythromycin, 2 g/day in four divided doses; azithromycin, 500 mg orally on day 1, then 250 mg/day thereafter; clarithromycin, 1 g/day orally in two divided doses; or doxycycline, 200 mg/day in two divided doses. Rifampin should be added to one of the preceding drugs for treatment of life-threatening disease in an immunocompromised host. However, no controlled studies that confirm these recommendations have been published. Each should be given for at least 3 to 4 months. The lesions, fever, and systemic symptoms sometimes recur despite antibiotic therapy with agents to which the *Bartonella* organisms show in vitro susceptibility.

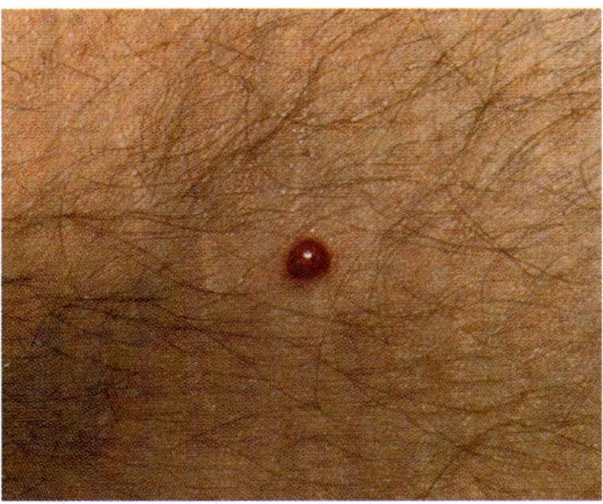

Figure 5 **A superficial cutaneous papular lesion of bacillary angiomatosis is shown. Skin lesions also arise in a dermal or subcutaneous location.**

CAT-SCRATCH DISEASE

Cat-scratch disease is generally a benign, self-limited regional lymphadenitis that is preceded by a local cat scratch or bite. Although lymph nodes may suppurate and the disease may smolder for months, most cases are mild and are not brought to medical attention.[65] Occasionally, cat-scratch disease disseminates and involves visceral organs, especially in immunocompromised patients. The granulomatous tissue response that typifies this disease contrasts with the angioproliferative lesions that characterize bacillary angiomatosis-peliosis even though *B. henselae* is associated with both diseases.

Etiology

Small pleomorphic gram-negative bacilli were first demonstrated in the lymph nodes of patients with cat-scratch disease in 1983 by means of the Warthin-Starry stain. These bacteria were also found at primary inoculation sites in the skin. From a few samples of tissue from patients with classic cat-scratch disease, a fastidious organism was cultivated and later named *Afipia felis*; however, detection of this organism was not consistently demonstrated, and by 1992, evidence began to accumulate incriminating *B. henselae* in the etiology of this disease.

Three types of data associate *B. henselae* with cat-scratch disease: serologic, molecular (PCR-based DNA detection), and cultivation. On IFA testing, 82% to 88% of patients thought to have cat-scratch disease have detectable serum IgG directed against *Bartonella* species at dilutions of 1:64 or greater.[66] From 3.6% to 6% of healthy control subjects and approximately 18% of asymptomatic cat owners demonstrate similar levels of anti-*Bartonella* antibodies. PCR has detected *Bartonella* species or *B. henselae* DNA in 74% to 84% of the lymph nodes of patients thought to have cat-scratch disease.[67] *B. clarridgeiae* has been implicated in one case of this disease.[68] No evidence of *B. quintana* and only rare evidence of *A. felis* DNA have been found in these tissues.[69] Finally, *B. henselae* has been cultivated from the lymph nodes of patients thought to have cat-scratch disease.

Epidemiology

More than 22,000 cases of cat-scratch disease, with more than 2,000 hospitalizations, occur annually in the United States, mostly in the fall and winter.[65,70] The more frequent association of kittens than adult cats with cat-scratch disease may reflect at least two factors: kittens are more likely to scratch and bite, and cats younger than 1 year are more likely to have *B. henselae* bacteremia.[63]

Cats appear to be a reservoir for *B. henselae* and *B. clarridgeiae*.[63,71] Cats that have been implicated in transmitting the disease have not been ill. Cases of cat-scratch disease may occur in clusters within households or, occasionally, within geographic regions.[70,72] A cat is usually present in households in which family outbreaks occur, but disease transmission is usually limited to several weeks.

Pathophysiology

Cat-scratch disease is an important cause of unilateral lymphadenopathy that has four stages: (1) areas of reticular cell hyperplasia and follicular hypertrophy appear in the peripheral node; (2) these areas progress to small granulomas associated with epithelioid and, occasionally, giant cells; (3) microabscesses form in the centers of the granulomas as a result of necrosis; and (4) the microabscesses coalesce to form gross areas of suppuration. The histopathologic findings in the inoculation papule include a central area of necrosis surrounded by a mantle of histiocytes and lymphocytes.

The early microscopic patterns resemble those of Hodgkin's disease or sarcoidosis. In the microabscess stage, the lesions may resemble those of tularemia, brucellosis, lymphogranuloma venereum, pyogenic bacterial lymphadenitis, various fungal infections, or infection with atypical mycobacteria, *Mycobacterium tuberculosis*, or *Yersinia* species. Prominent caseous necrosis surrounded by epithelioid cells may suggest mycobacterial disease.

Clinical Features

In more than 50% of patients with cat-scratch disease, a visible primary skin lesion develops at the inoculation site 3 to 14 days after the scratch. The papule is often inconspicuous, nonpruritic, and erythematous; it may become inflamed, pustular, or crusted and may persist for several weeks. Regional lymphadenopathy without lymphangitis appears 1 to 3 weeks after the scratch. Mild systemic symptoms, such as low-grade fever, malaise, headache, and abdominal pain, usually begin a few weeks after the cat scratch, when lymph node enlargement first becomes apparent.

The principal, and sometimes only, clinical manifestation is prominent solitary or regional adenopathy. Most often, a single node in the axilla or the neck is involved.[73] The inflamed nodes are often as large as golf balls and somewhat tender; the overlying skin displays mild erythema and edema. The nodes are frequently movable but may become fixed if gross suppuration has developed. Lymphadenopathy persists for 2 weeks to 8 months and regresses spontaneously. In 5% to 10% of patients, gross suppuration develops and occasionally drains spontaneously; healing occurs with minimal scarring.

An unusual manifestation of cat-scratch disease (seen in 2% to 10% of cases) is oculoglandular involvement (Parinaud's syndrome). The inoculation site is commonly on the palpebral conjunctiva and less often on the ocular conjunctiva, both of which may become infected. A nontender ocular lesion may appear; it measures 3 to 5 mm and is gray or yellowish. Little, if any, exudate develops. This primary ocular lesion persists for a few weeks and then heals without scarring. Unilateral involvement of the preauricular node, sometimes accompanied by ipsilateral cervical adenopathy, is the other component of this syndrome.

Complications rarely arise during the course of cat-scratch disease in an otherwise healthy person. Disseminated infection may involve the liver, spleen, lymph nodes, bone marrow, lower respiratory tract, and eye. Neurologic manifestations of headache, obtundation, convulsions, and coma may appear abruptly 1 to 5 weeks after initial symptoms. Patients usually show improvement within several days. Seventy-five percent of patients with neurologic abnormalities are found to have essentially normal CSF; the remainder have pleocytosis (up to 100 cells, predominantly mononuclear). The electroencephalogram almost always shows diffuse abnormalities during the acute phase of CNS involvement.

Diagnosis

The serum IFA test for anti-*Bartonella* antibodies may be helpful in corroborating a clinical diagnosis of cat-scratch disease[66]; however, significant levels of IgM and IgG probably will not appear for at least several weeks and 1 to 2 months, respectively. Testing of paired serum samples, drawn at least 6 weeks apart, is recommended because some persons, especially those who have frequent contact with cats, have significant anti-*Bartonella* antibody levels (see above). Most *Bartonella* serologic tests cannot reliably identify the offending species.

Isolation of *B. henselae* from specimens from patients with cat-scratch disease is rare. PCR assays for *Bartonella* DNA yield positive results in approximately 75% of lymph node samples,[67] but these assays are not widely available. The cat-scratch disease skin test is no longer recommended, and the antigen preparation is no longer available.

Differential Diagnosis

In its early stages, cat-scratch disease may resemble infectious mononucleosis or toxoplasmosis. If an affected lymph node suppurates, the fluctuant process may suggest a pyogenic bacterial origin; if suppuration occurs in the neck, a cystic hygroma, branchial cleft cyst, or thyroglossal duct cyst may be present. Cultivation methods and special stains help distinguish mycobacterial disease, tularemia, and fungal infections (e.g., coccidioidomycosis, histoplasmosis, and sporotrichosis) from cat-scratch disease. Involvement of the external eye and preauricular lymph node suggests various other causes of Parinaud's syndrome, including tularemia, the uveoparotid fever of sarcoidosis, and tuberculosis. Tularemia, however, is often associated with exposure to rabbits, and patients with uveoparotid fever have uveal tract, rather than conjunctival, involvement. Inguinal node involvement may suggest that lymphogranuloma venereum or primary syphilis is present. Dark-field examination of any primary lesion and serologic tests may be helpful in making the diagnosis. In patients who exhibit minimal inflammatory features and have had no history of cat scratches or other cat contact, a lymphoproliferative disorder should be considered; lymph node biopsy may be necessary for diagnosis.

Treatment

In almost all patients, cat-scratch disease is self-limited, runs a benign course over several months, and requires no treatment other than analgesics, local heat, and reassurance. Antibiotics have little proven value in most cases of cat-scratch disease in otherwise healthy persons. A small randomized, double-blind, prospective trial suggested that azithromycin speeds the resolution of this disease.[74] Immunocompromised patients or those with disseminated disease are usually given antibiotics, but data clearly supporting their efficacy for such patients are lacking. If the affected node becomes increasingly tender and fluctuant, needle aspiration (rather than incisional drainage) is the preferred form of treatment.

Acknowledgments

Figure 2 Slide courtesy of Dr. Mark Lebwohl, Mount Sinai Medical Center, New York, New York.

Figure 3 Slide courtesy of Dr. P. Joanne Cornbleet, Stanford University School of Medicine, Stanford, California.

Figure 4 Slide courtesy of Dr. Don Regula, Stanford University School of Medicine, Stanford, California.

Figure 5 Photograph courtesy of Dr. Clay J. Cockerell, University of Texas Southwestern Medical Center, Dallas.

References

1. Azad AF, Beard CB: Rickettsial pathogens and their arthropod vectors. Emerg Infect Dis 4:179, 1998

2. Winkler HH: Rickettsia species (as organisms). Annu Rev Microbiol 44:131, 1990

3. Eremeeva ME, Silverman DJ: Effects of the antioxidant α-lipoic acid on human umbilical vein endothelial cells infected with *Rickettsia rickettsii*. Infect Immunol 66:2290, 1998

4. Clifton DR, Goss RA, Sahni SK, et al: NF-κB–dependent inhibition of apoptosis is essential for host cell survival during *Rickettsia rickettsii* infection. Proc Natl Acad Sci USA 95:4646, 1998

5. Walker DH: Rocky Mountain spotted fever: a seasonal alert. Clin Infect Dis 20:1111, 1995

6. Kirk JL, Fine DP, Sexton DJ, et al: Rocky Mountain spotted fever: a clinical review based on 48 confirmed cases, 1943–1986. Medicine (Baltimore) 69:35, 1990

7. Dalton MJ, Clarke MJ, Holman RC, et al: National surveillance for Rocky Mountain spotted fever, 1981–1992: epidemiologic summary and evaluation of risk factors for fatal outcome. Am J Trop Med Hyg 52:405, 1995

8. Sexton DJ, Corey GR: Rocky Mountain "spotless" and "almost spotless" fever: a wolf in sheep's clothing. Clin Infect Dis 15:439, 1992

9. Conlon PJ, Procop GW, Fowler V, et al: Predictors of prognosis and risk of acute renal failure in patients with Rocky Mountain spotted fever. Am J Med 101:621, 1996

10. Tzianabos T, Anderson BE, McDade JE: Detection of *Rickettsia rickettsii* DNA in clinical specimens by using polymerase chain reaction technology. J Clin Microbiol 27:2866, 1989

11. Dumler JS, Gage WR, Pettis GL, et al: Rapid immunoperoxidase demonstration of *Rickettsia rickettsii* in fixed cutaneous specimens from patients with Rocky Mountain spotted fever. Am J Clin Pathol 93: 410, 1990

12. Westerman EL: Rocky Mountain spotless fever: a dilemma for the clinician. Arch Intern Med 142:1106, 1982

13. Kirkland KB, Wilkinson WE, Sexton DJ: Therapeutic delay and mortality in cases of Rocky Mountain spotted fever. Clin Infect Dis 20:1118, 1995

14. Kass EM, Szaniawski WK, Levy H, et al: Rickettsialpox in a New York City hospital, 1980 to 1989. N Engl J Med 331:1612, 1994

15. La Scola B, Raoult D: Laboratory diagnosis of rickettsioses: current approaches to diagnosis of old and new rickettsial diseases. J Clin Microbiol 35:2715, 1997

16. Bella-Cueto F, Font-Creus B, Sequia-Porta F: Comparative, randomized trial of one-day doxycycline versus 10-day tetracycline therapy for Mediterranean spotted fever. J Infect Dis 155:1056, 1987

17. Williams SG, Sacci JB Jr, Schriefer ME, et al: Typhus and typhus-like rickettsiae associated with opossums and their fleas in Los Angeles County, California. J Clin Microbiol 30:1758, 1992

18. Schriefer ME, Sacci JB Jr, Dumler JS, et al: Identification of a novel rickettsial infection in a patient diagnosed with murine typhus. J Clin Microbiol 32:949, 1994

19. Dumler JS, Taylor JP, Walker DH: Clinical and laboratory features of murine typhus in south Texas, 1980 through 1987. JAMA 266:1365, 1991

20. Perine PL, Chandler BP, Krause DK, et al: A clinico-epidemiological study of epidemic typhus in Africa. Clin Infect Dis 14:1149, 1992

21. Raoult D, Ndihokubwayo JB, Tissot-Dupont H, et al: Outbreak of epidemic typhus associated with trench fever in Burundi. Lancet 352: 353, 1998

22. Murray ES, Baehr G, Shwartzman G, et al: Brill's disease: I. Clinical and laboratory diagnosis. JAMA 142:1059, 1950

23. Green CR, Fishbein D, Gleiberman I: Brill-Zinsser: still with us (letter). JAMA 264:1811, 1990

24. Silpapojakul K, Ukkachoke C, Krisanapan S, et al: Rickettsial meningitis and encephalitis. Arch Intern Med 151:1753, 1991

25. Watt G, Chouriyagune C, Ruangweerayud R, et al: Scrub typhus infections poorly responsive to antibiotics in northern Thailand. Lancet 348:86, 1996

26. Raoult D, Marrie T: Q fever. Clin Infect Dis 20:489, 1995

27. Baca OG, Li YP, Kumar H: Survival of the Q fever agent *Coxiella burnetii* in the phagolysosome. Trends Microbiol 2:476, 1994

28. McCaul TF, Dare AJ, Gannon JP, et al: In vivo endogenous spore formation by *Coxiella burnetii* in Q fever endocarditis. J Clin Pathol 47: 978, 1994

29. Spelman DW: Q fever: a study of 111 consecutive cases. Med J Aust 1:547, 1982

30. Tissot-Dupont H, Raoult D, Brouqui P, et al: Epidemiologic features and clinical presentation of acute Q fever in hospitalized patients: 323 French cases. Am J Med 93:427, 1992

31. Raoult D, Bollini G, Gallais H: Osteoarticular infection due to *Coxiella burnetii*. J Infect Dis 159:1159, 1989

32. Brouqui P, Tissot-Dupont H, Drancourt M, et al: Chronic Q fever: ninety-two cases from France, including 27 cases without endocarditis. Arch Intern Med 153:642, 1993

33. Tobin MJ, Cahill N, Gearty G, et al: Q fever endocarditis. Am J Med 72:396, 1982

34. Soriano F, Camacho MT, Ponte C, et al: Serological differentiation between acute (late control) and endocarditis Q fever. J Clin Pathol 46: 411, 1993

35. Fournier P-E, Marrie TJ, Raoult D: Diagnosis of Q fever. J Clin Microbiol 36:1823, 1998

36. Stein A, Raoult D: Detection of *Coxiella burnetii* by DNA amplification using polymerase chain reaction. J Clin Microbiol 30:2462, 1992

37. Levy PY, Drancourt M, Etienne J, et al: Comparison of different antibiotic regimens for therapy of 32 cases of Q fever endocarditis. Antimicrob Agents Chemother 35:533, 1991

38. Rikihisa Y: The tribe Ehrlichieae and ehrlichial diseases. Clin Microbiol Rev 4:286, 1991

39. Fritz CL, Glaser CA: Ehrlichiosis. Infect Dis Clin North Am 12:123, 1998

40. Bakken JS, Dumler JS, Chen SM, et al: Human granulocytic ehrlichiosis in the upper midwest United States: a new species emerging? JAMA 272:212, 1994

41. Dumler JS, Bakken JS: Ehrlichial diseases of humans: emerging tick-borne infections. Clin Infect Dis 20:1102, 1995

42. Statewide surveillance for ehrlichiosis—Connecticut and New York, 1994–1997. MMWR Morb Mortal Wkly Rep 47:476, 1998

43. Standaert SM, Dawson JE, Schaffner W, et al: Ehrlichiosis in a golf-oriented retirement community. N Engl J Med 333:420, 1995

44. Schwartz I, Fish D, Daniels TJ: Prevalence of the rickettsial agent of human granulocytic ehrlichiosis in ticks from a hyperendemic focus of Lyme disease (letter). N Engl J Med 337:49, 1997

45. Nadelman RB, Horowitz HW, Hsieh T-C, et al: Simultaneous human granulocytic ehrlichiosis and Lyme borreliosis. N Engl J Med 337:27, 1997

46. Katavolos P, Armstrong PM, Dawson JE, et al: Duration of tick attachment required for transmission of granulocytic ehrlichiosis. J Infect Dis 177:1422, 1998

47. Fishbein DB, Dawson JE, Robinson LE: Human ehrlichiosis in the United States, 1985 to 1990. Ann Intern Med 120:736, 1994

48. Bakken JS, Krueth J, Wilson-Nordskog C, et al: Clinical and laboratory characteristics of human granulocytic ehrlichiosis. JAMA 275:199, 1996

49. Horowitz HW, Kilchevsky E, Haber S, et al: Perinatal transmission of the agent of human granulocytic ehrlichiosis. N Engl J Med 339:375, 1998

50. Dumler JS, Bakken JS: Human granulocytic ehrlichiosis in Wisconsin and Minnesota: a frequent infection with the potential for persistence. J Infect Dis 173:1027, 1996

51. Magnarelli LA, Dumler JS, Anderson JF, et al: Coexistence of antibodies to tick-borne pathogens of babesiosis, ehrlichiosis, and Lyme borreliosis in human sera. J Clin Microbiol 33:3054, 1995

52. Goodman JL, Nelson C, Vitale B, et al: Direct cultivation of the causative agent of human granulocytic ehrlichiosis. N Engl J Med 334: 209, 1996

53. Everett ED, Evans KA, Henry RB, et al: Human ehrlichiosis in adults after tick exposure: diagnosis using polymerase chain reaction. Ann Intern Med 120:730, 1994

54. Anderson BE, Neuman MA: *Bartonella* spp. as emerging human pathogens. Clin Microbiol Rev 10:203, 1997

55. Spach DH, Koehler JE: *Bartonella*-associated infections. Infect Dis Clin North Am 12:137, 1998

56. Spach DH, Kanter AS, Dougherty MJ, et al: *Bartonella (Rochalimaea) quintana* bacteremia in inner-city patients with chronic alcoholism. N Engl J Med 332:424, 1995

57. Jackson LA, Spach DH, Kippen DA, et al: Seroprevalence to *Bartonella quintana* among patients at a community clinic in downtown Seattle. J Infect Dis 173:1023, 1996

58. Raoult D, Fournier PE, Drancourt M, et al: Diagnosis of 22 new cases of *Bartonella* endocarditis. Ann Intern Med 125:646, 1996

59. Baorto E, Payne RM, Slater LN, et al: Culture-negative endocarditis due to *Bartonella henselae*. J Pediatr 132:1051, 1998

60. Relman DA, Loutit JS, Schmidt TM, et al: The agent of bacillary angiomatosis: an approach to the identification of uncultured pathogens. N Engl J Med 323:1573, 1990

61. Koehler JE, Quinn FD, Berger TG, et al: Isolation of *Rochalimaea* species from cutaneous and osseous lesions. N Engl J Med 327:1625, 1992

62. Koehler JE, Sanchez MA, Garrido CS, et al: Molecular epidemiology of bartonella infections in patients with bacillary angiomatosis-peliosis. N Engl J Med 337:1876, 1997

63. Koehler JE, Glaser CA, Tappero JW: *Rochalimaea henselae* infection: a new zoonosis with the domestic cat as reservoir. JAMA 271:531, 1994

64. Slater LN, Welch DF, Hensel D, et al: A newly recognized fastidious gram-negative pathogen as a cause of fever and bacteremia. N Engl J Med 323:1587, 1990

65. Jackson LA, Perkins BA, Wenger JD: Cat scratch disease in the United States: an analysis of three national databases. Am J Public Health 83:1707, 1993

66. Dalton MJ, Robinson LE, Cooper J, et al: Use of *Bartonella* antigens for serologic diagnosis of cat-scratch disease at a national referral center. Arch Intern Med 155:1670, 1995

67. Bergmans AMC, Groothedde JW, Schellekens JFP, et al: Etiology of cat scratch disease: comparison of polymerase chain reaction detection of *Bartonella* (formerly *Rochalimaea*) and *Afipia felis* DNA with serology and skin tests. J Infect Dis 171:916, 1995

68. Kordick DL, Hilyard EJ, Hadfield TL, et al: *Bartonella clarridgeiae*, a newly recognized zoonotic pathogen causing inoculation papules, fever, and lymphadenopathy (cat scratch disease). J Clin Microbiol 35: 1813, 1997

69. Giladi M, Avidor B, Kletter Y, et al: Cat scratch disease: the rare role of *Afipia felis*. J Clin Microbiol 36:2499, 1998

70. Hamilton DH, Zangwill KM, Hadler JL, et al: Cat-scratch disease—Connecticut, 1992–1993. J Infect Dis 172:570, 1995

71. Jameson P, Greene C, Regnery R, et al: Prevalence of *Bartonella henselae* antibodies in pet cats throughout regions of North America. J Infect Dis 172:1145, 1995

72. Encephalitis associated with cat scratch disease—Broward and Palm Beach counties, Florida, 1994. Centers for Disease Control and Prevention. MMWR Morb Mortal Wkly Rep 43:909, 1994

73. Carithers HA: Cat-scratch disease: an overview based on a study of 1,200 patients. Am J Dis Child 139:1124, 1985

74. Bass JW, Freitas BC, Freitas AD, et al: Prospective randomized double blind placebo-controlled evaluation of azithromycin for treatment of cat-scratch disease. Pediatr Infect Dis J 17:447, 1998

27 Infections Due to Mycoplasmas

David A. Relman, M.D.

Mycoplasmas are the smallest known free-living organisms. Their genome is roughly half the size of that of other bacteria and has been completely characterized for two species, *Mycoplasma pneumoniae* and *M. genitalium*.[1] The characterization of *M. genitalium*, which has only 580,070 base pairs and 468 predicted proteins, has helped define the minimal set of genes necessary for cellular life.[2]

At least 13 *Mycoplasma* species, two *Acholeplasma* species, and one *Ureaplasma* species have been isolated from humans with varying frequency; most of these species are thought to be normal inhabitants of oral and urogenital mucous membranes.[3] Only three species, *M. pneumoniae*, *M. hominis*, and *U. urealyticum*, have been shown conclusively to be pathogenic in humans. *M. pneumoniae* is the species most clearly demonstrated to cause disease in humans. The respiratory tract is its primary site of involvement. The other two species are associated with a variety of genitourinary tract disorders. Evidence also implicates a fourth species, *M. genitalium*, as a cause of genitourinary tract disease in humans. Several *Mycoplasma* species have been detected in the blood and visceral tissues of persons infected with HIV type 1 (HIV-1). The hypothesis that these organisms may act as cofactors in the development of AIDS remains unproved.[4]

Mycoplasmas have been implicated in a variety of other diseases, from asthma[5] to arthritis.[6] Confirming an etiologic role of mycoplasmas in such diseases is difficult because these organisms do not necessarily elicit a major inflammatory response in the host, and they tend to be almost ubiquitous in the human body; they can be found in the blood and in a variety of tissues in healthy persons. It may be inappropriate to presume that mycoplasmas detected in an ill person have a causative role in the disease.

Unlike other bacteria, mycoplasmas lack a rigid cell wall. Their limited biosynthetic capabilities are reflected in their paucity of genes for synthesis of amino acids, nucleotides, folic acid, fatty acids, and sterols. As a result, they are highly dependent on host cells for their survival. Mycoplasmas are also saprophytes that are ubiquitous among plants, animals, and insects.

Mycoplasmas can be cultivated in either broth or agar culture medium that has been supplemented with yeast extract and 20% horse serum. On solid culture medium, most species form colonies that exhibit a typical so-called fried-egg appearance; that is, the central portion of the colony penetrates deep into the agar and is surrounded by secondary superficial growth. Under both aerobic and anaerobic conditions, *M. pneumoniae* grows more slowly than the other mycoplasmas: it takes 1 to 2 weeks before colonies can be detected on initial isolation. These colonies do not exhibit the typical fried-egg pattern but rather have a more homogeneous appearance. Because *Ureaplasma* species produce tiny colonies on solid medium, they were originally called T-strains or T-mycoplasmas; they are distinguished from *Mycoplasma* species by their ability to metabolize urea. All mycoplasmas are resistant to antibiotics such as the penicillins and the cephalosporins (whose site of action is the bacterial cell wall) and the sulfonamides (which block folic acid synthesis), but they are generally susceptible to the macrolides and the tetracyclines.

Pneumonia and Other Respiratory Tract Diseases

EPIDEMIOLOGY

Although *M. pneumoniae* respiratory tract infections occur sporadically throughout the world, they are endemic to crowded urban areas and military, university, and closed populations. In a study of a large urban community, 15% of all pneumonias were caused by *M. pneumoniae*.[7] Among civilian adults, *M. pneumoniae* accounts for at least 4%

to 9% of all cases of community-acquired pneumonia that require hospitalization.[8] These figures probably underestimate the morbidity caused by this agent, because in the majority of such persons who are infected, only pharyngitis or tracheobronchitis develops.[9] Incidence rates are age specific and are highest in children between 5 and 14 years of age. Although the incidence of *M. pneumoniae* pneumonia is lower in older children and young adults, as many as 50% of all pneumonias in persons in these age groups are caused by *M. pneumoniae*.[10] In military recruits, 20% to 40% of all cases of pneumonia are caused by *M. pneumoniae*. Attack rates are also high in college students. Infection rates and the likelihood of severe disease, however, are lower in middle-aged and elderly persons.

Epidemic outbreaks of *M. pneumoniae* respiratory tract disease occur periodically in large urban populations as well as in closed groups. During these epidemics, the incidence of *M. pneumoniae* pneumonia may triple. In some urban populations, epidemics are cyclic, occurring every 4 to 7 years, and may be protracted.[10] Unlike endemic *M. pneumoniae* pneumonia, which has no seasonal predilection, these epidemics tend to occur in the fall.

M. pneumoniae is the only *Mycoplasma* species that has clearly been established as a cause of human respiratory tract disease, although *M. genitalium* has been isolated from the respiratory tract in mixed infections with *M. pneumoniae*, an organism with which *M. genitalium* can be confused.[11] *M. pneumoniae* infection can be asymptomatic; in one study, during a period of maximum disease incidence, the organism was cultivated from the pharynges of 13.5% of healthy people.[12] *M. pneumoniae* infection can also cause various clinical syndromes, such as pneumonia, tracheobronchitis, and pharyngitis.

Mycoplasma pneumonia has traditionally been designated an atypical pneumonia. Other pneumonias in this category include viral pneumonia, Q fever, psittacosis, and *Chlamydia pneumoniae* pneumonia. *Mycoplasma* pneumonia was also called Eaton agent pneumonia and cold agglutinin-positive primary atypical pneumonia. Recent studies have shown that the term atypical is a misnomer, however. In fact, so-called atypical pneumonias may be epidemiologically and clinically indistinguishable from pneumococcal pneumonia.[13] To further blur the distinction, *M. pneumoniae* may play a contributory role in cases of community-acquired pneumonia involving other respiratory pathogens. Coinfection with *Streptococcus pneumoniae* and *M. pneumoniae* has been reported.[14]

ETIOLOGY

M. pneumoniae is transmitted by infected respiratory secretions. Spread of *Mycoplasma* pneumonia from one person to another usually requires close and prolonged contact. This requirement contrasts with the relative ease with which disease caused by some of the respiratory viruses is spread. Occasionally, an outbreak of *M. pneumoniae* pneumonia appears that has an abrupt onset and spreads rapidly; each of these outbreaks may be linked to a single, common source.[15]

Secondary cases of *M. pneumoniae* infection are typically found within families in which disease has been introduced by an index patient, usually a school-age child. Intrafamily spread of infection has been reported in approximately two thirds of families in which an index case of *M. pneumoniae* pneumonia appeared. The disease has an incubation period of 2 to 4 weeks and characteristically spreads slowly within a family, where it may persist for several months [*see Figure 1*]. Manifestations vary and include asymptomatic infection, pharyngitis, tracheobronchitis, and pneumonia. Intrafamily attack rates may be as high as 84% in children and 41% in adults.

PATHOGENESIS, PATHOLOGY, AND IMMUNITY

M. pneumoniae penetrates mucociliary secretions by means of gliding motility and adheres firmly to the surface of respiratory epithelial cells.[16] Adherence is mediated by a specialized terminal attachment organelle, on the surface of which are located the p1 protein, a specific adhesin, and the p30 protein, a putative adhesin.[17] *M. genitalium* expresses a protein immunologically related to p1 (p140) that is believed to be a functional counterpart. Multiple unlinked, incomplete copies of the genes that encode these adhesins constitute approximately 5% of the *Mycoplasma* genome; it has been proposed that recombination between gene copies generates antigenically variant proteins that avoid host immune recognition.[18] Once attached to the respiratory epithelium, *M. pneumoniae* multiplies extracellularly and causes local host cell damage and ciliary stasis; the organism does not seem to invade eukaryotic cells. *M. fermentans, M. pirum,* and *M. penetrans,* which enter eukaryotic cells in vitro, are exceptions. The mechanisms that produce host cell damage are unclear but may be related to *Mycoplasma*-generated hydrogen peroxide and superoxide anions, leading to oxidative host cell injury. *M. pneumoniae* can be cultured from pharyngeal secretions 8 weeks or more after the clinical onset of illness,

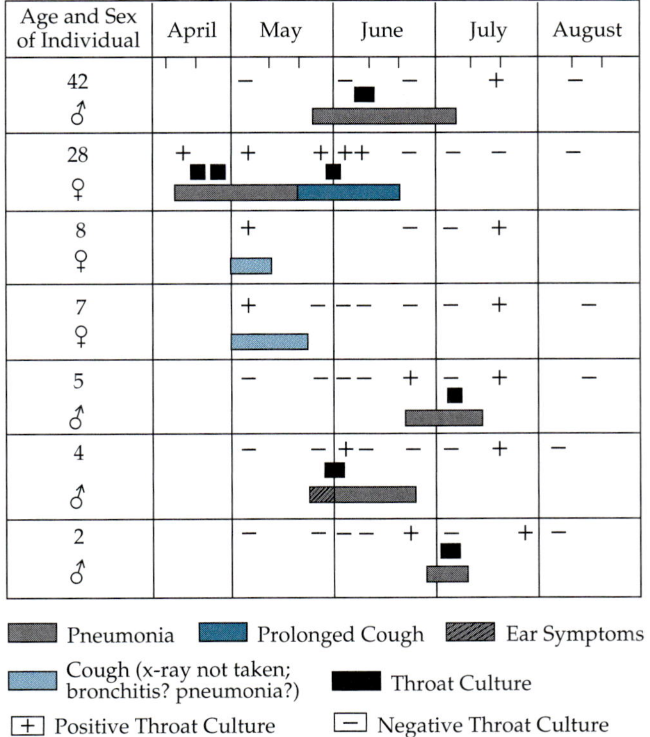

Figure 1 **During a 5-month period, a *Mycoplasma pneumoniae* infection spread through seven members of a family. Positive throat cultures were obtained in all seven individuals, but clinically documented pneumonia was observed in only five. Pneumonia was treated with tetracycline. In the other two infected individuals, coughs developed during the period in which their throat cultures were positive, suggesting the possibility of *Mycoplasma*-induced bronchitis or pneumonia; however, radiologic confirmation of the diagnosis was not obtained. A prolonged cough followed the episode of pneumonia in one patient, and ear symptoms were observed in another. Positive throat cultures were obtained in six of seven cases after cessation of therapy and disappearance of symptoms.**

even in the presence of circulating antimycoplasmal antibody and often despite effective antimicrobial therapy. On rare occasions, *M. pneumoniae* has been cultured from extrapulmonary sites, including blood and cerebrospinal, pericardial, and synovial fluids.[10]

Study of the pathology of human *Mycoplasma* pneumonia is limited because the disease has an extremely low mortality (< 0.1%). The few cases studied have shown primarily interstitial pneumonia, a mononuclear-type alveolar exudate, acute bronchiolitis, and bronchiolitis obliterans.[19]

M. pneumoniae infection in humans provokes a specific immune response that results in the production of secretory IgA and circulating IgG antibodies. Naturally acquired humoral immunity is associated with partial protection against reinfection; in particular, the immunity that follows more severe *M. pneumoniae* infections (e.g., pneumonia) is more protective and longer lasting than that which follows mild infection.[20] The protective value of antibody-mediated immunity against *M. pneumoniae* infection is emphasized by the observation that persons with hypogammaglobulinemia are unusually susceptible to infection by *Mycoplasma* and *Ureaplasma* species.[21] Bona fide second attacks of *M. pneumoniae* pneumonia have been reported occasionally, however, both in immunocompetent and in immunodeficient individuals. The ability of *M. pneumoniae* and other mycoplasmas to trigger antiself immune responses is an area of active research.[18]

DIAGNOSIS

Clinical Manifestations

M. pneumoniae infections have an incubation period of 20 to 23 days in naturally occurring cases but an incubation period of only 8 to 10 days in studies of human infection. Approximately 20% of *M. pneumoniae* infections are asymptomatic.[9] Clinically apparent *M. pneumoniae* infections generally produce tracheobronchitis or an upper respiratory tract syndrome that is commonly characterized by pharyngitis, fever, and headache. Pneumonia, however, is the best-described clinical manifestation of *M. pneumoniae* infection and occurs in 3% to 13% of persons who are infected.[9]

Although *Mycoplasma* pneumonia may begin with a sore throat, the most common presenting symptom is cough. Headache, malaise, chills, and a temperature of 37.8° to 40.0° C (100° to 104° F) are present in the majority of patients. In a smaller percentage, nasal symptoms occur. Cough is often nonproductive. Purulent sputum is produced in some patients, however; and in rare instances, the sputum is blood streaked. In most patients, the onset is subacute (occurring over several days), but in some, it is quite abrupt and associated with high fever.

Fine or medium rales are present in the majority of patients with *Mycoplasma* pneumonia; bronchial breath sounds are noted less frequently. In many patients, however, pneumonia can be diagnosed only on chest x-ray. Pleural rubs are rare, as are pleural effusions that are of sufficient magnitude to be detected on physical examination.

Symptoms usually clear within 1 to 3 weeks after the onset of illness, even without treatment. In about 20% of patients, symptoms and radiologic abnormalities persist for at least a month. The physical findings may last even longer. Relapse and recurrence are reported to occur infrequently.

Although *M. pneumoniae* pneumonia is usually a benign, self-limited disease, pulmonary complications may occur and, on rare occasions, result in death. Fulminant disease may occur more often in young, previously healthy adults.[19] Multilobar involvement, lung abscess, massive pleural effusion, acute respiratory distress syndrome (ARDS), and diffuse interstitial fibrosis have been described. At particular risk for these complications are immunodeficient patients and children with sickle cell disease or other hemoglobinopathies.[10] Although bacterial superinfection is a well-known complication of influenza virus infection, it is unusual after *M. pneumoniae* infection.

A variety of nonrespiratory complications involving many organ systems may occur during the course of *M. pneumoniae* respiratory infections.[3,10,22] The pathogenic mechanism responsible for these complications is unclear, but possible mechanisms include metastatic infection, autoimmune phenomena, and toxin production. In some cases of extrapulmonary *M. pneumoniae* disease, respiratory disease may be absent.

Symptoms and objective findings associated with the ear and tympanic membrane may be noted in 20% to 30% of cases of *M. pneumoniae* pneumonia. Because direct cultures rarely if ever grow *M. pneumoniae,* there is little evidence to support the old belief that this organism is the cause of otitis media, with or without bullous myringitis.[23]

Cold agglutinin-induced hemolysis is one of the most frequent nonrespiratory manifestations of *Mycoplasma* pneumonia. It has been suggested that *M. pneumoniae* interacts with and alters the erythrocyte I antigen, changing it to an immunogen; as a result, complement-fixing, temperature-sensitive IgM antibodies are produced that are directed against erythrocyte I antigens. Although up to 83% of patients with *M. pneumoniae* infection may have a positive direct Coombs test finding and reticulocytosis, clinically significant hemolysis is rare.[24] When anemia does occur, it begins suddenly in the second or third week of illness, and the agglutinin titer is high (> 1:512). Jaundice is common, and hemoglobinuria occurs in severe cases. The process is usually self-limited, lasting a few weeks.

Neurologic disease is reportedly the most common nonpulmonary manifestation of *M. pneumoniae* infection.[25] A wide spectrum of neurologic manifestations has been reported. The most common ones include meningoencephalitis, encephalitis, polyradiculopathy (including Guillain-Barré syndrome), and aseptic meningitis; the less common neurologic manifestations include cranial neuropathy, acute psychosis, cerebellar ataxia, and transverse myelitis. The pathogenesis of these neurologic complications is unclear; *M. pneumoniae* organisms have been recovered only rarely from cerebrospinal fluid. However, in a larger percentage of cases, *M. pneumoniae* DNA has been detected with polymerase chain reaction testing.[26] Persistent deficits, such as seizure disorders, and an overall mortality of 10% have been reported when neurologic disease has complicated *M. pneumoniae* infection.

Gastrointestinal symptoms of *M. pneumoniae* infection occur in 12% to 44% of patients; symptoms include nausea, vomiting, and diarrhea. Hepatitis and pancreatitis have been detected but are probably rare. Erythema multiforme is the most important skin eruption associated with *M. pneumoniae* infection, especially when it presents with involvement of two or more mucous membranes and systemic toxicity (the Stevens-Johnson syndrome).[27] Cases of myocardial disease, pericardial disease, arthralgias, and arthritis have been attributed to this pathogen.[3,28]

Laboratory Testing

The leukocyte count is normal in most patients with *Mycoplasma* pneumonia. In 10% to 25% of patients, it ranges from 10,000 to 20,000/mm^3.

About 50% to 60% of patients with *M. pneumoniae* pneumonia show a fourfold or greater rise in the cold agglutinin titer for human type O erythrocytes or have a single titer of 1:128 or higher. The more severe the illness, the more likely that an increase in cold agglutinins will be observed. Low titers (< 1:32) may occur with infectious mononucleosis and with pneumonias caused by adenovirus or influenza virus. Titers of 1:128 or greater are more specific, however, and are highly suggestive of *M. pneumoniae* infection. The physician can screen for the presence of cold agglutinins by means of a simple bedside test.[29] Four to five drops of blood are added to a Vacutainer tube containing sodium citrate (blue-top tube in most hospitals). The tube is immersed in ice water for 30 seconds and then tilted so that the blood runs down the side. Definite flocculation that disappears after the tube is incubated at 37° C for 3 to 5 minutes indicates a positive reaction. This bedside screening test correlates well with cold agglutinin titers of 1:64 or greater.

Sputum smears from patients with *Mycoplasma* pneumonia reveal large mononuclear cells and some granulocytes. Occasionally, some patients raise grossly purulent sputum that on microscopic examination shows large numbers of polymorphonuclear leukocytes.

Radiologic abnormalities of primary atypical pneumonias of all etiologies are similar and are seen 1 to 5 days after the onset of symptoms. These abnormalities consist of patchy alveolar infiltrates that usually involve one of the lower lobes; atelectatic and reticular changes that extend from the hilus and are usually confined to one segment or lobe are also seen. Occasionally, upper lobe infiltrates are apparent, which may suggest tuberculosis. On rare occasions, extensive consolidation of a lobe or a diffuse interstitial pulmonary process is evident. Hilar adenopathy and pneumatocele formation are rare complications. Clinically evident pleural effusions are uncommon in *Mycoplasma* pneumonia, but lateral decubitus views reveal that up to 20% of patients have small, transient effusions.

Laboratory diagnosis of an *M. pneumoniae* infection in a patient with primary atypical pneumonia is established by (1) the finding of a rising or already high titer of cold agglutinins, (2) the isolation of *M. pneumoniae* from sputum or throat culture on special media, or (3) the results of specific serologic tests, such as complement fixation (the most practical test),[30] indirect immunofluorescence, and enzyme-linked immunosorbent assays (ELISAs) for specific IgM and IgG antibodies in paired serum samples. Current serologic tests have several inadequacies. For example, IgM antibodies may not be produced during reinfection in older patients (i.e., persons older than 40 years with preexisting anti–*M. pneumoniae* IgG antibodies).[31] In addition, most serologic tests do not distinguish between *M. pneumoniae* and *M. genitalium*. None of these tests is likely to provide positive confirmation of the diagnosis early in the illness; therefore, therapeutic decisions must be based on clinical and radiologic findings and on results of the Gram stain of the sputum and routine sputum culture.

Direct detection of nucleic acids, using PCR, is an important step forward in the diagnosis of *M. pneumoniae* infections.[32] PCR allows a rapid and specific diagnosis to be made during the first week of clinical illness. The combination of nasopharyngeal PCR testing and IgM ELISA has been recommended as the most sensitive and rapid approach to diagnosis of *M. pneumoniae* infection in children.[33] PCR-based methods have been developed for all of the clinically relevant mycoplasmas; however, they are not yet widely available outside of research and reference laboratories.

DIFFERENTIAL DIAGNOSIS

Nonlobar pneumonia with a subacute onset and nonpurulent sputum suggests primary atypical pneumonia. Typical bacterial pneumonia (e.g., bronchopneumonia caused by pneumococcus, *Escherichia coli*, or *Haemophilus influenzae*) should be ruled out on the basis of the peripheral leukocyte count, Gram stain of the sputum, and sputum culture. Primary atypical pneumonias other than *Mycoplasma* pneumonia that should be considered are the pneumonias associated with psittacosis, *C. pneumoniae* infection [see 28 Diseases Due to *Chlamydia*], Q fever, tularemia, pertussis, and infection by adenoviruses or influenza, parainfluenza, or respiratory syncytial viruses. Epidemiologic features are important clues to a diagnosis of psittacosis, Q fever, or tularemia. An upper lobe infiltrate in a patient with blood-streaked sputum may initially suggest tuberculosis.

In sporadic cases of Legionnaires disease, the radiologic and clinical picture can be identical to that in *M. pneumoniae* pneumonia, and it may not be possible to establish the diagnosis unless cultures, specialized immunofluorescent staining, or DNA probe methods are available. Serologic testing of acute and convalescent sera and bacterial antigen detection in urine also can confirm a diagnosis of Legionnaires disease [see 21 Infections Due to *Haemophilus, Moraxella, Legionella, Bordetella,* and *Pseudomonas*].

TREATMENT

The treatment of mycoplasmal infection generally requires classes of antibiotics that are falling out of favor for the empirical treatment of pneumonia. The possibility of *M. pneumoniae* deserves particular consideration in a patient with community-acquired pneumonia who has failed to respond to an empirically prescribed antibiotic (e.g., a cephalosporin) that is ineffective against mycoplasmas.

A macrolide or tetracycline is the antibiotic of choice for *M. pneumoniae* pneumonia. A macrolide (e.g., erythromycin or clarithromycin) is preferable in children because it does not stain teeth.[34] These drugs are effective in that they decrease the duration of fever and malaise, length of hospitalization, and duration of radiologic abnormalities. In one study of military trainees with serologically confirmed *M. pneumoniae* pneumonia, treatment with oral erythromycin for 7 days reduced mean duration of fever from 4.2 days to 2.4 days, hospitalization from 14.1 days to 7.0 days, and radiologic abnormalities from 14.8 days to 7.2 days. Cough often persists despite antibiotic use.

Erythromycin is usually administered to adults in an oral dosage of 250 to 500 mg four times daily. The dosage of tetracycline is 250 to 500 mg orally four times daily. Clarithromycin and azithromycin appear to be as effective as erythromycin in the treatment of *M. pneumoniae* pneumonia and less likely to cause adverse gastrointestinal effects, but they are more expensive.[34] Antimicrobial resistance has not been clinically important in the treatment of *M. pneumoniae* infections, as it has in the treatment of diseases caused by genital mycoplasmas. Treatment with appropriate antibiotics does not eradicate *M. pneumoniae*; in 30% to 40% of infected volunteers, treatment does not prevent continued shedding, which in some patients persists for 3 to 8 weeks or longer. Supportive therapy for patients with clinically significant cold agglutinin hemolytic anemia should include maintenance of an environmental temperature above the thermal amplitude of the cold agglutinin (usually 30° to 34° C).

Genitourinary Tract Infections

Of the more than eight species of mycoplasmas and ureaplasmas that have been cultured repeatedly from the human genitourinary tract, only *M. hominis*, *M. genitalium*, and *U. urealyticum* are strongly associated with disease.[35,36] Because the lower genitourinary tract of healthy infants and of adults (especially those who are sexually active or pregnant) is frequently colonized by these organisms, it has been difficult to prove them to be the cause of infection simply on the basis of positive cultures. Despite this difficulty, there is evidence that *M. hominis*, *M. genitalium*, and *U. urealyticum* are causally associated with several clinical syndromes. A variety of other syndromes are more loosely associated with these organisms. In practice, only a few clinical situations mandate the use of specific antimicrobial therapy directed against the genital mycoplasmas.

NONGONOCOCCAL URETHRITIS

About 40% of men who experience an initial episode of nongonococcal urethritis have infection caused by *C. trachomatis* [see 28 Diseases Due to *Chlamydia*].[37] In many cases of *Chlamydia*-negative nongonococcal urethritis (negative culture and negative serology), *U. urealyticum* may be the causative agent, as judged by (1) the presence of larger numbers of *U. urealyticum* organisms in *Chlamydia*-negative cases than in *Chlamydia*-positive cases; (2) the production of urethritis in human volunteers and nonhuman primates by intraurethral inoculation of *U. urealyticum* clinical isolates; and (3) the differential response to sulfisoxazole therapy (in one study, all 13 cases of *Chlamydia*-positive, *Ureaplasma*-negative nongonococcal urethritis responded, whereas only 14 of 30 *Chlamydia*-negative, *Ureaplasma*-positive cases responded).[37] *C. trachomatis* is susceptible to sulfonamides, but *U. urealyticum* is not. Such evidence suggests that *U. urealyticum* is the cause of at least some initial episodes of *Chlamydia*-negative nongonococcal urethritis in men—perhaps as many as 15% to 25% of these episodes.[38] Other studies have implicated *U. urealyticum* as a cause of the acute urethral syndrome in some women; this organism may also cause chronic voiding symptoms in women, which may be mistaken for interstitial cystitis.[39] It is possible that factors such as *U. urealyticum* serotype, strain-specific virulence determinants, or host factors will explain why positive cultures are not better correlated with evidence of clinical infection.

M. hominis does not appear to have a primary etiologic role in nongonococcal urethritis. However, it does appear that *M. genitalium* causes nongonococcal urethritis. One group of investigators found *M. genitalium* DNA in *C. trachomatis*–negative samples from 22% of heterosexual men with nongonococcal urethritis but from only 4% of asymptomatic control subjects.[40] Other studies have confirmed the disproportionate detection rates of *M. genitalium* in patients with nongonococcal urethritis.

Treatment

Doxycycline, 100 mg orally two times daily for 7 days, has been the treatment of choice for nongonococcal urethritis; this antibiotic seems to be equally effective in eliminating symptoms in men infected by *M. genitalium* and *C. trachomatis*.[41] Erythromycin, 250 to 500 mg orally four times daily for 7 days, has been an alternative and is the treatment of choice for pregnant women. Azithromycin, 1 g orally as a single dose, is now considered to be as effective as doxycycline for empirical treatment of nongonococcal urethritis; this conclusion applies equally well to cases associated with *U. urealyticum* and to cases associated with *C. trachomatis*.[38] Sexual contacts of an index case should be treated at the same time as the index case.

Approximately 30% of individuals with nongonococcal urethritis have persistent or recurrent symptoms despite antimicrobial therapy.[42] Tetracycline resistance has increased in recent decades and has been reported in as much as one third of clinical *U. urealyticum* isolates.[43] Resistant strains are known to cause persistent urethritis; however, they are usually sensitive to treatment with erythromycin, and the illness generally responds to this antibiotic therapy. Erythromycin-resistant *U. urealyticum* isolates arise in vivo, but their prevalence and significance are unclear.[44] Other causes of treatment failure include poor compliance with medications, reinfection, disease caused by *Trichomonas vaginalis*, herpes simplex virus, prostatitis, and noninfectious etiologies.

UPPER URINARY TRACT INFECTION

On the basis of culture and serologic data, *M. hominis* has been demonstrated to play an etiologic role in acute pyelonephritis, accounting for approximately 5% of cases.[45] However, the same association cannot be made for *U. urealyticum*. Efforts to implicate the urease of *U. urealyticum* in the formation of bladder and renal calculi have not yielded convincing evidence.

PELVIC INFLAMMATORY DISEASE

Microbiologic and serologic evidence of *M. hominis* infection can be found in a majority of women with pelvic inflammatory disease (PID).[46] In most of these cases, the organism occurs as part of a polymicrobial infection, but isolation of *M. hominis* from laparoscopic cultures of fallopian tubes in women with acute salpingitis has been reported, and the organism may be responsible for a few cases of PID on its own.[47] The prevalence of *M. hominis* involvement in PID may vary with global geographic location.

As is the case with infection caused by *C. trachomatis*, upper genital tract infection caused by *M. hominis* may often be mildly symptomatic or clinically silent. For this reason, it remains unclear how large a role *M. hominis* plays in the development of acute salpingitis and its sequelae. In contrast, *U. urealyticum* is isolated far less frequently than *M. hominis* from women with PID.

Treatment

The recommended treatment protocols for PID in the United States include tetracycline, ofloxacin, or clindamycin to provide activity against *C. trachomatis* and anaerobes. These drugs are also effective against *M. hominis*, although the tetracyclines are the drugs of choice. As with *U. urealyticum*, tetracycline-resistant clinical isolates of *M. hominis* are becoming increasingly prevalent.[48] Erythromycin has no activity against *M. hominis*.

POSTABORTION AND POSTPARTUM FEVER

Positive blood cultures and concurrent seroconversion have implicated *M. hominis* as the primary pathogen in approximately 10% of women who have fever after abortion.[35] Antimicrobial therapy is not usually required for this self-limiting infection. *M. hominis* is also a cause of fever after vaginal childbirth. Studies have indicated that this organism is responsible for 5% to 10% of cases of fever that occur more than 24 hours after delivery.[49] Women with vaginal colonization by *M. hominis* who have low or absent mycoplasmacidal antibody titers may be predisposed to postpartum fever, probably caused by endometritis. Specific therapy is not warranted in most of these cases.

OTHER CONDITIONS ASSOCIATED WITH MYCOPLASMAS

M. hominis rarely causes brain abscess, wound infection, poststernotomy mediastinitis,[50] neonatal meningitis, and other nongenitourinary infections.[51,52] These infections are more common in immunocompromised or hypogammaglobulinemic persons. *U. urealyticum* and *M. hominis* can cause septic arthritis in immunodeficient patients,[35] and *U. urealyticum* probably causes chorioamnionitis and neonatal pneumonitis.[53] It is unclear whether there are causal relations between the mycoplasmas *U. urealyticum* and *M. hominis* and infertility (male and female),[54] spontaneous abortion,[55] premature labor and low birth weight,[56] and chronic lung disease (including bronchopulmonary dysplasia[57]) in premature infants.[53] Although difficult to diagnose, *Mycoplasma* chorioamnionitis may be a better predictor of adverse pregnancy outcome than is lower genital tract colonization. Routine culture and treatment for *U. urealyticum* in these patients are not recommended.

ASSOCIATION OF MYCOPLASMAS WITH AIDS

Several *Mycoplasma* species have been cultivated from, or otherwise detected in, the blood and various internal and mucosal sites of HIV-infected individuals, leading to speculation that these organisms may play a pathogenic role in AIDS. In 1989, a strain (incognitus) of *M. fermentans* was detected directly in necrotic tissue lesions from 22 patients with AIDS and from six patients with no evidence of HIV-1 infection who later died of the *Mycoplasma* infection.[58,59] In a study that used PCR methodology, *M. fermentans* DNA sequences were amplified from the blood of 11 of HIV-seropositive patients but from none of the 26 HIV-seronegative persons.[60] *M. fermentans* is not the only *Mycoplasma* species associated with HIV-infected hosts. *M. pirum* and *M. penetrans* have each been cultivated more often from the urine of HIV-seropositive persons than from the urine of HIV-negative persons.[61] In addition, specific antibody responses to *M. penetrans* have been detected more frequently in HIV-seropositive hosts[62,63]; however, these studies have not carefully addressed the confounding role of sexual activity in *M. penetrans* transmission.

Investigators who favor a possible pathogenic role for these mycoplasmas point to some of their biologic features to support this speculation. *M. pirum* and *M. penetrans* have a tiplike structure that appears to mediate attachment and entry into host cells.[18] In addition, *M. fermentans* enhances the cytotoxicity of HIV-1 for T cell and monocytic cell lines in vitro.[64,65] Nevertheless, infection by these organisms does not predict clinical stage of HIV infection.[60,66] Other studies indicate that these mycoplasmas are found with equal frequency in healthy HIV-negative persons and in symptomatic HIV-positive persons.[67] One group of investigators have argued that *M. fermentans* cannot be important in the development of most AIDS cases because only a small proportion of AIDS patients have serologic evidence of infection by this organism, and these investigators have also argued that there is no association between the presence of *M. fermentans* and the rate of HIV disease progression.[68] Additional well-controlled studies are essential before any conclusions regarding the specificity and relevance of coinfection with mycoplasmas and HIV-1 can be reached.

Acknowledgment

Figure 1 Al Miller.

References

1. Himmelreich R, Plagens H, Hilbert H, et al: Comparative analysis of the genomes of the bacteria *Mycoplasma pneumoniae* and *Mycoplasma genitalium*. Nucleic Acids Res 25:701, 1997

2. Mushegian AR, Koonin EV: A minimal gene set for cellular life derived by comparison of complete bacterial genomes. Proc Natl Acad Sci USA 93:10268, 1996

3. Taylor-Robinson D: Infections due to species of *Mycoplasma* and *Ureaplasma*: an update. Clin Infect Dis 23:671, 1996

4. Blanchard A: Mycoplasmas and HIV infection, a possible interaction through immune activation. Wien Clin Woehenschr 109:590, 1997

5. Esposito S, Principi N: Asthma in children: are chlamydia or mycoplasma involved? Paediatr Drugs 3:159, 2001

6. Gilroy CB, Keat A, Taylor-Robinson D: The prevalence of *Mycoplasma fermentans* in patients with inflammatory arthritides. Rheumatology (Oxford) 40:1355, 2001

7. Foy HM, Kenny GE, Cooney MK, et al: Long-term epidemiology of infections with *Mycoplasma pneumoniae*. J Infect Dis 139:681, 1979

8. Mufson MA, Chang V, Gill V, et al: The role of viruses, mycoplasmas and bacteria in acute pneumonia in civilian adults. Am J Epidemiol 86:526, 1967

9. Clyde WA Jr: Clinical overview of typical *Mycoplasma pneumoniae* infections. Clin Infect Dis 17(suppl 1):S32, 1993

10. Broughton RA: Infections due to *Mycoplasma pneumoniae* in childhood. Pediatr Infect Dis 5:71, 1986

11. Baseman JB, Dallo SF, Tully JG, et al: Isolation and characterization of *Mycoplasma genitalium* strains from the human respiratory tract. J Clin Microbiol 26:2266, 1988

12. Gnarpe J, Lundback A, Sundelof B, et al: Prevalence of *Mycoplasma pneumoniae* in subjectively healthy individuals. Scand J Infect Dis 24:161, 1992

13. Gupta SK, Sarosi GA: The role of atypical pathogens in community-acquired pneumonia. Med Clin North Am 85:1349, 2001

14. Toikka P, Juven T, Virkki R, et al: *Streptococcus pneumoniae* and *Mycoplasma pneumoniae* coinfection in community-acquired pneumonia. Arch Dis Child 83:413, 2000

15. Broome CV, LaVenture M, Kaye HS, et al: An explosive outbreak of *Mycoplasma pneumoniae* infection in a summer camp. Pediatrics 66:884, 1980

16. Krause DC: *Mycoplasma pneumoniae* cytadherence: unravelling the tie that binds. Mol Microbiol 20:247, 1996

17. Hu PC, Cole RM, Huang YS, et al: *Mycoplasma pneumoniae* infection: role of a surface protein in the attachment organelle. Science 216: 313, 1982

18. Baseman JB, Tully JG: Mycoplasmas: sophisticated, reemerging, and burdened by their notoriety. Emerg Infect Dis 3:21, 1997

19. Chan ED, Welsh CH: Fulminant *Mycoplasma pneumoniae* pneumonia. West J Med 162:133, 1995

20. Foy HM, Kenny GE, Cooney MK, et al: Naturally acquired immunity to pneumonia due to *Mycoplasma pneumoniae*. J Infect Dis 147:967, 1983

21. Gelfand EW: Unique susceptibility of patients with antibody deficiency to mycoplasma infection. Clin Infect Dis 17 (suppl 1):S250, 1993

22. Ali NJ, Sillis M, Andrews BE, et al: The clinical spectrum and diagnosis of *Mycoplasma pneumoniae* infection. Mycoplasma Q J Med New Series 58:241, 1986

23. Roberts DB: The etiology of bullous myringitis and the role of mycoplasmas in ear disease: a review. Pediatrics 65:761, 1980

24. Cherry JD: Anemia and mucocutaneous lesions due to *Mycoplasma pneumoniae* infections. Clin Infect Dis 17(suppl 1):S47, 1993

25. Smith R, Eviatar L: Neurologic manifestations of *Mycoplasma pneumoniae* infections: diverse spectrum of diseases: a report of six cases and review of the literature. Clin Pediatr (Phila) 39:195, 2000

26. Bitnun A, Ford-Jones EL, Petric M, et al: Acute childhood encephalitis and *Mycoplasma pneumoniae*. Clin Infect Dis 32:1674, 2001

27. Tay YK, Huff JC, Weston WL: *Mycoplasma pneumoniae* infection is associated with Stevens-Johnson syndrome, not erythema multiforme (von Hebra). J Am Acad Dermatol 35:757, 1996

28. Kenney RT, Li JS, Clyde WA Jr, et al: Mycoplasmal pericarditis: evidence of invasive disease. Clin Infect Dis 17(suppl 1):S58, 1993

29. Griffin JP: Rapid screening for cold agglutinins in pneumonia. Ann Intern Med 70:701, 1969

30. Kenny GE, Kaiser GG, Cooney MK, et al: Diagnosis of *Mycoplasma pneumoniae* pneumonia: sensitivities and specificities of serology with lipid antigen and isolation of the organism on soy peptone medium for identification of infections. J Clin Microbiol 28: 2087, 1990

31. Petitjean J, Vabret A, Gouarin S, et al: Evaluation of four commercial immunoglobulin G (IgG)- and IgM-specific enzyme immunoassays for diagnosis of *Mycoplasma pneumoniae* infections. J Clin Microbiol 40:165, 2002

32. Ieven M, Goossens H: Relevance of nucleic acid amplification techniques for diagnosis of respiratory tract infections in the clinical laboratory. Clin Microbiol Rev 10:242, 1997

33. Ferwerda A, Moll HA, de Groot R: Respiratory tract infections by *Mycoplasma pneumoniae* in children: a review of diagnostic and therapeutic measures. Eur J Pediatr 160:483, 2001

34. Block S, Hedrick J, Hammerschlag MR, et al: *Mycoplasma pneumoniae* and *Chlamydia pneumoniae* in pediatric community-acquired pneumonia: comparative efficacy and safety of clarithromycin vs. erythromycin ethylsuccinate. Pediatr Infect Dis J 14:471, 1995

35. Taylor-Robinson D, Furr PM: Genital mycoplasma infections. Wien Klin Wochenschr 109:578, 1997

36. Taylor-Robinson D: *Mycoplasma genitalium*: an update. Int J STD AIDS 13:145, 2002

37. Bowie WR, Wang S, Alexander ER, et al: Etiology of nongonococcal urethritis: evidence for *Chlamydia trachomatis* and *Ureaplasma urealyticum*. J Clin Invest 59:735, 1977

38. Stamm WE, Hicks CB, Martin DH, et al: Azithromycin for empirical treatment of the nongonococcal urethritis syndrome in men. JAMA 274:545, 1995

39. Potts JM, Ward AM, Rackley RR: Association of chronic urinary symptoms in women and *Ureaplasma urealyticum*. Urology 55:486, 2000

40. Totten PA, Schwartz MA, Sjostrom KE, et al: Association of *Mycoplasma genitalium* with nongonococcal urethritis in heterosexual men. J Infect Dis 183:269, 2001

41. Deguchi T, Maeda S: *Mycoplasma genitalium*: another important pathogen of nongonococcal urethritis. J Urol 167:1210, 2002

42. Wong ES, Hooton TM, Hill CC, et al: Clinical and microbiological features of persistent or recurrent nongonococcal urethritis in men. J Infect Dis 158:1098, 1988

43. Chua KB, Ngeow YF, Ng KB, et al: *Ureaplasma urealyticum* and *Mycoplasma hominis* isolation from cervical secretions of pregnant women and nasopharyngeal secretions of their babies at delivery. Singapore Med J 39:300, 1998

44. Palu G, Valisena S, Barile MF, et al: Mechanisms of macrolide resistance in *Ureaplasma urealyticum*: a study on collection and clinical strains. Eur J Epidemiol 5:146, 1989

45. Thomsen AC: Occurrence and pathogenicity of *Mycoplasma hominis* in the upper urinary tract: a review. Sex Transm Dis 10(4 suppl):323, 1983

46. Kinghorn GR, Duerden BI, Hafiz S: Clinical and microbiological investigation of women with acute salpingitis and their consorts. Br J Obstet Gynaecol 93:869, 1986

47. Stacey CM, Munday PE, Taylor-Robinson D, et al: A longitudinal study of pelvic inflammatory disease. Br J Obstet Gynaecol 99:994, 1992

48. McCormack WM: Susceptibility of mycoplasmas to antimicrobial agents: clinical implications. Clin Infect Dis 17(suppl 1):S200, 1993

49. Moller BR: The role of mycoplasmas in the upper genital tract of women. Sex Trnsm Dis 10:281, 1983

50. Sielaff TD, Everett JE, Shumway SJ, et al: *Mycoplasma hominis* infections occurring in cardiovascular surgical patients. Ann Thorac Surg 61: 99, 1996

51. Madoff S, Hooper DC: Nongenitourinary infections caused by *Mycoplasma hominis* in adults. Rev Infect Dis 10:602, 1988

52. McMahon DK, Dummer JS, Pasculle AW, et al: Extragenital *Mycoplasma hominis* infections in adults. Am J Med 89:275, 1990

53. Waites KB, Crouse DT, Cassell GH: Systemic neonatal infection due to *Ureaplasma urealyticum*. Clin Infect Dis 17(suppl 1):S131, 1993

54. Stray-Pedersen B: Repercussion of mycoplasmas on male and female sterility. Acta Eur Fertil 16:101, 1985

55. Donders GG, Van Bulck B, Caudron J, et al: Relationship of bacterial vaginosis and mycoplasmas to the risk of spontaneous abortion. Am J Obstet Gynecol 183:431, 2000

56. Berman SM, Harrison HR, Boyce WT, et al: Low birth weight, prematurity, and postpartum endometritis. Association with prenatal cervical *Mycoplasma hominis* and *Chlamydia trachomatis* infections. JAMA 257:1189, 1987

57. Cassell GH, Waites KB, Watson HL, et al: *Ureaplasma urealyticum* intrauterine infection: role in prematurity and disease in newborns. Clin Microbiol Rev 6:69, 1993

58. Lo S-C, Dawson MS, Wong DM, et al: Identification of *Mycoplasma incognitus* infection in patients with AIDS: an immunohistochemical, in situ hybridization and ultrastructural study. Am J Trop Med Hyg 41:601, 1989

59. Lo S-C, Dawson MS, Newton PB, et al: Association of the virus-like infectious agent originally reported in patients with AIDS with acute fatal disease in previously healthy non-AIDS patients. Am J Trop Med Hyg 41:364, 1989

60. Hawkins RE, Rickman LS, Vermund SH, et al: Association of mycoplasma and human immunodeficiency virus infection: detection of amplified *Mycoplasma fermentans* DNA in blood. J Infect Dis 165:581, 1992

61. Lo S-C, Hayes MM, Wang RY-H, et al: Newly discovered mycoplasma isolated from patients infected with HIV. Lancet 338:1415, 1991

62. Wang RY-H, Shih JW-K, Grandinetti T, et al: High frequency of antibodies to *Mycoplasma penetrans* in HIV-infected patients. Lancet 340: 1312, 1992

63. Grau O, Slizewicz B, Tuppin P, et al: Association of *Mycoplasma penetrans* with human immunodeficiency virus infection. J Infect Dis 172:672, 1995

64. Lo S-C, Tsai S, Benish JR, et al: Enhancement of HIV-1 cytocidal effects in CD4+ lymphocytes by the AIDS-associated mycoplasma. Science 251:1074, 1991

65. Lemaitre M, Henin Y, Destouesse F, et al: Role of mycoplasma infection in the cytopathic effect induced by human immunodeficiency virus type 1 in infected cell lines. Infect Immun 60:742, 1992

66. Katseni VL, Gilroy CB, Ryait BK, et al: *Mycoplasma fermentans* in individuals seropositive and seronegative for HIV-1. Lancet 341:271, 1993

67. Hakkarainen K, Jansson E, Ranki A, et al: Serological responses to mycoplasmas in HIV-infected and non-infected individuals. AIDS 6: 1287, 1992

68. Ainsworth JG, Hourshid S, Easterbrook PJ, et al: *Mycoplasma* species in rapid and slow HIV progressors. Int J STD AIDS 11:76, 2000

28 Diseases Due to *Chlamydia*

Walter E. Stamm, M.D.

The chlamydiae are obligate intracellular bacteria that produce a wide variety of infections in many mammalian and avian species.[1] Three species of *Chlamydia* infect humans: *C. trachomatis, C. psittaci,* and *C. pneumoniae* [*see Table 1*]. *C. trachomatis* is exclusively a human pathogen and is transmitted from person to person via sexual contact, perinatal transmission, or close contact in households. *C. trachomatis* causes trachoma in arid developing parts of the world and is a major cause of sexually transmitted and perinatal infections worldwide. In the United States, *C. trachomatis* infection is the most common reportable infectious disease.[2] *C. psittaci,* in contrast, is more widely distributed in nature, producing genital, conjunctival, intestinal, or respiratory infections in many avian and mammalian species.[3] Humans are occasionally infected by avian strains after contact with infected birds, incurring a pneumonitis or a systemic infection termed psittacosis.

C. pneumoniae, the third chlamydial species that infects humans, was identified and characterized in the 1980s.[4] It is a fastidious organism that produces upper respiratory tract infection and pneumonitis in both children and adults.[5] Recent studies have also linked *C. pneumoniae* infection to atherosclerotic cardiovascular disease and perhaps to other illnesses, such as asthma and sarcoidosis.[6] Transmission is believed to occur via aerosol droplets; no animal reservoir has been identified.

All chlamydiae share a unique life cycle characteristic of the genus [*see Figure 1*].[7] The organism is transmitted in an extracellular nonreplicating form known as the elementary body. The elementary body adheres to and is phagocytosed into a host epithelial cell. Once inside the epithelial cell, the elementary body transforms into the intracellular replicative form of the organism, the reticulate body. Reticulate bodies divide by binary fission within membrane-bound vacuoles called inclusions. After approximately 36 hours, reticulate bodies condense into elementary bodies, the inclusion ruptures, and the elementary bodies disperse to infect adjacent epithelial cells or to be transmitted to other hosts. A unique feature of the chlamydial inclusion is its ability to resist lysosomal fusion; the mechanism of resistance is as yet unknown. The intracellular milieu also provides the organism with nutrients and serves as a refuge from host immune defense mechanisms.

Although chlamydiae were initially thought to be large viruses, they in fact possess both DNA and RNA, have a cell wall and ribosomes similar to those of gram-negative bacteria, and are inhibited by a variety of antimicrobials (see below).[7] *C. trachomatis, C. psittaci,* and *C. pneumoniae* all share a genus-specific lipopolysaccharide antigen. The commonly available complement fixation test for *Chlamydia* measures antibodies against this antigen. The three species can be differentiated serologically with the microimmunofluorescence test, which is directed against epitopes in the major outer membrane protein (MOMP).

Characteristically, chlamydial species produce chronic, persistent, and often asymptomatic infections of the epithelial lining of the eye, respiratory tract, and urogenital tract. Infection of epithelial cells induces secretion of cytokines and initiation of an innate immune response. Induction and persistence of a chronic inflammatory response may eventually result in fibrosis, scarring, and other chronic sequelae of infection.[8]

In cell cultures, chlamydia species are susceptible to many antimicrobials, including tetracycline, doxycycline, erythromycin, azithromycin, rifampin, clindamycin, ofloxacin, and levofloxacin. Although antibiotic-resistant strains of *Chlamydia* have been described, clinical antimicrobial resistance has yet to become a frequent problem in treating chlamydial infections.[9]

Diseases Due to *C. trachomatis*

Unlike *C. pneumoniae,* which appears to have only a single serotype, and *C. psittaci,* whose number of

Table 1 Comparative Features of *Chlamydia* species

Species	C. trachomatis	C. psittaci	C. pneumoniae
Natural hosts	Humans	Birds, mammals	Humans
Mode of transmission	Sexual; close personal contact; maternal/infant	Zoonotic	Respiratory droplets
Typical diseases	STDs, LGV, trachoma	Pneumonia, psittacosis	Upper respiratory infections, pneumonia, atherosclerotic vascular disease
Risk groups	STDs: sexually active adolescents and young adults Trachoma: young children in arid, unhygienic, crowded conditions	Bird fanciers, pet-shop workers, veterinarians, animal and poultry workers	Young children, older adults
Number of serotypes	18	Unknown	1

LGV—lymphogranuloma venereum STDs—sexually transmitted diseases

serotypes is unknown, *C. trachomatis* has at least 18 distinct serotypes (serovars).[10] These serotypes confer tissue tropism and disease specificity: serovars A, B, Ba, and C are associated with trachoma, whereas serovars D through K are associated with sexually transmitted and perinatally acquired infections. Serovars L1, L2, and L3 are more invasive than the other serovars, spread to lymphatic tissue, and grow readily in macrophages; they produce the clinical syndromes of lymphogranuloma venereum and hemorrhagic proctocolitis. In addition to these more commonly reported syndromes, *C. trachomatis* has been reported as an infrequent cause of other infections, including endocarditis, peritonitis, pleuritis, and periappendicitis.[11]

LABORATORY DIAGNOSIS

Laboratory testing for *C. trachomatis* has evolved considerably over the past decade. Four types of confirmatory procedures are now available: (1) direct microscopic examination of swabs or tissue scrapings utilizing fluorescent antibody staining (DFA); (2) cell culture isolation of the organism; (3) detection of chlamydial antigens or genes in specimens by immunologic means or nucleic acid amplification testing; and (4) serologic testing for antibodies to *C. trachomatis* [*see Table* 2].

Except in cases of inclusion conjunctivitis, DFA has largely been abandoned for diagnosis of chlamydial infection. Even in inclusion conjunctivitis, nucleic acid amplification testing of conjunctival smears is probably a better choice because of its higher sensitivity. Cell culture techniques for isolation of *Chlamydia* are not widely available and have numerous drawbacks: culture has exacting requirements for specimen transport and is technically demanding and expensive; moreover, its sensitivity is only 60% to 80% of that of newer diagnostic tests.[12] For those reasons, nonculture alternatives utilizing antigen or gene detection are the diagnostic methods of choice in most cases. The least expensive and most widely used of the nonculture tests are enzyme-linked immunoassays that detect chlamydial antigens on urethral or endocervical swabs. These tests, however, have limited sensitivity and specificity and cannot be used to test vaginal swabs or urine for *Chlamydia*.

The newer nucleic acid amplification tests, such as polymerase chain reaction (PCR), ligase chain reaction (LCR), and transcription-mediated amplification (TMA), are the most sensitive and specific of the currently available tests.[13] Uniquely, these tests have high accuracy even when used on specimens that contain only small numbers of organisms (e.g., first-void urine or vaginal swabs). The ability to use such specimens is of particular importance because their ease of collection facilitates patient compliance and community-based screening programs.

Serologic tests are of little value in the diagnosis of most chlamydial ocular or genital infections.[14] They are useful only in invasive syndromes such as pelvic inflammatory disease, epididymitis, lymphogranuloma venereum, and infant pneumonia, which are associated with significant increases in both microimmunofluorescence and complement-fixing antibodies.

SEXUALLY TRANSMITTED DISEASES

C. trachomatis is the most common bacterial cause of sexually transmitted disease (STD) in the United States, being responsible for an estimated four million cases a year.[2] The spectrum of illness

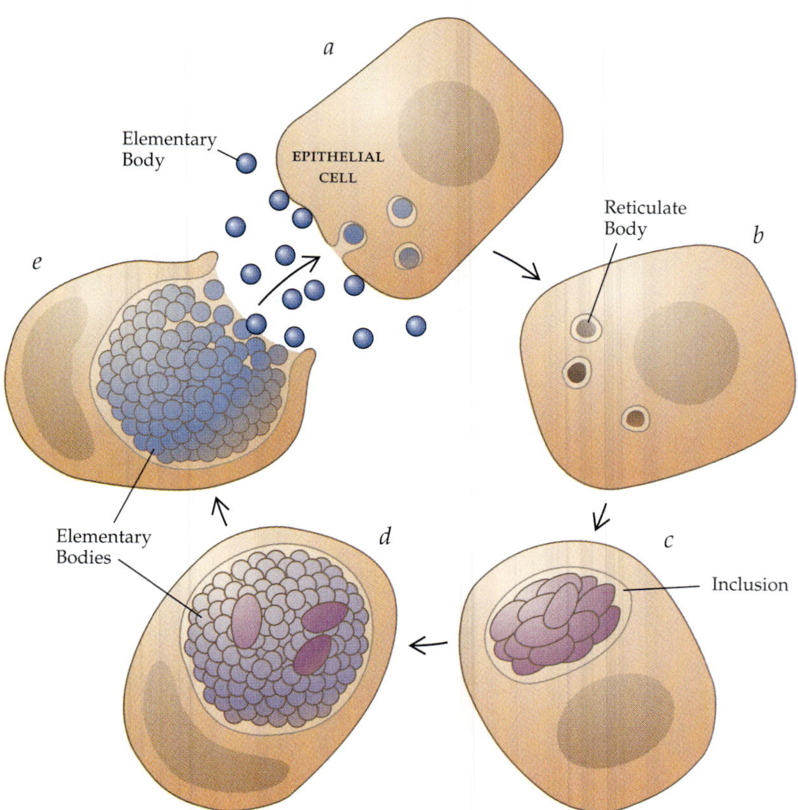

Figure 1 **(*a*) Chlamydiae are transmitted in an extracellular nonreplicating form known as the elementary body. The elementary body adheres to and is phagocytosed into a host epithelial cell. (*b*) Once inside the epithelial cell, the elementary body transforms into the intracellular replicative form of the organism, the reticulate body. (*c*) Reticulate bodies divide by binary fission within membrane-bound vacuoles called inclusions. (*d*) The reticulate bodies then reorganize into elementary bodies; multiplication stops. (*e*) After 35 to 40 hours, the inclusion ruptures, and elementary bodies are released to infect adjacent epithelial cells or to be transmitted to other hosts.**

attributable to these infections parallels that of gonococcal infection. In men, the most common syndromes are nongonococcal urethritis and acute epididymitis. In women, mucopurulent cervicitis, urethritis, bartholinitis, acute salpingitis, and perihepatitis are the syndromes most commonly seen. Inclusion conjunctivitis, proctitis, and Reiter syndrome affect both sexes.

Sexually transmitted *C. trachomatis* infection has a widespread distribution and a high incidence and prevalence in adolescents and young adults in the United States and Europe.[15] The age of peak incidence is the late teens and early 20s. Prevalence has been reported at 3% to 8% in general medical clinics and urban high schools, over 10% in asymptomatic military personnel undergoing routine physical examination, and as high as 15% to 20% in men and women attending STD clinics.[16,17] The highest prevalences of infection have been observed in persons who are single, have multiple sexual partners, are not using barrier contraception, report genital symptoms, have an infected sexual partner, or are attending a high-risk clinic such as an STD clinic. As many as 90% of infections in many settings may be asymptomatic and are thus discoverable only by screening. Recurrent chlamydial infections—often from untreated sexual partners—are common in high-risk groups.[18]

C. trachomatis initially infects the columnar epithelium of the genital tract and induces an inflammatory response that may persist for months or years. Serious sequelae, such as scarring of the fallopian tubes and damage to the upper genital tract,

Table 2 Clinical Characteristics of Common *C. trachomatis* Infections in Adults

	Infection	*Symptoms and Signs*	*Presumptive Diagnosis*	*Definitive Diagnosis*	*Treatment*
Men	Nongonococcal urethritis	Urethral discharge, dysuria	Urethral leukocytosis; no gonococci seen	Urine or urethral NAAT	Azithromycin, 1 g p.o. (single dose) *or* Doxycycline, 100 mg p.o., b.i.d., for 7 days
	Epididymitis	Unilateral epididymal tenderness, swelling; pain; fever; presence of NGU	Urethral leukocytosis; pyuria on urinalysis	Urine or urethral NAAT; urine culture	Outpatient: Ofloxacin, 300 mg b.i.d. for 10 days *or* Ceftriaxone, 1 g I.M., plus doxycycline, 100 mg p.o., b.i.d., for 7 days
	Proctitis	Rectal pain, discharge, bleeding; history of receptive anal intercourse	≥ 1 PMNs/OIF on rectal Gram stain; no gonococci seen	Rectal culture or DFA (NAAT untested)	Doxycycline, 100 mg p.o., b.i.d., for 7 days
	Conjunctivitis	Ocular pain, redness, discharge, simultaneous genital infection	Gram stain of conjunctival swab negative for bacterial pathogens; PMNs on smear	DFA or NAAT on conjunctival swab	Azithromycin, 1 g p.o. (single dose) *or* Doxycycline, 100 mg p.o., b.i.d., for 7 days
Women	Cervicitis	Mucopurulent cervical discharge; cervical bleeding; cervical edema	≥ 20 PMNs/OIF on cervical Gram stain	Urine or cervical NAAT	Azithromycin, 1 g p.o. (single dose) *or* Doxycycline, 100 mg p.o., b.i.d., for 7 days
	Urethritis	Dysuria, frequency; no hematuria	Pyuria on UA; negative urine Gram stain and culture	Urine, cervical, or urethral NAAT	Azithromycin, 1 g, p.o. (single dose) *or* Doxycycline, 100 mg p.o., b.i.d., for 7 days
	Salpingitis	Lower abdominal pain, adnexal pain, cervical motion tenderness	Evidence of mucopurulent cervicitis	Urine or cervical NAAT	Outpatient: Ofloxacin, 400 mg b.i.d., p.o., plus metronidazole, 500 mg p.o., b.i.d., for 14 days *or* Ceftriaxone, 250 g I.M. plus doxycycline, 100 mg p.o., b.i.d., for 14 days
	Conjunctivitis	Ocular pain, redness, discharge; simultaneous genital infection	Gram stain of conjunctival swab negative for bacterial pathogens; PMNs on smear	DFA or NAAT on conjunctival swab	Azithromycin, 1 g p.o. (single dose) *or* Doxycycline, 100 mg p.o., b.i.d., for 7 days

DFA—direct fluorescent antibody NAAT—nucleic acid amplification test NGU—nongonococcal urethritis OIF—oil-immersion field PMN—polymorphonuclear neutrophil UA—urinalysis

occur most often with repeated or persistent infections.[19] The mechanism through which repeated infection induces inflammation and subsequent complications is not clear. The *C. trachomatis* 60 kd heat shock protein has been implicated in these deleterious inflammatory responses and may induce antibodies that cross-react with human heat-shock protein. Other chlamydial proteins also may be important in this process.[20] Host genetic susceptibility may also play a role: persons with particular HLA haplotypes appear to be more susceptible to scarring with either genital or ocular infection.[21]

Nongonococcal Urethritis

Diagnosis Nongonococcal urethritis (NGU), the most common chlamydial urogenital infection in men, typically presents with burning pain on urination, urethral discharge, or urethral itching. A discharge from the urethra may be apparent on observation or may be visible only after stripping the urethra. The discharge is generally clear or mucoid, but it may be mucopurulent or purulent.[22] However, up to half of the men with *C. trachomatis* infection of the urethra will have no clinical manifestations of urethritis. Many of these patients will nevertheless have an increased number of leukocytes on Gram stain of a urethral smear. A presumptive diagnosis of NGU can be made on the basis of a leukocytic urethral exudate (≥ 4 polymorphonuclear leukocytes [PMNs] per 1,000× oil-immersion field) in the absence of concurrent gonococcal infection by Gram stain or culture [*see Table* 2]. About 40% of such cases of presumptive NGU are caused by *Chlamydia;* the remainder are caused by *Ureaplasma urealyticum, Mycoplasma genitalium,* and other microbes.[23] The specific diagnosis of chlamydial infection can be confirmed by a nucleic acid amplification assay such as PCR or LCR, an antigen detection test, or culture.

Treatment Men with presumed or confirmed NGU should be treated with oral doxycycline, 100 mg twice a day for 7 days, or azithromycin, 1 g orally as a single dose. The two regimens appear equally effective.[24] The azithromycin regimen offers the advantage of single-dose therapy but is considerably more expensive. Female partners of men with NGU should be examined and treated for presumed concomitant chlamydial infection.

Epididymitis

In 1% to 2% of men with chlamydial urethritis, the infection ascends in the genital tract to cause acute epididymitis. *C. trachomatis* is the major cause of acute epididymitis in heterosexual men younger than 35 years; other causes include *Neisseria gonorrhoeae* and, less commonly, urinary pathogens such as *Escherichia coli* or *Pseudomonas aeruginosa*.[25] Urinary pathogens are a more common cause of epididymitis in homosexual men who practice rectal intercourse and in men older than 35 years who have had urologic instrumentation or surgery.

Diagnosis Epididymitis caused by *C. trachomatis* typically presents as unilateral scrotal pain, fever, and epididymal tenderness and swelling. Testicular torsion should be excluded by a radionuclide scan or Doppler flow study if the diagnosis is in doubt.

Treatment In some patients, epididymitis may be mild enough to be treated on an outpatient basis with oral antibiotics. In other cases, hospitalization is required for management of pain and initiation of parenteral antibiotics. Initial empirical therapy with ofloxacin, 300 mg orally or intravenously twice daily, is recommended until the etiologic agent is identified [*see Table* 2].[26]

Mucopurulent Cervicitis

Endocervical infection with *C. trachomatis* is considered the female counterpart of male urethritis.[27]

Diagnosis *C. trachomatis* cervical infection is often clinically silent, although a careful speculum examination will reveal mucopurulent cervicitis in some cases. When clinical manifestations are present, they are nonspecific—for example, vaginal discharge, vaginal bleeding, lower abdominal pain, or dysuria. On examination, findings include a yellow or green mucopurulent discharge from the endocervical os, the presence of cervical ectropion, edema in the area of ectropion, and easily induced mucosal bleeding.[27] A Gram stain of the endocervical exudate typically shows large numbers of PMNs. Women with suspected mucopurulent cervicitis should be evaluated for both chlamydial and gonococcal infection [*see Table* 2].

Treatment Chlamydial mucopurulent cervicitis is best treated with a single dose of 1 g of azithromycin. This regimen is effective and safe. Although more expensive than doxycycline, azithromycin is cost-effective because adolescents often fail to complete a 7-day course of doxycycline.[28] Unlike doxycycline, azithromycin appears to be safe during pregnancy and is used by many practitioners for treatment of chlamydial mucopurulent cervicitis or cervical infection in pregnant women.[29] Sexual partners of women found to have chlamydial cervical infection or mucopurulent cervicitis should be examined and empirically treated for chlamydial infection.

Acute Urethral Syndrome in Women

In women presenting with dysuria, frequency, and pyuria, *C. trachomatis* is the pathogen that is most commonly identified if urine cultures fail to find *E. coli, Staphylococcus saprophyticus,* or other uropathogens.[30] Chlamydial infection should be considered to be the cause of so-called dysuria-pyuria syndrome when the urine culture does not demonstrate expected urinary bacterial pathogens, symptoms have been present for more than 7 days, the patient has a new sexual partner, or concomitant mucopurulent cervicitis is present on examination.[30,31]

Pelvic Inflammatory Disease

C. trachomatis is thought to account for about half of all cases of pelvic inflammatory disease (PID) in the United States.[32] Ascending intraluminal spread of *C. trachomatis* from the lower genital tract can produce endometritis, endosalpingitis, and pelvic peritonitis. On examination, evidence of mucopurulent cervicitis is generally found in women who have laparoscopically verified salpingitis due to *C. trachomatis*.

Diagnosis Chlamydial salpingitis often produces fewer clinical symptoms and signs than gonococcal or anaerobic salpingitis.[33] However, patients often present with lower abdominal pain, adnexal tenderness, vaginal discharge or bleeding, and uterine tenderness. They may or may not have fever.

Treatment Empirical treatment of PID must provide antimicrobial coverage for the major pathogens, including *C. trachomatis*, *N. gonorrhoeae*, and vaginal anaerobes [*see Table 2*]. Screening of high-risk young women for chlamydial cervical infection followed by treatment has been shown to prevent subsequent PID in a prospective cohort study.[34] Thus, chlamydial screening of all sexually active adolescent girls and women younger than 25 years with new sexual partners is strongly recommended.[35]

Complications Infertility and ectopic pregnancy are important sequelae of chlamydial tubal infection. Antecedent *C. trachomatis* PID has been linked to infertility from fallopian tube scarring. In more recent studies, demonstration of persistent, slowly replicating *C. trachomatis* in tubal tissue suggests that these patients may have chronic infection.

Perihepatitis, or Fitzhugh-Curtis syndrome, develops in a subset of women with chlamydial salpingitis. These patients present with right upper quadrant pain, fever, and often adnexal tenderness. The diagnosis can be established with an endocervical nucleic acid amplification test for chlamydia or by demonstration of high titers of antibody to *C. trachomatis*.

Acute Proctitis

Men who practice receptive anal intercourse may develop acute proctitis from *C. trachomatis* strains of serovars D through K or, rarely, L1 through L3.[36] Since 1998, chlamydial proctitis has been resurgent in homosexual and bisexual men in the United States.[37] These infections occasionally develop in heterosexual women. The severity of disease ranges from asymptomatic (which generally occurs in patients infected with serovars D through K) to severe (generally, serovars L1 through L3).

Diagnosis Patients with severe infection typically present with rectal pain, a rectal mucosal discharge, tenesmus, and rectal bleeding. Characteristically, a rectal Gram stain shows one or more PMNs per 1000× oil-immersion field and anoscopy demonstrates a mucopurulent discharge and easily induced mucosal bleeding.[36] The specific diagnosis can be made by rectal culture for *Chlamydia* or by a chlamydial DFA. The sensitivity and specificity of the newer nucleic acid amplification tests for rectal specimens has not been extensively studied, and these tests are not approved for this purpose.

Treatment Treatment regimens for chlamydial proctitis have not been extensively studied. Nevertheless, a 7-day regimen of doxycycline (100 mg b.i.d.) is recommended for cases caused by serovars D through K, and a 21-day course is recommended for cases caused by serovars L1 through L3 [*see Table 2*].

Reiter Syndrome

An unusual complication of chlamydial urethritis, Reiter syndrome (more recently termed reactive arthritis) consists of conjunctivitis, urethritis (or cervicitis in women), oligoarthritis, and characteristic lesions of the skin and mucous membranes. Although the pathogenesis of Reiter syndrome is obscure, more than 80% of affected patients have the HLA B27 haplotype, so a genetic predisposition is clearly involved.[38] Recent studies have found chlamydial antigens and genes in the involved joints, suggesting that viable *Chlamydia* organisms migrate from the urethra to the synovial tissue in these cases.

Lymphogranuloma Venereum

Lymphogranuloma venereum (LGV) is a sexually transmitted infection caused by *C. trachomatis* strains of the L1, L2, and L3 serovars. Typically, the disease begins with a transient primary genital lesion, followed by multilocular suppurative regional lymphadenopathy and, sometimes, hemorrhagic proctitis with associated regional lymphadenitis.[39] The acute phase of the disease is generally associated with fever, leukocytosis, and in some cases proctitis. Possible late complications include genital elephantiasis, rectal strictures, and fistulas of the penis, urethra, and rectum.

Epidemiology LGV occurs primarily in the second and third decades of life and is approximately four times more common in men than in women. Worldwide, the incidence is declining, but the disease is still endemic in parts of Asia, Africa, South America, and the Caribbean. The disease is rare in the United States, with only 186 cases reported in 1995. In the United States, many cases involve travelers or military personnel returning from endemic areas; most microbiologically confirmed cases have been in homosexual or bisexual men.[40]

Clinical manifestations The initial lesion of LGV in heterosexual persons is often a papule, vesicle, or ulcer on the penis or, in women, on the labia. This lesion typically heals without scarring. LGV strains of *C. trachomatis* have occasionally been recovered from these genital ulcers, as well as from the urethra of men or the endocervix of women who present with inguinal adenopathy. It is thus not entirely clear whether the most important primary site of infection is the skin lesion, the urethra, or the endocervix. Alternatively, primary anal or rectal infection may develop in men or women after receptive rectal intercourse.[41] Initial inoculation of the oral mucosa can also occur, leading to primary oral or pharyngeal lesions that may go unnoticed until adenopathy develops.

From the initial site of primary infection (urogenital, anal, rectal, or oral), the organism spreads to adjacent regional lymphatics. Typically, penile, vulvar, or anal infections spread to the inguinal and femoral lymph nodes. Rectal infection produces hypogastric and deep iliac lymphadenitis, whereas upper vaginal or cervical infection may result in obturator and iliac lymphadenitis. Heterosexual men with urogenital infection commonly display the so-called inguinal syndrome, which consists of painful inguinal lymphadenopathy developing approximately 2 to 6 weeks after the presumed exposure. Adenopathy generally is unilateral, with palpable enlargement of the iliac and femoral nodes on the same side as the enlarged inguinal nodes. Although the nodes may be discrete at first, they increasingly become matted, fluctuant, and suppurative. The overlying skin becomes fixed and inflamed and eventually develops multiple draining fistulas. Enlargement of lymph nodes both above and below the inguinal ligament may produce the so-called sign of the groove. On biopsy, the infected nodes have small abscesses surrounded by histiocytes. Spontaneous healing may occur after several months, but scarring and granulomatous masses often persist.

In the United States, LGV proctitis has increasingly been recognized in homosexual men. These patients present with rectal pain and mucopurulent bloody rectal discharge.[42] They often complain of tenesmus and such systemic signs and symptoms as fever, malaise, and weakness. Sigmoidoscopy reveals ulcerative proctocolitis with a purulent exudate and mucosal bleeding.

During the active development of regional lymphadenopathy, many patients experience extensive constitutional symptoms, including fever, chills, headache, meningismus, myalgia, and arthralgias. Complications may include arthritis, aseptic meningitis, encephalitis, hepatitis, and arthritis. If left untreated, rectal infections may eventually progress to perirectal abscesses, anal fistula, and fistulas involving the rectum, the vagina, the bladder, and the pelvic musculature. Rectal strictures are a late complication, as is elephantiasis due to associated lymphatic obstruction.[26]

Laboratory tests LGV is most readily diagnosed serologically. Both the LGV complement fixation test and the microimmunofluorescence test become strongly positive soon after the onset of lymphadenopathy. Alternatively, demonstration of *C. trachomatis* by culture or nucleic acid amplification tests from urethral or cervical specimens or from pus aspirated from buboes can confirm the diagnosis.

Differential diagnosis LGV must be differentiated from other sexually transmitted conditions that produce genital ulcers and associated adenopathy. These include genital herpes simplex virus (HSV) infection, syphilis, chancroid, and granuloma inguinale. The clinical presentation, epidemiologic circumstances, and specific laboratory testing can usually differentiate these conditions unambiguously.

Treatment Doxycycline, 100 mg orally twice daily for 21 days, is generally recommended for treatment of LGV, despite the absence of trials demonstrating its efficacy. Alternative agents include erythromycin and sulfonamides.

PERINATAL INFECTIONS

Depending on the population tested, 5% to 25% of pregnant women have *C. trachomatis* infection of the cervix. A high proportion of infants born to these infected women will acquire *C. trachomatis* infection during passage through the birth canal.[35] If not identified and treated, the infection may persist for months or years.[43]

Clinically apparent neonatal inclusion conjunctivitis develops in approximately 50% to 60% of infants with perinatally acquired *C. trachomatis* infection.[44] In addition, *C. trachomatis* can often be isolated from the rectum, vagina, and nasopharynx of these infants.[45] Approximately 10% of perinatally infected infants experience a distinctive afebrile pneumonitis-like syndrome.[46]

Neonatal chlamydial conjunctivitis typically develops 5 to 14 days after birth and generally presents as a mucopurulent ocular discharge. Other causes of neonatal conjunctivitis—such as *N. gonorrhoeae, Haemophilus influenzae, Streptococcus pneumoniae,* and HSV—should also be considered. The diagnosis can be readily confirmed by DFA of a conjunctival smear or by PCR or LCR testing of the discharge. Because infants tend to be infected at multiple sites, systemic therapy is indicated, generally with erythromycin, 50 mg/kg/day orally in four divided doses for 10 to 14 days.

To prevent neonatal infection, all pregnant women should be screened for *C. trachomatis* infection in the third trimester, preferably with a nucleic acid amplification test. Those women found to be infected should be treated with a single 1 g oral dose of azithromycin; amoxicillin, 500 mg orally three times a day for 7 days; or erythromycin base, 500 mg orally four times a day for 7 days.[47]

ADULT INCLUSION CONJUNCTIVITIS

Inclusion conjunctivitis caused by *C. trachomatis* is occasionally seen in adults.

Diagnosis

Adult chlamydial conjunctivitis usually arises from inadvertent inoculation of the conjunctiva in patients with sexually acquired chlamydial infection. These patients typically present with an acute unilateral follicular conjunctivitis. Associated preauricular adenopathy may be evident. Such cases must be distinguished from acute conjunctivitis due to other organisms, such as adenovirus, HSV, or bacterial pathogens. If not treated, the disease may persist for weeks to months, but it typically resolves without scarring or visual impairment. Approaches to diagnosis are the same as those used for neonatal conjunctivitis (see above).

Treatment

Systemic treatment is indicated to cure both the ocular and the genital infection. Treatment regimens are the same as for genital infection (see above). Sexual partners should be evaluated and treated to prevent reinfection.

TRACHOMA

C. trachomatis—specifically, serovars A, B, Ba, and C—is the source of trachoma, the major preventable cause of blindness throughout the world.

Epidemiology

Trachoma remains prevalent in arid portions of the developing world, especially North Africa and the Middle East. Trachoma was formerly endemic in Native Americans of the southwestern United States, but it has largely been eliminated from that population. Transmission of *C. trachomatis* in endemic areas is believed to occur via eye to hand to eye contact, as well as via contaminated towels and other fomites.[48] Flies and other insects also may play a role in transmission. Most infections take place in early childhood, particularly in areas marked by crowding, poor standards of cleanliness, and the lack of clean water. The overall incidence of trachoma, as well as its severity, has been reduced dramatically over the past 35 years, primarily because of improved sanitary conditions and greater availability of clean water.

Pathogenesis

Severe, chronic, blinding trachoma is generally associated with repeated reinfection or persistent infection by trachoma-causing strains of *C. trachomatis.*[49] The immune response to the *C. trachomatis* 60 kd heat shock protein appears to be strongly linked to the conjunctival scarring and pannus formation that causes blindness in trachoma. Host genetic factors are likely also to be important, because specific HLA types are more commonly found in persons with progressive trachoma.[50]

Diagnosis

Clinical manifestations Initially, trachoma presents as a conjunctivitis characterized by multiple lymphoid follicles. Infection generally begins in children between 1 and 4 years of age. Reinfection is common, as is asymptomatic infection.[51] With repeated episodes, the cornea becomes involved, with inflammatory infiltrates and pannus formation (superficial vascularization). Conjunctival scarring eventually develops and causes the eyelids to turn inward and abrade the eyeball.[52] Eventually, corneal epithelial ulceration occurs. Destruction of the lacrimal glands and ducts produces a dry eye.

Laboratory tests Trachoma can be diagnosed on clinical grounds in a patient from an endemic area with follicular conjunctivitis. The diagnosis can be confirmed with culture, DFA, or nucleic acid amplification testing of secretions.

Treatment

Antimicrobial treatment should be provided in the early phases of trachoma, when its impact is potentially greatest. Oral tetracycline (in older children and adults) or erythromycin for 4 to 8 weeks has been recommended. Azithromycin (20 mg/kg orally in a single dose) can be used but may be prohibitively expensive in the developing world. Topical antimicrobials can be used, but their effectiveness is uncertain.

Public health measures to control endemic trachoma have focused on improving hygienic conditions and making clean water available. More recently, mass treatment of villages with single-dose azithromycin or topical antimicrobials has been utilized. Personal cleanliness and a reduction in flies in a village may also be important.

Disease Due to *C. psittaci*

PSITTACOSIS

C. psittaci infects a wide variety of avian species, including parrots, parakeets, pigeons, finches, chickens, pheasants, and turkeys. Humans become infected through exposure to infected birds. Human infection is subacute, characterized by pneumonitis and a variety of systemic manifestations.[53]

Epidemiology

Parrots, parakeets, and budgerigars (so-called psittacine birds) are the most common sources of human psittacosis. However, human cases have also been attributed to pigeons, ducks, turkeys, chickens, and a variety of other bird species. Psittacosis is an occupational disease of pet-shop employees, pigeon fanciers, taxidermists, veterinarians, poultry workers, and others who work around birds. The actual incidence is unknown: 50 to 100 cases are reported each year in the United States,[54] but it is likely that many cases, especially milder ones, go undiagnosed and thus unreported.

Pathogenesis

C. psittaci can be isolated from the nasal secretions, excreta, tissues, and feathers of infected birds. The birds may be ill, but many show only minor evidence of infection; complete absence of symptoms is uncommon, however.

C. psittaci enters humans via the upper respiratory tract and spreads throughout the body via the bloodstream, localizing primarily in pulmonary alveolar macrophages and the endothelial cells of the liver and spleen.[55] A lymphocytic inflammatory response ensues in the lungs and at other sites of infection. Little is known of the pathogenesis of psittacosis at the cellular or molecular level.

Diagnosis

Clinical manifestations Psittacosis may vary in severity from a mild flulike illness to a fatal disease.[56] The incubation period is typically 7 to 14 days. Often, the illness begins abruptly, with shaking chills and fever. In other cases, onset is more gradual. Among the most common symptoms are a severe headache and a nonproductive cough. Systemic illness characterized by fever, malaise, myalgias, and chills is also common. Features that may help differentiate psittacosis from other pneumonic processes include the absence of signs of consolidation, absence of a pleural effusion, a relative bradycardia, absence of neutrophilia, splenomegaly, abnormal liver function tests, and a rash resembling the rose spots of typhoid fever (Horder spots). The course may be relatively benign and short-lived or severe and prolonged, with complications such as myocarditis, pericarditis, meningitis, or encephalitis.[57]

A history of a recent exposure to birds is most helpful. Other diseases that must be considered include influenza, other viral pneumonias, *M. pneumoniae*, Q fever, Legionnaires disease, and other bacterial or fungal pneumonias. With patients in whom pneumonia is not prominent, other systemic febrile illnesses such as brucellosis, leptospirosis, mononucleosis, hepatitis, or typhoid fever must be considered.

Laboratory tests In psittacosis, the white blood cell count is most commonly normal or decreased and the erythrocyte sedimentation rate is not elevated. Liver function tests may be abnormal. Changes on chest x-ray are typically nonspecific, with patchy infiltrates that may be lobar, wedge shaped, segmental, or nodular. The diagnosis of psittacosis is best confirmed by serologic studies, because *C. psittaci* is difficult to isolate from blood or infected secretions. In addition, the organism is hazardous to work with in the laboratory, and most clinical laboratories do not offer culture diagnosis. A fourfold rise in titer of complement-fixing antibody in acute and convalescent sera from a patient with a compatible clinical syndrome confirms the diagnosis.

Treatment

Tetracycline generally produces a rapid and dramatic response when initiated during the early phase of psittacosis.[58] Generally, 2 g daily given in four divided doses is sufficient. Treatment should be continued for at least 14 days after defervescence to prevent relapse of infection. An alternative to tetracycline is erythromycin. Although as many as 20% of patients died in the preantibiotic era, fewer than 5% of patients do not respond to therapy currently.

Diseases Due to *C. pneumoniae*

C. pneumoniae is a recently described species that, as its name indicates, is associated primarily with respiratory tract infections. Initially, *C. pneumoniae* strains were thought to be variants of *C. psittaci*, but subsequent studies have demonstrated that *C. pneumoniae* is a distinct species, on the basis of differences in small subunit ribosomal RNA sequence, morphology, and antigenic properties.[59] The organisms are fastidious and cannot be easily isolated from respiratory or other clinical specimens. *C. pneumoniae* from clinical specimens grows most effectively in HL cells and Hep 2 cells.[60]

EPIDEMIOLOGY

Because of the difficulty in isolating the organism, most epidemiologic studies have depended on microimmunofluorescence serologic studies. Such studies have indicated that *C. pneumoniae* infection is extremely prevalent, with approximately 40% to 50% of adults demonstrating seropositivity in almost all countries examined worldwide. Infections are uncommon until late childhood; the peak period of incidence appears to be between 10 and 20 years of age.[61] New infections or reinfections are acquired throughout life, however, with the seroprevalence continuing to increase throughout adult life. Serologic studies suggest that infections are more common in men than in women. Transmission is thought to occur from person to person via the respiratory route, much like *Mycoplasma* or respiratory viral infections. Most transmission occurs in schools or households. Well-described outbreaks of *C. pneumoniae* infection have also occurred in settings such as military barracks or school dormitories.[62]

PATHOGENESIS

Little is yet known about the molecular pathogenesis of *C. pneumoniae* infection. However, the organism is thought to initially infect the upper respiratory tract epithelium. In many individuals, long-lived, asymptomatic infection persists at these sites. Recent studies have demonstrated that after infection of respiratory tract epithelial cells and inflammatory cells, *C. pneumoniae* is likely transmitted throughout the body via macrophages in the bloodstream.[63] There is clear evidence that replication of the organism occurs in vascular endothelium and synovial membranes. As with *C. trachomatis*, the outer membrane protein of *C. pneumoniae* may induce host immune responses that cross-react with human proteins, resulting in autoimmune inflammatory damage to tissues.

DIAGNOSIS

Clinical Manifestations

C. pneumoniae, like other chlamydial species, can produce asymptomatic infection of the respiratory tract and endovascular tissues. *C. pneumoniae* was originally discovered as a cause of upper and lower respiratory tract infection, and the organism may produce a pneumonic illness somewhat like that produced by *Mycoplasma*, although few studies have utilized culture to confirm the presence of *C. pneumoniae* in infected tissues. Characteristically, patients with *C. pneumoniae* pneumonia have prominent antecedent upper respiratory infections and a mild illness with fever, nonproductive cough, and small segmental infiltrates on chest x-ray. Pleuritis and pleural effusion are uncommon. It is likely that *C. pneumoniae* also causes other respiratory infections, including bronchitis, pharyngitis, sinusitis, and otitis media, but this is less extensively studied.

In addition to respiratory diseases, *C. pneumoniae* has recently been associated in serologic studies with a wide range of other conditions, including myocarditis, pericarditis, aseptic meningitis, erythema nodosum, sarcoidosis, asthma, chronic fatigue syndrome, multiple sclerosis, and Alzheimer disease. At present, the validity of these associations remains uncertain; their significance must be demonstrated in further studies.

There is more convincing evidence linking *C. pneumoniae* infection with atherosclerotic vascular disease. More than 30 epidemiologic studies have clearly demonstrated a strong association between serologic evidence for *C. pneumoniae* infection and atherosclerotic disease of the coronary and other arteries.[64] These associations remain after adjustment for potential confounding variables. In addition, *C. pneumoniae* has been identified in atherosclerotic plaques by a variety of techniques, including electron microscopy, DNA hybridization, immunocytochemistry, and PCR.[65] The organism has also been cultured from atherosclerotic plaques, demonstrating the presence of viable *C. pneumoniae* in the vessel wall.[66] Studies in cell-culture systems and in animal models support the hypothesis that *C. pneumoniae* can infect vascular endothelial cells, including smooth muscle cells and macrophages. Animal models also support the contention that *C. pneumoniae* infection of the upper respiratory tract is followed by widespread dissemination of the organism to atheromatous lesions in vessels.[67] In animals, antimicrobial treatment appears to slow the progression of atherosclerotic lesions associated with *C. pneumoniae* infection. Human trials are now ongoing to ascertain whether treatment with antimicrobials can reduce the risk of atherosclerotic heart disease and other vascular diseases associated with *C. pneumoniae* infection.

Laboratory Tests

Confirmation of *C. pneumoniae* respiratory infection is difficult because cell culture techniques are not widely available and in any case are not very sensitive. PCR and DNA probes have been utilized in research laboratories but are not available through most clinical laboratories. Microimmunofluorescence studies showing an increase in antibody to *C. pneumoniae* between acute and convalescent sera provide a specific diagnosis, but this technique is available in only a small number of laboratories. Complement-fixing antibody can also be measured, but that does not distinguish *C. pneumoniae* infection from *C. psittaci* or *C. trachomatis* infection. Accurate diagnosis of *C. pneumoniae* infection likely will await development and implementation of a more accurate and convenient PCR technology.

TREATMENT

There have been no controlled trials to ascertain the best antimicrobial regimen for *C. pneumoniae* respiratory infections. In vitro, *C. pneumoniae* is inhibited by erythromycin, tetracycline, doxycycline, azithromycin, clarithromycin, and some fluoroquinolones, such as levofloxacin. Most experts recommend tetracycline (2 g daily in four divided doses) or doxycycline (100 mg b.i.d.) as initial therapy. Treatment should be given for at least 2 to 3 weeks. Many cases can be managed in the outpatient setting, although severe disease (especially in the elderly) may occasionally require hospitalization and ventilatory support.

The impact of antimicrobial therapy on either treatment or prevention of atherosclerotic cardiovascular disease is unknown. Antibiotics are not currently recommended for this indication.

Acknowledgment

Figure 1 Seward Hung.

References

1. Schachter J, Stamm WE: *Chlamydia*. Manual of Clinical Microbiology 7th ed. Murray PR, Baron EJ, Pfaller MA, et al, Eds. ASM Press, Washington, DC, 1999, p 795

2. Ten leading nationally notifiable infectious diseases—United States, 1995. MMWR Morb Mortal Wkly Rep 45:883, 1996

3. VanBuuren CE, Dorrestein GM, vanDijk JE: *C. psittaci* in birds: a review of the pathogenesis and histopathological features. Vet Q 16:38, 1994

4. Grayston JT, Kuo CC, Campbell LA, et al: *Chlamydiae pneumoniae* sp nov. for *Chlamydia* sp strain TWAR. Int J Syst Bacteriol 39:88, 1989

5. Grayston JT: Infections caused by *Chlamydia pneumoniae* strain TWAR. Clin Infect Dis 15:757, 1992

6. Grayston JT: Background and current knowledge of *Chlamydiae pneumoniae* and atherosclerosis. J Infect Dis 181(S3):S402, 2000

7. Schachter J: Biology of *Chlamydia trachomatis*. Sexually Transmitted Diseases, 3rd ed. Holmes KK, Mårdh P-A, Sparling PF, et al, Eds. McGraw-Hill, New York, 1999, p 391

8. Brunham RC: Human Immunity to Chlamydiae. *Chlamydia* Intracellular Biology, Pathogenesis, and Immunity. Stephens RS, Ed. ASM Press, Washington, DC, 1999, p 211

9. Stamm WE: Potential for antimicrobial resistance in *Chlamydia pneumoniae*. J Infect Dis 181(S3):S456, 2000

10. Lampe MF, Suchland RJ, Stamm WE: Nucleotide sequence of the variable domains within the major outer membrane protein gene from serovariants of *Chlamydia trachomatis*. Infect Immun 61:213, 1993

11. Jones RB: *Chlamydia trachomatis* (trachoma, perinatal infections, lymphogranuloma venereum, and other genital infections). Principles and Practice of Infectious Diseases, 4th ed. Mandell GL, Bennet JE, Dolin R, Eds. Churchill Livingstone, New York, 1995, p 1679

12. Stamm WE: *Chlamydia trachomatis*—the persistent pathogen: Thomas Parran Award lecture. Sex Transm Dis 28:684, 2001

13. Stamm WE: *Chlamydia trachomatis* infections: progress and problems. J Infect Dis 179:S380, 1999

14. Campbell LA, Marrazzo JM, Stamm WE, et al: Chlamydiae. Laboratory Diagnosis of Bacterial Infections. Cimolai N, Ed. Marcel Dekker, New York, 2001, p 795

15. *Chlamydia trachomatis* genital infections—United States, 1995. MMWR Morb Mortal Wkly Rep 46:193, 1997

16. Stamm WE: *Chlamydia trachomatis* infections of the adult. Sexually Transmitted Diseases, 3rd ed. Holmes KK, Mårdh P-A, Sparling PF, et al, Eds. McGraw-Hill, New York, 1999, p 407

17. Gaydos CA, Howell MR, Pare B, et al: *Chlamydia trachomatis* infections in female military recruits. N Engl J Med 339:739, 1998

18. Xu F, Schillinger JA, Markowitz LE, et al: Repeat *Chlamydia trachomatis* infection in women: analysis through a surveillance case registry in Washington State, 1993–98. Am J Epidemiol 152:1164, 2000

19. Hillis SE, Owens LM, Marchbanks PA, et al: Recurrent chlamydial infections increase the risks of hospitalization for ectopic pregnancy and pelvic inflammatory disease. Am J Obstet Gynecol 176:103, 1997

20. LaVerda D, Albanese LN, Ruther PE, et al: Seroreactivity of *Chlamydia trachomatis* Hsp10 correlates with severity of human genital tract disease. Infect Immun 68:303, 2000

21. Gaur LK, Peeling RW, Cheang M, et al: Association of *Chlamydia trachomatis* heat-shock protein 60 antibody and HLA class II DQ alleles. J Infect Dis 180:234, 1999

22. Stamm WE, Koutsky LA, Benedetti JK, et al: *Chlamydia trachomatis* urethral infections in men: prevalence, risk factors, and clinical manifestations. Ann Intern Med 100:47, 1984

23. Horner P, Thomas B, Gilroy CB, et al: Role of *Mycoplasma geni-*

talium and *Ureaplasma urealyticum* in acute and chronic nongonococcal urethritis. Clin Infect Dis 32:995, 2001

24. Martin DH, Mroczkowski TF, Dalu ZA, et al: A controlled trial of a single dose of azithromycin for the treatment of chlamydial urethritis and cervicitis. N Engl J Med 327:921, 1992

25. Berger RE, Kessler D, Holmes KK: Etiology and manifestations of epididymitis in young men: correlations with sexual orientation. J Infect Dis 155:1341, 1987

26. 1998 guidelines for treatment of sexually transmitted diseases. MMWR Morb Mortal Wkly Rep 47:1, 1998

27. Holmes KK, Stamm WE: Lower genital tract infection syndromes in women. Sexually Transmitted Diseases, 3rd ed. Holmes KK, Mårdh P-A, Sparling PF, et al, Eds. McGraw-Hill, New York, 1999, p 761

28. Haddix AC, Hillis SD, Kassler WJ: The cost-effectiveness of azithromycin for *Chlamydia trachomatis* infections in women. Sex Transm Dis 22:274, 1995

29. Bush MR, Rosa C: Azithromycin and erythromycin in the treatment of cervical chlamydial infection during pregnancy. Obstet Gynecol 84: 61, 1994

30. Stamm WE, Wagner KF, Amsel R, et al: Causes of the acute urethral syndrome in women. N Engl J Med 303:409, 1980

31. Stamm WE, Stapleton AE: Approach to the patient with urinary tract infections. Infectious Diseases, 2nd ed. Gorbach SL, Bartlett JG, Blacklow NR, Eds. WB Saunders Co, Philadelphia, 1997, p 943

32. Cates W Jr, Rolfs RT JR, Aral SO: Sexually transmitted diseases, pelvic inflammatory disease, and infertility: an epidemiologic update. Epidemiol Rev 12:199, 1990

33. Cates W Jr, Joesoef MR, Goldman MB: Atypical pelvic inflammatory disease: can we identify clinical predictors? Am J Obstet Gynecol 169:341, 1993

34. Scholes D, Stergachis A, Heidrich FE, et al: Prevention of pelvic inflammatory disease by screening for cervical chlamydia infection. N Engl J Med 334:1362, 1996

35. Nelson HD, Helfand M: Screening for chlamydial infection. Am J Prev Med 20(3S):95, 2001

36. Boisvert JF, Koutsky LA, Suchland RJ, et al: Clinical features of *Chlamydia trachomatis* rectal infection by serovar among homosexually active men. Sex Transm Dis 26:392, 1999

37. Resurgent bacterial STDs among men who have sex with men. King County, Washington 1997–1999. MMWR Morb Mortal Wkly Rep 48:773, 1999

38. Hughes RA, Keat AC: Reiter's syndrome and reactive arthritis: a current view. Semin Arthritis Rheum 24:190, 1994

39. Perrine PL, Stamm WE: Lymphogranuloma venereum. Sexually Transmitted Diseases, 3rd ed. Holmes KK, Mårdh P-A, Sparling PF, et al, Eds. McGraw-Hill, New York, 1999, p 425

40. Division of STD Prevention, Sexually Transmitted Disease Surveillance, 1995. U. S. Department of Health and Human Services, Public Health Service. Atlanta Centers for Disease Control and Prevention, 1996

41. Hopsu-Havu VK, Sonck CE: Infiltrative, ulcerative and fistular lesions of the penis due to lymphogranuloma venereum. Br J Vener Dis 49:193, 1973

42. Schachter J, Smith DE, Dawson CR, et al: Lymphogranuloma venereum. I. comparison of the Frei test, complement fixation test, and isolation of the agent. J Infect Dis 120:372, 1969

43. Bell TA, Stamm WE, Wang SP, et al: Chronic *Chlamydia trachomatis* infections in infants. JAMA 267:400, 1992

44. Hammerschlag MR, Anderka M, Semine DZ, et al: Prospective study of maternal and infantile infection with *Chlamydia trachomatis*. Pediatrics 64:142, 1979

45. Schachter J, Grossman M, Sweet RL, et al: Prospective study of perinatal transmission of *Chlamydia trachomatis*. JAMA 255:3374, 1986

46. Beem MD, Saxon EM: Respiratory-tract colonization and a distinctive pneumonia syndrome in infants infected with *Chlamydia trachomatis*. N Engl J Med 296:306, 1977

47. Cohen I, Veille JC, Calkins BM: Improved pregnancy outcome following successful treatment of chlamydial infection. JAMA 263:3160, 1990

48. Taylor HR: A trachoma perspective. Ophthalmic Epidemiol 8:69, 2001

49. Grayston JT, Wang SP, Yeh LJ, et al: Importance of reinfection in the pathogenesis of trachoma. Rev Infect Dis 7:717, 1985

50. Mabey D, Fraser-Hurt N: Trachoma. BMJ 323:218, 2001

51. West SK, Munoz B, Mkocha H, et al: Progression of active trachoma to scarring in a cohort of Tanzanian children. Ophthalmic Epidemiol 8:137, 2001

52. Bailey RL, Arullendran P, Whittle HC, et al: Randomized controlled trial of single-dose azithromycin in treatment of trachoma. Lancet 342: 453, 1993

53. Yung AP, Grayson ML: Psittacosis—a review of 135 cases. Med J Aust 148:228, 1988

54. Compendium of psittacosis (chlamydiosis) control, 1997. MMWR Morb Mortal Wkly Rep 46(RR-13):1, 1997

55. MacFarlane JT, MacRae AD: Psittacosis. Br Med Bull 39:163, 1983

56. Mason AB, Jenkins P: Acute renal failure in fulminant psittacosis. Respir Med 88:239, 1994

57. Shapiro DS, Kenney SC, Johnson M, et al: *Chlamydia psittaci* endocarditis diagnosed by blood culture. N Engl J Med 325:1192, 1992

58. Grayston JT, Campbell LA, Kuo CC, et al: A new respiratory tract pathogen: *Chlamydia pneumoniae* strain TWAR. J Infect Dis 161:618, 1990

59. Chi EY, Kuo CC, Grayston JT: Unique ultrastructure in the elementary body of *Chlamydia* sp. strain TWAR. J Bacteriol 169:3797, 1987

60. Saikku P: The epidemiology and significance of *Chlamydia pneumoniae*. J Infect Dis 25:27, 1992

61. Falsey AR, Walsh EE: Transmission of *Chlamydia pneumoniae*. J Infect Dis 168:493, 1993

62. Saikku P, Wang SP, Klumola M, et al: An epidemic of mild pneumonia due to an unusual strain of *Chlamydia psittaci*. J Infect Dis 151: 832, 1985

63. Boman J, Gaydos CA: Polymerase chain reaction detection of *Chlamydia pneumoniae* in circulating white blood cells. J Infect Dis 181 (suppl 3):S452, 2000

64. Danesh J, Collins R, Peto R: Chronic infections and coronary heart disease: Is there a link? Lancet 350:430, 1997

65. Taylor-Robinson D, Thomas BJ: *Chlamydia pneumoniae* in atherosclerotic tissue. J Infect Dis 181 (suppl 3):S437, 2000

66. Maass M, Bartels C, Engel PM, et al: Endovascular presence of viable *Chlamydia pneumoniae* is a common phenomenon in coronary artery disease. J Am Coll Cardiol 31:827, 1998

67. Moazed TC, Kuo CC, Grayston JT, et al: Evidence of systemic dissemination of *Chlamydia pneumoniae* via macrophages in the mouse. J Infect Dis 177:1322, 1998

29 Herpesvirus Infections

Martin S. Hirsch, M.D.

Human and Animal Herpesviruses

The herpes group of viruses is composed of at least eight human viruses and numerous animal viruses [see 34 Viral Zoonoses]. The human herpesviruses include herpes simplex virus types 1 and 2 (HSV-1 and HSV-2), varicella-zoster virus (VZV), cytomegalovirus (CMV), Epstein-Barr virus (EBV), and human herpesvirus types 6 (HHV-6), 7 (HHV-7), and 8 (HHV-8, also known as Kaposi sarcoma–associated herpesvirus [KSHV]).

All human herpesviruses are of similar size and morphology and are characterized by a core, 30 to 60 nm in diameter, that contains a double-stranded DNA genome; a nucleocapsid, 95 to 100 nm, that exhibits icosahedral symmetry; and a lipoprotein envelope with glycoprotein projections that has a diameter of 120 to 250 nm. All the human herpesviruses replicate primarily in cell nuclei. A protein envelope is added as the virus passes through the nuclear membrane.

Human herpesviruses share the properties of latency and reactivation. Members of the group can cause productive lytic infections, in which infectious virus is produced and cells are killed, or nonproductive lytic infections, in which viral DNA persists but complete replication does not occur and cells survive. After acute lytic infections, herpesviruses often persist in a latent form for years; periodic reactivations are followed by recurrent lytic infections. Sites of latency vary: HSV and VZV persist in neural ganglion cells, EBV persists in B cells, and CMV probably remains latent in many cell types. The sites of latency for HHV-6 and HHV-7 have not been identified, although both herpesviruses have been detected in salivary glands.

All human herpesviruses have a worldwide distribution [*see Sidebar* Herpesvirus Information on the Internet]. Considerable efforts are being directed toward the development of vaccines and antiviral agents that will be active against herpesviruses.

Herpes Simplex Virus

HSV-1 and HSV-2 can be distinguished by a variety of properties, including clinical and epidemiologic patterns, antigenicity, DNA base composition, biologic characteristics, and sensitivity to various physical and chemical stresses.[1] Advances in molecular biology technology have proved that HSV-1 and HSV-2 share certain antigens (e.g., glycoprotein B) but differ with respect to other antigens (e.g., glycoprotein G). Restriction enzyme analysis of HSV DNA is used to identify, or fingerprint, individual isolates.

EPIDEMIOLOGY

Humans are the only known natural hosts for HSV, although animals can readily be infected experimentally. HSV-1 primary infection occurs mainly in childhood, whereas HSV-2 infection occurs predominantly in sexually active adolescents and young adults. The prevalence of HSV-2–specific antibodies in the United States increases from less than 6% in those younger than 19 years to more than 25% in those older than 30 years.[2] In older age groups, changes in prevalence are negligible. Infection rates are influenced by race (the rate for African Americans is higher than that for whites) and sex (more women are infected than men).[2] The frequency of sexual contact with different partners correlates closely with the likelihood of contracting HSV-2 infection. In the United States, changes in sexual mores resulted in an age-adjusted seroprevalence of HSV-2 infection in the 1990s that was 30% higher than the seroprevalence in the 1970s; HSV-2 is now detectable in one of five persons older than 12 years of age.[2] Of new HSV-2 infections, approximately one third are symptomatic.[3] Prevalence of antibody to HSV-1 in different populations ranges from 30% to 100%.

Direct contact with infected secretions is the principal mode of transmission. HSV-1 is usually transmitted by an oral route and HSV-2 by a geni-

Herpesvirus Information on the Internet

General

http://www.nesfile.com/xlp.htm
Herpes Viruses Weekly

http://www.cdc.gov/nchstp/dstd/STD98TG.HTM
1998 Guidelines for Treatment of Sexually Transmitted Disease

http://www.cdc.gov/epo/mmwr/preview/mmwrhtml/00033634.htm
Recommended infection-control practices for dentistry

http://www.cdc.gov/epo.mmwr/preview/mmwrhtml/00001053.htm
Perspectives in disease prevention and health promotion: condoms for prevention of sexually transmitted diseases

http://www.cdc.gov/od/owh/whstd.htm
Office of Women's Health: Sexually Transmitted Diseases

http://www.cdc.gov/ncidod/focus/vol6no1/dvrd.htm
NCID Focus: DVRD initiates surveillance of acyclovir-resistant herpesvirus infections

http://www.nci.nih.gov/intra/dcs/HAMB/cidofovir.htm
Cidofovir

HSV

http://www.cdc.gov/nchstp/dstd/Genital_Herpes_facts.htm
Patient information on genital herpes

http://www.cdcgov/epo/mmwr/other/case_def/gen_h97.html
Case definition: genital herpes

VZV

http://www.cdc.gov/nip/manual/varicell/varicell.htm
Varicella

http://www.cdc.gov/epo/mmwr/preview/mmwrhtml/00022690.htm
ACIP recommendation: varicella-zoster immune globulin for chickenpox

http://www.cdc.gov/od/oc/media/fact/chickenp.htm
Facts abut chickenpox (varicella) from the CDC Office of Communications, Division of Media Relations

http://www.cdc.gov/nip/clinqa2/var.htm
Frequently asked questions about varicella and varicella vaccine

http://www.cdc.gov/nip/genqa/varicqa.htm
Patient information on varicella

http://www.cdc/gov/epo/mmwr/preview/rr4511.html
Recommendations and Reports-June 27, 1996/Vol. 45/No. RR-1-Preview (The first statement by the Advisory Committee on Immunization Practices [ACIP] on the use of live, attenuated varicella virus vaccine)

CMV

http://www.cdc.gov/nchstp/hiv_aids/pubs/brochure/oi_cmv.htm
Division of HIV/AIDS (DHAP)–HIV/AIDS Brochures: Cytomegalovirus (CMV) and You

http://www.cdc.gov/nchstp/hiv_aids/hivinfo/vfax/362302.htm
AIDS information: cytomegalovirus (CMV) infection and high-risk groups

Herpesvirus Simiae

http://www.cdc.gov/epo/mmwr/preview/mmwrhtml/00015936.htm
Guidelines for prevention of herpesvirus simiae (B virus) infection

tal route. Although virus titers are higher and transmission is more likely when lesions are present, asymptomatic excretion of the virus is common. HSV-2 shedding from the genital tract can occur in seropositive persons who have no history of genital HSV infection.[4] Thus, transmission occurs frequently, even in the absence of lesions. Spread of infection through contact with oral secretions may be an occupational hazard for respiratory care and dental care providers; thus, gloves should be worn when fingers are placed in patients' mouths. Autoinoculation to other skin sites also occurs, more often with HSV-2 than with HSV-1. Fomites, including toilet seats and towels, are not important modes of transmission. HSV-2 is transmitted more efficiently from males to females than from females to males.

Recurrences are frequent with both HSV-1 and HSV-2 infections, usually as a result of endogenous reactivation. In the United States, lip or perioral recurrences develop in 20% to 40% of the population. Precipitating factors are sunlight, wind, local trauma, fever, menstruation, and emotional stress. Ocular herpes is present in about 5% of all patients seen at ophthalmology clinics; 25% to 50% of ocular HSV infections recur within 2 years. Of all the primary cases of genital herpes in the United States each year, 60% to 80% will recur. Although most genital recurrences represent reactivation, exogenous reinfection can also occur. Clinically significant recurrences tend to decrease over time.[5]

PATHOGENESIS

After the initial replication of the virus in epithelial cells, cytolysis and local inflammatory reactions develop, resulting in the characteristic lesion—a superficial vesicle on an inflammatory base. Multinucleated cells and Cowdry type A inclusion bodies are present. Subsequent lymphatic spread to regional nodes and viremic spread to other organs may occur, depending on the immune competence of the host. Viremia can be demonstrated in malnourished children, in certain adults with depressed T cell–mediated immunity, and, occasionally, in immunocompetent persons.

After initial infection, HSV travels along sensory nerve pathways to ganglion cells, the site of latent infection. The viral DNA persists, only to become reactivated by certain stresses. After reactivation, the virus reverses its course and spreads peripherally by sensory nerve pathways. Once HSV reaches cutaneous sites, cell-to-cell spread occurs until host immune mechanisms limit further dissemination. Various mechanisms are engaged in host responses to HSV, including T cell and natural killer cell cytotoxicity, macrophage activation, production of antibody, and production of interferon.

CLINICAL SYNDROMES

Oral-Labial Herpes

In patients younger than 5 years, primary HSV-1 infection is most often asymptomatic; when symptomatic, it presents as gingivostomatitis or pharyngitis. After an incubation period of 2 to 12 days, fever and sore throat develop. Small vesicles are observed on the oral mucosa and pharynx. Mouth pain may be severe, breath is fetid, and cervical adenopathy is present. In adolescents and young adults, posterior pharyngitis and tonsillitis may be the primary problem. The differential diagnosis includes streptococcal pharyngitis, aphthous stomatitis, Stevens-Johnson syndrome, herpangina, and infectious mononucleosis. Symptoms and signs may persist for 10 to 21 days, and autoinoculation to other sites, such as fingers and eyes, is common. Oral shedding may persist for as long as 23 days (mean, 7 to 10 days).[1]

Recurrent herpes labialis is a shorter and milder affliction, often heralded by local pain or tingling for a few hours. HSV-1 oral-labial lesions recur more often than HSV-2 oral-labial lesions.[3] Vesicles appear most often on the vermilion border and are painful. The lesion is usually small (< 1 cm^2), and the progression from vesicle to ulcer to crust is rapid (< 96 hours). Healing is complete within 8 to 10 days. Systemic complaints are uncommon in recurrent herpes labialis.

Ocular Herpes

Most ocular herpetic infections are caused by HSV-1. Primary infections may present as unilateral follicular conjunctivitis, blepharitis, or corneal epithelial opacities. Healing is usually complete within 2 to 3 weeks. Recurrences may take the form of keratitis (more than 90% of cases are unilateral), blepharitis, or keratoconjunctivitis. Branching dendritic ulcers, usually detected by fluorescein staining, are virtually diagnostic and are often associated with diminished visual acuity. Deep stromal involvement may result in scarring, corneal thinning, and abnormal vascularization, with resultant blindness or rupture of the globe.

Genital Herpes

HSV-2 is the causative agent in 70% to 95% of primary genital herpesvirus infections. After an incubation period of 2 to 7 days, fever, malaise, and inguinal adenopathy develop; these symptoms are associated with the appearance of vesicular lesions. In men, lesions are often on the glans penis or penile shaft [*see Figure 1*]; in women, lesions may involve the vulva, perineum, buttocks, cervix, or vagina. The differential diagnosis includes syphilis, chancroid, Behçet syndrome, erythema multiforme, and candidiasis. In women, lesions rapidly ulcerate and become covered with exudate, with resultant vaginal discharge. Urethral involvement sometimes results in dysuria or urinary retention. Extragenital lesions develop during the course of primary infection in 10% to 18% of patients. Aseptic meningitis is not uncommon during primary genital herpes, and in rare instances, herpetic sacral radiculomyelitis occurs. Signs and symptoms of primary genital herpes often persist for several weeks before complete healing. Previous infection with HSV-1 may reduce the severity and duration of a first episode of genital herpes caused by HSV-2.

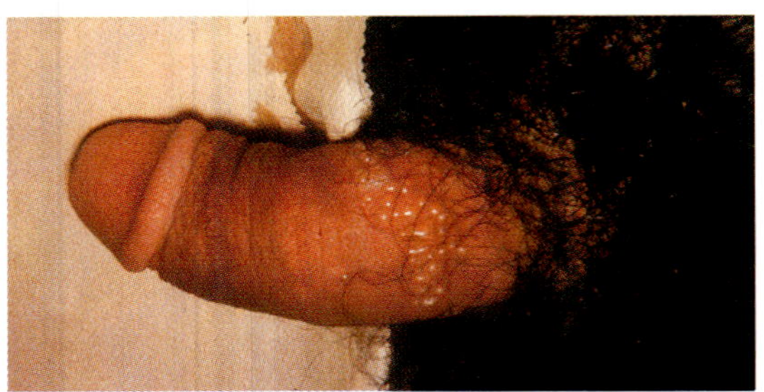

Figure 1 **Herpes simplex virus genital lesions in men often present as grouped vesicles on the penile shaft.**

Recurrent episodes of genital herpes are usually shorter and milder than primary episodes but still affect women more severely than men. HSV-2 genital lesions recur more often than those caused by HSV-1, and on rare occasions, the two can be found simultaneously in lesions.[6] After a variable prodrome of tenderness, itching, or tingling, lesions develop on the penis, labia minora, labia majora, perineum, mons pubis, or buttocks. Healing occurs in 6 to 10 days and is usually uncomplicated; frequent asymptomatic shedding occurs, however, particularly in women.[4,7] HSV-2 may also cause benign, recurrent lymphocytic meningitis that may be associated with recurrent genital lesions.[8]

Perianal and Anal Herpes

Perianal and anal HSV-2 infection is an important problem in male homosexuals. Pain, itching, tenesmus, discharge, fever, chills, sacral paresthesias, headache, and difficulty in urinating may all occur. Vesicles and ulcerations may lead to an erythematous cryptitis with inguinal adenopathy. Herpes proctitis is often prolonged and severe in patients with AIDS [*see Figure 2*].

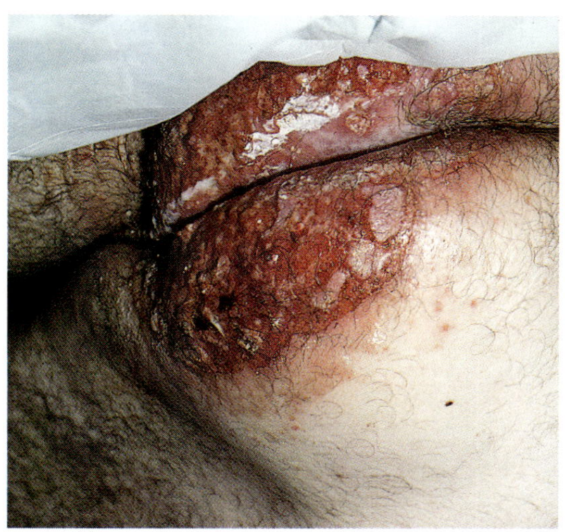

Figure 2 **Perianal herpes simplex infections in patients with compromised immunity may be severe and prolonged.**

Other Herpes Syndromes

Herpetic whitlow Primary finger infections, or whitlows, usually involve one digit and are characterized by intense itching or pain followed by the formation of deep vesicles that may coalesce [*see Figure 3*]. Among the general public, whitlows are most often caused by HSV-2, whereas among medical and dental personnel, HSV-1 is the principal culprit. The lesions gradually resolve in 2 to 3 weeks, unless they are mistakenly incised, in which case healing may be delayed by secondary bacterial infection. Recurrent whitlows commonly appear and are sometimes associated with severe local neuralgia.

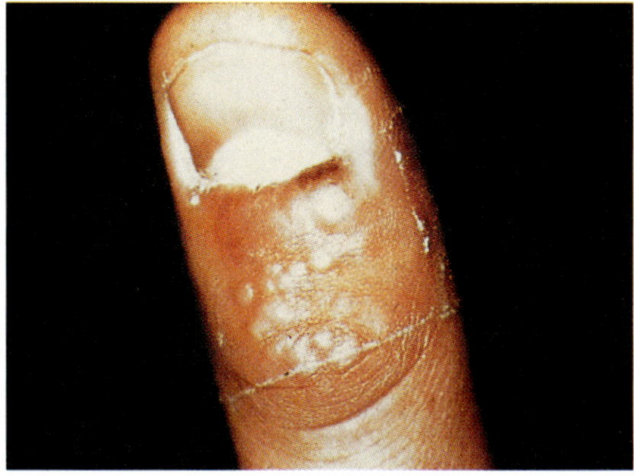

Figure 3 **Herpetic whitlows, which occur on fingers, are often misdiagnosed as staphylococcal infections.**

Neurologic complications Encephalitis, a severe form of HSV infection, is discussed elsewhere [see 35 Acute Viral Central Nervous System Diseases]. HSV-1 has also been implicated as an etiologic agent in Bell palsy[9] and in rare cases of recurrent self-limited meningitis (Mollaret meningitis).[10]

Infection in the immunocompromised host Disorders of T cell–mediated immunity are associated with more severe HSV infections. In clinical settings such as organ transplantation, lymphoreticular neoplasm, or AIDS, HSV infection is often slow to heal and may disseminate cutaneously or to visceral organs. Certain skin conditions, such as eczema and burns, are associated with cutaneous but not visceral dissemination. In rare instances, HSV infection during pregnancy or in the elderly is complicated by visceral dissemination, particularly to the liver. Intubation or catheterization of debilitated patients may facilitate the spread of infection; for instance, herpes esophagitis often complicates long-term use of nasogastric tubes.

Neonatal infection Between one in 2,500 and one in 10,000 births are complicated by HSV infection, usually HSV-2. Involvement can be localized or disseminated and results from transmission of the virus to the infant at the time of delivery, either by ascending infection after premature membrane rupture or by passage of the infant through an infected genital tract. The risk of transmission is increased in premature births, after prolonged membrane rupture, and with the use of fetal scalp monitor electrodes. About 40% to 50% of infants born to mothers with primary infections are at risk for the development of severe disease, whereas fewer than 8% of those born to women with recurrent herpes are at risk for severe disease.[11,12] Maternal infection is often asymptomatic at the time of delivery, and asymptomatic shedding may occur in women with no known history of genital herpes. In women with a history of genital HSV infection, genital HSV can be detected at delivery in approximately 2% by use of tissue culture and in 14% by use of polymerase chain reaction (PCR) techniques.[13]

Infection becomes apparent several days to weeks after delivery. Newborns often present with vesicles or conjunctivitis, or a syndrome resembling neonatal sepsis may be evident. Neurologic signs such as seizures, cranial nerve palsies, and lethargy often predominate and are accompanied by cerebrospinal fluid pleocytosis. Disseminated infection may involve the liver, lungs, or adrenal glands. If untreated, disseminated or central nervous system infection is fatal in more than 70% of patients, whereas localized disease is generally self-limited. Treatment has greatly reduced the mortality from severe infection [see 35 Acute Viral Central Nervous System Diseases].

DIAGNOSIS

A variety of tissue culture systems support the replication of HSV, and virus isolation from specimens collected early in the course of infection is the diagnostic method of choice. The characteristic cytopathic effect of the virus is often detectable within a period of 24 to 48 hours. Typing of isolates can be accomplished most readily by immunofluorescence with monoclonal antibodies directed against type-specific antigens. Scrapings or tissue specimens can sometimes be tested directly for herpesvirus antigens by immunofluorescence or immunohistochemistry. Alternatively, scrapings may be prepared by Giemsa or Wright stain and examined for the presence of multinucleated giant cells, which indicates infection with HSV or VZV. Serologic techniques may be useful in documenting primary HSV infection and in differentiating HSV-1 from HSV-2 infections, but they are seldom helpful in diagnosing recurrences. Differentiation between HSV-1 and HSV-2 seropositivity may identify women at unsuspected risk for primary infection with HSV-2 during pregnancy or those at risk for HSV-2 reactivation. PCR detection of HSV DNA in CSF has become the standard means of diagnosing HSV encephalitis. For patients with HSV encephalitis, PCR results are often positive within 24 hours of the onset of symptoms, and test results may remain positive during the first week of illness.[14] PCR techniques will likely become more widely used to diagnose other herpesvirus infections as well.

PREVENTION AND TREATMENT

HSV infection cannot yet be prevented by immunoglobulins or vaccines; however, prophylactic measures that prevent contact with the virus may help in avoiding primary infection. The best strategy for the prevention of neonatal herpes may be close physical examination at the time of labor.[15] Cesarean section is indicated to prevent perinatal infection when lesions consistent with the diagnosis of genital herpes are noted during labor. If primary genital herpes is detected during the third trimester of pregnancy, acyclovir for mother and newborn should be considered. Medical and dental personnel should wear gloves to prevent contact with infected areas. The use of condoms may prevent sexual transmission when either sexual partner has a history of genital HSV infection. Application of sunscreens to susceptible skin areas before exposure to ultraviolet light can prevent reactivation of HSV.

A number of nucleoside derivatives are active against primary and recurrent HSV infection; of these, acyclovir has become the standard of care, although the prodrug valacyclovir (which is converted to acyclovir) and famciclovir (which is converted to penciclovir) now provide alternative options. Either oral acyclovir, 200 mg five times daily, or intravenous acyclovir, 5 mg/kg three times daily, is recommended for treatment of primary genital herpes or mucocutaneous herpes (HSV-1 or HSV-2) in the immunocompromised host. Suppression of severe and frequently recurring genital herpes can also be accomplished by the administration of oral acyclovir (200 to 400 mg twice daily), oral famciclovir (250 mg twice daily), or oral valacyclovir (500 mg daily). Intravenous acyclovir, in a dosage of 10 mg/kg three times daily, is the treatment of choice for herpes encephalitis.

In immunocompromised persons and, in rare instances, in immunocompetent persons, acyclovir-resistant HSV-2 may lead to chronic progressive infections.[16] Intravenous foscarnet (40 mg/kg two to three times daily for 2 to 3 weeks) has been reported to be useful against acyclovir-resistant HSV-2 infection.[16,17] Topical preparations of foscarnet, cidofovir, and trifluridine are also under study for acyclovir-resistant HSV.[18–20]

Varicella-Zoster Virus

VZV is the causative agent of varicella (chickenpox) and herpes zoster (shingles). Because it is a strongly cell-associated member of the human herpesvirus group, it is difficult to detect or isolate in cell-free specimens. Its host range is largely limited to human cells. As with other herpesviruses, latency and reactivation are characteristic features of VZV.

EPIDEMIOLOGY

Varicella is a highly communicable disease of childhood. More than 90% of patients are children younger than 9 years; most adults have antibody to the virus. Infection is spread by respiratory droplets or by direct contact with active lesions. Fomites are not an important mode of transmission. Chickenpox occurs most frequently in the winter and the spring and spreads rapidly to susceptible household members. The incubation period ranges from 11 to 20 days.

Herpes zoster results from the reactivation of VZV infection. Varicella in one patient cannot produce herpes zoster in another; however, persons who are exposed to patients who have herpes zoster can contract varicella. There is no seasonal pattern for herpes zoster. The likelihood of reactivation is related to both age and immune status. The incidence of disease in patients older than 60 years is two to three times higher than that in younger persons. The incidence in immunosuppressed patients, particularly those with depressed T cell function (e.g., patients who have lymphomas, leukemias, organ transplants, or AIDS), is as much as 100 times higher than that in immunocompetent hosts.[21]

Herpes zoster occurs more frequently in patients with neoplasms. The risk of developing herpes zoster is 13% to 15% for patients with Hodgkin disease, 7% to 9% for patients with other lymphomas, and 1% to 3% for patients with solid tumors. Approximately 15% to 30% of patients with Hodgkin disease and herpes zoster exhibit significant dissemination; however, mortality in such patients is low. Localized and disseminated herpes zoster are more common in patients with advanced malignant disease who are receiving intensive chemotherapy or irradiation. The incidence of herpes zoster is also increased after organ or bone marrow transplantation and in patients with AIDS. Chronic, nonhealing VZV ulcers may persist for several months in patients with advanced HIV infection, and herpes zoster may be precipitated by the introduction of highly active antiretroviral therapy.

CLINICAL SYNDROMES

Varicella

After local replication of VZV at the site of virus entry, the virus is carried by blood leukocytes to focal skin areas and visceral organs. Replication at skin sites results in vesicle formation accompanied by degeneration of epithelial cells, accumulation of edema fluid, and infiltration of inflammatory cells; multinucleated giant cells containing intranuclear inclusions are present.

Clinical features Subclinical infections are rare (less than 4% of cases). Illness usually presents as a generalized vesicular eruption that is followed by a variable prodrome of headache, fever, and malaise. Vesicles often appear initially on the face or trunk [*see Figure 4*]. During the next 4 to 7 days, successive crops of lesions appear. Most childhood cases are uncomplicated and resolve in 7 to 10 days without producing scarring.

Complications In adolescents and adults, pneumonia may develop that is characterized by cough, tachypnea, and diffuse reticulonodular infiltrates, which may calcify with time. Pulmonary diffusion difficulties may persist for a period of weeks to months. Although varicella encephalopathies are uncommon, they can occur at any age and can take several forms; the presenting feature may be hyperexcitability, which can progress to coma or cerebellar ataxia. Other rare complications of varicella infection are Reye syndrome (fulminating encephalopathy and fatty liver), thrombocytopenia, arthritis, ocular involvement, carditis, gastrointestinal bleeding, nephritis, orchitis, and bacterial superinfection. A pregnant woman who contracts varicella during the first 20 weeks of pregnancy has a small (< 2%) risk of giving birth to an infant with congenital varicella syndrome, which includes limb hypoplasia, skin scarring, and ocular defects.[22]

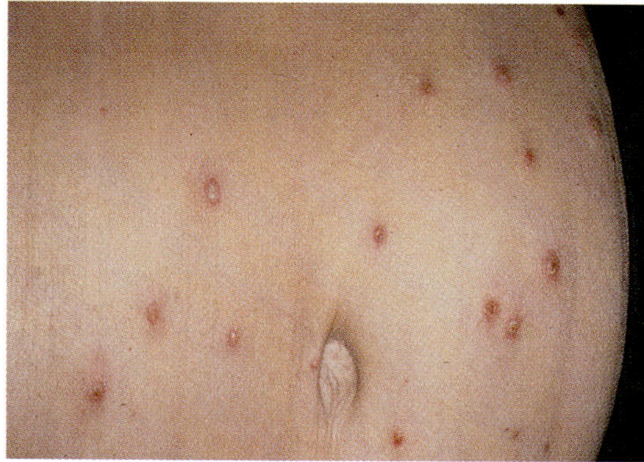

Figure 4 **The lesions characteristics of varicella-zoster virus infection often manifest initially on the face and trunk, and may present as maculopapules, vesicles, and scabs simultaneously.**

Disseminated disease is more likely to develop after varicella infection in children with leukemia, lymphoma, or Hodgkin disease. Visceral dissemination occurs in 20% to 35% of children with cancer who are receiving chemotherapy; mortality in such patients is 7% to 30%. Clinical reinfection, with resultant atypical generalized varicella, can occur in the severely immunocompromised host; such reinfection tends to be mild and self-limited.

Herpes Zoster

Herpes zoster occurs in patients previously infected with varicella. After an initial episode of varicella infection, the virus persists in neurons of sensory ganglia in a relatively quiescent, extrachromosomal, cytoplasmic state.[23,24] Both subclinical and clinical reactivations occur. Clinical VZV reactiva-

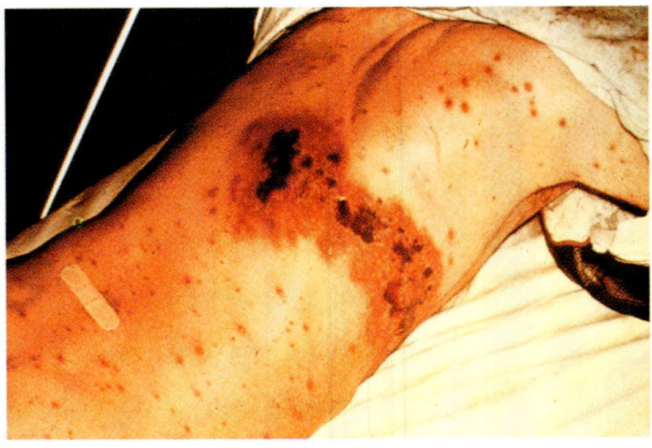

Figure 5 **Herpes zoster is most often thoracic and dermatomal in distribution. Cutaneous dissemination, as seen in this patient, as well as visceral dissemination may occur when immunity is severely compromised.**

tion is enhanced by many factors, including increasing age, immunosuppression, and local skin injury.

Clinical features Attacks of herpes zoster are often preceded by pain, which may persist for several days before lesions appear. The vesicular eruption is unilateral and most often appears on the thorax [*see Figure 5*]. Individual attacks are usually limited to one to three dermatomes, although a few isolated skin lesions at sites distant from this area are not uncommon. Vesicles surrounded by an erythematous base may continue to develop for several days; the lesions then dry and crust. Superinfections are common, and scarring can occur.

Complications The most common complication of herpes zoster is postherpetic neuralgia, which may be severe, particularly in the elderly. Postherpetic neuralgia may be refractory to treatment and persist for months to years. Other neurologic syndromes associated with herpes zoster are segmental myelitis, Guillain-Barré syndrome, and Ramsay Hunt syndrome.[24] Ramsay Hunt syndrome is an infection of the geniculate ganglion of the seventh cranial nerve, producing facial paralysis; vesicles on the eardrum and side of the tongue can also occur.

VZV encephalitis, another infrequent complication of herpes zoster, may present in two forms.[24] Large vessel encephalitis (granulomatous arteritis) occurs predominantly in immunocompetent persons; it is characterized by acute focal deficits that occur weeks after zoster of the contralateral trigeminal pattern of distribution. Angiography demonstrates segmental narrowing, primarily in the internal carotid and middle or anterior cerebral arteries. Microscopic examination shows arterial inflammation, multinucleated giant cells, and virus particles. Small vessel encephalitis occurs almost exclusively in immunocompromised persons and is characterized by headache, fever, mental changes, seizures, and focal deficits. Imaging studies show ischemic or hemorrhagic infarcts of gray and white matter, and CSF examination demonstrates mononuclear pleocytosis and both VZV DNA and VZV antibody.

DIAGNOSIS

Varicella and herpes zoster can usually be diagnosed solely on clinical grounds. Varicella is sometimes confused with disseminated herpes simplex, impetigo, insect bites, or scabies; on rare occasions, HSV infection presents with zosteriform eruptions. Diagnosis of VZV infection can be confirmed by virus isolation, direct immunofluorescence of lesions, PCR detection of viral DNA, or demonstration of a fourfold rise in antibodies to viral antigens. Herpes zoster provokes a more rapid and greater rise in antibodies than varicella.

PREVENTION AND TREATMENT

Nosocomial transmission of VZV has been reported. Thus, hospitalized patients with varicella or herpes zoster should be isolated to prevent spread of virus to other susceptible persons. Susceptible immunocompromised patients who are exposed to infected persons should receive prophylaxis with varicella-zoster immune globulin (one dose up to 4 days after exposure) to prevent or modify clinical illness. Small studies suggest that high-dose acyclovir (40 to 80 mg/kg for 7 days, beginning 7 to 9 days after exposure) or VZV vaccine (one dose on the day of exposure or up to 3 days after exposure) may also be useful in postexposure prophylaxis.[23] A live attenuated VZV vaccine is available in the United States and appears both safe and effective. It is recommended for persons older than 1 year who are in good health and have no history of clinical VZV infection.[25] A single subcutaneous dose is recommended for children 1 to 12 years of age, whereas two doses separated by 4 to 8 weeks are recommended for susceptible adolescents and adults. Because approximately 90 persons die each year in the United States as a result of complications of VZV infections, there is a need for better vaccination of susceptible populations.[26]

Considerable success in the treatment of VZV infections in immunocompromised hosts has been achieved with parenteral administration of acyclovir (for adults, 10 mg/kg every 8 hours). Comparative trials indicate that intravenous acyclovir is superior to vidarabine for treating herpes zoster in immunocompromised hosts.[27] High-dose oral acyclovir (800 mg five times daily), when begun early, may also shorten the course and reduce the severity of herpes zoster in otherwise healthy hosts.[28] Oral valacyclovir (1 g three times daily) or famciclovir (500 mg three times daily) may also be used. The use of corticosteroids in combination with acyclovir for the treatment of acute herpes zoster remains controversial.[29,30] Steroid use may be justified in persons older than 50 years who have no relative contraindications, such as diabetes, hypertension, or glaucoma.[23] Acyclovir resistance has been described in VZV isolates from patients with HIV infection who received long-term acyclovir therapy. Foscarnet (40 mg/kg every 8 hours) is the drug of choice for acyclovir-resistant VZV infections in immunocompromised hosts.[31] Acyclovir is also effective in reducing the severity and shortening the course of chickenpox in both children and adults who are immunologically competent. Whether young children with chickenpox should receive acyclovir is a source of controversy, although there is general agreement that the early treatment of adolescents and adults is beneficial. Famciclovir, acyclovir, and valacyclovir have similar effects on herpes zoster; famciclovir and valacyclovir can be administered less frequently but are more expensive.[32,33]

Postherpetic neuralgia is difficult to treat, particularly in elderly patients. Recommended treatments are topical anesthetics, oral analgesics, tricyclic antidepressants, and gabapentin.[21,34]

Cytomegalovirus

Although cytomegalic inclusion disease of infants was recognized as a clinical entity at the turn of the 20th century, the etiologic agent, CMV, was not isolated until the mid-1950s. CMV has since become recognized as a nearly ubiquitous virus that plays an important role in many diseases, including a form of mononucleosis and disseminated disease in the immunocompromised host.

EPIDEMIOLOGY

Transmission occurs by close contact with infected persons, most commonly by the sharing of secretions or leukocyte-containing blood products. CMV is shed in semen, cervical secretions, saliva, maternal milk, and urine. In late adolescence and adulthood, genital transmission is common. Primary infection in pregnant women may result in transplacental spread to the fetus, sometimes with devastating consequences. Approximately 1% of newborns in developed countries are infected with CMV, and the incidence is much higher in developing areas. Perinatal infection is also common because of spread from maternal milk or other secretions. Communal living and poor personal hygiene facilitate transmission. Spread of CMV in day care centers is increasing; the infected child often serves as a source of transmission to other family members. Blood transfusions and organ transplantation may also transmit CMV from an asymptomatic donor to a recipient.

PATHOGENESIS

Once infected, one probably carries the virus for life. Generally, such infections remain dormant, but reactivation occurs during periods of immune compromise. Reactivation is particularly common in patients with compromised T cell function (e.g., transplant recipients or patients with lymphoid neoplasms or AIDS). Reinfections with new strains of CMV can also occur in immunosuppressed patients.

In the fetus, primary infection may result in disseminated cytomegalic inclusion disease with numerous congenital abnormalities, in localized disease affecting the auditory system or the CNS, or in subclinical involvement. Perinatal infection is usually asymptomatic, although protracted interstitial pneumonitis, hepatitis, and failure to thrive may result.

Symptomatic disease is more likely to be produced by primary CMV infection than by viral reactivation. The sites of latent infection are poorly defined, although it appears likely that CMV persists in numerous cell types in many organs. If host immune responses become compromised, virus reactivation and increased replication can occur and result in various syndromes. CMV replication can further suppress immune responses, leading to profound lymphocyte hyporesponsiveness and severe opportunistic infections with protozoa (e.g., *Pneumocystis carinii* and *Toxoplasma gondii*), fungi, or bacteria. The mechanisms by which CMV replication inhibits host responses are complex and involve virus interactions with both host lymphocytes and monocyte-macrophages.

CLINICAL SYNDROMES

CMV Mononucleosis

Clinical features CMV mononucleosis occurs in patients of any age but is most common in sexually active young adults. A vigorous host T cell response may contribute to the syndrome, which is characterized by fever, malaise, fatigue, and myalgia. Headache and splenomegaly are also often present. Mild liver enzyme abnormalities are common, and atypical lymphocytes are present in the peripheral blood. Heterophile antibodies are not formed in response to CMV infection; however, mild immunologic abnormalities, including the presence of rheumatoid factor and antinuclear antibodies, are common.

Complications Occasionally, hemolytic anemia, thrombocytopenia, neurologic complications (e.g., Guillain-Barré syndrome), or other organ involvement (liver, lung) occurs and is severe.[35] Acute infections generally resolve in 2 to 4 weeks, but postviral asthenia and viral excretion often persist for months.

CMV Infection in the Immunocompromised Host

Clinical features CMV appears to be the most frequent and important viral pathogen in patients who have had organ transplants. Most commonly, such patients with CMV syndromes present with fever and leukopenia, which may progress to pneumonitis or, in rare instances, to disseminated disease. The period of highest risk is 1 to 4 months after transplantation and appears to be related to the degree of host immunosuppression. CMV may also increase the risk of graft loss after organ transplantation.[36] CMV pneumonia occurs in nearly 20% of marrow transplant recipients; mortality in such patients, if untreated, is about 90%.

CMV is recognized as an important pathogen in patients with AIDS. The virus often contributes to the immunosuppression observed in such patients and may cause disseminated disease affecting the eyes, GI tract, or CNS. At least 50% of patients with AIDS have CMV viremia, and 90% or more have evidence of CMV infection at autopsy.[37] Ulcers of the esophagus, stomach, small intestine, or colon may be present and may lead to bleeding or perforation.[38] It is critical to recognize CMV polyradiculopathy or encephalitis in this setting because this disorder is potentially reversible with therapy.[39,40] Similarly, CMV retinitis is an important treatable cause of blindness in patients with AIDS.[41] Early lesions consist of small white areas of retinal necrosis that progress in a centrifugal manner and are subsequently accompanied by hemorrhage, vessel sheathing, and retinal edema [*see Figure 6*]. CMV and HIV have been shown to potentiate each other's replication in vitro, and it is possible that such interactions occur in dually infected organs (e.g., the retina and brain of an AIDS patient who has CMV infection).

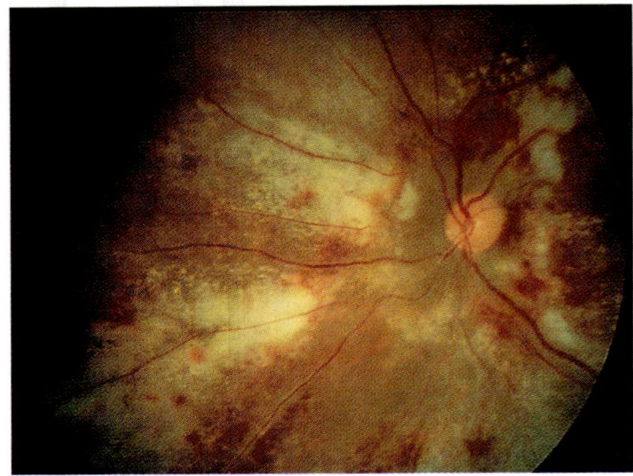

Figure 6 **Cytomegalovirus retinitis may result in hemorrhage exudates and, eventually, blindness.**

Two forms of CMV encephalitis are clinically and pathologically distinguishable in patients with AIDS: multifocal micronodular encephalitis, which resembles HIV encephalitis and presents with progressive dementia, and ventriculoencephalitis, which is characterized by acute cranial nerve deficits, ventriculomegaly, nystagmus, lethargy, and disorientation.[40,42]

DIAGNOSIS

CMV infection cannot be reliably diagnosed on clinical grounds alone. Virus can be isolated from a variety of secretions or infected tissues, but definitive identification can take several weeks. Use of shell vial centrifugation and immunocytochemical analysis for CMV early antigens can facilitate rapid diagnosis, as can the application of immunofluorescence or PCR-based assays to plasma or peripheral blood leukocytes.[43-45] Demonstration of viremia is a better indicator of acute infection than the detection of virus in urine or saliva. The use of PCR to detect CMV DNA in CSF is helpful in the diagnosis of CMV encephalitis and polyradiculopathy.[40,42]

PREVENTION AND TREATMENT

Several specific and nonspecific prophylactic measures to prevent CMV syndromes are under investigation. CMV immune globulin is useful in certain seronegative bone marrow and renal transplant recipients.[46] Matching of seronegative transplant or transfusion recipients with seronegative organ or blood donors may also reduce the likelihood of transmission. Use of blood that has been frozen and thawed, washed with saline, or filtered through cotton wool can prevent transfusion-associated CMV infection.

Ganciclovir, an analogue of deoxyguanosine, is effective in the treatment of CMV retinitis[41] and probably of other advanced CMV infections in immunocompromised hosts.[47] When it is administered intravenously (5 mg/kg twice daily for 14 to 21 days), stabilization or improvement is observed in more than 80% of patients with CMV retinitis. If immunocompromise persists, prolonged maintenance therapy (5 mg/kg daily) is required to maintain improvement, and drug-induced neutropenia is common. Maintenance therapy can be safely discontinued in patients with AIDS whose CD4 cell counts increase substantially with antiretroviral therapy, but relapses occur if CD4 cell counts fall below 50/mm^3.[48] Prophylactic or suppressive ganciclovir may also be useful in other high-risk patients, such as CMV-seropositive bone marrow or solid-organ transplant recipients. Oral ganciclovir was approved for use in the United States in 1995. Although blood levels of oral ganciclovir are inadequate for acute treatment of CMV retinitis, the drug may be useful for both prophylaxis and suppressive maintenance. Several regimens of parenteral or oral ganciclovir have proved useful in protecting susceptible transplant recipients.[49–51]

Foscarnet (90 mg/kg twice daily for 2 to 3 weeks, followed by 90 to 120 mg/kg daily) is also effective for CMV retinitis or GI disease,[47,52] and cidofovir (5 mg/kg weekly for 2 weeks, followed by 5 mg/kg every 2 weeks) may be useful in CMV retinitis.[53] Ganciclovir ocular implants in combination with oral ganciclovir (1.5 g 5 three times daily) is also effective for long-term therapy of CMV retinitis in persistently immunocompromised patients with HIV infection.[54] The combination of ganciclovir and foscarnet may be necessary for severe CNS infections in patients with AIDS.[55] Resistance to ganciclovir and other anti-CMV drugs may complicate prolonged therapy.[56–58]

Epstein-Barr Virus

EBV has a very limited cell tropism; its host range is generally restricted to human B cells and epithelial cells of the nasopharynx and uterine cervix. It is the cause of heterophile antibody-positive infectious mononucleosis and has been implicated in a variety of other disorders, including Burkitt lymphoma, nasopharyngeal carcinoma, and a variety of B cell and possibly T cell lymphoproliferative disorders.

EPIDEMIOLOGY

EBV is shed from the oropharynx in approximately 15% of the adult seropositive population at any given time. Shedding occurs much more frequently in patients with infectious mononucleosis and in immunocompromised persons, such as renal transplant recipients and patients with AIDS. Transmission requires close contact, usually oral to oral, with a person shedding EBV. On rare occasions, virus can be transmitted by other routes, including blood transfusion. EBV infection of the uterine cervix has been documented, and genital ulcerations have been observed in patients with infectious mononucleosis,[59] suggesting the possibility of genital transmission of EBV to sexual partners and newborns.

Antibody prevalence is related to socioeconomic status. In developing countries, most of the population is exposed at an early age. In the United States, approximately 50% of the population seroconvert by 5 years of age; there is also a high rate of seroconversion in adolescence and young adulthood. Clinical infectious mononucleosis develops primarily in persons who contract primary EBV infection when they are between 10 and 20 years of age; in younger persons, primary EBV infection is usually clinically inapparent. Thus, most cases of infectious mononucleosis occur in members of higher socioeconomic groups in developed countries, where viral transmission is often delayed until the patients are older than 10 years. Approximately 12% of susceptible college-age young adults seroconvert each year; about 50% of them acquire infectious mononucleosis.[60] As a result, EBV infection has important public health implications for young adult populations, including students and military personnel.

PATHOGENESIS

Infection is initiated by the binding of EBV envelope proteins gp350/120 to the cell surface molecule CD21. After initial replication in nasopharyngeal cells, EBV infects B cells, which apparently carry the virus to other parts of the body. In the nasopharynx, infectious virus is actively replicated. In contrast, in B cells, the viral genome is present, but mature infectious virus particles are not produced. The B cell may harbor EBV for prolonged periods. In cells in which EBV remains latent, its DNA exists as a circular episome; in cells in which infectious virus is produced, EBV DNA exists in a linear form. Infected B cells are referred to as immortalized (i.e., capable of continuous proliferation) and may produce a variety of antibodies as a consequence of polyclonal B cell activation. One of the antibodies they produce, the heterophile antibody, is a useful diagnostic marker of infection. Once infection is initiated, the host mounts a T cell response against new antigens on infected cells and a B cell antibody response against several EBV-associated antigens, including viral capsid antigen, early antigen, and Epstein-Barr nuclear antigen.[61] Antibody patterns vary according to the stage of infection and the syndrome expressed (*see below*).

CLINICAL FEATURES

Age and immunocompetence greatly influence the expression of EBV infection. Young children usually have asymptomatic or trivial infections and often do not produce heterophile antibodies. In the elderly, EBV infection may present as a persistent febrile syndrome in which the patient tests negative for heterophile antibodies. The most common clinical manifestation of primary EBV infection is infectious mononucleosis. Patients usually present with fever, pharyngitis, and lymphadenopathy. Hepatosplenomegaly, a palatal enanthema, periorbital edema, and jaundice are less common features. A maculopapular diffuse rash occurs in 10% of patients, particularly in patients who have been given ampicillin. Hematologic abnormalities include a peripheral blood lymphocytosis; usually more than 10% of the leukocytes in the peripheral blood consist of atypical lymphocytes. The total leukocyte count may be normal, low, or high; a relative and absolute neutropenia is observed in 60% to 90% of patients. Thrombocytopenia is also common, and hepatocellular enzymes are abnormal in about 90% of patients. Cryoproteins and antigranulocyte antibodies are frequently present but are usually of little clinical significance.

Most cases of infectious mononucleosis resolve in 1 to 3 weeks, although malaise and fatigue occasionally persist for several weeks to months. Complications of infectious mononucleosis can affect most organ systems. Tonsillar enlargement can be extreme, causing respiratory embarrassment. Splenic rupture is rare but must be considered when abdominal pain develops, particularly during the second and third weeks of illness. Patients with splenic rupture usually have left upper quadrant pain and tenderness, often accompanied by signs of peritoneal irritation and laboratory evidence of a falling hematocrit. Splenectomy may be required when a diagnosis of splenic rupture is confirmed, although splenic preservation is sometimes possible with intensive supportive care.[62]

COMPLICATIONS

Neurologic complications occur in fewer than 1% of patients with infectious mononucleosis; these complications include encephalitis, aseptic meningitis, transverse myelitis, Guillain-Barré syndrome, optic neuritis, and peripheral neuropathies. EBV encephalitis often presents as a cerebellitis, but it may mimic the temporal lobe presentation of herpes encephalitis [see 35 Acute Viral Central Nervous System Diseases]. Despite the severity of the neurologic complications, most patients with such complications recover completely.

Autoimmune hemolytic anemia mediated by cold agglutinins directed against i antigens may occur, usually during the second or third week of illness. Aplastic anemia, thrombocytopenia with bleeding, and severe granulocytopenia with superinfection are rare but potentially fatal complications. EBV has been detected in bone marrow specimens by in situ hybridization. Cardiac and pulmonary complications are rare. EBV-associated genital ulcers have also been described.[59] A chronic syndrome of fever and interstitial pneumonitis has been associated with persistent EBV infection and an inability to produce antibody to the viral nuclear antigen K polypeptide.[63]

Immunocompromised hosts are susceptible to overwhelming EBV lymphoproliferative syndromes. A familial X-linked disorder, Duncan disease, has been associated with fatal infectious mononucleosis as well as agammaglobulinemia and lymphoma. All of these disorders are apparently related to EBV infection in genetically predisposed persons. The gene involved encodes for a 128 amino acid protein that may be involved in T lymphocyte signal transduction.[64] Occasionally, in transplant recipients receiving cyclosporine and in patients with AIDS, overwhelming EBV infections develop that culminate in B cell lymphoproliferative syndromes.

The nature of the association of EBV with Burkitt lymphoma and nasopharyngeal carcinoma remains unresolved. Nearly all African patients with Burkitt lymphoma and East Asian patients with nasopharyngeal carcinoma have elevated EBV antibody titers, and EBV DNA is found in the tumors themselves. A single clonal form of EBV has been associated with nasopharyngeal carcinoma and with preinvasive lesions.[65] However, it is not clear whether or how the virus is involved in the etiology of these neoplasms.[66] EBV has also been associated with some cases of primary CNS B cell lymphoma, T cell lymphoma, smooth muscle tumors, lymphomatoid granulomatosis, and Hodgkin disease.[67–70]

DIAGNOSIS

In most cases of infectious mononucleosis, the diagnosis is confirmed by detection of heterophile antibodies and abnormalities in the blood, characterized by the presence of atypical lymphocytes that frequently account for more than 10% of the leukocytes in the peripheral blood. Heterophile antibodies, often detected with monospot or slide tests, are not directed against viral antigens but rather against erythrocyte antigens of a variety of species, including sheep, horses, and goats. These acute-phase reactants, present in about 90% of patients at some point during the illness, must be distinguished from naturally occurring Forssman antibodies and the antibodies present in patients with serum sickness; differentiation can be accomplished by proper absorption tests. Heterophile antibodies may be present at the onset of clinical illness or may appear later in the course of disease; they usually disappear 3 to 4 months after the onset of illness but may persist for longer periods. False positive reactions are rare.

For heterophile antibody–negative cases of infectious mononucleosis and for other EBV-associated syndromes, measurement of EBV-specific antibodies may be useful. Antibodies to viral capsid antigen appear early in the course of infection and are present in 85% of patients at the time of their initial physician visit. The presence of IgM antibodies to viral capsid antigen suggests acute infection, whereas IgG antibodies to viral capsid antigen indicate past infection. Antibodies to early antigen appear transiently during active infections and are also found in patients with the African variant of Burkitt lymphoma and in patients with nasopharyngeal carcinoma. Antibodies to Epstein-Barr nuclear antigen appear late in the course of illness and persist after recovery. Thus, the pattern of specific EBV antibody responses may indicate the stage of infection.

Cultures are usually not helpful in making a diagnosis. Although EBV can be isolated from the nasopharynx, culture techniques are cumbersome and time consuming.

TREATMENT

Treatment is supportive. The administration of corticosteroids may be helpful in certain situations, such as impending airway obstruction, severe thrombocytopenia, or hemolytic anemia. Short-course regimens (1 to 2 weeks) are adequate. Specific antiviral agents such as acyclovir or ganciclovir are not recommended for most EBV-related disorders.[71] Although intravenous acyclovir can reduce viral shedding in patients with infectious mononucleosis, clinical benefit appears to be minimal. Infusion of donor leukocytes has also been useful in some EBV-related lymphoproliferative diseases after bone marrow transplantation.[72]

Human Herpesvirus Type 6

In 1986, a newly recognized herpesvirus, HHV-6, was isolated from the peripheral blood leukocytes of six persons with various lymphoproliferative disorders.[73] It was initially designated human B lymphotropic virus but was renamed when subsequent studies demonstrated that the virus replicated in cells of T cell origin.[74] Two genetically distinct variants of HHV-6—HHV-6A and HHV-6B—are recognized, although disease is most commonly associated with HHV-6B infection.[75] HHV-6A may have greater neurotropism.[76] An immunomodulatory protein, CD46, is a cellular receptor for HHV-6.[77]

HHV-6 infection typically occurs during infancy as the level of maternal antibody wanes, although intrauterine infection can also occur.[78] As many as 80% of adults are seropositive for HHV-6. Infection can manifest as exanthema subitum (roseola infantum), a common illness characterized by fever followed by a rash or by a febrile illness without rash but often with febrile seizures.[79] HHV-6 has been associated with encephalitis,[80] and it has been suggested, though not proved, that HHV-6 is a causal agent in multiple sclerosis.[81] HHV-6 may be transmitted by saliva[82] and possibly by genital secretions[83] and may cause a mononucleosis-like syndrome.[84] In immunocompromised adults, HHV-6 may be associated with pneumonitis or disseminated disease.[85–87] There is no antiviral agent with proven clinical efficacy against HHV-6.

Human Herpesvirus Type 7

In 1990, another lymphotropic human herpesvirus, tentatively called HHV-7, was isolated from human T cells obtained from a healthy 26-year-old man.[88] Its role in human disease has not been established, although it appears frequently in the saliva of healthy adults.[89] Infection generally occurs by age 5, and approximately 90% of adults are seropositive.[90] The HHV-7 genome can also be detected in peripheral blood leukocytes and cervical secretions. HHV-7 may account for some cases of roseola or febrile seizures.[91,92] Although it has been suggested that both HHV-6 and HHV-7 are etiologic agents in chronic fatigue syndrome, supportive evidence is lacking.[93]

Human Herpesvirus Type 8

Several reports in late 1994 and 1995 provided convincing evidence of unique herpesvirus-like sequences in Kaposi sarcoma (KS) and body cavity–based lymphoma tissue from patients with AIDS.[94–97] Using representational difference analysis, researchers found that more than 90% of the KS tissue studied contained these sequences; appropriate control tissue tested negative, except for 15% of non-KS tissue from AIDS patients.[94] The same herpesvirus-like DNA sequences were subsequently reported in KS tissue from patients who did not have AIDS[95–97] and in lymph node biopsy specimens from patients with multicentric Castleman disease.[98]

HHV-8 has been propagated in cell cultures[99–101] and closely resembles a recently identified gamma herpesvirus of rhesus monkeys.[102] Several serologic assays have been developed.[103–105] One, which detects antibody to a latency-associated nuclear antigen, finds seropositivity in 1% to 2% of HIV-negative blood donors; in 30% of HIV-positive hemophiliacs, transfusion recipients, and women; and in more than 80% of patients with HIV infection and KS.

The clinical spectrum of diseases caused by HHV-8 is not well characterized. One patient developed fever, hepatosplenomegaly, angiolymphoid hyperplasia, and transient KS during seroconversion.[106] Molecular and serologic evidence strongly suggests a causal role for HHV-8 in KS and associations with body cavity–based lymphomas and multicentric Castleman disease.[94–97,104,105,107] Although it has been suggested that HHV-8 is associated with both multiple myeloma and sarcoidosis, confirmatory evidence is lacking. Studies of HHV-8 susceptibility to antiviral drugs suggest relative resistance to acyclovir and penciclovir but susceptibility to ganciclovir, foscarnet, and cidofovir.[108,109]

References

1. Whitley RJ, Kimberlin DW, Roizman B: Herpes simplex viruses. Clin Infect Dis 26:541, 1998

2. Fleming DT, McQuillan GM, Johnson RE, et al: Herpes simplex virus type 2 in the United States, 1976 to 1994. N Engl J Med 337:1105, 1997

3. Langenberg AGM, Corey L, Ashley RL, et al: A prospective study of new infections with herpes simplex virus type 1 and type 2. N Engl J Med 341:1432, 1999

4. Wald A, Zeh J, Selke S, et al: Reactivation of genital herpes simplex virus type 2 infection in asymptomatic seropositive persons. N Engl J Med 342:844, 2000

5. Benedetti JK, Zeh J, Corey L: Clinical reactivation of genital herpes simplex virus infection decreases in frequency over time. Ann Intern Med 131:14, 2000

6. Sucato G, Wald A, Wakabayashi E, et al: Evidence of latency and reactivation of both herpes simplex virus (HSV)-1 and HSV-2 in the genital region. J Infect Dis 177:1069, 1998

7. Wald A, Corey L, Cone R, et al: Frequent genital herpes simplex virus 2 shedding in immunocompetent women—effect of acyclovir treatment. J Clin Invest 99:1092, 1997

8. Tedder DG, Ashley R, Tyler KL, et al: Herpes simplex virus infection as a cause of benign recurrent lymphocytic meningitis. Ann Intern Med 121:334, 1994

9. Murakami S, Mizobuchi M, Nakashiro Y, et al: Bell palsy and herpes simplex virus: identification of viral DNA in endoneurial fluid and muscle. Ann Intern Med 124:27, 1996

10. Yamamoto LJ, Tedder DG, Ashley R, et al: Herpes simplex virus type 1 DNA in cerebrospinal fluid of a patient with Mollaret's meningitis. N Engl J Med 325:1082, 1991

11. Brown ZA, Vontver LA, Benedetti J, et al: Effects on infants of a first episode of genital herpes during pregnancy. N Engl J Med 317:1246, 1987

12. Prober CG, Corey L, Brown ZA, et al: The management of pregnancies complicated by genital infections with herpes simplex virus. Clin Infect Dis 15:1031, 1992

13. Boggess KA, Watts DH, Hobson AC, et al: Herpes simplex virus type 2 detection by culture and polymerase chain reaction and relationship to genital symptoms and cervical antibody status during the third trimester of pregnancy. Am J Obstet Gynecol 176:443, 1997

14. Wildemann B, Erhart K, Storch-Hagenlocher B, et al: Quantification of herpes simplex virus type 1 in DNA of cerebrospinal fluid of patients with herpes simplex encephalitis. Neurology 48:1341, 1997

15. Management of herpes in pregnancy. American College of Obstetricians and Gynecologists. ACOG Practice Bulletin 8, 1999, Washington, D.C.

16. Swetter SM, Hill EL, Kern ER, et al: Chronic vulvar ulceration in an immunocompetent woman due to acyclovir-resistant, thymidine kinase deficient herpes simplex virus. J Infect Dis 177:543, 1998

17. Safrin S, Crumpacker C, Chatis P, et al: A controlled trial comparing foscarnet with vidarabine for acyclovir-resistant mucocutaneous herpes simplex in the acquired immunodeficiency syndrome. N Engl J Med 325:551, 1991

18. Javaly K, Wohlfeiler M, Kalayjian R, et al: Treatment of mucocutaneous herpes simplex virus infections unresponsive to acyclovir with topical foscarnet cream in AIDS patients: a phase I/II study. J Acquir Immune Defic Syndr 21:301, 1999

19. Lalezari J, Schacker T, Feinberg J, et al: A randomized, double-blind, placebo-controlled trial of cidofovir gel for the treatment of acyclovir-unresponsive mucocutaneous herpes simplex virus infections in patients with AIDS. J Infect Dis 176:892, 1997

20. Kessler HA, Hurwitz S, Farthing C, et al: Pilot study of topical trifluridine for the treatment of acyclovir-resistant mucocutaneous herpes simplex disease in patients with AIDS (ACTG 172). AIDS Clinical Trials Group. J Acquir Immune Defic Syndr Hum Retrovirol 12:147, 1996

21. Kust RG, Straus SE: Postherpetic neuralgia-pathogenesis, treatment and prevention. N Engl J Med 335:32, 1996

22. Enders G, Miller E, Cradock-Watson J, et al: Consequences of varicella and herpes zoster in pregnancy: prospective study of 1739 cases. Lancet 334:1548, 1994

23. Cohen JI, Brunnell PA, Straus SE, et al: Recent advances in varicella-zoster virus infection. Ann Intern Med 130:922, 1999

24. Gilden DH, Kleinschmidt-DeMasters BK, LaGuardia JJ, et al: Neurologic complications of the reactivation of varicella-zoster virus. N Engl J Med 342:636, 2000

25. Centers for Disease Control and Prevention: Prevention of varicella: recommendations of the Advisory Committee for Immunization Practices (ACIP). MMWR Morb Mortal Wkly Rep 45(RR-11):1, 1996

26. Meyer PA, Seward JF, Jumaan AO, et al: Varicella mortality: trends before vaccine licensure in the United States, 1970–1994. J Infect Dis 182: 383, 2000

27. Shepp DH, Dandliker PS, Meyers JD: Treatment of varicella-zoster virus infection in severely immunocompromised patients: a randomized comparison of acyclovir and vidarabine. N Engl J Med 314: 208, 1986

28. Wood MJ, Shukla S, Fiddian AP, et al: Treatment of acute herpes zoster: effect of early (< 48 h) versus late (48–72 h) therapy with acyclovir and valaciclovir on prolonged pain. J Infect Dis 178(suppl 1):S81, 1998

29. Wood MJ, Johnson RW, McKendrick MW, et al: A randomized trial of acyclovir for 7 days or 21 days with and without prednisolone for treatment of acute herpes zoster. N Engl J Med 330:896, 1994

30. Whitley RJ, Weiss H, Gnann JW Jr, et al: Acyclovir with and without prednisone for the treatment of herpes zoster-a randomized placebo-controlled trial. Ann Intern Med 125:376, 1996

31. Breton G, Fillet AM, Katlama C, et al: Acyclovir-resistant herpes zoster in human immunodeficiency virus-infected patients: results of foscarnet therapy. Clin Infect Dis 27:1525, 1998

32. Tyring S, Barbarash RA, Nahlik JE, et al: Famciclovir for the treatment of acute herpes zoster: effects on acute disease and postherpetic neuralgia: a randomized, double-blind, placebo-controlled trial. Ann Intern Med 123:89, 1995

33. Beutner KL, Friedman DJ, Forszpaniak C, et al: Valaciclovir compared with acyclovir for improved therapy for herpes zoster in immunocompetent adults. Antimicrob Agents Chemother 39:1546, 1995

34. Rowbotham M, Harden N, Stacey B, et al: Gabapentin for the treatment of postherpetic neuralgia: a randomized controlled trial. JAMA 280:1837, 1998

35. Eddleston M, Peacock S, Juniper M, et al: Severe cytomegalovirus infection in immunocompetent patients. Clin Infect Dis 24:52, 1997

36. de Otoro J, Gavalda J, Murio E, et al: Cytomegalovirus disease as a risk factor for graft loss and death after orthotopic liver transplantation. Clin Infect Dis 26:865, 1998

37. Jacobson MA, Mills J: Serious cytomegalovirus disease in the acquired immunodeficiency syndrome (AIDS): clinical findings, diagnosis, and treatment. Ann Intern Med 108:585, 1988

38. Goodgame RW: Gastrointestinal cytomegalovirus disease. Ann Intern Med 119:924, 1993

39. Kim YS, Hollander H: Polyradiculopathy due to cytomegalovirus: report of two cases in which improvement occurred after prolonged therapy and review of the literature. Clin Infect Dis 17:32, 1993

40. Arribas JR, Storch GA, Clifford DB, et al: Cytomegalovirus encephalitis. Ann Intern Med 125:577, 1996

41. Jacobson M: Treatment of cytomegalovirus retinitis in patients with the acquired immunodeficiency syndrome. N Engl J Med 337:105,1997

42. McCutchan JA: Cytomegalovirus infections of the nervous system in patients with AIDS. Clin Infect Dis 20:747, 1995

43. Humar A, Wood S, Lipton J, et al: Effect of cytomegalovirus infection on 1-year mortality rates among recipients of allogeneic bone marrow transplants. Clin Infect Dis 26:606, 1998

44. Spector SA, Wong R, Hsia K, et al: Plasma cytomegalovirus (CMV) DNA load predicts CMV disease and survival in AIDS patients. J Clin Invest 101:497, 1998

45. Bowen EF, Emery VC, Wilson P, et al: Cytomegalovirus polymerase chain reaction viraemia in patients receiving ganciclovir maintenance therapy for retinitis. AIDS 12:605, 1998

46. Bowden RA, Sayers M, Flournoy N, et al: Cytomegalovirus immune globulin and seronegative blood products to prevent primary cytomegalovirus infection after marrow transplantation. N Engl J Med 314:1006, 1998

47. Whitley RJ, Jacobson MA, Friedberg DN, et al: Guidelines for the treatment of cytomegalovirus diseases in patients with AIDS in the era of potent antiretroviral therapy: recommendations of an international panel. International AIDS Society–USA. Arch Intern Med 158: 957, 1998

48. Torriani FJ, Freeman WR, Macdonald JC, et al: CMV retinitis recurs after stopping treatment in virological and immunological failures of potent antiretroviral therapy. AIDS 14:173, 2000

49. Jassal SV, Roscoe JM, Zaltsman JS, et al: Clinical practice guidelines: prevention of cytomegalovirus disease after renal transplanation. J Am Soc Nephrol 9:1697, 1998

50. Flechner SM, Avery RK, Fisher R, et al: A randomized prospective controlled trial of oral acyclovir versus oral ganciclovir for cytomegalovirus prophylaxis in high-risk kidney transplant recipients. Transplantation 66:1682, 1998

51. Turgeon N, Fishman JA, Basgoz N, et al: Effect of oral acyclovir or ganciclovir therapy after preemptive intravenous ganciclovir therapy to prevent cytomegalovirus disease in cytomegalovirus seropositive renal and liver transplant recipients receiving antilymphocyte antibody therapy. Transplantation 66:1780, 1998

52. Parente F, Bianchi Porro G: Treatment of cytomegalovirus esophagitis in patients with acquired immune deficiency syndrome: a randomized controlled study of foscarnet versus ganciclovir. The Italian Cytomegalovirus Study Group. Am J Gastroenterol 93:317, 1998

53. Lalezari JP, Holland GN, Kramer F, et al: Randomized, controlled study of the safety and efficacy of intravenous cidofovir for the treatment of relapsing cytomegalovirus retinitis in patients with AIDS. J Acquir Immune Defic Syndr Hum Retrovirol 17:339, 1998

54. Martin DF, Kuppermann BD, Wolitz RA, et al: Oral ganciclovir for patients with cytomegalovirus retinitis treated with a ganciclovir implant. Roche Ganciclovir Study Group. N Engl J Med 340:1063, 1999

55. Anduze-Faris BM, Fillet AM, Gozlan J, et al: Induction and maintenance therapy of cytomegalovirus central nervous system infection in HIV-infected patients. AIDS 14:517, 2000

56. Jabs DA, Enger C, Dunn JP, et al: Cytomegalovirus retinitis and viral resistance: ganciclovir resistance. J Infect Dis 177:770, 1998

57. Chou S, Marousek G, Parenti DM, et al: Mutation in region III of the DNA polymerase gene conferring foscarnet resistance in cytomegalovirus isolates from 3 subjects receiving prolonged antiviral therapy. J Infect Dis 178:526, 1998

58. Drew WL, Stampien MJ, Andrews J, et al: Cytomegalovirus (CMV) resistance in patients with CMV retinitis and AIDS treated with oral or intravenous ganciclovir. J Infect Dis 179:1352, 1999

59. Hudson LB, Perlman SE: Necrotizing genital ulcerations in a premenarcheal female with mononucleosis. Obstet Gynecol 92:642, 1998

60. Sawyer RN, Evans AS, Niederman JC, et al: Prospective studies of a group of Yale University freshmen: I. Occurrence of infectious mononucleosis. J Infect Dis 123:263, 1971

61. Cohen JI: Epstein-Barr virus and the immune system. JAMA 278: 510, 1997

62. Asgari MM, Begos DG: Spontaneous splenic rupture in infectious mononucleosis: a review. Yale J Biol Med 70:175, 1997

63. Schooley RT, Carey RW, Miller G, et al: Chronic Epstein-Barr virus infection associated with fever and interstitial pneumonitis: clinical and serologic features and response to antiviral chemotherapy. Ann Intern Med 104:636, 1986

64. Sayos S, Wu C, Morra M, et al: The X-induced lymphoproliferative-disease gene product SAP regulates signals induced through the co-receptor SLAM. Nature 395:462, 1998

65. Pathmanathan R, Prasad U, Sadler R, et al: Clonal proliferation of cells infected with Epstein-Barr virus in preinvasive lesions related to nasopharyngeal carcinoma. N Engl J Med 33:693, 1995

66. Razzouk BI, Srinivas S, Sample CE, et al: Epstein-Barr virus DNA recombination and loss in sporadic Burkitt's lymphoma. J Infect Dis 173:529, 1996

67. McClair KL, Leach CT, Jenson HB, et al: Association of Epstein-Barr virus with leiomyosarcomas in young people with AIDS. N Engl J Med 332:12, 1995

68. Lee ES, Locker J, Nalesnik M, et al: The association of Epstein-Barr virus with smooth-muscle tumors occurring after organ transplantation. N Engl J Med 332:19, 1995

69. Dockrell DH, Strickler JG, Paya CV: Epstein-Barr virus-induced T cell lymphoma in solid organ transplant recipients. Clin Infect Dis 26: 180, 1998

70. Haque AK, Myers JL, Hudnall SD, et al: Pulmonary lymphomatoid granulomatosis in acquired immunodeficiency syndrome: lesions with Epstein-Barr virus infection. Mod Pathol 11:347, 1998

71. Torre D, Tambini R: Acyclovir for treatment of infectious mononucleosis: a meta-analysis. Scand J Infect Dis 31:543, 1999

72. Papadopoulos EB, Ladanyi M, Emanuel D, et al: Infusions of donor leukocytes to treat Epstein-Barr virus-associated lymphoproliferative disorders after allogeneic bone marrow transplantation. N Engl J Med 330:1185, 1994

73. Salahuddin SZ, Ablashi DV, Markham PD, et al: Isolation of a new virus, HBLV, in patients with lymphoproliferative disorders. Science 234: 596, 1986

74. Lopez C, Pellett P, Stewart J, et al: Characteristics of human herpesvirus-6. J Infect Dis 157:1271, 1988

75. Inove N, Dambaugh TR, Pellett PE: Molecular biology of human herpesviruses 6A and 6B. Infect Agents Dis 2:343, 1994

76. Hall CB, Caserta MT, Schnabel KC, et al: Persistence of human herpesvirus 6 according to site and variant: possible greater neurotropism of variant A. Clin Infect Dis 26:132, 1998

77. Santoro F, Kennedy PE, Locatelli G, et al: CD46 is a cellular receptor for human herpesvirus 6. Cell 99:817, 1999

78. Ashshi AM, Cooper RJ, Klapper PE, et al: Detection of human herpesvirus 6 DNA in fetal hydrops. Lancet 335:1519, 2000

79. Hall CB, Long CE, Schnabel KC, et al: Human herpesvirus-6 infection in children: a prospective study of complications and reactivation. N Engl J Med 331:432, 1994

80. Ahtiluoto S, Mannonen L, Paetau A, et al: In situ hybridization detection of human herpesvirus 6 in multiple sclerosis. Pediatrics 105: 431, 2000

81. Hay KA, Tenser RB: Leukotropic herpesviruses in multiple sclerosis. Mult Scler 6:66, 2000

82. Levy J, Ferro F, Greenspan D, et al: Frequent isolation of HHV6 from saliva and high prevalence of the virus in the population. Lancet 335:1047, 1990

83. Leach CT, Newton ER, McParlin S, et al: Human herpesvirus 6 infection of the female genital tract. J Infect Dis 169:1281, 1994

84. Akashi K, Eizuru Y, Sumiyoshi Y, et al: Severe infectious mononucleosis-like syndrome and primary human herpesvirus 6 infection in an adult. N Engl J Med 329:168, 1993

85. Cone RW, Hackman RC, Huang MLW, et al: Human herpesvirus 6 in lung tissue from patients with pneumonitis after bone marrow transplantation. N Engl J Med 329:156, 1993

86. Knox KK, Carrigan DR: Disseminated active HHV-6 infections in patients with AIDS. Lancet 343:577, 1994

87. Singh N, Carrigan DR: Human herpesvirus-6 in transplantation: an emerging pathogen. Ann Intern Med 124:1065, 1996

88. Frenkel N, Schirmer EC, Wyatt LS, et al: Isolation of a new herpesvirus from human CD4+ T cells. Proc Natl Acad Sci USA 87:748, 1990

89. Wyatt LS, Frenkel N: Human herpesvirus 7 is a constitutive inhabitant of adult human saliva. J Virol 66:3206, 1992

90. Black JB, Pellett PE: Human herpesvirus 7. Rev Med Virol 9:245, 1999

91. Levy JA: Three new human herpes viruses (HHV 6, 7, and 8). Lancet 349:558, 1997

92. Hall CB: Human herpesviruses at sixes, sevens, and more. Ann Intern Med 127:481, 1997

93. Reeves WC, Stamey FR, Black JB, et al: Human herpesviruses 6 and 7 in chronic fatigue syndrome: a case-control study. Clin Infect Dis 31:48, 2000

94. Chang Y, Cesarman E, Pessin MS, et al: Identification of herpesvirus-like DNA sequences in AIDS-associated Kaposi's sarcoma. Science 266:1865, 1994

95. Moore PS, Chang Y: Detection of herpesvirus-like DNA sequences in Kaposi's sarcoma in patients with and those without HIV infection. N Engl J Med 332:1181, 1995

96. Cesarman E, Chang Y, Moore PS, et al: Kaposi's sarcoma–associated herpesvirus-like DNA sequences in AIDS-related body-cavity–based lymphomas. N Engl J Med 332:1186, 1995

97. Huang YQ, Li JJ, Kaplan MH, et al: Human herpesvirus-like nucleic acid in various forms of Kaposi's sarcoma. Lancet 345:759, 1995

98. Soulier J, Grollet L, Oksenhendler E, et al: Kaposi's sarcoma–associated herpesvirus-like DNA sequences in multicentric Castleman's disease. Blood 86:1276, 1995

99. Renne R, Zhong W, Herndier B, et al: Lytic growth of Kaposi's sarcoma-associated herpesvirus (human herpesvirus 8) in culture. Nat Med 2:342, 1996

100. Foreman KE, Friborg J Jr, Kong WP, et al: Propagation of a human herpesvirus from AIDS-associated Kaposi's sarcoma. N Engl J Med 336:163, 1997

101. Vierra J, Huang ML, Koelle DM, et al: Transmissible Kaposi's sarcoma–associated herpesvirus (human herpesvirus 8) in saliva of men with a history of Kaposi's sarcoma. J Virol 71:7083, 1997

102. Desrosiers RC, Sasseville VG, Czajak SC, et al: A herpesvirus of rhesus monkeys related to the human Kaposi's sarcoma–associated herpesvirus. J Virol 71:9764, 1997

103. Kedes DH, Ganem D, Ameli N, et al: The prevalence of serum antibody to human herpesvirus 8 (Kaposi sarcoma–associated herpesvirus) among HIV-seropositive and high-risk HIV-seronegative women. JAMA 277:478, 1997

104. Lennett E, Blackboum DJ, Levy JA: Antibodies to human herpesvirus type 8 in the general population and in Kaposi's sarcoma patients. Lancet 348:858, 1996

105. Gao SJ, Kingsley L, Hoover DR, et al: Seroconversion to antibodies against Kaposi's sarcoma–associated herpesvirus-related latent nuclear antigens before the development of Kaposi's sarcoma. N Engl J Med 335:233, 1996

106. Oksenhendler E, Cazals-Hatem D, Schulz TF, et al: Transient angiolymphoid hyperplasia and Kaposi's sarcoma after primary infection with human herpesvirus 8 in a patient with human immunodeficiency virus infection. N Engl J Med 338:1585, 1998

107. Rezza G, Andreoni M, Dorrucci M, et al: Human herpesvirus 8 seropositivity and risk of Kaposi's sarcoma and other acquired immunodeficiency syndrome-related diseases. J Natl Cancer Inst 91:1468, 1999

108. Kedes DH, Ganem D: Sensitivity of Kaposi's sarcoma–associated herpesvirus replication to antiviral drugs: implications for potential therapy. J Clin Invest 99:2082, 1997

109. Neyts J, De Clercq E: Antiviral drug susceptibility of human herpesvirus 8. Antimicrob Agents Chemother 41:2754, 1997

30 Measles, Mumps, Rubella, Parvovirus, and Poxvirus

Martin S. Hirsch, M.D.

Measles

Measles (rubeola) is a highly infectious disease caused by a paramyxovirus of worldwide distribution. The measles virus was once one of the most common and important global pathogens, but infections caused by this agent are now becoming rare in developed countries, where vaccine use is widespread. In areas where vaccines are not widely used, measles remains a major health problem. It is estimated that over 36 million cases of measles occur each year worldwide, resulting in one million deaths, approximately 50% of which occur in Africa.[1]

EPIDEMIOLOGY

Humans are the principal reservoirs of measles virus, which is spread by respiratory droplet aerosols produced by sneezing and coughing. The disease may be contagious from several days before the onset of rash to up to 5 days after lesions appear. The attack rate for exposed susceptible contacts may exceed 90%; asymptomatic infections are rare.

Vaccines have dramatically reduced the incidence of indigenous measles in the United States and have eliminated the disease altogether in some developed countries.[2] However, large outbreaks still occur among unvaccinated populations in developed countries (e.g., among certain religious groups in the Netherlands).[3]

Among undernourished children in developing countries, measles can cause a devastating illness, and case-fatality rates may reach or exceed 25%.[4] Before widespread vaccine use, epidemics occurred every 2 to 3 years in developed countries, and the illness developed in 95% of urban dwellers before they reached 15 years of age. Outbreaks occurred primarily in late winter and early spring. In 1989, the World Health Assembly instituted major efforts to reduce measles morbidity and mortality through implementation of control strategies. By 1996, estimated incidence and death rates were reduced by 78% and 88%, respectively.[1,5,6] In the Americas, between 1990 and 1996, the number of new measles cases decreased from 246,607 to 2,109 (a decrease of 99%) and vaccine coverage increased from 77% to 85%. In 1999, only 100 confirmed measles cases were reported in the United States, the lowest number on record.[7] Molecular epidemiologic studies suggest that most cases in the United States may now be imported.[8]

PATHOGENESIS

The portals of entry for measles virus include cells of the respiratory tract and possibly the conjunctivae. After undergoing local replication and spreading to regional lymph nodes, measles virus is disseminated to distant sites, particularly skin and mucous membranes, by a leukocyte-associated viremia. Lesions on mucous membranes (Koplik spots) appear as bluish-white specks on an erythematous base. Histologically, Koplik spots are composed of epithelioid giant cells with cytoplasmic and nuclear inclusions that contain microtubular aggregates; inflammatory cells and intercellular edema are present. Lesions of the skin also demonstrate inclusions and microtubular aggregates, suggesting that active viral replication occurs in skin as well as in mucous membranes. Infectious virus can be isolated from leukocytes, urine, conjunctivae, and respiratory secretions. Antibody appears in the serum as viremia ceases. Leukopenia may accompany the illness, together with lymphocyte hyporesponsiveness.

DIAGNOSIS

Clinical Features

Approximately 9 to 11 days after a person is initially exposed to the virus, malaise, fever, conjunctivitis, photophobia, periorbital edema, coryza, and cough develop. Cough may be severe, although generally nonproductive, and temperature may reach 40.6° C (105.1° F). Within 2 to 3

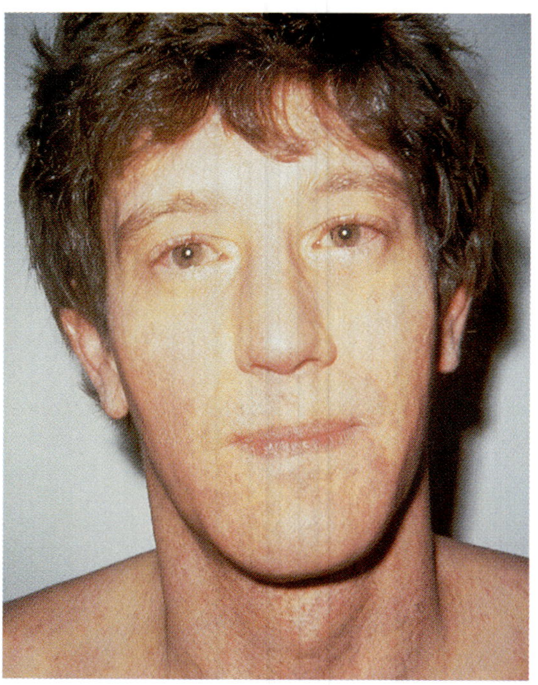

Figure 1 **A case of measles in a young man is characterized by maculopapular rash and conjunctivitis.**

days, Koplik spots may appear on the buccal mucosa and occasionally on the conjunctivae. The skin rash, which erupts 2 to 3 days later, usually appears at the hairline and spreads downward during the next 3 days as systemic symptoms subside [*see Figure 1*]. Lesion density is greatest above the shoulders, where macular lesions may coalesce. The rash lasts 4 to 6 days and then fades from the head downward. Desquamation may be present but is usually not severe. Complete recovery without scarring generally occurs within 7 to 10 days from the onset of the rash.

A severe atypical presentation of measles may appear in persons who were immunized between 1963 and 1967 with killed measles virus vaccine and who were later exposed to the wild virus. After a prodrome of fever, headache, abdominal pain, and myalgias, a rash develops on the hands and feet and advances toward the head. The eruption may be vesicular, urticarial, maculopapular, or hemorrhagic and is most prominent along body creases. Pneumonia, pleural effusion, and hilar lymphadenopathy are common in atypical measles. All persons vaccinated after 1967 received the live attenuated measles vaccine, which is rarely, if ever, associated with the atypical measles syndrome.

Laboratory Tests

In an epidemic setting, observation of the characteristic rash, fever, coryza, and conjunctivitis is sufficient to establish the diagnosis. However, as measles declines in prevalence, clinical acumen in diagnosis also diminishes. Multinucleated giant cells can often be detected in stained smears of nasal secretions, and measles antigen can be demonstrated in such cells by immunofluorescence. The virus can be isolated from nasal secretions or urine by cultivation of such materials on primate cell monolayers. A rise in hemagglutination inhibition antibodies during a period of 2 to 3 weeks confirms the diagnosis. Confirmation by measles-specific IgM enzyme immunoassay is also available.

DIFFERENTIAL DIAGNOSIS

Sporadic cases of measles must be differentiated from other viral exanthems, secondary syphilis, scarlet fever, and drug reactions. Atypical measles may resemble Rocky Mountain spotted fever, meningococcemia, or varicella.

COMPLICATIONS

Measles is usually benign and uncomplicated. Complications occur more commonly in adults, malnourished children, and immunocompromised patients. Measles is associated with severe pulmonary and neurologic complications in up to 80% of immunocompromised children and adults with cancer or HIV infection, with case-fatality rates of 40% to 70%; rash is absent in 30%.[9,10] Measles virus may further suppress host immune responses, leading to reactivation of latent tuberculosis or superimposition of new bacterial pneumonia, particularly among malnourished children.

Measles virus infection often involves the central nervous system, but clinically apparent encephalomyelitis is rare (one in every 1,000 to 2,000 measles patients).[2] CNS involvement may precede the rash but usually begins 4 to 7 days after the eruption appears. The onset of encephalomyelitis is often precipitous and is characterized by a rise in fever, sudden mental deterioration, and seizures; motor defects and cerebellar ataxia are common. An autoimmune demyelinating process may be involved in the pathogenesis of measles encephalomyelitis, which is fatal in about 10% of patients.

Subacute measles encephalitis may complicate measles in immunocompromised hosts 1 to 7 months after exposure; the patient has seizures and altered mental status, but results of cerebrospinal fluid analysis are normal.[11] Diagnosis may require brain biopsy for histology, immunocytochemical analysis, or polymerase chain reaction detection of viral RNA.[10] In rare instances, a subacute sclerosing panencephalitis occurs as a complication of measles in infected children younger than 2 years, but the panencephalitis develops after a latent period of several years. Other measles complications include thrombocytopenia with associated purpura or bleeding, myocarditis, pericarditis, hepatitis, and severe keratitis progressing to blindness.

TREATMENT AND PREVENTION

Therapy is mainly supportive. Ribavirin, either intravenous or aerosolized, has been proposed for certain complications (i.e., encephalitis or pneumonitis),[9,10] but controlled trials are lacking. Postexposure prophylaxis can be provided for high-risk patients (e.g., pregnant women and immunosuppressed children) by administering immunoglobulin intramuscularly at a dosage of 0.25 to 0.50 ml/kg body weight within 6 days after exposure.[12]

In vaccination guidelines in the United States, two immunizations are suggested for children before school enrollment to reduce the chance of primary vaccine failure. Vaccination is recommended for nonpregnant women of childbearing years and may be considered for institutionalized adults or individuals working in day care centers. Severely immunocompromised individuals should avoid measles vaccination because of the risk of vaccine-associated diseases, such as inclusion body encephalitis or pneumonitis.[13,14]

The effort to eradicate measles from the United States relies on identification and immunization of susceptible children, adolescents, and adults; on strict enforcement of more comprehensive school immunization requirements; and on strengthening of surveillance and outbreak-control measures.

Mumps

Mumps virus is a pleomorphic, enveloped, single-stranded RNA paramyxovirus capable of causing parotitis, epididymo-orchitis, and CNS disease. Because of widespread vaccination efforts, its role as a major cause of childhood morbidity has greatly diminished.

EPIDEMIOLOGY

Mumps virus has worldwide distribution, and infection is seen more commonly in winter and spring. Humans are the only natural host. Infection is uncommon in persons younger than 1 year, and congenital infection is rare but can lead to fetal loss in the first trimester.

A live mumps virus vaccine was approved for use in the United States in 1967; its use was facilitated by subsequent incorporation with measles and rubella (MMR) vaccine. Since its widespread use, mumps cases have fallen by over 99%, from 185,691 cases in 1968 to 906 cases in 1995.[12] Approximately 11% of cases are observed in children between 1 and 4 years of age, 52% in children between 5 and 14 years of age, and 11% in children older than 15 years.

PATHOGENESIS

Mumps virus spreads from person to person by direct contact with nasopharyngeal secretions. Virus is shed in saliva from as long as 6 days before to 5 days after clinical onset. Incubation ranges from 2 to 4 weeks (mean, 18 days). Initial replication occurs in the pharynx, followed by viremic dissemination. Both humoral and cell-mediated immune responses are induced and correlate with cessation of viremia and salivary virus excretion.

DIAGNOSIS

Clinical Features

Two thirds of cases are symptomatic, with initial symptoms of malaise and fever predominating. Painful swelling of the parotid gland is the characteristic feature of infection. It may be unilateral, and other salivary glands may be involved. However, parotitis occurs in only 30% to 40% of all cases of mumps virus infection.

An unvaccinated child who presents with tender parotitis generally has mumps; further diagnostic testing is not required. In older age groups, other entities (sarcoidosis, tumors, alcohol abuse, drug side effects, and other viral or bacterial infections) should be considered. In persons without parotitis who have orchitis, aseptic meningitis, encephalitis, or other obscure syndromes (e.g., myocarditis or pancreatitis), mumps should be considered [*see* Complications, *below*].

Laboratory Tests

Definitive diagnosis of mumps can be made by virus isolation from the oropharynx, CSF, or urine or by virus serology. Rapid detection by PCR techniques is now possible in some laboratories.[15]

COMPLICATIONS

Epididymo-orchitis occurs in up to 38% of postpubertal males with mumps and is usually unilateral. Subsequent sterility is uncommon, although testicular atrophy may occur.

CSF pleocytosis occurs in at least 50% of patients with mumps,[16] although symptomatic meningitis is less common. A lymphocytic pleocytosis is seen, with an elevated protein level and a normal to low (10%) glucose level. Symptomatic encephalitis occurs in one of 6,000 cases and presents as decreased consciousness and focal neurologic deficits. Most patients with encephalitis recover completely, although 0.5% to 2.3% of patients with mumps encephalitis may die. Other neurologic complications may include hydrocephalus; deafness; and rare cases of demyelinating disorders, transverse myelitis, Guillain-Barré syndrome, and cerebellar ataxia.[17] Deafness may be sudden, unilateral, and permanent.[12]

Pancreatitis, mastitis, and oophoritis have been observed in patients with mumps. Myocarditis occurs and in rare cases can be fatal.[18] Endocardial fibroelastosis, an infrequent sequela of myocarditis, has been associated with mumps infection.[19] Mumps can cause polyarticular or monoarticular arthritis; it generally affects adult males and is self-limited (usually less than 8 weeks).[20]

TREATMENT AND PREVENTION

Treatment of patients with mumps is largely supportive, although anti-inflammatory agents may be useful in cases of severe orchitis or arthritis. Administration of immune globulin does not prevent mumps and is not recommended. Prevention can be achieved in well over 90% of persons by the use of live attenuated mumps vaccine, administered twice as part of the recommended MMR vaccine regimen.[12]

Rubella

Rubella, or German measles, is usually a benign febrile exanthem, but when it occurs in pregnant women, it can produce major congenital malformations. The infective agent is a single-stranded RNA virus of the Togaviridae family.

EPIDEMIOLOGY

Humans are the only known natural hosts for the rubella virus, which appears to be spread by respiratory droplets. The virus is moderately contagious but less so than measles. Before a rubella vaccine was introduced in 1969, epidemics occurred in the United States at 6- to 9-year intervals, predominantly in children younger than 15 years. Since the widespread use of rubella vaccine, the incidence of rubella has decreased by 99%.[21] Outbreaks continue to occur, primarily among young adults in hospitals, colleges, prisons, and prenatal clinics, but no major epidemics have occurred in the United States since 1964. Susceptibility rates among young adults vary, with the greatest proportion of cases now seen among persons of Hispanic origin.[21,22] Approximately four confirmed cases of congenital rubella syndrome are reported in the United States annually.

PATHOGENESIS

Initially, the virus replicates in the nasopharynx and regional lymph nodes. After the virus invades the bloodstream, it may spread to the skin and distal organs or, transplacentally, to the developing fetus. The virus may be present in throat washings or blood for several days before the appearance of the rash and up to 2 weeks after its onset. In rare cases of rubella arthropathy, the virus may persist in peripheral leukocytes or in synovial cells for months to years.

A pregnant woman infected with rubella is at risk for transmitting the virus to her fetus. Damage to the fetus is most likely to occur if the mother is infected within the first 2 months of gestation (fetal abnormalities are observed in 40% to 85% of such cases).[23,24] Infection within the third month is associated with fetal defects in 20% to 40% of cases, whereas infection during the fourth month is associated with fetal defects in 10% of cases. Mechanisms of fetal damage are not clear but may include viral cytolysis, chromosomal breaks, reduced cell multiplication, and alteration of fetal blood supply. As a result, fetal growth may be retarded, and defects may develop in multiple organ systems. Despite the production of fetal antibodies, the rubella virus can persist in the fetus and newborn and be excreted for months to years after birth.

DIAGNOSIS

Clinical Features

After an incubation period of 12 to 23 days, a mild prodrome of malaise, headache, fever, and mild conjunctivitis may develop. Postauricular, suboccipital, and posterior cervical lymphadenopathy often precede the rash, which begins on the face and forehead. Within 1 to 5 days, the discrete maculopapular lesions spread over the trunk and extremities and may coalesce. The rash usually disappears within 3 days.

Laboratory Tests

The presence of rubella can be confirmed by virus isolation, by PCR detection, or by demonstration of seroconversion in response to rubella antigens. Virus isolation is often difficult because rubella virus does not cause cytopathic effects on the cell lines that are generally employed in diagnostic laboratories. Antibodies are often present shortly after rash appears and increase in titer during the next 2 to 3 weeks. Measurements of specific IgM antibodies to rubella virus are particularly useful in newborns: raised IgM levels denote recent infection and are specific for fetal infection because IgM antibodies do not cross the placenta. Elevated IgM antibodies may return to nondiagnostic levels by 3 to 6 months, and persistence of IgG antibodies beyond this period may also help diagnose neonatal infection.[21]

DIFFERENTIAL DIAGNOSIS

Rubella may be confused with other viral exanthems (e.g., those caused by enteroviruses, parvoviruses, or adenoviruses), scarlet fever, or drug eruptions.

COMPLICATIONS

The most common complications of rubella are arthropathies of the fingers, wrists, and knees; they occur predominantly in young women. Such arthropathies consist of arthralgia or frank arthritis, and recurring joint symptoms may persist for a year or more. Encephalitis and thrombocytopenia are rare complications of acute rubella. Encephalitis occurs in one in 6,000 cases,[12] and thrombocytopenia, which is sometimes associated with purpura or hemorrhage, occurs most often in children.

Congenital rubella syndrome, also a rare complication of acute rubella, may manifest itself as defects in one or many organ systems. Hearing impairment is the most common single defect (60%).[21] Heart malformations, particularly patent ductus arteriosus and peripheral pulmonic stenosis, are also common (45%), as are cataracts (25%), microcephaly (27%), and mental retardation (13%). Malformation of bone metaphyses may also be present, together with hepatosplenomegaly, thrombocytopenia, interstitial pneumonitis, myocarditis, and thrombocytopenic purpura. Congenitally infected infants are often of low birth weight (23%), and they excrete rubella virus for prolonged periods. Late complications may result from imbalances of cellular and humoral immunity, from immune complex deposition, or from prolonged viral replication. Diabetes mellitus and other endocrine abnormalities may be late complications of congenital rubella, as is subacute sclerosing panencephalitis.[25]

TREATMENT AND PREVENTION

Beyond the fetal period, rubella is mild and self-limited. Current treatment of congenital rubella syndrome is only supportive. Rubella vaccines are described elsewhere.

Pregnant women infected with rubella virus who are asymptomatic may still transmit rubella to their fetuses. Thus, testing of immune status is advisable for women of childbearing age and for hospital employees who have no history of rubella vaccination. About 10% to 15% of such persons are seronegative and should be vaccinated when not pregnant. Pregnancy should be delayed for 3 months after vaccination, although no cases of congenital rubella syndrome were seen in 321 women who were vaccinated within 3 months before or 3 months after conception.[12] Vaccine virus has, however, been isolated from aborted fetuses.

Parvovirus

Although only recently recognized as a human pathogen, parvovirus B19 is now appreciated as a cause of several syndromes in both children and adults. Parvovirus B19, a small (20 to 26 nm), single-stranded DNA virus, causes erythema infectiosum (fifth disease) in normal persons, aplastic crises in persons with underlying hemolytic disorders, chronic anemia in immunocompromised hosts, and fetal loss in pregnant women.[26–30]

EPIDEMIOLOGY

Parvovirus B19 infection occurs most commonly in school-age children in outbreaks during late winter and spring. Only 2% to 15% of preschool-age children have antibodies, but seroprevalence increases to 35% to 60% by 11 years to 19 years of age, and to greater than 75% in persons older than 50 years.[31] Respiratory transmission is likely and is facilitated by close contact. Hospital outbreaks have also been described and are often traced to patients with aplastic crises who carry large amounts of virus in blood and respiratory secretions.[32,33] Maternal infection can lead to fetal anemia, hydrops fetalis, heart failure, and death resulting in spontaneous abortion, most commonly 4 to 6 weeks after infection. When women are infected during the first 20 weeks of pregnancy, the risk of parvovirus-related fetal death is approximately 9% to 10%.[34,35] Routine antenatal screening is not recommended.[28,36]

PATHOGENESIS

Replication of parvovirus B19 has been demonstrated in human erythroid progenitor cells, and the receptor appears to be the P blood group antigen globoside, a neutral glycosphingolipid, which occurs in erythrocytes, erythroblasts, megakaryocytes, endothelial cells, placenta, and fetal liver and heart cells.[37] Expression of this glycosphingolipid in tissues helps to determine parvovirus B19 tropism.[38] Persons who lack erythrocyte P antigen (p phenotype) are naturally resistant to infection,[27,39] and the distribution of parvovirus in infected individuals is linked to the presence of the P antigen. Although little is known about the pathogenesis of parvovirus, antiviral antibodies—particularly those directed against the capsid protein VP1—appear to be responsible for viral clearance.

DIAGNOSIS

Clinical Features

The rash of erythema infectiosum usually appears without prodromal symptoms after an incubation period of 4 to 14 days. The exanthem progresses through three stages. Initially, a fiery-red rash develops on both cheeks (giving them the appearance of having been slapped), accompanied by relative pallor around the mouth. From 1 to 4 days later, an erythematous maculopapular eruption appears on the proximal extremities and spreads to the trunk in a lacelike, reticular pattern. The third stage, during which the eruption waxes and wanes, may persist for several weeks and may be precipitated by skin trauma, exposure to sunlight, or extremes of temperature. Arthralgia and arthritis are seen in up to 80% of infected adults; arthralgia is particularly common in women, may occur without rash, and may linger for weeks. Joint involvement is often symmetrical in the hands, wrists, knees, and ankles. Hemolytic anemias and encephalopathies are rare complications.

Laboratory Tests

Parvovirus-specific IgM antibodies usually appear within 3 days after symptoms develop; these antibodies persist for several weeks and then rapidly decline. IgG antibodies, however, persist for years. Viral DNA can also be detected in blood, tissues, and secretions, although culture techniques for virus isolation are unsatisfactory.

COMPLICATIONS

Transient aplastic crises associated with parvovirus B19 occur in patients who have sickle cell anemia, hereditary spherocytosis, thalassemia, and various other hemolytic anemias.[27] These aplastic crises are abrupt in onset and associated with giant pronormoblasts in the bone marrow. They generally last 1 to 2 weeks and go into remission spontaneously. In immunocompromised hosts (e.g., patients with HIV infection), acute infection may lead to viral persistence and chronic bone marrow suppression.[30] A significant proportion of patients with AIDS who develop severe anemia while receiving zidovudine (AZT) have persistent parvovirus infection.[40] Pneumonia, hepatitis, and myocarditis have also been associated with parvovirus infections in immunocompromised as well as immunocompetent adults and children.[41–46]

TREATMENT

Pooled human immune globulin contains anti-parvovirus B19 antibodies and has been used to treat persistent infections as well as acute exposures.[30] Prevention of nosocomial infections is of great concern: pregnant health care workers should not care for patients with aplastic crises. Droplet isolation is recommended for such patients, including the use of gowns, gloves, and masks during close contact. Because certain blood products (e.g., clotting factors) contain B19 DNA, screening of products, donors, and recipients has been suggested.[47]

Poxvirus Infections

Poxviruses are the largest (200 to 320 nm) and most complex human viruses. They replicate in cell cytoplasm and may produce eosinophilic cytoplasmic inclusion bodies. They preferentially infect skin epithelial cells and may cause a variety of human diseases. Smallpox (variola), once the most devastating and feared worldwide pestilence, has now been virtually eliminated. Other human poxvirus diseases include vaccinia, molluscum contagiosum, orf (contagious pustular dermatitis), and paravaccinia (milker's nodules).

SMALLPOX

A detailed discussion of smallpox is no longer needed, because no naturally acquired cases of smallpox have been observed since 1977 as a result of a global eradication effort that was initiated by the World Health Organization in the 1960s.[48] Several biologic features of the smallpox virus favored its eradication: only one serotype existed, a stable and effective vaccine had been developed, and there were no nonhuman reservoirs and no human carriers of the smallpox virus. Widespread use of smallpox vaccination, intense surveillance in previously endemic areas, and destruction of laboratory virus stocks have contributed to the current optimism that smallpox is now a disease of purely historical interest. The World Health Assembly recommended in May 1996 that all remaining virus stocks be destroyed in June 1999. However, the stocks have not been totally destroyed, and therefore, concerns related to the use of smallpox virus as a potential biological warfare agent have led to renewed interest in developing antiviral agents to combat its possible reemergence.[49,50]

VACCINIA

The exact origin of vaccinia virus is not clear, but it has long been used as the source of smallpox vaccines. In immunized persons, injection of vaccinia virus usually induces a localized papular eruption at the injection site. However, patients with compromised immune function or with skin conditions such as eczema may experience more severe disease after vaccination. Progressive generalized vaccinia, vaccinia gangrenosa, and eczema vaccinatum may complicate such disorders. Fortunately, smallpox vaccinations are no longer required or recommended for use in the United States or for international travel. There is no evidence that smallpox vaccination is beneficial when used in the treatment of recurrent herpes simplex, warts, or any other infection; moreover, the vaccine is contraindicated for these disorders. Nevertheless, because certain military personnel at home and abroad continue to be vaccinated, complicated human vaccinia infections may continue to occur. Vaccinia immune globulin and antiviral agents (e.g., thiosemicarbazones, idoxuridine, and interferons) have been suggested as possible therapies for vaccinia complications, but their effectiveness has not been established.

MOLLUSCUM CONTAGIOSUM

Molluscum contagiosum is characterized by multiple painless, pearly white nodules 2 to 5 mm in diameter with a central umbilication. They can appear anywhere on the body except the palms and soles [*see Figure 2*]. The nodules, which are most commonly found in anogenital regions, rupture easily and may be spread by sexual routes, by autoinoculation, or by close familial contact under conditions of poor hygiene. The infection has worldwide distribution, and incidence rates of clinically apparent infection range from 0.1% to 4.5%. Incubation periods vary from several days to several weeks, and lesions may clear rapidly or persist for up to 18 months. Lesions are common in patients with AIDS and may be severe.[51] Lesions near the eye may be complicated by chronic conjunctivitis or superficial keratitis.

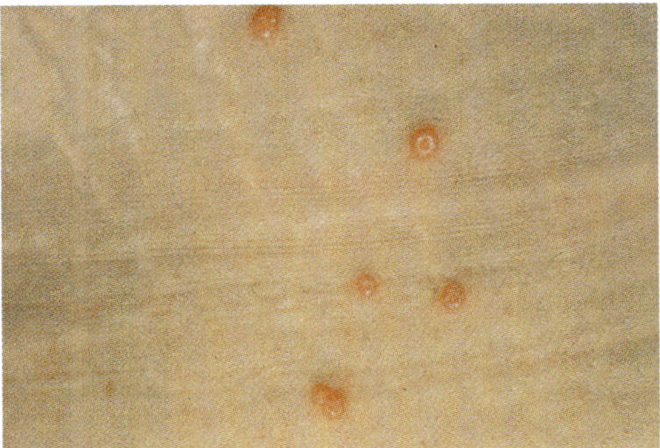

Figure 2 **The pearly white papular lesions of molluscum contagiosum shown here are 2 to 5 cm in diameter, with a central umbilication.**

The molluscum contagiosum virus (MCV) has been visualized by electron microscopy but has not been cultivated in vitro. Microscopic observation of large cytoplasmic inclusions, called molluscum bodies [*see Figure 3*], in appropriately stained, expressed lesion contents or histologic sections confirms a clinical diagnosis. Restriction endonuclease cleavage patterns of DNA from purified virus obtained from skin lesions indicate that there are two distinct MCV genotypes.[52]

The lesions resolve spontaneously without scarring. A small number of lesions can be removed by

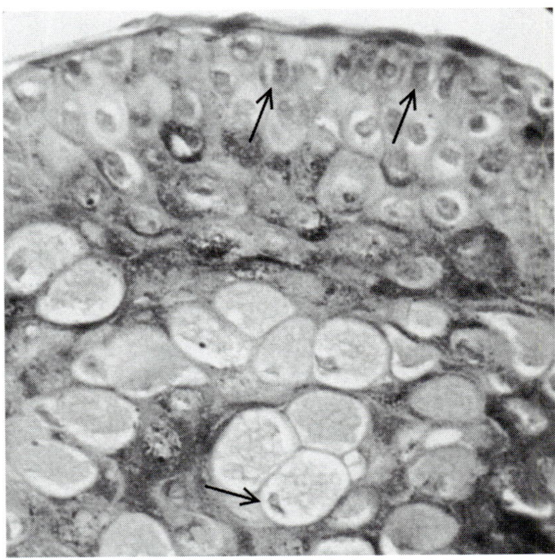

Figure 3 **Micrograph of a molluscum contagiosum lesion demonstrates basophilic molluscum bodies (arrows) in epidermal cell cytoplasm.**

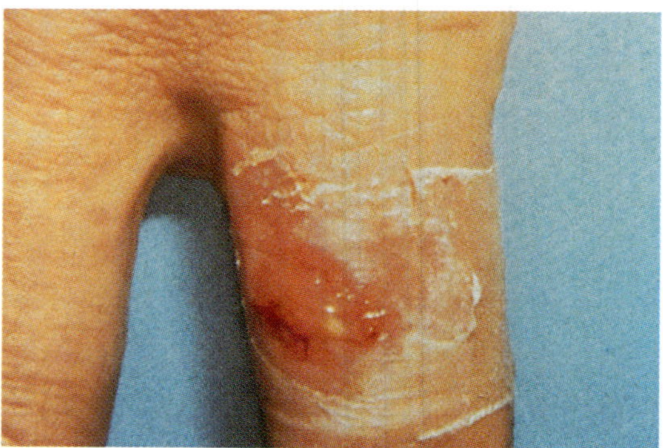

Figure 4 **Papillomatous lesions of orf (pustular dermatitis) can be observed on the finger of a sheep handler.**

gentle curettage or caustic chemicals if desired. No antiviral therapy or vaccine is available.

PARAVACCINIA, ORF, AND MONKEYPOX

Human paravaccinia, orf, and monkeypox infections result from direct contact with natural animal reservoirs of these agents; humans are only incidental hosts.

Paravaccinia is an infection that produces lesions on the teats and oral mucosa of calves and milk cows. When humans are infected by direct contact, so-called milker's nodules develop on the fingers or hands and occasionally are associated with lymphadenitis. Lesions develop during a period of 1 to 2 weeks and resolve in 3 to 8 weeks.

The orf virus causes papillomatous lesions (pustular dermatitis) on the mucous membranes and corneas of sheep. Lesions in humans [*see Figure 4*] are caused by direct contact with infected animals and resemble those caused by paravaccinia, although paravaccinia and orf viruses are distinct.

Human monkeypox infections occur sporadically in small villages in African tropical rain forests; monkeypox infections also occur in captive monkeys in European and North American laboratories. Smallpox-like diseases caused by monkeypox virus have been noted in central Africa in humans who live in close proximity to monkeys.[53,54] Although the primary reservoir for the monkeypox virus remains uncertain, humans appear to be incidental hosts for the virus. Person-to-person transmission has been described.[55]

Acknowledgments

Figures 1 and 4 Photographs courtesy of Dr. Howard Baden, Department of Dermatology, Massachusetts General Hospital, and Harvard Medical School, Boston.

Figure 2 Photograph courtesy of the American Academy of Dermatology.

Figure 3 Micrograph courtesy of Dr. George W. Hambrick, Department of Dermatology, New York Hospital, New York.

References

1. Advances in global measles control and elimination: summary of the 1997 international meeting. MMWR Morb Mortal Wkly Rep 47(RR-11):1, 1998

2. Norrby E, Kristensson K: Measles virus in the brain. Brain Res Bull 44:213, 1997

3. Measles outbreak—Netherlands, April 1999–January 2000. MMWR Morb Mortal Wkly Rep 49:299, 2000

4. Dollimore N, Cutts F, Binka FN: Measles incidence, case fatality, and delayed mortality in children with or without vitamin A supplementation in rural Ghana. Am J Epidemiol 146:646, 1997

5. Progress toward global measles control and elimination, 1990–1996. MMWR Morb Mortal Wkly Rep 46:893, 1997

6. de Quadros CA, Olivé JM, Hersh BS, et al: Measles elimination in the Americas: evolving strategies. JAMA 275:224, 1996

7. Measles—United States, 1999. MMWR Morb Mortal Wkly Rep 49:557, 2000

8. Bellini WJ, Rota PA: Genetic diversity of wild-type measles viruses: implications for global measles elimination programs. Emerging Infect Dis 4:29, 1998

9. Kaplan LJ, Daum RS, Smaron M, et al: Severe measles in immunocompromised patients. JAMA 267:1237, 1992

10. Mustafa MM, Weitman SD, Winick NJ, et al: Subacute measles encephalitis in the young immunocompromised host: report of two cases diagnosed by polymerase chain reaction and treated with ribavirin and review of the literature. Clin Infect Dis 16:654, 1993

11. Budka H, Urbanits S, Liberski PP, et al: Subacute measles virus encephalitis: a new and fatal opportunistic infection in a patient with AIDS. Neurology 46:586, 1996

12. Measles, mumps and rubella-vaccine use and strategies for elimination of measles, rubella and congenital rubella syndrome and control of mumps. MMWR Morb Mortal Wkly Rep 47(RR8):1, 1998

13. Bitnun A, Shannon P, Durward A, et al: Measles inclusion–body encephalitis caused by the vaccine strain of measles virus. Clin Infect Dis 29:855, 1999

14. Angel JB, Walpita P, Lerch RA, et al: Vaccine-associated measles pneumonitis in an adult with AIDS. Ann Intern Med 129:104, 1998

15. Boriskin YS, Booth JC, Yamada A: Rapid detection of mumps virus by the polymerase chain reaction. J Virol Methods 42:23, 1994

16. Hammer SM, Connolly KJ: Viral aseptic meningitis in the United States: clinical features, viral etiologies, and differential diagnosis. Curr Clin Top Infect Dis 12:1, 1992

17. Nussinovitch M, Volovitz B, Varsano I: Complications of mumps requiring hospitalization in children. Eur J Pediatr 154:732, 1995

18. Baandrup U, Mortensen SA: Fatal mumps myocarditis. Acta Med Scand 216:331, 1984

19. Ni J, Bowles NE, Kim YH, et al: Viral infection of the myocardium in endocardial fibroelastosis: molecular evidence for the role of mumps virus as an etiologic agent. Circulation 95:133, 1997

20. Gordon SC, Lauter CB: Mumps arthritis: a review of the literature. Rev Infect Dis 6:338, 1984

21. Reef SE, Plotkin S, Cordero JF, et al: Preparing for elimination of congenital rubella syndrome (CRS): summary of a workshop on CRS elimination in the United States. Clin Infect Dis 31:85, 2000

22. Rubella and congenital rubella syndrome—United States, 1994–1997. MMWR Morb Mortal Wkly Rep 46:350, 1997

23. Miller E, Craddock-Watson JE, Pollock TM: Consequences of confirmed maternal rubella at successive stages of pregnancy. Lancet 2:781, 1982

24. Munro ND, Sheppard S, Smithells RW, et al: Temporal relations between maternal rubella and congenital defects. Lancet 2:201, 1987

25. Townsend JJ, Baringer JR, Wolinsky JS, et al: Progressive rubella panencephalitis: late onset after congenital rubella. N Engl J Med 292: 990, 1975

26. Torok TJ: Parvovirus B19 and human disease. Adv Intern Med 37: 431, 1992

27. Carper E, Kurtzman GJ: Human parvovirus B19 infection. Curr Opin Hematol 3:111, 1996

28. Parvovirus, erythema infectiosum, and pregnancy. American Academy of Pediatrics Committee on Infectious Diseases. Pediatrics 85:131, 1990

29. Torok TJ: Human parvovirus B19 infection in pregnancy. Pediatr Infect Dis J 9:772, 1990

30. Frickhofen N, Abkowitz JL, Safford M, et al: Persistent B19 parvovirus infection in patients infected with human immunodeficiency virus type 1 (HIV-1): a treatable cause of anemia in AIDS. Ann Intern Med 113:926, 1990

31. Lin KH, You SL, Chen CJ, et al: Seroepidemiology of human parvovirus B19 in Taiwan. J Med Virol 57:169, 1999

32. Bell LM, Naides SJ, Stoffman P, et al: Human parvovirus B19 infection among hospital staff members after contact with infected patients. N Engl J Med 321:485, 1989

33. Pillay D, Patou G, Hurt S, et al: Parvovirus B19 outbreak in a children's ward. Lancet 339:107, 1992

34. Miller E, Fairley C, Cohen BJ, et al: Immediate and long-term outcome of human parvovirus B19 infection during pregnancy. Br J Obstet Gynaecol 105:174, 1998

35. Markenson GR, Yancey ML: Parvovirus B19 infections in pregnancy. Semin Perinatol 22:309, 1998

36. Guidozzi F, Ballot D, Rothberg AD: Human B19 parvovirus infection in an obstetric population: a prospective study determining fetal outcome. J Reprod Med 39:36, 1994

37. Brown KE, Anderson SM, Young NS: Erythrocyte P antigen: cellular receptor for B19 parvovirus. Science 262:114, 1993

38. Coding LLW, Koerner TAW, Naides SJ: Multiple glycosphingolipids determine the tissue tropism of parvovirus B19. J Infect Dis 172:1198,1995

39. Brown KE, Hibbs JR, Gallinella G, et al: Resistance to parvovirus B19 infection due to lack of virus receptor (erythrocyte P antigen). N Engl J Med 330:1192, 1994

40. Naides SJ, Howard EJ, Swack NS, et al: Parvovirus B19 infection in human immunodeficiency virus type 1–infected persons failing or intolerant to zidovudine therapy. J Infect Dis 168:101, 1993

41. Janner D, Bork J, Baum M, et al: Severe pneumonia after heart transplantation as a result of human parvovirus B19. J Heart Lung Transplant 13:336, 1994

42. Hillingso JG, Jensen IP, Tom-Peterson L: Parvovirus B19 and acute hepatitis in adults. Lancet 351:955, 1998

43. Sokal EM, Melchioir M, Cornu C, et al: Acute parvovirus B19 infection associated with fulminant hepatitis of favourable prognosis in young children. Lancet 352:1739, 1998

44. Enders G. Dotsch J, Bauer J, et al: Life-threatening parvovirus B19-associated myocarditis and cardiac transplantation as possible therapy: two case reports. Clin Infect Dis 26:355, 1998

45. Nigro G, Bastianon V, Colloridi V, et al: Human parvovirus B19 infection in infancy associated with acute and chronic lymphocytic myocarditis and high cytokine levels: reports of 3 cases and review. Clin Infect Dis 31:65, 2000

46. Morris CN, Smilack JD: Parvovirus B19 infection associated with respiratory distress. Clin Infect Dis 27:900, 1998

47. Lefrère J-J, Mariotti M, Thauvin M: B19 parvovirus DNA in solvent/detergent-treated antihaemophilia concentrates. Lancet 343:211, 1994

48. Barquet N, Domingo P: Smallpox: the triumph over the most terrible of the ministers of death. Ann Intern Med 127:635, 1997

49. Breman JG, Henderson DA: Poxvirus dilemmas—monkeypox, smallpox, and biologic terrorism. N Engl J Med 339:556, 1998

50. Institute of Medicine: Assessment of future scientific needs for live variola virus. Report of a committee on the assessment of future scientific needs for live variola virus. National Academy Press. Washington, DC, 1999

51. Schwartz MJ, Myskowski PL: Molluscum contagiosum in patients with human immunodeficiency virus infection: a review of twenty-seven patients. J Am Acad Dermatol 27:583, 1992

52. Scholz J, Rosen-Wolff A, Bugert J, et al: Molecular epidemiology of molluscum contagiosum. J Infect Dis 158:898, 1988

53. Jeziek Z, Szczeniowski M, Paluku KM, et al: Human monkeypox: clinical features of 282 patients. J Infect Dis 156:293, 1987

54. Heymann DL, Szczeniowski M, Esteves K: The resurgence of monkeypox in Africa. Br Med Bull 54:691, 1998

55. Human monkeypox: Kasai Oriental, Zaire, 1996–1997. MMWR Morb Mortal Wkly Rep 46:304, 1997

31 Respiratory Viral Infections

Frederick G. Hayden, M.D.
Michael G. Ison, M.D.

The respiratory tract can be infected by a diverse group of viruses that produce syndromes ranging in severity from mild colds to fulminant pneumonias. Respiratory viral infections are a leading cause of morbidity, hospitalization, and mortality throughout the world; influenza and pneumonia were the most prevalent infectious causes of death during the 20th century in the United States.[1] Respiratory viral infections are also the single most common cause of acute illness and physician visits in the United States and a leading cause of prescriptions for antibiotics.[2]

Epidemiology of Respiratory Viral Infections

The high prevalence of respiratory viral infections relates to the large number of infectious agents and serotypes, incomplete immunity with frequent reinfections, and, in the instance of influenza viruses, frequent changes in viral antigenicity. The frequency of viral respiratory illness is highest in children up to 4 years of age, gradually declines in teenaged individuals, rises again in parents exposed to children, and is generally lowest in the elderly.[3] In families, the average adult contracts two to four acute respiratory illnesses annually, about one quarter of which lead to physician contact. This age-related pattern reflects the gradual acquisition of immunity to some agents and the important role that children play in the transmission of infection. The major reservoir for most respiratory viruses is schoolchildren, who acquire infection in the classroom and introduce it into their homes.

The respiratory viruses show significant differences in seasonality and transmission patterns [*see Table 1*], but sporadic cases or nosocomial outbreaks can occur year-round. The presence or absence of a lipid-containing envelope affects viral survival in the environment. In temperate areas, the enveloped viruses, such as influenza virus, respiratory syncytial virus (RSV), and coronavirus, are characteristically prevalent during midwinter periods, whereas nonenveloped ones, such as rhinoviruses, are found most often in spring through fall. Although respiratory viruses spread from person to person, the relative importance of different routes depends on the virus. Large-droplet spread over short distances (< 1 m) appears common for many viruses. Viruses such as influenza virus and adenovirus spread efficiently in small-particle aerosols. Others, including rhinovirus and RSV, can spread by hand contact with contaminated skin and fomites, with subsequent inoculation onto the nasal mucosa or conjunctiva. A number of respiratory viruses, mainly RSV, influenza virus, and parainfluenza viruses, cause outbreaks of infection in closed populations, including hospitals, day care centers, and nursing homes. These outbreaks are associated with a high mortality in frail elderly or immunocompromised hosts.

Pathophysiology of Respiratory Viral Infection

INFECTIOUS AGENTS

Viruses that infect the respiratory tract can be divided into primary respiratory pathogens, whose transmission and replication are generally restricted to the human respiratory tract, and pathogens that affect the respiratory tract as part of a systemic or, sometimes, locally reactivated infection. The latter group includes three types of viruses: (1) those that cause pneumonia occasionally in healthy persons but more often in immunocompromised or pregnant persons, such as measles virus and varicella-zoster virus (VZV) [see 29 Herpesvirus Infections]; (2) those that primarily affect immunocompromised hosts, such as cytomegalovirus (CMV) [see 29 Herpesvirus Infections], herpes simplex virus (HSV) [see 29 Herpesvirus Infections], and, less frequently, human herpesvirus type 6; and (3) several viruses that cause uncommon but severe zoonotic infections, such as

Table 1 Epidemiologic Features of Principal Human Respiratory Viruses

Virus	*Incubation Period (days)*	*Principal Mode of Spread**	*Peak Seasonality*	*Nosocomial Pathogen*
Adenovirus	4–7	Aerosol, direct	Summer	Yes
Coronavirus	2–5	Droplet	Winter	Minor
Influenza A and B viruses	1–4	Aerosol	Winter	Major
Parainfluenza virus	3–6	Droplet	Types 1 and 2, fall; type 3, spring and summer	Yes
Respiratory syncytial virus	2–8	Hands, droplet	Late fall to spring	Major
Rhinovirus	1–5	Hands, droplet	Early fall, late spring	Yes

*Multiple routes of transmission (i.e., direct, fomites, large droplets, and small-particle aerosols) are possible for most respiratory viruses.

hantaviruses and zoonotic paramyxoviruses (e.g., Hendra and Nipah viruses). The primary respiratory viruses (adenovirus, coronavirus, influenza virus, parainfluenza virus, RSV, and rhinovirus) are similar in that they are distributed globally, they have the same mucosal sites of infection, and they are spread from person to person, but they differ in many important features, including viral composition, seasonality, pathogenesis of disease, and availability of vaccines and specific antiviral agents.

PATHOGENESIS OF INFECTION

Although the extent of viral replication correlates well with severity of illness for most respiratory viruses, the pathogenesis of infection differs for the various groups. Rhinovirus and coronavirus infections are largely limited to the upper respiratory tract, whereas influenza virus, RSV, parainfluenza virus, and adenovirus commonly infect lower airways as well. These viruses may also produce intra-alveolar inflammatory exudate with hemorrhage, hyaline membrane formation, and differing amounts of epithelial damage. Tracheobronchitis and damage to the respiratory epithelium are typical of influenza virus. RSV infection in young infants is associated with epithelial damage and desquamation, bronchial edema with inflammatory cells, and plugging of small airways. In contrast, damage to the nasal mucosa is modest during rhinovirus or coronavirus colds. Disease manifestations are associated with respiratory tract damage caused by the virus and with host responses to infection, including specific immunologic responses, release of host inflammatory mediators, and neurogenic reflexes. For example, increased levels of histamine, leukotriene C_4, eosinophilic cationic protein, and virus-specific IgE occur in the respiratory secretions of children with RSV bronchiolitis. Influenza is associated with increases in the levels of interleukin-6 (IL-6), interferon gamma, and tumor necrosis factor–α (TNF-α) in the nasal mucosa and the blood; correlations exist between viral replication, symptom expression, and IL-6 production.[4,5] In rhinovirus colds, concentrations of bradykinin, IL-1, IL-6, and IL-8 are increased in nasal secretions. In addition, respiratory viral infections may alter bacterial colonization patterns, increase bacterial adherence to respiratory epithelium, reduce mucociliary clearance, and alter bacterial phagocytosis by host cells. The impairment of host defenses may foster bacterial infection of areas that are normally sterile, such as the paranasal sinuses, middle ear, and lower respiratory tract.

For many respiratory viruses, the presence of neutralizing antibody in serum and respiratory secretions correlates with protection against infection. Generally, immunity is longer lasting and reinfection less common in virus groups with many serotypes (e.g., rhinovirus and adenovirus) than in those with only a few serotypes. Although reinfection is frequent with parainfluenza virus and RSV, severity generally decreases with each episode. In addition to humoral responses, cell-mediated immunity appears to be important for recovery from infection by certain respiratory viruses. In patients who have undergone bone marrow or solid-organ transplantation and in other highly immunocompromised hosts (e.g., patients with acute leukemia or AIDS), certain viruses can cause prolonged infection and can result in severe pulmonary disease; these viruses include parainfluenza virus, RSV, measles virus, adenovirus, and influenza virus.[6]

Table 2 Laboratory Methods for Diagnosis of Respiratory Viral Infections

Virus	*Specimen Source*	*Time to Isolation in Cell Culture (days)*	*Rapid Detection Methods and Molecular Techniques*	*Common Serologic Assays*
Adenovirus	Respiratory tract, throat, conjunctiva, urine, stool, blood	2–10	EIA, IF, RT-PCR, IC	CF
Coronavirus	Nasopharynx	Not routine	Not routine, RT-PCR, IF	Not routine (ELISA)
Influenza A and B viruses	Nasopharynx, throat, lower respiratory tract	2–5	EIA, IF, neuraminidase assay, RT-PCR	CF, HAI, ELISA
Parainfluenza virus	Nasopharynx, lower respiratory tract	3–14	IF, RT-PCR	CF, HAI, ELISA
Respiratory syncytial virus	Nasopharynx, lower respiratory tract	3–14	EIA, IF, RT-PCR	CF, ELISA, NT
Rhinovirus	Nasopharynx	2–7	Not routine, RT-PCR	Not routine (NT)

CF—complement fixation EIA—enzyme immunoassay ELISA—enzyme-linked immunosorbent assay HAI—hemagglutination inhibition IC—immunochromatography IF—immunofluorescence NT—neutralization RT-PCR—reverse transcriptase–polymerase chain reaction

Approach to the Diagnosis of Respiratory Viral Infections

GENERAL CONSIDERATIONS

In general, respiratory viruses cause acute, spontaneously resolving illnesses, although involvement of the lower airways and certain complications (e.g., otitis media, sinusitis, and exacerbations of asthma or COPD) are common. Clinical diagnosis is complicated for several reasons: infection with one of the respiratory viruses may result in a variety of clinical syndromes, each syndrome can result from infection with a range of viruses, and the syndromes often overlap. Consequently, clinical diagnosis is accurate only under certain circumstances, such as during an influenza epidemic or outbreaks of RSV bronchiolitis. The limited correlation between virus and syndrome emphasizes the importance of rapid virologic techniques for making a specific etiologic diagnosis, particularly in hospitalized or severely affected patients [*see Table* 2]. Data from community-based surveillance programs are also essential to improve the accuracy of the clinical diagnosis, as such data permit the physician to know which respiratory viral pathogens are circulating within the community.

LABORATORY DIAGNOSIS

Most respiratory viruses can be isolated from nose and throat swabs, nasal washes or aspirates, sputum, and other lower respiratory samples. Tests done on nasopharyngeal samples taken early in illness provide the most sensitive results. However, some respiratory viruses are slow growing [*see Table* 2], and most are present in lower titers in adults than in children, so samples from adults may require longer periods for isolation or have lower yields on rapid diagnostic tests. Because temperature fluctuations and freezing may cause loss of infectivity, samples should be transported at refrigerator temperatures (4° C) or on wet ice. Cell culture inoculation (shell vials) followed by antigen detection has a sensitivity of 80% or greater at 1 to 2 days for adenovirus, influenza virus, parainfluenza virus, and RSV.[7]

Immunofluorescence testing of exfoliated respiratory cells and enzyme immunoassay for viral antigens are reasonably sensitive, specific, and rapid techniques for detecting some respiratory viruses, particularly RSV and influenza virus.[8] Nucleic acid amplification techniques appear to be at least as sensitive as cell culture isolation. Simultaneous detection of respiratory viruses (influenza virus types A and B, RSV, parainfluenza virus types 1, 2, and 3) by the use of multiplex reverse transcriptase-polymerase chain reaction (RT-PCR) has good sensitivity,[9] and a commercial assay is available. Real-time quantitative RT-PCRs have been described, but their utility in clinical practice still needs to be determined.

Serologic diagnosis requires paired serum specimens and is intrinsically slower than direct methods. A variety of serologic techniques, such as neutralization, hemagglutination inhibition, complement fixation, and enzyme-linked immunosorbent assay (ELISA), are used to measure antibodies. Measurement of complement-fixation antibodies is generally less sensitive than the other methods and does not provide a serotype-specific diagnosis. Immunocompromised hosts often fail to develop diagnostic increases in antibody titers. The combined use of cultures, antigen detection, and serology provides the most conclusive identification of important respiratory viral pathogens in hospitalized adults.

Clinical Syndromes

COMMON COLDS

Diagnosis

The common cold is generally a mild illness of the upper respiratory tract, primarily affecting the nasopharynx and paranasal sinuses. Rhinoviruses, which cause about 50% of colds, and coronaviruses, which cause 10% to 20%, are the most important pathogens. RSV, parainfluenza virus, influenza virus, adenovirus, and some enteroviruses also cause colds.

Adults with rhinovirus colds typically have prominent upper respiratory tract symptoms (i.e., sneezing, nasal discharge, nasal obstruction, sore or scratchy throat, and cough) and often have headache but little fever or few systemic complaints other than malaise. Physical findings are nonspecific and include nasal discharge and mucosal erythema. Although generally absent in adults, lower respiratory tract manifestations (e.g., cough, sputum, and wheezing) do occur in about 60% of cases in elderly persons, and lower respiratory tract illness and fever are common in young children infected with rhinovirus.

The differential diagnosis of the common cold includes allergic rhinitis, bacterial nasopharyngitis in infants, and, in rare instances, nasal diphtheria or bacterial nasal infection in adults. Because nearly 50% of colds last longer than 1 week and 25% last up to 2 weeks, it is often unclear whether a complicating viral or bacterial sinusitis has occurred. More than 80% of uncomplicated colds have reversible sinus abnormalities demonstrable on computed tomography,[10] and sinusitis is an inherent part of rhinovirus colds. Fever, purulent nasal drainage, cough productive of purulent sputum, increasing symptoms or malaise after 1 week, localized facial pain, or maxillary toothache suggests a bacterial sinusitis.[11] Otitis media complicates approximately 2% of colds in adults and 5% of colds in children.[12]

Treatment

Treatment is directed toward specific symptoms. Saline nose drops may be helpful for relief from obstructing secretions, particularly in young children, and warm saline gargles reduce sore throat. Topical decongestants such as phenylephrine and the longer-acting oxymetazoline provide prompt relief of nasal obstruction but may be associated with rebound congestion and possibly throat irritation. Oral pseudoephedrine also provides partial relief of nasal obstruction but may cause anxiousness and insomnia in some patients. The oral decongestant phenylpropanolamine has been associated with an increased risk of stroke[13] and is no longer available as an over-the-counter medication. It is uncertain whether topical or oral vasoconstrictors alter the risks of bacterial complications. First-generation oral antihistamines, such as chlorpheniramine and clemastine, reduce sneezing and, to a lesser extent, rhinorrhea, but they are often associated with excess sedation. Nonsedating antihistamines such as loratadine and astemizole are not effective for colds in nonallergic persons. Intranasal ipratropium, a quaternary anticholinergic, reduces cold-associated rhinorrhea in about 30% of patients and may also reduce sneezing, but excess nasal drying may result in blood-tinged mucus.[14] Cough suppressants with codeine or dextromethorphan may be used if the cough is severe or disturbs sleep, but they should be used cautiously in patients with underlying chronic obstructive disease. Specific antiviral therapy is not currently available, but several investigational agents (e.g., pleconaril) show promise.[15] A number of other remedies (e.g., echinacea, zinc lozenges or nasal gels, and hot-air inhalation) are of unproven or doubtful value.[16–18]

PHARYNGITIS AND LARYNGITIS

Pharyngitis usually is associated with the same viruses that cause common colds and occurs concurrently, but it is also often a prominent complaint of persons with adenovirus and influenza virus infections. Enteroviruses are also important causes of fever and pharyngitis during the summer and early fall.

Diagnosis

Pharyngitis may be associated with characteristic clinical findings, such as palate vesicles and ulcers caused by coxsackievirus-induced herpangina, acute ulcerative stomatitis and pharyngitis caused by HSV, and exudative pharyngitis related to Epstein-Barr virus mononucleosis. Pharyngitis occurs with primary HIV infection and typically is associated with mucosal erosions and lymphadenopathy. Pharyngitis caused by group A streptococci and other bacteria (anaerobes, *Corynebacterium diphtheriae, Chlamydia pneumoniae,* and *Mycoplasma pneumoniae*) are generally not associated with acute rhinorrhea.

Treatment

In most cases of viral pharyngitis, treatment is symptomatic, although HSV stomatitis, particularly in immunocompromised patients, should be treated with specific antiviral therapy (e.g., acyclovir, famciclovir, or valacyclovir).

Hoarseness caused by laryngitis frequently occurs during acute viral infections and is more common during infections caused by viruses that invade the lower airways. Treatment is primarily voice rest.

ACUTE BRONCHITIS

Diagnosis

Acute bronchitis manifests itself as a severe or prolonged cough that is usually nonproductive or has scant mucoid sputum. Bronchitis can follow infection by any of the respiratory viruses, but especially those that affect the lower airways. Viral infections commonly cause exacerbation of preexisting airway disease, including chronic bronchitis, emphysema, asthma, and cystic fibrosis. HSV can cause bronchospasm and sometimes ulcerative tracheobronchitis in immunocompetent persons and, more often, immunocompromised persons. Cough production results from direct viral damage to the respiratory mucosa, release of inflammatory mediators, stimulation of airway irritant receptors, and increased production and decreased clearance of respiratory secretions. Infection may also enhance airway hyperreactivity, characterized by increased sensitivity to cold air and pollutants such as smoke.

The differential diagnosis of acute viral bronchitis includes bacterial, mycoplasmal, chlamydial, and pertussis infections.

Treatment

Treatment of acute bronchitis in otherwise healthy persons is directed at suppression of the cough with codeine or dextromethorphan, but these agents should be used cautiously in patients with underlying chronic obstructive disease. Antibiotics are generally not indicated.[19]

INFLUENZA SYNDROME

Diagnosis

The influenza syndrome is characterized by the rapid onset of constitutional symptoms that are associated with respiratory tract symptoms. Constitutional symptoms include fever, chills, prostration, muscle aches, and headache, which tend to dominate during the first several days of illness. Respiratory complaints are sore throat and cough. Persistent nonproductive cough, easy fatigability, and asthenia are common in the second week of illness.

Epidemic influenza A and B viruses are the principal causes of the influenza syndrome, but other respiratory viruses can cause similar clinical features.

Treatment

Treatment for influenza is usually symptomatic and includes bed rest, oral hydration, antipyretics, and antitussives. Specific antiviral therapy with the oral M2 inhibitors (amantadine or rimantadine) for influenza A virus infection or with the neuraminidase inhibitors (zanamivir and oseltamivir) for influenza A and B viruses is effective if given early in the course of illness.[20] Unlike the M2 inhibitors, early treatment with the neuraminidase inhibitors has been shown to reduce the risk of influenza-related complications and associated antibiotic use.[21,22] Fever should be treated in patients in whom it would contribute to disease, such as children with previous febrile convulsions or patients with preexisting cardiac disease. Aspirin should be avoided in pediatric patients because of its association with Reye syndrome.

CROUP

Diagnosis

Croup, or laryngotracheobronchitis, is a characteristic pediatric syndrome characterized by brassy or barking cough, inspiratory stridor, dyspnea, and hoarseness. Symptoms are often preceded by several days of upper respiratory tract illness and typically become worse at night. Croup is seen primarily in children younger than 5 years and is associated most closely with parainfluenza virus infections and less often with RSV, influenza viruses, adenoviruses, or rhinoviruses. Measles virus is an important cause of severe croup. Acute spasmodic croup is characterized by recurrent attacks precipitated by viral infections, allergies, or possibly other factors. The differential diagnosis of croup includes foreign-body aspiration or trauma, bacterial epiglottitis or tracheitis, localized abscess, and angioedema.

Inflammation of the larynx and trachea with subglottic narrowing causes localized obstruction, which is enhanced by inspiration related to the extrathoracic location of the obstruction and the compliance of the airway walls in children. In addition, inflammatory changes occur throughout the lower respiratory tract. Symptoms usually abate in 3 to 4 days and can be managed at home.

Treatment

Correction of hypoxemia is essential for hospitalized patients. Aerosolized racemic epinephrine provides transient benefit for those with persistent stridor. Systemic glucocorticoids appear to be effective in moderating the severity of illness and shortening hospitalization; inhaled steroids are beneficial in less severe cases.

BRONCHIOLITIS

Diagnosis

Bronchiolitis is an acute inflammatory disorder of the small airways, typically occurring in children younger than 2 years, and is characterized by airway obstruction with wheezing, hyperinflation, and atelectasis. It is associated most closely with RSV infection, which is detected in about 75% of infants hospitalized with bronchiolitis, and less often with parainfluenza viruses, influenza viruses, rhinoviruses, and adenoviruses. The peak incidence occurs in infants between 2 and 6 months of age, and over 80% of cases occur in the first year of life. Premature infants and young children with underlying pulmonary conditions have a high risk of developing RSV bronchiolitis. After several days of coryza and possibly fever, patients experience acute respiratory distress with wheezing, cough, and, often, inspiratory rales; apnea may occur in babies. Characteristic radiologic features are atelectasis and signs of hyperinflation. In mild cases, bronchiolitis symptoms resolve within several days, but prolonged or severe disease may occur in premature infants or those with underlying cardiopulmonary disorders. The major differential diagnosis is asthma, which is uncommon in children younger than 2 years.

The syndrome relates to viral destruction of the respiratory epithelium and associated peribronchiolar mononuclear inflammation, which is perhaps in part immunologically mediated. In the setting of disproportionately narrow airways in infants, bronchiolar obstruction causes distal collapse or air trapping and abnormal gas exchange.

Treatment

Correction of hypoxemia is the most important aspect of managing RSV bronchiolitis. Bronchodilators, glucocorticoids, and routine antibiotics are not of proven value. Aerosolized ribavirin therapy is available for selected infants hospitalized with RSV bronchiolitis or pneumonia, but it is an expensive intervention of uncertain value.[23]

REACTIVE AIRWAY DISEASE EXACERBATION

Respiratory viruses precipitate exacerbation of asthma and chronic obstructive pulmonary disease (COPD) in persons of all ages. Respiratory viral infections, half of which are rhinovirus infections, are associated with up to 85% of asthma exacerbations in schoolchildren.[24] Young children hospitalized with wheezing illness are in most cases infected with RSV, rhinoviruses, or parainfluenza viruses. Patients with COPD frequently have exacerbation of their disease as the result of respiratory viral infections. Approximately 25% of hospitalizations for COPD exacerbations have been associated with a documented respiratory tract viral infection; this percentage increases to 45% of COPD patients admitted between December and March.[25]

PNEUMONIA

Viral infections have been associated with at least 10% to 15% of community-acquired cases of pneumonia in hospitalized adults and with as many as one half of cases in hospitalized infants.[26] The relative importance of different viruses depends heavily on the geographic location of the outbreak, the season, and patient age and immune status. Influenza A and, less often, influenza B viruses are the most common cause of community-acquired viral pneumonia in adults and account for over one half of documented cases of community-acquired viral pneumonia in elderly persons. In children younger than 3 years, RSV accounts for about 50% of all patients hospitalized with pneumonia[27]; parainfluenza virus 3 is also prominent. Parainfluenza virus, adenovirus, rhinovirus, and coronavirus infections have been implicated as causes of pneumonia in children and adults. Respiratory viruses reach the lung by contiguous spread from the upper respiratory tract or inhalation of small-particle aerosols. Depending on the agent, nonrespiratory viruses infect the lung parenchyma by hematogenous dissemination (e.g., CMV, VZV,

HSV, and measles) or, less often, by contiguous spread from the tracheobronchial tree (e.g., HSV).

Diagnosis

The clinical and radiographic features of viral pneumonia are not distinctive. Unless a typical exanthem of measles or varicella is present, diagnosis of specific etiology requires appropriate virologic studies. Although viruses are considered to be atypical pneumonia pathogens in patients with normal white cell counts and diffuse patchy infiltrates, the clinical and radiologic appearance is often indistinguishable from that of bacterial infection, and mixed infections are common. Differentiation between pure viral pneumonias, mixed viral-bacterial pneumonias, and viral infections of the tracheobronchial tree with complicating bacterial pneumonia is usually not possible on clinical grounds.

Treatment

Management is primarily supportive; ventilatory support has improved the prognosis for patients with extensive viral pneumonia. Specific antiviral therapy for respiratory viruses is limited, and no controlled data for treating viral pneumonia are available. Amantadine or rimantadine are available to treat influenza A,[28] and neuraminidase inhibitors are active against both influenza A and B.[29,30] Combination therapies (e.g., an M2 inhibitor plus a neuraminidase inhibitor for influenza A) need further study. Inhaled ribavirin is available for RSV and possibly for parainfluenza virus and has been used intravenously for adenovirus, hantavirus, measles, and influenza virus infections. Specific immunoglobulins for RSV prevention and possibly for treatment are also available for high-risk patients. Individually, I.V. ribavirin, ganciclovir, and cidofovir have all been reported to be effective in the management of severe adenoviral infection.[31-33] New drugs active against rhinovirus are also in clinical development.

Pneumonia in Immunocompromised Hosts

Immunocompromised hosts are at risk for reactivation of latent viruses (e.g., HSV, CMV, or adenovirus) or acquisition of exogenous viruses; these concerns are particularly relevant for patients undergoing organ transplantation or experiencing chemotherapy-induced neutropenia and immunosuppression. In immunocompromised patients, bronchoalveolar lavages yield viruses in one half of acute pneumonia cases.[34] CMV is the most frequently recovered, accounting for more than 80% of isolates; fewer than 10% of isolates are HSV or various respiratory viruses.[35] In immunosuppressed patients, influenza viruses, parainfluenza viruses, RSV, and adenoviruses can cause severe pneumonia[36] that is often nosocomially acquired and usually associated with a preceding upper respiratory tract illness.[6] Rhinoviruses might also cause severe lower respiratory tract diseases in highly immunocompromised patients, such as myelosuppressed bone marrow transplant (BMT) recipients.[37] It seems prudent to delay chemotherapy or transplantation in the presence of an upper respiratory tract illness.

Intravenous acyclovir is recommended for patients with HSV or VZV pneumonia. Ganciclovir with or without immunoglobulin appears to be effective in reducing the mortality associated with CMV pneumonia in BMT recipients. Aerosolized ribavirin and immunoglobulin, if given early, may be effective for RSV pneumonia in such patients, and aerosolized and intravenous ribavirin have been used for adenovirus or severe measles. Cidofovir may be beneficial in adenoviral pneumonia.[31,38-40]

Infections Caused by Specific Agents

ADENOVIRUS

Adenoviruses cause a variety of respiratory tract syndromes, ranging from pharyngoconjunctival fever (often contracted while swimming in contaminated water) to severe pneumonia in infants, immunosuppressed patients, and, uncommonly, healthy adults. Epidemics of acute respiratory disease and pneumonia caused by adenovirus have been recognized for decades in military recruits and are expected to continue, given the cessation of immunization programs in the United States military.[41]

Epidemiology and Transmission

Adenovirus infections may be endemic or epidemic. Lower-numbered serotypes routinely infect infants and young children. Other types (e.g., types 3, 4, and 7) are acquired later in life and are typically associated with epidemic respiratory disease. In addition to transmission by direct contact with respiratory secretions or infectious aerosols, fecal-oral transmission occurs. Infection may be acquired by pharyngeal inoculation or conjunctival inoculation from contaminated water. Adenovirus infection occurs throughout the year but is often recognized during the summer in association with outbreaks of pharyngitis or bronchitis. Adenovirus probably accounts for about 5% of total acute respiratory infections in civilian adults. Nosocomial transmission, including clusters of pneumonia in chronic care facilities and large outbreaks of epidemic keratoconjunctivitis, is well documented.[42,43] Persistent infections occur in the tonsils and gastrointestinal tract; prolonged viral shedding is common in immunocompromised hosts and in the GI tract of children.

Classification and Pathogenesis

Adenoviruses are medium-sized (65 to 80 nm), nonenveloped, double-stranded DNA viruses, of which 49 antigenic types (divided into six subgroups) are associated with human infections. The protein coat of the virus is composed of hexagonal and pentagonal subunits (capsomers) with long fibers at each vertex, which are the sites of host cell attachment. Type-specific antigens, which give rise to neutralizing antibody, are present on the hexons and fibers of the capsid. The hexons also contain a group-specific antigen with cross-reactivity among most adenoviruses. Only about one half of serotypes cause disease. Immunity results from the presence of type-specific neutralizing antibody.

Diagnosis

Clinical features The incubation period for adenovirus infection of the respiratory tract is usually 4 to 7 days. Adenovirus respiratory disease typically causes a moderate to severe, sometimes exudative, pharyngitis and tracheobronchitis. Fever and systemic symptoms are often prominent, and rhinitis, cervical adenitis, and follicular conjunctivitis are common. Pharyngoconjunctival fever, usually associated with serotypes 3, 4, and 7, tends to manifest less frequent lower respiratory symptoms. In infants and young children, infections also cause a pertussislike syndrome, croup, and bronchiolitis.

Adenovirus pneumonia is similar to other viral pneumonias; it usually begins with pharyngitis, rhinitis, fever, and cervical adenopathy (conjunctivitis may or may not be present) and then spreads to involve the lower airways and lungs. Bilateral interstitial or alveolar infiltrates are common, although focal consolidation or effusion also occurs.

Laboratory tests The presence of cells with large basophilic, intranuclear inclusions (smudge cells) in lower respiratory biopsy specimens may provide early histopathologic diagnosis. A variety of serotypes have been recovered from stool, urine, and lower respiratory specimens of immunocompromised patients.[44] Rapid methods for virus detection include enzyme immunoassay (EIA), immunofluorescence (IF), antigen immunochromatography,[45] and RT-PCR.

Complications

Acute complications, which occur mainly in children and immunocompromised hosts, are leukopenia, lymphocytopenia, thrombocytopenia, rhabdomyolysis, disseminated intravascular coagulation, renal failure, and bacterial infection. Survivors may acquire restrictive lung disease, bronchiectasis, and, particularly in children, bronchiolitis obliterans. Mortality in BMT recipients with adenovirus pneumonia is as high as 60%.[46]

Adenoviruses are also associated with extrarespiratory infections, including epidemic keratoconjunctivitis, hepatitis and genitourinary infections in immunosuppressed hosts, myocarditis, arthritis, meningoencephalitis, and, especially in children, hemorrhagic cystitis, mesenteric adenitis, intussusception, and gastroenteritis. Adenovirus commonly complicates hematopoietic stem cell transplantation and is frequently associated with invasive disease. Invasive infections in this population are associated with poorer chance of survival.[47]

Treatment

Antiviral therapy of proven value is not available, but intravenous ribavirin, ganciclovir, cidofovir, and immunoglobulin have been used to treat severe infections. Treatment is otherwise supportive.

Prevention

Live-attenuated vaccines for adenovirus types 4 and 7 were used in the military but are not licensed for civilian use.[41,43] Other control measures are swimming-pool chlorination, careful hand washing, and, in the instance of nosocomial keratoconjunctivitis, use of gloves and proper sterilization of equipment.

CORONAVIRUSES

Epidemiology and Transmission

Coronaviruses are the second most frequently documented cause of common colds. Coronaviruses account for 4% to 15% of cases of acute respiratory disease annually and as many as 35% during peak periods. Most coronavirus infections occur in winter and early spring, but infections have been detected throughout the year. Immunity to infection is short-lived, and reinfection is common.

Classification and Pathogenesis

Coronaviruses are moderate-sized (100 to 150 nm), enveloped, single-stranded RNA viruses named for their distinctive club-shaped surface projections, which resemble a crown. Two antigenic types of human coronavirus (229E and OC43) have been recognized.

Diagnosis

Clinical features The incubation period of coronavirus colds ranges from 2 to 5 days, longer than that of rhinovirus colds. Infections produce a typical coryzal illness that is indistinguishable from colds caused by other viruses. Lower respiratory manifestations are pneumonia in children, military recruits, and possibly immunocompromised hosts and exacerbation of asthma in children and of chronic airway disease in adults. Reported associations with GI disease, including necrotizing enterocolitis in infants, are controversial.

Laboratory tests Virus isolation is impractical, and infection can be confirmed with serology or by detection of coronavirus RNA. Culture of virus in human embryonic trachea cells is the most sensitive cell culture system for recovering coronavirus, but other methods (serology, IF, and RNA detection with RT-PCR) are more practical.

Treatment

Effective antivirals or vaccines are unavailable. Intranasal interferon alfa is protective against experimental coronavirus colds. Treatment is symptomatic.

INFLUENZA VIRUS

Influenza A and B viruses cause annual outbreaks of illness affecting approximately 5% to 10% of adults, with higher rates in children. In the United States, influenza causes an average of over 20,000 deaths and 130,000 to 170,000 hospitalizations during each epidemic.[48] The appearance of a new strain for which most of the population lacks immunity can cause worldwide outbreaks, or pandemics. Pandemic strains are associated with global spread over months and with high attack rates in persons in all susceptible age groups. Three such pandemics occurred during the past century, the most severe of which was the Spanish influenza pandemic in 1918 and 1919, which caused 20 to 40 million deaths worldwide and over 500,000 deaths in the United States.

Epidemiology and Transmission

Epidemic influenza occurs annually in temperate areas, typically between the months of December and March in the Northern Hemisphere, and follows the reintroduction of virus each year. Influenza activity usually occurs in May through August in the Southern Hemisphere and can be year-round in the tropics. Regional outbreaks caused by a particular strain are usually short (6 to 8 weeks), although successive waves of infection by different influenza viruses can occur. Influenza activity in the community is marked by increased medical contacts for febrile respiratory illness, increased absenteeism from school and the workplace, subsequent increased hospitalizations for pneumonia and other cardiopulmonary disorders, and increased mortality. Pneumonia hospitalizations increase by two to five times in high-risk patients. Nearly 50% of excess hospitalizations and over 85% of deaths occur in persons 65 years of age and older.[49]

Aerosol spread by coughing is the usual mode of transmission of influenza viruses. Direct transmission of influenza A virus from animals, particularly swine and more recently chickens, to humans has been documented.[50] Aquatic fowl are the main reservoir for influenza A viruses in nature, although other species, including swine, horses, and marine mammals, are also infected by some subtypes. Swine are susceptible to infection with viruses from birds and humans and may serve as a "mixed vessel," providing an opportunity for the generation of new pathogenic viruses. In addition, direct transmission from birds to humans can occur, as documented in Hong Kong, where an avian influenza A H5N1 subtype virus caused 18 confirmed human infections and six deaths in 1997.[51] In the cluster of H5N1 avian virus in Hong Kong,[52] the source was domestic poultry, although human-to-human transmission may have occurred in several cases. Recently, avian H9N2 influenza virus infection has been documented in several children. Influenza H5N1 or other avian viruses may pose a reemerging pandemic threat in the future.

Classification and Pathogenesis

Influenza viruses belong to the orthomyxovirus family and consist of types A, B, and C. These medium-size (80 to 120 nm), enveloped, single-stranded RNA viruses contain eight gene segments (seven for influenza C). The segmented nature of the genome allows reassortment of RNA segments between two influenza viruses during dual infection and facilitates antigenic variation. Surface glycoprotein spikes possess either hemagglutinin or neuraminidase activity. Hemagglutinin mediates early events in replication, specifically cell attachment and fusion of virus and cell membranes. By cleaving terminal sialic acid residues and destroying the receptors recognized by hemagglutinin, neuraminidase promotes release of virus from infected cells and spread within the respiratory tract.

Influenza A viruses are further classified into subtypes on the basis of their surface proteins (15 hemagglutinins and nine neuraminidases are recognized in animal influenza viruses). Three A subtypes (H1N1, H2N2, and H3N2) have caused extensive human infections. Influenza C viruses have seven gene segments and lack a neuraminidase. Influenza viruses are named by the type, location of isolation, isolate number, year of recovery, and, for influenza A type viruses, the subtype (e.g., A/Texas/36/91[H1N1]).

The surface glycoproteins induce host humoral and cellular immune responses and are responsible for the changing antigenicity of influenza viruses. Two major types of antigenic change can occur: drift and shift. Antigenic drift refers to relatively minor changes in hemagglutinin and less often with neuraminidase that occur frequently (usually every few years) and sequentially in the setting of selective immunologic pressure in the population. Drift results from point mutations of the corresponding RNA segment. Antigenic shift occurs only in influenza A viruses and results from acquisition of a new gene segment for hemagglutinin with or without one for neuraminidase. This may occur through genetic reassortment during dual infections with human and animal influenza type A viruses, perhaps in intermediate hosts like swine, capable of replicating both human and avian viruses; by the reintroduction of a virus that has not circulated recently in the human population; or by direct transmission to humans of an animal influenza virus that could be capable of efficient human-to-human transmission.

Diagnosis

Clinical features The incubation period for influenza virus is short, averaging 2 days (range, 1 to 4 days). Classic influenza is distinguished by abrupt onset of prominent systemic symptoms, including fever, chills, headache, myalgia, malaise, and anorexia. Fever usually lasts for an average of 3 days in adults. Sore throat, dry cough, photophobia, and pain upon eye movement are frequent early in the illness. Mild conjunctivitis, clear nasal discharge, pharyngeal injection, and small, tender cervical lymph nodes are also common. As systemic illness abates, respiratory symptoms become more apparent. The most troubling respiratory symptom is protracted cough, which results from viral tracheobronchitis. Airway hyperactivity and abnormalities in pulmonary function may last weeks to several months in previously healthy persons. Exacerbations of asthma and other types of preexisting airway disease are often severe. Infections may be subclinical or cause milder illness, including colds.

Primary influenza virus pneumonia is a heterogeneous condition, ranging from mild disease with patchy infiltrates to rapidly fatal infection. Severe pneumonia generally accounts for 2% of influenza-associated pneumonia, but during pandemics, it can account for up to 20%; influenza A viruses cause more than 90% of cases.[53] As many as 40% of patients have had no prior underlying disease. It usually begins with typical influenza, followed within 1 to 3 days by rapidly progressive dyspnea, cyanosis, diffuse rales, and wheezing. Pleuritic chest pain and blood-tinged sputum or frank hemoptysis occurs. Patients with influenza virus pneumonia have a high mortality.

Laboratory tests Several rapid assays are commercially available in the United States to detect influenza A and B occurring together; some of these assays allow one to rapidly differentiate between influenza A and B [*see Table* 2]. The specificity of these assays is good to excellent, but the sensitivity varies between approximately 60% and 90%, depending on the sample type, the age of the patient, and the duration of the illness.[54] When viral pneumonia is present, Gram stain of sputum shows few to many polymorphonuclear leukocytes, but only rarely does it show bacteria. The chest radiograph shows bilateral infiltrates that may be diffuse interstitial infiltrates, perihilarlike pulmonary edema, or dense opacifications. Leukocytosis with left shift is variably present. A definitive diagnosis can have a significant impact on medical management. In a recent study in a pediatric population, detection of influenza A by EIA resulted in a decrease in antibiotic use, a decrease in duration of antibiotic use in hospitalized patients, and an increase in antiviral use.[55]

Complications

Secondary bacterial pneumonia should be suspected when fever, increasing cough, and sputum production develop after several days of improvement. *Streptococcus pneumoniae* is the most common bacterial pathogen, but *Staphylococcus aureus* is associated with up to 25% of cases and high mortality. *S. aureus* and certain other bacteria produce proteolytic enzymes that activate influenza hemagglutinin and enhance viral replication. *Haemophilus influenzae* and *Streptococcus pyogenes* are also recognized as causes of bacterial complications. Bacterial infections of the sinuses and ears are frequent. Toxic-shock syndrome and invasive meningococcal disease have also been known to occur secondary to influenza virus infection.

Uncommon complications are myositis with rhabdomyolysis, renal failure, disseminated intravascular coagulopathy, myocarditis, pericarditis, myelitis, Guillain-Barré syndrome, and Reye syndrome. Neurologic complications, including encephalopathy or encephalitis, although unusual, occur mainly in children.[50,56]

Treatment

Amantadine and rimantadine are active against influenza A only.[28] Oral amantadine and rimantadine reduce the duration of fever and symptoms of uncomplicated influenza A virus infection by 1 to 2 days and provide more rapid overall functional recovery. Effectiveness in preventing complications or treating severe illness in hospitalized patients is uncertain. Resistant virus may arise during treatment and be transmissible on close contact.[57]

A new class of compounds, the neuraminidase inhibitors, is active against influenza A and B viruses.[29] Currently, two neuraminidase inhibitors are available: inhaled zanamivir and oral oseltamivir. Inhaled zanamivir may rarely cause bronchospasm, which can sometimes be severe. Oseltamivir is associated with self-limited GI upset in about 10% to 15% of treated patients. Treatment of acute uncomplicated influenza in adults with inhaled zanamivir or oral oseltamivir provides symptomatic relief, reduces time to functional recovery, and decreases the likelihood of lower respiratory tract complications leading to antibiotic use.[21,22] In children 1 to 12 years of age, oseltamivir provides symptomatic relief and also reduces the likelihood of otitis media.[48] Resistance emergence appears to be very uncommon.

Treatment of influenza virus pneumonia is primarily supportive. With improved techniques of assisted ventilation, the survival rate exceeds 50%, although pulmonary fibrosis develops in some patients. Amantadine, rimantadine, and aerosolized or I.V. ribavirin, which is active against influenza A and B viruses, have been used with uncertain benefit. Although unstudied, the use of neuraminidase inhibitors in the treatment of influenza virus pneumonia, either alone or in combination with other agents, seems reasonable.

A listing of antiviral therapies for influenza is provided [*see Table 3*].

Prevention

Chemoprophylaxis Antiviral chemoprophylaxis with amantadine or rimantadine is about 70% to 90% effective in preventing illness caused by influenza A virus. Chemoprophylaxis can be used for several weeks' protection in persons immunized after influenza A activity has begun, throughout the season in those who cannot receive influenza vaccine (such as those with egg allergy) or who are unlikely to respond to the vaccine, or for protection of high-risk persons when the epidemic strain diverges significantly from the vaccine antigens. GI upset and minor, reversible side effects affecting the central nervous system (e.g., insomnia, dizziness, and difficulty with concentration) are associated with amantadine. Rimantadine appears to be of equal efficacy and is associated with a lower risk of CNS side effects.

The neuraminidase inhibitors are also effective for prophylaxis of influenza A and B infections. Both inhaled zanamivir[58,59] and oral oseltamivir[60,61] prevent influenza when used for seasonal prophylaxis or after exposure (e.g., for family or nursing home contacts), but only oseltamivir has been approved by the Food and Drug Administration for this indication. Oseltamivir has been found to be safe for treatment of children as young as 1 year of age[62]; inhaled zanamivir has been found to be safe in children as young as 5 years of age.

Immunization Current influenza vaccines are made from formalin-inactivated, egg-grown virus and are produced as whole-virus, split-virus, and purified surface antigen preparations. Their composition is reviewed annually and adjusted as necessary to reflect changes in antigenicity; current vaccines contain one influenza B and two influenza A (H1 and H3 subtypes) antigens.[48] The efficacy of these vaccines is 70% to 90% in young adults, especially when the vaccine antigen and the circulating strain are closely matched. Use of this vaccine in healthy working adults is associated with fewer upper respiratory illnesses and fewer visits to physicians' offices.[63] Immunization reduces influenza-related hospitalizations and mortality in ambulatory elderly patients by 40% to 60%.[64] Recently published data have demonstrated that wide-scale immunization of schoolchildren appears to reduce influenza-related mortality in older adults.[65] Although vaccine is less effective in infirm elderly and immunocompromised patients, vaccine provides partial protection against pneumonia and death. In elderly persons with chronic lung diseases, influenza vaccination has also been asso-

Table 3 Agents Used to Prevent and Treat Influenza[95,96]

Drug	*Dosage*		*Efficacy for Documented Influenza*		*Dosage Adjustment*	
	*Prophylaxis**	*Treatment†*	*Prophylaxis*	*Treatment*	*State*	*Dosage*
Amantadine	100 mg b.i.d.	100 mg b.i.d.	63% efficacy[95]	Shorter duration of fever and symptoms	C_{Cr} 30–50 C_{Cr} 15–30 C_{Cr} < 15 Hemodialysis Elderly	100 mg q.d. 100 mg q.o.d. 100 q.wk. 100 mg q.wk. ≤ 100 mg q.d.
Rimantadine	100 mg b.i.d. or 200 mg q.d.	100 mg b.i.d. or 200 mg q.d.	72%–83% efficacy[95]	Shorter duration of fever and symptoms	Severe hepatic dysfunction Elderly C_{Cr} < 10	100 mg q.d. 100 mg q.d. 100 mg q.d.
Zanamivir	2 puffs q.d.‡	2 puffs b.i.d.	67%–84% efficacy[96]	1 day faster recovery from illness (up to 2.5 day improvement in high-risk patients) Reduction in severity of illness, number of nights of disturbed sleep, and use of relief medications Reduction in complications that require antibiotic More rapid return to normal function	—	No dosage adjustments
Oseltamivir	75 mg q.d.	75 mg b.i.d.	87% efficacy[96]	24 to 36 hr faster recovery from illness Reduction in severity of illness, number of nights of disturbed sleep, and use of relief medications Reduction in complications that require antibiotic	C_{Cr} < 30 Age 1–13 yr < 15 kg 15–23 kg 23–40 kg > 40 kg	Treatment, 75 mg q.d. Prophylaxis, 75 mg q.o.d. 30 mg b.i.d. 45 mg b.i.d. 60 mg b.i.d. 75 mg b.i.d.

*Duration of prophylaxis depends on the clinical circumstances: 7–10 days after close contact for postexposure prophylaxis; 2 wk after immunization of an adult; 4–6 wk after a community outbreak; and at least 1 wk (preferably 2 wk) after the last case in outbreak control.
†First dose should be given within 48 hr of the onset of illness to be effective. Therapy should be continued for 5 days.
‡The Food and Drug Administration has not approved zanamivir for this indication.
C_{Cr}—creatinine clearance

ciated with substantial health benefits, including fewer hospitalizations and fewer deaths.[66]

The target groups for immunization are those at increased risk for influenza-related complications [*see Table 4*]. Administration is associated with soreness at the injection site in as many as one third of recipients, but fever or systemic reactions are uncommon in adults. Influenza vaccination does not adversely affect $CD4^+$ counts, HIV RNA levels, or progression to AIDS or death in HIV-infected patients.[67]

To improve vaccine efficacy, stimulate mucosal immunity, and enhance ease of administration, a live-attenuated cold-adapted vaccine has been developed for intranasal administration. In children, a trivalent cold-adapted vaccine was associated with an overall protection of about 90% against culture-confirmed influenza[68] and also protected against a drift variant of influenza virus. Such vaccines are comparable in effectiveness to inactivated vaccine in younger adults. Although still investigational, the live-attenuated cold-adapted vaccine is potentially applicable to wide segments of the population.

PARAINFLUENZA VIRUSES

Parainfluenza viruses are the most commonly recognized cause of croup, accounting for up to 75% of cases with a documented viral cause, and they are the second leading cause of lower respiratory tract disease resulting in hospitalization of infants. Natural infection with parainfluenza virus induces partial immunity that moderates disease severity. These viruses commonly reinfect older

Table 4 Indications for Administering Annual Influenza Vaccine*[60]

PERSONS AT INCREASED RISK FOR COMPLICATIONS

- All adults older than 50 yr
- Residents of nursing homes and other long-term care facilities that house persons of any age who have chronic medical conditions
- Patients with chronic cardiopulmonary disorders, including children with asthma
- Patients who have required regular medical follow-up or hospitalization during the preceding year because of chronic metabolic diseases (including diabetes), renal dysfunction, hemoglobinopathies, or immunosuppression (including immunosuppression caused by medication or by HIV)
- Children and teenagers (6 mo to 18 yr of age) who are receiving long-term aspirin therapy and therefore may be at risk for Reye syndrome
- Women who will be in the second or third trimester of pregnancy during influenza season

PERSONS WHO CAN TRANSMIT INFLUENZA TO THOSE AT HIGH RISK

- Physicians, nurses, and other health care workers in any facility that provides medical care
- Home care providers
- Household members of high-risk persons

OTHERS

- Persons who provide essential community services (e.g., police and firefighters)
- Students or other persons in institutional settings (e.g., schools and prisons) who may be considered for immunization to prevent disruption of routine activities
- Anyone who wishes to reduce the chance of acquiring influenza

*These are the current recommendations from the Advisory Committee on Immunization Practices, Centers for Disease Control and Prevention, Atlanta, Georgia.

children and adults to produce milder respiratory illness and colds.

Epidemiology and Transmission

Parainfluenza virus infections occur initially during childhood; type 3 virus infections often occur during infancy. Parainfluenza type 3 virus is an important cause of illness in infants younger than 6 months and is the most common type associated with disease in immunocompromised hosts. The incidence of croup and respiratory disease caused by type 1 or 2 virus infections is highest between the ages of 6 months and 5 years. Type 1 virus typically causes epidemics lasting several months, peaking in October or November of alternating years. Type 2 virus activity is more sporadic. Type 3 virus causes infections throughout the year, with outbreaks during the spring and summer.

Parainfluenza viruses are transmitted from person to person, either by direct contact with respiratory secretions or by large aerosol droplets. Transmission occurs readily in families, and reinfections in older children and adults are common. Outbreaks occur in nurseries, day care centers, and hospitals, with attack rates of 40% or higher in susceptible patients.

Classification and Pathogenesis

Human parainfluenza viruses are medium-sized (120 to 150 nm), enveloped RNA viruses belonging to the Paramyxoviridae family and are classified into four antigenically stable types (1, 2, 3, and 4); type 4 is further classified into subtypes A and B. Parainfluenza virus replicates in epithelial cells of the upper and lower respiratory tract, and antibodies to the two major envelope surface glycoproteins, namely the hemagglutinin-neuraminidase protein and the fusion protein, confer protection against infection. These proteins are necessary for attachment of virus to host cell receptors and membrane-fusing activity. Parainfluenza viruses type 1 and type 2, which cause croup and laryngitis, probably replicate principally in the major airways, whereas parainfluenza type 3 causes lower respiratory tract infections.

Diagnosis

Clinical features The incubation period of parainfluenza viruses is approximately 3 to 6 days. Virus replication is generally limited to the respiratory tract, although viremia and CNS infections[69] have been rarely documented. Initial infections cause fever, rhinitis, pharyngitis, laryngitis, croup, and bronchitis in children.

Laboratory tests Immunofluoresence of respiratory cells and RT-PCR have been used for rapid parainfluenza virus detection. Culture is generally slow and requires days to weeks. Serologic assays, including complement fixation, ELISA, and hemagglutination assays, are also used to make retrospective diagnosis.

Complications

In adults and older children, reinfections are frequently asymptomatic. Parainfluenza viruses cause serious lower respiratory tract disease, including exacerbations of chronic airway disease and pneumonia in adults. During periods of activity, about 2% to 3% of cases of community-acquired pneumonia in adults are linked to parainfluenza virus infection.[70] Severe pneumonia, sometimes in the absence of upper respiratory tract illness, occurs in immunosuppressed adults and children, particularly after BMT.[5]

Treatment

Specific antiviral therapy of proven value has not been established. Early treatment with aerosol ribavirin may benefit some immunocompromised patients with serious infections.

Prevention

An effective vaccine for parainfluenza virus infections is not yet available, but live-attenuated vaccines derived from either human or bovine parainfluenza viruses have been developed and appear safe and immunogenic in children.

RESPIRATORY SYNCYTIAL VIRUS

RSV is the major cause of lower respiratory tract disease in infants and young children, accounting for 45% to 90% of bronchiolitis cases and up to 40% of pneumonia cases. As many as 100,000 hospitalizations and 510 deaths of infants and children are attributed to RSV each year in the United States.[71] RSV is also increasingly recognized as a cause of lower respiratory tract disease in older adults and immunocompromised persons.[72,73] The number of RSV-related deaths in elderly adults is estimated to be 10-fold higher than in infants.[74] In elderly persons, it is estimated that RSV is associated with 2% to 9% of hospitalizations or deaths caused by pneumonia[72] and about 10% of hospitalizations for acute cardiopulmonary conditions.[71]

Epidemiology and Transmission

RSV causes prolonged outbreaks of infection from late fall to spring annually in temperate climates.[75] Most outbreaks peak between January and March in the Northern Hemisphere, but sporadic cases can occur year-round. Epidemics are associated with increased pediatric hospitalizations and deaths caused by lower respiratory tract illness. Essentially all children are infected within several years after birth. Immunity is incomplete, and reinfections in children and adults are common. Higher titers of circulating and mucosal antibody occur with successive infections and appear to be associated with milder illness.

RSV appears to be spread by large-particle aerosols during close personal contact and by hand contamination with self-inoculation of the eye or nose. RSV is a major nosocomial pathogen, and high attack rates occur during outbreaks in hospitals, transplantation units, day care centers, and geriatric homes.[76] Illness rates are commonly 20% to 50% among hospital staff and patients during epidemics. In households, secondary infection occurs in about one third of adults.

Classification and Pathogenesis

RSV is a paramyxovirus with surface glycoproteins that have neither hemagglutinin nor neuraminidase activity. The F protein is responsible for fusion of the viral envelope with the host cell membranes. Antibody against this protein neutralizes RSV infectivity and blocks syncytial cell formation. The G protein is responsible for attachment. Two major subgroups (A and B) are distinguished primarily by antigenic differences in the G glycoprotein, and multiple strains are recognized within each subgroup.

Diagnosis

Clinical features The average incubation period of RSV is 4 to 5 days but ranges up to 1 week. In infants and young children, almost all primary infections are symptomatic, and 40% or more are associated with bronchiolitis or pneumonia. Febrile upper respiratory tract illness and otitis media are common. Approximately 1% to 2% of infections result in hospitalization, and about 10% of hospitalized infants require ventilatory support. Mortality is usually less than 1% among previously healthy infants but is much higher in persons with primary immunodeficiency, persons undergoing cancer chemotherapy, and persons with preexisting pulmonary and heart disease.[77]

Most recurrent infections in adults are associated with upper respiratory tract illness. Adults typically experience coryza, pharyngitis, and cough, often with low-grade fever. Bronchitis, influenzalike illness, pneumonia, and exacerbations of asthma and chronic bronchitis also occur. Influenza and RSV infections are associated with similar clinical pictures and outcomes in the elderly.[71,75] Elderly adults hospitalized with RSV commonly manifest dyspnea, wheezing, and sputum production. Viral bronchopneumonia or secondary bacterial pneumonia appears to complicate a high proportion of RSV infections in such patients.

RSV causes severe lower respiratory tract disease in immunosuppressed patients, particularly BMT recipients and acute leukemia patients receiving chemotherapy.[6] Most cases are nosocomial; mortality exceeds 60% when pneumonia develops.

Rhinitis with sinusitis or otitis often precedes the development of pneumonia by several days and may provide a clue to diagnosis.

Laboratory tests Bronchoalveolar lavage with RSV antigen detection provides rapid diagnosis in pneumonia cases. Commercially available ELISAs are sensitive to RSV in children, but nasopharyngeal samples are an insensitive means of detecting RSV antigen in adults, owing to the fact that adults have low titers of virus in the upper respiratory tract. RT-PCR is also a sensitive technique to identify RSV. Serology is more sensitive than cell culture for diagnosis in adults but is slow because of the need for paired sera.[71]

Treatment

The value of aerosolized ribavirin in the management of RSV disease in hospitalized children remains controversial, and studies of its value in mechanically ventilated infants have yielded conflicting results.[22] Aerosolized ribavirin should be considered for infants hospitalized with RSV infections who are at high risk for severe or complicated illness (e.g., congenital heart disease, bronchopulmonary dysplasia, cystic fibrosis, and immunodeficiency), for those who are already severely ill, and for those who are younger than 6 weeks. Treatment with polyclonal immunoglobulins or monoclonal antibodies does not provide clear clinical benefit for RSV-infected infants and young children. Although ineffective as monotherapy, early combination therapy with aerosolized ribavirin and I.V. immunoglobulin appears to benefit immunosuppressed patients with RSV pneumonia.[78]

Prevention

Passive immunoprophylaxis by means of monthly intravenous administration of immunoglobulin containing high anti-RSV titers reduces the risk of severe RSV illness in high-risk children,[79] and polyvalent and monovalent preparations containing antibodies for F protein are approved for prophylaxis in premature infants and children with bronchopulmonary dysplasia.[80] No vaccine against RSV is available yet, but efficacy trials with live-attenuated, cold-adapted vaccine are ongoing in children and in elderly persons. Inactivated subunit vaccines are also being tested.

Interruption of nosocomial transmission may be facilitated by thorough hand washing,[81] decontamination of fomites, early identification and rapid isolation of infected infants and other potential RSV cases,[82] and cohorting of staff with infected infants.[83] Regular use of gowns, gloves, disposable eye-nose goggles, and possibly masks by hospital staff caring for infected children may further reduce the risk of nosocomial RSV spread.

RHINOVIRUS

Epidemiology and Transmission

Rhinoviruses cause approximately one infection per person a year in adults, and rates are even higher in children. Rhinovirus causes about 50% of colds in adults each year and up to 90% during the fall months.[84] Immunity to rhinovirus is type specific and relatively enduring after infection, although reinfection can occur. Rhinoviruses cause infections year-round but are most prevalent in early fall and late spring. The relative importance of fomite spread with hand contamination and self-inoculation into the eyes or nose and aerosols in rhinovirus transmission is uncertain under natural conditions.

Classification and Pathogenesis

Rhinoviruses are small (30 nm), nonenveloped viruses that belong to the Picornaviridae family. They have a single-stranded RNA genome and are composed of four structural proteins. Three of the proteins induce neutralizing antibodies and form the basis for serotyping. The large number of serotypes (> 110) makes the development of an effective vaccine unlikely. Nearly 90% of rhinovirus serotypes use intercellular adhesion molecule–1 as a common cellular receptor. Acid sensitivity and optimal growth at 32° to 34° C are thought to account for restriction of rhinovirus replication in the nasal mucosa and possibly the large airways.

Diagnosis

Clinical features The incubation period of rhinoviruses averages about 2 days (range, 1 to 5 days). Rhinovirus colds vary in severity from mild episodes characterized by 1 to 2 days of coryza or scratchy throat to illnesses with profuse rhinorrhea, pharyngitis, and subsequent bronchitis. Symptoms usually peak on the second and third days of illness, and the median duration is 1 week.

Rhinovirus infections are associated with more frequent lower respiratory tract illness in the elderly and with bronchospasm and protracted cough in persons with preexisting airway disease.[85,86] Rhinovirus is the major infectious cause of asthma exacerbations in children and in adults. In addition, rhinovirus infections are associated with acute sinusitis,[87] otitis media,[88] exacerbations of chronic bronchitis, and lower respiratory tract disease in infants and young children. In BMT recipients, rhinovirus infection has been associated with pneumonia and poor prognosis.

Laboratory tests No rapid diagnostic test is routinely available; detection is usually done by virus isolation and, more recently, by RT-PCR.[89]

Treatment

No antiviral therapy of proven clinical value is currently available, but interferons, capsid-binding antirhinoviral compounds such as pleconaril, and protease inhibitors are under investigation. Nonselective regimens such as high-dose vitamin C, inhalation of heated air, and zinc lozenges are of unproven value.

Prevention

Intranasal interferon alfa is effective for the prevention of rhinovirus infections but is associated with nasal irritation when used for more than 1 week. In households, a 1-week regimen of interferon prevents nearly 90% of rhinovirus colds in persons exposed to ill family members but does not reduce the risk of other respiratory viral infections.[90]

Barrier control measures may be beneficial, although tissues impregnated with virucides have proved disappointing in this regard. Hand washing and avoidance of finger-to-nose and finger-to-eye contact should reduce the risk of infection. The risk of nosocomial transmission of rhinovirus infections is also documented, emphasizing the importance of adherence to infection control measures in cases of upper respiratory tract illness.

HANTAVIRUS CARDIOPULMONARY SYNDROME

In May 1993, an outbreak of acute fatal respiratory illness was recognized in previously healthy adults residing in the southwestern United States. The causative agent was a hantavirus termed Sin Nombre virus,[91,92] for which the principal animal reservoir is the deer mouse, *Peromyscus maniculatus*. Human infections occur by inhalation of aerosols of infectious excreta. Several other agents of the hantavirus cardiopulmonary syndrome (HCPS) have been isolated from other rodent species in other parts of North and South America.[93]

Most HCPS cases have occurred in young to middle-aged adults with no underlying disease. The largest numbers of cases have occurred in New Mexico, Arizona, and California, but cases have also been identified throughout western North America and sporadically in the eastern United States. Person-to-person transmission of hantavirus has not been documented except in South America with Andes virus. The incubation period averages 12 to 16 days (range, 4 to 42 days). A history of exposure to a rural setting, rodents or their dwellings, or agricultural work may suggest the diagnosis.

The disease is primarily caused by increases in permeability of the pulmonary vascular endothelium that appears to be immune mediated. Serum antibodies are usually found at the time of presentation, which supports the presumption of an associated immunopathologic disease process. Microscopy shows intra-alveolar edema, scant signs of acute inflammation or hyaline membranes, and no necrosis. Viral antigen has been identified in capillary endothelial cells in many organs.

Diagnosis

HCPS begins with a prodromal phase that lasts 3 to 6 days. Fever and myalgia are almost always present; GI symptoms (i.e., nausea, vomiting, and pain) may be prominent. Upper respiratory tract symptoms are uncommon and suggest an alternative diagnosis. Productive cough occurs in approximately one fourth of cases. The pulmonary capillary leak and the development of noncardiogenic pulmonary edema lead to respiratory failure in 80% to 90% of patients within 1 to 2 days of hospitalization.[94] Unlike patients with bacterial sepsis, HCPS patients have hypotension and low cardiac output, and their systemic vascular resistance values may be normal or elevated. Hemoconcentration, thrombocytopenia, prolonged partial thromboplastin time, an elevated lactate dehydrogenase level, and an elevated aspartate aminotransferase level are common. Leukocytosis may be pronounced (> 25,000/mm^3) and is unusual in that both immature myeloid precursors and atypical lymphocytosis may be present. Specific diagnosis is made by serology, immunohistochemical staining of tissues, or RT-PCR for hantaviral RNA in blood or tissues.

Treatment

Treatment of HCPS entails correction of hypoxemia and hypotension. Specific antiviral therapy has been attempted with I.V. ribavirin, but its value for patients with HCPS is uncertain; a controlled trial is in progress. Corticosteroids are also of uncertain value. The mortality is about 50%; most deaths have been caused by intractable hypotension and associated dysrhythmia. In survivors, recovery is often very rapid and apparently complete.

Internet Resources for Respiratory Viral Infections

Adenovirus

National Respiratory and Enteric Virus Surveillance System

http://www.cdc.gov/ncidod/dvrd/nrevss/eadfeat.htm

Influenza Virus

World Health Organization

http://www.who.int/emc/diseases/flu

Centers for Disease Control and Prevention

http://www.cdc.gov/ncidod/diseases/flu/fluvirus.htm

National Foundation for Infectious Diseases

http://www.nfid.org/library/influenza

American Lung Association

http://www.lungusa.org/diseases/luninfluenz.html

Parainfluenza Viruses

National Respiratory and Enteric Virus Surveillance System

http://www.cdc.gov/ncidod/dvrd/nrevss/hpivfeat.htm

Respiratory Syncytial Virus

National Respiratory and Enteric Virus Surveillance System

http://www.cdc.gov/ncidod/dvrd/nrevss/rsvfeat.htm

American Lung Association

http://www.lungusa.org/diseases/rsvfac.html

Hantavirus

Centers for Disease Control and Prevention

http://www.cdc.gov/ncidod/diseases/hanta/hantvrus.htm

http://www.cdc.gov/ncidod/diseases/hanta/hps/index.htm

Hantavirus Reference Laboratory

http://www.thor.unm.edu/Hanta/website1.htm

American Lung Association

http://www.lungusa.org/diseases/hantavirus_factsheet.html

Prevention

There is currently no clinically available vaccine to prevent hantavirus infections. As a result, the only way to prevent infection is to prevent exposure to the virus by eliminating rodent harborage; by controlling rodent populations through the use of snap traps, rodenticides, or both; and by avoiding rodents when outdoors. In addition, it is advisable to air out infested spaces before cleanup, and then to spray areas of infestation as well as all excreta, nesting, and other materials with household disinfectant or 10% bleach solution; these materials should then be cleaned up, sealed in bags, and disposed of. Sweeping, vacuuming, or stirring dust should be avoided until the area is thoroughly wet with disinfectant.[94]

INTERNET RESOURCES

A listing of Internet resources with information about respiratory viral infections is provided [*see Sidebar* Internet Resources for Respiratory Viral Infections].

References

1. Amstrong GL, Conn LA, Pinner RW: Trends in infectious disease mortality in the United States during the 20th century. JAMA 281:61, 1999

2. Mainous AG, Hueston WJ: The cost of antibiotics in treating upper respiratory tract infections in a medical population. Arch Fam Med 7: 45, 1998

3. Monto AS: Studies of the community and family: acute respiratory illness and infection. Epidemiol Rev 16:351, 1994

4. Kaiser L, Fritz RS, Straus SE, et al: Symptom pathogenesis during acute influenza: interleukin-6 and other cytokine responses. J Med Virol (in press)

5. Hayden FG, Fritz R, Lobo MC, et al: Local and systemic cytokine responses during experimental human influenza A virus infection: relation to symptom formation and host defense. J Clin Invest 101:643, 1998

6. Sable CA, Hayden FG: Orthomyxoviral and paramyxoviral infections in transplant patients. Infect Dis Clin North Am 9:987, 1995

7. Olsen MA, Shuck KM, Sambol AR, et al: Isolation of seven respiratory viruses in shell vials: a practical and highly sensitive method. J Clin Microbiol 31:422, 1993

8. Hindiyeh M, Goulding C, Morgan H, et al: Evaluation of BioStar Flu OIA assay for rapid detection of influenza A and B viruses in respiratory specimens. J Clin Virol 17:119, 2000

9. Grondahl B, Puppe W, Hoppe A, et al: Rapid identification of nine microorganisms causing acute respiratory tract infections by single-tube multiplex reverse transcription-PCR: feasibility study. J Clin Microbiol 37:1, 1999

10. Gwaltney JM Jr, Phillips CD, Miller RD, et al: Computed tomographic study of the common cold. N Engl J Med 330:25, 1994

11. Kaiser L, Lew D, Hirschel B, et al: Effects of antibiotic treatment in the subset of common-cold patients who have bacteria in nasopharyngeal secretions. Lancet 347:1507, 1996

12. Arola M, Ruuskanen O, Ziegler T, et al: Clinical role of respiratory virus infection in acute otitis media. Pediatrics 86:848, 1990

13. Kernan WN, Viscoli CM, Brass LM: Phenylpropanolamine and the risk of hemorrhagic stroke. N Engl J Med 343:1826, 2000

14. Hayden FG, Diamond L, Wood PB, et al: Effectiveness and safety of intranasal ipratropium bromide in common colds: a randomized, double-blind, placebo-controlled trial. Ann Intern Med 125:89, 1996

15. Romero JR: Pleconaril: a novel antipicornaviral drug. Expert Opin Investig Drugs 10:369, 2001

16. Melchart D, Linde K, Fischer P, et al: Echinacea for preventing and treating the common cold. Cochrane Database Syst Rev (2):CD000530, 2000

17. Marshall I: Zinc for the common cold. Cochrane Database Syst Rev (2):CD001364, 2000

18. Vickers AJ, Smith C: Homoeopathic Oscillococcinum for preventing and treating influenza and influenza-like syndromes. Cochrane Database Syst Rev (2):CD001957, 2000

19. Gonzales R, Bartlett JG, Besser RE, et al: Principles of appropriate antibiotic use for treatment of uncomplicated acute bronchitis: background. Ann Intern Med 134:521, 2001

20. Bridges CB, Fukuda K, Cox NJ, et al: Prevention and control of influenza. Recommendations of the Advisory Committee on Immunization Practices (ACIP). MMWR Morb Mortal Wkly Rep 50(RR-4):1, 2001

21. Kaiser L, Keene ON, Hammond JMJ, et al: Impact of zanamivir on antibiotic use for respiratory events following acute influenza in adolescents and adults. Arch Intern Med 160:3234, 2000

22. Treanor JJ, Hayden FG, Vrooman PS, et al: Efficacy and safety of the oral neuraminidase inhibitor oseltamivir in treating acute influenza: a randomized controlled trial. US Oral Neuraminidase Study Group. JAMA 283:1016, 2000

23. Reassessment of the indications for ribavirin therapy in respiratory syncytial virus infections. American Academy of Pediatrics Committee on Infectious Diseases. Pediatrics 97:137, 1996

24. Folkerts G, Busse WW, Nijkamp FP, et al: Virus-induced airway hyperresponsiveness and asthma. Am J Respir Crit Care Med 157:1708, 1998

25. Glezen WP, Greenberg SB, Atmar RL, et al: Impact of respiratory virus infections on persons with chronic underlying conditions. JAMA 283:499, 2000

26. Greenberg SB: Viral pneumonia. Infect Dis Clin North Am 5:603, 1991

27. Loda FA, Clyde WA Jr, Glezen WP, et al: Studies on the role of viruses, bacteria, and *M. pneumoniae* as causes of lower respiratory tract infections in children. J Pediatr 72:161, 1968

28. Hayden FG, Aoki FY: Amantadine, rimantadine, and related agents. Antimicrobial Chemotherapy. Yu VL, Merigan TC, White NJ, et al, Eds. Williams & Wilkins, Baltimore, 1999, p 1344

29. Gubareva LV, Kaiser L, Hayden FG: Influenza virus neuraminidase inhibitors. Lancet 355:827, 2000

30. Hayden FG, Osterhaus AD, Treanor JJ, et al: Efficacy and safety of the neuraminidase inhibitor zanamivir in the treatment of influenza virus infections. N Engl J Med 337:874, 1997

31. Shetty AK, Gans HA, So S, et al: Intravenous ribavirin therapy for adenovirus pneumonia. Pediatr Pulmonol 29:69, 2000

32. Duggan JM, Farrehi J, Duderstadt S, et al: Treatment with ganciclovir of adenovirus pneumonia in a cardiac transplant patient. Am J Med 103:439, 1997

33. Safrin S, Cherrington J, Jaffe HS: Clinical uses of cidofovir. Rev Med Virol 7:145, 1997

34. Connolly MG Jr, Baugham RP, Dohn MN, et al: Recovery of viruses other than cytomegalovirus from bronchoalveolar lavage fluid. Chest 105:1775, 1994

35. Baughman RP: The lung in the immunocompromised patient. Infectious complications Part 1. Respiration 66:95, 1999

36. Rabella N, Rodriguez P, Labeaga R, et al: Conventional respiratory viruses recovered from immunocompromised patients: clinical considerations. Clin Infect Dis 28:1043, 1999

37. Ghosh S, Champlin R, Couch R, et al: Rhinovirus infections in myelosuppressed adult blood and marrow transplant recipients. Clin Infect Dis 29:528, 1999

38. Dagan R, Schwartz RH, Insel RA, et al: Severe diffuse adenovirus 7a pneumonia in a child with combined immunodeficiency: possible therapeutic effect of human immune serum globulin containing specific neutralizing antibody. Pediatr Infect Dis 3:246, 1984

39. DeVincenzo J: Pre-emptive ribavirin for 'RSV' in BMT. Bone Marrow Transplant 26:113, 2000

40. Goetz MB, Mathisen GE: Clinical course and treatment of adults with severe measles pneumonitis. Clin Infect Dis 21:443, 1995

41. Ludwig SL, Brundage JF, Kelley PW, et al: Prevalence of antibodies to adenovirus serotypes 4 and 7 among unimmunized US Army trainees: results of a retrospective nationwide seroprevalence survey. J Infect Dis 178:1776, 1998

42. Jernigan JA, Lowry BS, Hayden FG, et al: Adenovirus type 8 epidemic keratoconjunctivitis in an eye clinic: risk factors and control. J Infect Dis 167:1307, 1993

43. Uemura T, Kawashitam T, Ostuka Y, et al: A recent outbreak of adenovirus type 7 infection in a chronic inpatient facility for the severely handicapped. Infect Control Hosp Epidemiol 21:559, 2000

44. Hierholzer JC: Adenoviruses in the immunocompromised host. Clin Microbiol Rev 5:262, 1992

45. Tsutsumi H, Ouchi K, Ohsaki M, et al: Immunochromatography test for rapid diagnosis of adenovirus respiratory tract infections: comparison with virus isolation in tissue culture. J Clin Microbiol 37:2007, 1999

46. Couch RB, Englund JA, Whimbey E: Respiratory viral infections in immunocompetent and immunocompromised persons. Am J Med 102:2, 1997

47. Howard DS, Phillips II GL, Reece DE, et al: Adenovirus infections in hematopoietic stem cell transplant recipients. Clin Infect Dis 29:1494, 1999

48. Prevention and control of influenza: recommendations of the Advisory Committee on Immunization Practices (ACIP). MMWR Morb Mortal Wkly Rep 49(RR3):1, 2000

49. Lui KJ, Kendal AP: Impact of influenza epidemics on mortality in the United States from October 1972 to May 1985. Am J Public Health 77:712, 1987

50. Kaiser L, Hayden FG: Hospitalizing influenza in adults. Curr Clin Top Infect Dis 19:112, 1999

51. Claas EC, Osterhaus AD, van Beek R, et al: Human influenza A H5N1 virus related to a highly pathogenic avian influenza virus. Lancet 351:472, 1998

52. Subbarao K, Klimov I, Katz J, et al: Characterization of an avian influenza A (H5N1) virus isolated from a child with a fatal respiratory illness. Science 279:393, 1998

53. Oliveira EC, Marik PE, Colice G: Influenza pneumonia: a descriptive study. Chest 119:1717, 2001

54. Leonardi GP, Leib H, Birkhead GS, et al: Comparison of rapid detection methods for influenza A virus and their value in health-care management of institutionalized geriatric patients. J Clin Microbiol 32: 70, 1994

55. Noyola DE, Demmler GJ: Effect of rapid diagnosis on management of influenza A infections. Pediatr Infect Dis J 19:303, 2000

56. Fujimoto S, Kobayashi M, Uemura O, et al: PCR on cerebrospinal fluid to show influenza-associated acute encephalopathy or encephalitis. Lancet 352:873, 1998

57. Hayden FG: Amantadine and rimantadine: clinical aspects. Antiviral Drug Resistance. Richman DD, Ed. John Wiley & Sons, 1996, p 59

58. Monto AS, Robinson DP, Herlocher ML, et al: Zanamivir in the prevention of influenza among healthy adults: a randomized controlled trial. JAMA 282:31, 1999

59. Hayden FG, Gubareva LV, Monto AS, et al: Inhaled zanamivir for the prevention of influenza in families. N Engl J Med 343:1282, 2000

60. Hayden FG, Atmar RL, Schilling M, et al: Use of the selective oral neuraminidase inhibitor oseltamivir to prevent influenza. N Engl J Med 341:1336, 1999

61. Munoz FM, Galasso GJ, Gwaltney JM Jr, et al: Current research on influenza and other respiratory viruses: II international symposium. Antiviral Res 46:91, 2000

62. Whitley RJ, Hayden FG, Reisinger KS, et al: Oral oseltamivir treatment of influenza in children. Pediatr Infect Dis J 20:127, 2001

63. Nichol KL, Lind A, Margolis KL, et al: The effectiveness of vaccination against influenza in healthy, working adults. N Engl J Med 333: 889, 1995

64. Gross PA, Hermogenes AW, Sacks HS, et al: The efficacy of influenza vaccine in elderly persons: a meta-analysis and review of the literature. Ann Intern Med 123:518, 1995

65. Reichert TA, Sugaya N, Fedson DS, et al: The Japanese experience with vaccinating schoolchildren against influenza. N Engl J Med 344: 889, 2001

66. Nichol KL, Baken L, Nelson A: Relation between influenza vaccination and outpatient visits, hospitalization, and mortality in elderly persons with chronic lung disease. Ann Intern Med 130:397, 1999

67. Sullivan PS, Hanson DL, Dworkin MS, et al: Effect of influenza vaccination on disease progression among HIV-infected persons. AIDS 14:2781, 2000

68. Belshe R, Iacuzio D, Mendelman P, et al: Efficacy of a trivalent live attenuated intranasal influenza vaccine in children. N Engl J Med 338: 1405, 1998

69. Arisoy ES, Demmler GJ, Thakar S, et al: Meningitis due to parainfluenza virus type 3: report of two cases and review. Clin Infect Dis 17: 995, 1993

70. Marx A, Gary HE Jr, Marston BJ, et al: Parainfluenza virus infection among adults hospitalized for lower respiratory tract infection. Clin Infect Dis 29:134, 1999

71. Shay DK, Holman RC, Roosevelt GE, et al: Bronchiolitis-associated mortality and estimates of respiratory syncytial virus-associated deaths among US children 1979–1997. J Infect Dis 183:16, 2001

72. Falsey AR, Cunningham CK, Barker WH, et al: Respiratory syncytial virus and influenza A infections in the hospitalized elderly. J Infect Dis 172:389, 1995

73. Han LL, Alexander JP, Anderson LJ: Respiratory syncytial virus pneumonia among elderly: an assessment of disease burden. J Infect Dis 179:25, 1999

74. Navas L, Wang E, de Carvalho V, et al: Improved outcome of respiratory syncytial virus infection in a high-risk hospitalized population of Canadian children. Pediatric Investigators Collaborative Network on Infections in Canada. J Pediatr 121:348, 1992

75. Respiratory syncytial virus activity—United States, 1999–2000 season. MMWR Morb Mortal Wkly Rep 49:1091, 2000

76. Falsey AR, McCann RM, Hall WJ, et al: Acute respiratory tract infection in daycare centers for older persons. J Am Geriatr Soc 43:30, 1995

77. Holberg CJ, Wright AL, Martinez FD, et al: Risk factors for respira-

tory syncytial virus-associated lower respiratory illnesses in the first year of life. Am J Epidemiol 133:1135, 1991

78. Whimbey E, Champlin RE, Englund JA, et al: Combination therapy with aerosolized ribavirin and intravenous immunoglobulin for respiratory syncytial virus disease in adult bone marrow transplant recipients. Bone Marrow Transplant 16:393, 1995

79. Groothuis JR, Simoes EA, Levin MJ, et al: Prophylactic administration of respiratory syncytial virus immune globulin to high-risk infants and young children. The Respiratory Syncytial Virus Immune Globulin Study Group. N Engl J Med 329:1524, 1993

80. Palivizumab, a humanized respiratory syncytial virus monoclonal antibody, reduces hospitalization from respiratory syncytial virus infection in high-risk infants. The Impact-RSV Study Group. Pediatrics 102: 531, 1998

81. Contreras PA, Sami IR, Darnell ME, et al: Inactivation of respiratory syncytial virus by generic hand dishwashing detergents and antibacterial hand soaps. Infect Control Hosp Epidemiol 20:57, 1999

82. Karanfil LV, Conlon M, Lykens K, et al: Reducing the rate of nosocomially transmitted respiratory syncytial virus. Am J Infect Control 27:91, 1999

83. Madge P, Paton JY, McColl JH, et al: Prospective controlled study of four infection-control procedures to prevent nosocomial infection with respiratory syncytial virus. Lancet 340:1079, 1992

84. Arruda E, Pitkaranta A, Witek TJ, et al: Frequency and natural history of rhinovirus infections in adults during autumn. J Clin Microbiol 35:2864, 1997

85. Wald TG, Shult P, Krause P, et al: A rhinovirus outbreak among residents of a long-term care facility. Ann Intern Med 123:588, 1995

86. Nicholson KG, Kent J, Hammersley V, et al: Acute viral infections of upper respiratory tract in elderly people living in the community: comparative, prospective, population based study of disease burden. BMJ 315:1060, 1997

87. Pitkaranta A, Arruda E, Malmberg H, et al: Detection of rhinovirus in sinus brushings of patients with acute community-acquired sinusitis by reverse transcription-PCR. J Clin Microbiol 35:1791, 1997

88. Pitkaranta A, Virolainen A, Jero J: Detection of rhinovirus, respiratory syncytial virus, and coronavirus infections in acute otitis media by reverse transcriptase polymerase chain reaction. Pediatrics 102:291, 1998

89. Andeweg AC, Bestebroer TM, Huybreghs M, et al: Improved detection of rhinoviruses in clinical samples by using a newly developed nested reverse transcription-PCR assay. J Clin Microbiol 37:524, 1999

90. Hayden FG, Albrecht JK, Kaiser DL, et al: Prevention of natural colds by contact prophylaxis with intranasal alpha 2-interferon. N Engl J Med 314:71, 1986

91. Levy H, Simpson SQ: Hantavirus pulmonary syndrome. Am J Respir Crit Care Med 149:1710, 1994

92. Butler JC, Peters CJ: Hantavirus and hantavirus pulmonary syndrome. Clin Infect Dis 19:387, 1994

93. Schmaljohn C, Hjelle B: Hantaviruses: a global disease problem. Emerg Infect Dis 3:95, 1997

94. Update: Hantavirus pulmonary syndrome—United States, 1999. MMWR Morb Mortal Wkly Rep 48:521, 1999

95. Jefferson TO, Demicheli V, Deeks JJ, et al: Amantadine and rimantadine for preventing and treating influenza A in adults. Cochrane Database Syst Rev (2):CD001169, 2000

96. Jefferson T, Demicheli V, Deeks J, et al: Neuraminidase inhibitors for preventing and treating influenza in healthy adults. Cochrane Database Syst Rev (2):CD001265, 2000

32 Enteric Viral Infections

Nino Khetsuriani, M.D., Ph.D
Umesh D. Parashar, M.D., M.P.H.

Enterovirus Infections

Enteroviruses belong to the family Picornaviridae and include 65 currently recognized serotypes of polioviruses (types 1 to 3), coxsackieviruses A (types 1 to 22 and 24) and B (types 1 to 6), echoviruses (types 1 to 7, 9, 11 to 21, 24 to 27, and 29 to 33), and numbered enteroviruses (types 68 to 71 and 73).[1-3] Enteroviruses are small (approximately 30 nm), nonenveloped, single-stranded RNA-containing viruses with an icosahedral capsid composed of 60 subunits consisting of four structural proteins (VP1 to VP4). Enterovirus RNA is approximately 7.5 kb long and codes structural proteins, RNA polymerase, other polypeptides necessary for viral replication, and two untranslated regions at the 5' and 3' ends of the RNA molecule.

EPIDEMIOLOGY

Enteroviruses are among the most common viruses worldwide. In temperate climates, the incidence of enterovirus infections peaks during the summer and fall months (June through October in the United States), whereas in the tropics, transmission occurs year-round.

Several enterovirus serotypes commonly cocirculate in the community, and predominant serotypes tend to change over time. The serotypes most commonly reported in the United States included echovirus 9, coxsackievirus B5, echovirus 30, coxsackieviruses A9 and B2 (from 1993 to 1996[4]), and echoviruses 30, 11, 9, 6, and 7 (from 1997 to 1999[5]). The appearance of new predominant enterovirus serotypes is often accompanied by large-scale outbreaks. For example, large outbreaks of aseptic meningitis were reported in 2001, when previously rare echoviruses 13 and 18 became the predominant serotypes in the United States.[6]

Illnesses associated with enteroviruses affect predominantly children, but persons of any age may be susceptible. In addition to young age, predisposing factors for enterovirus illness include male sex, lower socioeconomic status, residence in urban areas, poor sanitation, large household size, and crowded living conditions.[7]

No animal reservoir for human enteroviruses exists. However, large amounts of enteroviruses are excreted by infected persons, and the enteroviruses are universally found in the environment (e.g., in sewage; surface water, such as rivers, lakes, and other reservoirs; and seawater). The lack of a lipid envelope and the presence of a dense protein capsid allow enteroviruses to survive in the environment for long periods, especially at low temperatures. Enteroviruses are inactivated by extreme heat, ultraviolet light, drying, and chlorine. A high concentration of organic matter prevents inactivation of enteroviruses by chlorine.[8]

Enteroviruses are most often transmitted from person to person by the fecal-oral or the respiratory route, but transmission by fomites also occurs. Young children are the most important transmitters of enteroviruses and are often the index case in family or school outbreaks.

PATHOGENESIS

Enteroviruses gain entry into the host cell after binding to specific cellular receptors. Several different receptors with tropism to different serotypes have been identified. Initial virus replication takes place in submucosal lymphatic tissues of the pharynx and the gut (Peyer patches). The virus then spreads to the regional lymph nodes, enters the bloodstream ("minor" viremia), and reaches the reticuloendothelial system (deep lymph nodes, bone marrow, spleen, and liver). If viral replication is not contained by host defense mechanisms at this stage, symptomatic infection occurs, resulting in "major" viremia and dissemination of the virus to target organs. Certain enteroviruses (e.g., polioviruses) may spread along neural pathways as well. Tissue tropism of the serotype determines target organs for further replication. The histopathologic lesions in target organs consist of inflammation and necrosis of various degrees.

The incubation period usually is 3 to 7 days (range, 1 to 35 days). Shorter incubation periods are observed in children and for certain specific enterovirus infections (e.g., upper respiratory illnesses and acute hemorrhagic conjunctivitis).

Excretion of enteroviruses by an infected individual starts at the end of the incubation period, and patients are most infectious shortly before and after onset of illness. Depending on the stage of the infection and the clinical syndrome, enteroviruses are found in oropharyngeal secretions, stool, cerebrospinal fluid, blood, and vesicular fluids. In immunocompetent hosts, the period of enterovirus shedding in oropharyngeal secretions and circulation in the blood or CSF usually does not exceed 1 week, but fecal excretion may persist for up to 2 months after infection, even after clinical symptoms resolve. Long-term persistence of enteroviruses (in some cases, for several years) may occur in individuals with impaired humoral immunity.[9–11]

IMMUNITY

Immunity to enteroviruses is long lasting and serotype specific and is primarily mediated by humoral mechanisms. Primary infection results in an IgM response and is followed by IgG and IgA production. Secondary infections induce an anamnestic response, resulting in high antibody titers. Circulating IgG and IgM antibodies have a neutralizing effect on enteroviruses during the extracellular phase of replication, and secretory IgA antibodies mediate local mucosal immunity. The importance of antibodies in providing protective immunity against enteroviruses is emphasized by the occurrence of severe chronic enterovirus infections in patients with defective humoral immunity.[9–11]

CLINICAL SYNDROMES

The vast majority of enterovirus infections are clinically inapparent or result only in a minor febrile illness. A smaller proportion of infected individuals develop more serious diseases, and on relatively rare occasions, conditions with substantial sequelae or fatal outcome may occur.

Of host factors influencing the clinical outcome of enterovirus infection, age and the degree of immunocompetence are the most important. Agent factors, such as serotype or intratypic strain of the virus and tissue tropism, are also important. The organ systems and tissues in which symptoms of enterovirus infections manifest themselves include the respiratory system, central nervous system, heart, skin, muscles, and gastrointestinal tract, depending on preferential target organs for a given serotype. Associations between distinctive clinical syndromes and serotypes have been established [*see Table 1*], but there is considerable overlap.

Minor Febrile Illness

Enteroviruses are a common cause of febrile illness, particularly during the summer and fall months. Fever may be the sole symptom, or infection may be accompanied by rashes or respiratory symptoms (the "summer cold"); in infants, symptoms include irritability, lethargy, anorexia, vomiting, and diarrhea. Because of the need to rule out potentially serious bacterial infections, a high proportion of infants with enteroviral febrile illness require evaluation for bacterial sepsis or meningitis.[12]

Aseptic Meningitis

Aseptic meningitis is the most common CNS illness associated with enteroviruses; enteroviruses account for more than 90% of cases of aseptic meningitis for which a causative organism is identified.[13] Patients experience acute onset of fever, headache, nuchal rigidity, photophobia, nausea, and vomiting. The fever may be biphasic, subsiding for several days and then recurring; development of meningeal symptoms occurs after recurrence of fever. A variable degree of lethargy, irritability, and drowsiness may be present, but considerable changes in mental status are uncharacteristic. Meningeal signs may not be obvious in young infants. Other manifestations of enterovirus infection, such as respiratory symptoms, exanthems, enanthems, or myalgia, are often present.

Examination of the CSF reveals a mild to moderate pleocytosis, with a predominance of lymphocytes (usually < 1,000 cells/ml^3). In some patients—particularly young children—polymorphonuclear cells may be predominant initially, with the subsequent development of lymphocytosis. In rare cases, CSF cell counts are normal. CSF glucose levels are normal; protein levels may be normal or elevated.

Symptoms usually resolve in about 1 week, although CSF pleocytosis may persist for some time thereafter. Severe illness and fatal outcome are uncommon except in the immediate neonatal period. Recovery is usually complete, and there are no significant sequelae.

Table 1 Diseases Associated with Enteroviruses

Disease	*Associated Enteroviruses**					*Clinical Features*
	Polio	*Coxs (Group A)*	*Coxs (Group B)*	*Echo*	*Numbered EV*	
Febrile illness	+	+	+	+	+	Mild, transient, febrile illness with or without rash or respiratory symptoms; resolves within a few days
Neurologic illnesses						
Aseptic meningitis	+	+	+ (Coxs B5)	+ (Echo 30, 9, 11, 6, 4, 7, 13, 18)	+ (EV 71)	Acute onset of fever, severe headache with meningeal irritation; meningeal symptoms in young infants may not be obvious CSF findings: mild to moderate pleocytosis (< 1,000 cells/mm^3) that is predominantly lymphocytic; rarely, normal cell counts; an initial predominance of polymorphonuclear cells in CSF with a subsequent shift to lymphocytosis may be observed, particularly in young children; CSF glucose level, normal; protein level, normal or elevated; CSF bacterial cultures, negative; enteroviruses often are detected in CSF by culture or PCR; often accompanied by other symptoms of enteroviral infection (respiratory symptoms, rashes, or myalgia) Usually resolves with no neurologic deficits in about 1 wk; illness and convalescence in adults may last longer
Encephalitis	+	+	+ (Coxs B5)	+ (Echo 30, 11, 6, 9, 24)	+ (EV 71)	Clinical presentation of meningoencephalitis; symptoms of aseptic meningitis plus confusion, lethargy, seizures; rarely, coma, cerebellar ataxia, choreiform movements, and paresthesias; diffuse encephalitis more common than focal; CSF profile similar to that of aseptic meningitis Outcome usually favorable; residual neurologic deficits uncommon; severe illness and deaths mostly in neonates and with EV 71 infection
Paralytic illness	+	+ (Coxs A7)	+	+	+ (EV 70, 71)	Usually preceded or accompanied by febrile illness Poliomyelitis: acute, usually asymmetrical, rapidly progressive flaccid paralysis; decreased or absent deep tendon reflexes; normal sensory function; respiration and swallowing may be compromised; the extent of paralysis depends on the location of CNS damage (spinal, bulbar, or spinobulbar forms) Muscle weakness associated with nonpolio enteroviruses usually milder than polio and transient; other manifestations of enteroviral infection common Residual permanent paralysis occurs in paralytic poliomyelitis but is rare after infection with nonpolio enteroviruses Death: in fewer than 10% of patients with poliomyelitis, mostly in patients with bulbar involvement; fatal bulbar involvement with nonpolio enteroviruses uncommon
Skin/mucosal syndromes						
Nonspecific rashes		+	+	+ (Echo 9, 11, 16)	+	Variety of exanthems and enanthems (e.g., maculopapular, roseoliform, vesicular), rarely as a sole manifestation of enteroviral illness; resolve within a few days

(*continued*)

Table 1 (continued)

Disease	Associated Enteroviruses*					Clinical Features
	Polio	*Coxs (Group A)*	*Coxs (Group B)*	*Echo*	*Numbered EV*	
Herpangina		+ (Coxs A10, 16, 2, 4, 5, 8)				Acute onset; fever, headache, malaise, sore throat with 10 to 12 vesicular enanthems, usually ulcerating, on soft palate, anterior tonsillar pillars, or posterior pharynx Self-limiting illness; complete recovery in a few days
Hand, foot, and mouth disease		+ (Coxs A16)			+ (EV 71)	Benign illness with acute onset; fever and mild pharyngitis 1 to 2 days before rash onset; lesions initially maculopapular but evolve into whitish-gray tender, flat, often oval vesicles; lesions on oral mucosa, dorsal surface of hands and feet, sometimes buttocks; peripheral distribution of rash on the limbs Recovery usually complete in a few days; CNS complications with fatalities observed in outbreaks of hand, foot, and mouth disease caused by EV 71
Muscle diseases						
Myopericarditis		+ (Coxs A4, A16)	+ (All serotypes)	+ (Echo 9, 22)		Both myocardium and pericardium are affected, but signs of either myocarditis or pericarditis predominate Dyspnea, chest pain, fever, malaise; ECG abnormalities (ST segment elevation, nonspecific ST segment and T wave abnormalities, ventricular tachyarrhythmias and heart block); cardiomegaly; serum levels of myocardial enzymes frequently elevated Severity varies; permanent myocardial injury possible in approximately 30% of cases; may later lead to chronic dilated cardiomyopathy Deaths in acute period rare (< 5%), mostly in patients with severe myocardial involvement; mortality in neonates approximately 50%
Pleurodynia			+			Synonyms: epidemic myalgia, Bornholm disease Attacks of spasmodic paroxysmal pain of variable intensity in the chest or upper abdomen with fever, which subsides as the pain recedes; pain usually more intense in adults; affected muscles painful by palpation; may be swollen; chest auscultation and x-ray normal Usually resolves within 1 wk; multiple relapses possible
Systemic infections						
Neonatal systemic infection			+ (All serotypes)	+ (Echo 11)		Overwhelming sepsislike illness Initial symptoms (fever, poor feeding, irritability, lethargy, hypotonus, and vomiting) are followed by multiple organ involvement; dominant syndromes include encephalomyocarditis (severe myocarditis, often accompanied by heart failure, and meningoencephalitis) and hemorrhage-hepatitis (overwhelming hepatitis with hepatic failure and DIC) High mortality (50% to 83%); most deaths within 1 wk of onset; the risk of fatal outcome highest with onset in infants younger than 2 wk

Table 1 (continued)

Disease	Polio	Coxs (Group A)	Coxs (Group B)	Echo	Numbered EV	Clinical Features
	*Associated Enteroviruses**					
Chronic EV infection in immunocompromised host				+		Occurs in patients with B cell defects; chronic, persistent infection of CNS (meningoencephalitis), skeletal muscles (dermatomyositis-like syndrome), and other organs Progressive course; outcome usually fatal
Acute hemorrhagic conjunctivitis		+ (Coxs A24 variant)			+ (EV 70)	Acute eye pain, photophobia, swelling of eyelids, subconjunctival hemorrhages; transient corneal involvement possible Complete recovery in less than 10 days; permanent poliolike paralysis with onset after a few weeks of the EV 70 illness has been described
Respiratory illnesses		+ (Coxs A21, A24)	+ (Coxs B2)	+ (Echo 11, 9, 4, 18)	+ (EV 71)	Acute febrile illness; both upper (coryza, pharyngitis) and lower (bronchitis, tracheobronchitis, bronchiolitis, pneumonia) respiratory manifestations occur Course usually benign with complete recovery, except in neonatal systemic illness; fatal pulmonary edema observed in Southeast Asian outbreaks of EV 71
Diarrhea		+	+	+ (Echo 11, 14, 18)		Diarrhea usually febrile, accompanying other symptoms of enterovirus infection; recovery complete

*The most commonly associated serotypes are indicated in parentheses. More common serotypes are listed first.
CNS—central nervous system Coxs—coxsackievirus CSF—cerebrospinal fluid DIC—disseminated intravascular coagulation Echo—echovirus EV—enterovirus PCR—polymerase chain reaction Polio—poliovirus

Encephalitis

Enteroviral encephalitis results from progression of enteroviral meningitis; therefore, most patients with enteroviral encephalitis have symptoms of meningoencephalitis. Meningoencephalitis usually starts as aseptic meningitis, but it is accompanied by changes in mental status or cerebral involvement, characterized by somnolence, lethargy, generalized or focal seizures, and psychiatric symptoms. Coma, cerebellar ataxia, choreiform movements, and paresthesias are rare. Diffuse symptoms are more common than focal symptoms. The outcome is favorable in the majority of cases, but severe residual neurologic damage and death have been reported. In neonates, the disease is part of a systemic illness. In such patients, the disease follows a much more severe course; the prognosis is guarded, and there is a higher risk of neurologic sequelae and death.[14] In recent years in Southeast Asia, fulminant, rapidly fatal bulbar encephalitis has occurred in young children during outbreaks of enterovirus 71 infection.[15,16]

Poliomyelitis and Poliolike Paralytic Illness

Muscle paralysis is primarily associated with poliovirus infection but has also been observed, sometimes in outbreaks, with several nonpolio enterovirus infections, such as infections with coxsackievirus A7, enteroviruses 70 and 71, and several echoviruses. Through successful immunization programs, control of poliomyelitis has been achieved in numerous countries worldwide, including the entire Western Hemisphere, but wild polioviruses continue to circulate in some countries of sub-Saharan Africa and Southeast Asia. It is likely that the large-scale Polio Eradication Initiative, led by the World Health Organization since 1988, will result in global polio eradication in the near future[17]; until that occurs, there remains a risk of importation of poliomyelitis into the United States.

Paralysis in poliomyelitis results from the replication of polioviruses in the anterior horn of the spinal cord or in the brain stem, causing the destruction of motor neurons. Depending on the location of the damage, spinal, bulbar, or spinobulbar forms of poliomyelitis may occur. Clinical hallmarks of paralytic poliomyelitis include the acute onset of flaccid, usually asymmetrical, rapidly progressive paralysis that is more severe proximally than distally and that is characterized by decreased or absent deep tendon reflexes without sensory loss. Respiration and swallowing may be compromised if respiratory muscles, cranial nerves, or respiratory centers are affected. Death occurs in fewer than 10% of cases; the majority of deaths involve cases of bulbar poliomyelitis. Recovery of muscle function takes place during the first few months after disease onset, but some degree of permanent paralysis usually remains.

Paralysis associated with nonpolio enterovirus infections results more from inflammatory changes than motor neuron destruction; therefore, it is usually milder and transient, rarely resulting in residual paresis. Fatal bulbar involvement is uncommon.

Myopericarditis

Carditis caused by enteroviruses (predominantly group B coxsackieviruses) occurs mostly in newborns, adolescents, and young adults and usually affects both pericardium and myocardium. Electrocardiographic abnormalities of varying degree, ranging from ST segment elevation or nonspecific ST segment and T wave abnormalities to ventricular tachyarrhythmias and heart block, are present. Cardiomegaly caused by pericardial effusion or acute cardiac dilatation is common. Serum levels of myocardial enzymes are frequently elevated. Death in the acute period is rare (< 5%) and mostly occurs in patients with severe myocardial involvement. Most patients recover without complications, but permanent myocardial injury occurs in about 30% of cases. Residual damage includes persistent ECG abnormalities, cardiomegaly, and chronic congestive heart failure and may later lead to dilated cardiomyopathy.[18,19]

Pleurodynia

Pleurodynia is characterized by attacks of spasmodic paroxysmal pain in the chest or upper abdomen accompanied by fever, which subsides as the pain recedes. The intensity of pain varies and is usually greater in adults. Affected muscles are painful on palpation and may be swollen. Normal auscultatory examination and chest x-ray are helpful in the differential diagnosis. The disease resolves within 1 week, but some patients experience multiple relapses.

Exanthems and Enanthems

Skin and mucosal lesions seldom appear as a sole presentation of enterovirus infection. Maculopapular rashes are most commonly associated with echoviruses; they appear simultaneously with fever, and they spread from the face to the chest, neck, and extremities. Roseoliform rashes appear on the face and upper chest after defervescence. Of the vesicular rashes, the most distinctive clinical syndrome is hand, foot, and mouth disease. This disease is most often caused by coxsackievirus A16, but it can also be caused by enterovirus 71. Most cases of hand, foot, and mouth disease occur in children, who present with fever, vesicular lesions in the mouth, and macular rash on the limbs and sometimes buttocks; these lesions may later become vesicular. The disease generally resolves in a few days, but CNS complications with fatalities occurred in Southeast Asia during large outbreaks of hand, foot, and mouth disease caused by enterovirus 71.[15,16,20] The most common example of enterovirus enanthems is herpangina, a common illness of young children that is characterized by fever, sore throat, and vesicular enanthems on the soft palate; symptoms resolve within a few days.

Neonatal Systemic Infection

In most cases, enterovirus infections in infants are benign, self-limited illnesses similar to those observed in older persons. In some neonates, especially during the first 2 weeks of life, enteroviruses may cause an overwhelming sepsislike illness.[21,22] In most cases, infection is transmitted from the sick mother (either transplacentally or during delivery), but nosocomial infections, including nursery outbreaks, also occur.

The initial symptoms associated with neonatal enteroviral sepsis are nonspecific and include fever, poor feeding, irritability, lethargy, hypotonia, and vomiting. There subsequently occurs involvement of multiple organs, notably the heart, CNS, liver, lungs, pancreas, and adrenal glands. The dominant features of the encephalomyocarditis syndrome, which is associated with group B coxsackieviruses, are severe myocarditis, often accompanied by heart failure, and meningoencephalitis. The leading clinical features of the hemorrhage-hepatitis syndrome, predominantly associated with echovirus 11, are overwhelming hepatitis with hepatic failure and disseminated intravascular coagulation. Neonatal enteroviral sepsis is often fatal (reported case fatality ranges from 50% to 83%), and most deaths occur within 1 week of onset.[14,21,22]

Chronic Enterovirus Infection in Immunocompromised Hosts

Neutralizing antibodies play a critical role in the immune response to enteroviruses. Thus, in patients with inherited or acquired defects of humoral immunity, enteroviruses often persist; this results in chronic infections of the CNS, skeletal muscles, and the GI system. Most commonly, the condition occurs in children with X-linked agammaglobulinemia, but it may also develop in children with severe combined immunodeficiency syndrome and, rarely, in bone marrow transplant recipients.[9–11] Chronic progressive meningoencephalitis is the predominant clinical feature. More than half of patients experience a dermatomyositis-like syndrome. Chronic hepatitis is commonly present. The course of illness is progressive; although periodic improvements may occur, the overall prognosis is poor, and the disorder is usually fatal.[11]

Acute Hemorrhagic Conjunctivitis

From 1969 through the 1980s, there occurred an explosive pandemic of millions of cases of acute hemorrhagic conjunctivitis caused by coxsackievirus A24 variant and enterovirus 70. The disease is highly contagious; unlike other enteroviruses, the primary mode of transmission is direct introduction of the virus into the eye by fingers or fomites. The symptoms include eye pain, photophobia, swelling of eyelids, and characteristic subconjunctival hemorrhages of various intensity. The symptoms initially affect one eye and then spread to the other. The disease usually resolves in less than 10 days. Corneal involvement may occur but is transient and leaves no permanent scars. A permanent poliolike paralysis has been reported in persons who had recently had acute hemorrhagic conjunctivitis caused by enterovirus 70.

Other Illnesses

The respiratory syndromes in enterovirus infections involve both upper and lower respiratory tracts and ranges from the so-called summer cold to pneumonia. These infections are usually mild, except when associated with systemic illness in neonates. Fatal pulmonary edema, apparently of neurogenic origin, was reported to have occurred in association with the 1998 outbreak of enterovirus 71 infection in Taiwan.[20]

GI symptoms are often associated with other manifestations of enterovirus infections. In young children, outbreaks of febrile diarrhea associated with some echoviruses have been described, but in general, enteroviruses are not a major cause of gastroenteritis.

Enteroviruses are also known to cause hepatitis and pancreatitis, usually as part of generalized infection. An association of enterovirus infections, particularly group B coxsackievirus infection, with type 1 (insulin-dependent) diabetes mellitus has been suggested, but no conclusive evidence is available.[23]

DIAGNOSIS

Isolation of the virus with subsequent serotyping has traditionally been the gold standard for laboratory diagnosis of enterovirus infections. Most enteroviruses can be grown in susceptible cell lines and identified by observing a characteristic cytopathic effect, but for almost all group A coxsackieviruses, inoculation of suckling mice is needed. The use of several cell lines and multiple specimen types from the patient increases the diagnostic yield. However, viral culture is relatively insensitive, laborious, and time consuming; these factors limit the utility of viral culture for patient care.[24–26]

The most widely accepted method for the identification of individual enterovirus serotypes is neutralization reaction, using intersecting pools of internationally standardized antisera. Immunofluorescence assay with monoclonal antibodies is also available for several common enteroviruses.

Compared with viral culture for enterovirus detection, reverse transcriptase polymerase chain reaction (RT-PCR) assays have been shown to be more sensitive, as specific, and much more rapid. These assays have been used increasingly in clinical practice over the past few years, with demonstrated clinical utility, particularly for the diagnosis of enterovirus meningitis.[12,26–28] The primers most often used in enterovirus RT-PCR have broad specificity for enteroviruses in general; this precludes serotype identification, but specific primers for individual serotypes are being developed. Molecular typing by sequence analysis, based on the close correlation of the serotype with the nucleotide sequence of the *VP1* gene, is a new modality for enterovirus identification.[29]

Detection of the virus in normally sterile sites (e.g., CSF, blood, pericardial fluid, tissue specimens) is considered diagnostic. Because enteroviruses are ubiquitous and because asymptomatic infections commonly occur, positive results from testing of nonsterile sites (e.g., stool sample, throat swab) should be interpreted with caution.

Serology has a limited role in the diagnosis of enterovirus infections; it is helpful only if paired sera are available for testing. Demonstration of a greater than fourfold increase in titers of antibodies against the implicated serotype is indicative of recent infection. Of various serologic methods, virus neutralization reaction is preferred.

TREATMENT

Most patients with enterovirus infections recover uneventfully after a few days of supportive care, but patients with potentially serious illnesses require intensive support. No antiviral therapy for enterovirus infections has yet been approved by the Food and Drug Administration. In limited clinical trials and in compassionate use cases, pleconaril (ViroPharma Inc., Exton, Pennsylvania), one of the candidate drugs with broad antipicornavirus activity, has been shown to have some benefit for enteroviral meningitis and chronic enterovirus infection of immunodeficient hosts.[30] The drug is available from the manufacturer for compassionate use in life-threatening illnesses caused by enteroviruses.

Immunoglobulin preparations are used both for treatment and prophylaxis of enterovirus infections in patients with humoral immunodeficiencies.[9,11] The occurrence of chronic enterovirus meningoencephalitis has declined notably since the introduction of regular prophylactic immunoglobulin treatment. The benefit for patients with established chronic enterovirus meningoencephalitis is less clear. Most commonly, immunoglobulin preparations are administered intravenously. Results of intramuscular and intrathecal administration are mixed.[9,11] Intravenous immunoglobulin is sometimes used for neonatal enterovirus infections, but the data on the effectiveness of this therapy are limited.[31]

PREVENTION AND CONTROL

Two types of highly effective vaccines—inactivated poliovaccine (IPV) and live, attenuated oral poliovaccine (OPV)—are available for prevention and control of poliovirus infection. Since 2000, IPV has been the recommended vaccine for routine use in the United States, but an emergency stockpile of OPV is maintained by the Centers for Disease Control and Prevention for use in the event of outbreaks.[32]

In the absence of vaccines, prevention and control of nonpolio enteroviral illnesses are primarily accomplished through adherence to good personal hygiene (e.g., thorough hand washing, especially after diaper changes). To prevent neonatal infections, routine infection-control measures in neonatal nurseries must be strictly enforced, and pregnant women near term should be advised to avoid contact with patients with known or suspected enterovirus infections. Control of enterovirus transmission is complicated by the fact that the majority of infections are asymptomatic and by the relatively long duration of viral shedding. For similar reasons, the effectiveness of isolation of symptomatic persons is questionable.

Viral Gastroenteritis

Viral gastroenteritis occurs in two distinct epidemiologic forms: sporadic disease that commonly affects children, and epidemic disease that afflicts both children and adults. Sporadic, childhood viral gastroenteritis is primarily caused by rotaviruses (group A), human caliciviruses (including both Norwalk-like viruses and Sapporo-like viruses), enteric adenoviruses, and astroviruses. Epidemic viral gastroenteritis is caused most often by Norwalk-like viruses.

Rotavirus

In 1973, Bishop and colleagues visualized by electron microscopy a 70 nm triple-layered virus in the duodenal epithelium of children with diarrhea.[33] This virus, designated as rotavirus because of its morphologic appearance (in Latin, *rota* means wheel), belongs to the family Reoviridae; its genome consists of 11 segments of double-stranded RNA. The segmented genome of rotavirus allows reassortment during coinfection, a property that has been utilized in the development of rotavirus vaccines and is probably important in virus evolution. There are seven major groups of rotavirus (groups A to G); human illness is caused by rotaviruses of groups A, B, and C. Two outer capsid proteins, the glycoprotein (G protein) and the protease-cleaved protein (P protein), determine the serotype specificity and form the basis of the binary classification (G and P types) of rotaviruses. Both G protein and P protein induce neutralizing antibodies.

EPIDEMIOLOGY

Rotaviruses are ubiquitous, infecting 95% of children worldwide by the time they are 3 to 5 years of age.[34] Neonatal infections, although common, are often asymptomatic. The incidence of clinical illness peaks in children 4 to 23 months of age. Globally, rotaviruses are the most common agents of severe childhood gastroenteritis; they are estimated to cause about one third of all gastroenteritis hospitalizations and 500,000 deaths a year.[35] Rotavirus infections of adults are usually subclinical but occasionally cause illness in parents of children with rotavirus diarrhea and in immunocompromised individuals, the elderly, and travelers.

In temperate climates, rotavirus disease predominantly occurs during the fall and winter months. A recent study from Japan showed that, unlike in children, rotavirus diarrhea in adults did not show significant winter seasonality.[35] In the United States, rotavirus activity peaks in the Southwest in autumn (October through December) and migrates across the continent, peaking in the Northeast during spring (March through May).[36] In tropical settings, rotavirus disease occurs year-round.

During episodes of diarrhea, rotaviruses are shed in large amounts in stool; fecal shedding detectable by antigen enzyme immunoassays usually subsides within a week but may persist for more than 30 days in immunocompromised persons. Viral shedding may be detected for longer periods using more sensitive assays, such as PCR. Transmission of rotavirus occurs predominantly through the fecal-oral route. Transmission through respiratory secretions, person-to-person contact, or contaminated environmental surfaces has been postulated.

In humans, most rotavirus diseases, including endemic childhood diarrhea, are caused by group A rotaviruses. Group B rotaviruses have caused large epidemics of severe gastroenteritis in China since 1982 and have also been identified in India.[37,38] Group C rotaviruses have been associated with epidemic gastroenteritis worldwide, and some studies indicate a possible association with extrahepatic biliary atresia in infants.[39]

Rotavirus strains that infect animals differ from those that infect humans. Although some strains of human rotavirus possess a high degree of genetic homology with animal strains, animal-to-human transmission is uncommon.

PATHOGENESIS

Rotaviruses infect the mature enterocytes in the middle or upper villous epithelium of the small intestine. Ultimately, the epithelium becomes necrotic and sloughs off. The loss of absorptive villous epithelium coupled with proliferation of secretory crypt cells reverses the inherent absorptive state of the epithelium, resulting in secretory diarrhea. Levels of brush-border enzymes characteristic of differentiated cells (e.g., sucrase and lactase) are reduced, leading to the accumulation of unmetabolized disaccharides in the gut lumen, with consequent osmotic diarrhea. The toxinlike effect of a nonstructural rotavirus protein, NSP4, increases intracellular calcium through the opening of a cation channel, causing an efflux of chloride and, thus, sodium and water, contributing to the secretory diarrhea.[40] Furthermore, rotavirus appears to evoke intestinal fluid secretion through activation of the enteric nervous system.[41]

IMMUNITY

Protection against rotavirus disease is correlated with the presence of virus-specific secretory IgA antibodies in the feces and serum.[42,43] Because virus-specific IgA is short-lived at the intestinal surface, complete protection against natural rotavirus disease is only temporary. Memory B and T cells in the lamina propria are believed to be important in reducing the severity of disease resulting from reinfection.[44]

DIAGNOSIS

Clinical Manifestations

The clinical spectrum of rotavirus infection ranges from subclinical illness to severe gastroenteritis associated with life-threatening dehydration. The onset of illness is abrupt; vomiting frequently precedes the development of diarrhea. Up to one third of patients may have a temperature greater than 39° C (102.2° F). GI symptoms generally resolve in 3 to 6 days.

Respiratory symptoms have been observed in children with rotavirus infection, as have symptoms of CNS involvement, but these associations have not been well studied.[45] Rotavirus infection has been observed in patients with a variety of other clinical syndromes, including sudden infant death syndrome, Reye syndrome, necrotizing enterocolitis, intussusception, Kawasaki syndrome, disseminated intravascular coagulation, and Crohn disease. A causal relationship has not been confirmed between any of these syndromes and rotavirus infection.

In immunodeficient children, rotavirus can cause a protracted diarrhea with prolonged viral excretion and, in rare instances, can disseminate systemically and cause hepatic infection.[46]

Laboratory Tests

Illness caused by rotavirus is difficult to distinguish clinically from that caused by other enteric viruses. Because a large number of viruses are shed in feces, the diagnosis usually can be confirmed by using one of a wide variety of commercial immunoassays or by techniques for detecting viral RNA, such as gel electrophoresis, probe hybridization, or RT-PCR.

TREATMENT AND PREVENTION

Treatment relies primarily on replacement of fluids and electrolytes; antibiotics and antimotility agents should be avoided.[47] Although oral rehydration therapy is successful in most children, intravenous fluid replacement may be required for children who have severe dehydration or are unable to tolerate oral therapy. A variety of other therapeutic agents have been evaluated, including probiotics,[48] bismuth salicylate,[49] and enkephalinase inhibitors,[50] but their therapeutic roles are not clearly defined.

Efforts to develop rotavirus vaccines were initiated when it became apparent that the incidence of disease in less developed countries was similar to that in industrialized countries and that, therefore, improvements in hygiene and sanitation were unlikely to interrupt viral transmission.[51] In 1998, only 25 years after the identification of rotavirus in humans, a live, attenuated rotavirus vaccine (Rotashield, Wyeth Laboratories, Marietta, Pennsylvania) with 80% efficacy against severe rotavirus disease was licensed in the United States and was recommended for routine immunization of infants. This vaccine was withdrawn, however, in 1999, after it was confirmed that its use was associated with intussusception.[52] Efforts are ongoing to develop other rotavirus vaccines with improved safety profiles.

Norwalk and Related Human Caliciviruses

In 1972, using immune electron microscopy, Kapikian and colleagues identified the 27 nm Norwalk agent in stool filtrates of a volunteer challenged with fecal specimens from patients affected by an outbreak of gastroenteritis.[53] Several related but genetically and antigenically diverse single-stranded RNA viruses of positive polarity measuring 27 to 35 nm were subsequently identified; these organisms are currently classified as Norwalk-like viruses, in the family Caliciviridae. The Caliciviridae family also includes the Sapporo-like viruses, which cause gastroenteritis in children and adults, and Lagovirus and Vesivirus, neither of which is pathogenic for humans.

EPIDEMIOLOGY

Recent studies indicate that infections with the Norwalk and related caliciviruses are more common than previously believed; a majority of children and nearly all adults demonstrate antibodies to these viruses. Acquisition of antibody occurs at an earlier age in developing countries, as would be expected, given the presumed fecal-oral mode of transmission of these viruses. Although their role in sporadic illness in children and adults is still being defined, the Norwalk-like viruses are clearly recognized as the most common cause of epidemics of gastroenteritis worldwide.[54] Epidemics occur throughout the year and are often linked to consumption of fecally contaminated water and foods; often, food and water become contaminated by an infectious food handler. Dispersion of virus through direct contact, vomitus, or airborne droplets has been postulated in situations in which an alternative mode of transmission cannot be established.

PATHOGENESIS

Because no animal model exists for calicivirus gastroenteritis, the data on pathogenesis of disease arise exclusively from studies of human volunteers. After challenge of volunteers with either Norwalk virus or Hawaii virus, which is a related calicivirus, biopsy demonstrates lesions in the proximal small intestine; these lesions are characterized by villus shortening, crypt hyperplasia, and infiltration of the lamina propria by polymorphonuclear cells and lymphocytes.[55] The lesions persist for at least 4 days after the person's symptoms disappear and are associated with malabsorption of carbohydrates and fats and a decreased level of brush-border enzymes. No changes are observed in the stomach or colon, but gastric motor function is delayed, which probably contributes to the characteristic nausea and vomiting.[56]

IMMUNITY

Approximately 50% of persons challenged with Norwalk virus become ill and acquire short-term homologous immunity (i.e., immunity against the same strain) that is correlated with serum antibody levels; immunity does not appear to persist for longer than 2 years.[57] Some reports indicate, paradoxically, that persons with higher levels of preexisting antibody to Norwalk virus are more susceptible to illness.[58]

DIAGNOSIS

Clinical Manifestations

Gastroenteritis caused by Norwalk virus and related enteric caliciviruses occurs with sudden onset after a viral incubation period of 12 to 48 hours. The illness generally lasts 12 to 60 hours and is characterized by nausea, vomiting, abdominal cramps, and diarrhea. In children, vomiting is more prevalent than diarrhea, whereas in adults, diarrhea is more prevalent. Constitutional symptoms, such as headache, fever, chills, and myalgias, are frequently reported. Death is rare and usually occurs from severe dehydration in vulnerable persons, such as the elderly with debilitating health conditions.

Laboratory Tests

Cloning and sequencing of the genome of Norwalk virus and a few other human caliciviruses has allowed the development of sensitive detection methods based on PCR amplification and Southern blot analysis; strains can be further characterized by sequencing of nucleotide products. Expression of capsid proteins in a recombinant baculovirus vector produces virus-like particles that have been used to develop immunoassays. However, diagnostic assays are not widely available.

TREATMENT AND PREVENTION

Treatment is generally not required, because the disease is self-limited.[47] Rehydration may be required for patients with volume depletion.

Epidemic prevention relies on situation-specific measures, such as control of contamination of food and water, prevention of the handling of food by persons who are ill, and reduction of person-to-person spread through good personal hygiene. Calicivirus vaccines are being developed and may be particularly useful for groups for whom the impact of short-term morbidity from gastroenteritis is great (e.g., military troops) or those who are at high risk for severe disease (e.g., the elderly in nursing homes).

Other Viral Agents of Gastroenteritis

Enteric adenoviruses have double-stranded DNA and measure 70 to 80 nm; they belong to the family Adenoviridae. Serotypes 31, 40, and 41 cause approximately 10% of diarrheal illness in young children. Unlike their counterparts that cause respiratory illness, enteric adenoviruses are difficult to cultivate in cell lines. Their detection requires use of immunoassays to the adenovirus hexon antigen and subsequent serotyping using monoclonal antibodies.

Astroviruses have positive-sense, single-stranded RNA and measure 28 to 30 nm; they belong to the family Astroviridae. Although at least seven different serotypes have been identified, strains of serotype 1 are most common. Preliminary epidemiologic studies indicate that astroviruses may be important causes of mild to moderate diarrhea in children, causing half as many illnesses as rotavirus.[59] The availability of simple immunoassays to detect virus in fecal specimens and of molecular methods to confirm and further characterize strains will allow for a more comprehensive assessment of the etiologic role of these agents in endemic childhood diarrhea.

Other viruses, including toroviruses, picobirnaviruses, coronaviruses, pestiviruses, and parvoviruses, have been identified in the feces of patients with diarrhea, but their etiologic role has not been well studied. It appears from preliminary studies that some of these agents, such as picobirnaviruses, may be important causes of diarrhea in HIV-infected persons.[60,61]

References

1. Oberste MS, Maher K, Kilpatrick DR, et al: Molecular evolution of the human enteroviruses: correlation of serotype with VP1 sequence and application to picornavirus classification. J Virol 73:1941, 1999

2. Stanway G, Joki-Korpela P, Hyypia T: Human parechoviruses: biology and clinical significance. Rev Med Virol 10:57, 2000

3. Oberste M, Schnurr D, Maher K, et al: Molecular identification of new picornaviruses and characterization of a proposed enterovirus 73 serotype. J Gen Virol 82:409, 2001

4. Nonpolio enterovirus surveillance—United States, 1993–1996. MMWR Morb Mortal Wkly Rep 46:748, 1997

5. Enterovirus surveillance—United States, 1997–1999. MMWR Morb Mortal Wkly Rep 49:913, 2000

6. Echovirus type 13—United States, 2001. MMWR Morb Mortal Wkly Rep 50:777, 2001

7. Morens MM, Pallansch MA: Epidemiology. Human Enterovirus Infections. Rotbart HA, Ed. ASM Press, Washington, DC, 1995, p 3

8. Feachem R, Garelick H, Slade J: Enteroviruses in the environment. Trop Dis Bull 78:185, 1981

9. O'Neil KM, Pallansch MA, Winkelstein JA, et al: Chronic group A coxsackievirus infection in agammaglobulinemia: demonstration of genomic variation of serotypically identical isolates persistently excreted by the same patient. J Infect Dis 157:183, 1988

10. Galama JM, de Leeuw N, Wittebol S, et al: Prolonged enteroviral infection in a patient who developed pericarditis and heart failure after bone marrow transplantation. Clin Infect Dis 22:1004, 1996

11. McKinney RE Jr, Katz SL, Wilfert CM: Chronic enteroviral meningoencephalitis in agammaglobulinemic patients. Rev Infect Dis 9:334, 1987

12. Byington CL, Taggart WE, Carrol KC, et al: A polymerase chain reaction-based epidemiologic investigation of the incidence of nonpolio enteroviral infections in febrile and afebrile infants 90 days and younger. Pediatrics 103:E27, 1999

13. Rotbart HA: Viral meningitis. Semin Neurol 20:277, 2000

14. Modlin JF: Update on enterovirus infections in infants and children. Adv Pediatr Infect Dis 12:155, 1996

15. Chan LG, Parashar UD, Lye MS, et al: Deaths of children during an outbreak of hand, foot, and mouth disease in Sarawak, Malaysia: clinical and pathological characteristics of the disease. For the Outbreak Study Group. Clin Infect Dis 31:678, 2000

16. Huang CC, Liu CC, Chang YC, et al: Neurologic complications in children with enterovirus 71 infection. N Engl J Med 341:936, 1999

17. Progress toward global poliomyelitis eradication, 2000. MMWR Morb Mortal Wkly Rep 50:320, 2001

18. Smith WG: Coxsackie B myopericarditis in adults. Am Heart J 89: 34, 1970

19. Helin M, Savola J, Lapinleimu K: Cardiac manifestations during a coxsackie B5 epidemic. BMJ 3:97, 1968

20. Chang LY, Lin TY, Hsu KH, et al: Clinical features and risk factors of pulmonary oedema after enterovirus-71-related hand, foot, and mouth disease. Lancet 354:1862, 1999

21. Modlin JF: Perinatal echovirus infection: insights from a literature review of 61 cases of serious infection and 16 outbreaks in nurseries. Rev Infect Dis 8:918, 1986

22. Abzug MJ, Levin MJ, Rotbart HA: Profile of enterovirus disease in the first two weeks of life. Pediatr Infect Dis J 12:820, 1993

23. Graves PM, Norris JM, Pallansch MA, et al: The role of enteroviral infections in the development of IDDM: limitations of current approaches. Diabetes 46:161, 1997

24. Sawyer MH: Enterovirus infections: diagnosis and treatment. Pediatr Infect Dis J 18:1033, 1999

25. Tanel RE, Kao SY, Niemiec TM, et al: Prospective comparison of culture vs genome detection for diagnosis of enteroviral meningitis in childhood. Arch Pediatr Adolesc Med 150:919, 1996

26. Romero JR: Enteroviruses: diagnosis, screening, and surveillance. Infect Med 16(suppl D):11, 1999

27. Santos AP, Costa EV, Oliveira SS, et al: RT-PCR based analysis of cell culture negative stools samples from poliomyelitis suspected cases. J Clin Virol 23:149, 2002

28. Hamilton MS, Jackson MA, Abel D: Clinical utility of polymerase chain reaction testing for enteroviral meningitis. Pediatr Infect Dis J 18:533, 1999

29. Oberste MS, Maher K, Kilpatrick DR, et al: Typing of human enteroviruses by partial sequencing of VP1. J Clin Microbiol 37:1288, 1999

30. Romero JR: Pleconaril: a novel antipicornaviral drug. Expert Opin Investig Drugs 10:369, 2001

31. Abzug MJ, Keyserling HL, Lee ML, et al: Neonatal enterovirus infection: virology, serology, and effects of intravenous immune globulin. Clin Infect Dis 20:1201, 1995

32. Poliomyelitis prevention in the United States: updated recommendations of the Advisory Committee on Immunization Practices (ACIP). MMWR Morb Mortal Wkly Rep 49[RR-5]:1, 2000

33. Bishop RF, Davidson GP, Holmes IH, et al: Virus particles in epithelial cells of duodenal mucosa from children with viral gastroenteritis. Lancet 2:1281, 1973

34. Parashar UD, Bresee JS, Gentsch JR, et al: Rotavirus. Emerg Infect Dis 4:561, 1998

35. Nakajima H, Nakagomi T, Kamisawa T, et al: Winter seasonality and rotavirus in adults. Lancet 357:1950, 2001

36. Torok TJ, Kilgore PE, Clarke MJ, et al: Visualizing geographic and temporal trends in rotavirus activity in the United States, 1991 to 1996. National Respiratory and Enteric Virus Surveillance System Collaborating Laboratories. Pediatr Infect Dis J 16:941, 1997

37. Fang ZY, Ye Q, Ho MS, et al: Investigation of an outbreak of adult diarrhea rotavirus in China. J Infect Dis 160:948, 1989

38. Krishnan T, Sen A, Choudhury JS, et al: Emergence of adult diarrhoea rotavirus in Calcutta, India (letter). Lancet 353:380, 1998

39. Riepenhoff-Talty M, Gouvea V, Evans MJ, et al: Detection of group C rotavirus in infants with extrahepatic biliary atresia. J Infect Dis 174: 8, 1996

40. Ball JM, Tian P, Zeng CQ, et al: Age-dependent diarrhea induced by a rotaviral nonstructural glycoprotein. Science 272:101, 1996

41. Lundgren O, Peregrin AT, Persson K, et al: Role of the enteric nervous system in the fluid and electrolyte secretion of rotavirus diarrhea. Science 287:491, 2000

42. Coulson BS, Grimwood K, Hudson IL, et al: Role of coproantibody in clinical protection of children during reinfection with rotavirus. J Clin Microbiol 30:1678, 1992

43. Matson DO, O'Ryan ML, Herrera I, et al: Fecal antibody responses to symptomatic and asymptomatic rotavirus infections. J Infect Dis 167: 577, 1993

44. Offit PA: Host factors associated with protection against rotavirus disease: the skies are clearing. J Infect Dis 174(suppl 1):S59, 1996

45. Lynch M, Lee B, Azimi P, et al: Rotavirus and central nervous system symptoms: cause or contaminant? Case reports and review. Clin Infect Dis 33:932, 2001

46. Gilger MA, Matson DO, Conner ME, et al: Extraintestinal rotavirus infections in children with immunodeficiency. J Pediatr 120:912, 1992

47. Farthing MJ: Treatment of gastrointestinal viruses. Novartis Found Symp 238:289, 2001

48. Szajewska H, Mrukowicz JZ: Probiotics in the treatment and prevention of acute infectious diarrhea in infants and children: a systematic review of published randomized, double-blind, placebo-controlled trials. J Pediatr Gastroenterol Nutr 33(suppl 2):S17, 2001

49. Figueroa-Quintanilla D, Salazar-Lindo E, Sack RB, et al: A controlled trial of bismuth subsalicylate in infants with acute watery diarrheal disease. N Engl J Med 1993

50. Salazar-Lindo E, Santisteban-Ponce J, Chea-Woo E, et al: Racecadotril in the treatment of acute watery diarrhea in children. N Engl J Med 343:463, 2000

51. Bresee J, Glass RI, Ivanoff B, et al: Current status and future priorities for rotavirus vaccine development, evaluation and implementation in developing countries. Vaccine 17:2207, 1999

52. Murphy TV, Gargiullo PM, Massoudi MS, et al: Intussusception among infants given an oral rotavirus vaccine. N Engl J Med 344:564, 2001

53. Kapikian AZ, Wyatt RG, Dolin R, et al: Visualization by immune electron microscopy of a 27-nm particle associated with acute infectious nonbacterial gastroenteritis. J Virol 10:1075, 1972

54. Parashar UD, Monroe SS: "Norwalk-like viruses" as a cause of foodborne disease outbreaks. Rev Med Virol 11:243, 2001

55. Schreiber DS, Blacklow NR, Trier JS: The mucosal lesion of the proximal small intestine in acute infectious nonbacterial gastroenteritis. N Engl J Med 288:1318, 1973

56. Meeroff JC, Schreiber DS, Trier JS, et al: Abnormal gastric motor function in viral gastroenteritis. Ann Intern Med 92:370, 1980

57. Graham DY, Jiang X, Tanaka T, et al: Norwalk virus infection of volunteers: new insights based on improved assays. J Infect Dis 170:34, 1994

58. Johnson PC, Mathewson JJ, DuPont HL, et al: Multiple-challenge study of host susceptibility to Norwalk gastroenteritis in US adults. J Infect Dis 161:18, 1990

59. Glass RI, Noel J, Mitchell D, et al: The changing epidemiology of astrovirus-associated gastroenteritis: a review. Arch Virol Suppl 12:287, 1996

60. Grohmann GS, Glass RI, Pereira HG, et al: Enteric viruses and diarrhea in HIV-infected patients. Enteric Opportunistic Infections Working Group. N Engl J Med 329:14, 1993

61. Giordano MO, Martinez LC, Rinaldi D, et al: Diarrhea and enteric emerging viruses in HIV- infected patients. Aids Res Hum Retroviruses 15:1427, 1999

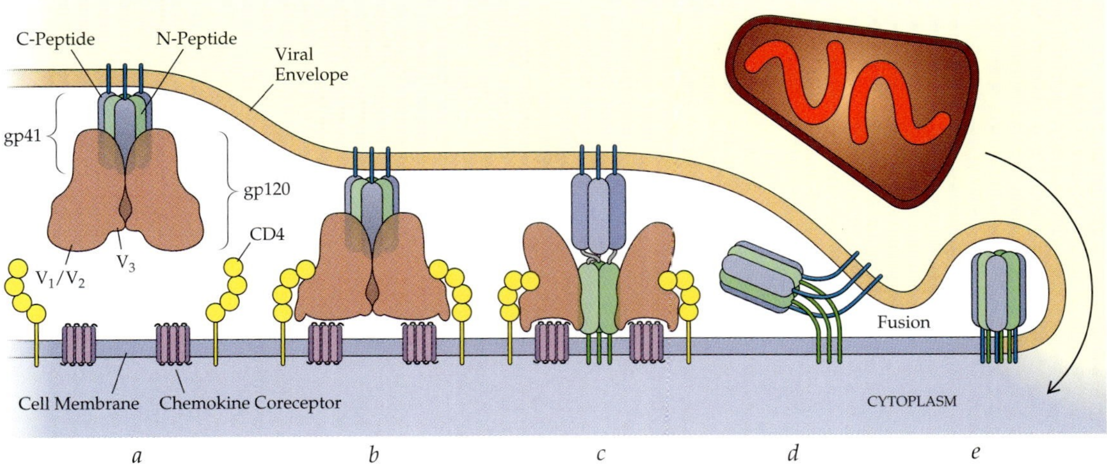

Figure 2 **Illustrated is the binding of HIV-1 with a CD4+ T cell. In unbound virions, gp41 exists in a stable, nonfusogenic conformation in which the fusion peptides are buried within the envelope trimer complex (*a*). When gp120 binds to the CD4 receptor, a conformational change exposes the chemokine receptor attachment site on gp120 (either CXC chemokine receptor–4 [CXCR4] or CC chemokine receptor–5 [CCR5]) (*b*). This in turn triggers a transition of gp41 to the prehairpin intermediate (*c*), with exposure of the fusion peptide attached to the trimeric coiled-coil N-peptide region. The fusin peptide inserts into the target membrane (*c*). In this form, the C-peptide has not associated with the N-peptide because of continued association with gp120; at this stage, the intermediate gp41 polypeptide is vulnerable to C-peptide inhibition (e.g., T-20). When the C-peptide region binds to the N-peptide region coiled-coil, the complex adopts a helical conformation of the fusion-active hairpin, which brings the two membranes into apposition (*d*). The precise mechanism of membrane fusion is not clear, but after fusion is complete, the fusion peptide and transmembrane segment of gp41 lie in the same membrane (*e*). A similar mechanism presumably applies to the fusion of a cell infected with HIV-1 that expresses viral envelope on the plasma membrane surface with an uninfected CD4+ T cell, which leads to syncytium formation among infected and uninfected cells in vitro.[12,132]**

are located at the 5' and 3' terminal ends of the genome. All retroviruses are terminally redundant and contain identical sequences, called long terminal repeats (LTRs). The coding sequences include the *gag* gene, which encodes group-specific structural antigens; the *pol* gene, which encodes RNA-dependent DNA polymerase or reverse transcriptase, integrase, and protease; and the *env* gene, which encodes envelope structural proteins. The *gag* gene encodes a precursor polypeptide that is cleaved by viral-encoded protease to form several internal structural proteins—namely, matrix protein (MA), capsid protein (CA), and nucleic acid binding protein (nucleocapsid, or NC).[4]

In addition, the 3' end of the *gag* gene reading frame overlaps with the *pol* gene reading frame to encode for the virus-specific protease. The *pol* gene encodes for a precursor polypeptide that is cleaved by the virus-specific protease enzyme to form three enzymes: protease, reverse transcriptase, and integrase. The *env* gene encodes for a 160 kd precursor protein, which is cleaved posttranscriptionally into two noncovalently associated envelope glycoproteins during transport through the endoplasmic reticulum and the Golgi complex by host proteases, termed furins. The first env protein is gp120, which is a highly charged glycoprotein that is external to the viral envelope; gp120 binds to cell-specific viral receptors (e.g., CD4+ T cell receptor in the case of HIV) and ancillary coreceptors (e.g., chemokine receptors for HIV-1). There are five domains of the *env* gene—V1 through V5. Some of these are highly variable (of these domains, the V3 loop is the most highly variable). These variable domains are responsible for defining multiple variants or quasispecies that contribute to viral evasion from neutralizing antibodies produced by the host in response to viral infection. The second env protein, gp41, is a hydrophobic transmembrane glycoprotein that anchors the oligomeric surface subunit glycoprotein to the viral envelope membrane. The virion surface is studded with approximately 72 knobs; each is composed of three heterodimers of the gp120env/gp41env complex.[7,11] Fusion of the retroviral envelope with the target cell plasma membrane is facilitated by the transmembrane glycoprotein through conformational change mediated by a helix coiled-coil mechanism. This mechanism is present in enveloped viruses other than retroviruses (e.g., influenzavirus)[12] [*see Figure 2*].

Table 2 Genes and Proteins of HIV[13]

Gene	*Gene Product*	*Size (kd)*	*Function*
gag	Capsid matrix protein	p17	Interacts with gp41; binds cyclophilin A in the virion
	Nucleocapsid core protein	p24	Forms nucleocapsid along with p6
	Nucleocapsid core protein	p6	Forms nucleocapsid along with p24; binds to vpr
	Nucleic acid binding protein	p7	Binds to viral RNA
		p1, p2	Cleavage products of gag precursor protein
pol	Protease	p10	Proteolytic cleavage of gag, pol, and env precursor polypeptides
	Reverse transcriptase	p66/51	Polymerase and ribonuclease H activity (p66 only)
	Integrase	p32	Integration of viral DNA (vDNA) into host cell chromosome
env	Envelope protein	gp120	Trimeric external envelope protein; glycosylated protein with five variable domains (V1 through V5) and four invariant regions (C1 through C4); binds to CD4 receptor and chemokine coreceptor
	Transmembrane protein	gp41	Trimeric protein that attaches gp120 to virion envelope; facilitates fusion of the viral envelope with the cell plasma membrane; each molecule is composed of two α-helical regions that form a six-helix bundle; coiled-coil state is basis for "spring-loaded" interaction that leads to virus cell fusion
vif	Virion infectivity protein	p23	Efficient cell free transmission; required for proper assembly of nucleoprotein core
vpr	Viral protein R	p15	Enhances viral replication in primary cells; G2/M phase arrest; nuclear localization in cell; transports vDNA in preintegration complex to the nucleus; virion-associated protein
tat	*Trans*-activator of transcription	p14	Major viral *trans*-activator
rev	Regulator of expression of virion protein	p19	Enhances expression of unspliced and singly spliced RNA molecules; regulates transport of messenger RNA; shuttles back and forth between nucleus and cytoplasm
*vpu**	Viral protein U	p15-16	Enhances release of virion from cells; downregulates CD4 on cell
nef	Negative regulatory factor	p27	Inhibits or enhances viral replication, depending on strain and cell type; downregulates CD4 and MHC class I receptor
vpx†	Virion protein X	p25	Packaged into the virion

*HIV-1 only.
†HIV-2 only.

The complexity of the human retroviruses is best exemplified by the array of viral proteins that are responsible for regulating viral replication and the host cell response to infection.[4,7] HTLV-I has a region between the *env* gene and the 3' LTR that encodes for two regulatory proteins, tax and rex, which are produced from messages that are spliced differently from distinct overlapping reading frames. The tax protein induces the expression of cell transcription factors that alter host cell gene expression, and the rex protein regulates the expression of viral messenger RNA (mRNA). The HIV viruses have a larger genome than HTLV. In addition, HIV has a larger translated region (regulatory genes) between the *pol* and *env* genes, which encode portions of several regulatory proteins that depend on the overlapping open reading frame (ORF) into which the mRNA is spliced.

These retroviral regulatory proteins express the following functions[13,14] [*see Table 2*]. The tat protein augments the expression of virus from the LTR region. The rev protein regulates RNA splicing and RNA transport, or both, in HIV and may function in a manner similar to that of the rex protein in HTLV. The nef protein downregulates CD4 protein, which is the cellular receptor for HIV; it alters host T cell activation pathways by decreasing major histocompatibility complex (MHC) class I antigen expression; and it enhances viral infectivity. The vif protein is necessary for the proper assembly of the

HIV nucleoprotein core; without the vif protein, viral cDNA is not efficiently produced. The vpr protein (in HIV-1) and the vpx protein (in HIV-2) facilitate transport of the viral cDNA into the nucleus and cause an arrest in the G_2 stage of the cell cycle, which is necessary for optimal viral infection. As such, the vpr protein appears to facilitate the infection of nondividing cells by HIV, a property not shared by HTLV. The vpu protein promotes the degradation of CD4 protein in the endoplasmic reticulum and stimulates the release of virions from infected cells.

PATHOGENETIC TRYPTIC

The biologic properties of the human retroviruses, summarized above, orchestrate a viral pathogenesis tryptic defined by latency, transformation, and cytopathicity; this process occurs through two replication phases [*see Figure 3*]. In the first replication phase, the viral-encoded proteins that are packed within the virion nucleocapsid enter the cell; this eventually results in the formation of the integrated cDNA provirus. In the second replication phase, the enzymatic machinery of the host cell is utilized to replicate the viral RNA genome and to transcribe and translate viral proteins from the provirus. With the exception of retroviral latency, the pathogenesis tryptic leads to cell dysfunction (and sometimes cell death), with eventual immunosuppression and clinical disease. Both HTLV-I and HTLV-II immortalize primary human peripheral blood T cells in vitro. Immortalization is defined as interleuken-2 (IL-2)–dependent, long-term growth in culture. Subsequently, cells become fully transformed—that is, they are subject to continuous cell proliferation in the absence of IL-2. Cellular transformation is an early step in the pathogenic process of HTLV and is distinct from oncogenesis or malignancy.[4] As such, HTLV transformation of T cells results in a pool of proliferating cells that are not oncogenic themselves but that provide a population from which a malignant clone may subsequently arise.[4] This accounts for the long latent period between infection and tumor development in HTLV disease. In contrast, HIV does not transform the infected cell but rather produces a cytopathic effect that results in cell dysfunction and, eventually, cell death.

The first phase of viral replication starts when the retrovirus binds to a specific cell receptor, which for HIV is the CD4 molecule on the cell surface and an associated chemokine coreceptor.[15] The HTLV receptors have not been characterized; however, cellular targets for HTLV-I include several types of T cells, the primary one being the $CD4^+$ T cell. HTLV-II preferentially infects $CD8^+$ T cells.[16] The retroviral nucleocapsid complex enters the cell cytoplasm, and the viral genomic RNA is reverse-transcribed to a slightly longer, double-stranded cDNA molecule that actively enters the nucleus as a nucleoprotein-preintegration complex and integrates permanently at a single random site in the cell chromosome. The integration of linear viral cDNA occurs during division of the cell; as such, nondividing cells are generally resistant to retroviral infection. However, the one exception to this is HIV, which is able to infect resting cells (the G_1 phase of the cell cycle), albeit less efficiently than activated cells in the S phase of the cell cycle. The inhibition of reverse transcription by combinations of nucleotide, nucleoside, or nonnucleoside reverse transcriptase inhibitors (NNRTIs) is a cornerstone of current HIV-1 therapeutics.[10]

The second replication phase begins with the production of viral genomic RNA and mRNA and protein synthesis; the production of mRNA and protein synthesis occur almost exclusively through the enzymatic machinery of the host cell under the influence of viral gene regulatory products. Processing of virion proteins begins in the endoplasmic reticulum and Golgi complex. Virion assembly begins at the plasma membrane, and the nascent virions are released from the cell surface through budding. The budding viral envelope, which has a phospholipid composition different from that of the plasma membrane of the cell, may incorporate some cell membrane surface proteins (e.g., β_2-microglobulin and MHC class I and II proteins), along with virus-specific glycoproteins.[6,7] Extracellular HIV undergoes further maturation by continued proteolytic cleavage of the nucleocapsid polypeptide, which results in the mature infectious virion with a distinctive cone-shaped nucleocapsid core. The inhibition of viral protease through virus-specific protease inhibitor therapy, in combination with reverse transcriptase inhibitor therapy, is an important aim of current antiretroviral therapeutics. However, inhibition of reverse transcriptase with combinations of nucleoside reverse transcriptase inhibitors (NRTIs) and NNRTIs is equally efficacious in many cases.[10]

Pathogenesis of Retroviral Infection

The clinical consequences of retrovirus infection reflect a precarious balance between the type of

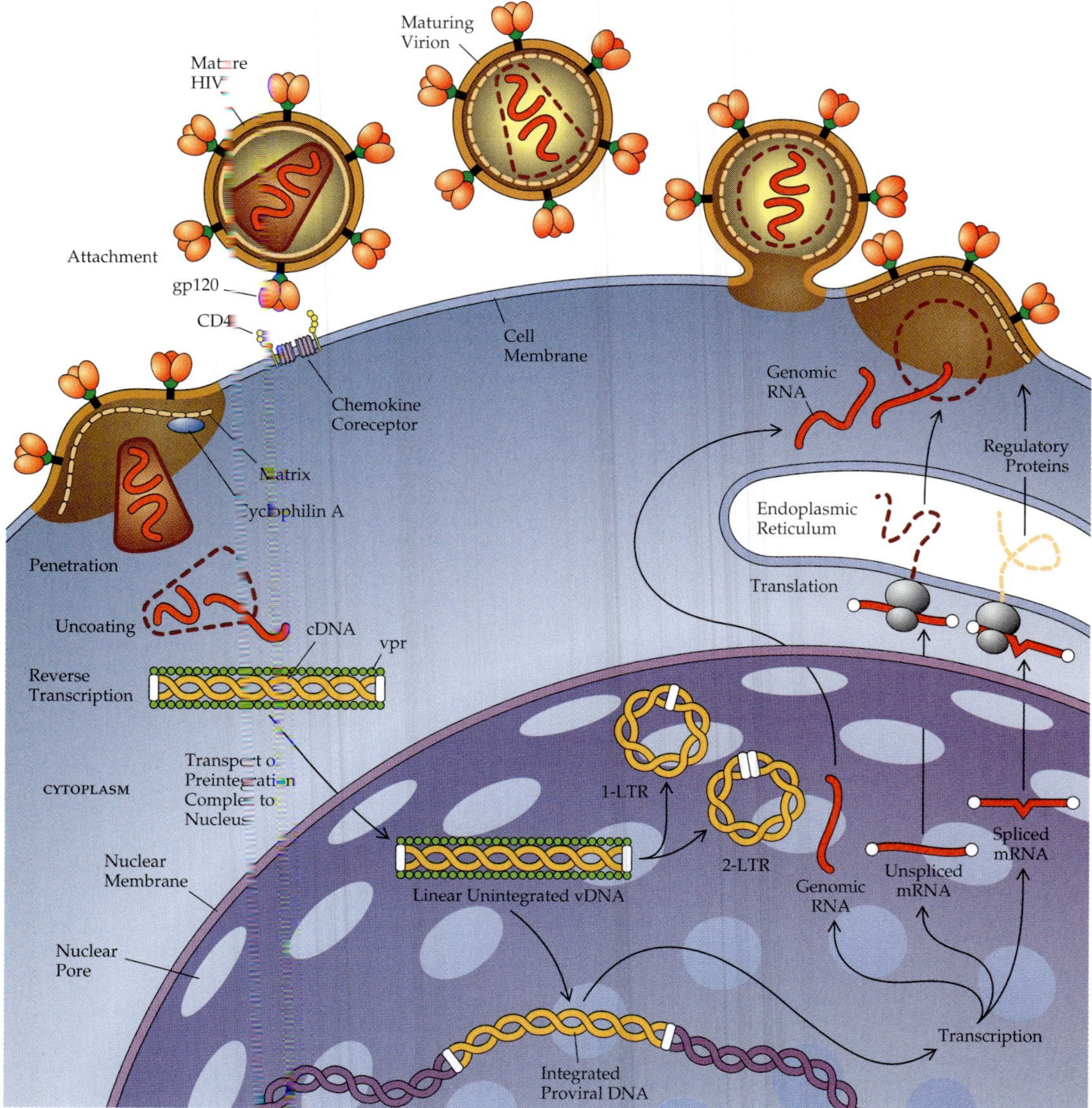

Figure 3 **Illustrated is the replication cycle of HIV-1. The virus must first attach to the CD4 receptor and chemokine coreceptor on the cell surface [*see Figure* 2]. After fusion of the viral envelope with the plasma membrane of the target cell, the nucleocapsid undergoes uncoating, which is facilitated by the presence of cyclophilin A. The viral RNA genome is reverse-transcribed to double-stranded viral DNA (vDNA), which enters the nucleus as a preintegration complex that contains vpr protein and integrase. Only linear vDNA is capable of integrating randomly into the host chromosome; other forms of partially transcribed linear vDNA fragments and 1-long-terminal repeat (LTR) and 2-LTR circularized, episomal vDNA are not capable of integration. The integrated linear vDNA (now termed the provirus) serves as the template for viral transcription. Transcription of the proviral DNA template yields genomic viral RNA, and alternative messenger RNA (mRNA) splicing creates spliced viral mRNA species that encode the viral accessory proteins and the unspliced viral mRNA species that encode the viral structural polyproteins [*see Table* 2]. All of the transcripts are exported to the cytoplasm, where translation processing and assembly begins to occur in the endoplasmic reticulum and Golgi complex. The viral polypeptides, protease, viral RNA, and other constituents of the viral core condense at areas of the plasma membrane that have already accumulated viral envelope proteins (gp120/gp41). Budding of the virion ensues, and the immature virion nucleocapsid core undergoes further proteolytic maturation in the extracellular milieu.[133]**

invading retrovirus, its tropism for specific cells and tissues, and the patient's natural and acquired resistance. The pathophysiologic model of retrovirus infection can be approached by understanding viral mechanisms of infection, latency and persistence, cell injury, and immune system evasion and modulation. Some aspects of this model are shared by other RNA and DNA viruses; other aspects are unique to the human retroviruses.

VIRAL ENTRY, TARGET CELL TROPISM, AND VIRUS RECEPTOR INTERACTIONS

Human retrovirus transmission requires parenteral or intimate mucous membrane exposure to the virus. Transmission by fomites is unlikely because the viral envelope of retroviruses is easily damaged in the environment by exposure to high temperatures, detergents, and chemical disinfectants and through drying. The concentration of virus in body fluids to which a person is exposed is a very important determinant of transmission.[17] For HIV, the blood level of virus may or may not reflect the virus level in genital fluids and breast milk.[18–20]

Receptors

The cellular receptor for HTLV has not been identified. Only T cells are productively targeted by HTLV, but infection of B cells and other cell types has been detected. Much more is known about the manner by which HIV enters the host cell. Susceptible cells must be available for the process of adsorption, penetration, and uncoating of the virus to occur. The receptor for HIV is the CD4 molecule, which is present on T cells and defines the subset of CD4+ helper-inducer T cells. The HIV-1 gp120env protein binds specifically to the CD4 receptor; in addition, other cell surface proteins, such as the chemokine receptors, serve as essential coreceptors for different strains of HIV.[15]

Coreceptors

The HIV-1 coreceptors belong to the superfamily of protein-coupled receptors that bind guanosine triphosphate (GTP). These receptors have a characteristic structure of seven transmembrane segments and are coupled with the G protein.[21] The two principal HIV-1 coreceptors, CC chemokine receptor–5 (CCR5) and CXC chemokine receptor–4 (CXCR4), and their chemokine ligands are involved in diverse biologic processes, such as immunomodulation, inflammation, hematopoiesis, and organogenesis.[22] Three cytokines released by CD8+ T cells—RANTES (regulated on activation, normal T cell expressed and secreted), macrophage inflammatory protein–1α (MIP-1α), and MIP-1β—bind to the CCR5 receptor and may suppress HIV macrophage tropic virus. Similarly, stromal cell–derived factor–1α (SDF-1α), which is the natural ligand for CXCR4, and AMD-3100, which is a small molecule inhibitor of SDF-1α, can inhibit R4 virus.[23,24] Clinical development of AMD-3100 was abandoned in May 2001 because of possible cardiac toxicity and limited efficacy. It has been proposed that aberrant signaling through binding of gp120env with the chemokine receptors may cause apoptosis and contribute to the decrease in the CD4+ T cell count in patients with AIDS.[25]

Infection with strains of virus that recognize the CXCR4 coreceptor generally results in cell fusion or syncytium formation in vitro; such strains are termed syncytium-inducing (SI), T-tropic, or R4 strains. Strains of virus that recognize the CCR5 coreceptor generally result in infection without syncytium formation in vitro; such strains are termed non–syncytium-inducing (NSI), monocytotropic, or R5 strains. Dual-tropic strains are able to use both chemokine coreceptors. Other chemokine receptors have also been shown to facilitate HIV infection of susceptible cells in vitro.[26] Thus, chemokine coreceptor use may be a determinant of viral virulence and disease progression.[27] For example, a 32-base-pair deletion in the *CCR5* gene, which is found as a homozygous mutation in less than 1% of the Western European white population, prevents surface expression of the truncated CCR5 receptor protein. This deletion is associated with slower progression of HIV-1 infection and a decrease in HIV-1 infection of peripheral mononuclear blood cells in vitro.[28] Even heterozygosity for this gene defect, which is observed in 20% of Western European whites, may provide some degree of protection against disease progression.[28–30]

HIV-1 gp120env also binds to a dendritic cell-specific C-type lectin DC-SIGN (dendritic cell–specific intracellular adhesion molecule–grabbing nonintegrin), which is highly expressed on dendritic cells in mucosal tissues.[31] DC-SIGN does not function as a receptor per se for viral entry into dendritic cells; rather it promotes infection of T cells that express CD4 and chemokine receptors.[32] As such, DC-SIGN efficiently captures HIV-1 in the periphery, stabilizes the virus, and facilitates its transport to secondary lymphoid organs rich in CD4+ T cell targets.[31]

HIV infection is associated with a loss of CD4 antigen on the infected T cell and ultimately leads to the death of the infected T cell. This in turn contributes to a decrease in the ratio of CD4+ T cells to CD8+ T cells—a hallmark of HIV-induced immunosuppression. However, the CD4+ T cell is not the only type of cell subject to infection by HIV. Other cells, such as the monocyte-macrophage, express CD4 molecules and probably disseminate HIV to target organs. In addition, monocyte-macrophages serve as a reservoir for HIV and other lentiviruses. Other cells can be infected with HIV in vitro, including Langerhans cells of the skin, follicular dendritic cells, and several others, some of which do not express the CD4 antigen. For example, astrocytes, oligodendrocytes, M cells of the enteric mucosa, and epithelial cells of the intestine and vagina all express galactosylceramide or a related glycolipid receptor that may act as an alternative virus receptor for gp120env.[33,34]

LATENCY AND PERSISTENCE

For any virus infection to persist, viral gene expression must be restricted to some extent. Three patterns of restricted viral expression are known; all three patterns are important for retroviral infections.[35] The first pattern, latent infection, is characterized by intermittent episodes of acute or subclinical disease; in latent infection, no virus is detectable between episodes. An example of latent infection is herpes simplex virus infection, which is characterized by episodic subclinical shedding. Latent infection may be particularly important for patients infected with HTLV or HIV-1 whose plasma levels of viral RNA have been suppressed below detectable levels through use of antiretroviral therapy. Latent infection must be differentiated from clinical latency, which occurs in the presence of ongoing viral replication.

The second pattern of restricted viral expression is chronic infection. In chronic infection, the virus is usually demonstrable but disease is absent. An example of chronic infection is cytomegalovirus infection. The chronic pattern of infection is seen in approximately one half of the patients infected with HIV-1 who are treated with antiretroviral drugs. In these patients, the plasma levels of HIV-1 RNA are persistently low as a result of potent antiretroviral therapy (HIV-1 RNA counts are greater than 50 RNA copies/ml of plasma but are less than 5,000 copies/ml). However, unlike untreated patients, these patients experience a sustained increase in CD4+ T cells and improved clinical status.

The third pattern of restricted viral expression is persistent infection. This pattern is characterized by a long incubation period with slowly increasing amounts of virus, eventually leading to symptomatic disease. Examples are subacute sclerosing panencephalitis associated with measles virus infection and hepatitis C virus (HCV) infection. This pattern is often seen in HTLV infection, which is characterized by a low probability of developing clinical disease over the infected person's lifetime (the probability is from 5% to 10%) and a period lasting decades in which the patient is asymptomatic. This pattern is also seen in patients with HIV-1 infection; in these patients, the median time to the development of AIDS is approximately 10 years.

Infections with the lentiviruses, particularly HIV, have features characteristic of all three patterns but are best described as persistent and cytopathic. HTLV infections have the characteristic features of latent and persistent infections, but in addition, the infected cell may be transformed.

Both the HIV and HTLV cDNA become integrated with the genome of the infected host cell at a single random site to establish the provirus as a permanent chromosomal resident.[4] In addition, most of the HIV cDNA remains in an extrachromosomal state, either as linear cDNA fragments or as circularized forms (neither of which are replicatively competent). The degree of viral transcription and translation depends on the stage of differentiation of the infected CD4+ T cell. That stage, in turn, is probably related to exogenous antigen stimulation and the action of cytokines (e.g., IL-2) and viral regulatory proteins (e.g., the vpr protein), which promote cell differentiation and activation of viral promotors (e.g., nuclear factor–κB [NF-κB] inducible transcription factors). Integration of human retroviruses differs from that of certain animal retroviruses in that no transforming genes (oncogenes) are associated with the viral genome, and the proviral genome is not regularly inserted next to a host-transforming gene. Moreover, clinically important human retroviruses are exogenous and are not transmitted in germ cells, as are some endogenous vertebrate retroviruses and the clinically unimportant HERVs [*see Table 1*].

CYTOPATHICITY

The cytopathic destruction of lymphoid cells is a characteristic of lentivirus infection in general. In a minority of patients with HIV, an initial period of intense viral replication is followed by an acute and rapidly progressive disease; in most patients with HIV, however, this initial period of viral replication is followed by a period of persistent infection, with clinical disease developing only after a prolonged period. In some patients in whom disease progression is very slow, chronic infection can develop, and the development of such chronic infection is a viable long-term clinical objective of antiretroviral therapy.

The clinical manifestations of HIV are governed by cell and tissue tropism; the clinical signs and symptoms of infection arise directly or indirectly from viral replication within these cells and tissues. The sine qua non of HIV infection is $CD4^+$ T cell depletion, immunosuppression, and the development of opportunistic infections and malignancies. This depletion of $CD4^+$ T cells occurs not only by direct viral replication and cell lysis but also through other mechanisms. For example, HIV env-induced cell fusion may result in syncytia formation; cell surface expression of the *Fas* gene and programmed cell death (apoptosis); aberrant signaling through chemokine receptors; arrest of proliferation at the G_2 phase of the cell cycle, with cytopathic ballooning of the cells; and antibody-dependent or cell-mediated depletion induced by the binding of gp120env. In addition, the functional responses of T cells, such as signaling, are impaired both in vitro and in vivo because of the binding of gp120env with the CD4 molecule.[36]

A number of other cellular and lymphoid abnormalities are observed in persons infected with HIV, including abnormal B cell immunity and humoral immunity, monocyte-macrophage dysfunction, and immune defects in natural killer cells, among many observed immunologic defects.[36] Moreover, the follicular dendritic cells (FDCs) may play a key role in maintaining a large reservoir of protected infectious virus particles on the dendritic cell surface; although these cells do not appear to be infected, the presence of virus particles on the cell surface results in chronic immune activation and cytokine secretion, which leads to further virus replication and dissemination. Eventually, the FDCs are destroyed, which in turn leads to the destruction of the lymphoid architecture and the evolution of clinical disease.[36] In many instances, lymphoid architecture may be partially restored after prolonged antiretroviral therapy.

GENOMIC DIVERSITY

HIV undergoes active and continuous replication in the infected person, with infected cells dying after approximately 2 days.[37,38] The level of plasma HIV particles remains relatively constant for each infected person because of the balance between rapid production and clearance of virions. To maintain this steady-state level of HIV RNA, there are an estimated one billion infectious events every day in the untreated person with HIV infection. As such, the large number of replication cycles—estimated to be 300 cycles or more a year—provide ample opportunity for the virus to develop genetic diversity as a primary defense against immune and antiretroviral therapy suppression of replication. For example, within the *env* gene, localized regions of extraordinary hypervariability are interspersed with well-conserved (i.e., nonvariable) regions. One such hypervariable region is the V3 loop, which is a target for neutralizing antibodies. The force driving this variability is probably caused by selective pressure from the host's immune system.

This variability within HIV *env* gene contrasts with the relative genetic stability of HTLV. The mutation rate in the HIV *env* gene is one million times greater than that of DNA viruses and 10 to 100 times greater than that of other retroviruses; this results in a production of so-called quasispecies and is comparable only to the variability noted for another RNA virus, HCV. This extraordinary *env* gene hypervariability is associated with amino acid changes of as much as 35% or more among divergent HIV-1 isolates. Variation arises during reverse transcription of viral RNA to cDNA, a step that is highly prone to error, that lacks proofreading (i.e., correction of transcriptional copying errors) because the RNA template is destroyed by RNase H, and that leads to substitutions and misreading, which may result in the modification of several biologic properties, including tissue tropism, virulence, replication rate, and susceptibility to antiretroviral agents. In addition, recombination between different subtypes has been shown to be an important mechanism for generating diversity. Ultimately, continued genetic diversity of HIV may allow the virus to evade containment by the immune system.[39]

Origins of Human Retroviruses

The extent to which different human and primate retroviruses are related can be determined by comparing nucleic acid sequences through a process called phylogenetic analysis. Through such analysis, the human retroviruses have been shown to be phylogenetically related to the retroviruses of Old World primates. The closest viral relative of HTLV-I is the simian T cell lymphotropic virus type I (STLV-I), which was identified as an agent of naturally occurring infection in many species of Old World monkeys and great apes. Antecedent infection of the human population probably occurred from three geographically distinct interspecies transmission events; once established, the virus followed the migratory patterns of people around the world.[40] Moreover, recent studies have convincingly shown that there have been three separate interspecies transfers of the lentivirus simian immunodeficiency virus (SIV_{cpz}) from chimpanzees (*Pan troglodytes*) to humans; these transmission events occurred within the past century and resulted in the establishment of HIV-1 groups M, N, and O.[41,42] Similarly, HIV-2 has its origin with multiple interspecies transfers of SIV_{smm} from the primate sooty mangaby (*Cerocebus atys*) to man and to primates in captivity (e.g., SIV_{mac} in the rhesus monkey *Macaca mulatta*).

Human T Cell Lymphotropic Viruses

Retroviruses cause many animal malignancies and characteristically immortalize cells in vitro. In humans, the prototype retroviruses associated with malignant transformation are HTLV-I (and possibly HTLV-II). HTLV-I causes adult T cell leukemia (ATL); direct infection of the central nervous system results in a spastic or ataxic myelopathy termed tropical spastic paraparesis, also referred to as HTLV-I–associated myelopathy (HAM). HTLV-II was first isolated from a patient with a T cell variant of hairy-cell leukemia; it may be associated with certain neurologic, hematologic, and dermatologic diseases, but unequivocal evidence that HTLV-II is the etiologic agent is lacking.[43,44]

HTLV-I and HTLV-II have similar genomic organizations and share approximately 60% nucleotide homology[45] [*see Figure 2*]. The *gag* gene encodes for the structural proteins p19, p24, and p15. The *pol* gene encodes for the protease and the reverse transcriptase. The *env* gene encodes for the external envelope and transmembrane glycoproteins gp46 and gp21. The spliced regulatory proteins tax and rex and the other three open reading frames constitute the 9 kb genome. The gag and env proteins are most immunogenic; the antibodies to these proteins are commonly detected by enzyme immunoassay (EIA) and Western blot (WB) assay.

EPIDEMIOLOGY

HTLV-1 has a worldwide distribution; prevalence rates range from 5% to 27%, with the higher rates occurring in certain populations in which HTLV-1 is highly endemic.[46] HTLV-II is endemic in several Native American populations in the Americas and in Pygmy tribes in central Africa; in these populations, prevalence rates range from 7% to 9%.[44] In the United States, the seroprevalence rates of HTLV-I and HTLV-II range from 7% to 49% in injection drug users and prostitutes.[46] Early serologic and epidemiologic studies are confusing, because these studies were unable to effectively differentiate between HTLV-I and HTLV-II; however, this problem has been corrected through the use of more specific recombinant peptide–based WB and nucleic acid amplification methods.[47]

CLASSIFICATION OF HTLV SUBTYPES

The HTLV genome is highly conserved, but greater nucleotide convergence in the LTRs has made possible the development of restriction fragment length polymorphism (RFLP) testing. Through such testing, it is possible to classify both HTLV-I and HTLV-II into genotypic subtypes, and valuable information on viral transmission has become available.[47] There are five major molecular and geographic subtypes of HTLV-I: cosmopolitan (worldwide), Japanese, West African, Central African, and Melanesian.[48] There are three HTLV-II subtypes that reflect population clustering rather than geographic clustering: IIa, IIb, and IIc. Subtype IIa is found in injection drug users worldwide; subtype IIb is found primarily in Native Americans; and subtype IIc is found in Brazilian tribes.[49]

OVERVIEW OF LABORATORY DIAGNOSIS OF HTLV

Screening of blood donors for HTLV-I and HTLV-II is now routinely used in the United States, Canada, several Caribbean countries, Europe, and Japan.[47] The primary screening assay is the EIA; WB assay is used for confirmatory testing. However, EIA cannot distinguish between HTLV-I and HTLV-II infections because of the significant protein homology between the two viruses. Importantly, antibodies to HTLV do not cross-react with HIV proteins. After repeatedly positive results on EIA, the diagnosis of HTLV infection is confirmed if antibodies to two gene products (gag and env proteins) are detected on WB assay. For example, a specimen demonstrating antibody reactivity to p24gag and to pg46env or gp61/68env, or both, is considered to be positive for HTLV-I or HTLV-II. For specimens that test positive on EIA and that react with any of the WB bands but that do not meet this criterion, results are considered indeterminate. Specimens that test positive on EIA but that display no immunoreactivity to any of the HTLV WB bands are considered to be negative for antibodies to HTLV-I and HTLV-II, and the result of the EIA is considered to be false positive. To better differentiate between HTLV-I and HTLV-II, the WB assay has been modified to contain type-specific recombinant proteins from the external glycoprotein of HTVL-I (rgp46envI) and HTLV-II (rgp46envII) as well as a truncated recombinant peptide, rp21e, from the transmembrane glycoprotein gp21env. In one study, persons with indeterminate WB assay profiles (i.e., persons who did not demonstrate antibody reactivity to p24, p19, or rp21e) who did not have risk factors for HTLV infection were shown by polymerase chain reaction amplification not to be infected with either HTLV-I or HTLV-II.[50] Such indeterminate WB assay results appear to represent antibodies to other viral and cellular antigens that cross-react with HTLV proteins. Nevertheless, blood donors with indeterminate results are deferred and their blood is excluded for transfusion purposes.

PCR has become the reference method for determining infectious status; for validating serologic assays; for distinguishing between HTLV-I and HTLV-II; for studying in vivo viral load and tissue distribution; and for further evaluating patients with risk factors for HTLV infection whose serologic status is either indeterminate or negative.[47] PCR is also an important method of testing infants for HTLV infection, because their serologic status may be unclear, owing to the presence of passively transferred maternal antibodies. In addition, PCR is important for the detection of infection in the window period between exposure, infection, and seroconversion.[47]

HTLV-I

HTLV-I is the etiologic agent of adult T cell leukemia/lymphoma (ATL) and a chronic progressive inflammatory neurologic degenerative disorder known as tropical spastic paraparesis or, more commonly, HTLV-I–associated myelopathy (HAM). However, this virus has been implicated in several other disorders, including an inflammatory arthropathy, uveitis, polymyositis, infectious dermatitis in children, pulmonary disorders, and Sjögren syndrome. There are provocative but unproven associations of HTLV-I with mycosis fungoides and Sézary syndrome. This discussion focuses on ATL and HAM because of the established etiologic linkage to HTLV-I.

EPIDEMIOLOGY

HTLV-I is endemic in southwestern Japan and Okinawa, where more than one million persons are infected. HTLV-I infection is also prevalent in Taiwan, the Caribbean basin (including areas of South America and the southeastern United States, central Africa, Israel, and the Arctic, where seroprevalence rates range from 5% to 27% in adults.[46] In the United States, HTLV seroprevalence rates range from 0.025% in blood donors to 7% to 49% in injection drug users and prostitutes.[46] The incidence rates of seroconversion associated with HTLV are estimated to be 1.09 per 100,000 persons per year.[51] HTLV-I infection is transmitted from mother to child; perinatally; sexually; through breast milk and blood transfusions; and from contaminated needles.[52] In the United States, where blood donors are screened for HTLV, the risk of transmitting HTLV through a unit of blood is estimated to be 1 in 641,000 (95% confidence interval, 256,000 to 2,000,000).[51]

The distribution of both ATL and HAM overlaps the distribution of HTLV-I, with more than 95% of affected persons having serologic evidence of HTLV-I infection. Although early serologic studies suggested that HTLV-I infections were common in injection drug users, confirmatory serologic assays that reliably distinguish between HTLV-I and HTLV-II have subsequently shown that the majority of HTLV infections in injection drug users are HTLV-II infections.[53] The development of ATL in persons infected by blood products is rare; however, 20% of patients with HAM acquire HTLV-I infection from contaminated blood. In ATL, there is a latent period between infection and the emergence of disease of 20 to 30 years or more; in contrast, HAM has a shorter median latency of approximately 3 years, but the latency period can be as long as 20 to 30 years.

Cross-sectional studies have suggested that coinfection with HTLV-I and HIV-1 results in an acceleration of clinical immunosuppression and shortened survival. However, prospective studies of dual infection are not available, and other factors associated with dual infection could be responsible for the clinical findings. Of interest, dual infection with HTLV-I and HIV-1 may affect the interpretation of the results of immunophenotyping because coinfection alters the relationship between CD4+ T cell count and HIV-1 disease stage. As such, patients infected with HIV-1 who have a higher than expected CD4+ T cell count for a given level of clinical immunosuppression should be tested for HTLV-I infection.[16]

PATHOGENESIS

The pathophysiologic basis of HTLV-I disease is less well known than that of HIV-1. Unlike HIV-1, the cellular receptor for HTLV-I has not been identified. CD4+ T cells are productively infected by HTLV-I, but some other cell types, including B cells and CD8+ T cells, are infected occasionally. Like HIV-1, the reverse-transcribed viral cDNA integrates randomly into the host cell to establish the provirus, but in contrast to HIV-1, HTLV-I establishes a latent infection with infrequent expression of viral gene products. As such, HTLV-I has a very low level of disease penetrance; the transformation of an infected cell is a rare event, and the cumulative lifetime risk of developing ATL is 1% to 5% in persons infected with HTLV-I. The latent period from infection to clinical disease is estimated to be 30 to 50 years[54]; most persons with ATL appear to have acquired the infection in childhood.[55]

In contrast to many of the animal retroviruses, and in particular avian retroviruses, HTLV-I does not contain a transforming oncogene. Moreover, the integrated provirus does not locate at a unique site in the genome that would result in the expression of a cellular gene (proto-oncogene), as does, for example, the classical avian leukosis virus, which causes B cell leukemia in birds by inducing the expression of the proto-oncogene *myc*. The only viral gene product expressed in tumor cells transformed by HTLV-I in vivo is tax, a 40 kd protein with exons on either side of the *env* gene. In contrast, the infection of CD4+ T cells in vitro results in transformed cells that produce complete, infectious HTLV-I virions. Tax protein induces the expression of a wide range of host cell proteins, including transcription factors and cytokines (IL-2, tumor necrosis factor [TNF], and others). However, it is not known how this induction of host cell factors leads to neoplastic transformation, and no consistent chromosomal abnormalities have been reported in ATL. The discordant observations between the in vitro and in vivo milieus are a recurrent theme in understanding the complex biology of human retroviral disease.

The pathogenesis of HAM is virus induced. Interestingly, patients with HAM generally have high proviral levels in the blood and a stronger immune response to HTLV-I, with higher antibody titers in the cerebrospinal fluid than in the serum. It has been proposed that the pathology of CNS disease may result from an autoimmune destruction of neuronal tissue by viral-specific CD8+ T cells. HTLV-I has also been associated with uveitis, arthropathy, and infective dermatitis; each of these conditions probably has an autoimmune/inflammatory pathogenesis.[16]

CLINICAL FEATURES AND DIAGNOSIS

HTLV-I–Induced Adult T Cell Leukemia/Lymphoma

Four clinical presentations of ATL have been described: acute, lymphomatous, chronic, and smoldering.[54] All of these malignancies are characterized by the monoclonal expansion of CD4+ T cells that contain HTLV-I provirus and rearrangements of clonal T cell receptor genes. HTLV-I virions are not recovered directly from the infected T cells, but viral tax protein is expressed in vivo. The molecular pathogenesis of this retroviral-induced neoplasm has not been fully elucidated.

Acute ATL Acute ATL accounts for approximately 60% to 80% of cases of ATL. Patients experience a short clinical prodrome, with an average of 2 weeks between the onset of symptoms and diagnosis. ATL has an aggressive natural history; median survival is 6 months. The clinical picture is characterized by rapidly progressive skin lesions (40% of cases ranging from maculopapular rashes to tumorous lesions), pulmonary infiltrates, diarrhea, hypercalcemia (seen in 50% of cases), elevated lactate dehydrogenase (LDH) and alkaline phosphatase levels, and lymphocytosis with pleomorphic mononuclear cells (termed flower cells) that contain lobulated, cloven-hoof–shaped nuclei. The skin lesions may be difficult to distinguish from those in mycosis fungoides and Sézary syndrome. The pulmonary lesions may be the result of a leukemic infiltrate or an opportunistic infection, such as *Pneumocystis carinii* infection or fungal infections. Diarrhea is almost always associated with an opportunistic infection. Hepatosplenomegaly may be present. Lytic bone lesions are common; the lesions are patchy and are composed of osteolytic cells without osteoblastic activity. Leptomeningeal involvement associated with weakness, altered mental status, paresthesias, and headache is found in approximately 10% of patients. The cerebrospinal fluid protein level is usually normal. The diagnosis is confirmed by a finding of malignant cells in the CSF.

Lymphomatous ATL Lymphomatous ATL accounts for approximately 20% of cases of ATL. Lymphomatous ATL is similar to acute ATL but differs in that lymphadenopathy is present and there is an absence of circulating, morphologically abnormal lymphocytes. The diagnosis may be suspected on the basis of the patient's geographic birthplace and the presence of skin lesions and hypercalcemia. The diagnosis is confirmed by

HTLV-I serologic testing or the detection of the integrated provirus on PCR testing.

Chronic ATL Chronic ATL accounts for approximately 15% of cases of ATL. This form of ATL is characterized by normal serum levels of calcium, elevated levels of LDH, and the absence of bony involvement or involvement of the CNS or gastrointestinal tract. The median survival for these patients is 2 years. Chronic ATL may progress to acute ATL.

Smoldering ATL Smoldering ATL accounts for fewer than 5% of cases of ATL. Although fewer than 5% of the circulating lymphocytes display the morphologic abnormalities characteristic of ATL or an integrated HTLV-I provirus, there is no hypercalcemia, adenopathy, or hepatosplenomegaly. The CNS, bones, and GI tract are not involved, but typical skin lesions and pulmonary infiltrates may be present. The median survival for patients with the smoldering form of ATL is 5 years or longer.

HTLV-1–Associated Myelopathy/Tropical Spastic Paraparesis

HAM is a slowly progressive thoracic myelopathy that leaves one third of patients bedridden within 10 years of diagnosis.[56] HAM affects women disproportionately for reasons that are not understood.

The onset of symptoms in HAM is insidious; symptoms include weakness or stiffness in one or both legs, back pain, and urinary incontinence. Peripheral neuropathy is usually mild. Physical findings include spastic paraparesis or paraplegia with hyperreflexia, ankle clonus, and extensor plantar responses (Babinski reflex). Cognitive function is usually spared, and cranial nerve involvement is distinctly unusual. Demyelinating lesions are seen in the white matter and paraventricular regions of the brain and spinal cord; the clinical presentation may thus resemble multiple sclerosis or the myelopathy of HIV infection. The pathologic changes in HAM include symmetrical degeneration of the lateral columns, corticospinal tracts, and posterior columns. An inflammatory infiltrate is present on the spinal meninges, and spinal cord parenchyma shows evidence of myelin destruction, similar to that in multiple sclerosis. HTLV-I provirus is usually not found in the cells of the CNS parenchyma, but it may be detected in a few CSF-associated lymphocytes. Although a high proviral serum level of HTLV-I is an important risk factor in the development of HAM, the presence of provirus in the blood is not sufficient to cause disease, and the immunopathogenesis of HAM is probably associated with host genetic factors.

PREVENTION AND TREATMENT

The principles of prevention of HIV infection also apply to the prevention of HTLV infection—avoidance of breast-feeding, if possible; screening of blood donors for HTLV antibody; safe sexual practice; and the avoidance of sharing or reusing of needles.

There is no proven, effective therapy for either ATL or HAM.[55,57] Unlike with HIV disease, disease progression of ATL and HAM is not associated with HTLV-I replication; as a result, antiretroviral drugs have not been effective in the treatment of these diseases. The neoplasm is responsive to combination chemotherapy that is used against other forms of lymphoma, but patients usually experience relapse within 1 year of initial remission. The combination of interferon alfa and zidovudine (AZT) is effective therapy and is associated with less toxicity than standard lymphoma regimens; however, the effectiveness of this regimen is most likely the result of the cytotoxic effects of AZT rather than its antiretroviral activity. Anecdotal cases involving the successful use of allogeneic bone marrow transplantation have been reported. Patients with chronic ATL or smoldering ATL should be treated for opportunistic infections and observed for progression to acute ATL, at which time chemotherapy should be initiated. In ATL, hypercalcemia is generally controlled with glucocorticoid therapy and cytotoxic therapy of the neoplasm. In HAM-associated inflammation, glucocorticoids reduce inflammation and may improve uveitis, but antiretroviral therapies are not effective. Danazol, an androgenic steroid, has been reported to benefit women with HAM-associated urinary and fecal incontinence.

HTLV-II

HTLV-II is endemic in certain Native American tribes of North and South America. The modes of transmission are the same as for HTLV-I, although HTLV-II is less readily transmitted sexually than HTLV-I. Because of the similarity in biologic properties between the two viruses and because of the initial inability to distinguish the two viruses serologically, the two viruses were grouped together in early studies. The seroprevalence of HTLV-II in injection drug users in several metropolitan drug treatment programs in the United States was approximately 20%.[58] Approximately 3% of these persons were infected with both HTLV-II and HIV-1. Women are significantly more likely to be infected with HTLV-II than men, a feature of the disease that may reflect the more efficient sexual transmission of HTLV-II from men to women than from women to men.

Although HTLV-II was isolated from a patient with a T cell variant of hairy-cell leukemia,[1] the virus has not been unequivocally associated with a particular disease. Nevertheless, evidence is slowly accumulating that HTLV-I may play a role in certain degenerative neurologic, hematologic, and dermatologic diseases. No effective therapy exists for HTLV-II infection.

HIV

The pathogenesis, epidemiology, clinical features, and treatment of HIV-1 infection are described elsewhere [see 14 HIV and AIDS]. This subsection discusses the principles of laboratory diagnosis and the basis for the laboratory monitoring of HIV-1 infection. It is important that therapy be individualized on the basis of a thorough understanding of the host-virus relationship in the individual patient (see above). In this regard, an understanding of the use of the laboratory for diagnosing and monitoring HIV-1 disease is critical.[59]

LABORATORY DIAGNOSIS

Serologic Diagnosis

The HIV-1 testing algorithm recommended by the United States Public Health Service consists of initial screening with an EIA licensed by the Food and Drug Administration, followed by testing of repeatedly reactive specimens with an FDA-licensed supplemental test (i.e., WB assay or immunofluorescent assay).[60] Although EIAs are highly sensitive and specific, the positive predictive value of EIA is highly dependent on the seroprevalence of HIV-1 antibody in the population from which the individual is being tested. As such, use of both EIA and a supplementary test increases the likelihood of detecting HIV-1 infection. For maximum diagnostic accuracy, the laboratory HIV test results should always be interpreted by the clinician in conjunction with the clinical and epidemiologic history of the person being tested. At this time, FDA-licensed HIV nucleic acid detection kits are not approved for diagnosis or for supplemental testing but only for disease monitoring (see below).

Enzyme immunoassays The current generation of EIAs have shortened the estimated antibody-negative window period of primary infection to approximately 1 month or less.[61] The specificities of the current commercial EIAs are over 99.5%.[62] False positive reactions arise from nonspecific cross-reacting antibodies in the serum of persons with underlying immunologic disease and of those who are gravid, who have received multiple transfusions, or who have recently received an immunization.[63] Several EIAs that may be used to screen for both HIV-1 and HIV-2 antibody are commercially available.

Immunoblot WB assay detects the serum antibodies directed against specific HIV proteins of varying molecular weights after separation of the viral proteins by gel electrophoresis and blotting onto nitrocellulose paper. WB assay detects antibodies to the following specific HIV-1 proteins: core (p17gag, p24gag, and the precursor p55gag); polymerase (p31pol, p51pol, and p66pol); and envelope (gp41env and gp120env/160env). The reported analytic specificity of the WB assay is 97.8%.[60] A WB assay is interpreted as being negative when no antibody-antigen band is present; it is interpreted as being positive when antibodies are present to core proteins (p24gag), envelope proteins (gp41env or gp120env/160env), and, in some cases, polymerase proteins (p31pol). Although several organizations have proposed criteria for interpreting WB assay reactivity, the Centers for Disease Control and Prevention (CDC) endorses interpretative criteria that require the presence of antibodies to two of the three following proteins: p24gag, gp41env, and gp120env/160env.[60]

Regardless of the HIV-1 antibody seroprevalence, a reactive EIA and confirmatory WB assay together have a positive predictive value of greater than 99.99%.[64] In the blood-donor population, approximately 10 of 10,000 persons (0.1%) who are without risk for HIV-1 infection will have repeatedly reactive results on the HIV-1 EIA. Eight of those 10 low-risk persons with repeatedly reactive results on the HIV-1 EIA will have negative results on the HIV-1 WB assay, and two will have indeterminate results. False positive results for HIV-1 antibody (i.e., both EIA and WB assay are reactive for a person who is not infected with HIV-1) are extremely rare (less than one in 100,000 persons screened).[64] Therefore, an indeterminate WB assay result is more common than a false positive WB assay result.[65]

With the increased use of HIV-1 antibody screening in low-risk populations, including health care workers, it is essential that HIV-1 test results be interpreted accurately. Between 4% and 20% of serum samples that are repeatedly reactive on HIV-

1 EIA are interpreted as indeterminate on WB assay.[66] Indeterminate WB assays (IWB assays) in persons infected with HIV-1 may result from early formation of antibody against viral core antigens during primary infection. IWB assays may also occur in conjunction with early detection of HIV-1 antibody by the more sensitive third-generation EIAs. IWB assays rarely occur as a result of the loss of core-specific antibody late in infection because of severe immunosuppression.[67,68] The presence of cross-reacting antibody to HIV-2 has been implicated as a cause of positive results in HIV-1 testing. False positive results on both EIA and WB assay are extremely uncommon, occurring with a frequency of fewer than one in 135,000 tests.[64]

The following recommendations have been proposed for the clinical management of patients with an IWB assay result.[63] Low-risk individuals who have a nonreactive result on repeat testing with EIAs do not need further follow-up. High-risk individuals should be followed serologically for at least 6 months; this is especially important for those with a p24gag band on WB assay. Such a result may reflect the presence of HIV-1 antibody in conjunction with early seroconversion. The early, selective use of supplemental tests for HIV-1 proviral cDNA or plasma RNA may help determine the infection status of high-risk individuals before full seroconversion occurs.[63,66,69] Seroconversion is usually identified within 3 months of primary infection through the use of appropriate supplemental testing.[61] Importantly, negative supplemental test results may help alleviate the anxiety associated with an indeterminate HIV-1 serologic result.[66]

Rapid serologic testing Rapid, reliable, and less expensive alternatives to the use of EIA with a confirmatory WB assay have been sought for use in acute care settings, emergency departments, clinics for sexually transmitted disease, medical field settings, and developing countries. Consideration should be given to the introduction of rapid screening for HIV-1 antibody in certain clinical settings, such as clinics for sexually transmitted disease; such measures would greatly enhance testing programs by preventing delays in the counseling of seronegative patients and by providing preliminary results to seropositive patients.[70] These preliminary results may encourage patients to return for confirmatory testing and to adopt risk-reducing behaviors sooner than they would if following the currently accepted testing algorithms.[71] In addition, the use of rapid screening for HIV-1 after occupational exposure to blood will reduce the duration of antiretroviral prophylaxis therapy for the exposed health care worker, thus minimizing drug-related toxicity and cost and alleviating anxiety sooner should the test result prove negative.[72,73] Rapid serologic testing will likely become the standard of diagnostic care; physicians and other health care professionals should become familiar with the indications for rapid testing.

Detection of HIV-1 subtypes HIV-1 groups and subtypes differ with regard to their diagnostic properties on both serologic and nucleic acid assays. As such, reagents in diagnostic kits have been modified to ensure optimal sensitivity and specificity for antibodies to viruses of groups M and O. Current clinical HIV-1 antibody testing does not distinguish between the various HIV-1 subtypes. However, from an epidemiologic perspective, distinguishing these subtypes by nucleic acid sequencing is very important for understanding the global spread of HIV-1.

As mentioned previously, HIV-1 strains are divided into three groups: M, O, and, most recently, N.[74] To date, in the United States, infection with group O is uncommon, and no group N infections have been reported.[75] Neutral variation in HIV-1 strains of group M has led to a further subdivision of these viruses into nine geographically distributed subtypes, or clades, designated A through K. Subtype B is the most common subtype in the United States and Europe; subtypes A and C are prominent in Africa and Asia. In addition, there are four major circulating recombinant forms: AE is prevalent in Southeast Asia; AG, in west and central Africa; AGI, in Cyprus and Greece; and AB, in Russia. However, the circulating recombinant forms are expanding in number as more full-genome sequences of HIV-1 become available (e.g., FD, from the Democratic Republic of Congo; BC, from China; and several additional complex recombinants that combine three or more subtypes). Although there are differences in the biologic properties of these subtypes (e.g., there is a low frequency of syncytium-inducing phenotype in subtype C), the overall data are too limited to support any strong influence of subtype on either disease progression or transmission.

Because most of the primer pairs for HIV-1 cDNA PCR amplification have been optimized for group B viruses (see below), it is not surprising that HIV-1 cDNA PCR may also fail to detect HIV-1 group O and some subtypes of groups M and N. To accommodate this deficiency, primer pair modifications have been incorporated into the recent Roche Amplicor HIV-1 DNA and Roche Monitor

HIV-1 RNA assays (version 1.5).[76] Because of the large number of *pol*-specific synthetic oligonucleotide target probes used by the branched-chain DNA (bDNA) assay, detection of group O and different group B subtypes has not been a problem for the bDNA assay.[77]

Detection of HIV-2 antibodies HIV-2 infection is less geographically dispersed than HIV-1 infection; the epidemic of HIV-2 is primarily focused in West Africa, and is common in the epidemic in India. In the United States, only a relatively few cases of HIV-2 have been reported. In blood donors in the United States, HIV-2 is extremely rare; only three cases of HIV-2 were detected in screening 74 million blood donations through June 1995.[78] Of the 62 persons reported with HIV-2 infection in the United States, 44 (71%) were born in, had traveled to, or had a sex partner from western Africa. Nevertheless, diagnosis of HIV-2 infection will continue to be an emerging problem in the United States and many other countries, and antibody screening for both viruses is warranted.

HIV-1 and HIV-2 genomes have about 60% homology in conserved genes, such as *gag* and *pol*, and 35% to 45% homology in the *env* gene.[79] The core proteins of HIV-1 and HIV-2 display frequent cross-reactivity, whereas the envelope proteins are more type specific. Despite this cross-reactivity, it has been estimated that the first- and second-generation EIAs used in the United States for screening of blood donors for HIV-1 detect 55% to 91% of HIV-2 infections.[80] The WB assay that is used to detect HIV-1 antibodies may yield positive, negative, or indeterminate results when used to assess sera known to be positive for HIV-2 (when the WB assay is used to confirm a positive result on EIA for HIV-2, p26gag and gp36env correspond to their HIV-1 counterparts p24gag and gp41env, respectively).

Laboratory Detection of HIV-1

The methods of direct detection of HIV-1 include the use of culture, antigen detection, and detection of nucleic acid. Each method has a specific role to play: use of culture is important in research; use of antigen detection is important to public health; and detection of nucleic acid is important for individual patient care. Near the beginning of the HIV-1 pandemic, viral culture and antigen detection were used to evaluate the effectiveness of antiretroviral therapy. However, both methods were replaced by more sensitive and precise methods involving the quantification of viral RNA in plasma through nucleic acid amplification or signal amplification. Nevertheless, both culture and antigen detection continue to have useful roles.

Viral culture Use of mixed-lymphocyte coculture for the detection of HIV-1 is a specialized procedure that has extremely high specificity but lower sensitivity in patients with high $CD4^+$ T cell counts, as compared to methods used to detect viral nucleic acid (see below).[81,82] Use of HIV-1 culture is restricted primarily to research laboratories because of its lower sensitivity than currently available nucleic acid detection methods, cost, time constraints, and highly specialized, technical nature. However, interest is being shown in the use of HIV-1 coculture for assessing viral containment after potent antiretroviral therapy[83]; HIV-1 coculture may also be useful for obtaining primary clinical HIV-1 isolates to study viral syncytium-inducing phenotype and drug-susceptibility phenotype[84] and for assessing viral fitness.[85]

Measurement of HIV-1 p24 antigen With the advent of nucleic acid amplification methods for the monitoring of HIV-1, the measurement of HIV-1 p24 antigen has a much more limited role than it once did. Currently, the primary use of p24 antigen detection is to identify patients who are in the antibody-negative window period of acute HIV-1 infection. Although antigen detection is a less expensive alternative to viral RNA detection in this setting, both the determination of viral RNA levels and the culturing of peripheral blood mononuclear cells are significantly more sensitive than detection of p24 antigenemia,[86] even with the added sensitivity of p24 antigen acid dissociation.[87] However, a tyramide signal-amplification-boosted EIA for quantification of p24 antigen has been reported to have equivalent sensitivity to viral RNA reverse transcriptase polymerase chain reaction (RT-PCR) amplification at 200 to 400 copies/ml.[87,88] Currently, the greatest use of p24 antigen testing is for screening the United States blood supply. This screening program was introduced in 1996 and has been augmented by a plasma HIV-1 RNA screening assay[89,90] to further lower the residual risk of HIV-1 infection, which is estimated to be less than one in 500,000 units (95% confidence interval, 200,000 to 2,800,000).[51]

Detection of viral nucleic acid Commercially available methods for the detection of viral nucleic acid (proviral cDNA or viral RNA) are specific and sensitive and are an effective method for identifying those persons who are infected but who have not undergone seroconversion.[86,91] These methods are also useful in identifying infected infants[92] and in resolving indeterminate HIV-1 antibody serology.[66] In addition, the quantification of plasma viral RNA has assumed a critically important clinical role in assessing disease prognosis and response to antiretroviral therapy.[93–97]

Qualitative HIV-1 DNA PCR amplification is the most commonly used assay for the diagnosis of HIV-1 infection in neonates and infants.[98,99] The Roche Amplicor HIV-1 test (Roche Diagnostic Systems, Inc.) is the only FDA-licensed commercial kit available for clinical use.

The major advantages of HIV-1 DNA PCR over culture are its increased sensitivity and more rapid reporting time (the reporting time is 1 day, as compared to 2 to 4 weeks). There is always a risk of false positive reactivity caused by contamination of the specimen with amplicons (so-called carry-over product contamination) or by specimen handling errors[69,99,100–102]; carryover contamination is decreased somewhat by the use of the uracyl *N*–glycosylase enzyme in the commercial assay. False negative results can also occur because of inhibition of the PCR reaction by either hemoglobin or heparin or because there are fewer target cells in the assay than expected. To control for the latter and improve the precision of the assay, testing for HIV-1 DNA should include concurrent amplification of a cell-associated host gene, such as *HLA-DQ* or the β-globin gene. Diagnostic laboratories should participate in a quality-assurance program to ensure that problems with sensitivity and specificity are quickly identified.[103]

RT-PCR amplification is generally more sensitive than p24 antigen EIA in detecting plasma HIV-1 RNA.[86–88,91] As such, there is much interest in using plasma HIV-1 RNA in diagnostic testing.[69,100,104] As mentioned (see above), HIV-1 RNA has augmented HIV-1 p24 antigen screening; it will likely replace HIV-1 p24 antigen screening of donor blood in the United States after its use has been validated. However, the HIV-1 RNA assays that are commercially available are not currently licensed for use in screening. To avoid incorrectly diagnosing a patient as having HIV-1, the HIV-1 RNA assay should be used diagnostically only as a supplemental test for detecting antibody-negative acute infection. In this particular diagnostic setting, a positive result on HIV-1 RNA assay (particularly one that indicates a viral RNA level of fewer than 1,000 copies/ml) should be confirmed by either another nucleic acid technology (preferably, HIV-1 DNA PCR) or HIV-1 p24 antigen EIA or HIV-1 culture, if available.[100,102,105,106] Alternatively, one can again test for the development of HIV-1–specific antibody, which should be present shortly after viral RNA reaches detectable levels.[107] The presence of HIV-1 RNA in the absence of other laboratory findings requires a correlation with the medical and epidemiologic history and a confirmatory repeat blood test for HIV-1.[100–102,106]

HIV-1 RNA Quantitative Assays

The diversity of viral subtypes of HIV-1 necessitates the use of molecular assays capable of measuring viral RNA concentrations independently of viral sequence or subtype.[10-] First-generation viral RNA quantification assays were designed for optimal performance with subtype B, which predominates in Europe and North America. However, the entry of nonsubtype B virus into these areas and the discovery of intersubtype recombinant viruses complicate nucleic acid-based testing.[109] Currently, there are four commercial assays available for quantifying HIV-1 subtype B RNA in ethylenediaminetetraacetic acid (EDTA)–anticoagulated plasma. The current versions of these assays are capable of quantifying a broader range of HIV-1 subtypes than earlier tests.[108] Because these assays are not equivalent, patients should be followed clinically with repeated viral RNA testing using the same manufacturer's assay. Some of the benefits and limitations of viral RNA testing can be better appreciated if the clinician is somewhat familiar with the viral RNA assays that are currently available for clinical use.

The nucleic acid sequence–based amplification (NASBA) (NucliSens QT HIV-1 RNA assay, Organon Teknika, Advanced BioScience Laboratories) assay involves first obtaining nucleic acid through isolation by lysis and binding of the viral RNA to silica dioxide microparticles. The next step involves isothermal amplification (so-called target amplification) through use of the reverse transcriptase RNase H and T7 RNA polymerase. Three internal calibrators are added to the specimen; these are adsorbed along with the specimen before lysis. Amplification covers approximately 1,500 base-pairs in the *gag* and *pol* genes. Detection is by means of chemiluminescence. The sensitivity of the assay is approximately 100 RNA copies/ml; the quantitation limit is 500 copies/ml; and the linear dynamic range is up to 10,000,000 RNA copies/ml.

The bDNA assay (Versant HIV-1 RNA 3.0 assay, Bayer Corp.) is a nonisotopic sandwich nucleic acid hybridization assay that uses a series of target probes of the *pol* gene to hybridize the viral RNA target onto a series of capture probes on the surface of the microwell plate. The bDNA amplifier molecules are hybridized onto the captured viral RNA target. Multiple alkaline phosphatase label probes are attached to the bDNA amplifier molecules to amplify the signal after adding a specific substrate (so-called signal amplification); detection is by chemiluminescence. An external standard curve is used to calculate the HIV-1 RNA copy number. The detection and quantitation levels are approximately 50 to 100 RNA copies/ml, with a linear dynamic range up to 750,000 RNA copies/ml.[110]

The RT-PCR amplification assay (Roche Amplicor HIV-1 Monitor Test, Roche Diagnostic Systems) is the only FDA-licensed assay for assessing HIV-1 disease prognosis. The assay uses the recombinant *Thermus thermophilus* (rTth) enzyme, which serves to catalyze both reverse transcription and DNA amplification of a 142 base *gag* gene sequence in a single reaction tube. An internal quantitative standard is used to adjust for recovery and to calculate the final HIV-1 RNA copy number. The assay has an analytic sensitivity of 200 RNA copies/ml and a quantitation limit of 400 RNA copies/ml, with a dynamic range up to 750,000 RNA copies/ml. A centrifugation step (Amplicor HIV-1 Monitor Ultrasensitive specimen preparation protocol, Roche Molecular Systems) can be used to concentrate virus and thus increase the sensitivity of the assay to 50 copies/ml, and the quantitation limit is 200 copies/ml.[111]

Detection of Antiretroviral Susceptibility Genotype and Phenotype

Incomplete inhibition of HIV-1 replication in vivo may arise because of patient noncompliance with therapy, inadequate potency of the chosen regimen, poor drug absorption, drug-drug interactions, inadequate activation of the antiretroviral drug, or infection with drug-resistant virus variants[112] [see 14 HIV and AIDS]. This incomplete inhibition may result in the emergence of drug-resistant HIV-1 variants and thus is an important cause of therapy failure.[113] An assessment of drug resistance may be helpful in selecting subsequent antiretroviral therapy, but this has not been rigorously proved. Nevertheless, assays for drug resistance testing in HIV-1 infection are now available, and clinical studies suggest that viral drug resistance correlates with poor virologic response to new therapy.[114] It is recommended that interpretation be made by specialists who are expert in this area, given the complexity of results and assay limitations.[115]

Antiretroviral drug susceptibility is determined either phenotypically by assessing for the susceptibility of the virus (or viral recombinant) ex vivo or genotypically by assessing for mutations that confers resistance. There are two phenotypic approaches: the first approach tests the sensitivity of the proviral population present in the peripheral blood mononuclear cells of the patient; the second approach generates recombinant fragments of the virus that contain *pol* genes obtained from the viral RNA or from the proviral DNA.[116,117] There are several genotypic approaches: DNA sequencing of the entire viral population or clones; selective PCR assay; determination of point mutations; differential probe hybridization; EIA modification of the oligoligase detection reaction assay; and a commercially available HIV-1 reverse transcription line probe assay.[118] Genotypic changes may not always correlate with changes in drug susceptibility of the clinical isolate.[119] Before these techniques can be applied effectively in the clinic, much still needs to be learned about the correlation between genotype and phenotype and the effect of these phenotypic and genotypic approaches on clinical outcome in patients who receive antiretroviral therapy.[120] Nevertheless, despite the recommendation by some experts for the wider use of susceptibility testing in clinical practice,[115,121,122] most decisions to start or change therapy are based on the viral RNA level, $CD4^+$ T cell count, and previous antiretroviral drug history. In addition, the patient should be carefully educated about the importance of compliance with and adherence to the prescribed therapy regimen.[112,123]

Assessment of disease progression is discussed elsewhere [see 14 HIV and AIDS].

Monitoring of Infection

In general, nadir responses in plasma viral RNA occur in most patients 4 to 12 weeks after initiation of potent antiretroviral therapy. With some potent antiretroviral regimens, plasma viral RNA levels will decrease to less than 500 RNA copies/ml by 16 weeks in 60% to 80% of patients and to less than 50 viral RNA copies/ml by 24 weeks in approximately 70%. Previous antiretroviral therapy is a factor affecting the decrease in viral RNA levels.[94,124] For patients who show a stable response, continued monitoring at intervals of 3 to 4 months seems warranted; more frequent monitoring is warranted if the plasma viral RNA level approaches a value that would cause a change in therapy. It is advisable to plot the plasma viral RNA values on a $\log_{10}$ scale; plasma viral RNA levels should be reassessed only when values exceed the upper 95% confidence interval for the expected variation in plasma viral RNA level (that is, 0.5 $\log_{10}$ RNA copies/ml above the mean nadir response value) and only if such a change in viral RNA levels would necessitate a change in therapy.[125]

By current consensus guidelines, the goal of therapy is to reduce the plasma viral RNA level to an undetectable amount, which is now fewer than 50 RNA copies/ml.[10] Other targets of therapy are a durable reduction in the plasma viral RNA level by at least threefold (0.5 $\log_{10}$) or more from pretherapy levels[125,126] and a reduction in plasma viral RNA level to below 1,000 copies/ml.[9] Although there are only limited data from controlled clinical trials that carefully delineate the decrease in risk of disease progression associated with decreases in the plasma viral RNA levels to less than 1,000 copies/ml,[9] a preliminary analysis of 1,083 patients from the AIDS Clinical Trials Group 320 Study Team showed that only seven of 126 clinical events (5.6%) were associated with a preceding plasma HIV-1 level lower than 500 copies/ml; for the remaining 119 clinical events, the plasma viral RNA level was higher than 500 copies/ml.[94] Nevertheless, many investigators believe that the target for therapy should be at least one $\log_{10}$ value lower than this (i.e., < 50 RNA copies/ml).[10] Occasional blips in detectable levels of viral RNA do not appear to adversely affect outcome. The "as low as you can go" concept in HIV treatment is an appealing virologic concept that has been repeated so often as to have been accepted as the standard. Whether this concept pertains to a chronic viral infection such as HIV-1 requires careful validation by controlled clinical trials. This is particularly important with regard to the treatment of asymptomatic patients with HIV-1 who have a CD4+ T cell count greater than 500 cells/μl; in such patients, the possibility of long-term toxicity associated with the use of potent drug combinations that contain protease inhibitors needs to be weighed against the relatively small clinical benefit derived from reducing plasma viral RNA levels to the lowest level possible.

In addition to reducing plasma viral RNA levels, therapy should also lead to a stabilization of the CD4+ T cell count at or above the expected level of biologic variation; the absolute number of CD4+ T cells should be increased by more than 30%, or the proportion of lymphocytes that are CD4+ T cells should increase by more than 3%. Interpretation of any given reduction in the level of plasma HIV-1 RNA depends on the treatment response of the CD4+ T cell count. To determine clinical response to therapy, changes in both the viral RNA level and the CD4+ T cell count must be considered because of the interaction between them.[127] In an analysis of several clinical studies primarily of nucleoside therapy, patients who did not experience a reduction in the plasma HIV-1 RNA level but who did experience a reduction in the CD4+ T cell count had a 30% greater risk of clinical progression over 2 years than patients who had an increase in CD4+ T cells above pretherapy levels.[9]

An important goal of antiretroviral therapy is to provide an improved sense of patient well-being and to minimize adverse effects. Therefore, in establishing as a target the lowest plasma viral RNA level, consideration must be given to previous antiretroviral drug exposure; in addition, therapy compliance, tolerability of the regimen, and long-term toxicity of the therapy regimen must be weighed.

Use of plasma viral RNA to define therapeutic failure A precise definition of therapeutic failure cannot be based on viral RNA level alone. Such a definition should embrace as a minimum the clinical status of the patient, the tolerability of the antiretroviral regimen, the CD4+ T cell count, and the plasma viral RNA level. The failure of the plasma viral RNA level to decrease by at least 30-fold (1.5 $\log_{10}$) or more from baseline after 4 to 8 weeks of therapy is generally considered a suboptimal virologic response.[9] In addition, many clinicians consider the inability to lower plasma viral RNA to undetectable levels (< 50 RNA copies/ml) after 12 to 24 weeks of therapy to be evidence of therapeutic failure.[10] Lowering viral RNA to undetectable levels is considered a benchmark of success because of the possibility of the development of drug resistance, which can arise when viral replication occurs in the presence of selective pressure by antiretroviral drug regimens.[128] However, many patients fail to achieve undetectable viral RNA levels or experience a rebound in viral RNA after starting antiretroviral therapy.[94,124] Although the pretherapy plasma viral RNA level is itself an independent risk factor for disease progression, the relative benefit of a decline in plasma viral RNA is the same regardless of the level of viral RNA before therapy. For example, a 1 $\log_{10}$ decline in the viral RNA level from 10^5 to 10^4 RNA copies/ml represents the same relative 72% reduction in risk as a change from 10^4 to 10^3 RNA copies/ml.[9] However, these two pretherapy plasma HIV RNA levels confer different relative hazards of disease progression, after controlling for baseline CD4+ T cell count and therapy assignment.[9]

Viral resistance It has been somewhat arbitrarily established that any sustainable 0.5 $\log_{10}$

(threefold) increase in plasma viral RNA level above the therapy-induced plasma viral RNA nadir that is not attributable to intercurrent infection, vaccination, incomplete adherence to the antiretroviral therapy regimen, decreased absorption of antiretroviral drugs, altered drug metabolism, drug-drug interactions, or testing methodology likely represents viral failure caused by the emergence of drug-resistant HIV variants.[10,115] Although genotypic and phenotypic changes associated with drug resistance in vitro are not always synonymous with clinical drug failure in practice, retrospective and prospective clinical data on the predictive value of these tests have supported their adjunctive use in the selection of the antiretroviral regimen to employ next after virologic failure.[114,115] The correct interpretation of viral susceptibility is complicated by the complexity of the mutational patterns, the potential for undetected subpopulations of mutant virus, and residual effects of previous antiretroviral therapy. Thus, the practicing clinician should be cautious about using viral genotypic or phenotypic susceptibility analysis until definitive, prospective clinical trial data are available. Until such data are available, the clinical decision as to when to initiate or change therapy for a patient with HIV should be individualized and should depend primarily on the viral RNA level and CD4+ T cell count, not antiretroviral resistance test results alone.[112]

Discordant viral RNA and CD4+ T cell responses The plasma viral RNA level may increase while the CD4+ T cell count remains stable or continues to rise in response to therapy.[129] This discordance occurs in approximately 14% or more of patients who receive antiretroviral therapy.[9] For many patients, the discordant response is associated with a decrease in disease progression; this raises into question the wisdom of changing antiretroviral therapy solely on the basis of plasma viral RNA response.[130] In the absence of clinical trial data, if the plasma viral RNA level increases in a sustained manner during therapy to either less than 0.5 $\log_{10}$ above the plasma viral RNA therapy nadir or 5,000 (3.7 $\log_{10}$) copies/ml, whichever is less, then it might be prudent to observe carefully for a further deterioration in CD4+ T cell count or clinical progression before considering a change of therapy. A sustained increase in the plasma viral RNA level that exceeds these criteria warrants a reassessment of the antiretroviral regimen for adherence and possible therapy failure because of antiretroviral drug resistance. A more aggressive approach would be to consider a switch in therapy warranted if plasma viral RNA remains at detectable levels.[10] Neither approach, however, has received adequate validation in a controlled clinical trial.

Acknowledgment

Figures 1 through 3 Seward Hung.

References

1. Kalyanaraman VS, Sarngadharan MG, Robert-Guroff M, et al: A new subtype of human T-cell leukemia virus (HTLV-II) associated with a T-cell variant of hairy cell leukemia. Science 218:571, 1982

2. Poiesz BJ, Ruscetti FW, Reitz MS, et al: Isolation of a new type C retrovirus (HTLV) in primary uncultured cells of a patient with Sézary T-cell leukaemia. Nature 294:268, 1981

3. Linial M, Weiss RA: Other human and primate retroviruses. Fields Virology Vol. 2: Knipe DM, Howley MD, Eds. Lippincott Williams & Wilkins, Philadelphia, 2001, p 2123

4. Goff SP: Retroviridae: the retroviruses and their replication. Fields Virology Vol. 2: Knipe DM, Howley MD, Eds. Lippincott Williams & Wilkins, Philadelphia, 2001, p 1871

5. Weiss RA, Griffiths D, Takeuchi Y, et al: Retroviruses: ancient and modern. Arch Virol 15(suppl):171, 1999

6. Arthur LO, Bess JW Jr, Sowder RC 2nd, et al: Cellular proteins bound to immunodeficiency viruses: implications for pathogenesis and vaccines. Science 258:1935, 1992

7. Luciw PA: Human immunodeficiency viruses and their replication. Fields Virology Vol. 2: Fields BN, Knipe DM, Howley PM, Eds. Lippincott–Raven, Philadelphia, 1996, p 1881

8. Sherry B, Zybarth G, Alfano M, et al: Role of cyclophilin A in the uptake of HIV-1 by macrophages and T lymphocytes. Proc Natl Acad Sci USA 95:1758, 1998

9. Marschner IC, Collier AC, Coombs RW, et al: Use of changes in plasma levels of human immunodeficiency virus type 1 RNA to assess the clinical benefit of antiretroviral therapy. J Infect Dis 177:40, 1998

10. Carpenter CC, Cooper DA, Fischl MA, et al: Antiretroviral therapy in adults: updated recommendations of the International AIDS Society–USA Panel. JAMA 283:381, 2000

11. Wyatt R, Kwong PD, Desjardins E, et al: The antigenic structure of the HIV gp120 envelope glycoprotein. Nature 393:705, 1998

12. Chan DC, Kim PS: HIV entry and its inhibition. Cell 93:681, 1998

13. Streicher HZ, Reitz MSJ, Gallo RC: Human immunodeficiency viruses. Mandell, Douglas, and Bennett's Principles and Practice of Infectious Diseases 5th ed, Vol. 2: Mandel GL, Bennett JE, Donlin R, Eds. Churchill Livingstone, New York, 2000, p 1874

14. Emerman M, Malim MH: HIV-1 regulatory/accessory genes: keys to unraveling viral and host cell biology. Science 280:1880, 1998

15. Feng Y, Broder CC, Kennedy PE, et al: HIV-1 entry cofactor: functional cDNA cloning of a seven-transmembrane, G protein-coupled receptor. Science 272:872, 1996

16. Cleghorn FR, Blattner WA: Human T-cell lymphotropic virus and HTLV infection. Sexually Transmitted Diseases. Holmes KK, Sparling PF, Mårdh PA, et al, Eds. McGraw-Hill, New York, 1999, p 259

17. Quinn TC, Wawer MJ, Sewankambo N, et al: Viral load and heterosexual transmission of human immunodeficiency virus type 1. Rakai Project Study Group. N Engl J Med 342:921, 2000

18. Coombs RW, Speck CE, Hughes JP, et al: Association between culturable human immunodeficiency virus type 1 (HIV-1) in semen and HIV-1 RNA levels in semen and blood: evidence for compartmentalization of HIV-1 between semen and blood. J Infect Dis 177:320, 1998

19. Shepard RN, Schock J, Robertson K, et al: Quantitation of human immunodeficiency virus type 1 RNA in different biological compartments. J Clin Microbiol 38:1414, 2000

20. Pillay K, Coutsoudis A, York D, et al: Cell-free virus in breast milk of HIV-1-seropositive women. J Acquir Immune Defic Syndr 24:330, 2000

21. Berger EA, Murphy PM, Farber JM: Chemokine receptors as HIV-1 coreceptors: roles in viral entry, tropism, and disease. Annu Rev Immunol 17:657, 1999

22. Premack BA, Schall TJ: Chemokine receptors: gateways to inflammation and infection. Nat Med 2:1174, 1996

23. Bleul CC, Farzan M, Choe H, et al: The lymphocyte chemoattrac-

tant SDF-1 is a ligand for LESTR/fusin and blocks HIV-1 entry. Nature 382:829, 1996

24. Donzella GA, Schols D, Lin SW, et al: AMD3100, a small molecule inhibitor of HIV-1 entry via the CXCR4 co-receptor. Nat Med 4:72, 1998

25. Herbein G, Mahlknecht U, Batliwalla F, et al: Apoptosis of CD8+ T cells is mediated by macrophages through interaction of HIV gp120 with chemokine receptor CXCR4. Nature 395:189, 1998

26. Pleskoff O, Treboute C, Brelot A, et al: Identification of a chemokine receptor encoded by human cytomegalovirus as a cofactor for HIV-1 entry. Science 276:1874, 1997

27. Connor RI, Sheridan KE, Ceradini D, et al: Change in coreceptor use correlates with disease progression in HIV-1-infected individuals. J Exp Med 185:621, 1997

28. Huang Y, Paxton WA, Wolinsky SM, et al: The role of a mutant CCR5 allele in HIV-1 transmission and disease progression. Nat Med 2: 1240, 1996

29. Michael NL, Louie LG, Rohrbaugh AL, et al: The role of CCR5 and CCR2 polymorphisms in HIV-1 transmission and disease progression. Nat Med 3:1160, 1997

30. Michael NL, Chang G, Louie LG, et al: The role of viral phenotype and CCR-5 gene defects in HIV-1 transmission and disease progression. Nat Med 3:338, 1997

31. Geijtenbeek TB, Kwon DS, Torensma R, et al: DC-SIGN, a dendritic cell-specific HIV-1-binding protein that enhances trans-infection of T cells. Cell 100:587, 2000

32. Geijtenbeek TB, Torensma R, van Vliet SJ, et al: Identification of DC-SIGN, a novel dendritic cell–specific ICAM-3 receptor that supports primary immune responses. Cell 100:575, 2000

33. Albright AV, Strizki J, Harouse JM, et al: HIV-1 infection of cultured human adult oligodendrocytes. Virology 217:211, 1996

34. Delezay O, Koch N, Yahi N, et al: Co-expression of CXCR4/fusin and galactosylceramide in the human intestinal epithelial cell line HT-29. AIDS 11:1311, 1997

35. Ahmed R, Morrison LA, Knipe DM: Persistence of viruses. Fields Virology Vol. 2: Fields BN, Knipe DM, Howley PM, Eds. Lippincott–Raven, Philadelphia, 1996, p 219

36. Koenig S, Fauci AS: Immunology of human immunodeficiency virus. Sexually Transmitted Diseases. Holmes KK, Sparling PF, Mårdh PA, et al, Eds. McGraw-Hill, New York, 1999, p 231

37. Ho DD, Neumann AU, Perelson AS, et al: Rapid turnover of plasma virions and CD4 lymphocytes in HIV-1 infection. Nature 373: 123, 1995

38. Wei X, Ghosh SK, Taylor ME, et al: Viral dynamics in human immunodeficiency virus type 1 infection. Nature 373:117, 1995

39. Mortara L, Letourneur F, Gras-Masse H, et al: Selection of virus variants and emergence of virus escape mutants after immunization with an epitope vaccine. J Virol 72:1403, 1998

40. Liu HF, Goubau P, Van Brussel M, et al: The three human T-lymphotropic virus type I subtypes arose from three geographically distinct simian reservoirs. J Gen Virol 77:359, 1996

41. Gao F, Bailes E, Robertson DL, et al: Origin of HIV-1 in the chimpanzee *Pan troglodytes troglodytes.* Nature 397:436, 1999

42. Korber B, Muldoon M, Theiler J, et al: Timing the ancestor of the HIV-1 pandemic strains. Science 288:1789, 2000

43. Zehender G, De Maddalena C, Osio M, et al: High prevalence of human T cell lymphotropic virus type II infection in patients affected by human immunodeficiency virus type 1-associated predominantly sensory polyneuropathy. J Infect Dis 172:1595, 1995

44. Hall WW, Ishak R, Zhu SW, et al: Human T lymphotropic virus type II (HTLV-II): epidemiology, molecular properties, and clinical features of infection. J Acquir Immune Defic Syndr Hum Retrovirol 13:S204,1996

45. Franchini G: Molecular mechanisms of human T-cell leukemia/ lymphotropic virus type I infection. Blood 86:3619, 1995

46. Kaplan JE, Khabbaz RF: The epidemiology of human T-lymphotropic virus type I and II. Rev Med Virol 3:137, 1993

47. Dezzutti CS, Lal RB: Human T-cell lymphotropic virus types I and II. Manual of Clinical Microbiology. Murray PR, Baron KJ, Pfaller MA, et al, Eds. American Society for Microbiology, Washington, DC, 1999, p 871

48. Vidal AU, Gessain A, Yoshida M, et al: Phylogenetic classification of human T cell leukaemia/lymphoma virus type I genotypes in five major molecular and geographical subtypes. J Gen Virol 75:3655, 1994

49. Eiraku N, Novoa P, da Costa Ferreira M, et al: Identification and characterization of a new and distinct molecular subtype of human T-cell lymphotropic virus type 2. J Virol 70:1481, 1996

50. Lal RB, Rudolph DL, Coligan JE, et al: Failure to detect evidence of human T-lymphotropic virus (HTLV) type I and type II in blood donors with isolated gag antibodies to HTLV-I/II. Blood 80:544, 1992

51. Schreiber GB, Busch MP, Kleinman SH, et al: The risk of transfusion-transmitted viral infections. The Retrovirus Epidemiology Donor Study. N Engl J Med 334:1685, 1996

52. Green PL, Chen SY: Human T-cell leukemia virus types 1 and 2. Fields Virology Vol. 2: Knipe DM, Howley PM, Eds. Lippincott Williams & Wilkins, Philadelphia, 2001, p 1941

53. Schreiber GB, Murphy EL, Horton JA, et al: Risk factors for human T-cell lymphotropic virus types I and II (HTLV-I and -II) in blood donors. NHLBI Retrovirus Epidemiology Donor Study. J Acquir Immune Defic Syndr Hum Retrovirol 14:263, 1997

54. Shimoyama M: Diagnostic criteria and classification of clinical subtypes of adult T-cell leukaemia-lymphoma: a report from the Lymphoma Study Group (1984–87). Br J Haematol 79:428, 1991

55. Ifthikharuddin JJ, Rosenblatt JD: Human T-cell lymphotropic virus types I and II. Mandell, Douglas, and Bennett's Principles and Practice of Infectious Diseases 5th ed, Vol 2. Mandel GL, Bennett JE, Donlin R, Eds. Churchill Livingstone, New York, 2000, p 1862

56. Roman GC, Roman LN: Tropical spastic paraparesis: a clinical study of 50 patients from Tumaco (Colombia) and review of the worldwide features of the syndrome. J Neurol Sci 87:121, 1988

57. Blattner WA: Human lymphotropic viruses: HTLV-I and HTLV-II. Clinical Virology. Richman DD, Whitley RJ, Hayden FG, Eds. Churchill Livingstone, New York, 1997, p 683

58. Robert-Guroff M, Weiss SH, Giron JA, et al: Prevalence of antibodies to HTLV-I, -II, and -III in intravenous drug abusers from an AIDS endemic region. JAMA 255:3133, 1986

59. Coombs RW: Clinical laboratory diagnosis of HIV-1 and use of viral RNA to monitor infection. Holmes KK, Sparling PF, Mårdh PA, et al, Eds. McGraw-Hill, New York, 1999, p 973

60. Interpretive criteria used to report western blot results for HIV-1-antibody testing—United States. MMWR Morb Mortal Wkly Rep 40: 692, 1991

61. Zaaijer HL, van Exel-Oehlers P, Kraaijeveld T, et al: Early detection of antibodies to HIV-1 by third-generation assays. Lancet 340:770, 1992

62. Ascher DP, Roberts C: Determination of the etiology of seroreversals in HIV testing by antibody fingerprinting. J Acquir Immune Defic Syndr 6:241, 1993

63. Celum CL, Coombs RW, Jones M, et al: Risk factors for repeatedly reactive HIV-1 EIA and indeterminate western blots: a population-based case-control study. Arch Intern Med 154:1129, 1994

64. Burke DS, Brundage JF, Redfield RR, et al: Measurement of the false positive rate in a screening program for human immunodeficiency virus infections. N Engl J Med 319:961, 1988

65. Celum CL, Coombs RW: Indeterminate HIV-1 western blots: implications and considerations for wide-spread HIV testing. J Gen Intern Med 7:640, 1992

66. Celum CL, Coombs RW, Lafferty W, et al: Indeterminate human immunodeficiency virus type 1 western blots: seroconversion risk, specificity of supplemental tests, and an algorithm for evaluation. J Infect Dis 164:656, 1991

67. Montagnier L, Brenner C, Chamaret S, et al: Human immunodeficiency virus infection and AIDS in a person with negative serology. J Infect Dis 175:955, 1997

68. Zaaijer HL, Bloemer MH, Lelie PN: Temporary seronegativity in a human immunodeficiency virus type 1-infected man. J Med Virol 51:80, 1997

69. Brown AE, Jackson B, Fuller SA, et al: Viral RNA in the resolution of human immunodeficiency virus type 1 diagnostic serology. Transfusion 37:926, 1997

70. Kassler WJ, Dillon BA, Haley C, et al: On-site, rapid HIV testing with same-day results and counseling. AIDS 11:1045, 1997

71. Irwin K, Olivo N, Schable CA, et al: Performance characteristics of a rapid HIV antibody assay in a hospital with a high prevalence of HIV infection. CDC-Bronx-Lebanon HIV Serosurvey Team. Ann Intern Med 125:471, 1996

72. Beltrami EM, Williams IT, Shapiro CN, et al: Risk and management of blood-borne infections in health care workers. Clin Microbiol Rev 13:385, 2000

73. Public Health Service guidelines for the management of health-care worker exposures to HIV and recommendations for postexposure prophylaxis. MMWR Morb Mortal Wkly Rep 47:1, 1998

74. Simon F, Mauclere P, Roques P, et al: Identification of a new human immunodeficiency virus type 1 distinct from group M and group O. Nat Med 4:1032, 1998

75. Sullivan PS, Do AN, Ellenberger D, et al: Human immunodeficiency virus (HIV) subtype surveillance of African-born persons at risk for group O and group N HIV infections in the United States. J Infect Dis 181:463, 2000

76. Michael NL, Herman SA, Kwok S, et al: Development of calibrated viral load standards for group M subtypes of human immunodeficiency virus type 1 and performance of an improved AMPLICOR HIV-1 MONITOR test with isolates of diverse subtypes. J Clin Microbiol 37:2557, 1999

77. Coste J, Montes B, Reynes J, et al: Comparative evaluation of three assays for the quantitation of human immunodeficiency virus type 1 RNA in plasma. J Med Virol 50:293, 1996

78. Onorato IM, O'Brien TR, Schable CA, et al: Sentinel surveillance for HIV-2 infection in high-risk US populations. Am J Public Health 83: 515, 1993

79. Guyader M, Emerman M, Sonigo P, et al: Genome organization and transactivation of the human immunodeficiency virus type 2. Nature 326:662, 1987

80. Busch MP, Petersen L, Schable C, et al: Monitoring blood donors for HIV-2 infection by testing anti-HIV-1 reactive sera. Transfusion 30: 184,1990

81. Coombs RW, Collier AC, Allain JP, et al: Plasma viremia in human immunodeficiency virus infection. N Engl J Med 321:1626, 1989

82. Ho DD, Moudgil T, Alam M: Quantitation of human immunodeficiency virus type 1 in the blood of infected persons. N Engl J Med 321: 1621, 1989

83. Finzi D, Hermankova M, Pierson T, et al: Identification of a reservoir for HIV-1 in patients on highly active antiretroviral therapy. Science 278:1295, 1997

84. D'Aquila RT, Johnson VA, Welles SL, et al: Zidovudine resistance and HIV-1 disease progression during antiretroviral therapy. AIDS Clinical Trials Group Protocol 116B/117 Team and the Virology Committee Resistance Working Group. Ann Intern Med 122:401, 1995

85. Picchio GR, Valdez H, Sabbe R, et al: Altered viral fitness of HIV-1 following failure of protease inhibitor-based therapy. J Acquir Immune Defic Syndr 25:289, 2000

86. Schacker T, Collier AC, Hughes J, et al: Clinical and epidemiologic features of primary HIV infection. Ann Intern Med 125:257, 1996

87. Schupbach J, Tomasik Z, Nadal D, et al: Use of HIV-1 p24 as a sensitive, precise and inexpensive marker for infection, disease progression and treatment failure. Int J Antimicrob Agents 16:441, 2000

88. Ledergerber B, Flepp M, Boni J, et al: Human immunodeficiency virus type 1 p24 concentration measured by boosted ELISA of heat-denatured plasma correlates with decline in CD4 cells, progression to AIDS, and survival: comparison with viral RNA measurement. J Infect Dis 181:1280, 2000

89. Yerly S, Pedrocchi M, Perrin L: The use of polymerase chain reaction in plasma pools for the concomitant detection of hepatitis C virus and HIV type 1 RNA. Transfusion 38:908, 1998

90. Sun R, Jayakar H, Yeh S, et al: Experience with PCR screening. Dev Biol Stand 102:81, 2000

91. Phair JP, Margolick JB, Jacobson LP, et al: Detection of infection with human immunodeficiency virus type 1 before seroconversion: correlation with clinical symptoms and outcome. J Infect Dis 175:959, 1997

92. Shearer WT, Quinn TC, LaRussa P, et al: Viral load and disease progression in infants infected with human immunodeficiency virus type 1. Women and Infants Transmission Study Group. N Engl J Med 336:1337, 1997

93. Coombs RW, Welles SL, Hooper C, et al: Association of plasma human immunodeficiency virus type 1 RNA level with risk of clinical progression in patients with advanced infection. AIDS Clinical Trials Group (ACTG) 116B/117 Study Team. J Infect Dis 174:704, 1996

94. Hammer SM, Squires KE, Hughes MD, et al: A controlled trial of two nucleoside analogues plus indinavir in persons with human immunodeficiency virus infection and CD4 cell counts of 200 per cubic millimeter or less. AIDS Clinical Trials Group 320 Study Team. N Engl J Med 337:725, 1997

95. Katzenstein DA, Hammer SM, Hughes MD, et al: The relation of virologic and immunologic markers to clinical outcomes after nucleoside therapy in HIV-infected adults with 200 to 500 CD4 cells per cubic millimeter. AIDS Clinical Trials Group Study 175 Virology Study Team. N Engl J Med 335:1091, 1996

96. O'Brien WA, Hartigan PM, Martin D, et al: Changes in plasma HIV-1 RNA and CD4+ lymphocyte counts and the risk of progression to AIDS. Veterans Affairs Cooperative Study Group on AIDS. N Engl J Med 334:426, 1996

97. Welles SL, Jackson JB, Yen-Lieberman B, et al: Prognostic value of plasma human immunodeficiency virus type 1 (HIV-1) RNA levels in patients with advanced HIV-1 disease and with little or no prior zidovudine therapy. J Infect Dis 174:696, 1996

98. Bremer JW, Lew JF, Cooper E, et al: Diagnosis of infection with human immunodeficiency virus type 1 by a DNA polymerase chain reaction assay among infants enrolled in the Women and Infants' Transmission Study. J Pediatr 129:198, 1996

99. Owens DK, Holodniy M, McDonald TW, et al: A meta-analytic evaluation of the polymerase chain reaction for the diagnosis of HIV infection in infants. JAMA 275:1342, 1996

100. Owens DK, Holodniy M, Garber AM, et al: Polymerase chain reaction for the diagnosis of HIV infection in adults: a meta-analysis with recommendations for clinical practice and study design. Ann Intern Med 124:803, 1996

101. Frenkel LM, Mullins JI, Learn GH, et al: Genetic evaluation of suspected cases of transient HIV-1 infection of infants. Science 280:1073, 1998

102. Schwartz DH, Laeyendecker OB, Arango-Jaramillo S, et al: Extensive evaluation of a seronegative participant in an HIV-1 vaccine trial as a result of false-positive PCR. Lancet 350:256, 1997

103. Brambilla D, Leung S, Lew J, et al: Absolute copy number and relative change in determinations of human immunodeficiency virus type 1 RNA in plasma: effect of an external standard on kit comparisons. J Clin Microbiol 36:311, 1998

104. Steketee RW, Abrams EJ, Thea DM, et al: Early detection of perinatal human immunodeficiency virus (HIV) type 1 infection using HIV RNA amplification and detection. New York City Perinatal HIV Transmission Collaborative Study. J Infect Dis 175:707, 1997

105. Weber B, Fall EH, Berger A, et al: Reduction of diagnostic window by new fourth-generation human immunodeficiency virus screening assays. J Clin Microbiol 36:2235, 1998

106. Rich JD, Merriman NA, Mylonakis E, et al: Misdiagnosis of HIV infection by HIV-1 plasma viral load testing: a case series. Ann Intern Med 130:37, 1999

107. Schacker TW, Hughes JP, Shea T, et al: Biological and virologic characteristics of primary HIV infection. Ann Intern Med 128:613, 1998

108. Jagodzinski LL, Wiggins DL, McManis JL, et al: Use of calibrated viral load standards for group M subtypes of human immunodeficiency virus type 1 to assess the performance of viral RNA quantitation tests. J Clin Microbiol 38:1247, 2000

109. Robertson DL, Sharp PM, McCutchan FE, et al: Recombination in HIV-1. Nature 374:124, 1995

110. Collins ML, Irvine B, Tyner D, et al: A branched DNA signal amplification assay for quantification of nucleic acid targets below 100 molecules/ml. Nucleic Acids Res 25:2979, 1997

111. Mulder J, Resnick R, Saget B, et al: A rapid and simple method for extracting human immunodeficiency virus type 1 RNA from plasma: enhanced sensitivity. J Clin Microbiol 35:1278, 1997

112. Kartsonis NA, D'Aquila RT: Clinical monitoring of HIV-1 infection in the ERA of antiretroviral resistance testing. Infect Dis Clin North Am 14:879, 2000

113. Brown AJ, Richman DD: HIV-1: gambling on the evolution of drug resistance? Nat Med 3:268, 1997

114. Durant J, Clevenbergh P, Halfon P, et al: Drug-resistance genotyping in HIV-1 therapy: the VIRADAPT randomised controlled trial. Lancet 353:2195, 1999

115. Hirsch MS, Brun-Vezinet F, D'Aquila RT, et al: Antiretroviral drug resistance testing in adult HIV-1 infection: recommendations of an International AIDS Society—USA Panel. JAMA 283:2417, 2000

116. Nijhuis M, Schuurman R, Boucher CA: Homologous recombination for rapid phenotyping of HIV. Curr Opin Infect Dis 10:474, 1997

117. Hertogs K, de Bethune MP, Miller V, et al: A rapid method for simultaneous detection of phenotypic resistance to inhibitors of protease and reverse transcriptase in recombinant human immunodeficiency virus type 1 isolates from patients treated with antiretroviral drugs. Antimicrob Agents Chemother 42:269, 1998

118. Schuurman R: State of the art of genotypic HIV-1 drug resistance. Curr Opin Infect Dis 10:480, 1997

119. Larder BA, Kemp SD, Harrigan PR: Potential mechanism for sus-

tained antiretroviral efficacy of AZT-3TC combination therapy. Science 269:696, 1995

120. Brun-Vezinet F, Boucher C, Loveday C, et al: HIV-1 viral load, phenotype, and resistance in a subset of drug-naive participants from the Delta trial. The National Virology Groups; Delta Virology Working Group and Coordinating Committee. Lancet 350:983, 1997

121. Hirsch MS, Conway B, D'Aquila RT, et al: Antiretroviral drug resistance testing in adults with HIV infection: implications for clinical management. International AIDS Society—USA Panel. JAMA 279:1984, 1998

122. Rodriguez-Rosado R, Briones C, Soriano V: Introduction of HIV drug-resistance testing in clinical practice. AIDS 13:1007, 1999

123. Andrews L, Friedland G: Progress in HIV therapeutics and the challenges of adherence to antiretroviral therapy. Infect Dis Clin North Am 14:901, 2000

124. Gulick RM, Mellors JW, Havlir D, et al: Treatment with indinavir, zidovudine, and lamivudine in adults with human immunodeficiency virus infection and prior antiretroviral therapy. N Engl J Med 337:734, 1997

125. Brambilla D, Reichelderfer PS, Bremer JW, et al: The contribution of assay variation and biological variation to the total variability of plasma HIV-1 RNA measurements. The Women Infant Transmission Study Clinics; Virology Quality Assurance Program. AIDS 13: 2269, 1999

126. Paxton WB, Coombs RW, McElrath MJ, et al: Longitudinal analysis of quantitative virologic measures in human immunodeficiency virus-infected subjects with ≥ 400 CD4 lymphocytes: implications for applying measurements to individual patients. National Institute of Allergy and Infectious Diseases AIDS Vaccine Evaluation Group. J Infect Dis 175:247, 1997

127. Grabar S, Le Moing V, Goujard C, et al: Clinical outcome of patients with HIV-1 infection according to immunologic and virologic response after 6 months of highly active antiretroviral therapy. Ann Intern Med 133:401, 2000

128. Martinez-Picado J, DePasquale MP, Kartsonis N, et al: Antiretroviral resistance during successful therapy of HIV type 1 infection. Proc Natl Acad Sci U S A 97:10948, 2000

129. Reichelderfer PS, Coombs RW: Cartesian coordinate analysis of viral burden and CD4+ T-cell count in human immunodeficiency virus type-1 infection. Antiviral Res 38:131, 1998

130. Ledergerber B, Egger M, Opravil M, et al: Clinical progression and virological failure on highly active antiretroviral therapy in HIV-1 patients: a prospective cohort study. Swiss HIV Cohort Study. Lancet 353:863, 1999

131. Fauci AS, Longo DL: The human retroviruses. Harrison's Principles of Internal Medicine, 15th ed., Vol. 1. Braunwald E, Fauci A, Kasper D, et al. McGraw-Hill, New York, 2001, p 1131

132. Moore JP, Binley J: HIV: envelope's letters boxed into shape. Nature 393:630, 1998

133. Furtado MR, Callaway DS, Phair JP, et al: Persistence of HIV-1 transcription in peripheral blood mononuclear cells in patients receiving potent antiretroviral therapy. N Engl J Med 340:1614, 1999

34 Viral Zoonoses

Duane J. Gubler, SC.D.
Lyle R. Petersen, M.D., M.P.H.

Zoonoses are human diseases caused by pathogens that normally infect animals. About 534 zoonotic viruses from eight taxonomic families have been identified, 120 of which are known to cause human illness [*see Tables 1 and 2*]. The natural hosts of zoonotic viruses are usually unaffected by the viruses. Infection in humans may cause no obvious illness, a nonspecific viral syndrome, or more severe illness that generally falls into one of three categories: hemorrhagic fever, encephalitis, or rash arthralgia [*see Table 1*].

Transmission of Zoonotic Viruses

Zoonotic viruses replicate in the reservoir animal host and are usually transmitted to humans by direct contact or the bite of a hematophagous (blood-sucking) arthropod. Transmission by direct contact normally involves a bite by the infected reservoir animal or handling of the animal's tissues or materials contaminated by the animal's body fluids. Most viral zoonoses require a blood-sucking arthropod for transmission to humans. Mosquitoes are the most important arthropod vectors, followed by ticks, sandflies, and midges. Arthropod vector–borne viruses are called arboviruses and are maintained in complex life cycles involving a nonhuman primary vertebrate host and a primary arthropod vector [*see Figure 1*]. The arthropod vector usually becomes infected when it ingests virus while feeding on the blood of a viremic animal. Virus replicates in the arthropod tissues, ultimately infecting the salivary glands. The arthropod then transmits the virus to a new host when it injects infective salivary fluid while taking a blood meal. This extrinsic incubation period (time between ingestion and transmission of the virus) is usually 8 to 12 days, depending on environmental factors, the virus, and the vector species.

Arthropod-borne viruses generally remain undetected until humans encroach on the natural enzootic focus or until the virus escapes the primary cycle via a secondary vector or vertebrate host. Although humans may become ill, they are generally considered dead-end hosts because they do not develop sufficient viremia to infect feeding vectors and thus do not contribute to the transmission cycle. Notable exceptions include dengue, yellow fever, chikungunya, and Ross River virus infection [*see Table 1*].

Hemorrhagic Fevers

Hemorrhagic fevers are diseases, generally viral, that often cause extensive bleeding in humans. Specific laboratory diagnosis of hemorrhagic fevers usually requires special serologic or virologic tests, such as enzyme-linked immunosorbent assays (ELISAs) to detect virus-specific immunoglobulin M (IgM) or immunoglobulin G (IgG) antibody, or other tests such as hemagglutination-inhibition, complement fixation, and neutralization tests on paired serum samples taken during the acute and convalescent phases of illness. Some viruses produce viremia [*see Table 1*] and can be isolated from, or detected in, the acute-phase serum or cerebrospinal fluid by polymerase chain reaction (PCR) or immunohistochemistry (IHC) testing of autopsy tissues. Clinicians who suspect a hemorrhagic fever in one of their patients can have samples sent through their state health department to the Centers for Disease Control and Prevention (CDC) for testing.

VIRUSES OF THE FAMILY FLAVIVIRIDAE

Dengue Fever

The dengue virus complex (family Flaviviridae, genus *Flavivirus*) consists of four antigenically related serotypes (DEN-1, DEN-2, DEN-3, and DEN-4). Although there is extensive cross-reactivity between dengue virus serotypes in serologic tests,

Table 1 Important Viral Zoonoses That Cause Human Disease

Family/Virus	*Vector*	*Vertebrate Host*	*Ecology*	*Disease in Humans*	*Geographic Distribution*	*Epidemics*
Togaviridae						
Chikungunya*	Mosquitoes	Humans, primates	U,† S, R	SFI	Africa, Asia	Yes
Ross River*	Mosquitoes	Humans, marsupials	R,† S, U	SFI	Australia, South Pacific	Yes
Mayaro*	Mosquitoes	Birds	R, S, U	SFI	South America	Yes
O'nyong-nyong*	Mosquitoes	?	R	SFI	Africa	Yes
Sindbis	Mosquitoes	Birds	R	SFI	Asia, Africa, Australia, Europe, Americas	Yes
Eastern equine encephalitis	Mosquitoes	Birds	R	SFI, ME	Americas	Yes
Western equine encephalitis	Mosquitoes	Birds, rabbits	R	SFI, ME	Americas	Yes
Venezuelan equine encephalitis*	Mosquitoes	Rodents	R	SFI, ME	Americas	Yes
Barmah Forest*	Mosquitoes	?		SFI	Americas	Yes
Flaviviridae						
Dengue I–IV*	Mosquitoes	Humans, primates	U,† S, R	SFI, HF	Worldwide in tropics	Yes
Yellow fever*	Mosquitoes	Humans, primates	R,† S, U	SFI, HF	Africa, South America	Yes
Kyasanur Forest disease*	Ticks	Primates, rodents, camels	R	SFI, HF, ME	India, Saudi Arabia	No
Omsk hemorrhagic fever	Ticks	Rodents	R	SFI, HF	Asia	No
Japanese encephalitis	Mosquitoes	Birds	R,† S	SFI, ME	Asia	Yes
Murray Valley encephalitis	Mosquitoes	Birds	R	SFI, ME	Australia	Yes
Rocio	Mosquitoes	Birds	R	SFI, ME	South America	Yes
St. Louis encephalitis	Mosquitoes	Birds	R,† S, U	SFI, ME	Americas	Yes
West Nile encephalitis	Mosquitoes	Birds	R,† S, U	SFI, ME	Asia, Africa, North America, Europe	Yes
Tick-borne encephalitis	Ticks	Rodents	R	SFI, ME	Europe, Asia	No
Bunyaviridae						
Sandfly fever*	Sandflies	?	R	SFI	Europe, Africa, Asia	Yes
Rift Valley fever*	Mosquitoes	?	R	SFI, HF, ME	Africa	Yes
La Crosse encephalitis	Mosquitoes	Rodents	R,† S	SFI, ME	North America	No
California encephalitis	Mosquitoes	Rodents	R	SFI, ME	North America, Europe, Asia	Yes
Crimean-Congo hemorrhagic fever*	Ticks	Rodents	R	SFI, HF	Europe, Asia, Africa	Yes
Oropouche*	Midges	?	R,† S, U	SFI	Central and South America	Yes
Hemorrhagic fever with renal syndrome		Rodents	R, S	SFI, HF	Asia, Europe	Yes
Hantavirus pulmonary syndrome		Rodents	R	SFI, HF	United States, Central and South America	Yes
Arenaviridae						
Lassa fever		Rodents	R	SFI, HF	Africa	Yes
Venezuelan hemorrhagic fever		Rodents	R	SFI, HF	Venezuela	Yes
Bolivian hemorrhagic fever		Rodents	R	SFI, HF	Bolivia	Yes
Argentine hemorrhagic fever		Rodents	R	SFI, HF	Argentina	Yes
Filoviridae						
Ebola	?	?	R	SFI, HF	Africa	Yes
Marburg	?	?	R	SFI, HF	Africa	Yes
Rhabdoviridae						
Rabies		Bats, dogs, raccoons	R, S, U	SFI, ME	Global	No
Paramyxoviridae						
Nipah		Pigs, ?bats	R	SFI, ME	Malaysia	Yes
Reoviridae						
Colorado tick fever	Ticks	Rodents, small mammals	R	SFI, ME	Western United States, Canada	No

*Arboviruses that produce significant human viremia.
†The most important ecology.
HF—hemorrhagic fever ME—meningoencephalitis R—rural S—suburban SFI—systemic febrile illness U—urban

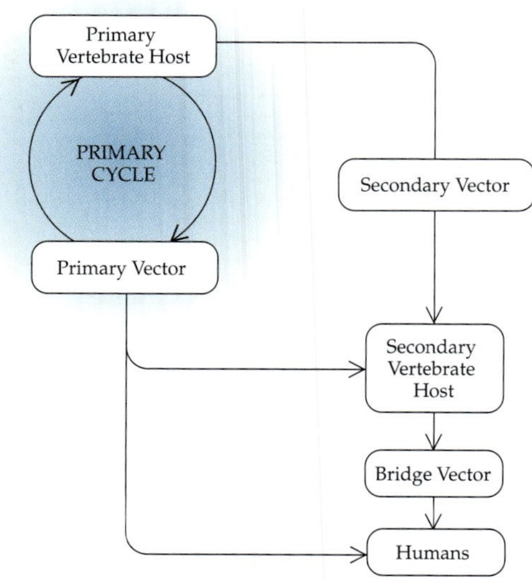

Figure 1 **Generalized arbovirus maintenance cycle.**

there is no lasting cross-protective immunity in humans; cross-protection lasts for only a few months. Thus, individuals can have as many as four dengue infections in their lifetime, one from each serotype.[1]

Epidemiology All four dengue virus serotypes have a worldwide distribution in the tropics and are maintained in tropical rain forests of Asia and Africa in a mosquito-monkey-mosquito cycle and in most tropical urban centers in a mosquito-human-mosquito transmission cycle.[1] The forest cycle is not considered important in terms of public health. A map of countries reporting dengue can be found at www.cdc.gov/ncidod/dvbid/dengue/index.htm. In many urban centers, multiple virus serotypes cocirculate (hyperendemicity). An estimated 50 to 100 million infections occur annually. The principal mosquito vector is *Aedes aegypti*, an African species that spread around the world during the 17th, 18th, and 19th centuries via the slave trade and shipping industry. *A. aegypti* became well adapted to living in intimate association with humans and is a highly efficient epidemic vector in urban settings. Secondary vectors include other *Aedes (Stegomyia)* species such as *A. albopictus, A. polynesiensis*, and *A. scutellaris*. These secondary vector species can transmit dengue viruses during outbreaks, but they are more important as maintenance vectors.

Diagnosis In the United States, dengue fever should be suspected in a traveler who falls abruptly ill within 2 weeks of returning from the tropics. Infection with dengue viruses can be inapparent or can cause a spectrum of clinical illness ranging from a mild, nonspecific viral syndrome to classic dengue fever to severe and fatal hemorrhagic disease. The classic form usually affects adults and older children;

Table 2 Principal Hantaviruses That Cause Human Disease

Virus	*Disease*	*Geographic Distribution*	*Primary Host in Nature*
Dobrava	HFRS (severe)	Balkans	*Apodemus flavicollis* (yellow-necked field mouse)
Hantaan	HFRS (severe)	Asia	*Apodemus agrarius* (striped field mouse)
Puumala	HFRS (mild)	Northern, western, central Europe; Balkans; Russia	*Clethrionomys glareolus* (red bank vole)
Seoul	HFRS (moderate)	Principally Southeast Asia, probably worldwide	*Rattus norvegicus, R. rattus* (common rat, Norway rat)
Andes	HPS (renal)	Argentina	*Oligoryzomys longicaudatus* (long-tailed pygmy rice rat)
Bayou	HPS (renal)	United States	*Oryzomys palustris* (rice rat)
Black Creek Canal	HPS (renal)	United States	*Sigmodon hispidus* (cotton rat)
Juquitiba	HPS	Brazil	Host unknown
Laguna Negra	HPS	Paraguay, Bolivia	*Calomys laucha* (vesper mouse)
Lechiguanas	HPS (renal)	Argentina	*Oligoryzomys* (long-tailed mouse)
Monongahela	HPS	United States	*Peromyscus leucopus* (white-footed mouse)
New York	HPS	United States	*Peromyscus leucopus* (white-footed mouse)
Oran	HPS (renal)	Argentina	*Oligoryzomys longicaudatus* (long-tailed pygmy rice rat)
Sin Nombre	HPS	North America	*Microtus pennsylvanicus* (meadow vole)

HFRS—hemorrhagic fever with renal syndrome HPS—hantavirus pulmonary syndrome in young children, the illness is usually mild but may be severe. After an infective mosquito bite, there is an incubation period of 3 to 14 days (average, 4 to 7 days), followed by the sudden onset of fever (which is often biphasic—with 2 to 5 days of fever, followed by a 1- to 2-day afebrile period, and then 1 to 2 days of fever), severe headache, chills, retro-orbital pain, and generalized, severe pain in the muscles and joints. A maculopapular rash generally appears on the trunk between the third and fifth days of illness and spreads to the face and extremities. Nausea, vomiting, lymphadenopathy, anorexia, constipation, and altered taste sensation are common. Occasionally, petechiae are seen on the dorsum of the feet, legs, hands, axillae, and palate late in the illness. The illness generally lasts 5 to 7 days, after which recovery is complete, although convalescence may be prolonged. Leukopenia with a relative lymphocytosis and thrombocytopenia may occur. Liver enzyme levels may be elevated, and hemorrhagic manifestations may occur. Neurologic manifestations such as encephalopathy and seizures may occur during the disease's febrile stage.[2,3]

Diagnosis of dengue infections should be based on clinical signs and symptoms and on epidemiologic information such as travel history. Laboratory testing is useful only for confirmation of the clinical diagnosis. The IgM-capture ELISA is the serologic test of choice for dengue infection.

Treatment and prevention Treatment of dengue fever is supportive; there are no antiviral agents that are effective for the disease. Prevention consists of environmental control (*see below*).

Dengue Hemorrhagic Fever

Epidemiology Dengue hemorrhagic fever (DHF) is a severe form of dengue infection that is most commonly observed in children younger than 15 years in Southeast Asia and in all age groups in the Americas and the Pacific region.[4]

Pathogenesis The pathogenesis of DHF is still not well understood. Classic DHF with a vascular leak syndrome may have a unique immunopathologic basis that is associated with enhancement of viral infection of mononuclear phagocytes in patients with dengue antibodies from a previous infection with a different serotype (heterologous antibody).[5] Infection of mononuclear phagocytes stimulates the release of vasoactive mediators, leading to a cascade of events that result in increased vascular permeability.

Although the risk of DHF is higher in patients experiencing a second dengue infection, DHF also occurs in patients who have primary infections, which suggests that heterologous dengue antibody (previous infection) is not a prerequisite for DHF. Furthermore, some strains of dengue viruses cannot be enhanced in vitro. Both field evidence and laboratory evidence support a more prominent role of viral factors in the pathogenesis of DHF and suggest that virus strain and serotype are also important risk factors for severe disease.[1,3,5–8] Hemorrhage may occur without vascular leakage, suggesting another pathogenetic mechanism.[3,9]

Diagnosis DHF is characterized by sudden onset of fever, usually lasting 2 to 7 days, and nonspecific signs and symptoms.[1] The critical stage of DHF occurs between 24 hours before and 24 hours after the patient's temperature falls to or below normal. During this time, hemorrhagic manifestations usually occur, and signs of circulatory failure may appear. The patient may become restless or lethargic, experience acute abdominal pain, and have cold extremities and oliguria, usually on or after the third day of illness. Clinical laboratory tests at this time will show thrombocytopenia (platelet count < 100,000/mm^3), a low serum total protein level, a low albumin level, and a rise in hematocrit secondary to plasma leakage from the vascular compartment. Another indication of vascular leakage is pleural effusion. Loss of intravascular volume may result in hypovolemia, shock, and death if not corrected. The most common hemorrhagic manifestations are skin hemorrhages, but epistaxis, bleeding gums, gastrointestinal hemorrhage, and hematuria may occur.

Treatment and prevention Early diagnosis and prompt management with fluid replacement therapy can substantially reduce case-fatality rates.[10] Initial management and treatment decisions should not be delayed pending results of serologic tests. Clinical laboratory tests should be used to monitor vascular leakage.[10]

There is no vaccine for dengue/DHF, although significant progress is being made toward the development of live attenuated and recombinant candidate vaccines using infectious clone technology.[11] Currently, disease prevention depends exclusively on mosquito control and personal protective measures such as mosquito repellents.

Yellow Fever

Epidemiology Yellow fever (YF) virus (family Flaviviridae, genus *Flavivirus*) is believed to have originated in Africa. The disease is now present in tropical America and Africa but does not occur in

Asia. Like dengue, YF virus has two transmission cycles: jungle and urban. The jungle or forest transmission cycle involves canopy-dwelling mosquitoes and monkeys. The urban cycle involves humans as the vertebrate host and *A. aegypti* as the principal vector. In the past 30 years, *A. aegypti* has reinvaded Central and South America, putting the American tropics at the highest risk for urban epidemics of yellow fever in over 50 years. Epidemics in Africa often occur in moist savanna regions, involving forest or peridomestic *Aedes* mosquitoes and humans as viremic hosts. In dry areas and urban centers where water storage practices promote the breeding of domestic *A. aegypti*, this mosquito is responsible for epidemic transmission. Several hundred thousand people are infected yearly, and outbreaks are frequent. Cases among unvaccinated travelers are rare; however, since 1996, six travelers have died in the United States and Europe of yellow fever acquired in South America and Africa.

Diagnosis YF varies from an inapparent infection to a deadly fulminating hemorrhagic disease. Three clinical stages are commonly recognized: infection, remission, and intoxication.[12,13] After an incubation period of 3 to 10 days, the period of infection begins with sudden onset of fever, rigors, headache, and backache. In severe cases, the patient is intensely ill and restless, with flushed face, swollen lips, bright-red tongue, congested conjunctivae, and bleeding. There may be bradycardia relative to fever (Faget sign). This stage is followed after 2 to 3 days by a brief period of remission. Remission is often not obvious. The period of intoxication occurs on the third to sixth day after illness onset in about 15% of patients. This period consists of moderate or severe disease with jaundice. Fever returns with relative bradycardia, along with nausea, vomiting, a hemorrhagic diathesis, hypotension, albuminuria, oliguria, and anuria. Most patients with severe disease will have leukopenia, thrombocytopenia, elevated levels of serum creatinine and liver enzymes, and coagulation defects. The jaundice, which gives the disease its name, is generally apparent only in convalescing patients. In fatal cases, death usually occurs within 7 to 10 days; case-fatality rates vary widely, but they can exceed 50% in clinically ill patients.[14] At autopsy, the organs most affected are the liver, spleen, kidneys, and heart. Typically, the liver shows midzonal hyaline necrosis and Councilman inclusion bodies.

Initial diagnosis of yellow fever should be based on clinical signs and symptoms and on epidemiologic information such as vaccination history and recent travel to an endemic area. Laboratory diagnosis is made by detection of virus, viral antigen, or viral nucleic acid or made by serologic examination. Virus is often isolated from blood during the first 4 days of illness. Serologic tests may be negative during the first week of illness. Diagnostic testing for yellow fever may be obtained by request to the CDC through state and local health departments.

Treatment and prevention Treatment is supportive. Yellow fever is an international reportable disease, and immunization is required for travelers to many countries of sub-Saharan Africa and tropical America. The live, attenuated 17D vaccine, delivered as a single 0.5 ml subcutaneous dose, is highly effective. Immunity is probably lifelong, but for travel certification, revaccination is recommended every 10 years. Information about indications for yellow fever vaccine and requirements for international travel are available at www.cdc.gov/travel/reference.htm.[15] For patients who require immunization, the locations of designated yellow fever vaccination centers can be obtained through local health departments in most areas.

Although the 17D vaccine is one of the safest vaccines, rare cases of severe and fatal infection from vaccination have been reported, and the elderly may experience a higher incidence of serious adverse events.[16–18] Persons with documented egg allergy should not be immunized or should be skin-tested with the vaccine. The vaccine must not be given to children younger than 6 months, in whom there is a risk of postvaccinial encephalitis, and it is best to delay vaccination until 9 months of age. On theoretical grounds, persons with immunosuppression, including those with clinical AIDS, should not be immunized. Immunization during pregnancy is generally contraindicated.

Other Flaviviruses

Other hemorrhagic diseases caused by flaviviruses include Kyasanur Forest disease in India and Saudi Arabia and Omsk hemorrhagic fever in Russia [*see Table 1*]. Both are tick-borne diseases and are rare in comparison with disease from mosquito-borne flaviviruses.

VIRUSES OF THE FAMILY BUNYAVIRIDAE

Crimean-Congo Hemorrhagic Fever

Epidemiology and etiology Crimean-Congo hemorrhagic fever (CCHF) virus (family Bunyaviridae, genus *Nairovirus*) is transmitted by ticks, primarily of the genus *Hyalomma*, over a broad geographic range that includes sub-Saharan Africa, eastern Europe and Russia, the Middle East, and western China.[13] Humans become infected after a tick bite; after parenteral exposure to, or contact with, blood from acutely ill patients[19]; or, on occasion, after the slaughter of sick domestic animals. Disease may be seasonal in humans, reflecting the natural abundance of ticks.

Diagnosis In the United States, CCHF should be suspected in a traveler who falls abruptly ill less than 2 weeks after returning from an endemic area. The incubation period for CCHF is 3 to 7 days for nosocomial infections and up to 12 days for those infected by a tick bite, followed by abrupt onset of fever, headache, myalgia, weakness, nausea, and vomiting. This initial phase may last 2 to 3 days, followed by remission of several hours' duration in one third to two thirds of patients. The second phase of illness is associated with hemorrhagic manifestations, which may last from 3 days to as long as 10 days and includes, most commonly, petechiae over the chest and abdomen, epistaxis, ecchymoses, bleeding from puncture sites, melena, and hematuria. Those surviving the hemorrhagic phase enter a convalescence phase characterized by normalization of fever, cessation of hemorrhages, occasionally transient hair loss, and prolonged fatigue and dizziness. Mortality ranges from 9% to 40%.

Treatment and prevention Treatment is supportive and focuses on the hemorrhagic manifestations. The antiviral drug ribavirin has been administered to a limited number of patients with apparent success.[19] Persons in endemic areas should take protective measures to prevent exposure to infected ticks, and barrier methods should be used in hospitals where patients with suspected CCHF are being treated.

Hantavirus Infections

Hantaviruses (family Bunyaviridae, genus *Hantavirus*) are rodent-borne viruses causing human diseases known as hemorrhagic fever with renal syndrome (HFRS) in Europe and Asia and as hantavirus pulmonary syndrome (HPS) in the Americas.[20,21] The prototype hantavirus is Hantaan virus, which causes epidemic hemorrhagic fever in China and Korea, but many different hantaviruses are now recognized. Hantaviruses are maintained in nature by chronic infection of rodent hosts, and each is principally associated with a specific rodent host [*see Table 2*]. Humans are infected after aerosol exposure to infectious excreta or occasionally by bites. Apparent human-to-human transmission was noted in one outbreak with the Andes virus.[22]

The incidence of hantavirus infections in humans often fluctuates with rodent densities and human activities that increase contact with contaminated materials. Commonly infected are military personnel on field maneuvers, shepherds, woodcutters, campers, and others involved in outdoor activities.

Hemorrhagic fever with renal syndrome Along with Hantaan virus, other hantaviruses causing HFRS are Seoul virus, Puumala virus, and Dobrava/Belgrade virus. Classic HFRS caused by Hantaan or Dobrava virus infection has a variable incubation period and is characterized by five phases: (1) a febrile phase of 3 to 7 days with fever, malaise, headache, abdominal pain, nausea, vomiting, facial flushing, petechiae, and conjunctival hemorrhage; (2) a hypotensive phase of a few hours to 3 days, when hypotension, shock, blurred vision, hemorrhagic signs, and a drop in blood pressure occur; (3) an oliguric phase of 3 to 7 days during which oliguria or anuria predominates and hemorrhagic manifestations may worsen; (4) a diuretic phase of days to weeks, when polyuria predominates; and (5) a prolonged convalescence phase of weeks to months.[20,21] Mortality in classic HFRS results from shock, multiorgan hypoperfusion, or uremia and ranges from 5% to 10%. Infection with Puumala virus or Seoul virus produces milder disease, with lower mortality. Serology is the main diagnostic tool, but it should be used only for confirmatory retrospective diagnosis.[20,21]

Early treatment with ribavirin may reduce hemorrhage, renal failure, and mortality in HFRS.[23] Commercially available inactivated vaccines for Hantaan virus or bivalent Hantaan/Seoul virus vaccines are produced in Korea and China; other vaccines are in development.[24] Control of HFRS relies on reduction of human-rodent contact through good sanitation and waste management, rodent control, and rodent-proofing buildings.

Hantavirus pulmonary syndrome Since its discovery in 1993 during an outbreak in the southwestern United States, several hundred cases of HPS have been identified in the Americas.[20] The Sin Nombre virus, which is carried by deer mice, caused the initial outbreak; subsequently, a number of related hantaviruses hosted by other sigmodontine rodents have been identified as a cause of human disease [*see Table 3*].

Diagnosis HPS should be suspected on the basis of the clinical picture, clinical laboratory results, and radiologic findings; confirmation of diagnosis is by serologic testing. Diagnostic

Table 3 Arenaviruses That Cause Significant Human Illness

Virus	*Disease*	*Geographic Distribution*	*Primary Host in Nature*
Lymphocytic choriomeningitis virus	Lymphocytic choriomeningitis	Americas, Europe, parts of Asia	*Mus musculus* (house mouse)
Lassa virus	Lassa fever	West Africa	*Mastomys* species (rodent)
Junin virus	Argentine hemorrhagic fever	Argentina	*Calomys musculinus* (rodent)
Machupo virus	Bolivian hemorrhagic fever	Bolivia	*Calomys callosus* (rodent)
Guanarito virus	Venezuelan hemorrhagic fever	Venezuela	*Zygodontomys brevicauda* (rodent) *Sigmodon alstoni* (?) (rodent)
Sabia virus	Hemorrhagic fever	Brazil	Unknown

information about HPS, including instructions on submitting suspected HPS specimens for serologic testing, can be obtained from the CDC at www.cdc.gov/ncidod/diseases/hanta/hps/index.htm.

The incubation period of HPS probably ranges from 9 to 33 days. Clinical disease can be divided into four phases: febrile, cardiopulmonary, diuretic, and convalescent.[25] The febrile phase, typically lasting 3 to 5 days, is characterized by fever, myalgia, and malaise. Headache, dizziness, anorexia, nausea, vomiting, and diarrhea may occur. The cardiopulmonary phase is marked by pulmonary edema and shock. Once pulmonary edema develops, rapid onset of circulatory compromise and hypoxia often leads to death. During the diuretic phase, pulmonary edema clears, along with resolution of fever and shock. The convalescent phase may last several months; complete recovery is the rule. Renal insufficiency has been reported with the Sin Nombre virus and is a more constant feature of many of the newly recognized American hantaviruses causing HPS, suggesting that HPS and HFRS are not as clinically distinct as previously thought. Thrombocytopenia is almost universally present. Mortality is approximately 40% but varies with the infecting virus.

Treatment of patients with HPS remains supportive. Early intensive care management is important, with prompt correction of electrolyte, pulmonary, and hemodynamic abnormalities. Vaccines are in development.[24] Despite its in vitro activity against Sin Nombre virus, ribavirin failed to produce a dramatic reduction in case fatality in an open-label trial.

Rift Valley Fever

Epidemiology and etiology Rift Valley fever (RVF) is caused by the RVF virus (family Bunyaviridae, genus *Phlebovirus*). First described from the Rift Valley of Kenya during a fatal epizootic in sheep in 1931, RVF is a mosquito-borne disease affecting domestic ungulates, especially goats and sheep.[13] Large epizootics occur during periods of heavy rainfall. Humans become infected through the bite of an infected mosquito, by infectious aerosols when sick animals are slaughtered, or by occupational exposure (e.g., veterinarians attending to infected animals). Large human outbreaks have occurred in sub-Saharan Africa, Egypt, and more recently on the Saudi Arabian peninsula.[13] RVF is a potential agent of bioterrorism.

Diagnosis The incubation period in humans is 2 to 6 days, followed by abrupt onset of fever, headache, chills, and malaise. Uncomplicated illness usually resolves within 2 to 3 days. Retinitis, hemorrhagic fever, and encephalitis occur in rare instances.

Treatment and prevention Treatment is supportive, although the antiviral drug ribavirin has been effective in the treatment of related viruses of the family Bunyaviridae and deserves further investigation. Inactivated and live attenuated vaccines have been produced for use in domestic animals and appear to be efficacious. No vaccine is commercially available for use in humans, although an experimental inactivated vaccine has been used to protect select populations at risk for laboratory or occupational exposure.[13]

VIRUSES OF THE FAMILY ARENAVIRIDAE

Significant human illnesses caused by Arenaviridae viruses include lymphocytic choriomeningitis; Lassa fever; and Argentine, Bolivian, and Venezuelan hemorrhagic fever. Arenaviruses are transmitted directly to humans after close rodent-human contact, such as touching objects or eating food contaminated with rodent excreta [*see Table 4*]. Human-to-human transmission of Lassa fever has occurred. Several of the arenaviruses are considered potential agents of bioterrorism.

Table 4 Viral Zoonoses Endemic in the United States

Disease	*Region*	*Vector/Host*	*Clinical Manifestations*
Colorado tick fever	Mountainous areas of western states	Wood ticks	Flulike illness, rash, leukopenia
Eastern equine encephalitis	Focal locations along eastern seaboard, Gulf Coast, and some midwestern states	Mosquitoes	Mild flulike illness to encephalitis
Hantavirus pulmonary syndrome	Most prevalent in southwestern states	Deer mice and other rodents (aerosol exposure to infected excreta, or bites)	Febrile, cardiopulmonary, diuretic, and convalescent phases
La Crosse virus	Widespread; most prevalent in rural upper Midwest	Mosquitoes	Mild flulike illness to encephalitis, often with focal seizures
Powassan virus encephalitis	Northeastern states	*Ixodes* ticks	Encephalitis, with localizing neurologic signs and convulsions
Rabies	All except Hawaii	Wild carnivores, bats	Encephalomyelitis
St. Louis encephalitis	All lower 48 states; epidemics in Midwest and Southeast	Mosquitoes	Febrile headache to encephalitis
West Nile virus infection	Eastern states	Mosquitoes	Febrile illness to encephalitis
Western equine encephalitis	Western states	Mosquitoes	Mild flulike illness to encephalitis

Diagnosis

Arenaviral infections typically begin with fever, malaise, headache, and GI symptoms. More severe cases may involve the heart, lungs, liver, and kidneys. Fulminant and often fatal hemorrhagic shock occurs in a minority of cases (e.g., about 20% of hospitalized Lassa fever patients). Lassa fever is especially severe in pregnant women, often causing death in both mother and fetus. Hearing loss (of varying degrees) is a common sequela of Lassa fever, even in mild cases.

Several cases of Lassa fever have been imported into Europe, Japan, and the United States in recent years. Consequently, the clinician should consider the diagnosis in patients who experience a febrile illness within 3 weeks after travel to endemic countries in West Africa (Nigeria, Guinea, Liberia, and Sierra Leone). South American arenaviruses should be considered in the differential diagnosis of hemorrhagic fever in patients with a history of travel to that region. Because its symptoms are varied and nonspecific, arenavirus infection can be confirmed by serology, most commonly with ELISA, which can be requested from the CDC through state and local health departments.

Treatment and Prevention

The antiviral drug ribavirin reduces mortality from Lassa fever, especially if started within the first 6 days after the onset of fever. Ribavirin may be of value in the treatment of other arenaviral infections as well, although significant clinical experience is lacking for full validation of efficacy.[26] A live, attenuated vaccine of proven efficacy has been developed for Junin virus and is available in Argentina.[27]

VIRUSES OF THE FAMILY FILOVIRIDAE

Marburg and Ebola viruses are among the most severe and mysterious viral pathogens to emerge in the 20th century.[28] Filoviruses share common morphology as long, pleomorphic rods but are antigenically and genetically distinct. Current understanding of these agents is largely restricted to investigations of human outbreaks and limited experimental studies conducted at the few laboratories worldwide able to safely handle filoviruses. There is no vaccine or effective chemotherapy for any known filovirus. Marburg and Ebola viruses are considered potential agents of bioterrorism.

Marburg Virus

African green monkeys, *Cercopithecus aethiops*, imported from Uganda for use in research and vaccine production, were the source of the initial 31-person outbreak that led to the discovery of the Marburg virus in 1967. Human fatality was 23%. Only three detected recurrences of Marburg virus have been identified, all in humans traveling in rural Africa.[28] The ecology of Marburg virus remains virtually unknown.

Ebola Virus

Epidemiology At least 1,000 persons have died from Ebola virus infection since its discovery in Sudan in 1976. Of the four known genetic subtypes of Ebola virus—Zaire, Côte d'Ivoire, Sudan, and Ebola-Reston—the first three have been associated with human disease in West and central Africa.[28] Ebola-Reston was discovered in macaques imported from the Philippines for medical research.[29] Occupational exposure to Ebola-Reston from nonhuman primates is infrequent and results in asymptomatic infection.[30]

The natural history of Ebola virus remains a mystery. Outbreaks of Ebola hemorrhagic fever are associated most often with the introduction of the virus into the community by one infected person, followed by dissemination by person-to-person transmission, often within medical facilities.[31]

Diagnosis Ebola virus infection has an incubation period of approximately 6 days, which is commonly followed by two clinical phases.[32] Early symptoms include fever, asthenia, diarrhea, nausea and vomiting, anorexia, abdominal pain, headaches, arthralgia, and back pain. Bilateral conjunctivitis, nonpruritic rash, and sore throat with odynophagia, when present, suggest Ebola virus infection. The second phase, characterized by hemorrhagic manifestations, neuropsychiatric abnormalities, and oligoanuria, portends a worse outcome. In recent outbreaks, bleeding occurred in a minority of patients.[28,31] Mortality during outbreaks typically exceeds 50%.

Clinical diagnosis is challenging, because the presentation is nonspecific. To exclude other infections, patients with clinical manifestations consistent with Ebola virus infection should have a blood smear examination for malaria, a blood culture, and a stool culture if they have bloody diarrhea. ELISA, PCR, and virus isolation can be used to confirm Ebola virus infection within a few days of the onset of symptoms. Detailed diagnostic information is available from the CDC at www.cdc.gov/ncidod/dvrd/spb/mnpages/dispages/ebola.htm.

Treatment and prevention Treatment is supportive. Outbreak control rests on initiation of case finding, case isolation, and other infection-control practices, including barrier nursing procedures.[28,31]

Encephalitis

Viral encephalitis is caused by a number of arboviruses belonging to the families *Flaviviridae, Togaviridae, Bunyaviridae*, and *Reoviridae*, as well as other zoonotic viruses. Specific laboratory diagnosis of encephalitis from zoonotic viruses requires special serologic tests, such as hemagglutination-inhibition, complement fixation, and neutralization tests. ELISAs are used to detect virus-specific IgM or IgG antibody in serum or CSF samples. As with the flaviviruses, serologic tests must be cautiously interpreted, because there is considerable serologic cross-reactivity among many of these viruses of the same genus. Viruses can also be isolated and detected by PCR or immunohistochemistry in autopsy tissue. Assistance with serologic diagnosis can be obtained from the CDC at www.cdc.gov/ncidod/dvbid/index.htm and through state and local health departments.

VIRUSES OF THE FAMILY BUNYAVIRIDAE

La Crosse Encephalitis

Epidemiology La Crosse (LAC) virus (family Bunyaviridae, genus *Bunyavirus*) is the most pathogenic member of the California encephalitis serogroup, which includes the California encephalitis, trivittatus, snowshoe hare, and Jamestown Canyon viruses. LAC is maintained in a cycle involving *A. triseriatus* mosquitoes and a number of mammalian hosts, including the eastern chipmunk, tree squirrels, and foxes.

Human infections occur in the central and eastern United States, mostly as sporadic cases in school-age children from July through September [*see Table 2*].[33]

Diagnosis Most infections are asymptomatic. After an incubation period of 3 to 7 days, headache, fever, and vomiting develop. Seizures are a presenting finding in about half of cases and focal neurologic abnormalities in about one fifth.[33] The combination of fever, focal signs, and focal seizures may mimic herpes simplex encephalitis. Mortality is 1%. About 10% of children have residual neurologic sequelae, including focal neurologic deficits and decreased intelligence. Diagnosis can be confirmed serologically by the CDC on request of state and local health departments.

Treatment and prevention Treatment is supportive; management of cerebral edema and seizures is important [see 35 Acute Viral Central Nervous System Diseases]. Ribavirin has been used, but efficacy is unproved.[33] Prevention rests on avoidance of mosquito bites.

VIRUSES OF THE FAMILY FLAVIVIRIDAE

Japanese Encephalitis

Epidemiology Japanese encephalitis (JE) is the most important global cause of arboviral encephalitis; more than 45,000 cases are reported annually. JE virus (family Flaviviridae, genus *Flavivirus*) is widespread throughout Asia. In recent years, the disease has been detected in Australia and other areas in the Pacific region. Epidemics occur in late summer in temperate regions, but the virus is enzootic and occurs throughout the year in many tropical areas of Asia. JE virus is maintained in a natural enzootic cycle involving *Culex* mosquitoes and water birds. The virus is transmitted to humans by *Culex* mosquitoes, primarily *C. tritaeniorhynchus* and related species, which breed in rice fields. Pigs are the primary amplifying hosts in the peridomestic environment.

Diagnosis Only about one in 250 infections results in symptomatic illness. The incubation period of JE is 5 to 14 days. Symptomatic illness is primarily seen in children. Mild clinical illness, such as aseptic meningitis and simple febrile illness with headache, usually goes undetected. In severe cases, the onset of symptoms is usually sudden, with fever, headache, and vomiting. The illness resolves in 5 to 7 days if there is no central nervous system involvement. Patients with CNS involvement commonly are lethargic, with expressionless faces, and have sensory and motor disturbances affecting their speech, eyes, and limbs. They may have confusion and delirium progressing to coma; in children, convulsions are sometimes a presenting sign. Weakness and paralysis may affect any part of the body. Neck rigidity and a positive Kernig sign are found, and reflexes are abnormal. Signs of extrapyramidal involvement are characteristic. Initial leukocytosis is followed by leukopenia. Mortality is 5% to 30%, with higher case-fatality rates in young children. Approximately one third of patients who recover have neurologic sequelae. The diagnosis can be confirmed serologically by the CDC on request of state and local health departments.

Prevention A formalin-inactivated mouse brain vaccine prepared with the Nakayama strain of JE virus is used internationally. Vaccination is recommended to residents in JE-endemic areas and to certain travelers to those areas. The risk to travelers is generally low, but vaccination is recommended for visitors to endemic or epidemic areas during the transmission season, especially when potential exposure will be prolonged and when there is a high likelihood of exposure to vectors.[34] Treatment is supportive. One case study suggested that recombinant interferon alfa may improve clinical outcome.[35] More information on JE is available at www.cdc.gov/ncidod/dvbid/jencephalitis/index.htm. Mosquito control and improved animal husbandry and rice-growing practices are needed to decrease transmission risk in endemic areas.

Murray Valley Encephalitis

Epidemiology Murray Valley encephalitis (MVE) virus (family Flaviviridae, genus *Flavivirus*) was first isolated in 1951. MVE occurs only in Australia and New Guinea.[36] Like other flaviviruses, MVE virus is believed to be maintained in a natural cycle involving water birds and *Culex* mosquitoes. Viremia has not been documented in humans, who are likely dead-end hosts.

Diagnosis Only one in 1,000 to 2,000 infections results in clinical illness. Clinical illness resembles Japanese encephalitis. Illness is characterized by sudden onset of fever, headache, nausea and vomiting, anorexia, and myalgias, followed by drowsiness, malaise, irritability, mental confusion, and meningismus. In severe cases, there may be hyperactive reflexes, spastic paresis, convulsions, coma, and death. Of patients with neurologic disease, approximately one third die and one quarter have residual neurologic deficits.

Prevention There is no vaccine for MVE virus. Prevention relies on mosquito control and avoidance of mosquito bites.

Saint Louis Encephalitis

Epidemiology St. Louis encephalitis (SLE) virus (family Flaviviridae, genus *Flavivirus*) is prevalent throughout the Western Hemisphere from Canada to Argentina. In North America, the infection is maintained between wild birds and *Culex* mosquitoes. Although clinical illness has been sporadically reported throughout much of this region, most infections occur in North America during epidemics, which occur sporadically in the Midwest and Southeast.

Diagnosis The ratio of infection to clinical illness is high, ranging from 800 to 1 in children younger than 10 years to 85 to 1 in persons older than 60 years. Illness ranges from fever with headache to aseptic meningitis to encephalitis. Advanced age is the strongest risk factor for both symptomatic disease and severity of encephalopathy. SLE should be considered in the differential diagnosis of adult viral encephalitis cases during summer months in the United States. After an incubation period of 4 to 21 days, the illness begins with fever, headache, chills, nausea, and dysuria. Within 1 to 4 days, CNS signs appear, with meningismus, tremor, abnormal reflexes, ataxia, cranial nerve palsies, convulsions (especially in children), stupor, and coma. About 25% of very young infants have residual mental deficits, personality changes, muscle weakness, and paralysis. Overall, the case-fatality rate is about 6%, but the disease is generally milder in children (case-fatality rate of those younger than 5 years is 1%). The diagnosis can be confirmed serologically by the CDC on request of state and local health departments.

Treatment and prevention Treatment is supportive; no specific therapy is available. No vaccine is available. Prevention is aimed at mosquito-bite avoidance and mosquito abatement.

Tick-Borne Encephalitis

Epidemiology and etiology Tick-borne encephalitis (TBE) is caused by two closely related viruses of the family Flaviviridae, genus *Flavivirus*.[37] The eastern subtype of the TBE virus is transmitted by *Ixodes persulcatus* and causes Russian spring-summer encephalitis, which occurs from Eastern Europe to China. The western subtype is transmitted by *I. ricinus* and causes Central European encephalitis, which occurs from Scandinavia in the north to Greece and Serbia and Montenegro in the south. Of the two subtypes, Russian spring-summer encephalitis is the more severe infection, having a mortality of 5% to 20%, compared with less than 2% for the western subtype. Both viruses are maintained in natural cycles involving a variety of mammals and ticks. Human exposure occurs through work or recreational activities in the spring and summer months in temperate zones and in fall and winter in the Mediterranean, when the ticks are most active. Infection may also occur through the ingestion of raw milk or cheese from cows, sheep, or goats.

Diagnosis The incubation period of TBE is usually 7 to 14 days. The western subtype typically produces a biphasic illness. Infection usually presents as a mild, influenzalike illness lasting 2 to 7 days, followed by an afebrile or relatively asymptomatic period lasting 2 to 10 days. Approximately one third of patients then develop higher fevers with aseptic meningitis or meningoencephalitis. The eastern subtype usually progresses without an asymptomatic phase. Permanent paresis develops in 2% to 10% of patients with the western subtype and in 10% to 25% of patients with the eastern subtype. Although cases have been confirmed in United States citizens who visited enzootic areas, this is rare. Infections can be confirmed serologically by the CDC on request of state and local health departments.

Treatment and prevention Treatment of TBE is supportive. Inactivated vaccines against both eastern and western subtypes of TBE viruses are available in Europe, but they are not commercially available in the United States.[37] Prevention strategies include avoiding tick bites and pasteurizing milk.

West Nile Virus

Epidemiology and etiology West Nile (WN) virus (family Flaviviridae, genus *Flavivirus*), first isolated in 1937 in the West Nile district of Uganda, has historically had a wide geographic distribution in Africa, Asia, the Middle East, and Europe.[38,39] The virus was first recognized in the Western Hemisphere during an epizootic among birds and horses and a human encephalitis outbreak in the New York City area in 1999.[40] By 2002, the virus's known geographic distribution extended to southeastern Canada, the Grand Cayman Islands, and throughout the eastern United States. Up-to-date maps of the virus's spread in the United States are available at www.cdc.gov/ncidod/dvbid/westnile/surv&control.htm. The virus has a natural maintenance cycle involving wild birds and *Culex* mosquitoes and is thought to spread via migrating birds.[38,39] Human infections result from infectious mosquito bites; there is no evidence of animal-to-human or human-to-human transmission of West Nile virus. From the 1950s to the 1970s, human outbreaks were reported infrequently, mostly in the Middle East. However, since the mid-1990s, outbreaks of neurologic disease in humans and horses, with an increase in death rates, may have marked the evolution of a new WN virus variant.[38,39] In temperate climates, infection incidence peaks during late summer and early fall; however, year-round transmission is possible in more tropical areas.

Diagnosis The incubation period of WN virus ranges from 3 to 14 days. Serologic surveys during recent outbreaks suggest that approximately 20% of persons who are infected develop a systemic febrile illness.[41] Fever; headache; myalgia; GI complaints; and an erythematous macular, papular, or morbilliform skin rash are common symptoms.[38–40] Lymphadenopathy may be present, but it has been reported less frequently in recent outbreaks. Overall, fewer than 1% of infected persons develop encephalitis.[41] Older persons are at increased risk for meningitis or encephalitis, and once these complications develop, such individuals have a higher case-fatality rate and incidence of residual neurologic deficits.[40] Of note, muscle weakness and flaccid paralysis, when present, may provide a clue to a WN virus etiology. Overall, case-fatality rates in severe cases are about 10%. The diagnosis is most efficiently confirmed serologically; testing can be obtained through state and local health departments.

Treatment and prevention Treatment of WN virus is supportive. Prevention relies on mosquito control and protection from mosquito bites. There is no human vaccine for WN virus. An equine vaccine has recently become available.

Powassan Virus

Powassan virus (family Flaviviridae, genus *Flavivirus*) is related to the Eastern Hemisphere's tick-borne encephalitis viruses. It was thought to be a rare cause of encephalitis in eastern Canada and the northern United States; however, WN virus surveillance has increased the recognition of this pathogen.[42] The case-fatality rate is 5% to 10%, with a high incidence of residual neurologic dysfunction in survivors. Serologic surveys indicate an antibody prevalence of 1% to 4%. The virus is transmitted between *Ixodes* ticks and rodents; humans become infected via tick bites. The clinical features are those of viral encephalitis, with localizing neurologic signs and convulsions. There is no specific treatment or vaccine.

VIRUSES OF THE FAMILY TOGAVIRIDAE

Eastern Equine Encephalitis

Epidemiology Eastern equine encephalitis (EEE) virus (family Togaviridae, genus *Alphavirus*) is widely distributed throughout North, Central, and South America and the Caribbean; however, little is known about the epidemiology of EEE outside North America. In the United States, human infections are usually sporadic and small outbreaks occur each summer, mostly in the upper Midwest and along the Atlantic and Gulf Coasts. In North America, wild birds and *Culiseta melanura* (a mosquito found in swamp areas that support cedar, red maple, and loblolly bay trees) maintain the virus.

Diagnosis The incubation period of EEE exceeds 1 week, and onset is abrupt, with high fever. About 2% of infected adults and 6% of infected children develop encephalitis. EEE causes the most severe of the arboviral encephalitides, with a mortality of 50% to 75%. Symptoms and signs include dizziness, decreasing level of consciousness, tremors, seizures, and focal neurologic signs. Death can occur within 3 to 5 days after onset. Sequelae, which are common in nonfatal encephalitis, include convulsions, paralysis, and mental retardation. Illness from EEE in South America is less severe. Infection can be confirmed serologically by the CDC on request of state and local health departments.

Treatment and prevention No specific treatment is available. Prevention focuses on avoidance of mosquito bites and mosquito control in suburban areas. Inactivated vaccines have been used successfully in horses, and an inactivated vaccine has been used in laboratory workers or others at high risk of exposure, but it is not commercially available.

EEE is a potential agent of bioterrorism through the aerosol route.

Venezuelan Equine Encephalitis

In the Venezuelan equine encephalitis (VEE) virus (family Togaviridae, genus *Alphavirus*) complex, six subtypes (I-VI) have been identified. Five antigenic variants exist in subtype I (IAB, IC, ID, IE, IF). These subtypes and variants are classified as epizootic or enzootic, based on their apparent virulence and epidemiology. Epizootic variants of subtype I (IAB and IC) cause equine epizootics and are associated with more severe human disease. Enzootic strains (ID-F, II [Everglades], III [Mucambo, Tonate, Paramana], IV [Pixuna], V [Cabassou], VI [unnamed]) do not cause epizootics in horses, but they may produce sporadic disease in man. Epizootic strains are transmitted by many different types of mosquitoes; enzootic strains are transmitted by culicine mosquitoes. VEE has a widespread geographic distribution, from Florida to South America, where it is an important veterinary and public health problem. Focal outbreaks occur periodically, but occasionally, large regional epizootics occur, with thousands of equine and human infections.

VEE is infectious via aerosols, making it an occupational risk to certain laboratory workers and a potential agent of bioterrorism.

Diagnosis After an incubation period of 1 to 6 days, there is a brief febrile illness of sudden onset, characterized by malaise, nausea or vomiting, headache, and myalgia. Fewer than 0.5% of adults and fewer than 4% of children develop encephalitis. Long-term sequelae and fatalities are uncommon.

Treatment and prevention Treatment is supportive. Effective prevention of both human and equine disease can be accomplished by immunizing horses and other equine animals, which serve as the primary amplification host for the epizootic VEE viruses and without which there would be little human disease. During epidemics, mosquito vectors can be controlled by insecticides. Live attenuated and inactivated vaccines have been used for laboratory workers; however, human vaccines are not commercially available.

Western Equine Encephalitis

Western equine encephalitis (WEE) virus (family Togaviridae, genus *Alphavirus*) is a complex of closely related viruses found in North and South America. Flooding, which increases breeding of culicine mosquitoes, may precipitate summer outbreaks of WEE. Large outbreaks in humans and horses occurred in the western United States in the 1950s and 1960s; however, a declining horse population, equine vaccination, and improved vector control have reduced disease incidence. The younger the patient, the greater the likelihood of symptomatic infection: the ratio of asymptomatic to symptomatic infection is less than one in 1,000 in adults but increases to 1:1 in infants.

Diagnosis After an incubation period of about 7 days, headache, vomiting, stiff neck, and backache are typical in WEE. In children, restlessness and irritability are seen, and convulsions are common. Neurologic sequelae are relatively common in infants, but they are rare in older children and adults. The case-fatality rate is 3% to 7%. The diagnosis can be confirmed serologically by the CDC on request of state and local health departments.

Treatment and prevention No specific treatment is available for WEE. Prevention focuses on mosquito control and personal measures to avoid mosquito bites. Inactivated vaccine is available for horses. Although inactivated vaccine has been used for laboratory staff and others at high risk of exposure, it is not commercially available for use in humans. WEE is a potential agent of bioterrorism through the aerosol route.

VIRUSES OF THE FAMILY RHABDOVIRIDAE

Rabies

Epidemiology The rabies virus (family Rhabdoviridae, genus *Lyssavirus*) occurs worldwide. Dogs remain the major source of human rabies worldwide. In the United States, however, vaccination has sharply limited canine rabies, and consequently, wildlife rabies has increased in importance. About 90% of all reported cases of animal rabies in the United States now occur in wildlife, particularly wild carnivores (e.g., skunks, raccoons, foxes, coyotes, and bobcats) and bats.[43,44] The major wildlife reservoir for rabies in the United States is the raccoon, which accounts for 50% of all reported cases of rabies in animals.[45] Raccoon rabies is the most prevalent in the eastern states; skunk rabies is predominant in the central and western states.[43] Rodents (e.g., squirrels, hamsters, guinea pigs, gerbils, chipmunks, rats, and mice) and lagomorphs (rabbits and hares) are rarely infected and have not been identified as sources of human rabies in the United States.[44] In the United States since 1990, indigenous rabies virus variants associated with insectivorous bats and foreign canine rabies virus variants have accounted for 30 of the 32 human cases. Although 74% of the 32 cases since 1990 have been attributed to bat-associated variants of the virus, a history of a bite was established in only two cases.[46]

Etiology and pathogenesis In most cases of rabies, an infected animal inoculates saliva containing rabies virus into the patient, and the virus may replicate in muscle cells near the bite. After replication, the virus spreads via retrograde axoplasmic flow in unmyelinated motor or sensory nerves to the CNS. It then replicates in the brain before moving via the nerves into other tissues, including the salivary glands, from which it can be shed.

Clinical manifestations The infectivity of rabies virus varies with the site and mode of transmission. A bite on the face presents a 60% chance of disease; a bite on the hand or arm reduces the chance of disease to between 15% and 40%, and a bite on the leg presents only a 3% to 10% chance of disease. The risk of disease from a bite is almost 50 times greater than the risk from scratches by a rabid animal. The virus can be inhaled, which accounts for rabies in laboratory workers exposed to viral aerosols and in a few explorers of bat-infested caves.

The incubation period of rabies ranges from 12 days to many years and probably averages 30 to 90 days or less. The clinical course is quite variable. The initial clinical presentation is a prodromal phase typically lasting a day or two. It is marked by pain and paresthesias in the area of the bite, GI and upper respiratory symptoms, irritability, apprehension, and a sense of impending death. Hydrophobia and aerophobia occur in some patients and, like the history of a bite, call attention to this disease. Thereafter, the patient enters an excitation state, marked by hyperventilation, hyperactivity, disorientation, and even seizures. During the next few days, the patient becomes lethargic and begins to show paralysis, particularly in areas innervated by the cranial nerves and in the somatic muscles, bladder, and bowels. Gradual involvement of cardiac muscles and paralysis of respiratory muscles lead to death. Rabies virus infection in humans is uniformly fatal once symptoms occur.

Diagnosis Rabies should be considered if classic signs of hydrophobia, aerophobia, and excited behavior are present or in any case of encephalitis or myelitis of unknown etiology, even in the absence of an exposure history. The CSF shows nonspecific elevation in levels of leukocytes and protein, as occurs in other viral encephalitides. Fluorescent antibody staining, virus isolation, and reverse transcriptase/PCR constitute the most accurate means of diagnosing rabies infection.[47] Circulating antibodies may be detected in unvaccinated persons as early as the sixth day of illness and usually appear within the first 2 weeks after infection. Rabies virus can be isolated from the second day through the second week of illness from a throat swab or saliva sample, as well as from tears, urine sediment, and CSF.

Treatment and prevention Three rabies vaccines are currently available in the United States: human diploid cell rabies vaccine (HDCV), rabies vaccine absorbed (RVA), and purified chick embryo cell vaccine (PCEC).[43] Each is licensed for preexposure or postexposure vaccination. Clinical trials with RVA and PCEC have demonstrated immunogenicity equivalent to that of HDCV.[43] Corticosteroids, other immunosuppressing agents and conditions, and antimalarials may interfere with the development of active immunity after vaccination. Preexposure prophylaxis is indicated for persons in high-risk groups such as certain laboratory workers, persons whose occupation puts them in frequent contact with animal species at risk for having rabies, and certain international travelers.[43]

Disease onset can be prevented by prompt postexposure prophylaxis. Postexposure prophylaxis begins with immediate and thorough washing of all bite wounds with soap and water and irrigation with a virucidal agent such as a povidone-iodine solution. Previously unimmunized persons should receive human rabies immunoglobulin and rabies vaccine. Guidelines for the indications and dosing schedules for postexposure prophylaxis are available from the CDC at www.cdc.gov/ncidod/dvrd/rabies.[44] Local or state public health officials should be consulted if questions arise about the need for rabies prophylaxis.

At present, therapy for clinical rabies is supportive. In unvaccinated patients, the disease is invariably fatal. A patient with rabies or suspected rabies should be kept in isolation, and standard infection control precautions should be followed, although laboratory-confirmed person-to-person transmission has not been documented.

VIRUSES OF THE FAMILY PARAMYXOVIRIDAE

Nipah Virus

Nipah virus (family Paramyxoviridae) is closely related to the Hendra virus which has rarely caused fever, pneumonia, and encephalitis in persons exposed to ill horses in Australia. Nipah virus was newly discovered during an outbreak involving 265 persons, with 105 deaths in 1998 and 1999 in Malaysia.[48,49] Most affected persons had contact with live pigs and were pig farmers. A small associated outbreak occurred in Singapore in 11 abattoir workers exposed to imported Malaysian pigs.[50]

Diagnosis The incubation period is unknown, but more than 90% of the hospitalized Malaysian patients had contact with pigs in the previous 2 weeks. Among hospitalized patients, fever was almost invariably present, with headache, dizziness, and vomiting common presenting symptoms. Predominant neurologic symptoms were decreased level of consciousness, segmental myoclonus, meningismus and seizures. Pneumonia was noted in 25% of the patients in Singapore, but it was not prominent in Malaysian patients. The diagnosis can be confirmed serologically by viral culture or by detection of viral nucleic acid.

Treatment Treatment is supportive. An open-label trial suggested that ribavirin reduced mortality.[51] Prevention is avoidance of pig farms.

VIRUSES OF THE FAMILY REOVIRIDAE

Colorado Tick Fever

The Colorado tick fever virus (family Reoviridae, genus *Coltivirus*) is transmitted to humans in the western United States and Canada mainly by the wood tick, *Dermacentor andersoni*. Human incidence corresponds to the wood tick's geographic distribution in mountainous areas at elevations of 4,000 to 10,000 ft. Transmission occurs from March to September, but it peaks from April to June.

Diagnosis The mean incubation period for Colorado tick fever virus is 3 to 4 days. In 90% of cases, the patient reports a tick bite or tick exposure. Fever, chills, myalgias, and prostration are common presenting symptoms. A petechial or maculopapular rash occurs in 15% of patients. Although acute symptoms last about a week, fever may recur several days later. Fatigue is often prolonged. Meningitis or encephalitis develops in 5% to 10% of children; fatal cases with hemorrhage and shock have been rarely reported. Leukopenia is very common. The virus infects marrow erythrocytic precursors, which accounts for the ability to recover the virus from peripheral blood up to 6 weeks after illness onset. Transmission via blood transfusion has been reported. The diagnosis can also be confirmed serologically by the CDC on request through state and local health departments.

Treatment Treatment is supportive. Prevention rests on avoiding tick bites in endemic areas.

Rash Arthralgia

VIRUSES OF THE FAMILY TOGAVIRIDAE

Several alphaviruses belonging to the family Togaviridae can cause a viral syndrome associated with rash and arthralgias or arthritis. Diagnosis requires serologic testing of paired acute-phase and convalescent-phase serum. Virus can also be isolated from or detected in acute-phase serum samples.

There are no vaccines available for general use against alphaviruses. Prevention depends on mosquito control and decreasing exposure to mosquitoes.

Barmah Forest Virus

Barmah Forest (BF) virus (family Togaviridae, genus *Alphavirus*) causes sporadic disease and epidemics in Australia.[36] Clinically, BF virus causes a Ross River virus–like illness, but the rash tends to be more florid and true arthritis is less common. Outbreaks have coincided with Ross River virus outbreaks, and BF virus has been identified in the same mosquito species as Ross River virus.[36]

Chikungunya

Chikungunya (CHIK) virus (family Togaviridae, genus *Alphavirus*) is found in Africa and Asia and is transmitted by *Aedes* mosquitoes. In urban settings, the virus is transmitted from human to human via *A. aegypti* mosquitoes. Explosive urban epidemics occur during the rainy season. The native name for the disease means "doubled up," because of the excruciating joint pains.

Diagnosis In patients with chikungunya, after an incubation period of 2 to 4 days, there is a sudden onset of fever and crippling joint pains, accompanied by chills, flushed face, headache, myalgias, backache, and photophobia. Arthralgias are polyarticular, are migratory, and mostly involve the small joints. Papular or maculopapular skin rashes, typically on the trunk and limbs, occur usually during the second to fifth day of illness. The clinical picture resembles that of dengue fever, with which chikungunya is often confused.[52] Most infections are probably asymptomatic. Arthralgias may last several months. In Asia, but not Africa, mild hemorrhagic manifestations have been reported; CHIK virus is not a cause of severe hemorrhagic disease. The diagnosis can be confirmed serologically by the CDC on request through state and local health departments. Confirmation by culture or detection of viral nucleic acid is possible early in illness.

Treatment There is no specific treatment for CHIK virus. Anti-inflammatory drugs may relieve arthralgia. Chloroquine phosphate has been used for refractory arthralgias. Prevention depends on mosquito control and decreasing mosquito exposure.

Mayaro Virus

Mayaro (MAY) virus (family Togaviridae, genus *Alphavirus*) is closely related to CHIK virus and causes a similar illness. The virus has been isolated from mosquitoes (mostly *Haemagogus*) in various countries in the Caribbean and South America. Little is known about the natural history of the disease. MAY causes febrile illness with headache, backache, myalgias, epigastric pain, chills, nausea, photophobia, arthralgias, and maculopapular rash. Polyarthritis occurs and may persist for several weeks. Cases of MAY disease have recently been imported into the United States.[53] MAY infection should be considered in the differential diagnosis in patients with a recent travel history to South America. Diagnosis can be confirmed serologically at the CDC by request through state and local health departments.

O'nyong-nyong

O'nyong-nyong (ONN) virus (family Togaviridae, genus *Alphavirus*) was first isolated during an epidemic in Uganda in 1959 and spread to an estimated two million people in neighboring countries by 1962. Another ONN virus epidemic began in south-central Uganda in 1996.[54] ONN is transmitted to humans by *Anopheles* and other mosquitoes. Clinically, ONN fever is similar to CHIK, although fever is less pronounced and lymphadenopathy is more common in ONN.

Ross River Fever

Ross River virus (family Togaviridae, genus *Alphavirus*) has caused so-called epidemic polyarthritis in Australia, southwestern Pacific Islands, and Fiji.[36] Several species of *Aedes* and *Culex* mosquitoes are important vectors.[36] The natural maintenance cycle of Ross River virus is not fully known. Humans have significant viremia, and the virus may follow a human-mosquito-human transmission cycle.[55]

After an incubation period of 2 to 21 days, the illness begins suddenly with myalgia and marked arthralgias in the small joints of the hands and feet. True arthritis occurs in over 40% of patients. A maculopapular rash occurs in 50% of patients within 2 days after onset. Myalgia, headache, anorexia, nausea, and tenosynovitis are common, but temperature is only slightly elevated. Arthralgia frequently persists for several weeks or longer—sometimes for longer than a year.

VIRUSES OF THE FAMILY FLAVIVIRIDAE

Dengue

In addition to their role in hemorrhagic fever (see above), dengue viruses are a common cause of rash and arthralgia.

OTHER VIRUSES CAUSING RASH AND ARTHRALGIA

There are a number of other viral zoonoses that cause similar nonspecific febrile illness in humans, but they occur infrequently or are rare. These include Igbo-Ora (family Togaviridae, genus *Alphavirus*) in Africa; Sindbis and Sindbis-like viruses (family Togaviridae, genus *Alphavirus*) in Africa, Asia, Australia, and Europe; Group C arboviruses (family Bunyaviridae, genus *Bunyavirus*) in South America; Oropouche (family Bunyaviridae, genus *Bunyavirus*) in South and Central America; Sandfly fever (family Bunyaviridae, genus *Phlebovirus*) in the Mediterranean, Middle East, West Asia, and South America; Zika virus (family Flaviviridae, genus *Flavivirus*) in Africa and Asia; and vesicular stomatitis virus (family Rhabdoviridae, genus *Vesiculovirus*) in the Americas.

Miscellaneous Viral Zoonoses

MONKEY B VIRUS DISEASE

Monkey B virus (*Herpesvirus simiae* or B virus) causes persistent latent infections in at least 70% of captive adult macaques. Monkey B virus disease in humans usually results from macaque bites or scratches; most documented infections have occurred in laboratory personnel working with apparently healthy rhesus, cynomolgus, or African green monkeys or their tissues, including kidney cell cultures.[56] Human infection from a mucocutaneous exposure to the eye and one human-to-human transmission have been reported. In humans, monkey B virus causes acute ascending myelitis and fulminant meningoencephalitis, which leads to death within days.

Infection can be diagnosed in humans by demonstrating a rise in antibody titer and by isolating the virus from the CNS. Cardiopulmonary support is the most important aspect of management. Human infection carries a high mortality; however, patients treated early with intravenous acyclovir or ganciclovir have survived. Significant neurologic residua are common in survivors. Monkey handlers should wear protective clothing and a face mask.[57] Bites, scratches, or mucosal surfaces exposed to macaque biologic materials should be cleansed thoroughly.[55] Postexposure management should include referral to a medical consultant knowledgeable about monkey B virus.

RUMINANT AND PRIMATE POXVIRUS DISEASES

Several ruminant and primate poxviruses rarely cause human illness. Cowpox (vaccinia virus) is an orthopoxvirus related to variola. In humans, it produces vesicular lesions on the hands. Generalized infections are rare. Monkeypox, the only other orthopoxvirus of significance to humans, is enzootic in monkeys and squirrels in western and central Africa; infection in humans is sporadic and produces a vesicular rash similar to variola. Secondary infections occur, and the case-fatality rate is 1.5%.[58] Tanapox virus is a yatapoxvirus that causes vesicular lesions in monkeys along the Tana River in Kenya and Zaire. It produces a monkeypoxlike illness in humans. The parapoxviruses produce disease in humans through direct contact with infected animals. These include bovine papular stomatitis virus, milkers' nodule (pseudocowpox) in cattle, and orf in sheep and goats. Infection results in vesicles that progress to pustules and scabbing at the site of contact with the original infected species or contaminated objects.

NEWCASTLE DISEASE VIRUS INFECTION

Newcastle disease is an often fatal systemic infection of poultry that is caused by a paramyxovirus. The virus is occasionally transmitted to humans from infected birds or in the laboratory, presumably by direct inoculation. In humans, the illness appears as acute, sometimes hemorrhagic conjunctivitis without corneal involvement. It can be accompanied by lymphangitis, headache, malaise, and chills but is usually self-limited. Patients recover within 2 weeks.

VESICULAR STOMATITIS VIRUS INFECTION

Vesicular stomatitis virus is a rhabdovirus whose structure resembles that of rabies virus. The agent is responsible for oral ulcers in cattle. Occasionally, laboratory workers become infected and experience fever, vesicular enanthemas, headache, and myalgias.

FOOT-AND-MOUTH DISEASE

Foot-and-mouth disease is a highly infectious viral infection of cloven-hoofed animals. The causative agent of the disease is aphthovirus, a member of the family Picornaviridae that is indistinguishable morphologically from rhinovirus. Persons contacting infected animals occasionally have fever, vesicular lesions on the hands, and an increase in neutralizing and complement-fixing titers. The infection is mild and transient, but relapses occur.

References

1. Gubler DJ: Dengue and dengue hemorrhagic fever. Clin Microbiol Rev 11:480, 1998

2. Pancharoen C, Thisyakorn U: Neurological manifestations in dengue patients. Southeast Asian J Trop Med Public Health 32:341, 2001

3. Sumarmo , Wulu H, Jahja E, et al: Clinical observations on virologically confirmed fatal dengue infections in Jakarta, Indonesia. Bull World Health Organ 61:693, 1983

4. Rigau-Perez JG, Vorndam AV, Clark GG: The dengue and dengue-hemorrhagic fever epidemic in Puerto Rico, 1994–1995. Am J Trop Med Hyg 64:67, 2001

5. Kurane I, Takasaki T: Dengue fever and dengue hemorrhagic fever: challenges of controlling an enemy still at large. Rev Med Virol 11:301, 2001

6. Trent DW, Grant JA, Monath TP, et al: Genetic variation and microevolution of dengue 2 virus in Southeast Asia. Virology 172:523, 1989

7. Corwin AL, Larasati RP, Bangs MJ, et al: Epidemic dengue transmission in southern Sumatra, Indonesia. Trans R Soc Trop Med Hyg 95:257, 2001

8. Rosen L: The emperor's new clothes revisited and reflections on the pathogenesis of dengue hemorrhagic fever. Am J Trop Med Hyg 26:337, 1977

9. Krishnamurti C, Kalayanarooj S, Cutting MA, et al: Mechanisms of hemorrhage in dengue without circulatory collapse. Am J Trop Med Hyg 65:840, 2001

10. Dengue haemorrhagic fever: diagnosis, treatment, control, 2nd ed. WHO Technical Report Series, World Health Organization, Geneva, Switzerland, 1997

11. Kinney RM, Huang CY: Development of new vaccines against dengue fever and Japanese encephalitis. Intervirology 44:176, 2001

12. Monath TP: Yellow fever. The Arboviruses: Epidemiology and Ecology Vol. V.: CRC Press, Boca Raton, Florida, 1988

13. Lacy MD, Smego RA: Viral hemorrhagic fevers. Adv Pediatr Infect Dis 12:21, 1996

14. Nasidi A, Monath TP, DeCock K, et al: Urban yellow fever epidemic in western Nigeria, 1987. Trans R Soc Trop Med Hyg 83:401, 1989

15. Centers for Disease Control and Prevention: Health information for the international traveler 2001–2002. Atlanta: US Department of Health and Human Services, Public Health Service, 2001

16. Chan RC, Penney DJ, Little D, et al: Hepatitis and death following vaccination with 17D-204 yellow fever vaccine. Lancet 358:121, 2001

17. Martin M, Tsai TF, Cropp B, et al: Fever and multisystem organ failure associated with 17D-204 yellow fever vaccination: a report of four cases. Lancet 358:98, 2001

18. Martin M, Weld LH, Tsai TF, et al: Advanced age a risk factor for illness temporally associated with yellow fever vaccination. Emerg Infect Dis 7:945, 2001

19. Fisher-Hoch SP, Khan JA, Rehman S, et al: Crimean-Congo haemorrhagic fever treated with oral ribavirin. Lancet 346:472, 1995

20. Escutenaire S, Pastoret PP: Hantavirus infections. Rev Sci Tech 19: 64, 2000

21. McCaughey C, Hart CA: Hantaviruses. J Med Microbiol 49:587, 2000

22. Wells RM, Estani SS, Yadon ZE, et al: An unusual hantavirus outbreak in southern Argentina: person-to-person transmission? Emerg Infect Dis 3:171, 1997

23. Huggins JW, Hsiang CM, Cosgriff TM, et al: Prospective, double-blind, concurrent, placebo-controlled clinical trial of intravenous ribavirin therapy of hemorrhagic fever with renal syndrome. J Infect Dis 164:1119, 1991

24. Hooper JW, Li D: Vaccines against hantaviruses. Curr Top Microbiol Immunol 256:171, 2001

25. Enria DA, Briggiler , Pini N, et al: Clinical manifestations of New World hantaviruses. Curr Top Microbiol Immunol 256:117, 2001

26. McCormick JB, King IJ, Webb PA, et al: Lassa fever: effective therapy with ribavirin. N Engl J Med 314:20, 1986

27. Maiztegui JI, McKee KT Jr, Barrera Oro JG, et al: Protective efficacy of a live attenuated vaccine against Argentine hemorrhagic fever. J Infect Dis 177:277, 1998

28. Peters CJ, LeDuc JW: An introduction to Ebola: the virus and the disease. J Infect Dis 179(suppl 1):ix, 1999

29. Jahrling PB, Geisbert TW, Dalgard DW, et al: Preliminary report: isolation of Ebola virus from monkeys imported to USA. Lancet 335: 502, 1990

30. Miranda ME, Ksiazek TG, Retuya TJ, et al: Epidemiology of Ebola (subtype Reston) virus in the Philippines, 1996. J Infect Dis 179(suppl 1): S115, 1999

31. Outbreak of Ebola hemorrhagic fever—Uganda, August 2000–January 2001. MMWR Morb Mortal Wkly Rep 50:73, 2001

32. Bwaka MA, Bonnet MJ, Calain P, et al: Ebola hemorrhagic fever in Kikwit, Democratic Republic of the Congo: clinical observations in 103 patients. J Infect Dis 179(suppl 1):vii, 1999

33. McJunkin JE, de los Reyes EC, Irazuzta JE, et al: La Crosse encephalitis in children. N Engl J Med 344:801, 2001

34. Inactivated Japanese Encephalitis Virus Vaccine. Recommendations of the Advisory Committee on Immunization Practices (ACIP). MMWR Morb Mortal Wkly Rep 42(RR-1):1, 1993

35. Harinasuta C, Nimmanitya S, Titsyakom U: The effect of interferon-alpha A on two cases of Japanese encephalitis in Thailand. Southeast Asian J Trop Med Public Health 16:332, 1985

36. Mackenzie JS, Broom AK, Hall RA, et al: Arboviruses in the Australian region. Commun Dis Intell 22:93, 1998

37. Dumpis U, Crook D, Oksi J: Tick-borne encephalitis. Clin Infect Dis 28:882, 1999

38. Petersen LR, Roehrig JT: West Nile virus: a reemerging global pathogen. Emerg Infect Dis 7:611, 2001

39. Marfin AA, Guler DJ: West Nile encephalitis: an emerging disease in the United States. Clin Infect Dis 33:1713, 2001

40. Nash D, Mostashari F, Fine A, et al: The outbreak of West Nile virus infection in the New York City area in 1999. N Engl J Med 344: 1807, 2001

41. Mostashari F, Bunning ML, Kitsutani PT, et al: Epidemic West Nile encephalitis, New York, 1999: results of household-based seroepidemiologic survey. Lancet 358:261, 2001

42. Outbreak of Powassan encephalitis—Maine and Vermont, 1999–2000. MMWR Morb Mortal Wkly Rep 50:761, 2001

43. Krebs JW, Smith JS, Rupprecht CE, et al: Mammalian reservoirs and epidemiology of rabies diagnosed in human beings in the United States, 1981–1998. Ann NY Acad Sci 916345, 2000

44. Human rabies prevention—United States, 1999. Recommendations of the Advisory Committee on Immunization Practices (ACIP). MMWR Morb Mortal Wkly Rep 48(RR-1):1, 1999

45. Update: raccoon rabies epizootic, United States, 1996. MMWR Morb Mortal Wkly Rep 45:1117, 1997

46. Human rabies—California, Georgia, Minnesota, New York, and Wisconsin, 2000. MMWR Morb Mortal Wkly Rep 49:1111, 2000

47. Noa DL, Drenzek CL, Smith JS, et al: Epidemiology of human rabies in the United States, 1980 to 1996. Ann Intern Med 128:922, 1998

48. Goh KJ, Tan CT, Chew NK, et al: Clinical features of Nipah virus encephalitis among pig farmers in Malaysia. N Engl J Med 342:1229,2000

49. Chua KB, Bellini J, Rota PA, et al: Nipah virus: a recently emergent deadly paramyxovirus. Science 288:1432, 2000

50. Paton NI, Leo YS, Zaki SR, et al: Outbreak of Nipah-virus infection among abattoir workers in Singapore. Lancet 354:1253, 1999

51. Chong HT, Kamarulzaman A, Tan CT, et al: Treatment of acute Nipah encephalitis with ribavirin. Ann Neurol 49:810, 2001

52. Carey DE: Chikungunya and dengue: a case of mistaken identity? J Hist Med Allied Sci 26:243, 1971

53. Tesh RB, Watts DM, Russell KL et al: Mayaro virus disease: an emerging mosquito-borne zoonosis in tropical South America. Clin Infect Dis 28:67, 1998

54. Kiwanuka N, Sanders EJ, Rwaguma EB, et al: O'nyong-nyong fever in South-Central Uganda, 1996–1997: clinical features and validation of a clinical case definition for surveillance purposes. Clin Infect Dis 29: 1243, 1999

55. Gubler DJ: Transmission of Ross River virus by *Aedes polynesiensis* and *Aedes aegypti*. Am J Trop Med Hyg 30:1303, 1981

56. Ostrowski SR, Leslie MJ, Parrott T, et al: B-virus from pet macaque monkeys: an emerging threat in the United States? Emerg Infect Dis 4: 117, 1998

57. Holmes GP, Chapman LE, Stewart JA, et al: Guidelines for the prevention and treatment of B-virus infections in exposed persons. The B Virus Working Group. Clin Infect Dis 20:421, 1995

58. Human monkeypox-Kasai Oriental, Democratic Republic of Congo, February 1996-October 1997. MMWR Morb Mortal Wkly Rep 46:1168, 1997

35 Acute Viral Central Nervous System Diseases

Donald H. Gilden, M.D.

Etiology

Viral infections of the central nervous system produce aseptic meningitis, encephalitis, and sometimes vasculopathy. Although nearly all the viruses discussed in this subsection are capable of producing both meningitis and encephalitis, one form of these two diseases usually predominates. Viruses that most often cause acute aseptic meningitis include the enteroviruses (coxsackievirus, echovirus, and nonparalytic polioviruses) and the influenza and parainfluenza viruses (especially mumps virus). Herpes simplex virus type 2 (HSV-2) and, occasionally, HSV type 1 (HSV-1) cause recurrent meningitis. Viruses that primarily produce acute encephalitis include the herpesviruses (HSV-1, varicella-zoster virus [VZV], and Epstein-Barr virus [EBV]), the togaviruses (St. Louis encephalitis virus, the California encephalitis virus group, the equine encephalitis viruses, and Colorado tick fever virus), the arenaviruses (lymphocytic choriomeningitis virus [LCM]), and the adenoviruses.

The time of year that an infection occurs may be a clue for a clinician attempting to identify the causative virus [*see Table 1*]. For example, enterovirus infections occur in the summer and account for most cases of aseptic meningitis. Mumps and other parainfluenza virus infections and influenza virus infection most often present in the winter, although they may occur at any time of year. Togavirus infection occurs in the late summer and autumn (the mosquito and tick season); LCM infection presents in the early winter (when mice come indoors); and chickenpox (varicella) occurs predominantly in the spring. All HSV infections can occur at any time of year.

Clinical Manifestations of Viral Aseptic Meningitis and Encephalitis

Aseptic meningitis is associated with headache, fever, and stiff neck. Irritability and alterations in state of consciousness may occur, although these symptoms are more common in encephalitis. Patients may suffer sore throat, photophobia, abdominal discomfort, focal paresthesias, diplopia, and nausea and vomiting. An erythematous maculopapular rash results from enterovirus (echovirus or coxsackievirus) infection; a vesicular eruption

Table 1 Important Clinical Features of the Major Virus Infections of the Nervous System

Virus	*Seasons*	*Major Acute Presentation*	*Brain Imaging*
Herpes simplex virus type 1	All	Encephalitis	Medial temporal lobe
Varicella-zoster virus	All*	Localized herpes zoster, postherpetic neuralgia, encephalitis with focal deficit	Multifocal pale and hemorrhagic infarction
Enterovirus	Summer	Aseptic meningitis	Normal; possible effacement
HIV	All	Aseptic meningitis, subacute encephalitis	Atrophy; diffuse white matter attenuation
Arthropod-borne encephalitis	Summer and fall	Encephalitis	Normal; possible effacement

*Although chickenpox (varicella) occurs mostly in the spring, zoster develops at any time of the year.

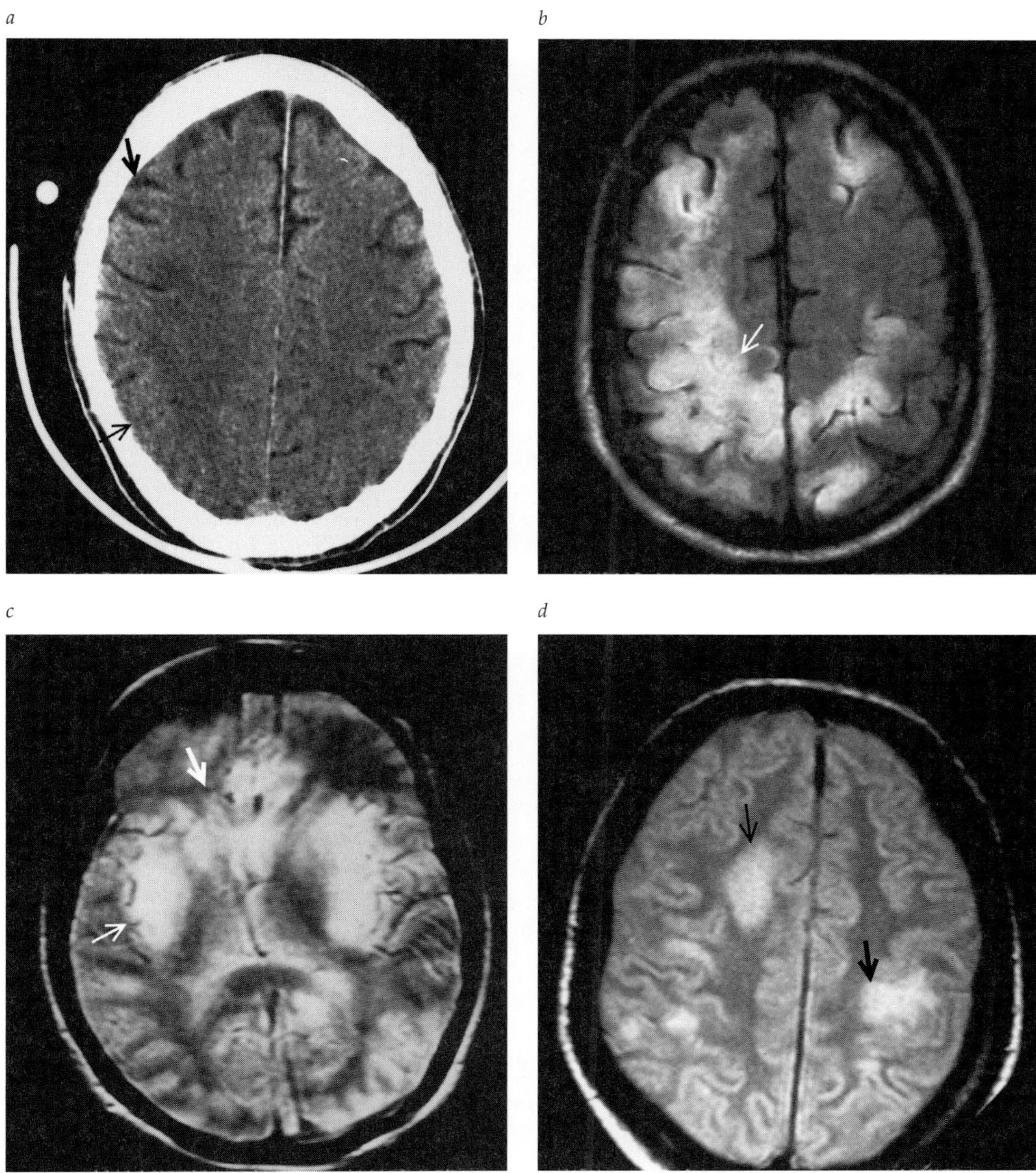

Figure 1 (*a*) CT changes that occur in most viral encephalitides. Brain computed tomography scan demonstrates relative effacement of sulci posteriorly in both hemispheres (thin arrow), compared with normal sulcal spaces anteriorly (thick arrow). (*b*) MRI changes that occur in most viral encephalitides. T_2-weighted inversion recovery (fluid-attenuated inversion recovery [FLAIR]) magnetic resonance imaging brain scan of the same patient demonstrates areas of increased signal in both hemispheres, with the increased signal being greater on the right and even more so posteriorly (arrow), reflecting increased water content in mildly swollen brain. (*c*) Herpes simplex virus encephalitis. T_2-weighted MRI brain scan demonstrates bilateral involvement of temporal lobes. The exaggerated signal does not extend beyond the insular cortex (thin arrow) but does involve the cingulate gyrus (thick arrow). (*d*) Varicella-zoster virus encephalitis. Proton-density brain MRI scan shows multiple areas of infarction in both hemispheres, particularly involving white matter (thin arrow) and extending to gray-white matter junctions (thick arrow).

suggests coxsackievirus or a herpesvirus infection. Stretching the irritated nerve roots may elicit pain. For example, in the recumbent patient, the Kernig sign is pain produced by attempts to extend the leg after flexion of the thigh. The Brudzinski sign is flexion of the thighs when the head is passively flexed onto the chest. These signs of meningeal irritation appear more often in nonviral and bacterial meningitis, however.

Clinical symptoms and signs of viral encephalitis include insomnia, lethargy, mental status changes, seizures, aphasia, and hemiplegia. Focal deficit is most common in HSV and VZV encephalitis and less common in cytomegalovirus (CMV) or EBV encephalitis. Brain imaging is usually normal but may reveal effacement [*see Figure 1a*] and increased water content [*see Figure 1b*], which is indicative of brain swelling.

Table 2 Nonviral Causes of Meningitis and Encephalitis

Behçet syndrome
Brucella infection
Cryptococcosis
Cysticerosis
Fungus
Granulomatous angiitis
Histoplasmosis
Leptospirosis (Weil disease)
Lyme disease
Mollaret meningitis*
Mycoplasma infection
Rocky Mountain spotted fever
Sarcoidosis
Syphilis
Systemic lupus erythematosus
Toxoplasmosis
Tuberculosis
Uveomeningoencephalitis (Vogt-Koyanagi-Harada syndrome)†
Whipple disease
Sulfonamides and nonsteroidal anti-inflammatory drugs‡

*Many cases are herpesvirus infections when studied by polymerase chain reaction.
†This may be viral if not autoimmune.
‡These agents mimic granulomatous meningitis.

Diagnosis of Viral Meningitis and Encephalitis

Clinical symptoms and signs alone usually cannot establish a specific diagnosis of viral meningitis or encephalitis, and nonviral causes of meningitis and encephalitis can be confused clinically with viral infections[1] [*see Table 2*]. Careful examination of the cerebrospinal fluid is the mainstay of diagnosis of viral meningitis or encephalitis. Characteristically, the CSF is clear and features a predominantly mononuclear pleocytosis and normal glucose content. Initially, the CSF may contain polymorphonuclear leukocytes. The CSF cell count is usually below 100 cells/mm^3; it may be higher with enteroviral infections, however, and the CSF may contain thousands of mononuclear cells after mumps and LCM virus infections. The CSF protein concentration is usually normal or mildly elevated. Bacteria are not found on a Gram stain, and CSF cultures are sterile. A mild depression in the CSF glucose content develops in approximately one third of patients with meningitis caused by mumps or LCM virus; this drop in CSF glucose occurs less often after enterovirus infection. In rare instances, the CSF glucose content is depressed in aseptic meningitis caused by HSV or VZV.

Most important is that a mononuclear pleocytosis with hypoglycorrhachia (low CSF glucose content) occurs in some nonviral forms of meningitis, necessitating prompt treatment; such nonviral forms include tuberculous (TB) or fungal meningitis, carcinomatous or lymphomatous meningitis, and about 30% of cases of sarcoid meningitis. Furthermore, viral aseptic meningitis may be mimicked by granulomatous meningitis (TB, fungal, sarcoid, and toxoplasmic meningitides), leptospiral infection (Lyme disease), *Brucella* infection, *Mycoplasma* pneumonia, sulfonamide or nonsteroidal anti-inflammatory drug toxicity, and various vasculitides.

Laboratory methods that are used to identify the causative agent of viral meningitis and encephalitis include polymerase chain reaction detection of viral RNA or DNA in the CSF, culturing virus from the CSF, antigen or antibody detection in the CSF, serologic tests (e.g., enzyme immunoassays and Western blot assay), and brain biopsy[1] [*see Table 3*].

Nonspecific Treatment of Viral CNS Infections

Bed rest is indicated for patients with viral CNS infection. If a patient has recently traveled to an area endemic for highly contagious agents that are spread by direct patient contact (e.g., Ebola virus), isolation procedures should be followed until the cause of the illness is established. Most other agents that cause viral meningitis and encephalitis present no special dangers to medical personnel—

Table 3 Viral Diagnosis of Aseptic Meningitis Syndrome and Encephalitis

Virus	*Tissue Culture*	*Antigen/ Antibody Detection in CSF**	*PCR*
Adenovirus	×		
Cytomegalovirus	×	×	×[60,61]
Enteroviruses	×	×	×[5]
Epstein-Barr virus		×	×[39]
Herpes simplex virus type 1	×	×	×[17,18]
Herpes simplex virus type 2	×	×	×[14,15]
HIV		×	
Influenza		×	
Measles		×	
Mumps		×	
Poliovirus	×	×	
Varicella-zoster virus	×	×	×[62]

*Results are not usually available during acute disease.

as long as antiviral precautions for blood products are followed—or to others. The patient's airway can be protected by repeated suctioning and, if necessary, by endotracheal intubation or tracheostomy. Nutritional support is important, but only conscious patients with intact brain stem function should receive oral feedings. All others should be fed by parenteral or nasogastric techniques. Patients should be monitored closely for secondary infections, especially of the urinary tract and lungs. Passive range-of-motion exercises and use of foot boards or Styrofoam boots will minimize contractures. Frequent turning decreases the risk of bedsores. Patients with encephalitis may develop the syndrome of inappropriate antidiuretic hormone secretion and become water intoxicated, which can lead to deepening coma and, sometimes, seizures. Serum and urine electrolytes and urine output should be monitored frequently. Encephalitis is treated by restricting fluid intake and, in rare instances, with hypertonic saline solution. Headache is a frequent problem and can be treated with acetaminophen, ibuprofen, and codeine; occasionally, meperidine (50 mg every 4 to 5 hours) is used. Most viruses are thermolabile, and modest temperature elevation may serve as a natural defense mechanism; but fever can be treated with acetaminophen if necessary. Specific viruses that cause aseptic meningitis, encephalitis, or both may also require particular treatment regimens.

Viruses That Cause Meningitis or Encephalitis

ENTEROVIRUSES

Enteroviruses are the most common cause of viral aseptic meningitis. Most, but not all, cases of enterovirus infection occur in children. Epidemics are common. The Picornaviridae family comprises nearly 70 distinct serotypes. People acquire enteroviruses primarily by the fecal-oral route and occasionally by the respiratory route. Fever is often biphasic. The first phase is associated with constitutional and gastroenterologic symptoms. After resolution of these symptoms, the fever may reappear with other signs and symptoms of meningeal irritation.[2] Almost all patients with enterovirus meningitis are immunocompetent. However, agammaglobulinemic enterovirus-infected persons may develop a chronic meningitis or meningoencephalitis that lasts years, and the outcome is often fatal.[3] The CSF contains between 50 and 1,000 cells, which are predominantly mononuclear. Elevated CSF protein levels are common. The CSF glucose content is usually normal, but hypoglycorrhachia has been reported.[4] The optimal time to culture virus from the CSF is 8 to 18 days after infection; PCR amplification of the conserved region of enterovirus is possible.[5] Enterovirus antibodies appear in the CSF at the end of the second week and persist longer than 1 month.

In rare instances, enteroviruses cause focal encephalitis. In addition, enterovirus infections have been associated with ataxia, opsoclonus and myoclonus,[6] and parkinsonism. In the 1998 enterovirus 71 epidemic in Taiwan, the main neurologic complication was rhombencephalitis. Myoclonic jerks were the most common initial symptoms, and MRI usually showed evidence of brain stem involvement.[7] Enteroviral infections may lead to myelitis and, occasionally, neuropathy (e.g., cranial nerve palsies). Since the eradication of poliovirus in Brazil, enterovirus 71 has emerged as a cause of persistent flaccid paralysis.[8] Chronic progressive echovirus and coxsackievirus meningoencephalitides in hypogammaglobulinemic and agammaglobulinemic persons have been treated successfully with immunoglobulin.[9]

POLIOVIRUS

Although immunization has nearly eradicated encephalomyelitis caused by type 1 poliovirus, a case of encephalomyelitis with oral-facial dyskinesias and quadriplegia was attributed to type 3 poliovirus on the basis of positive stool cultures and high neutralizing serum titers.[10]

MUMPS

The widespread use of attenuated vaccines to prevent childhood virus infections that include attenuated mumps virus as a component has dramatically reduced the incidence of mumps and mumps meningitis. Recent outbreaks of mumps meningitis have been traced to the use of incompletely attenuated mumps virus strains.

Mumps virus is a paramyxovirus that is transmitted by respiratory droplets. After the initial mucosal infection, viremia can lead to viral infection of many organs, including the heart and, in particular, the glands. The association of aseptic meningitis with parotitis, pancreatitis (abdominal pain and increased serum amylase levels), or oophoritis (abdominal pain and ovarian tenderness on pelvic examination) is a clue that mumps virus is the causative agent. One study revealed that as many as 23% of patients with mumps may develop aseptic meningitis, whereas encephalitis occurs in only one in 6,000 cases.[11] Months of persistent pleocytosis[12] and a low CSF glucose content or chronic encephalomyelitis[13] may follow mumps meningitis. Because mumps virus replicates in ependymal cells, aseptic meningitis may be followed by aqueductal stenosis and hydrocephalus months to years after an otherwise benign case of aseptic meningitis. Mumps meningoencephalitis is rarely fatal.

HERPES SIMPLEX VIRUS TYPE 2

HSV-2 Aseptic Meningitis

HSV-2 aseptic meningitis is the main neurologic complication of HSV-2, which causes genital herpes. In the United States, HSV-2 is the third most common cause of aseptic meningitis and accounts for approximately 5% of all cases. Unlike viral meningitides that have a seasonal association, HSV-2 meningitis occurs at any time of the year. The typical symptoms and signs are headache, fever, stiff neck, and a CSF with a marked lymphocytic pleocytosis. Meningitis may be preceded by genital or pelvic pain, and the astute clinician who suspects HSV-2 meningitis will ask about recent pelvic inflammatory disease symptoms or associated penile or scrotal pain. The workup for suspected HSV-2 meningitis should include a careful search for vesicular lesions over the external genitalia and a pelvic examination for lesions in the vaginal vault or cervix. PCR has revealed that the primary agent causing benign recurrent lymphocytic meningitis is HSV-2.[14,15] Occasionally, HSV-1 is the culprit, as evidenced by the detection by PCR of HSV-1 DNA in the CSF of patients with benign recurrent lymphocytic meningitis.[16] HSV-2 meningitis is self-limited, and treatment with acyclovir is not required.

HSV-2 Encephalitis

HSV-2 encephalitis is a rare disease; it occurs most often in newborns and, in rare instances, in immunocompromised adults. In both these populations, CNS infection by HSV-2 is diffuse, unlike the focal, medial temporal, and orbital frontal lesions observed in cases of HSV-1 infection. Nevertheless, seizures, alterations in state of consciousness, and focal neurologic deficit-common clinical features of HSV-1 encephalitis-also characterize HSV-2 encephalitis. AIDS predisposes a person to HSV-2 encephalitis, which frequently occurs in association with CNS infection by such other opportunistic agents as cytomegalovirus. HSV-2 encephalitis is treated with 15 to 30 mg/kg/day of acyclovir. After 10 to 14 days of intravenous acyclovir treatment, AIDS patients with HSV encephalitis may require indefinite maintenance on oral acyclovir or famciclovir to prevent further reactivation.

HERPES SIMPLEX VIRUS TYPE 1

HSV-1 Encephalitis

Unlike most viral encephalitides, HSV-1 encephalitis is focal. HSV replication in the medial temporal lobe and orbital surface of the frontal lobe, with accompanying inflammation, produces the characteristic clinical picture. Fever, headache, lethargy, irritability, and confusion are typical. Seizures (major motor, complex partial, focal, and even absence attacks) affect approximately 40% of patients. If the dominant temporal lobe is involved, aphasia and focal motor or sensory deficits develop. Progressive hemorrhagic necrosis and temporal lobe edema may lead to uncal herniation, the most common features of which are tachycardia, hyperventilation, flexor (and later extensor) posturing, and a dilated pupil (usually on the side of the herniated temporal lobe).

Because HSV becomes latent and periodically reactivates to produce recurrent herpes labialis, the misconception exists that HSV encephalitis is usually protracted or chronic. Although survivors of HSV encephalitis may have a permanent seizure disorder, mental changes, aphasia, or motor deficit, the onset of neurologic disease is usually acute or subacute, as in other viral encephalitides, and early treatment is crucial to a favorable outcome. Before acyclovir became available for treatment, approximately two thirds of patients with HSV encephalitis died.

The CSF is usually abnormal in HSV encephalitis. The CSF opening pressure is often elevated and may be very high if there is brain swelling and impending temporal lobe herniation. Clinicians usually perform the CSF examination in the first few days of illness, before there is significant brain swelling, to decrease the potential for herniation after lumbar puncture. The electroencephalogram and imaging studies may demonstrate features highly suggestive of HSV encephalitis, often obviating subsequent lumbar punctures. CSF pleocytosis is observed in more than 90% of patients, although its absence at initial evaluation does not rule out HSV encephalitis. The CSF cell count ranges from 4 to 755 cells/mm^3, and more than 200 cells/mm^3 may be present weeks after the onset of disease. The predominant cell type is mononuclear. Although unusual in other viral encephalitides, in HSV encephalitis, red blood cells (RBCs) are often present in the CSF, which may also be xanthochromic; this presumably reflects the hemorrhagic nature of brain lesions. Instead of attributing the presence of RBCs in CSF to a so-called traumatic tap, the astute clinician may use this finding to support the presumptive diagnosis of HSV encephalitis.

The majority of HSV encephalitis cases show elevated CSF protein and IgG indexes. In rare instances, hypoglycorrhachia occurs. Increased levels of antibody to HSV, suggestive of recent infection, may be found in serum and CSF; increased anti-HSV antibody ratios of CSF and serum may help diagnose HSV encephalitis. Unfortunately, increased antibody titers are not usually detected until 2 weeks or longer after the onset of disease; thus, their practical value lies more in retrospective presumptive diagnosis than in identifying acute encephalitis. Although HSV can often be isolated from cerebral biopsy or autopsy material, the isolation of HSV from CSF during acute disease is exceptional. PCR detection of HSV-1 DNA in the CSF is both sensitive and specific and has become the gold standard in suspected cases of HSV encephalitis.[17,18]

Electroencephalography Early in disease, background disorganization with generalized or focal slowing occurs, predominantly over the involved temporal region.[19] Within days, widespread, periodic, stereotyped sharp-wave and slow-wave complexes develop, usually at regular intervals of 2 to 3 seconds.[20] Bilateral periodic complexes appear if both sides of the brain are involved. Although these features can be seen in other CNS disorders (e.g., tumor, abscess, syphilis, infarct), their presence in the clinical setting of fever and rapidly progressive neurologic disease provides strong presumptive evidence for HSV encephalitis.

Imaging studies Computed tomographic scanning shows hypodense lesions involving the medial temporal regions.[21] An important diagnostic clue is a sharp transition from the hypodense temporal lesion to the normal basal ganglia.[22] Edema and mass effect occur in 80% of cases, and contrast enhancement appears in more than 50% of cases.

Magnetic resonance imaging reveals a decrease in T_1 and an increase in T_2 [*see Figure 1c*], and the signal abnormality includes a larger area of brain than CT scanning usually demonstrates. Unlike CT scanning, MRI of the temporal lobes is not subject to artifact from the petrous and sphenoid bones, which often obscure the temporal fossa.[23] A comparison of CT and MRI in four cases of HSV encephalitis showed that temporal lobe inflammation was obvious on MRI days before changes were visible on CT.[24]

Other viral and bacterial infections, cerebral abscess, tumor, and stroke can mimic the clinical features of HSV encephalitis. A focal area of decreased density and increased vascularity that extends into subcortical areas is consistent with the cerebritis that heralds frank abscess formation and helps distinguish evolving abscess from HSV encephalitis. Ring-enhancing lesions characteristic of cerebral abscess or tumor are not seen in the first few days of HSV encephalitis. Glioma and infarct are not likely to be associated with fever, and brain imaging reveals that they are not restricted to the medial temporal lobe.

Treatment Patients with HSV encephalitis should be treated with intravenous acyclovir, 15 to 30 mg/kg/day in three divided doses for at least 10 days. Early institution of acyclovir has reduced the mortality, which ranged between 60% and 70%, to slightly lower than 30%.[25] Generally, early treatment (before coma ensues) is associated with a more favorable outcome. Acyclovir appears to be safe; only mild hematologic, hepatic, and renal function abnormalities have been reported, although relapses after acyclovir therapy have been documented.[26]

Cerebral edema may be the most frequent cause of death resulting from HSV encephalitis. Treatment involves reducing the total fluid intake to between one half and two thirds of that required for maintenance and elevating the patient's head to 30 degrees. Edema is treated by intubation and hyperventilation to bring the partial pressure of carbon dioxide to 25 mmol/L. This reduces increased intracranial pressure (ICP) by constricting the intracranial vasculature. After 24 hours, hyperventilation is less effective. Steroids and osmotic agents may also control brain swelling. The benefits of a short course of steroids in instances of cerebral edema and impending herniation outweigh the small risk of potentiating HSV infection. Dexamethasone is administered intravenously at an initial dose of 10 mg, then 4 to 8 mg every 4 to 5 hours for the next 3 days. Incipient herniation may be managed with osmotic diuretics. Mannitol is given in repeated doses of 0.25 to 2.0 g/kg. The serum osmolality should be monitored closely and kept below 310 mOsm/L. The effectiveness of mannitol decreases with repeated use, and rebound increases in ICP may occur.

Anticonvulsants are used to treat seizures. For initial seizures, diazepam may be administered intravenously in doses of 2 mg/min for a maximum total dose of 15 to 20 mg; alternatively, lorazepam may be administered intravenously in doses of 2 mg/min for a maximum total dose of 5 to 10 mg. These treatments are followed by a loading dose of phenytoin (18 to 20 mg/kg) given intravenously no faster than 50 mg/min. Maintenance doses of phenytoin average between 300 and 400 mg/day. The clinician should guide therapy according to blood levels, side effects, and absence of seizures. Anticonvulsants should be continued for several months after the acute illness. No controlled studies exist on the prophylactic use of steroids or anticonvulsants in HSV encephalitis.

HSV Neuropathy (Zosteriform Eruption)

Numerous reports document a dermatomal distribution of pain and sensory loss in association with zosteriform eruption. The syndrome is usually characterized by a prodrome of diffuse neuralgia, often with malaise and fever, followed within a few days by vesicular eruption.[27] Most reports describe lesions on the face in one or more areas served by the trigeminal nerve. Zosteriform eruptions attributed to HSV have also been described on the trunk, extremities, and genitalia. A first episode may be confused with herpes zoster, but recurrent episodes of dermatomal neuralgic pain and zosteriform eruptions are almost always caused by HSV. One report of recurrent sciatica associated with HSV is particularly interesting.[28]

Although the clinical entity of HSV neuropathy is now well documented, more information is needed about each HSV type. Because there are regions of homology between HSV-1 and HSV-2 and because antibody typing was done before the development of monoclonal antibodies, the exact type of HSV responsible for each disease is still unknown. Clinicians attribute herpes lesions above the neck to the reactivation of HSV-1, whereas lesions below the waist are attributed to the reactivation of HSV-2. Future serotyping with monospecific polyclonal or monoclonal antibodies and DNA analysis of herpes isolates by PCR with primers specific for HSV-1 or HSV-2 will identify whether herpes neuropathy is caused primarily by HSV-1 or HSV-2.

Most accounts of HSV neuropathy were made before the development of acyclovir or famciclovir. Because each drug will probably reduce the number of days that patients have pain and rash, treatment with oral acyclovir (800 mg five times daily) or famciclovir (500 mg three times daily) for 7 to 10 days is reasonable. Neither HSV-1 nor HSV-2 can be eradicated by antiviral therapy. Rather, resolution of acute disease is followed by a return of the herpesvirus to the latent state and the potential for future reactivation.

VARICELLA-ZOSTER VIRUS

VZV causes chickenpox (varicella) in childhood and becomes latent in dorsal root ganglia. Reactivation decades later produces shingles (herpes zoster), the most common cause of virus-induced neurologic disease in adults. The incidence of herpes zoster in the United States is 131 per 100,000 persons per year; approximately 50% of persons 80 years of age and older have had herpes zoster once. Herpes zoster and its attendant complications [*see Figure 2*] are more common in immunocompromised patients, especially persons with AIDS, and elderly populations. A continuing increase in the number of elderly persons will result in greater herpes zoster–associated morbidity and mortality.

Herpes Zoster

Herpes zoster is characterized by pain and vesicular rash on an erythematous base in one to three dermatomes (localized zoster). Approximately 300,000 cases of herpes zoster are seen annually. It occurs eight to 10 times more frequently in persons older than 60 years. Fewer than 10% of cases of herpes zoster are recurrent. Although chickenpox occurs primarily in the spring, herpes zoster occurs at any time of the year. There is no sex bias. Most herpes zoster cases reflect VZV reactivation from the dorsal root ganglia. In rare instances, cases of

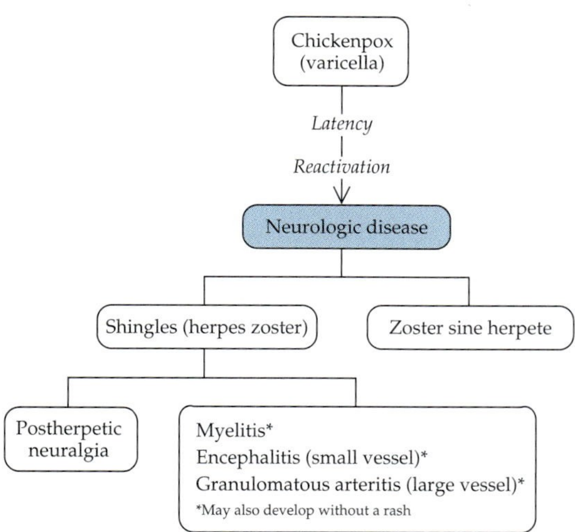

Figure 2 **The neurologic complications of varicella-zoster virus reactivation.**

herpes zoster are clustered in time, supporting the notion that herpes zoster can be acquired by exogenous reinfection. Herpes zoster strikes immunocompromised patients more frequently than those with intact immune systems. Before the AIDS era, herpes zoster occurred most often in bone marrow transplant recipients and patients with leukemia, particularly those who had received radiation therapy; herpes zoster developed at the irradiated site. In my experience, long-term, low-dose steroid therapy also predisposes patients to the serious complications of VZV reactivation, including postherpetic neuralgia (PHN), disseminated herpes zoster, and herpes zoster encephalitis.

Clinical features Herpes zoster pain is severe, deep, burning, and jabbing and usually lasts 4 to 6 weeks. Examination reveals both hypesthesia and hyperpathia in a dermatomal distribution with mixed hypopigmentation and hyperpigmentation. Except for its longer duration, acute herpes zoster pain does not differ from the pain of PHN. Herpes zoster may involve any dermatome. The trunk, represented by 12 pairs of thoracic ganglia, is the most frequently involved site. The face, which is supplied by the trigeminal nerve, is involved more often than any single thoracic dermatome, however.

Trigeminal distribution of herpes zoster most frequently occurs in the ophthalmic branch. Cranial neuropathies often occur weeks or months after cutaneous signs, perhaps because of microinfarction of cranial nerves from occlusion of the vasa vasorum. The blood supply of the cranial nerves is part of the carotid circulation. Because trigeminal afferent nerves innervate the large extracranial and intracranial blood vessels, virus can also spread along ganglionic afferent fibers to small vessels supplying cranial nerves, in a manner similar to that proposed to explain the pathogenesis of VZV-induced granulomatous arteritis. Peripheral facial weakness, an abnormality of the cranial nerves, is often associated with vesicles in the ear (herpes zoster oticus); the combination of these conditions constitutes the Ramsay Hunt syndrome.

Herpes zoster in cervical or lumbosacral dermatomes may be associated with muscle weakness. The incidence of herpes zoster paresis varies from as low as 0.5% to as high as 31%. Bladder and bowel dysfunction are often associated with a sacral distribution of herpes zoster.

Treatment of acute herpes zoster The treatment of acute herpes zoster is controversial. Oral acyclovir at a dosage of 800 mg taken five times daily or famciclovir at a dosage of 500 mg taken three times daily during acute disease reduces the duration of rash but does not decrease either acute or long-term pain (PHN). Because the sensitivity of VZV in vitro to acyclovir is less than that of HSV, the clinician may need to treat acute herpes zoster with higher doses of acyclovir and for a longer duration than is currently used.

Complications of herpes zoster infection Postherpetic neuralgia, defined as pain persisting longer than 4 to 6 weeks after the appearance of herpes zoster rash, is the most common complication of herpes zoster. Age is the most important factor in predicting the development of PHN. The incidence of PHN is 46.9% in patients 60 years of age and older[29] and varies from 0% to 15% in patients younger than 60 years; most of these cases occur in patients between 50 and 60 years of age. PHN is slightly more common in women than in men, but in both sexes, it occurs more often after an ophthalmic distribution of herpes zoster.

Analgesics are used to reduce the pain of PHN; narcotics are avoided, if possible. Starting with 25 mg at night, amitriptyline can be gradually increased to 150 mg daily. Side effects include postural hypotension, confusion, and urinary retention. Carbamazepine may help, but doses in excess of 600 mg daily are usually required, and side effects of sleepiness, confusion, and unsteadiness, particularly in the elderly, may be intolerable. Carbamazepine should be started at doses of 100 mg daily and gradually increased by 100 mg every third day until pain decreases. Transcutaneous electrical nerve stimulation units, nerve blocks, and rhizotomy do not usually provide long-term relief. Local application of capsaicin, triethanolamine salicylate (Aspercreme), or Flex-all 454 is useful if the agent is applied alternatively throughout the day and before sleep.

Studies linking PHN with VZV persistence[30] provide a rationale to treat with high-dose acyclovir for more than 10 days to reduce the virus burden. Further studies are needed to determine whether acyclovir, with or without steroids, initiated at the onset of herpes zoster prevents PHN and whether short-term, high-dose acyclovir is an effective treatment for PHN.

Zoster Sine Herpete

Prolonged radicular pain without rash is sometimes thought to be zoster sine herpete. Until recently, investigators lacked support that zoster sine herpete is caused by viral infection. This nosologic entity was verified in two men, ages 62 and 66, who developed radicular pain that persisted for years. The pain did not differ from that of PHN. VZV DNA, but not HSV DNA, was found in the CSF of both men 5 to 8 months after the onset of pain.[31] Treatment with intravenous acyclovir, 10 to 15 mg/kg every 8 hours for 14 days, followed by oral acyclovir, relieved pain in both patients.

VZV Encephalitis and Arteritis

CNS disease is the most alarming complication of herpes zoster. Two conditions predominate: small vessel encephalitis, primarily in immunocompromised individuals, and large vessel granulomatous arteritis in immunocompetent patients.

Small vessel herpes zoster encephalitis Small vessel herpes zoster encephalitis is the most common form of CNS involvement. Disease develops on a background of cancer, immunosuppression,[32] and AIDS. Neurologic disease is subacute, and death is common. Herpes zoster encephalitis presents as headache, fever, vomiting, mental changes, seizures, and focal deficit. Because VZV encephalitis is predominantly a small vessel vasculopathy, brain imaging reveals large and small ischemic or hemorrhagic infarcts-often both-of cortex and subcortical gray and white matter [*see Figure 1d*]. Deep-seated white-matter lesions often predominate and are ischemic or demyelinative. The demyelinative lesions are smaller and less coalescent than those seen in progressive multifocal leukoencephalopathy. The CSF shows a mild to moderate pleocytosis (predominantly mononuclear), normal or mildly elevated concentrations of CSF protein, and a normal CSF glucose content-findings that do not differ significantly from herpes zoster without encephalitis. Hypoglycorrhachia has been reported in herpes zoster meningoencephalitis.[33] Treatment of herpes zoster encephalitis includes acyclovir at a dosage of 15 to 30 mg/kg/day in three divided doses for 10 days. Longer treatment may be necessary in severely immunocompromised patients.

Large vessel herpes zoster granulomatous arteritis The salient feature of this form of VZV-induced CNS disease is an acute focal deficit that develops weeks or months after a contralateral trigeminal distribution of herpes zoster. Stroke results from a necrotizing arteritis, primarily of large cerebral arteries. One comprehensive review showed that most patients with large vessel encephalitis were older than 60 years and that there was no sex bias.[34] The mean onset of neurologic disease was 7 weeks, and the longest interval between the onset of herpes zoster and the onset of neurologic disease was 6 months. Transient ischemic attacks and mental symptoms were common. Twenty-five percent of patients died. The majority of patients had CSF pleocytosis, usually fewer than 100 cells (predominantly mononuclear), oligoclonal bands, and increased CSF IgG. Besides contralateral hemiplegia, ipsilateral central retinal artery occlusion and posterior circulation involvement have been described. Angiographic examination has revealed focal constriction and segmental narrowing, primarily in middle cerebral, internal carotid, and anterior cerebral arteries. Microscopic examination has revealed a necrotizing arteritis (primarily involving the intima and adventitia), inflammation with multinucleated giant cells, VZV antigen, Cowdry type A inclusions, and herpesvirus particles. Most herpes zoster-associated granulomatous angiitis infarcts are pale,[35] but hemorrhagic infarction also occurs. Afferent trigeminal ganglionic fibers to both intracranial and extracranial blood vessels provide an anatomic pathway for the spread of virus.

Clinicians do not have a definitive treatment for large vessel herpes zoster encephalitis, because it is not clear whether disease is exclusively viral, a virus-induced immunopathology, or both. Nevertheless, on the basis of pathologic changes, a strong case can be made for using acyclovir (to kill persistent replicating virus) and steroids (for their anti-inflammatory effect).

EPSTEIN-BARR VIRUS

EBV causes infectious mononucleosis and has been implicated as a cause of nasopharyngeal carcinoma and Burkitt lymphoma. EBV is ubiquitous. Primary infection of most humans usually occurs in childhood or adolescence. By 30 years of age, more than 90% of adults have antibody to EBV. Despite the prevalence of EBV infection, neurologic disease is rare. The most common presentation is meningoencephalitis, which is often associated with acute cerebellar ataxia. More serious meningoencephalopathy, presenting as athetosis and chorea or as stupor and coma, has been described. In a fascinating case of acute demyelinating encephalopathy after EBV infection, a patient presented with behavioral abnormalities, visual illusions, and a seizure.[36] EBV mononucleosis may also be followed by recurrent aseptic meningitis. Chronic active EBV infection has been associated with calcification in the basal ganglia.[37] EBV-associated cranial neuropathies,[38] including acute autonomic neuropathy,[39] have been described. Detection of EBV DNA in CSF has been used to diagnose infection in the peripheral[39] and central nervous systems.[40] There is no specific treatment.

CYTOMEGALOVIRUS

CMV produces neurologic disease, primarily in infants, as part of the clinical spectrum of congenital CMV infection. Although most congenital CMV infections are asymptomatic, many carriers develop sensorineural hearing loss and intellectual handicaps. Other neurologic complications of congenital infections include microcephaly, seizures, hypotonia, and spasticity. Lethargy and coma may follow a severe case of CMV meningoencephalitis.

In immunocompetent adults, the most common neurologic complication of CMV infection is the Guillain-Barré syndrome. The association was made on the basis of the following findings: the isolation of CMV from buffy coat of blood, the development of CMV IgM antibodies in serum,[41] and the demonstration of a fourfold or greater alteration in complement-fixing antibody to CMV in 21 of 92 patients with acute polyneuritis.[42] CMV infection has also been associated with acute brachial plexopathy.[43]

Until the AIDS era, CMV infection of the CNS was rare. A few cases of CMV encephalitis in immunocompetent adults were characterized by mental status changes and pyramidal signs. Because the natural history of CMV encephalitis in immunocompetent persons is not known, no treatment protocols have been established. However, two patients with presumptive CMV encephalitis, verified by the isolation of CMV from CSF and urine, were treated with vidarabine and responded well.[44] In contrast to the rare occurrences of CMV infection in the immunocompetent adult, CMV infections in the immunocompromised population, particularly AIDS patients, are common. CMV has now emerged as an important cause of encephalitis, myelitis, and polyradiculitis. CMV encephalitis was first documented in renal transplant[45] and bone marrow transplant recipients; an interesting case of CMV vasculitis and retinitis in a lymphoma patient receiving multiple cytotoxic and anti-inflammatory drugs was also reported.[46] In AIDS patients, CMV is the most common opportunistic infectious agent found in the nervous system. Complications include retinitis, encephalitis,[47] progressive myelitis, and polyradiculopathy. CMV encephalitis is usually subacute and characterized by headache, seizures, progressive dementia, and diffuse weakness. Thus, neurologic deficit may be diffuse, focal, or both.

Like other herpesviruses, CMV can establish a latent infection in persons with intact immune systems. The lymphoid system is the most likely site for viral latency. The source of CMV encephalitis may be circulating lymphocytes. Perhaps because of the ill-defined clinical picture, the diagnosis of CMV encephalitis has been made at autopsy in most cases. The CSF may show a neutrophilic or mononuclear pleocytosis, elevated protein concentration, and depressed glucose content, but these findings are hardly specific, particularly in immunosuppressed patients. MRIs may show enhancement in the ventricular ependyma, a finding that is highly suggestive of CMV ventriculitis or encephalitis. Focal disease has been attributed to CMV vasculitis or foci of demyelination. Characteristic owl-eyed cytomegalic inclusions and CMV-specific antigens have been found in the CNS and blood vessels of AIDS patients with subacute encephalopathy. Complicating the picture, however, is the additional presence of HIV or HSV-2. Thus, the attribution of specific symptoms and signs to CMV is difficult. The organism can occasionally be isolated from the CSF of AIDS patients.

Of particular interest is the occurrence in AIDS patients of a CMV polyradiculoneuropathy. Disease often begins insidiously as a cauda equina syndrome with paresthesias and distal weakness (which is usually asymmetrical), incontinence, and sacral-distribution sensory loss. CSF pleocytosis is usually present; either polymorphonuclear leukocytes or mononuclear cells may predominate; CSF protein concentration may be elevated; hypoglycorrhachia may be present; and, occasionally, CMV is isolated from CSF. Postmortem examination reveals inflammation, necrosis, and focal vasculitis of nerve roots, with typical CMV intranuclear and intracytoplasmic inclusions.[48]

Ganciclovir and foscarnet demonstrate high activity against CMV, although formal trials have not been performed to establish dosage or treatment length. Measurement of viral load in the CSF by PCR is a potential way to assess therapeutic efficacy. CMV infections of the nervous system are currently best treated with intravenous ganciclovir, 5 mg/kg every 12 hours for 2 weeks, followed by maintenance therapy of 5 mg/kg of ganciclovir daily. Patients may need maintenance therapy for life to prevent relapse. Oral ganciclovir was recently approved for maintenance therapy in AIDS patients. The recommended maintenance dosage is 1,000 mg three times daily with food or 500 mg six times daily every 3 hours with food. The main side effect of ganciclovir is neutropenia. The drug should be stopped if the total white cell count falls below 750 cells/mm^3.

RETROVIRUS

HIV infects the meninges early and persists in the CNS after primary infection. Aseptic meningitis affects 5% to 10% of HIV-infected patients just before seroconversion or after a mononucleosis-like syndrome that is characterized by headache, fever, altered mental status, and focal or generalized seizures. HIV infection is verified by the presence of p24 antigen in serum or the CSF, and proof of infection is aided by evidence of seroconversion 1 or 2 months later. Acute meningoencephalitis is usually self-limited, although slowly progressive HIV encephalitis with mental status changes and motor deficit may follow [see 14 HIV and AIDS].

INFLUENZA VIRUS

Acute encephalitis has been reported during the height of influenza epidemics. Mental and motor deficits (including ataxia) and a CSF lymphocytic pleocytosis, in association with rising complement-fixing and hemagglutination-inhibiting antibody titers to influenza virus, provide presumptive evidence of influenza encephalitis.[49]

ARTHROPOD-BORNE ENCEPHALITIS VIRUS

Arthropod-borne viruses include the virus families Togaviridae (alphaviruses and flaviviruses), Bunyaviridae, and Orbiviridae-all RNA viruses. Humans are infected by mosquito bites or ticks. Mosquitoes are infected by biting infected horses or birds. Human infection occurs in the summer and early fall. Human epidemics often follow epidemics in horses, the migration of infected birds, and the infection of rodents. Typical symptoms and signs of infection include headache, photophobia, myalgia, fever, lethargy, confusion, and seizures. Tremor and focal deficit may develop. The CSF pattern is the same as in aseptic meningitis. A specific diagnosis can be verified by the following means: virus isolation from CSF, the production of encephalitis in suckling mice inoculated with infected CSF, the development of a cytopathic effect in tissue culture cells inoculated with infected CSF, the detection of virus-specific antibody in CSF, the presence of virus-specific IgM during acute disease, or a rising titer of virus-specific IgG in sera during the acute and convalescent stages of the disease.

In the United States, the most common arbovirus infection is St. Louis encephalitis (SLE), followed by Western equine encephalitis (WEE), California virus encephalitis, and Eastern equine encephalitis (EEE). SLE is transmitted mostly by mosquitoes. Nervous system infections usually produce encephalitis, although aseptic meningitis occurs in about 15% of cases. Prominent opsoclonus and tremulousness[50] and brain stem involvement have been described. Nearly all SLE cases are self-limited, although approximately 3% to 4% of cases are fatal.

In 1999, an outbreak of encephalitis accompanied by severe weakness and axonal neuropathy occurred in New York. Initial serologic analysis attributed disease to SLE virus in five of six patients. More extensive molecular analysis, however, identified the virus responsible as a Kunjin/West Nile–like flavivirus, part of the Japanese encephalitis virus serogroup.[51] Neither the Kunjin nor the West Nile virus had been previously reported in the Americas. In October 1999, the Centers for Disease Control and Prevention positively identified the causative etiologic agent as West Nile virus.[52]

The bunyaviruses are transmitted by mosquitoes and cause California encephalitis; La Crosse virus is the most common. Nearly all cases occur in children. Although encephalitis is usually mild, 50% of victims have seizures, and focal deficits and focal EEG abnormalities are seen in 20% to 40% of patients.[53] More than 50% of patients with EEE die, and mental, visual, auditory, speech, and motor deficits remain in more than 80% of survivors. MRI often reveals focal increased signal intensity in the basal ganglia and thalamus[54] that distinguishes EEE from HSV encephalitis. WEE has a case-fatality rate of approximately 10%; it is more severe in infants and children and may produce transient parkinsonism.[55] Powassan encephalitis is caused by a flavivirus transported by ticks. Orbivirus infection causes Colorado tick fever. Arbovirus encephalitis has no specific treatment.

ADENOVIRUSES

Adenoviruses are large DNA viruses that usually cause outbreaks of acute respiratory illness, keratoconjunctivitis, and, occasionally, pneumonia. Different adenovirus serotypes produce meningoencephalitis. Although the incidence of CNS disease after adenovirus infection is unknown, the mortality after CNS infection ranges from 26% to 38%.[56] A fascinating case of subacute focal encephalitis in an immunocompromised man from whom type 32 adenovirus was isolated from the brain has been described.[57]

ARENAVIRUSES

The arenaviruses are RNA viruses endemic in rodents. Human infection, which occurs mostly in South America and Africa, produces various hemorrhagic fevers that are often fatal. In the United States, the most common arenavirus infection is produced by lymphocytic choriomeningitis virus (LCM). Infection is acquired from mice, pet hamsters, and laboratory personnel working with the virus. Most cases present as aseptic meningitis, but fatal meningoencephalitis also occurs. A recent report described LCM preceded by a lupuslike syndrome that included rash and the presence of a circulating anticoagulant.[58] As with mumps, orchitis and parotitis may develop concurrently with CNS disease[59]; profound mononuclear pleocytosis and hypoglycorrhachia are also produced. A specific diagnosis can be made by observing the development of choriomeningitis in weanling or adult mice inoculated intracerebrally with infected CSF or by observing the development of LCM-specific antibody in the serum or CSF of infected humans.

Acknowledgments

Figure 1a Courtesy of Dr. Elliott Sandberg, Department of Radiology, the University of Colorado School of Medicine, Denver.
Figure 1d From "The vasculopathy of varicella-zoster virus encephalitis," by C. Amlie-Lefond, B. K. Kleinschmidt-DeMasters, R. Mahalingam, et al, in *Annals of Neurology* 37:784, 1995. Used by permission.

References

1. Greenberg SB: Viral meningitis and encephalitis. Office Practice of Neurology. Samuels MA, Feske S, Eds. Churchill Livingstone, New York, 1996, p 403

2. Wilfert CM, Lehrman SN, Katz SL: Enteroviruses and meningitis. Pediatr Infect Dis 2:333, 1983

3. McKinney RE Jr, Katz SL, Wilfert CM: Chronic enteroviral meningoencephalitis in agammaglobulinemic patients. Rev Infect Dis 9:334, 1987

4. Malcom BS, Eiden JJ, Hendley JO: ECHO virus type 9 meningitis simulating tuberculous meningitis. Pediatrics 65:725, 1980

5. Rotbart HA, Levin MJ, Villarreal LP: Use of subgenomic poliovirus DNA hybridization probes to detect the major subgroups of enteroviruses. J Clin Microbiol 20:1105, 1984

6. Kuban KC, Ephros MA, Freeman FL, et al: Syndrome of opsoclonus-myoclonus caused by coxsackie B3 infection. Ann Neurol 13:69, 1983

7. Huang C-C, Liu C-C, Chang Y-C, et al: Neurologic complications in children with enterovirus 71 infection. N Engl J Med 341:936, 1999

8. da Silva EE, Winkler MT, Pallansch MA: Role of enterovirus 71 in acute flaccid paralysis after the eradication of poliovirus in Brazil. Emerg Infect Dis 2:231, 1996

9. Geller TJ, Condie D: A case of protracted coxsackie virus meningoencephalitis in a marginally immunodeficient child treated successfully with intravenous immunoglobulin. J Neurol Sci 129:131, 1995

10. Rosenberg RN, Chadwick DL: Oral-facial dyskinesia and quadriplegia associated with poliomyelitis virus type 3. Am J Dis Child 126: 699, 1973

11. Russell RR, Donald JC: The neurological complications of mumps. Br Med J 2:27, 1958

12. Azimi PH, Shaban S, Hilty MD, et al: Mumps meningoencephalitis: prolonged abnormality of cerebrospinal fluid. JAMA 234:1161, 1975

13. Vaheri A, Julkunen I, Koskiniemi M-L: Chronic encephalomyelitis with specific increase in intrathecal mumps antibody. Lancet 2:685, 1982

14. Cohen BA, Rowley AH, Long CM: Herpes simplex type 2 in a patient with Mollaret's meningitis: demonstration by polymerase chain reaction. Ann Neurol 35:112, 1994

15. Tedder DG, Ashley R, Tyler KL, et al: Herpes simplex virus infection as a cause of benign recurrent lymphocytic meningitis. Ann Intern Med 121:334, 1994

16. Yamamoto LJ, Tedder DG, Ashley R, et al: Herpes simplex virus type 1 DNA in cerebrospinal fluid of a patient with Mollaret's meningitis. N Engl J Med 325:1082, 1991

17. Aurelius E, Johansson B, Sköldenberg B, et al: Rapid diagnosis of herpes simplex encephalitis by nested polymerase chain reaction assay of cerebrospinal fluid. Lancet 337:189, 1991

18. Lakeman FD, Whitley RJ: Diagnosis of herpes simplex encephalitis: application of polymerase chain reaction to cerebrospinal fluid from brain-biopsied patients and correlation with disease: National Institute of Allergy and Infectious Diseases Collaborative Antiviral Study Group. J Infect Dis 171:857, 1995

19. Westmoreland BF: The EEG in cerebral inflammatory processes. Electroencephalography, 2nd ed. Niedermeyer E, Lopes da Silva FH, Eds. Urban & Schwarzenberg, Baltimore-Munich, 1987, p 261

20. Smith JB, Westmoreland BF, Reagan TJ, et al: A distinctive clinical EEG profile in herpes simplex encephalitis. Mayo Clin Proc 50:469, 1975

21. Dutt MK, Johnston IDA: Computed tomography and EEG in herpes simplex encephalitis. Arch Neurol 39:99, 1982

22. Zimmerman RD, Russell EJ, Leeds NE: CT in the early diagnosis of herpes simplex encephalitis. Am J Radiol 134:61, 1980

23. ter Penning B: Inflammatory disease of the brain and spine. Craniospinal Magnetic Resonance Imaging. Pomeranz SJ, Ed. WB Saunders, Philadelphia, 1989, p 436

24. Schroth G, Gawehn J, Thron A, et al: Early diagnosis of herpes simplex encephalitis by MRI. Neurology 37:179, 1987

25. Whitley RJ, Alford CA, Hirsch MS, et al: Vidarabine versus acyclovir therapy in herpes simplex encephalitis. N Engl J Med 314:144, 1986

26. Knezevic W, Carrol WM: Relapse of herpes simplex encephalitis after acyclovir therapy. Aust N Z J Med 13:625, 1983

27. Krohel GB, Richardson JR, Farrell DF: Herpes simplex neuropathy. Neurology 26:596, 1976

28. Morris HH III, Peters BH: Recurrent sciatica associated with herpes simplex: case report. J Neurosurg 41:97, 1974

29. Rogers RS, Tindall JP: Geriatric herpes zoster. J Am Geriatr Soc 19: 495, 1971

30. Mahalingam R, Wellish M, Brucklier J, et al: Persistence of varicella-zoster virus DNA in elderly patients with postherpetic neuralgia. J Neurovirol 1:130, 1995

31. Gilden DH, Wright RR, Schneck SA, et al: Zoster sine herpete, a clinical variant. Ann Neurol 35:530, 1994

32. Horton B, Price RW, Jimenez D: Multifocal varicella-zoster virus leukoencephalitis temporally remote from herpes zoster. Ann Neurol 9:251, 1981

33. Reimer LG, Reller LB: CSF in herpes zoster meningo-encephalitis. Arch Neurol 38:668, 1981

34. Hilt DC, Buchholz D, Krumholz A, et al: Herpes zoster ophthalmicus and delayed contralateral hemiparesis caused by cerebral angiitis: diagnosis and management approaches. Ann Neurol 14:543, 1983

35. Kuroiwa Y, Furukawa T: Hemispheric infarction after herpes zoster ophthalmicus: computed tomography and angiography. Neurology 31: 1030, 1981

36. Paskavitz JF, Anderson CA, Filley CM, et al: Acute arcuate fiber demyelinating encephalopathy following Epstein-Barr virus infection. Ann Neurol 38:127, 1995

37. Morita M, Tsuge I, Matsuoka H, et al: Calcification in the basal ganglia with chronic active Epstein-Barr virus infection. Neurology 50:1485, 1998

38. Salazar A, Martinez H, Sotelo J: Ophthalmoplegic polyneuropathy associated with infectious mononucleosis (letter). Ann Neurol 13:219, 1983

39. Bennett JL, Mahalingam R, Wellish MC, et al: Epstein-Barr virus–associated acute autonomic neuropathy. Ann Neurol 40:453, 1996

40. Tselis A, Duman R, Storch GA, et al: Epstein-Barr virus encephalomyelitis diagnosed by polymerase chain reaction: detection of the genome in the CSF. Neurology 48:1351, 1997

41. Kabins S, Keller R, Peitchel RT, et al: Acute idiopathic polyneuritis caused by cytomegalovirus. Arch Intern Med 136:100, 1976

42. Dowling P, Menonna J, Cook S: Cytomegalovirus complement fixation antibody in Guillain-Barré syndrome. Neurology 27:1153, 1977

43. Duchowny M, Caplan L, Siber G: Cytomegalovirus infection of the adult nervous system. Ann Neurol 5:458, 1979

44. Phillips CA, Fanning WL, Gump DW, et al: Cytomegalovirus encephalitis in immunologically normal adults: successful treatment with vidarabine. JAMA 238:2299, 1977

45. Schneck SA: Neuropathological features of human organ transplantation: I. Probable cytomegalovirus infection. J Neuropathol Exp Neurol 24:415, 1965

46. Koeppen AH, Lansing LS, Peng S-K, et al: Central nervous system vasculitis in cytomegalovirus infection. J Neurol Sci 51:395, 1981

47. Laskin OL, Stahl-Bayliss CM, Morgello S: Concomitant herpes simplex virus type 1 and cytomegalovirus ventriculoencephalitis in acquired immunodeficiency syndrome. Arch Neurol 44:843, 1987

48. Eidelberg D, Sotrel A, Vogel H, et al: Progressive polyradiculopathy in acquired immune deficiency syndrome. Neurology 36:912, 1986

49. Horner FA: Neurologic disorders after Asian influenza. N Engl J Med 258:983, 1958

50. Estrin WJ: The serological diagnosis of St Louis encephalitis in a patient with the syndrome of opsoclonia, body tremulousness, and benign encephalitis. Ann Neurol 1:596, 1977

51. Briese T, Xi-Yu J, Huang C, et al: Identification of a Kunjin/West Nile–like flavivirus in brains of patients with New York encephalitis. Lancet 354:1261, 1999

52. Update: West Nile virus encephalitis—New York, 1999. MMWR Morb Mortal Wkly Rep 48:944, 1999

53. Balfour HH Jr, Siem RA, Bauer H, et al: California arbovirus (La Crosse) infections: I. Clinical and laboratory findings in 66 children with meningoencephalitis. Pediatrics 52:680, 1973

54. Deresiewicz RL, Thaler SJ, Hsu L, et al: Clinical and neuroradiographic manifestations of eastern equine encephalitis. N Engl J Med 336:1867, 1997

55. Schultz DR, Barthal JS, Garrett C: Western equine encephalitis with rapid onset of parkinsonism. Neurology 27:1095, 1977

56. Similä S, Jouppila R, Salmi A, et al: Encephalomeningitis in children associated with an adenovirus type 7 epidemic. Acta Paediatr Scand 59: 310, 1970

57. Chou SM, Roos R, Burrell R, et al: Subacute focal adenovirus encephalitis. J Neuropathol Exp Neurol 32:34, 1973

58. Schanen A, Gallou G, Hincky J-M, et al: A rash, circulating anticoagulant, then meningitis. Lancet 351:1956, 1998

59. Lewis JM, Utz JP: Orchitis, parotitis and meningoencephalitis due to lymphocytic-choriomeningitis virus. N Engl J Med 265:776, 1961

60. Wolf DG, Spector SA: Diagnosis of human cytomegalovirus central nervous system disease in AIDS patients by DNA amplification from cerebrospinal fluid. J Infect Dis 166:1412, 1992

61. Cinque P, Vago L, Brytting M, et al: Cytomegalovirus infection of the central nervous system in patients with AIDS: diagnosis by DNA amplification from cerebrospinal fluid. J Infect Dis 166:1408, 1992

62. Amlie-Lefond C, Kleinschmidt-DeMasters BK, Mahalingam R, et al: The vasculopathy of varicella zoster virus encephalitis. Ann Neurol 37: 784, 1995

Table 1 Stages of HIV Dementia (AIDS Dementia Complex)[1]

Stage	*Characteristics*
0 (normal)	Normal mental and motor function
0.5 (subclinical)	Minimal or equivocal symptoms; no impairment of work; can perform tasks of daily life; few, if any, neurologic signs; and normal motor function
1 (mild)	Mild but unequivocal evidence of functional and intellectual impairment, although able to perform all but the most demanding tasks of work or daily life; ambulatory without assistance
2 (moderate)	Incapacitated for work but able to perform basic tasks of daily life; may need unilateral assistance for walking (cane)
3 (severe)	Major intellectual dysfunction, with slowing of mental processes or severe motor disability, requiring bilateral assistance for ambulation
4 (end stage)	Nearly vegetative, with minimal intellectual and social comprehension; nearly mute and paraparetic or paraplegic

well-controlled studies is that cognitive deterioration is not a feature of the relatively asymptomatic period between primary infection and the decline in the CD4+ T cell count,[7] even though there is active viral replication in the peripheral tissue.[8,9]

HIVD is a subcortical dementia, and psychomotor slowing, apathy, and such motor symptoms as ataxia and paralysis can precede memory loss and the deterioration of language function. In its end stages [*see Table 1*], persons with HIVD may be nearly vegetative.

The diagnosis of HIVD depends on the exclusion of other causes of dementia in an HIV-infected patient. Cerebrospinal fluid abnormalities (i.e., elevated protein, decreased cell count, and intrathecal synthesis of HIV antibody) are characteristic of HIV infection but are not specific for HIVD. The presence of HIV in the CSF is also not diagnostic of HIVD, as both cell-free and cell-associated virus can be cultured from the CSF of persons who do not manifest CNS symptoms. However, there may be a rough correlation between the level of viral RNA in the CSF and the incidence of HIVD. Magnetic resonance imaging studies have indicated that HIVD is associated with global atrophy of the brain, but a high background of atrophy is present in many persons with AIDS; thus, this finding is more useful for research than for diagnosis. Similarly, some metabolic abnormalities detectable with magnetic resonance spectroscopy point to neuronal destruction but cannot yet be used diagnostically.

Pathologic Features

The major neuropathologic findings associated with HIVD are (1) multinucleated giant cell encephalitis (MGCE) [*see Figure 2*], (2) HIV leukoencephalopathy (myelin pallor and other white matter changes), and (3) astrocytosis and perhaps neuronal dropout. MGCE, which is the most specific neuropathologic finding in HIVD, is present in approximately 25% of persons who have been diagnosed clinically and is characterized by microglial syncytia that may contain HIV-specific nucleic acid and antigens. MGCE is characteristically more prominent in the basal ganglia and other subcortical regions. Myelin pallor—which, as the name implies, is defined by decreased uptake of histochemicals by the CNS white matter—is present in 33% of patients with HIVD, but it is a less specific finding than MGCE and may be caused by alterations of the blood-brain barrier. Alternatively, white matter pallor may represent a low-level infection of oligodendrocytes by either HIV or, conceivably, another pathogen, such as human herpesvirus type 6 (HHV-6).

The most striking feature of the neuropathology of HIVD is the discordance between the histologic findings and the clinical disease. For example, in one study, neither MGCE nor diffuse pallor was present in 50% of the patients, and even in cases with morphologic findings, the abnormalities were

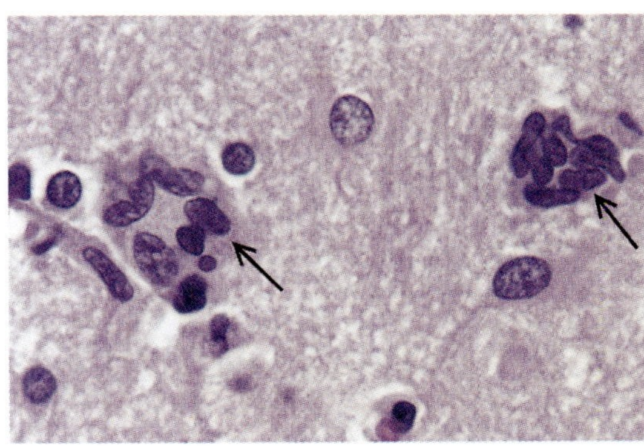

Figure 2 **Pathology of HIV dementia. Multinucleated giant cells (arrows) formed by the fusion of HIV-infected microglia or macrophages are the most specific finding in HIV dementia. Other pathologic changes (not shown) include astrocytosis and myelin pallor.**

frequently relatively unimpressive.[10] This implies that the symptoms associated with HIVD, although clearly associated with viral infection of microglia and the formation of microglial syncytia, are ultimately the result of a process in which a mild infection of one cell type is amplified by unknown mechanisms.

TREATMENT

There is increasing evidence that successful treatment of HIV infection brings improvement in HIVD,[2] although some studies suggest that HAART has less of an effect on HIVD than it has in other conditions associated with AIDS.[11] In view of the viral loads present in brain,[12] it will be critical to develop strategies that eliminate HIV from microglial cells. Otherwise, CNS involvement may thwart recent successes in reducing virus burden in the plasma and lymphoid tissue.

HTLV-I Myelopathy

The entity known as HTLV-I–associated myelopathy (HAM), which was initially described in Japanese patients, is the same disease as tropical spastic paraparesis (TSP), which occurs in the Caribbean. Epidemiologic studies have firmly established the association between HTLV-I infection and the development of this slowly progressive neurologic syndrome. However, HAM is a relatively rare complication of HTLV-I, with an incidence roughly comparable to that of adult T cell leukemia, another rare condition associated with HTLV-I.

DIAGNOSIS

HAM is characterized by the development of signs of spinal cord dysfunction, including paraparesis and urinary incontinence. Sensory changes are less common. In persons seropositive for HTLV-I, the diagnosis is based on the exclusion of space-occupying lesions by MRI of the spinal cord, which may instead be atrophic. Additionally, the T_2-weighted images (T_2 refers to the spin-spin, or transverse, relaxation time) may demonstrate areas of increased signal intensity in the spinal cord and, occasionally, above the foramen magnum; these findings may resemble the radiologic findings associated with multiple sclerosis, although these entities are clearly distinct. The CSF of patients with HAM may demonstrate high protein and oligoclonal bands, indicative of intrathecal antibody synthesis. Cells resembling those of adult T cell leukemia may also be present in the CSF. Patients with HAM will usually have a progressive course, leading to lower limb paralysis and, possibly, arm involvement. HAM is rarely fatal, however.

Autopsy studies have revealed low levels of HTLV-I in the spinal cord of HAM patients, indicating that direct cytolysis by virus infection is probably not the cause of the myelopathy.[13] The pathogenesis is generally thought to be, at the very least, associated with infiltration of the spinal cord by $CD8^+$ T cells.[14,15] Those patients infected with HTLV-I in whom this complication develops have a robust cytolytic T cell response to the viral protein tax.[16] These cytolytic T cells may mediate the neurologic dysfunction by attacking neuroglial cells minimally infected with HTLV-I. Alternatively, a neural antigen resembling the viral tax protein may be the target of an autoimmune attack.

TREATMENT

Because of the lack of evidence that direct viral infection mediates HAM, most therapeutic trials have been directed toward reduction of the immune attack on the CNS. To date, there is no established therapy for HAM, but some patients show improved neurologic function with high doses of intravenous steroids.

Transmissible Spongiform Encephalopathies

The spongiform encephalopathies, a group of neurologic disorders in humans and other mammals, are characterized by (1) subacute, progressive deterioration of neurologic function, involving several regions of the neuraxis (cognitive and motor dysfunction are most common, although other systems may also be involved); (2) spongiform neuropathologic changes in the affected areas of the CNS; (3) experimental transmissibility to either the same or a related species, with long incubation periods, typically many months or years; and (4) no evidence of conventional transmissible agents such as viruses.

In humans, the spongiform encephalopathies include both sporadic and genetic forms of CJD, Gerstmann-Sträussler syndrome (GSS), kuru disease (a spongiform encephalopathy associated with ritual endocannibalism of the Fore tribe in the remote highlands of New Guinea), and familial fatal insomnia (FFI). Parallel diseases in other species are scrapie of sheep, transmissible mink encephalopathy, and chronic wasting disease in deer and elk in the United States.[17] Spongiform diseases have been experimentally transmitted to mice and hamsters from sheep tissues, to monkeys and chimpanzees from human tissues, and acci-

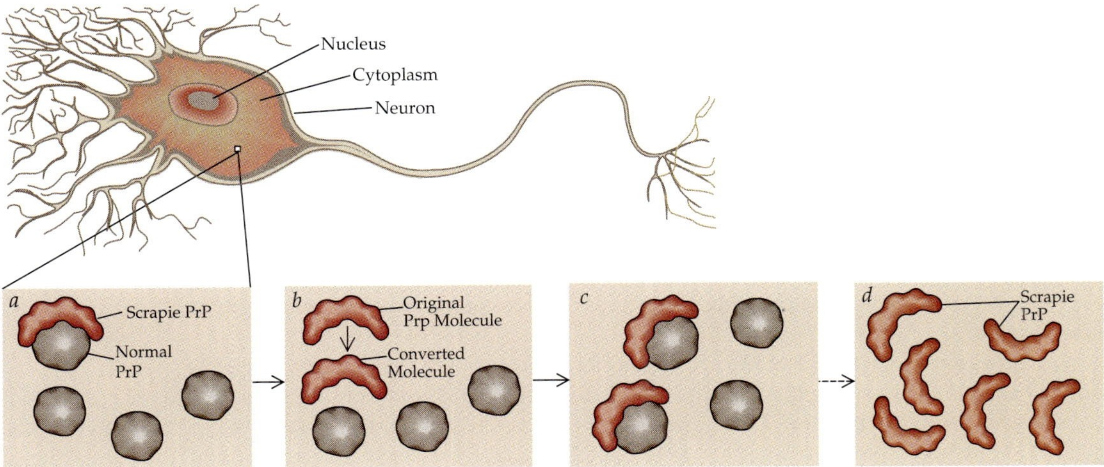

Figure 3 **Propagation of scrapie PrP in neurons of the brain apparently occurs via a domino effect on an internal membrane. A favored hypothesis holds that the process begins (*a*) when one molecule of scrapie (red) contacts a normal PrP molecule (brown) and (*b*) induces it to refold into the scrapie conformation. Then, the scrapie particles attack other normal PrP molecules (*c*). Those molecules, in turn, attack other normal molecules and so on (broken arrow) until scrapie PrP accumulation reaches dangerous levels (*d*).**

dentally to dairy cows (bovine spongiform encephalopathy [BSE], or mad-cow disease) by dietary supplementation with processed organs from infected sheep. Although there are species barriers, the spongiform diseases are generally considered to be caused by similar processes.

CJD and scrapie had been described for many years when transmission of the human form of the disease was first accomplished by intracerebral inoculation of primates with CNS tissues from patients dying of kuru.[18] Kuru disappeared with the cessation of cannibalistic practices, and human-to-human transmission of CJD and other spongiform encephalopathies is now limited to rare cases of accidental transplantation of an organ from a diseased person or parenteral exposure to CJD tissues through contaminated instruments.[19]

PRION HYPOTHESIS OF PATHOGENESIS

Initially championed by Prusiner and colleagues and now widely accepted, the prion hypothesis provides a model for the transmission of CJD and other spongiform encephalopathies. The hypothesis is based on the unquestionable presence of a protease resistant, pathogenic form of an endogenous protein (prion protein, or PrP) in the brains of all affected species.[20,21] The natural form of the protein, PrP^c, is a glycosylated protein of unknown function containing lengthy coils (α-helices). In the brains of affected mammals, PrP^c appears to misfold into a structure with a high concentration of β-pleated sheets, a protein conformation that promotes the formation of crystals [*see Figure 3*]. The misfolded protein (PrP^{Sc}, or scrapie PrP) is deposited in amyloid fibrils, or plaques, in the diseased brain. Together with the spongy appearance of the diseased brain [*see Figure 4*], these proteinaceous deposits are characteristic of the neuropathology of all the spongiform encephalopathies, although the extent of the deposit varies among the conditions.

Evidence supporting PrP involvement in the spongiform diseases includes experiments in which mice were genetically engineered to delete (knock out) the PrP gene. These mice became resis-

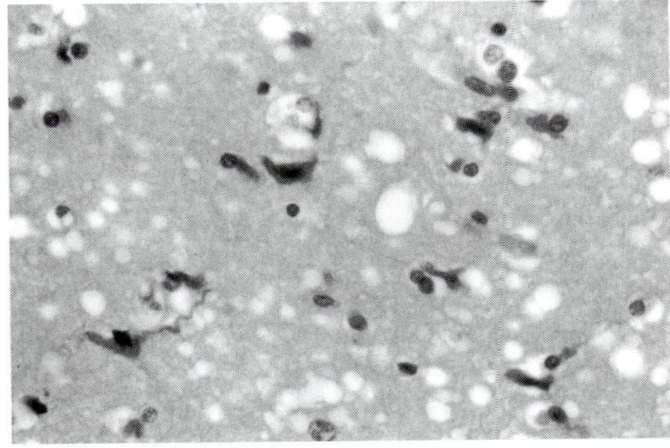

Figure 4 **Spongiform change is characteristic in the brain of a patient with Creutzfeldt-Jakob disease.**

tant to scrapie-infected brain and did not develop any spongiform changes, even after high concentrations of scrapie-infected tissue were injected intracerebrally. In contrast, transgenic mice that were engineered to express the PrP gene from other species, including humans, became particularly susceptible to the diseased brain harvested from the species supplying the transgene.[22] As there are species barriers to the transmission of spongiform change, these latter experiments suggest that the transgene is responsible for the disease process.

How does a protein devoid of nucleic acid function act as an infectious agent and encode its own replication in diseased brain? One scheme proposes that a misfolded PrP^{Sc} serves as a seed, which combines with PrP^{c} from normal tissue [*see Figure 3*]. This interaction induces PrP^{c} to change at least a portion of its α-helical structure into a structure composed primarily of β-pleated sheets. Because the β-pleated sheet–rich PrP^{Sc} is less soluble, the reaction is driven in a single direction. The initial aggregate then expands through the recruitment of additional PrP^{c} molecules, producing an insoluble deposition that is presumably injurious to neurons and neuroglia.

In this mechanism, the source of the seed PrP^{Sc} in spontaneously occurring spongiform encephalopathy is unknown. In a condition such as BSE, in which the disease appears to be transmitted by feeding diseased sheep tissues to cows, the seed protein would have to have been ingested and somehow transmitted to the brain from peripheral tissue. The spleen and other lymphoid organs are known to harbor scrapie infectivity; therefore, circulating lymphoid cells in the CNS are prime, though unproven, candidates for this neuroinvasion. Extensive epidemiologic surveys have not supported a role for blood transfusion in the transmission of CJD.

CREUTZFELDT-JAKOB DISEASE

Diagnosis

The diagnosis of CJD is based on clinical findings. The most important finding is a progressive dementia (occurring over weeks to months, rather than years, which is more typical of dementia in Alzheimer disease). This rapid cognitive deterioration should alert a clinician to the potential diagnosis of CJD. In addition, patients may complain of insomnia, fatigue, and problems with vision. In some instances, persons with CJD may be cortically blind. Neurologic examination shows evidence of pyramidal tract involvement and occasional muscle atrophy. Myoclonus (a jerky reaction, particularly prominent after a startle) is an important physical finding, but its absence does not rule out CJD. Other findings include cerebellar ataxia and seizures.

No single test can confirm the diagnosis of CJD, but commonly used diagnostic studies include examination of the CSF for an abnormal protein (14-3-3 protein) and electroencephalography, which may demonstrate characteristic triphasic forms.[23,24]

Treatment

CJD is uniformly fatal, usually within 2 years of onset. In vitro studies suggest a possible therapeutic role for antimalarial agents and phenothiazines,[25] but clinical studies have yet to be performed.

NEW-VARIANT CJD

Bovine spongiform encephalopathy, a spongiform encephalopathy that occurred primarily in the United Kingdom, is associated with the consumption of protein supplements derived from ruminant tissue by cows. Aggressive management of potentially infected herds has reduced the incidence of BSE. However, a variant form of CJD (new-variant CJD, or nvCJD), appearing in young adults and with characteristic neuropathologic findings, has been temporally associated with the appearance of BSE in the United Kingdom. Reliable diagnostic criteria for nvCJD have been formulated.[26] Because there are insufficient epidemiologic data to rule out potential transmission of nvCJD through blood products, the Food and Drug Administration recommends that persons who lived in the United Kingdom for more than 6 months between 1980 and 1996 and persons suspected of nvCJD not donate blood or blood products. However, no cases of nvCJD have been reported in the United States,[27] and current epidemiologic estimates suggest that the United Kingdom epidemic will be less widespread than initially predicted by some experts.[28]

GENETIC DISEASES ASSOCIATED WITH PRP MUTATIONS

In humans, the spongiform diseases include, in addition to spontaneous or accidentally transmitted CJD, genetic forms of CJD and even rarer conditions, such as GSS and FFI.[29,30] In GSS, which is transmitted as an autosomal dominant trait, the affected persons develop ataxia, followed by dementia; patients with FFI are unable to sleep. All these conditions can be transmitted to susceptible nonhuman primates by inoculation of diseased tissues. Remarkably, these conditions have been associated with mutations in the PrP gene, and in one series of experiments, mice engineered with the GSS mutation developed spongiform changes.[30] The mutations on the PrP gene are thought to be involved in promoting the conversion to a misfolded, insoluble state.

The existence of diseases that are simultaneously genetic and infectious and the association of mutations in the PrP gene with these diseases provide strong evidence in support of the prion hypothesis, although the hypothesis initially met with considerable skepticism because it violates the central dogma of molecular biology.[31] One experiment that has not yet been performed is the in vitro synthesis of a pure protein capable of serving as a seed for the development of spongiform disease; many groups are involved in this endeavor.

Progressive Multifocal Leukoencephalopathy

PML is a disease of the brain white matter—characterized by progressive motor deterioration, loss of vision, incontinence, and eventually dementia—that is caused by a papovavirus-related DNA virus, termed JC. PML was first described in patients with immunodeficiency caused by hematologic malignancies or by therapy for the prevention of transplant rejection. PML remained a very rare condition, however, until the appearance of AIDS. Before the widespread use of HAART, epidemiologic studies indicated that between 1% and 5% of HIV-infected persons would eventually develop PML. In many HIV-infected persons, the development of PML heralds the onset of immunodeficiency and is the AIDS-defining illness; in others, it is a complication associated with other opportunistic infections.

PATHOGENESIS

Oligodendrocytes, which are the cells responsible for the manufacture and maintenance of myelin, are the principal target of JC virus. Therefore, oligodendroglial cytolysis is the principal pathogenic mechanism in PML, and it leads to the characteristic severe demyelination. The initial event in the development of PML appears to be the rise of a microscopic focus of oligodendroglial infection, from which virus spreads centrifugally to involve large segments of the white matter. Astrocytes, as well as some oligodendrocytes, demonstrate bizarre morphologic changes similar to those associated with CNS neoplasia. There is little involvement of the gray matter or neurons in PML, and any involvement that does occur may reflect cytolysis of adjacent oligodendrocytes, perhaps through the recruitment of microglia and macrophages.[32]

JC Virus and Its Role in the Pathogenesis of PML

JC virus is related to, but clearly distinct from, other polyomaviruses.[33] A large percentage of the adult population in the United States (70% to 90%) has antibodies against JC virus, indicating that this is a common infection, but no diseases have been attributed to the primary infection.

The evidence of widespread infection and the isolation of JC virus from the urine of some immunosuppressed patients are consistent with the hypothesis that PML represents the reactivation of a latent DNA virus. The reservoir organ has not been identified, however. The absence of JC virus DNA in the brains of normal persons suggests that JC virus remains latent in other tissue. Lymphocytes, lymphoid organs, and kidneys have been considered prime candidates because JC virus has been detected in these tissues by PCR or has been isolated from these tissues.[34,35] However, the JC virus isolated from the peripheral tissue of nonimmunosuppressed persons (the archetypal virus) differs from that isolated from patients with PML in the regions responsible for the regulation of viral expression.[36] One intriguing hypothesis, which may explain these findings, is that the archetypal virus is modified by deletion or duplication and is thus converted into a neurotropic form that is carried into the brain in infected B cells.

DIAGNOSIS

The diagnosis of PML should be considered in any person with a subacute, progressive illness involving motor function and cognition in the setting of known or presumed immunodeficiency (e.g., AIDS or malignancy). Most cases exhibit features of white matter involvement, including ataxia, visual defects, and weakness. In rare cases, PML occurs in otherwise healthy persons. PML should be strongly suspected if MRIs show confluent areas of increased signal intensity in the T_2-weighted images [*see Figure 5*]. These areas, which respect the boundaries between gray matter and white matter, may be hypointense in the T_1-weighted images (T_1 refers to the spin-lattice, or longitudinal, relaxation time). The CSF is usually normal in PML; CSF pleocytosis, when present, is usually mild.

Pathologic examination of PML-diseased brain shows dramatic changes in the subcortical white matter. Traditionally, the definitive diagnosis of

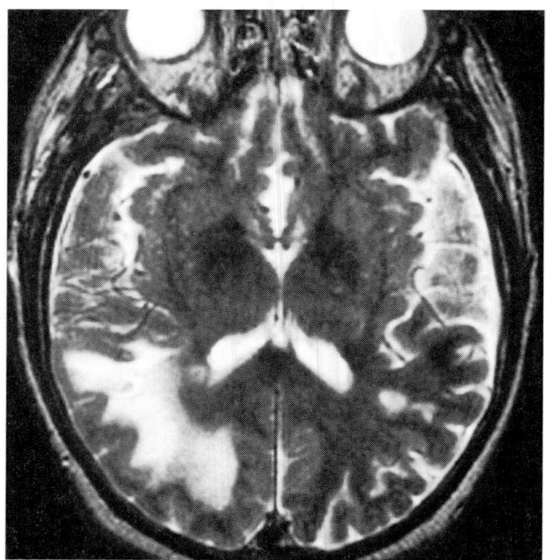

Figure 5 **Magnetic resonance imaging in progressive multifocal leukoencephalopathy. T_2-weighted MRI of a patient with progressive multifocal leukoencephalopathy (PML) demonstrates characteristic changes in the subcortical white matter of the right occipitoparietal region (increased intensity). As is typical of this disease, the abnormalities respect the gray matter–white matter junction, which accounts for the outline of the cortical sulci.**

PML has required a brain biopsy. However, biopsy has been largely superseded by the use of PCR to detect JC virus in the CSF.[37,38] The frequency of false positive reactions is low, and it has been estimated that CSF PCR has a sensitivity and specificity greater than 90%.[38]

TREATMENT

Improved outcomes in PML have recently been reported in AIDS patients treated with HAART.[39] Adjunctive treatment with cidofovir may also be beneficial, although the evidence for this is anecdotal.[40]

Subacute Sclerosing Panencephalitis

Subacute sclerosing panencephalitis (SSPE) is a rare sequela of measles infection (one per 100,000 cases). SSPE can also result from vaccination with a live, attenuated strain of measles, but the rate of development is at least 10 times less than that associated with wild-type measles infection. A similar disorder, progressive rubella paraencephalitis, is caused by rubella virus.

SSPE presents as a progressive encephalitis that develops several years after measles infection. The condition appears to result from a mutation in the measles virus that affects virus packaging, so the virus can spread only by fusion between adjacent infected and uninfected cells. This may explain viral persistence despite a strong humoral response.

There is no established therapy for SSPE, and its outcome is nearly always fatal.

Acknowledgments

Figure 2 Dimitry Schidlovsky.
Figure 3 Dimitry Schidlovsky. Adapted from "The Prion Diseases," by S. Prusiner, in Scientific American 272(1):48, 1995.
Figure 4 Dr. E. Lavi, Department of Pathology and Laboratory Medicine, University of Pennsylvania.

References

1. McArthur JC, Selnes OA, Glass JD, et al: HIV dementia, incidence, and risk factors. HIV, AIDS and the Brain. Price RW, Perry SW, Eds. Raven Press, New York, 1994, p 251

2. Sacktor N, Lyles RH, Skolasky R, et al: HIV-associated neurologic disease incidence changes: Multicenter AIDS Cohort Study, 1990–1998. Neurology 56:257, 2001

3. Achim CL, Wang R, Miners DK, et al: Brain viral burden in HIV infection. J Neuropathol Exp Neurol 53:284, 1994

4. Epstein LG, Gendelman HE: Human immunodeficiency virus type 1 infection of the nervous system: pathogenetic mechanisms. Ann Neurol 33:429, 1993

5. Bagasra O, Lavi E, Bobroski L, et al: Cellular reservoirs of HIV-1 in the central nervous system of infected persons: identification by the combination of in situ polymerase chain reaction and immunohistochemistry. AIDS 10:573, 1996

6. Takahashi K, Wesselingh SL, Griffin DE, et al: Localization of HIV-1 in human brain using polymerase chain reaction/in situ hybridization and immunohistochemistry. Ann Neurol 39:705, 1996

7. McArthur JC, Cohen BA, Selnes OA, et al: Low prevalence of neurological and neuropsychological abnormalities in otherwise healthy HIV-1 infected persons: results from the multicenter AIDS cohort study. Ann Neurol 26:601, 1989

8. Embretson J, Zupancic M, Ribas JL, et al: Massive infection of helper lymphocytes and macrophages by HIV during the incubation period of AIDS. Nature 362:359, 1993

9. Mellors JW, Rinaldo CR, Gupta P, et al: Prognosis in HIV-1 infection predicted by the quantity of virus in plasma. Science 272:1167, 1996

10. Glass JD, Fedor H, Wesselingh SL, et al: Immunocytochemical quantitation of human immunodeficiency virus in the brain: correlations with dementia. Ann Neurol 38:755, 1995

11. Dore GJ, Correll PK, Li Y, et al: Changes to AIDS dementia complex in the era of highly active antiretroviral therapy. AIDS 13:1249, 1999

12. Johnson RT, Glass JD, McArthur JC, et al: Quantitation of human immunodeficiency virus in brains of demented and nondemented patients with AIDS. Ann Neurol 39:392, 1996

13. Kuroda Y, Matsui M, Kikuchi M, et al: In situ demonstration of the HTLV-I genome in the spinal cord of a patient with HTLV-I myelopathy. Neurology 44:2295, 1994

14. Jacobson S: Human T-lymphotropic virus, type-I myelopathy: an immunopathologically mediated chronic progressive disease of the central nervous system. Curr Opin Neurol 8:179, 1995

15. Höllsberg P, Hafler DA: What is the pathogenesis of human T-cell lymphotropic virus type I-associated myelopathy/tropical spastic paraparesis (editorial)? Ann Neurol 37:143, 1995

16. Elovaara I, Koenig S, Brewah AY, et al: High HTLV-I specific precursor cytotoxic T cell (CTL) responses to tax in HTLV-I infected patients with neurological disease. J Immunol 156:3874, 1993

17. Belay ED, Gambetti P, Schonberger LB, et al: Creutzfeldt-Jakob disease in unusually young patients who consumed venison. Arch Neurol 58:1673, 2001

18. Brown P, Gibbs CJ, Rodgers-Johnson P, et al: Human spongiform encephalopathy: the NIH series of 300 cases of experimentally transmitted disease. Ann Neurol 35:513, 1994

19. Brown P, Cervenakova L, Goldfarb LG, et al: Iatrogenic Creutzfeldt-Jakob disease: an example of the interplay between ancient genes and modern medicine. Neurology 44:291, 1994

20. Prusiner SB: Molecular biology of prion disease. Science 252:1515, 1991

21. Mastrianni JA, Nixon R, Layzer R, et al: Prion protein conformation in a patient with sporadic fatal insomnia. N Engl J Med 340:1630, 1999

22. Telling GC, Scott M, Hsiao KK, et al: Transmission of Creutzfeldt-Jakob disease from humans to transgenic mice expressing chimeric human-mouse prion protein. Proc Natl Acad Sci USA 91:9936, 1994

23. Zerr I, Bodemer M, Gefeller O, et al: Detection of 14-3-3 protein in the cerebrospinal fluid supports the diagnosis of Creutzfeldt-Jakob disease. Ann Neurol 43:32, 1998

24. Zerr I, Schulz-Schaeffer WJ, Giese A, et al: Current clinical diagnosis in Creutzfeld-Jakob disease: identification of uncommon variants. Ann Neurol 48:323, 2000

25. Korth C, May BC, Cohen FE, et al: Acridine and phenothiazine derivatives as pharmacotherapeutics for prion disease. Proc Natl Acad Sci USA 98:9836, 2001

26. Will RG, Zeidler MN, Stewart GE, et al: Diagnosis of new variant Creutzfeldt-Jakob disease. Ann Neurol 47:575, 2000

27. Tan L, Williams MA, Khan MK, et al: Risk of transmission of bovine spongiform encephalopathy to humans in the United States: a report of the Council on Scientific Affairs. American Medical Association. JAMA 281:2330, 1999

28. Valleron AJ, Boelle PY, Will R: Estimation of epidemic size and incubation time based on age characteristics of vCJD in the United Kingdom. Science 294:1726, 2001

29. Hsiao K, Baker HF, Crow TJ, et al: Linkage of a prion protein missense variant to Gerstmann-Sträussler syndrome. Nature 338:342, 1989

30. Chapman J, Arlazoroff A, Goldfarb LG, et al: Fatal insomnia in a case of familial Creutzfeldt-Jakob disease with the codon 200Lys mutation. Neurology 46:758, 1996

31. Parchi P, Castellani R, Capellari S, et al: Molecular basis of phenotypic variability in sporadic Creutzfeldt-Jakob disease. Ann Neurol 39: 767, 1996

32. Major EO, Amemiya K, Tornatore CS, et al: Pathogenesis and molecular biology of progressive multifocal leukoencephalopathy, the JC virus-induced demyelinating disease of the human brain. Clin Microbiol Rev 5:49, 1992

33. ZuRhein GM, Chou S-M: Particles resembling papova viruses in human cerebral demyelination disease. Science 148:1477, 1965

34. Tornatore C, Berger JR, Houff SA, et al: Detection of JC virus DNA in peripheral lymphocytes from patients with and without progressive multifocal leukoencephalopathy. Ann Neurol 31:454, 1992

35. Dubois V, Lafon M-E, Ragnaud J-M, et al: Detection of JC virus DNA in the peripheral blood leukocytes of HIV-infected patients. AIDS 10:353, 1996

36. Daniel AM, Swenson JJ, Mayreddy RPR, et al: Sequences within the early and late promoters of archetype JC virus restrict viral DNA replication and infectivity. Virology 216:90, 1996

37. Weber T, Turner RW, Frye S, et al: Progressive multifocal leukoencephalopathy diagnosed by amplification of JC virus–specific DNA from cerebrospinal fluid. AIDS 8:49, 1994

38. McGuire D, Barhite S, Hollander H, et al: Virus DNA in cerebrospinal fluid of human immunodeficiency virus–infected patients: predictive value for progressive multifocal leukoencephalopathy. Ann Neurol 37:395, 1995

39. Albrecht H, Hoffmann C, Degen O, et al: Highly active antiretroviral therapy significantly improves the prognosis of patients with HIV-associated progressive multifocal leukoencephalopathy. AIDS 12:1149, 1998

40. De Luca A., Giancola ML, Ammassari A, et al: Potent anti-retroviral therapy with or without cidofovir for AIDS-associated progressive multifocal leukoencephalopathy: extended followup of an observational study. J Neurovirol 7:364, 2001

37 Mycotic Infections

Carol A. Kauffman, M.D.

Overview of Endemic Mycosis

The endemic mycoses (histoplasmosis, blastomycosis, coccidioidomycosis, and sporotrichosis) are caused by fungi that share several important characteristics but differ greatly in other respects. The fungi are all dimorphic, existing as molds in the environment and as either yeasts or spherules in tissues. Each organism occupies a different ecological niche; infection is directly related to exposure to the mycelial or mold phase of the organism in the environment. These fungi are true pathogens in that they are capable of causing infection in otherwise healthy individuals. The severity of infection is determined both by the extent of the exposure to the organism and by the immune status of the patient. Three of the four organisms (*Histoplasma capsulatum, Blastomyces dermatitidis,* and *Coccidioides immitis*) are inhaled, have the propensity to disseminate hematogenously, and are able to reactivate years later; the fourth organism, *Sporothrix schenckii*, usually causes primary infection after cutaneous inoculation and does not reactivate. Although many of the disease manifestations overlap, each of the four has its own distinctive characteristics.

The endemic mycoses mimic many common infections involving lungs, skin, and other organs, and frequently, the diagnosis of fungal infection is not entertained; this is especially true for patients who present outside of the areas endemic for these specific mycoses. Because of an increase in travel and leisure activities over the past several decades, patients often present with illness outside endemic areas. When faced with an elderly retiree who spends winters in Arizona and who has developed fever, headache, and visual complaints, a physician who practices in Ohio and who may have never seen coccidioidomycosis must remember that this fungal infection causes chronic meningitis. Similarly, an AIDS patient with fever, hepatosplenomegaly, and pancytopenia who lives in Seattle but who spent his childhood in Arkansas and has not returned there for the past 20 years may well be experiencing reactivation of disseminated histoplasmosis.

The most useful diagnostic tests differ for each of the endemic mycoses, but as a general rule, histopathologic demonstration of the fungi in biopsy specimens is the most expeditious way to make a diagnosis, especially in a severely ill patient; growth of the organism in vitro is definitive. For most patients with an endemic mycosis, treatment will be with an azole antifungal agent. For those who are severely ill, initial therapy with amphotericin B followed by consolidation therapy with an azole is standard.

A review of antifungal agents and guidelines for their use in the treatment of mycotic infections is found after the descriptions of specific manifestations of each endemic mycosis [*see* Antifungal Therapy, *below*].

Histoplasmosis

EPIDEMIOLOGY

H. capsulatum is a dimorphic fungus that every year infects hundreds of thousands of individuals in the United States. The organism is endemic in the Mississippi and Ohio River valleys and Central America. Soil containing high concentrations of bird or bat guano supports the profuse growth of the mycelial phase of *H. capsulatum*. Exposure typically occurs as a result of activities that generate aerosols containing the organism. Although most cases are sporadic and the exact source of exposure is unknown, many point-source outbreaks have been well described in association with disruption of soil; the cleaning of attics, bridges, or barns; tearing down old structures laden with guano; and spelunking.[1-3] Massive outbreaks of infection with *H. capsulatum* occurred when urban demolition exposed hundreds of thousands of people to the organism.[1]

Infection is very common in the endemic area, most persons having been infected before adulthood.

PATHOGENESIS

During the mycelial phase of the organism's life cycle, the microconidia are inhaled into the alveoli, causing a localized pulmonary infection. Neutrophils and macrophages phagocytize the organism, which converts to the yeast phase; the organism is then able to survive and travel within the macrophage. Spread to the hilar and mediastinal lymph nodes ensues, and hematogenous dissemination subsequently occurs throughout the reticuloendothelial system before specific immunity has developed. After several weeks, cell-mediated immunity that is specific for *H. capsulatum* activates macrophages, which then kill the organism.[4] Of all the human mycoses, histoplasmosis exemplifies best the pivotal importance of the cell-mediated immune system. The corollary of this observation is that most patients with severe infection are those with cellular immune deficiencies.

The extent of disease is determined by the number of conidia that are inhaled and the immune response of the host. A healthy individual may develop severe life-threatening pulmonary infection if a large number of conidia are inhaled. This might occur during demolition or renovation of an old building or as a result of spelunking in a heavily infested cave. Conversely, a small inoculum can cause severe pulmonary infection or progress to acute symptomatic disseminated histoplasmosis in a patient with advanced HIV infection whose cell-mediated immune system is unable to contain the organism.

Most persons who have been infected experience asymptomatic dissemination; only rarely will this lead to symptomatic acute or chronic disseminated histoplasmosis. However, by virtue of this dissemination, latent infection can persist for a lifetime. Reactivation of quiescent infection can occur years later if immunosuppression occurs.[5] Reinfection has also been documented, though rarely, in persons previously known to have had histoplasmosis. Such reinfection almost always occurs in the setting of exposure to a heavy inoculum of *H. capsulatum* conidia.

CLINICAL PRESENTATIONS

Pulmonary Histoplasmosis

Infection is asymptomatic in the vast majority of persons who have been infected with *H. capsulatum*. Most patients who have symptomatic pulmonary infection will have a self-limited illness characterized by fever, chills, and cough that is usually nonproductive; such infection is often associated with anterior chest discomfort, myalgias, arthralgias, and fatigue. A patchy lobar or multilobar nodular infiltrate is noted on chest radiography.[6] The diagnosis is usually not made in individual cases until the patient fails to respond to several courses of antibiotics given for atypical pneumonia.

The diagnosis of acute pulmonary histoplasmosis is more easily made when the patient has been involved in an outbreak.[2] A careful history of the patient's activities as well as the patient's colleagues' activities—especially if the history reveals participation in outdoor activities, activities around a demolition site, or spelunking several weeks before the onset of symptoms—may point to histoplasmosis. High spiking fever, prostration, dyspnea, and cough are prominent in severe cases in which the number of conidia inhaled is large. Diffuse nodular infiltrates are noted on the chest radiograph, and development of the acute respiratory distress syndrome (ARDS) can ensue.

In patients with cell-mediated immune deficiencies, including those who have advanced HIV infection, those with a hematologic malignancy, those who have received a transplant, and those who are receiving immunosuppressive medications, pulmonary infection is more severe than in otherwise healthy patients. Although pulmonary infection may be the only manifestation of histoplasmosis, in most immunosuppressed patients, pulmonary involvement is merely one component of widespread dissemination.[7] Prostration, fever, chills, marked dyspnea, and hypoxemia are prominent, and chest radiographs show diffuse infiltrates.

Chronic cavitary pulmonary histoplasmosis is a progressive, fatal form of histoplasmosis that usually develops in older patients who have chronic obstructive pulmonary disease (COPD). Typical symptoms include fever, fatigue, anorexia, weight loss, cough that is productive of purulent sputum, and hemoptysis.[8,9] On chest radiography, infiltrates can be either unilateral or bilateral and are almost always located in the upper lobes. Cavities may be multiple and are frequently quite large; extensive fibrosis occurs in the lower lobes.[6]

Disseminated Histoplasmosis

Hematogenous dissemination typically occurs in immunosuppressed patients and young children early in the course of infection with *H. capsulatum*. Patients who have HIV infection and whose

CD4+ T cell counts are less than 150 cells/mm^3 are at great risk for acquiring histoplasmosis, which almost always presents as disseminated infection. Symptoms and signs of acute disseminated histoplasmosis include chills, fever, malaise, anorexia, weight loss, dyspnea, hepatosplenomegaly, and skin and mucous membrane lesions. Pancytopenia, diffuse pulmonary infiltrates seen on chest radiographs, and blood cultures that yield *H. capsulatum* are common.[7,10] Adrenal insufficiency may also be present.

A chronic progressive disseminated form of histoplasmosis that occurs mostly in middle-aged to elderly men who have no known immunosuppressive illness is characterized by fever, night sweats, weight loss, and fatigue.[11] Patients appear chronically ill and frequently have hepatosplenomegaly, mucocutaneous ulcerations, and signs of adrenal insufficiency. Typical findings include an increase in the erythrocyte sedimentation rate, an elevation in the alkaline phosphatase level, pancytopenia, and diffuse pulmonary infiltrates seen on chest radiograph. If not diagnosed and treated appropriately, this form of histoplasmosis is fatal.

DIAGNOSIS

Culture

The definitive diagnostic test for histoplasmosis is growth of *H. capsulatum* in culture, which, unfortunately, may take as long as 6 weeks.[5] Sputum, bronchoalveolar lavage fluid, or tissue biopsy material should be sent to the laboratory for culture. For those patients who have evidence of dissemination, cultures of blood are useful. The best yield is with the lysis-centrifugation system (Isolator aerobic blood culture system, Wampole Laboratories). The laboratory should be informed that pulmonary histoplasmosis is a diagnostic consideration, so that a special medium that decreases the growth of commensal fungi, such as *Candida,* can be used for the culture of pulmonary samples. As soon as growth of a mold has been detected, a DNA probe specific for *H. capsulatum* confirms the identity of the organism.

Serologic Studies

In contrast to several other endemic mycoses, serology plays an important adjunctive role in the diagnosis of histoplasmosis.[12] Both complement fixation (CF) and immunodiffusion (ID) tests are available. ID is more specific than CF (> 95% specificity versus 85% to 90%); both are only modestly sensitive (75% to 85% sensitivity). False negative serologic test results occur in immunosuppressed patients who cannot mount an antibody response. However, most patients with pulmonary histoplasmosis are not immunosuppressed, and thus, in this group, antibody tests are helpful.

Patients with chronic cavitary pulmonary histoplasmosis almost always have an elevated CF antibody titer (> 1:32), and either an M precipitin band or both H and M precipitin bands are seen on ID in these patients. In a patient with acute pneumonia, a documented fourfold increase in CF titer or the appearance of an M precipitin band on ID establishes the diagnosis of histoplasmosis. Serologic tests are less definitive in patients with mediastinal lymphadenopathy and should always be confirmed by tissue biopsy. False positive test results, especially false positive results on CF, occur in patients with lymphoma, tuberculosis, sarcoidosis, and other fungal infections, all of which may present as mediastinal masses. In most patients with the chronic disseminated form of histoplasmosis, both precipitin and CF antibodies are present.

Antigen Tests

Enzyme immunoassays for the detection of *H. capsulatum* polysaccharide antigen in urine and serum are extremely helpful in AIDS patients who have disseminated infection and a large fungal burden.[13,14] They are less useful for patients with pulmonary histoplasmosis; antigen is detected in only about 20% of patients with pulmonary histoplasmosis. Cross-reactivity occurs in a small number of patients with blastomycosis, paracoccidioidomycosis, and penicilliosis.

Tissue Biopsy

For an acutely ill person, evidence of *H. capsulatum* on tissue biopsy allows the physician to make the diagnosis of histoplasmosis in a timely fashion.[5] The organisms appear as distinctive, fairly uniformly shaped, oval budding yeasts 2 to 4 µm in diameter. Tissue biopsy is most useful for the diagnosis of disseminated disease; bone marrow, liver, and mucocutaneous lesions reveal many organisms [*see Figure 1a and 1b*]. For most patients with acute pulmonary histoplasmosis, biopsy is not indicated unless the patient is severely ill. For patients with chronic pulmonary histoplasmosis or granulomatous mediastinitis, biopsy of lung or lymph nodes may reveal the organism. Routine hematoxylin-eosin staining will not show the tiny *H. capsulatum* yeasts; biopsy material must be stained with methenamine-silver stain, periodic acid–Schiff stain, or both. In contrast to larger

a

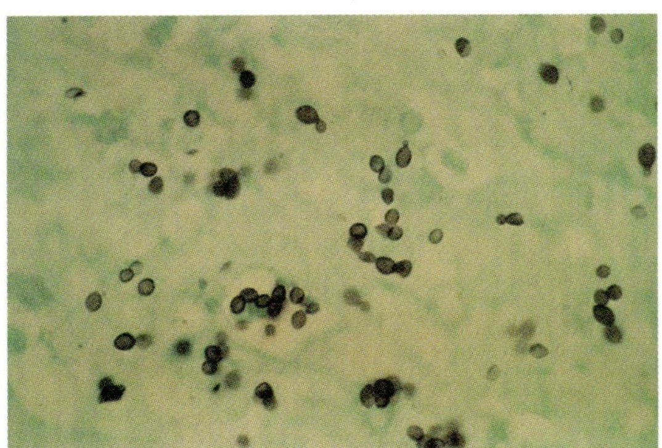

b

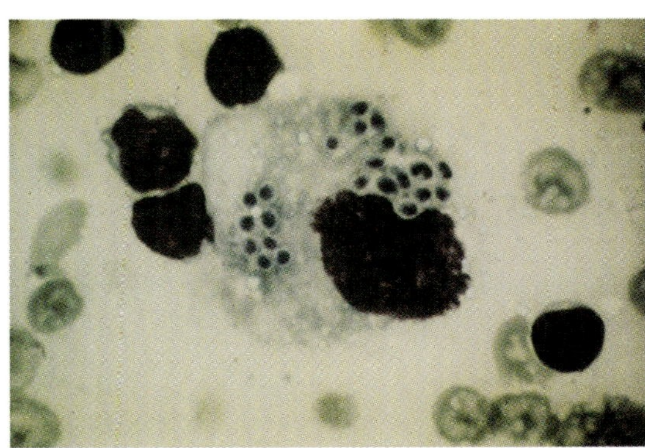

Figure 1 **Shown are biopsy samples from an elderly man with chronic progressive disseminated histoplasmosis. (*a*) Tongue ulcer stained with methenamine-silver stain shows several budding yeast forms measuring 2 to 4 μm. (*b*) A smear from a lung biopsy sample, which is stained with Giemsa stain, shows small intracellular yeasts inside a macrophage.**

yeasts, such as *B. dermatitidis,* it is extremely unusual to find *H. capsulatum* on cytologic examination of sputum or bronchoalveolar lavage fluid.

Skin Tests

Skin tests with histoplasmin antigen are not useful for the diagnosis of histoplasmosis in individual patients. In the endemic area, as many as 85% of adults have positive results on skin testing because of previous exposure to the organism; cross-reactions occur in those with other fungal infections, especially blastomycosis; and negative test results occur frequently in patients who have severe infection.

DIFFERENTIAL DIAGNOSIS

Acute pulmonary histoplasmosis is most difficult to differentiate from acute pulmonary blastomycosis. The clinical and radiographic findings of these two diseases are similar, the regions in which these diseases are endemic overlap, and the CF antibody tests for the two organisms show cross-reactivity. For either disease, culture of the causative organism from sputum is diagnostically definitive. However, results of sputum cultures are often negative for patients with acute pneumonia caused by either fungus. Treatment, fortunately, is the same for the two diseases. Atypical pneumonias caused by *Mycoplasma, Legionella,* and *Chlamydia* are included in the differential diagnosis of acute pulmonary histoplasmosis. Hilar and mediastinal lymphadenopathy, which is very common with histoplasmosis, is uncommon in patients with atypical pneumonia caused by these other organisms.

Chronic pulmonary histoplasmosis mimics tuberculosis in regard to symptoms, signs, and radiographic findings. Other chronic fungal pneumonias, especially blastomycosis and sporotrichosis, and nontuberculous mycobacterial infections also must be differentiated from this form of histoplasmosis. Sputum culture and serology are most useful in differentiating these infections.

Patients with acute disseminated histoplasmosis can present with a sepsis syndrome associated with ARDS and disseminated intravascular coagulation that is indistinguishable from sepsis of any bacterial or viral etiology. Helpful findings supporting the diagnosis of histoplasmosis are pancytopenia, diffuse nodular pulmonary infiltrates, and hepatosplenomegaly; the hematology laboratory may make the diagnosis when they find small yeasts inside white cells on the peripheral smear. In AIDS patients, the main infections that must be excluded are those caused by cytomegalovirus, *Mycobacterium avium* complex, and *M. tuberculosis.* Biopsy of involved tissues should be performed as soon as possible to help differentiate between these conditions. Culture of blood by means of lysis-centrifugation (Isolator system) for fungus and *Mycobacteria* and use of urinary antigen testing for *H. capsulatum* are very helpful diagnostic tests in this circumstance.

Patients with chronic disseminated histoplasmosis usually present with fever of unknown origin. The disease that mimics histoplasmosis most closely is miliary tuberculosis; lymphoma, brucellosis, and sarcoidosis also must be excluded. Serology is helpful, but histopathologic evidence of yeasts in tissue granulomas and confirmatory culture of the organism from bone marrow, mucous membrane lesions, or liver are definitive. It should be emphasized that the diagnosis of sarcoidosis requires firm evidence that the patient does not have histoplasmosis or tuberculosis; corticosteroid use for the treatment of suspected sarcoidosis in patients who in fact have histoplasmosis frequently leads to defervescence for a short period, followed by further worsening of the infection.[15]

TREATMENT

Guidelines for the treatment of histoplasmosis have recently been published by the Mycoses Study Group and the Infectious Diseases Society of America.[16] Efficacy has been defined primarily by open-label trials in patients with and without AIDS and through anecdotal experience[17–22]; there are no studies that directly compare azoles with amphotericin B. The only blinded, randomized treatment trial studied liposomal amphotericin B versus amphotericin B deoxycholate in a very restricted patient population: AIDS patients with severe disseminated histoplasmosis.[23] In spite of the lack of controlled treatment trials, it is clear that for the treatment of most patients with histoplasmosis, itraconazole is the drug of choice.[18–20] Fluconazole should be considered a second-line agent; primary response rates are lower for fluconazole in patients with and without AIDS, and relapse rates for AIDS patients receiving fluconazole are higher than those noted in previous studies with itraconazole.[21,22] If a patient does not tolerate itraconazole, fluconazole can be used, but the dosage should be 400 to 800 mg daily. Side effects, drug absorption, and drug-drug interactions are important considerations in antifungal therapy, particularly in long-term regimens such as those frequently required for AIDS patients [*see* Antifungal Therapy, *below*].

Pulmonary Histoplasmosis

Treatment recommendations are based on the type of histoplasmosis and the immune status of the host.[16] Treatment is generally not recommended for patients with acute pulmonary histoplasmosis; in fact, the diagnosis is often not made until after the patient's symptoms have resolved. However, if the patient remains symptomatic after 4 weeks, therapy with itraconazole, 200 mg daily for 6 to 12 weeks, is recommended. Children with acute pulmonary histoplasmosis should be treated with itraconazole, 5 to 7 mg/kg/day.

Although pneumonia resolves without treatment in most patients with acute outbreak-related histoplasmosis, those with severe infection should receive treatment. Immunosuppressed patients with acute pulmonary histoplasmosis should always be treated. Initial therapy should be administration of amphotericin B, 0.7 mg/kg/day. After a favorable response is noted, which usually occurs quite soon after initiation of therapy, therapy can be changed to oral itraconazole. Treatment should continue until the infiltrate has resolved.

Antifungal therapy is required for all patients with chronic pulmonary histoplasmosis.[8,16] Itraconazole, 200 mg once or twice daily for 12 to 24 months, is the treatment of choice. Even with appropriate antifungal therapy, outcome is poor.

Disseminated Histoplasmosis

All patients with symptomatic disseminated histoplasmosis should receive antifungal therapy.[11,16] Patients with acute disseminated disease who have only mild to moderate symptoms and most patients with chronic progressive disseminated histoplasmosis should be treated with itraconazole, 200 mg twice daily; this recommendation applies both to patients with AIDS and to those who do not have AIDS. For patients who do not have AIDS, a total of 12 months of therapy is usually adequate, but the length of therapy will be determined by the patient's clinical course; this is especially true for patients with chronic progressive disease. Patients who have AIDS should initially receive itraconazole twice daily for 12 weeks; after that period, they should receive a maintenance course of long-term suppressive therapy with itraconazole, 200 mg daily.[20]

Young infants, who frequently have overwhelming infection, and immunosuppressed patients with moderately severe to severe symptoms should be treated initially with amphotericin B, 0.7 to 1.0 mg/kg/day. For most adults, therapy can be changed to itraconazole after they become afebrile and are able to take oral medications. Infants should receive a full course of amphotericin B because experience with itraconazole is limited in this population group. When therapy is with amphotericin B deoxycholate only, the total dose should be 35 mg/kg.[16]

In a blinded, randomized clinical trial, liposomal amphotericin B, 3 mg/kg/day, was found to be superior to amphotericin B deoxycholate, 0.7 mg/kg/day, for initial treatment of AIDS patients who had severe disseminated histoplasmosis. In this study, the 51 patients receiving liposomal amphotericin B became afebrile sooner than the 22 receiving amphotericin B deoxycholate ($P = 0.01$); in addition, mortality was decreased and toxicity was lessened in the liposomal amphotericin B arm.[23] However, it is not clear whether these results should affect clinical decision making regarding the treatment of disseminated histoplasmosis in patients who do not have AIDS. The main drawback to the use of the liposomal formulation of amphotericin B is that it is extremely costly in comparison with the standard formulation.

COMPLICATIONS

Granulomatous mediastinitis is an uncommon complication of pulmonary histoplasmosis in which lymphadenopathy persists for months.[5] The enlarged nodes can erode into the esophagus; can lead to the formation of tracheoesophageal fistulas; and can cause traction diverticula. Chest radiography and CT scanning reveal enlarged hilar and mediastinal lymph nodes; necrosis and calcium deposition in the nodes are commonly noted on CT scan. Mediastinoscopy and biopsy reveal caseous material, which may contain a few yeastlike organisms typical of *H. capsulatum*. In most patients, the disease follows a self-limited, although protracted, course, and patients do not develop fibrosing mediastinitis. Patients may benefit from itraconazole, 200 mg twice daily, but there are no clinical trials proving efficacy.[16]

Fibrosing mediastinitis is a rare complication of pulmonary histoplasmosis in which an excessive amount of fibrosis develops in the mediastinal lymph nodes in response to infection.[24,25] The exuberant fibrous tissue entraps the great vessels, causing heart failure, pulmonary emboli, and superior vena cava syndrome. Odynophagia, dyspnea, cough, wheezing, and hemoptysis are commonly noted. There is no effective therapy for this progressive disease.

Pericarditis is a self-limited illness that occurs as an inflammatory response to acute pulmonary histoplasmosis.[5] Pleural effusions and mediastinal lymphadenopathy are commonly noted with pericarditis. The pericardial fluid is exudative. Drainage is required if tamponade occurs, but this is rare. Pericarditis should be treated with nonsteroidal anti-inflammatory drugs; corticosteroids should be used for severe cases. Antifungal agents should not be used.[16] The long-term outcome is excellent; only rarely has constrictive pericarditis occurred.

PROGNOSIS

Most patients with histoplasmosis respond quite well to antifungal agents. Even patients with advanced AIDS respond quickly and completely to therapy and continue to do well as long as they receive suppressive therapy with an azole. Patients with chronic progressive disseminated histoplasmosis usually experience a return to their baseline function, but it often takes months for this to occur. The patients who do poorly are those whose underlying illness precludes a return to normal function. For example, patients with chronic cavitary pulmonary histoplasmosis frequently have progressive respiratory insufficiency because of their severe underlying emphysema and the fibrosis caused by the fungal infection.

Blastomycosis

EPIDEMIOLOGY

Although the dimorphic fungus *B. dermatitidis* is present in many diverse geographic areas worldwide, most cases of blastomycosis are reported from the south central and north central United States.[26] The endemic area for blastomycosis overlaps that for histoplasmosis but extends further north into Wisconsin, Minnesota, and the southern portions of the Canadian provinces of Manitoba, Saskatchewan, and Alberta. Most cases are reported from Arkansas, Mississippi, and Kentucky.

The ecology of *B. dermatitidis* is not as well understood as that of the other endemic mycoses. It is assumed that the natural niche is soil, but the yield of soil cultures is quite low. Most cases occur sporadically, but several well-described outbreaks have helped define the presumed natural habitat.[27,28] The largest outbreak to date involved 95 students in northern Wisconsin who camped along a beaver pond and explored a beaver lodge.[27] Decomposed wood on the pond bank and samples from the lodge yielded *B. dermatitidis*.

Most, but certainly not all, patients who develop blastomycosis are men who have an outdoor occupation or hobby. Cases have been described in hunters and their dogs; in these cases, it is presumed that the hunters and their dogs were exposed to the same environmental source. For most sporadic cases, the source of exposure to the fungus is unknown.

PATHOGENESIS

Most patients with blastomycosis have no underlying illnesses, but the disease is more severe in immunosuppressed patients.[29] Blastomycosis is acquired by inhaling the conidia of *B. dermatitidis* into the alveoli. The organisms change to the yeast form in the lungs and then reproduce by budding. The immune response to *B. dermatitidis* appears to include both neutrophils and cell-mediated immune mechanisms involving T cells and macrophages.

Even though a major clinical manifestation of blastomycosis is cutaneous lesions, blastomycosis is only very rarely spread through inoculation. Examples of such cases include accidental inoculation in laboratory workers, conjugal inoculation from a genital lesion, and inoculation from the bite of an infected dog. The organism travels to the skin and other common target organs, including osteoarticular structures and the genitourinary tract, by the hematogenous route. Most persons infected with *B. dermatitidis* are asymptomatic or have mild pulmonary symptoms. Hematogenous dissemination occurs without clinical manifestations, and only later do patients present with skin lesions in the absence of other obvious organ involvement.

CLINICAL PRESENTATIONS

Pulmonary Blastomycosis

Blastomycosis begins as a pulmonary infection, but many patients never develop symptoms, and others have an acute illness with fever, cough, and a pulmonary infiltrate that is diagnosed as an atypical pneumonia. Overwhelming pulmonary disease with ARDS can occur; this appears to be more common in older adults.[30] Whether severe infection occurs because the patient has been exposed to a large number of conidia or has a defect in his or her immune response has not been clarified.

A more common presentation is a subacute to chronic pulmonary infection that is clinically and radiographically similar to tuberculosis. Fever, night sweats, weight loss, and fatigue are common symptoms. Cough, sputum production, hemoptysis, and dyspnea are noted. The lesions may be cavitary, nodular, fibrotic, or masslike in appearance.[31,32] Hilar and mediastinal lymphadenopathy and pleural effusions are uncommonly seen.

Disseminated Blastomycosis

Many patients with blastomycosis have no pulmonary symptoms.[26,31] They present with cutaneous lesions that are well circumscribed, nonpainful papules, nodules, or plaques that often become verrucous and develop punctate drainage areas in the center. The lesions are common on the face and extremities but can appear anywhere. There may be only a single lesion, or there may be multiple lesions. An uncommon manifestation seen mostly in immunocompromised patients is the appearance of hundreds of acute pustular lesions associated with widespread visceral involvement and an acute downhill course.

Additional manifestations of disseminated blastomycosis include prostatitis, septic arthritis, osteomyelitis, laryngeal and oropharyngeal nodules, and, less commonly, central nervous system involvement. Genitourinary involvement may be asymptomatic, or it may be associated with signs of prostatism. Although osteoarticular infection can be associated with a contiguous skin lesion, bone involvement often occurs at sites distant from the cutaneous lesions. It is helpful to obtain a bone scan for all patients with disseminated blastomycosis because of the propensity of the organism to seed into bone and because osteomyelitis requires prolonged antifungal therapy. All patients with manifestations of dissemination, even patients with only one skin lesion, need to be treated with systemic antifungal therapy to prevent progression of disease.[33]

DIAGNOSIS

Culture

The most definitive method for diagnosing blastomycosis is growth of the organism from an aspirate, tissue biopsy, sputum, or body fluid.[34] For patients with disseminated blastomycosis, urine obtained before and after prostatic massage should be sent for fungal culture. *B. dermatitidis* generally takes several weeks to grow at room temperature. Once growth has occurred, highly specific and sensitive DNA probes are used to rapidly identify the mold as *B. dermatitidis*.

Biopsy and Cytologic Studies

Biopsy specimens of skin lesions characteristically show pseudoepitheliomatous hyperplasia; when distinctive, large, thick-walled yeasts with a single broad-based bud are seen, a firm diagnosis of blastomycosis can be made before the results of cultures are known. In patients who have pulmonary lesions, the distinctive yeast forms should be sought on potassium hydroxide (KOH) preparations or Papanicolaou stains performed for cytologic examination of sputum or bronchoalveolar lavage fluid and on lung biopsy specimens [*see Figure 2a and 2b*].

Serologic Studies

Standard CF and ID serologic assays for blastomycosis are neither sensitive nor specific. Several

a

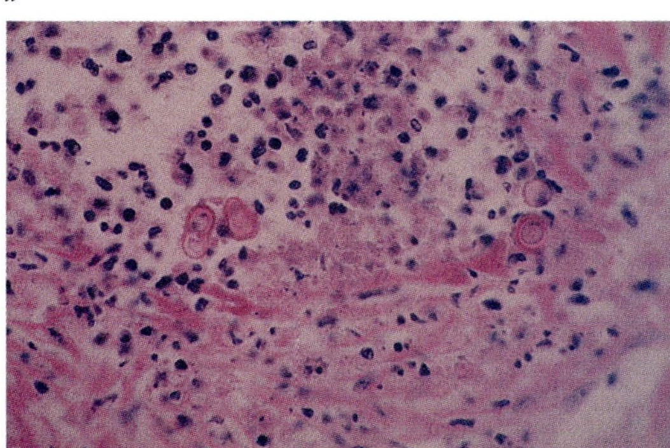

b

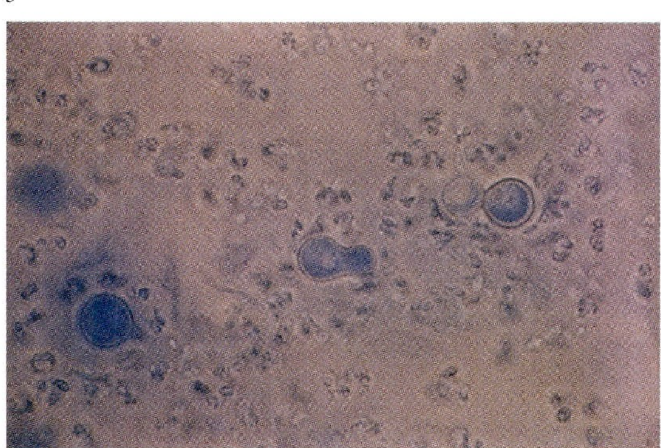

Figure 2 **Thick-walled, broad-based budding yeasts typical for *B. dermatitidis* are seen on biopsy material; they allow a definitive diagnosis of blastomycosis. (*a*) A lung biopsy specimen is stained with periodic acid–Schiff stain. The patient presented with a mass lesion in the right lower lobe and was initially thought to have lung carcinoma. (*b*) Purulent material was aspirated from one of numerous skin lesions in a patient with disseminated blastomycosis. Lactophenol cotton blue stain was used to prepare the slide.**

different enzyme immunoassays have been developed that enhance both specificity and sensitivity,[34] but they are not currently available.

DIFFERENTIAL DIAGNOSIS

The skin lesions of blastomycosis clinically mimic those caused by mycobacteria, especially nontuberculous mycobacteria; other fungal infections, especially coccidioidomycosis or paracoccidioidomycosis; mycosis fungoides; the lesions associated with bromide use; and atypical pyoderma granulosum. The histopathologic characteristics of pseudoepitheliomatous hyperplasia occur in response to other chronic infections and to bromoderma. Culture of biopsy material is of crucial importance in differentiating between these conditions.

Acute pulmonary blastomycosis is almost always misdiagnosed as a bacterial or atypical pneumonia and is then treated with antibiotics. Development of skin lesions is a strong clue suggesting blastomycosis. The masslike pulmonary lesion that is frequently noted with blastomycosis is usually thought to be lung cancer until biopsy results are reported. Likewise, lesions in the upper airways, which are usually firm and nodular, are frequently assumed to be squamous cell carcinoma until biopsy is performed. The clinical and radiographic signs and symptoms of patients with chronic pulmonary blastomycosis are indistinguishable from those associated with tuberculosis, histoplasmosis and other fungal infections, and sometimes sarcoidosis. Histopathologic studies and culture studies from biopsy material are most important in differentiating between these conditions.

TREATMENT

Guidelines for the treatment of blastomycosis have been published by the Mycoses Study Group under the auspices of the Infectious Diseases Society of America.[33] The current recommendations are based on several multicenter, nonrandomized, open-label treatment trials and a few retrospective and prospective reports from individual institutions.[17,18,35,36] There have been no trials comparing amphotericin B with azoles for the treatment of blastomycosis.

In general, patients with pulmonary or disseminated forms of blastomycosis can be treated in a similar manner. Those patients who have mild to moderate illness should be treated with an azole; patients who have severe blastomycosis, either pulmonary or disseminated, and all patients with CNS involvement should receive amphotericin B as initial therapy.[33]

Itraconazole is the drug of choice for the treatment of mild to moderate blastomycosis.[18,33] Although lesions often begin to resolve within the first month of therapy, treatment should be continued for 6 to 12 months to achieve a mycologic cure and to prevent relapse. The usual dosage is 200 mg once or twice daily for 6 to 12 months. Children with blastomycosis should be treated with itraconazole, 5 to 7 mg/kg/day. Osteoarticular involvement requires therapy for at least a year. Fluconazole is not as effective as itraconazole for blastomycosis.[35,36] However, if a patient is unable to take itraconazole because of drug interactions or problems with absorption, fluconazole can be used; the dosage should be high—a total daily dosage of 400 to 800 mg given in once-daily or twice-daily doses for 6 to 12 months.

Amphotericin B should be reserved for patients who have severe blastomycosis, are immunosuppressed, or have CNS involvement.[33] The daily dosage is 0.7 to 1.0 mg/kg until a total of 1 to 2 g has been given. An alternative and preferred approach is to first administer amphotericin B until the patient has improved and then to switch to itraconazole, 200 mg twice daily, for a total of 6 to 12 months of therapy.

Side effects, drug absorption, and drug-drug interactions are important considerations in the use of antifungal therapy [*see* Antifungal Therapy, *below*].

PROGNOSIS

In patients with pulmonary and cutaneous manifestations of blastomycosis who undergo treatment with itraconazole, the clinical and mycologic response rates are 90% to 95%.[18] If relapse occurs, a second treatment with itraconazole is generally successful. Most reported deaths from blastomycosis occur early in the course of disease in patients who present with overwhelming pneumonia and ARDS. The outcome for patients with osteoarticular infection is good, but antifungal therapy should be given for at least a year to effect a cure.

Coccidioidomycosis

EPIDEMIOLOGY

The dimorphic fungus *Coccidioides immitis*, the cause of coccidioidomycosis, occupies the most specific ecological niche of the endemic mycoses commonly seen in the United States.[37,38] The organism grows in the semiarid desert regions known as the Lower Sonoran Life Zone, which encompasses portions of California, Arizona, New Mexico, Nevada, and western Texas. The organism is also found in discrete areas of Central and South America.

The mycelial form of the organism produces arthroconidia, which can be widely dispersed and are highly infectious. Although persons who work outdoors are at highest risk for infection, the wide dispersal of arthroconidia ensures that most of the people who live in the endemic areas become infected before they reach adulthood. In recent years, as the allure of the sun belt has increased, there has been an increase in coccidioidomycosis in older adults. When patients with coccidioidomycosis were subjected to a case-control analysis, the greatest risk factor for the development of infection was a recent move into an area endemic for *C. immitis*.[39]

Periodic outbreaks of coccidioidomycosis in the endemic area have been reported; these outbreaks are probably related to environmental cycles of rain and drought in the desert.[40] Severe infection can follow massive exposure, as might occur during participation in activities such as anthropologic excavations, in which many arthroconidia are dispersed. In addition, catastrophic massive dust storms and earthquakes have been linked to the spread of *C. immitis* to areas far beyond those normally considered endemic for the disease.[40,41]

PATHOGENESIS

Coccidioidomycosis is acquired after the arthroconidia are inhaled into the alveoli. In the lung, the arthroconidia undergo morphologic changes that result in the formation of spherules, which are large (20 to 80 μm), thick-walled structures that become filled with huge numbers of endospores. When filled, the spherule ruptures, releasing the endospores, each of which forms a new spherule and thus propagates the infection. *C. immitis* does not form yeasts in tissues, as do other endemic mycoses.

The primary host defense against *C. immitis* is cell-mediated immunity. Neutrophils are present in most lesions but are ineffective at eradicating spherules. In hosts with deficient T cell immunity, such as patients with AIDS, the organism has the propensity to disseminate widely by the hematogenous route. Not yet elucidated is the reason for the well-known observation that dark-skinned races are at high risk for dissemination and severe infection. The highest risk appears to be among African Americans; higher but less dramatic risks for dissemination are also noted in persons from the Philippines, Native Americans, and Hispanics. Women who develop primary coccidioidomycosis while pregnant, especially in the third trimester, are also at increased risk for disseminated infection.

CLINICAL PRESENTATIONS

Pulmonary Coccidioidomycosis

Most persons with acute infection with coccidioidomycosis have no symptoms or have symptoms that are seen in many types of pneumonias, such as fever, nonproductive cough, chest pain, dyspnea, fatigue, myalgias, and arthralgias. Chest radiographs show a patchy pneumonitis. Erythema nodosum occurs during acute pulmonary coccidioidomycosis in as many as 25% of women and a smaller percentage of men and is a clue to the diagnosis. For most otherwise healthy patients, acute pulmonary coccidioidomycosis is a self-limited infection.

In rare cases, when exposure to the organism is extensive or the host is immunosuppressed, acute overwhelming pneumonia, characterized by high fevers, hypoxemia, and diffuse reticulonodular infiltrates, is seen. This is most commonly noted in patients with advanced HIV infection; in many cases, the pulmonary symptoms are merely one manifestation of widely disseminated infection.

It is estimated that fewer than 5% of patients will have residual manifestations of the acute pulmonary infection.[38] Other than nodules or coccidioidomas, the most common manifestations are cavitary lesions that persist for months to years. These are generally asymptomatic, solitary, thin-walled, peripherally located lesions. Although almost half of these cavities will resolve, for some patients they can last for years and cause hemoptysis, with or without the presence of a mycetoma; they rarely rupture into the pleura. Chronic progressive coccidioidal pneumonia is rare but is more likely to occur in older patients who have COPD and diabetes mellitus; this form of coccidioidomycosis mimics tuberculosis or chronic cavitary histoplasmosis clinically and radiographically.[42]

Disseminated Coccidioidomycosis

As with other endemic mycoses, hematogenous dissemination of *C. immitis* is probably common and mostly asymptomatic. However, approximately one in every 200 people will develop symptoms of extrapulmonary coccidioidomycosis.[37] The manifestations of extrapulmonary infection with *C. immitis* are protean; they may be focal and related to only one organ system that has been seeded, or they may be systemic. The sites involved most often are skin, bones, subcutaneous tissues, and the meninges. In a recent study, risk factors for disseminated disease included African-American race, low socioeconomic status, and pregnancy.[42] Other studies have noted an increased risk of dissemination in patients with hematologic malignancies, those who have received an organ transplant, and, not surprisingly, those with AIDS.[37,38]

The skin lesions of coccidioidomycosis are typically papular or pustular initially and then become plaquelike or verrucous; facial lesions are common. Ulceration can occur, but drainage is usually minimal. Subcutaneous abscesses are commonly noted in disseminated coccidioidomycosis. Sinus tracts form, and they may drain intermittently for years. There often is underlying osteomyelitis contiguous with these subcutaneous abscesses. Bony lesions may be single or multiple and can appear in any area of the body; vertebral involvement is particularly common. Although skin and soft tissue abscesses respond fairly well to antifungal therapy, osteomyelitis and coccidioidal arthritis are characterized by an indolent, relapsing course in spite of antifungal therapy.

C. immitis can infect any organ system, but the most dreaded complication of dissemination is meningitis. Chronic progressive meningeal infection is typically concentrated in the basilar area. Meningitis may be only one of several manifestations of severe disseminated coccidioidomycosis, or it may be the sole manifestation of coccidioidomycosis. The symptoms include headache, cranial nerve palsies, and signs of increased intracranial pressure. Vasculitis occurs throughout the brain in a minority of patients with coccidioidal meningitis, and spinal cord involvement at any level of the spinal cord is not uncommon. If not treated, this form of coccidioidomycosis is fatal in virtually all patients within 2 years of diagnosis. Even with treatment, which must be lifelong, the outcomes are poor.

DIAGNOSIS

Culture

The definitive diagnostic test is growth of the organism. The mold phase of *C. immitis* grows within several days to a week on most laboratory media. DNA probes can identify the organism very specifically once growth has occurred. Also very helpful is histopathologic identification of the very distinctive large spherules of *C. immitis* in tissue biopsy, on cytologic preparations from body fluids, and even on KOH smears from sputum or from purulent material of an abscess [*see Figure 3*].

Serologic Studies

Serology is quite helpful in the diagnosis of various forms of coccidioidomycosis, as discussed in several excellent reviews.[38,43] For serologic tests to be as useful as possible, it is important that they be sent to a reference laboratory that is experienced in performing fungal serologic analyses. Early appearance of IgM antibodies, detected through an ID test, is helpful for the diagnosis of acute coccidioidomycosis, but this test is not always sensitive enough to detect early infection. An enzyme immunoassay

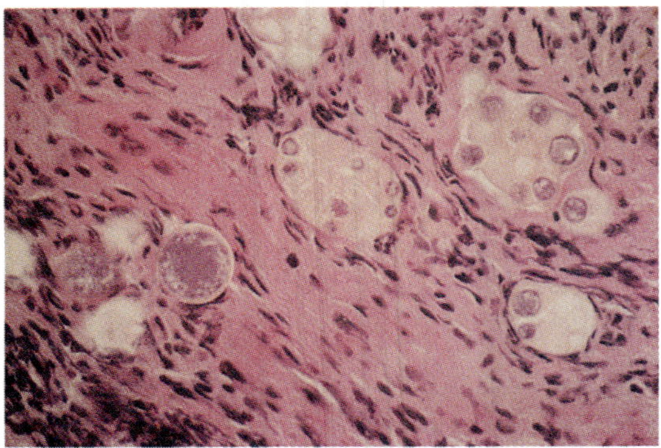

Figure 3 **Shown is a transbronchial lung biopsy specimen, stained with hematoxylin-eosin stain, from a patient with advanced HIV infection and diffuse reticulonodular pulmonary infiltrates. Large spherules (measuring 60 to 80 µm) of *C. immitis* in various stages of maturation are evident.**

that is not standardized appears to be more sensitive, but false positive results are common. For patients with chronic infections and to follow the course of infection, an IgG CF assay is generally used. A decrease in the CF antibody titer or reversion to a negative titer is associated with a good clinical response, and a stable high (> 1:16) titer or a rising titer is a poor prognostic sign. A positive CF antibody titer obtained on cerebrospinal fluid is diagnostic of coccidioidal meningitis; cultures of CSF very infrequently yield *C. immitis*.

Skin Tests

Skin testing with coccidioidal antigens is helpful for the diagnosis of acute infection in a person who has just entered an endemic area, but it is of little benefit for residents of endemic areas. A negative skin test result in a patient with known coccidioidomycosis implies absence of cell-mediated immunity and portends a poor prognosis.

DIFFERENTIAL DIAGNOSIS

Coccidioidomycosis mimics many other infections. Acute pulmonary coccidioidomycosis is often diagnosed as an atypical pneumonia caused by a virus, *Mycoplasma*, or *Chlamydia*. Chronic cavitary pneumonia is radiographically similar to tuberculosis and other endemic mycoses. The diffuse pulmonary infiltrates seen in immunosuppressed patients are no different from those noted in patients with *Pneumocystis carinii* infection, histoplasmosis, tuberculosis, nocardiosis, and many other infections. The importance of tissue biopsy for histopathology and culture in these settings cannot be overemphasized.

The cutaneous lesions can appear similar to those seen in patients with blastomycosis, or they can mimic squamous or basal cell carcinomas. The bone involvement associated with coccidioidomycosis, which is frequently accompanied by subcutaneous abscesses, is typical of that seen in patients with blastomycosis or tuberculosis. The differential diagnosis of chronic coccidioidal meningitis includes tuberculosis, other fungal infections (cryptococcosis, histoplasmosis, and, rarely, sporotrichosis or blastomycosis), and sarcoidosis and other disorders of noninfectious etiology.

TREATMENT

The Mycoses Study Group and the Infectious Diseases Society of America have recently published guidelines for the treatment of coccidioidomycosis.[44] Except for one recently completed randomized, blinded comparative trial,[45] the appropriate treatment for various forms of coccidioidomycosis has been defined by open-label, nonrandomized, multicenter trials and anecdotal experience from experienced clinicians who practice in areas endemic for coccidioidomycosis.[37,38,45–49] In contrast to the other endemic mycoses, either fluconazole or itraconazole can be used to treat coccidioidomycosis. A head-to-head, blinded, randomized comparison of fluconazole and itraconazole (each given in dosages of 400 mg daily for 1 year) showed no overall statistically significant difference in efficacy between the drugs.[45] However, for skeletal coccidioidomycosis, itraconazole was significantly superior to fluconazole (the response rates were 70% versus 30% after 1 year of therapy).[45]

Side effects, drug absorption, and drug-drug interactions are important considerations in the use of antifungal therapy [*see* Antifungal Therapy, *below*].

Pulmonary Coccidioidomycosis

Most patients with acute pulmonary coccidioidomycosis do not require therapy with an antifungal agent, and in fact, most are not seen by a physician or the diagnosis is not made until after improvement has occurred. For patients with symptoms lasting 3 to 4 weeks who show no sign of improvement, therapy with either itraconazole, 200 mg twice daily, or fluconazole, 400 mg daily, for 3 to 6 months is recommended.[44] Any patient with underlying immunosuppression, especially immunosuppression associated with HIV infection, solid-organ or stem cell transplantation, or corticosteroid therapy, should be treated because the risk of dissemination is high. Pregnant women are also at risk for dissemination and should be treated. However, azoles cannot be used in pregnant women; rather, amphotericin B, which is safe in pregnancy, is required. Consideration should be given for treatment of African-American and Filipino patients because of the high risk of dissemination in these populations.

When diffuse pulmonary infiltrates are present, patients should receive amphotericin B, 0.7 mg/kg/day initially, followed by azole therapy, for a total of at least 1 year of therapy. Patients who have chronic cavitary coccidioidomycosis should receive therapy with itraconazole, 200 mg twice daily, or fluconazole, 400 mg daily for 1 to 2 years, depending on the patient's response. However, patients with asymptomatic cavities are often observed, and treatment with an azole is begun only if the cavities increase in size or complications such as rupture into the pleural cavity have occurred or seem imminent. Surgical removal of cavities is preferred if the patient is a good operative candidate.

Disseminated Coccidioidomycosis

Disseminated coccidioidomycosis should always be treated. Patients who are seriously ill require therapy with amphotericin B, 0.7 mg/kg/day; patients with mild to moderate symptoms can be treated with an azole.[44] Treatment should be given for at least 1 year; for some patients, especially those with HIV infection and African Americans, lifelong azole therapy may be required to prevent relapse.

The most difficult form of coccidioidomycosis to treat is meningitis. The preferred treatment is fluconazole; the dosage probably should be 800 mg daily, although initial studies of this therapy employed doses of only 400 mg daily.[48,49] Itraconazole has been reported to be as effective as fluconazole, but experience with itraconazole is limited and most physicians prefer fluconazole. Approximately 20% to 25% of patients will not respond to fluconazole. Amphotericin B administered by both the intravenous and the intrathecal routes is used for those in whom fluconazole therapy fails. Intrathecal amphotericin B is not well tolerated. Repeated administration of amphotericin B into the lumbar area leads to arachnoiditis, and this is an inefficient method of delivering drug to the basilar meninges. Ideally, the drug should be administered into the cistern, but most physicians cannot perform this procedure. An alternative method is delivery through an intraventricular reservoir, but this method also does not deliver drug to the basilar meninges as efficiently as intracisternal injection. Therapy must be individualized and must be given for life.[49]

PROGNOSIS

Of all the endemic mycoses, infection with *C. immitis* is the least responsive to currently available antifungal agents. Success rates with azoles are highest in patients with soft tissue infections (approximately 70% of such patients respond after 12 months of therapy); success rates are lower in patients with chronic pulmonary infection (response rates of 50% to 60% are seen in these patients).[45–47] Relapses are more common with coccidioidomycosis than with other endemic mycoses. For patients with chronic relapsing disease, who are often of African-American descent, lifelong azole therapy may be required. For patients with meningitis, cures are rare, and suppressive therapy must be continued indefinitely.[49]

Sporotrichosis

EPIDEMIOLOGY

The dimorphic fungus *Sporothrix schenckii* is found worldwide. The environmental niches for the organism include sphagnum moss, decaying vegetation, hay, and soil. Infection is seen most often in persons whose vocation or avocation brings them into contact with the environment. Landscaping, rose gardening, Christmas tree farming, topiary production, baling hay, and motor vehicle accidents have all been associated with sporotrichosis.[50–52] Less commonly, pulmonary sporotrichosis results from inhalation of *S. schenckii* conidia from soil. Cases of sporotrichosis usually occur sporadically, but outbreaks have been described. The largest outbreak in the United States involved 84 patients in 25 states and was traced back to conifer seedlings that had been packed in sphagnum moss from Wisconsin.[50]

S. schenckii can also be acquired through exposure to animals that are either infected or are able to passively transfer the organism from soil through scratching or biting. A variety of animals have been reported to transmit sporotrichosis, but cats with ulcerated skin lesions appear to be the most infectious. Clusters of sporotrichosis involving families and veterinarians caring for infected cats have been described.[53]

PATHOGENESIS

Sporotrichosis typically develops in an otherwise healthy person who becomes exposed to the fungus while outdoors. The typical clinical picture is that of localized cutaneous or lymphocutaneous disease. After inoculation of *S. schenckii* conidia, the organism converts to the yeast form, which reproduces by budding. Strains that grow poorly at temperatures higher than 35° C tend to be found in fixed cutaneous lesions; these strains do not have the ability to spread along lymphatics, as do most strains of *S. schenckii*.[54]

In patients with underlying illnesses, including alcoholism, diabetes mellitus, COPD, and HIV infection, *S. schenckii* can disseminate to involve osteoarticular structures, lungs, meninges, and other organs. Neutrophils and macrophages are able to ingest and kill the yeast phase of *S. schenckii* in the presence of nonimmune human serum. A role for cell-mediated immunity as a host defense against *S. schenckii* is suggested by the observation that sporotrichosis is more severe in those with HIV infection.[55]

CLINICAL PRESENTATIONS

Lymphocutaneous Sporotrichosis

Days to weeks after cutaneous inoculation of the fungus, a papule develops at the site of inoculation. The primary lesion can become nodular, but most often, it ulcerates. The drainage is not grossly purulent and has no odor, and the lesion is not terribly painful. Similar lesions subsequently occur along the lymphatic channels proximal to the original lesion. A fixed cutaneous lesion that is verrucous or ulcerative and that is not associated with lymphatic extension can also occur.[56]

Visceral Sporotrichosis

Pulmonary sporotrichosis occurs most often in middle-aged men who have COPD and abuse alcohol.[57] In contrast to most forms of sporotrichosis, systemic symptoms, including fever, night sweats, weight loss, and fatigue, are common. Dyspnea, cough, purulent sputum, and hemoptysis are common respiratory symptoms. A chest radiograph shows unilateral or bilateral upper lobe cavities with variable amounts of fibrosis and nodular lesions.

Osteoarticular sporotrichosis is found most often in middle-aged men and occurs more frequently in patients with alcoholism.[58] Although some patients experience osteoarticular involvement after local inoculation, this form of infection most often develops through hematogenous spread. Infection may involve one joint or multiple joints. The joints most commonly affected are the knee, elbow, wrist, and ankle. Isolated cases of bursitis and tenosynovitis, sometimes presenting as nerve entrapment syndromes, have been reported.

S. schenckii has rarely been reported to cause localized infection of the meninges, pericardium, eye, perirectal tissues, larynx, breast, epididymis, spleen, liver, bone marrow, or lymph nodes.[54] Disseminated sporotrichosis is very uncommon, with cases occurring primarily in patients with advanced HIV infection.[55] Most patients have widespread ulcerative cutaneous lesions and may or may not have visceral dissemination.

DIAGNOSIS

Culture

Growth of *S. schenckii* from material aspirated from a lesion, a tissue biopsy specimen, sputum, or body fluid is the most sensitive method for establishing a diagnosis of sporotrichosis. Growth of the mold phase of *S. schenckii* is usually evident a few days after inoculation onto Sabouraud agar. Synovial tissue provides a better yield than synovial fluid.

Biopsy

Histopathologic examination of biopsy material shows a mixed granulomatous and pyogenic process. The organisms often are not visualized, even with special stains for fungi, because they are rarely present in large numbers. When visualized, *S. schenckii* yeasts are 3 to 5 µm in diameter; they are oval to cigar-shaped and may show multiple buds.

Serologic Studies

Serology is less useful in the diagnosis of sporotrichosis than in histoplasmosis and coccidioidomycosis. A tube agglutination test is available at the Centers for Disease Control and Prevention; however, the sensitivity and specificity of this assay has not been established.

DIFFERENTIAL DIAGNOSIS

The differential diagnosis of lymphocutaneous sporotrichosis includes atypical mycobacterial infections, especially *M. marinum* infections; *Nocardia* infections, particularly *N. brasiliensis* infections; *Leishmania brasiliensis* infections; and tularemia.[59] Both clinically and radiographically, pulmonary sporotrichosis mimics tuberculosis; nontuberculous mycobacterial infections; other fungal infections, especially histoplasmosis; and sarcoidosis. Osteoarticular sporotrichosis is often thought to have a bacterial etiology and is often treated with antibiotics, to no avail. Growth of the organism in culture is the most important method of differentiating between these conditions.

TREATMENT

Guidelines for the management of the various forms of sporotrichosis have recently been published by the Mycoses Study Group and the Infectious Diseases Society of America.[60] No comparative randomized, blinded treatment trials have been performed comparing various antifungal agents for the treatment of sporotrichosis. The guidelines are based entirely on open treatment trials and anecdotal experience.[58,61–64] Because most *S. schenckii* infections are subacute to chronic and are localized, oral antifungal agents are preferred; amphotericin B is reserved for the uncommon visceral infections.

Lymphocutaneous Sporotrichosis

Itraconazole is the drug of choice for lymphocutaneous sporotrichosis.[60] The usual dose is 200 mg/day. Treatment should continue for several weeks after all lesions have disappeared, usually for a total of 3 to 6 months.[58,62,63] Fluconazole is less active against *S. schenckii* but may be effective when a daily dose of 400 mg is used.[64] Saturated solution of potassium iodide (SSKI) is also effective and is much less costly than therapy with an azole. The initial dose is 5 to 10 drops three times daily in water or juice; the dose is increased each week to a maximum of 40 to 50 drops three times daily. SSKI is difficult for many patients to administer and tolerate; side effects include a metallic taste, salivary gland swelling, rash, and fever.[61]

Terbinafine appears to be effective for sporotrichosis, but few patients have been treated with this agent to date.[65] Local hyperthermia, induced by a variety of different warming devices or baths, also has been used with minimal side effects for localized cutaneous sporotrichosis.[66]

Visceral Sporotrichosis

For a seriously ill patient with pulmonary sporotrichosis, amphotericin B, 0.7 to 1.0 mg/kg/day, should be used as initial therapy.[60] After the patient has shown improvement, therapy can be changed to itraconazole, 200 mg twice daily. Azole therapy should be continued for at least 1 to 2 years. For patients who are not acutely ill, therapy can be initiated with itraconazole, 200 mg twice daily.[58] Surgical resection has proved to be useful for patients who have focal lesions and whose pulmonary function is adequate to withstand a lobectomy.[61]

Almost all patients who have osteoarticular sporotrichosis can be treated with itraconazole, 200 mg twice daily.[60] Therapy should continue for 1 to 2 years.[58] Other azoles are less effective, and SSKI is ineffective. Intravenous amphotericin B is rarely required.

Amphotericin B, 0.7 to 1.0 mg/kg/day, is the drug of choice for disseminated sporotrichosis, including meningeal infection.[60] Itraconazole, 200 mg twice daily, can be used in those patients with disseminated skin lesions and other nonmeningeal manifestations as soon as the patient's condition has stabilized. AIDS patients with disseminated sporotrichosis should receive lifelong maintenance therapy with itraconazole, 200 mg daily.[55]

PROGNOSIS

The success rate for treatment of lymphocutaneous sporotrichosis is 90% to 100%, but it is much lower for all other forms of the disease. This is undoubtedly related partly to delays in diagnosis and partly to the underlying diseases of the hosts who have noncutaneous forms of sporotrichosis. Joint function after cure of sporotrichal arthritis is often poor, and pulmonary function after treatment of pulmonary sporotrichosis is often marginal. The outcome of disseminated sporotrichosis in patients with HIV infection has been poor,[55] but almost all reports are from studies conducted before the era of highly active antiretroviral therapy. Presumably, combination antifungal therapy and highly active antiretroviral therapy would improve the prognosis.

Antifungal Therapy

For treatment of the endemic mycoses, the choice of azoles or amphotericin B is dependent on the severity of the infection and the underlying conditions and the immune status of the host. In general, most mild to moderately ill patients can be very effectively treated with an azole; most severely ill patients should receive amphotericin B as initial therapy.[67] Induction amphotericin B therapy can almost always be followed by consolidation therapy with an azole. The length of therapy is measured in months to years and is obviously managed primarily in the outpatient setting. For some patients (e.g., those with AIDS), lifelong maintenance therapy is required to prevent relapse. Thus, issues of compliance, absorption, and drug-drug interactions assume great importance in current treatment regimens for the endemic mycoses.

USE OF AZOLES TO TREAT ENDEMIC MYCOSES

There are three azole antifungal agents currently available: ketoconazole, itraconazole, and fluconazole. Ketoconazole, which is available only in tablet form, is used infrequently now because of its greater toxicity, poor absorption, and modest spectrum of antifungal activity when compared with the other azoles.[68] However, it is still used for some patients who require long-term therapy with an azole because it is much less expensive than itraconazole and fluconazole. For most patients, itraconazole has supplanted ketoconazole because it is both more effective and better tolerated. Fluconazole is less active than itraconazole against most of the endemic mycoses,[21,22,35,36,64] and except for coccidioidomycosis,[45,48] it is a second-line agent. The newer azoles, voriconazole, posaconazole, and ravuconazole, have not been studied for the treatment of the endemic mycoses, with the exception of a very small trial that used posaconazole for the treatment of coccidioidomycosis. These agents are not indicated for the treatment of the endemic mycoses at this time.

Side Effects

Idiosyncratic, non–dose-related hepatitis, which can sometimes be severe, occurs rarely with all azoles.[68,69] Before therapy is started, liver enzyme and bilirubin levels should be measured; they should be measured again after several weeks of therapy and then every 1 to 2 months in patients receiving long-term therapy. Mild elevations in the levels of alanine aminotransferase (ALT) or aspartate aminotransferase (AST) (i.e., a twofold to threefold increase over normal levels) do not require discontinuance of the drug, but such increases do require very careful follow-up. If the ALT and AST levels continue to rise, the drug should be discontinued. If therapy with an azole is required, another azole can be cautiously given after the ALT and AST levels return to normal, but liver enzyme levels should be assessed weekly, and the drug must be stopped if the ALT and AST levels rise threefold or more while the patient is receiving the second azole.

It is uncommon for hypertension, edema, and hypokalemia to occur with itraconazole therapy; such side effects usually occur in older adults and require discontinuance of the drug.[70] Whether these effects are related to the recently described myocardial dysfunction noted with itraconazole has not yet been elucidated.[71]

Rash and nausea can occur with all azoles. Long-term therapy with fluconazole has been associated with alopecia, which is reversible when the drug is discontinued.[72] All azoles are contraindicated during pregnancy; teratogenicity in animals has been noted, and several cases of fetal malformations have been reported in women taking fluconazole during pregnancy.[73]

Absorption Issues

Both ketoconazole and itraconazole require gastric acid for absorption, and the capsule formulation of itraconazole also requires food for absorption. Therefore, histamine receptor antagonists (H_2 receptor blockers), antacids, and proton pump inhibitors cannot be administered to patients receiving these agents.[68] Older adults, who are often achlorhydric, may not absorb these agents well. For the treatment of endemic mycoses, itraconazole is commonly used at a daily dose of 400 mg; regardless of whether solution or capsules are prescribed, the drug should be administered in twice-daily doses of 200 mg, rather than a once-daily dose of 400 mg, to achieve appropriate serum drug levels. At doses higher than 200 mg, decreased absorption of the drug occurs.

The oral-suspension formulation of itraconazole was developed specifically to overcome the poor absorption characteristics of the capsules. The suspension requires neither acid nor food for absorption. When taken on an empty stomach, absorption is approximately 30% better than when the capsule formulation is given with both food and acid.[74] Although compliance with long-term use of the oral suspension may be difficult, the suspension is preferred to ensure adequate serum levels. In patients with serious infection and those who do not respond to therapy, serum itraconazole levels should be obtained at a reference mycology laboratory to ensure that absorption is adequate.

Use of the intravenous formulation of itraconazole, solubilized in cyclodextrins, avoids absorption problems.[75] The intravenous formulation has been approved for use for periods of only 2 weeks because of concerns about the nephrotoxicity of the cyclodextrin vehicle, which is used to solubilize the drug. The intravenous formulation cannot be given if the rate of creatinine clearance is less than 30 ml/min. The dosage of the intravenous formulation is 200 mg twice daily for 2 days, followed by 200 mg daily for the next 12 days; intravenous therapy is usually followed by treatment with the oral suspension.

Fluconazole, which is nearly 100% bioavailable, has none of the absorption problems that have been so troublesome with itraconazole. It distrib-

Table 1 Effects of Concomitantly Administered Drugs on Serum Levels of Azoles

Drug Affecting Azole Serum Level	*Effects That Other Drugs Have on Azole Serum Levels*		
	Ketoconazole	*Itraconazole*	*Fluconazole*
Antituberculous drugs			
Rifampin	Decreased	Decreased	Decreased
Rifabutin	None known	Decreased	No effect
Isoniazid	Decreased	None known	None known
Anticonvulsants			
Phenytoin	Decreased	Decreased	None known
Carbamazepine	None known	Decreased	None known
Gastric acid-lowering agents*			
Antacids	Decreased	Decreased	No effect
H_2 receptor blockers	Decreased	Decreased	No effect
Proton pump inhibitors	Decreased	Decreased	No effect
Sucralfate	Decreased	None known	No effect

*Gastric acid-lowering agents should not be used with ketoconazole or itraconazole capsules; if necessary, they can be used with itraconazole suspension.

utes into most body compartments, including the eye and the CSF; is excreted as active drug in the urine; and can be given in a once-daily dose.

Drug-Drug Interactions

The azoles interact with many other drugs primarily through their interactions with cytochrome P-450 3A4 but also to a lesser extent through their interactions with several of the other cytochrome enzymes and with P-glycoprotein.[69] These interactions can be serious and even life-threatening. It is absolutely essential that the patient's concomitant medications be reviewed and the package insert read before use of any azole for the treatment of any fungal infection. Major interactions for the azoles are detailed [*see Tables 1 and 2*].

Itraconazole and ketoconazole have the most drug-drug interactions, but fluconazole shares several significant interactions. Increased serum levels of warfarin, phenytoin, and oral hypoglycemic agents occur when azoles are given with these commonly used drugs. Itraconazole increases serum levels of digoxin in some but not all patients. Thus, serum levels of these agents must be closely monitored in those receiving an azole.

Itraconazole and ketoconazole should never be given to patients receiving cholesterol-lowering agents, such as simvastatin and lovastatin, because of the potential for life-threatening rhabdomyolysis, nor should these agents be given to those receiving midazolam or triazolam because of the possibility of markedly increased sedation. Coadministration of an azole with cisapride, astemizole, or terfenadine is contraindicated because azoles potentiate the prolongation of the QT interval that is induced by these drugs.

Several commonly used drugs have the effect of inducing the metabolism of the azoles and thus decreasing serum azole concentrations and diminishing effectiveness. This has been reported with rifampin, phenytoin, and carbamazepine.

USE OF AMPHOTERICIN B TO TREAT ENDEMIC MYCOSES

Amphotericin B is fungicidal against a broad range of fungi. The major drawbacks are the need for intravenous administration and the inherent toxicity of the drug.[76] Some, but not all, of the infusion-related reactions to amphotericin B can be minimized with the use of preinfusion medications[77]; however, nephrotoxicity will almost always develop during the course of therapy with this agent.[78]

In an attempt to decrease the toxicity of amphotericin B, the drug has been incorporated into liposomes and other lipid delivery vehicles. Three formulations are currently available: liposomal amphotericin B (AmBisome, L-AmB); amphotericin B lipid complex (Abelcet, ABLC); and amphotericin B colloidal dispersion (Amphotec or Amphocil, ABCD). Each differs from the others and from amphotericin B deoxycholate with regard to composition, pharmacologic parameters, toxicity, recommended dosages, and cost.[79,80] All of these preparations are clearly less nephrotoxic than amphotericin B deoxycholate, and two of the three

Table 2 Effects of Azoles on Serum Levels of Other Drugs

Drug Affected by Azole	*Effects That Azoles Have on Other Drugs' Serum Levels*		
	Ketoconazole	*Itraconazole*	*Fluconazole*
Immunosuppressants			
Cyclosporine	Increased*	Increased*	Increased*
Tacrolimus	Increased*	Increased*	Increased*
Anticonvulsants			
Phenytoin	Increased*	Increased*	Increased*
Carbamazepine	Increased*	Increased*	Increased*
Antihistamines			
Loratadine	Increased	None known	None known
Terfenadine	Increased†	Increased†	No effect
Astemizole	Increased†	Increased†	None known
Sedatives			
Triazolam	Increased*	Increased*	Increased*
Midazolam	Increased*	Increased*	Increased*
Cholesterol-lowering agents			
Lovastatin	None known	Increased†	None known
Simvastatin	None known	Increased†	None known
Antiretroviral agents			
Indinavir	Increased	None known	None known
Saquinavir	Increased	None known	None known
Ritonavir	Increased	Increased	Increased
Nelfinavir	Increased	None known	None known
Antituberculous drugs			
Rifampin	Decreased	None known	None known
Isoniazid	Decreased	None known	None known
Rifabutin	None known	Increased	Increased
Other drugs			
Cisapride	Increased†	Increased†	Increased†
Warfarin	Increased*	Increased*	Increased*
Digoxin	None known	Increased*	None known
Sulfonylureas	Increased*	Increased*	Increased*
Quinidine	Increased†	Increased†	None known

*Significant interaction; monitoring of drug serum levels, clinical status, or both is required.
†Life-threatening interaction; these agents should not be used together.

cause fewer infusion-related reactions than amphotericin B deoxycholate. However, they are all much more costly than standard amphotericin B. Because of cost considerations, many hospitals restrict the use of these preparations to patients who have preexisting renal disease or have developed some degree of renal failure related to amphotericin B deoxycholate administration (as evidenced, for example, by a serum creatinine level of more than 2 or 3 mg/dl).

Other than two studies that show liposomal amphotericin B to be superior to amphotericin B deoxycholate for the treatment of severe histoplasmosis in AIDS patients and for the empirical treatment of febrile neutropenic patients,[23,81] there is little evidence to suggest that lipid formulations of amphotericin B are more efficacious than the standard formulation. Thus, for most patients, a lipid formulation of amphotericin B will not be used as a first-line antifungal agent but will be reserved for patients who cannot tolerate amphotericin B deoxycholate.

Nephrotoxicity

Nephrotoxicity is seen in most patients receiving amphotericin B. Diminished creatinine clearance is the major manifestation, but profound hypokalemia, hypomagnesemia, or both are also common. Patients with underlying renal disease show a more rapid rise in creatinine levels than

Table 3 Administration of Amphotericin B for Treatment of the Endemic Mycoses

General Guidelines

- Do not use in-line filters; no need to cover drug while infusing
- Use central I.V. catheter if at all possible. With peripheral I.V. catheter, 1,000 units of heparin can be added to the drug in an attempt to decrease phlebitis
- Dilute drug to a concentration of 0.1 mg/ml
- For the initial dose, infuse very slowly for the first 20 minutes and assess for the rare occurrence of anaphylaxis or arrhythmias
- Infuse drug over 2 to 4 hours; for patients with infusion-related reactions, slower infusion times are often better tolerated; for others, 2-hr infusion times are appropriate
- For subacute or chronic infections, start with 0.2 mg/kg and increase daily by the same increment until the desired daily dose is reached; use pretreatment medications only if required
- For life-threatening infections, give the desired daily dose within the first 24 hr; preinfusion medications should be given before the first dose because reactions are frequent

Measures to Decrease Infusion-Related Reactions (chills, fever, nausea and vomiting, headache, myalgia)

- Medications before beginning infusion of amphotericin B: acetaminophen (650 mg p.o.), diphenhydramine (50 mg p.o.), prochlorperazine (25 mg p.o. for nausea and vomiting), and meperidine (50–75 mg I.V. or I.M. for rigors); administer hydrocortisone (25–50 mg I.V.) if reactions do not improve with the above drugs

Measures to Reduce Nephrotoxicity

- Assess volume status before treatment; stop diuretics, if possible; do not restrict sodium
- Before each dose, infuse 500 ml 0.9% saline over 1 hr

Required Laboratory Studies to Assess Toxicity

- Baseline creatinine, blood urea nitrogen, potassium, magnesium levels; blood count, liver function tests
- Monitor creatinine, blood urea nitrogen, potassium, magnesium levels every other day
- Monitor blood count weekly; repeat liver function tests if clinically indicated

patients with normal renal function. Use of other nephrotoxic drugs, such as aminoglycosides, cisplatinum, cyclosporine, or tacrolimus, should be avoided when amphotericin B is being used.

Sodium loading is now routinely employed in an attempt to decrease nephrotoxicity[82] [*see Table 3*]. Potassium and magnesium losses can be large and can contribute to other organ dysfunction; for this reason, electrolytes should be monitored carefully, and electrolytes should be replaced as soon as the serum levels show even a slight decrease. In many patients, intravenous repletion is ultimately required to keep pace with the renal loss. Early oral repletion will obviate the need for intravenous repletion in many patients.

Infusion-related Reactions

Infusion-related reactions are the most common adverse events experienced by patients receiving amphotericin B. Chills or rigors, fever, nausea, headache, and myalgias occur in the majority of patients treated with amphotericin B. Most of these side effects can be diminished by prescribing a variety of medications before infusion of amphotericin B[77] [*see Table 3*].

Patients with life-threatening infections that require immediate treatment with large doses of amphotericin B are more likely to have infusion-related reactions. Pretreatment medications should be given before the first dose of amphotericin B in these patients. For others who have subacute to chronic infections, the dosage of amphotericin B can be increased gradually over a few days, decreasing the risk of immediate reactions.

Other Side Effects

Most patients receiving amphotericin B develop a normocytic, normochromic anemia, but transfusion is rarely required.[83] Other side effects, including leukopenia, thrombocytopenia, hepatotoxicity, neuropathy, and acute pulmonary edema, are rare.

The author has received grant or research support from Pfizer, Inc., and participates in the speakers' bureaus for Fujisawa Healthcare, Inc.; Ortho Biotech Products, L.P.; and Pfizer, Inc.

References

1. Wheat J: Histoplasmosis: experience during outbreaks in Indianapolis and review of the literature. Medicine (Baltimore) 76:339, 1997

2. Cano M, Hajjeh RA: The epidemiology of histoplasmosis: a review. Semin Respir Infect 16:109, 2001

3. Jones TF, Swinger GL, Craig AS, et al: Acute pulmonary histoplasmosis in bridge workers: a persistent problem. Am J Med 106:480, 1999

4. Newman SL: Cell-mediated immunity to *Histoplasma capsulatum*. Semin Respir Infect 16:102, 2001

5. Wheat LJ, Kauffman CA: Histoplasmosis. Infect Dis Clin North Am (in press)

6. Gurney JW, Conces DJ Jr: Pulmonary histoplasmosis. Radiology 199: 297, 1996

7. Wheat LJ, Connolly-Stringfield PA, Baker RL, et al: Disseminated histoplasmosis in the acquired immune deficiency syndrome: clinical findings, diagnosis and treatment, and review of the literature. Medicine (Baltimore) 69:361, 1990

8. Goodwin RA Jr, Owens FT, Snell JD, et al: Chronic pulmonary histoplasmosis. Medicine (Baltimore) 55:413, 1976

9. Wheat LJ, Wass J, Norton J, et al: Cavitary histoplasmosis occurring during two large urban outbreaks: analysis of clinical, epidemiologic, roentgenographic, and laboratory features. Medicine (Baltimore) 63:201, 1984

10. Johnson PC, Khardori N, Najjar AF, et al: Progressive disseminated histoplasmosis in patients with acquired immunodeficiency syndrome. Am J Med 85:152, 1988

11. Goodwin RA Jr, Shapiro JL, Thurman GH, et al: Disseminated histoplasmosis: clinical and pathologic correlations. Medicine (Baltimore) 59:1, 1980

12. Wheat LJ: Laboratory diagnosis of histoplasmosis: update 2000. Semin Respir Infect 16:131, 2001

13. Wheat LJ, Kohler RB, Tewari RP: Diagnosis of disseminated histoplasmosis by detection of *Histoplasma capsulatum* antigen in serum and urine specimens. N Engl J Med 314:83, 1986

14. Durkin MM, Connolly PA, Wheat LJ: Comparison of radioimmunoassay and enzyme-linked immunoassay methods for detection of *Histoplasma capsulatum* var. *capsulatum* antigen. J Clin Microbiol 35:2252:1997

15. Gulati M, Saint S, Tierney LM Jr: Impatient inpatient care. N Engl J Med 342:37, 2000

16. Wheat J, Sarosi G, McKinsey D, et al: Practice guidelines for the management of patients with histoplasmosis. Clin Infect Dis 30:688, 2000 http://www.journals.uchicago.edu/IDSA/guidelines

17. Dismukes WE, Cloud G, Bowles C, et al: Treatment of blastomycosis and histoplasmosis with ketoconazole: results of a prospective randomized clinical trial. Ann Intern Med 103:861, 1985

18. Dismukes WE, Bradsher RW Jr, Cloud GC, et al: Itraconazole therapy for blastomycosis and histoplasmosis. Am J Med 93:489, 1992

19. Wheat J, Hafner R, Korzun AH, et al: Itraconazole treatment of disseminated histoplasmosis in patients with the acquired immunodeficiency syndrome. Am J Med 98:336, 1995

20. Wheat J, Hafner R, Wulfsohn M, et al: Prevention of relapse of histoplasmosis with itraconazole in patients with the acquired immunodeficiency syndrome. Ann Intern Med 118:610, 1993

21. McKinsey DS, Kauffman CA, Pappas PG, et al: Fluconazole therapy for histoplasmosis. Clin Infect Dis 23:996, 1996

22. Wheat J, MaWhinney S, Hafner R, et al: Treatment of histoplasmosis with fluconazole in patients with acquired immunodeficiency syndrome. Am J Med 103:223, 1997

23. Johnson PC, Wheat LJ, Cloud GA, et al: Safety and efficacy of liposomal amphotericin B compared with conventional amphotericin B for induction therapy of histoplasmosis in patients with AIDS. Ann Intern Med (in press)

24. Davis AM, Pierson RN, Loyd JE: Mediastinal fibrosis. Semin Respir Infect 16:119, 2001

25. Sherrick AD, Brown LR, Harms GF, et al: The radiographic findings of fibrosing mediastinitis. Chest 106:484, 1994

26. Pappas PG: Blastomycosis. Seminars in Respiratory and Critical Care Medicine 18:217, 1997

27. Klein BS, Vergeront JM, Weeks RJ, et al: Isolation of *Blastomyces dermatitidis* in soil associated with a large outbreak of blastomycosis in Wisconsin. N Engl J Med 314:529, 1986

28. Baumgardner DJ, Buggy BP, Mattson BJ, et al: Epidemiology of blastomycosis in a region of high endemicity in north central Wisconsin. Clin Infect Dis 15:629, 1992

29. Pappas PG, Threlkeld MG, Bedsole GD, et al: Blastomycosis in immunocompromised patients. Medicine (Baltimore) 72:311, 1993

30. Meyer KC, McManus EJ, Maki DG: Overwhelming pulmonary blastomycosis associated with the adult respiratory distress syndrome. N Engl J Med 329:1231, 1993

31. Bradsher RW: Histoplasmosis and blastomycosis. Clin Infect Dis 22(suppl):S102, 1996

32. Sheflin JR, Campbell JA, Thompson GP: Pulmonary blastomycosis: findings on chest radiographs in 63 patients. AJR Am J Roentgenol 154:1177, 1990

33. Chapman SW, Bradsher RW Jr, Campbell GD Jr, et al: Practice guidelines for the management of patients with blastomycosis. Clin Infect Dis 30:679, 2000. http://www.journals.uchicago.edu/IDSA/guidelines

34. Areno JP IV, Campbell GD Jr, George RB: Diagnosis of blastomycosis. Semin Respir Infect 12:252, 1997

35. Pappas PG, Bradsher RW, Chapman SW, et al: Treatment of blastomycosis with fluconazole: a pilot study. Clin Infect Dis 20:267, 1995

36. Pappas PG, Bradsher RW, Kauffman CA, et al: Treatment of blastomycosis with higher doses of fluconazole. Clin Infect Dis 25:200, 1997

37. Stevens DA: Coccidioidomycosis. N Engl J Med 332:1077, 1995

38. Galgiani JN: Coccidioidomycosis. West J Med 159:153, 1993

39. Leake JAD, Mosley DG, England B, et al: Risk factors for acute symptomatic coccidioidomycosis among elderly persons in Arizona, 1996–1997. J Infect Dis 181:1435, 2000

40. Kirkland TN, Fierer J: Coccidioidomycosis: a reemerging infectious disease. Emerg Infect Dis 2:192, 1996

41. Schneider E, Hajjeh RA, Spiegel RA, et al: A coccidioidomycosis outbreak following the Northridge, Calif, earthquake. JAMA 277:904,1997

42. Rosenstein NE, Emery KW, Werner SB, et al: Risk factors for severe pulmonary and disseminated coccidioidomycosis: Kern County, California, 1995–1996. Clin Infect Dis 32:708, 2001

43. Pappagianis D, Zimmer BL: Serology of coccidioidomycosis. Clin Microbiol Rev 3:247, 1990

44. Galgiani JN, Ampel NM, Catanzaro A, et al: Practice guidelines for the treatment of coccidioidomycosis. Clin Infect Dis 30:658, 2000 http://www.journals.uchicago.edu/IDSA/guidelines

45. Galgiani JN, Catanzaro A, Cloud GA, et al: Comparison of oral fluconazole and itraconazole for progressive, nonmeningeal coccidioidomycosis: a randomized, double-blind trial. Ann Intern Med 133:676,2000

46. Graybill JR, Stevens DA, Galgiani JN, et al: Itraconazole treatment of coccidioidomycosis. Am J Med 89:282, 1990

47. Catanzaro A, Galgiani JN, Levine BE, et al: Fluconazole in the treatment of chronic pulmonary and nonmeningeal disseminated coccidioidomycosis. Am J Med 98:249, 1995

48. Galgiani JN, Catanzaro A, Cloud GA, et al: Fluconazole therapy for coccidioidal meningitis. Ann Intern Med 119:28, 1993

49. Dewsnup DH, Galgiani JN, Graybill JR, et al: Is it ever safe to stop azole therapy for *Coccidioides immitis* meningitis? Ann Intern Med 124: 305, 1996

50. Coles FB, Schuchat A, Hibbs JR, et al: A multistate outbreak of sporotrichosis associated with sphagnum moss. Am J Epidemiol 136:475, 1992

51. Hajjeh R, McDonnell S, Reef S, et al: Outbreak of sporotrichosis among tree nursery workers. J Infect Dis 176:499, 1997

52. Dooley DP, Bostic PS, Beckius ML: Spook house sporotrichosis: a point-source outbreak of sporotrichosis associated with hay bale props in a halloween haunted house. Arch Intern Med 157:1885, 1997

53. Reed KD, Moore FM, Geiger GE, et al: Zoonotic transmission of sporotrichosis: case report and review. Clin Infect Dis 16:384, 1993

54. Kauffman CA: Sporotrichosis. Clin Infect Dis 29:231, 1999

55. Bolao F, Podzamczer D, Ventin M, et al: Efficacy of acute phase and maintenance therapy with itraconazole in an AIDS patient with sporotrichosis. Eur J Clin Microbiol Infect Dis 13:609, 1994

56. Pappas PG, Tellez I, Deep AE, et al: Sporotrichosis in Peru: description of an area of hyperendemicity. Clin Infect Dis 30:65, 2000

57. Pluss JL, Opal SM: Pulmonary sporotrichosis: review of treatment and outcome. Medicine (Baltimore) 65:143, 1986

58. Sharkey-Mathis PK, Kauffman CA, Graybill JR, et al: Treatment of sporotrichosis with itraconazole. Am J Med 95:279, 1993

59. Kostman JR, DiNubile MJ: Nodular lymphangitis: a distinct but often unrecognized syndrome. Ann Intern Med 118:883, 1993

60. Kauffman CA, Hajjeh R, Chapman SW: Practice guidelines for the management of patients with sporotrichosis. Clin Infect Dis 30:684, 2000 http://www.journals.uchicago.edu/IDSA/guidelines

61. Kauffman CA: Old and new therapies for sporotrichosis. Clin Infect Dis 21:981, 1995

62. Restrepo A, Robledo J, Gómez I, et al: Itraconazole therapy in lymphangitic and cutaneous sporotrichosis. Arch Dermatol 122:413, 1986

63. Conti Díaz IA, Civila E, Gezuele E, et al: Treatment of human cutaneous sporotrichosis with itraconazole. Mycoses 35:153, 1992

64. Kauffman CA, Pappas PG, McKinsey DS, et al: Treatment of lymphocutaneous and visceral sporotrichosis with fluconazole. Clin Infect Dis 22:46, 1996

65. Pappas PG, Bustamante B, Nolasco D, et al: Treatment of lymphocutaneous sporotrichosis with terbinafine: results of a randomized double-blind trial (abstr 648). 39th Annual Meeting of the Infectious Diseases Society of America, San Francisco, October, 2001

66. Hiruma M, Kawada A, Noguchi H, et al: Hyperthermic treatment of sporotrichosis: experimental use of infrared and far infrared rays. Mycoses 35:293, 1992

67. Dismukes WE: Introduction to antifungal drugs. Clin Infect Dis 30: 653, 2000

68. Como JA, Dismukes WE: Oral azole drugs as systemic antifungal therapy. N Engl J Med 330:263, 1994

69. Kauffman CA, Carver PL: Use of azoles for systemic antifungal therapy. Adv Pharmacol 39:143, 1997

70. Kauffman CA: Fungal infections in older adults. Clin Infect Dis 33:550, 2001

71. Ahmad SR, Singer SJ, Leissa BG: Congestive heart failure associated with itraconazole. Lancet 357:1766, 2001

72. Pappas PG, Kauffman CA, Perfect J, et al: Alopecia associated with fluconazole therapy. Ann Intern Med 123:354, 1995

73. Pursley TJ, Blomquist IK, Abraham J, et al: Fluconazole-induced congenital anomalies in three infants. Clin Infect Dis 22:336, 1996

74. Barone JA, Moskovitz BL, Guarnieri J, et al: Enhanced bioavailability of itraconazole in hydroxypropyl-β cyclodextrin solution versus capsules in healthy volunteers. Antimicrob Agents Chemother 42: 1862, 1998

75. Stevens DA: Itraconazole in cyclodextrin solution. Pharmacotherapy 19:603, 1999

76. Gallis HA, Drew RH, Pickard WW: Amphotericin B: 30 years of clinical experience. Rev Infect Dis 12:308, 1990

77. Goodwin SD, Cleary JD, Walawander CA, et al: Pretreatment regimens for adverse events related to infusion of amphotericin B. Clin Infect Dis 20:755, 1995

78. Kauffman CA: Amphotericin B. Seminars in Respiratory and Critical Care Medicine 18:281, 1997

79. Hiemenz JW, Walsh TJ: Lipid formulations of amphotericin B: recent progress and future directions. Clin Infect Dis 22(suppl 2):S133, 1996

80. Wong-Beringer A, Jacobs RA, Guglielmo BJ: Lipid formulations of amphotericin B: clinical efficacy and toxicities. Clin Infect Dis 27:603, 1998

81. Walsh TJ, Finberg RW, Arndt C, et al: Liposomal amphotericin B for empirical therapy in patients with persistent fever and neutropenia. N Engl J Med 340:764, 1999

82. Branch RA: Prevention of amphotericin B-induced renal impairment: a review of the use of sodium supplementation. Arch Intern Med 148:2389, 1988

83. Lin AC, Goldwasser E, Bernard EM, et al: Amphotericin B blunts erythropoietin response to anemia. J Infect Dis 161:348, 1990

38 Mycotic Infections in the Compromised Host

Jo-Anne van Burik, M.D.

Opportunistic fungal infections have become increasingly important over the past 20 years, paradoxically because advances in medical practice have improved the survival of debilitated and immunosuppressed patients. Opportunistic fungal pathogens may originate as human commensals (e.g., *Candida albicans*) or have an environmental reservoir (e.g., *Aspergillus fumigatus*). They may have yeast (budding, unicellular) or mold (branching, tubular hyphal cell) phenotypes. Timely diagnosis of opportunistic fungal infection depends on understanding host characteristics, environmental risk factors, clinical presentation, and diagnostic testing. In treatment, correction of predisposing conditions can be as important as the use of antifungal medication. Localized infections may require surgery. Immunocompromised patients require either prophylaxis or early empirical treatment during high-risk periods.

Candidiasis

EPIDEMIOLOGY

C. albicans is a yeast that is virtually ubiquitous in humans. Acquired at or soon after birth, it becomes part of the normal flora of the gastrointestinal and vaginal tracts. In healthy persons, overgrowth of *Candida* at those commensal sites is a common cause of minor skin and mucous membrane infections—notably, oral candidiasis, diaper rash in infants, and vaginal candidiasis in women. In persons with immune system aberrations or iatrogenic factors that predispose to infection, candidal infections can become invasive; the organism may enter the bloodstream and disseminate to normally sterile tissues.

C. albicans has the best adherence mechanisms of the various *Candida* species and is therefore the predominant yeast colonizing the mouth, gut, and vagina. Treatment with systemic antifungal drugs may result in the replacement of *C. albicans* by other candidal species and their appearance as opportunistic pathogens. This phenomenon has grown with the wider use of such agents. In particular, *C. glabrata* and *C. krusei* bloodstream infections have become more common since the introduction of fluconazole in the early 1990s.[1] Other *Candida* species regarded as frequent human pathogens include *C. parapsilosis, C. tropicalis, C. lusitaniae, C. dubliniensis,* and *C. guilliermondii.*[2] *C. lusitaniae* is notable for resistance to amphotericin. *C. parapsilosis* is notable for nosocomial transmission from an exogenous source, such as hyperalimentation fluids. In a hospital, a series of infections with the same non-*albicans Candida* species in several patients over a short period of time suggests a common nosocomial point source.

ETIOLOGY

Candidal infection often reflects a combination of environmental and host defense factors; this is especially true of localized mucocutaneous infection from overgrowth of commensal *C. albicans.* Wearing diapers or dentures provides an environment conducive to candidal growth, as does antibiotic treatment that reduces the commensal bacteria that normally help keep *Candida* in check. Host factors include the normal life phases of infancy and pregnancy (especially third trimester) and pathologic conditions such as vitamin deficiencies and malnourishment, diabetes and other endocrine abnormalities, congenital or acquired defects in cell-mediated immunity, and malignancy. Iatrogenic contributors include radiotherapy, systemic or inhaled steroids, and other immunosuppressive medications.[3]

PATHOGENESIS

Candida can reach normally sterile tissues through iatrogenic means: contamination of plastic catheters may lead to localized infection, such as peritonitis from peritoneal dialysis catheters and cystitis or upper urinary tract infection from urinary (Foley) catheters.[4] Alternatively, *Candida* may spread from colonized surfaces to contiguous tissues. Depending on the original site, such invasion can lead to esophagitis, sinusitis, mastoiditis, and, in rare cases, primary pneumonia. A breakdown of gastrointestinal mucosa through damage from cancer chemotherapy, radiation, trauma, or concurrent viral ulcers may allow a commensal *Candida* strain to gain access to the bloodstream. Tissue abscesses from hematogenous dissemination can form in the lung, brain, liver, spleen, kidney, bone, joints, heart valves, skin, and eye. In short, *Candida* infections can affect almost every organ system in the body.

DIAGNOSIS

Clinical Manifestations

Oropharyngeal candidiasis Patients with oropharyngeal candidiasis may complain of sore throat or raw tongue; eating may be so uncomfortable that patients lose weight. Pseudomembranous candidiasis (thrush) presents as loosely adherent white patches and plaques on the buccal mucosa, palate, oropharynx, or tongue. Erythematous candidiasis presents as redness without pseudomembranes. An erythematous, smooth plaque on the dorsal surface of the tongue characterizes median rhomboid glossitis. Angular cheilitis presents as erythema, maceration, and fissuring at the corners of the mouth.

Gastrointestinal candidiasis Esophageal candidiasis causes painful swallowing, a feeling of obstruction on swallowing, and substernal or retrosternal chest pain. Thrush may also be evident.[5] Candidiasis elsewhere in the GI tract presents as pain in the abdominal quadrant where the affected organs are located.

Genital candidiasis Candidal vaginitis may present as intense pruritus of the vulva and a cervical discharge that can vary from scant to thick and white. There may be edema of the vulva and erythema of the vagina and labia that extends onto the perineum.

Balanitis can begin as itching or burning, with vesicles or white patches on the penis. Plaques may extend onto the thighs, buttocks, and scrotum.

Diaper rash *Candida* diaper rash causes itching and maceration in the perianal area that may spread to the entire skin region of diaper contact. Satellite lesions may be present. Girls may have a vaginal discharge.

Hematogenous candidiasis Patients with hematogenous *Candida* infection and major organ involvement may have fever, with or without additional manifestations in the organ system involved (central nervous system, lungs, heart, urinary tract, bones, joints, liver, spleen, gallbladder, or eyes). Even in the absence of ocular symptoms, patients with positive blood cultures for *Candida* should have a dilated eye examination to look for the white cotton ball–like chorioretinitis lesions of hematogenous *Candida* endophthalmitis, which can result in permanent blindness unless treated appropriately.

Laboratory Tests

Candidal lesions can be so distinctive that diagnosis does not require testing. When the appearance is uncertain, pseudomembranes should be scraped and sent for staining and culture. Fungal forms (4 to 6 μm oval yeast cells, pseudohyphae, and hyphae) can be visualized using 40× to 100× magnification after staining with potassium hydroxide—with or without calcofluor—and with Gram stain. Culture plates specific for yeast include bromo-cresol green and Sabouraud dextrose agar, although candidal organisms are easily cultured on blood agar. In immunosuppressed patients, endoscopy specimens from esophageal and other GI sites should be submitted for viral culture in addition to fungal culture, because such patients can have concurrent herpesvirus infections.

Diagnosis of hematogenous and major organ candidiasis requires culture of blood, radiographic imaging of the organ system involved, and culture of any localized fluid collections. Blood culture is used for diagnosis of fungemia, catheter-related infection, vascular infection, endocarditis, and liver and spleen infection. Even repeated cultures—both of blood and of biopsy tissue—are often negative in visceral (hepatosplenic) candidiasis, however.[6]

The current generation of automated blood culture systems has improved the ability to detect *Candida*, and *Candida* species are now the fourth most common nosocomial bloodstream isolate. When culture growth is noted, a germ tube test can be performed to distinguish *C. albicans* from other species of *Candida*. The organism is inoculated into serum and incubated for 2 to 3 hours at 37° C. If an elongated hypha (a germination tube) is seen extending from the yeast, the species is *C. albicans*. Antifungal susceptibility testing should be requested for the first bloodstream isolate from a new infection episode.

DIFFERENTIAL DIAGNOSIS

In patients with mucocutaneous manifestations that do not fit the classic picture of *C. albicans* infection, non-*albicans* candidal species, bacteria, mold, and viruses need to be considered. Bacterial infection is especially likely in patients with findings such as abscesses or fever, whereas viral infection may be present in those with ulcerations of the mucosal surface. Infections in severely debilitated patients may have multiple copathogens. Candidiasis must also be distinguished from noninfectious syndromes such as aphthous ulcers.

TREATMENT

Active Infection

Management of candidal infections should include attempts to correct any factors that can predispose to candidal overgrowth. In some cases, this will involve local measures: with diaper rash, for example, the affected areas should be kept dry. Other cases require general measures, such as tighter control of glucose levels in diabetic patients or minimizing the number and dosage of antibacterial or immunosuppressive medications.

Antifungal drug therapy for candidiasis may be topical or systemic[7] [*see Table 1*]. For mucocutaneous infections in particular, it is important to try topical agents before giving systemic ones. The use of topical agents can prevent the replacement of *C. albicans* with other candidal strains and the development of drug resistance, and it avoids the side effects of systemic treatment.

When systemic treatment is required, fluconazole is often the drug of choice for *C. albicans* infections. *C. glabrata* infections should be considered fluconazole resistant and treated with a different agent until sensitivities are known. Importantly, *C. krusei* is innately resistant to fluconazole, so infections caused by this organism should be treated with amphotericin.

Adjunctive measures are important in controlling severe candidal infections and in boosting the immune function of severely debilitated patients. For patients with catheter-related infections, strong consideration should be given to catheter removal from any affected site (intravascular, genitourinary, and peritoneal) if possible. Neutropenic patients may benefit from colony-stimulating factors or neutrophil transfusions. In patients with a central venous catheter, infections accompanied by tenderness or erythema along the catheter tunnel tract may require surgical debridement of the tract. Macroabscesses may require surgical drainage or debulking. Patients with recurrent positive cultures despite both systemic medication and adjunctive measures should be reexamined clinically and radiologically to look for an occult focus of *Candida* organisms, such as an infected thrombus or abscess.

Prophylaxis

Secondary pharmacologic prophylaxis for mucocutaneous infection may be started in patients who have experienced several episodes of thrush (in advanced AIDS) or vaginitis (in pregnancy). Profoundly neutropenic patients with sufficient mucosal breakdown to provide portals of entry for *Candida* into the bloodstream require primary pharmacologic prophylaxis until the mucosal barriers have recovered their protective function. Examples of such mucosal barrier breakdown include, but are not limited to, mucositis during bone marrow transplant procedures, GI graft versus host disease (GVHD), and viral gastroenteritis. Prophylactic medications can be topical or systemic, depending on the site involved and the patient's tolerance of individual agents.

The use of antifungal chemotherapy can shift GI yeast flora from *C. albicans* to fluconazole-resistant species. For that reason, candidal infections that manifest during fluconazole prophylaxis require culture and sensitivity testing to determine definitive treatment.

PROGNOSIS

Fortunately, most candidal infections are readily manageable, as long as further diagnostic investigation (e.g., susceptibility testing and radiography) is pursued for poorly responsive infections. Morbidity and mortality remain highest for hematogenous and major-organ candidiasis.

Cryptococcosis

EPIDEMIOLOGY

Cryptococcus neoformans is a yeast that is widely distributed in nature. Environmental sources include aged pigeon droppings, pigeon nesting areas, dust, and eucalyptus trees.[8] However, most people exposed to environmental sources do not experience symptomatic disease. Suppressed cell-mediated immunity is the most important risk factor for symptomatic infection; currently, AIDS patients with $CD4^+$ T cell counts below 100/mm^3 account for 80% to 90% of cases of clinical cryptococcosis. In the United States, the prevalence of cryptococcosis in AIDS patients is 5% to 10%. Person-to-person transmission has not been documented other than through transplanted organs.

Table 1 Treatment of Infections Caused by *Candida* Species

Infection	*Drug*	*Dosage*	*Relative Efficacy*	*Cost*	*Comments*
Denture stomatitis	Fluconazole	100–400 mg p.o. daily for 1–14 days	First-choice agent	100 mg p.o., q.d.: $10–19.99/day	Remove dentures at night
Gingivo-stomatitis	Nystatin	Swish 4–6 ml of 100,000 units/ml q.i.d., or suck 200,000-unit lozenges q.i.d. daily for 2 wk	First-choice topical agent	5 ml p.o., q.i.d.: $1–1.49/day	—
	Clotrimazole	Suck 10 mg troches five times daily for 2 wk	Alternative topical agent	$3–3.99/day	Less bitter than nystatin
	Gentian violet	Apply 1% solution to oropharynx once, repeat weekly as needed	Alternative topical agent	30 ml: $1	Stains tissue
	Fluconazole	100–400 mg p.o. daily for 1–14 days	First-choice systemic agent	100 mg p.o., q.d.: $10–19.99/day	May lead to replacement of *C. albicans* with other *Candida* strains
	Itraconazole	100 mg p.o., b.i.d., or 200 mg daily of oral solution for 14 days	Alternative systemic agent	100 mg p.o., q.d.: $100–149.99/mo; 100 mg q.d. oral solution: $200–299.99/mo	Capsule absorption improved by acidic stomach contents
	Amphotericin	0.5 mg/kg I.V. daily for 2 wk beyond the last clinical symptoms, then once or twice weekly as maintenance	Alternative systemic agent	50 mg I.V. q.d.: $10–19.99/day	—
Sinusitis/ mastoiditis	Fluconazole	400–800 mg p.o. or I.V. daily for 3 wk	First-choice agent	200 mg p.o., q.d.: $20–29.99/day; 200 mg I.V. q.d.: $80–89.99/day	—
	Amphotericin	0.5 mg/kg I.V. daily for 3 wk	Alternative agent	50 mg I.V. q.d. $10–19.99/day	—
	Itraconazole	200 mg p.o. or I.V. b.i.d., or 400 mg daily of oral solution for 3 wk	Alternative agent	200 mg p.o., q.d.: $200–299.99/mo	Capsule absorption improved by acidic stomach contents
Pneumonia	Amphotericin	0.5 mg/kg I.V. daily for 2 wk ± 50 mg nebulized daily	First-choice agent	50 mg I.V. q.d.: $10–19.99/day	—
	Fluconazole	400–800 mg p.o. or I.V. daily for 2 wk	Alternative agent	200 mg p.o., q.d.: $20–29.99/day; 200 mg I.V. q.d.: $80–89.99/day	—
	Itraconazole	200 mg p.o. or I.V. b.i.d., or 400 mg daily of oral solution for 2 wk	Alternative agent	200 mg p.o., q.d.: $200–299.99/mo	Capsule absorption improved by acidic stomach contents
	Flucytosine	25 mg/kg p.o., q.i.d., for duration of amphotericin therapy	Adjunct to amphotericin	1 g p.o., q.i.d.: $10–19.99/day	Follow levels and adjust dose for renal insufficiency

(*continued*)

Table 1 (continued)

Infection	*Drug*	*Dosage*	*Relative Efficacy*	*Cost*	*Comments*
Meningitis					Remove foreign bodies
	Amphotericin	0.7–1.0 mg/kg I.V. daily for 2–6 wk ± 1 mg intrathecal or intraventricular daily	First-choice agent	50 mg I.V. q.d.: $10–19.99/day	—
	Flucytosine	37.5 mg/kg p.o., q.i.d., for duration of amphotericin therapy	Adjunct to amphotericin	1 g p.o., q.i.d.: $10–19.99/day	Follow levels and adjust dose for renal insufficiency
	Fluconazole	400–800 mg p.o. or I.V. daily for duration of risk factors that led to infection	First-choice agent	200 mg p.o., q.d.: $20–29.99/day; 200 mg I.V. q.d.: $80–89.99/day	May be used for maintenance after amphotericin
Brain macroabscess	—	See meningitis; continue therapy until lesion has resolved	—	—	Debulk or drain abscess
Esophageal infection	—	Continue therapy for 2 wk after clinical resolution	—	—	—
	Fluconazole	100–400 mg p.o. daily	First-choice systemic agent	100 mg p.o., q.d.: $10–19.99/day	—
	Itraconazole	100–200 mg p.o., b.i.d., or 200–400 mg daily of oral solution	Alternative agent	100 mg p.o., q.d.: $100–149.99/mo; 200 mg p.o., q.d.: $200–299.99/mo; 100 mg q.d. oral solution: $200–299.99/mo	Capsule absorption improved by acidic stomach contents
	Amphotericin	0.5 mg/kg I.V. daily	Alternative agent	50 mg I.V. q.d.: $10–19.99/day	—
Liver/spleen infection					Correct neutropenia
	Amphotericin	0.5–1.0 mg/kg I.V. daily until fevers have resolved and lesions appear smaller on CT scan	First-choice agent	50 mg I.V. q.d.: $10–19.99/day	—
	Fluconazole	6–12 mg/kg p.o. or I.V. daily for the duration of lesions on serial CT scans	First-choice agent	200 mg p.o., q.d.: $20–29.99/day; 200 mg I.V. q.d.: $80–89.99/day	May be used for maintenance after amphotericin
Spleen infection	—	See liver/spleen infection, above	—		May require splenectomy
Peritoneum infection					Remove peritoneal catheter
	Amphotericin	0.5–1.0 mg/kg I.V. daily until fevers have resolved and peritoneal fluid appears less infected, for a minimum of 2 wk	First-choice agent	50 mg I.V. q.d.: $10–19.99/day	—
	Fluconazole	6–12 mg/kg p.o. or I.V. daily until fevers have resolved and peritoneal fluid appears less infected, for a minimum of 2 wk	First-choice agent	200 mg p.o., q.d.: $20–29.99/day; 200 mg I.V. q.d.: $80–89.99/day	May be used for maintenance after amphotericin

Cystitis, uncomplicated					Remove urinary catheter
	Fluconazole	200 mg p.o. or I.V. on first day, then 100 mg p.o. daily for 4 more days	First-choice agent	200 mg p.o., q.d.: $20–29.99/day; 200 mg I.V. q.d.: $80–89.99/day	If poor response, rule out fungus ball in renal pelvis
	Amphotericin	Bladder irrigation with 5 mg in 100 ml water at 42 ml/hr for 1–2 days, or 0.3 mg/kg I.V. once	Alternative agent	50 mg I.V. q.d.: $10–19.99/day	If poor response, rule out fungus ball in renal pelvis
Pyelonephritis	Amphotericin	0.5–1.0 mg/kg I.V. daily for 2 wk, or longer if fevers have not resolved	First-choice agent	50 mg I.V. q.d.: $10–19.99/day	Resolve concomitant nephrolithiasis
Renal/perinephric abscess	Amphotericin	0.5–1.0 mg/kg I.V. daily until scan shows resolution of abscess	First-choice agent	50 mg I.V. q.d.: $10–19.99/day	Drain abscess
Vulva/cervix infection					Stop antibacterial agents
	Clotrimazole	One applicator per vagina each evening for 3–7 days	First-choice topical agent	200 mg vaginal tablet: $3–3.99	—
	Gentian violet	Apply 0.25%–1% solution to vagina 2–3 times daily for 3 days	Alternative topical agent	30 ml 1% solution: $1	Stains tissue
	Fluconazole	100–400 mg p.o. daily for 1–14 days	First-choice systemic agent	100 mg p.o., q.d.: $10–19.99/day	—
	Itraconazole	100 mg p.o., b.i.d, or 200 mg daily of oral solution for 14 days	Alternative systemic agent	100 mg q.d.: $100–149.99/mo; 100 mg q.d. oral solution: $200–299.99/mo	Capsule absorption improved by acidic stomach contents
Balanitis/balanoposthitis					Reduce predisposing factors
	Clotrimazole	1% cream applied twice daily for 1 wk	First-choice topical agent	24 g: $8–8.99	—
	Fluconazole	Single oral 150-mg dose	First-choice systemic agent	100 mg p.o., q.d.: $10–19.99/day	—
Diaper/perianal rash					Keep affected area dry
	Nystatin	Cream or powder applied after every diaper change for 1 wk	First-choice topical agent	15 g cream: $0.72; 15 g powder: $14.69	—
	Miconazole	Ointment applied after every diaper change for 1 wk	First-choice topical agent	30 g topical 2% cream: $20–29.99	—
Osteomyelitis/septic arthritis					May require surgery
	Amphotericin	0.5–1.0 mg/kg I.V. daily for 4–12 wk	First-choice agent	50 mg I.V. q.d.: $10–19.99/day	Follow ESR
	Flucytosine	25 mg/kg p.o., q.i.d., for duration of amphotericin therapy	Adjunct to amphotericin	1 g p.o., q.d.: $10–19.99/day	Follow levels and adjust dose for renal insufficiency
	Fluconazole	6–12 mg/kg p.o. daily for 1–6 mo	Maintenance	100 mg p.o., q.d.: $10–19.99/day	Follow ESR

(continued)

Table 1 (continued)

Infection	*Drug*	*Dosage*	*Relative Efficacy*	*Cost*	*Comments*
Endocarditis/ pericarditis					May require surgery
	Amphotericin	0.5–1.0 mg/kg I.V. daily, often continued for 6–10 wk after corrective surgery	First-choice agent	50 mg I.V. q.d.: $10–19.99/day	Follow ESR
	Flucytosine	25–37.5 mg/kg p.o., q.i.d., for duration of amphotericin therapy	Adjunct to amphotericin	1 g p.o., q.i.d.: $10–19.99/day	Follow levels and adjust dose for renal insufficiency
	Fluconazole	6–12 mg/kg p.o. daily for 1–6 mo	Maintenance	100 mg p.o., q.d.: $10–19.99/day	Follow ESR
Chronic mucocutaneous candidiasis	Ketoconazole	400 mg p.o. daily for 3–9 mo	—	$100–149.99/mo	Take with food
Folliculitis	Fluconazole	100–400 mg p.o. daily for 1–6 wk	First-choice agent	100 mg p.o., q.d.: $10–19.99/day	—
	Econazole	1% cream rubbed into affected area twice daily	Adjunctive agent	15 g: $10–19.99	—
	Ketoconazole	400 mg p.o. daily for 1–6 wk	Alternative agent	$100–149.99/mo	Take with food
	Itraconazole	200 mg p.o. daily for 1–6 wk	Alternative agent	$200–299.99/mo	—
Paronychia/ onychomycosis					Avoid moisture
	Fluconazole	6–12 mg/kg p.o. daily for 2–6 mo	First-choice agent	100 mg p.o., q.d.: $10–19.99/day	—
	Itraconazole	200 mg p.o. daily for 2–6 mo	Alternative agent	$200–299.99/mo	Capsule absorption improved by acidic stomach contents
Keratitis					May require adjunctive penetrating keratoplasty
	Natamycin	1 drop 5% suspension every 1–2 hr for first 2 days, then decrease gradually over 3 wk	First-choice agent	15 ml: $106	—
	Fluconazole	0.2% topical, 1 drop to affected eye q. 5 min for four doses for 4–6 wk	Alternative agent	—	Must be prepared by pharmacy
Endophthalmitis	Amphotericin	Intravitreal 0.005–0.010 mg in 0.1 ml once, with repeat dosing based on ophthalmologic opinion	Ophthalmologist will make decision to use	—	Must be prepared by pharmacy; advanced vitreitis may require systemic amphotericin and/or vitrectomy

					Halt fungemia
Systemic infection	Amphotericin	0.5–1.0 mg/kg I.V. daily for 7 days after the last positive blood culture, then switch to fluconazole 6–12 mg/kg p.o. daily for 7 additional days; fluconazole may be continued longer if neutropenia has not resolved; if the *Candida* species recovered is resistant to fluconazole, continue amphotericin for a total of 14 days after the last positive blood culture	First choice for patients who are neutropenic, deteriorating, or otherwise unstable	50 mg I.V. q.d.: $10–19.99/day	Use lipid formulation, not generic, for patients with nephrotoxicity or infusion toxicity; remove catheters and replace at new sites; check for metastatic lesions (e.g., endophthalmitis)
	Fluconazole	6–12 mg/kg I.V. or p.o. daily for 14 days after the last positive culture	First choice for stable patients who are not neutropenic	200 mg p.o., q.d.: $20–29.99/day; 200 mg I.V. q.d.: $80–89.99/day	Remove catheters and replace at new sites; check for metastatic lesions (e.g., endophthalmitis)

Note: Major pathogens include *C. albicans*, *C. tropicalis*, *C. parapsilosis*, and *C. pseudotropicalis*. *C. lusitaniae* and *C. guilliermondii* are usually resistant to amphotericin. *C. glabrata* and *C. krusei* are usually resistant to fluconazole.

ESR — erythrocyte sedimentation rate

ETIOLOGY

Cryptococcus infection begins with the inhalation of aerosolized organisms and localized proliferation with pulmonary invasion. In immunocompetent individuals, pulmonary infection may be asymptomatic and resolve spontaneously. Immunocompromised persons may have an acute, symptomatic pulmonary infection, which may disseminate by hematogenous spread—most often to the CNS, but also to the skin, soft tissue, genitourinary tract, bone, or joints. In organ transplant recipients who receive tacrolimus as their primary immunosuppressive agent, however, only a minority of cryptococcal infections involve the CNS.[9] Cryptococcal CNS infection may become symptomatic while pulmonary infection clears because cerebrospinal fluid lacks several soluble anticryptococcal factors that are present in serum, such as complement components. Rarely, *Cryptococcus* can be directly inoculated through intact skin as a route of infection.

PATHOGENESIS

C. neoformans is a round or oval yeastlike structure, 4 to 6 μm in diameter, that grows well at body temperature. A large protective polysaccharide capsule surrounds each cell. The highly negative surface charge may contribute to resistance to leukocyte phagocytosis.

DIAGNOSIS

Clinical Manifestations

CNS infection Cryptococcosis of the CNS may present as mild and nonspecific complaints, such as persistent headache, nausea, dizziness, ataxia, impaired memory and judgment, irritability, somnolence, clumsiness, confusion, and obtundation. Patients may or may not have fever, and most have minimal or no nuchal rigidity. Papilledema is noted in up to one third of cases and cranial nerve palsies in about one fifth. If the cranial nerves become involved, patients may experience decreased visual acuity, diplopia, facial numbness or weakness, or catastrophic vision loss.[10] As the disease progresses, seizures may occur.

Respiratory infection Pulmonary cryptococcosis may present as cough, dyspnea, blood-streaked sputum, and a dull ache in the chest.

Cutaneous infection Skin lesions may be single or multiple and commonly begin as painless lesions of the face or scalp. Skin lesions may take the form of erythematous or umbilicated papules, pustules, acneiform lesions, indurated plaques, palpable purpura, soft subcutaneous masses, sinus tracts, cellulitis, vesicles, or large ulcers with undermined edges.

Prostatic infection Prostatic cryptococcosis may present as a peripheral prostatic nodule. Patients often have no symptoms.

Laboratory Tests

Routine blood studies remain normal in cryptococcosis. Lumbar puncture is indicated in immunosuppressed patients with CNS abnormalities; characteristic findings include elevated opening pressure, depressed glucose level, increased protein concentration, and lymphocytic pleocytosis. The latex agglutination test detects antigen in CSF or serum in more than 90% of patients with cryptococcal meningitis, whereas India ink smear of CSF detects cryptococci in 25% to 60%.

In cryptococcal CNS infection, CT or MRI scans of the head may be normal or reveal hydrocephalus, cerebral edema or atrophy, or a focal space-occupying mass lesion. Gelatinous cryptococcal pseudocysts may appear as nonenhancing lesions.

In pulmonary cryptococcosis, chest x-rays most often show one or more circumscribed masses or nodules, often in the upper lobes, without hilar involvement. Less common radiographic patterns include segmental pneumonia, single thick-walled cavities, pleural effusion, and miliary disease.

Antigen titers in either serum or CSF can be used to follow the course of disease, but a lack of standardization among manufacturers of cryptococcal antigen tests means that reliable results can be obtained only if the same kit is used for serial measurements. For definitive diagnosis of cryptococcosis, positive antigen results must be confirmed by culture. Sputum cultures are often negative, however, and may be falsely positive. A sequestered focus of active infection in the prostate can be diagnosed by culture of urine obtained after prostatic massage. Bone lesions appear on radiographic studies as round, lytic lesions.

DIFFERENTIAL DIAGNOSIS

CNS cryptococcosis may resemble coccidioidomycosis, histoplasmosis, tuberculosis, brucellosis, syphilis, viral meningoencephalitis, meningeal metastases, sarcoidosis, and chronic benign lymphocytic meningitis. Cryptococcomas may resemble pyogenic, nocardial, or mold-associated abscesses; tuberculosis; toxoplasmosis; hemorrhage; or lymphoma or other neoplasms. Pulmonary cryptococcosis may be indistinguishable from tuberculosis,

Table 2 Treatment of Infections Caused by *Cryptococcus* Species

Infection Site	*Drug*	*Dosage*	*Relative Efficacy*	*Cost*	*Comments*
CNS	Amphotericin	0.7–1.0 mg/kg I.V. daily for AIDS patients, 0.5–0.8 mg/kg I.V. daily for non-AIDS patients; continue for 2–6 wk	First-choice agent	50 mg I.V. q.d.: $10–19.99/day	Continue until patient is stable and afebrile
	Flucytosine	37.5 mg/kg p.o., q.i.d., for duration of amphotericin therapy	Adjunct to amphotericin	1 g p.o., q.i.d.: $10–19.99/day	Adjust dose for renal insufficiency
	Fluconazole	6 mg/kg p.o. daily for 8–10 wk, then 3 mg/kg for duration of suppressed cell-mediated immunity	Maintenance/ prophylaxis	100 mg p.o., q.d.: $10–19.99/day	—
Pulmonary	Fluconazole	6 mg/kg I.V. or p.o. daily for 2–6 mo	First-choice agent	200 mg p.o., q.d.: $20–29.99/day; 200 mg I.V. q.d.: $80–89.99/day	—
	Amphotericin	0.5–1.0 mg/kg I.V. daily for 2–6 wk, then change to fluconazole	Alternative agent	50 mg I.V. q.d.: $10–19.99/day	—

histoplasmosis, pneumocystosis, and neoplasm. Cutaneous cryptococcosis may resemble comedones, acne, lipoma, syphilis, tuberculosis, sarcoidosis, molluscum contagiosum, and basal cell carcinoma. Bone lesions resemble those of other mycoses and tuberculosis.

TREATMENT

In patients with cryptococcal CNS infection, therapy begins with intravenous amphotericin B plus oral flucytosine.[11] Once the patient is clinically stable and afebrile, which usually takes 2 to 6 weeks, those agents are replaced with fluconazole. After 8 to 10 weeks of maintenance therapy, fluconazole is continued at a reduced dose for the duration of suppressed cell-mediated immunity, to prevent relapse.[12] Pulmonary disease can be treated with amphotericin or fluconazole [*see Table 2*]. Secondary prophylaxis for pulmonary disease is often not indicated in patients whose immunosuppression is not severe.

COMPLICATIONS

Elevated CSF pressure in CNS cryptococcosis is associated with blindness and death. An absolute pressure under 250 to 300 mm H_2O can be maintained by removing CSF to decrease pressure by 50%.[13] Hydrocephalus can lead to permanent loss of cognitive function even in patients whose infection is considered cured. Relief of hydrocephalus with a shunt is vital to ensure an optimal outcome.[14]

Subclinical secondary prostatic foci may arise subsequent to therapy, even in patients who did not have prostatic involvement initially. These foci can be a source of recurrent systemic infection.

PROGNOSIS

In CNS cryptococcosis, a good prognosis is associated with normal mental status, a CSF leukocyte level of more than 20 cells/mm^3, and a CSF cryptococcal antigen titer of less than 1:1,024. Even in patients who respond to therapy initially, up to 40% may have residual neurologic defects and up to 25% of the 40% may relapse.

For HIV-negative patients who had cryptococcosis between 1990 and 1996, overall mortality was 30% and attributable mortality 12%. Significant predictors of mortality included age greater than 60 years, hematologic malignancy, and organ failure.[15] For solid-organ-transplant recipients, renal failure at the time of hospital admission has been identified as an independent predictor of death.[9]

Pneumocystosis

EPIDEMIOLOGY

Common and apparently harmless in the lungs of healthy persons, *Pneumocystis carinii* can cause pneumonia in those with prolonged lymphopenia. AIDS patients remain the single largest group at risk, although prophylaxis has markedly reduced the incidence of the disease in that population. The risk of *Pneumocystis* pneumonia is also higher in the setting of primary immune deficiencies, severe malnutrition (which accounted for epidemics in Central Europe during World War II), organ transplantation, and long-term corticosteroid treatment with monthly doses above 20 mg of prednisone or the equivalent. For solid-organ-transplant (except lung transplant) recipients, the incidence of *P. carinii* pneumonia is highest during the first year after transplantation.[16]

ETIOLOGY

Once *P. carinii* is inhaled, it attaches to lung epithelial cells. Host immune defects in humoral and cellular immunity allow unchecked replication of the organism. In the absence of CD4+ T cells, alveolar macrophages are unable to contain infection.

Uncommonly, *P. carinii* infection spreads beyond the lungs. Patients receiving aerosolized pentamidine as prophylaxis are at risk for upper lung lobe and extrapulmonary disease, because this is primarily a topical treatment; the aerosol does not penetrate into the less well ventilated portions of the lungs, and the drug is not absorbed into the circulation. Sites of extrapulmonary involvement include lymph nodes, abdominal organs, bone marrow, eyes, and thyroid.[17]

PATHOGENESIS

Although *Pneumocystis* was formerly classified as a protozoan, nucleic acid comparison studies have identified this organism as a fungus. Pulmonary infection focuses on the interstitium and the alveoli.

DIAGNOSIS

Clinical Manifestations

Most patients with *Pneumocystis* pneumonia have a fever.[18] Tachypnea and tachycardia are common in acutely ill patients. Clinical manifestations may develop insidiously and may not interfere with the person's daily routine initially. Consequently, some patients present with several weeks of pulmonary symptoms, including dyspnea, nonproductive cough, hypoxemia, chest pain, and hemoptysis. Nevertheless, lung auscultation may reveal only scant abnormal findings.

Laboratory Tests

Chest x-rays show bilateral infiltrates in most patients. Patients who have received aerosolized pentamidine as prophylaxis but experienced breakthrough infection are more likely to have disease confined to the apices.[17]

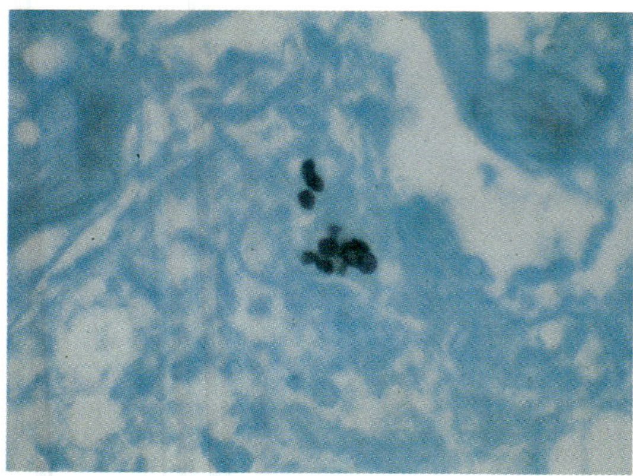

Figure 1 **Cysts of *Pneumocystis*, which stain black and measure approximately 4 to 5 μm, are visible on a methenamine-silver stain of a cytospin preparation from a bronchoscopic alveolar lavage fluid sample.**

Methenamine-silver staining of induced sputum or bronchoscopic alveolar lavage specimens can usually confirm the diagnosis [*see Figure 1*]. At 4 μm in diameter, the cysts of *Pneumocystis* are similar in size to the 5 μm cysts of *Histoplasma.* Pulse oximetry and arterial blood gases are among the methods for testing the level of oxygenation that are used to evaluate disease severity and monitor progression.

DIFFERENTIAL DIAGNOSIS

Any immunocompromised patient with respiratory symptoms, fever, and an abnormal chest radiograph should be considered to have pneumocystosis. Nevertheless, many other infectious agents and noninfectious diseases can mimic *P. carinii* pneumonia.

TREATMENT

Active Infection

The treatment of choice for *P. carinii* infection is high-dose intravenous trimethoprim-sulfamethoxazole (TMP-SMX). Severely hypoxemic patients should receive adjunctive corticosteroid therapy.[19] Approximately 25% of patients receiving high-dose TMP-SMX have a poor therapeutic response or hypersensitivity reactions. Alternative treatment regimens include pentamidine, trimethoprim-dapsone, clindamycin-primaquine, trimetrexate-leucovorin, and atovaquone [*see Table 3*].

Prophylaxis

Primary prophylaxis is indicated for HIV and organ-transplant patients whose CD4+ T cell count

Table 3 Treatment and Prophylaxis of *Pneumocystis carinii* Pneumonia

	Drug	*Dosage*	*Relative Efficacy*	*Cost*	*Comments*
Treatment					All treatments last 21 days
	Trimethoprim-sulfamethoxazole (TMP-SMX)	Two double-strength tablets p.o., or 5 mg/kg of the trimethoprim component I.V. q. 8 hr	First-choice agent	800/160 p.o., b.i.d.: $0.10–0.24/day	Rash or fever in 19% of patients
	Corticosteroid (oral prednisone or I.V. prednisolone)	40 mg b.i.d. for 5 days, then 40 mg daily for 5 days, then 20 mg daily for 11 days; administer 30 min before TMP-SMX	Adjunctive agent	20 mg p.o., q.d.: < $5/mo	If arterial oxygen pressure < 70 mm Hg or arterial-alveolar gradient > 35 mm Hg
	Pentamidine	4 mg/kg I.V. daily	Alternative agent	300 mg I.V. q.d.: $100–149.99/day	—
	Trimethoprim-dapsone	Trimethoprim 5 mg/kg p.o., t.i.d., and dapsone 100 mg p.o. daily	Alternative agent	TMP, 100 mg p.o., b.i.d.: $0.25–0.49/day; dapsone, 100 mg p.o., b.i.d.: $0.25–0.49/day	Rash or fever in 10% of patients
	Clindamycin-primaquine	Clindamycin 300–450 mg p.o., q.i.d., or 600 mg I.V. q. 8 hr, and primaquine base 15 mg p.o. daily	Alternative agent	Clindamycin, 300 mg: $329.50/100 capsules	Rash or fever in 21% of patients
	Atovaquone	750 mg suspension p.o., b.i.d.	Alternative agent	$20–29.99/day	Take with food
	Trimetrexate-leucovorin	Trimetrexate 45 mg/m² I.V. daily; leucovorin 20 mg/m² q. 6 hr for 3 days after trimetrexate	Alternative agent	Trimetrexate: $97.85/5 ml; leucovorin 25 mg: $194.87/100 tabs	—
Prophylaxis		Discontinue when CD4+ count > 200/mm³ for 3 mo			
	Trimethoprim-sulfamethoxazole	One double-strength or single-strength tablet, minimum three times per week but usually taken daily	First-choice agent	800/160 p.o., b.i.d.: $0.10–0.24/day	Provides cross-protection for toxoplasmosis and some bacteria
	Dapsone	100 mg p.o. daily	Alternative agent	100 mg p.o., b.i.d.: $0.25–0.49/day	Well tolerated if glucose-6-phosphatease levels are normal
	Pentamidine	300 mg in 6 ml sterile water by aerosol every 4 wk	Alternative agent	300 mg nebulized: $150–199.99	Breakthrough disease occurs in upper lung lobes
	Atovaquone	1,500 mg p.o. daily	Alternative agent	$20–29.99/day	Take with food
	Dapsone-pyrimethamine-leucovorin	Once weekly: dapsone 200 mg p.o.; pyrimethamine 75 mg p.o.; leucovorin 25 mg p.o.	Alternative agent	Dapsone, 100 mg: $15.93/100 tabs; pyrimethamine, $36.01/100 tabs; leucovorin, 25 mg: $174.87/100 tabs	Provides cross-protection for toxoplasmosis

is below 200/mm³, and secondary prophylaxis is indicated for those with a history of *P. carinii* pneumonia. In HIV-infected patients who respond to highly active antiretroviral therapy, recent evidence demonstrates that primary and secondary *Pneumocystis* prophylaxis can be safely discontinued once the CD4+ T cell count has remained above 200/mm³ for more than 3 months.[20]

TMP-SMX is the first choice for pharmacologic prophylaxis. Along with reducing pneumocysto-

Table 4 Desensitization of Adult Patients with Sulfa Allergy*

TMP-SMX Preparation	*Day*	*Dose (ml)*	*SMX Equivalent (mg)*
Pediatric oral suspension (40 mg/200 mg per 5 ml), 1 ml diluted with 9 ml normal saline, to equal 4 mg SMX/ml	1	0.25	1
	2	0.5	2
	3	1	4
	4	2	8
	5	4	16
Pediatric oral suspension, full strength	6	0.5	20
	7	1	40
	8	2	80
	9	4	160
Single-strength tablet	10–30	One tablet	400

Note: If the patient has had no reaction after 30 days of continuous therapy, the full dose can be given.
*This is only one of numerous sulfa desensitization regimens. Many hospital pharmacies have their own regimen and will provide the patient with a kit containing premeasured doses, if the physician writes a prescription for sulfa desensitization.
TMP-SMX — Trimethoprim-sulfamethoxazole

sis, it has the added benefit of providing protection against toxoplasmosis, salmonellosis, *Haemophilus* infection, and staphylococcal infection.[21] The dosage for TMP-SMX prophylaxis is specific to different immunocompromised patient populations.

There is a significant incidence of adverse reactions to TMP-SMX (rash, nausea, and, in rare cases, myelosuppression or cholestasis). However, because of its superior efficacy and low cost, desensitization should be attempted before switching to a second-choice agent in patients who experience side effects from TMP-SMX [*see Table* 4]. Other options for prophylaxis include dapsone, aerosolized pentamidine, atovaquone, and trimetrexate[22] [*see Table* 3]. Breakthrough infection with *P. carinii* may occur despite prophylaxis, especially in patients who have unrecognized poor compliance with a regimen of TMP-SMX or high-dose dapsone (100 mg daily).

PROGNOSIS

Prognosis is related to the degree of hypoxemia at presentation, degree of infiltrates on chest radiographs, elevated lactate dehydrogenase level, the presence of copathogens, prior lung damage, severity of the underlying disease, and general markers of debility. Spontaneous pneumothorax is associated with a poor prognosis.

Aspergillosis

Aspergillus is an environmental saprobe whose spores (conidia) readily become airborne. Conidia of *A. fumigatus,* the principal *Aspergillus* species involved in human infection, are the ideal size for deposition into lungs and sinuses, with a diameter of 2 to 5 µm. *Aspergillus* thrives in wet areas such as crawl spaces, basements, and water-treatment facilities. Renovations may result in the release of spore-bearing dust. Potted plants and marijuana have been suggested as sources of spores.

After it is inhaled, *Aspergillus* can cause a localized infection that may result in allergic or invasive disease. Allergic bronchopulmonary aspergillosis (ABPA) and invasive aspergillosis are the two major clinical variants.

ALLERGIC BRONCHOPULMONARY ASPERGILLOSIS

Epidemiology

ABPA affects patients with a hypersensitive immune status, such as those with atopy, asthma, extrinsic alveolitis, and cystic fibrosis.[23] Genetic determinants of immune response are thought to help explain why ABPA develops in only some patients with those conditions. ABPA is equally distributed between males and females with asthma and probably also cystic fibrosis. Diagnosis is usually made in the late teenage years or in the 20s.

Etiology

In susceptible individuals, exposure to *Aspergillus* antigens causes the formation of IgE antibodies directed at the antigen. Reexposure will then result in mast cell degranulation and eosinophilic infiltration, with wheezing and fleeting pulmonary infiltrates.

Pathogenesis

Aspergillus does not invade tissue in ABPA; rather, it colonizes pulmonary secretions. The severity of ABPA probably varies with the intensity of exposure to spores, the species of *Aspergillus* involved, and the immune status of the host. Initially, fungal spores are trapped within thick bronchial mucus. As the fungus proliferates, the bronchi fill with mucus and become dilated; fungal hyphae can be identified in mucoid impactions. ABPA has been divided into five stages [*see Table* 5]. Patients do not necessarily progress through these stages in linear fashion.[24]

Table 5 Clinical Stages of Allergic Bronchopulmonary Aspergillosis

Stage	*Clinical Findings*	*IgE Level*	*Eosinophilia*	Aspergillus fumigatus *Precipitating Antibodies*	*Chest Films*
I – Active	Asthma	Extremely elevated	Extreme	Present	Infiltrates
II – Remission	Normal	Below active levels but not normal	None	± Slightly elevated	Clear
III – Exacerbation	Asthma	Twice normal	Extreme	Not followed	Infiltrates
IV – Corticosteroid dependent	Tapering steroid therapy worsens asthma	Usually elevated but may be normal	—	Not followed	Central bronchiectasis
V – Fibrotic	Dyspnea, cyanosis, rales, clubbing, cor pulmonale	—	—	Not followed	Fibrosis

Note: IgE levels and eosinophilia are less often followed in patients with stage IV or V disease.

Diagnosis

Clinical manifestations Patients with ABPA may have cough, wheezing, expectoration of sputum containing brown plugs, fever, weight loss, dyspnea, malaise, pleuritic chest pain, sweats, and hemoptysis.

Lung auscultation in patients with active, recurrent, or corticosteroid-dependent disease (stages I, III, or IV) gives variable results, ranging from normal to localized rales in areas of consolidation to wheezes. In fibrotic disease (stage V), patients may have digital clubbing or cyanosis.

Laboratory tests Primary criteria for a diagnosis of ABPA include episodic bronchial obstruction (asthma), immediate skin reactivity to *A. fumigatus* antigen, precipitating antibodies against *A. fumigatus* antigen, increased total serum IgE concentration (> 1,000 ng/ml), history of transient or fixed pulmonary infiltrates, peripheral blood eosinophilia, and central bronchiectasis. Secondary criteria include *A. fumigatus* in sputum, history of expectoration of brown plugs or flecks, and late skin reactivity to *Aspergillus* antigen. Eosinophilia has diurnal variation and may decrease with steroid use or during remission (stage II). Pulmonary function tests are useful in defining the stage of disease and underlying asthmatic activity.

Differential Diagnosis

Allergic bronchopulmonary syndromes can be triggered by molds other than *A. fumigatus*. Allergic fungal sinusitis is histologically identical to ABPA; if caused by *A. fumigatus*, serologic findings will be positive in the absence of asthma and lower respiratory findings.

Treatment

Active infection Treatment for ABPA is systemic corticosteroids, supplemented with oral itraconazole [*see Table 6*]. Itraconazole reduces the burden of colonizing fungal organisms, thereby decreasing chronic antigen stimulation, permitting a lower corticosteroid dose, and decreasing future recurrences of ABPA.[25,26] Measures of clinical response can be followed serially and include decreasing serum IgE concentration, improvement in exercise tolerance and pulmonary function, and resolution of pulmonary infiltrates.

Corticosteroid-dependent (stage IV) patients will have disabling wheezing and dyspnea after oral corticosteroids are tapered or stopped. Patients with fibrotic disease (stage V) require supplemental oxygen and moderate doses of alternate-day prednisone.

Prophylaxis Serum IgE levels should be monitored monthly for 2 years and then every 2 months in patients who have had ABPA. Pulmonary function tests should be performed annually. An increase in serum IgE above remission levels should prompt an evaluation for exacerbation.

INVASIVE ASPERGILLOSIS

Epidemiology

Invasive aspergillosis typically occurs during periods of immune suppression, including neutro-

Table 6 Treatment of Disease Caused by *Aspergillus* Species

Disease	*Drug*	*Dosage*	*Relative Efficacy*	*Cost*	*Comments*
Allergic broncho-pulmonary aspergillosis	Corticosteroid (prednisone)	0.5 mg/kg daily for 2 wk, then 0.5 mg/kg every other day for 3 mo, then taper to discontinuance over another 3 mo	First-choice agent	20 mg p.o., q.d.: < $5/mo	Follow serum IgE monthly
	Itraconazole	200 mg p.o., b.i.d., for 4 mo	Adjunct to amphotericin	200 mg p.o., q.d.: $200–299.99/mo	Capsule absorption improved by acidic stomach contents
Invasive aspergillosis	Amphotericin	1.0–1.5 mg/kg I.V. daily for 2–12 wk, then switch to maintenance therapy	First-choice agent	50 mg I.V. q.d.: $10–19.99/day	Use lipid formulation, not generic, for patients with nephrotoxicity or infusion toxicity
	Itraconazole	200–300 mg p.o., b.i.d., for 2–12 mo or duration of clinical disease	Maintenance or alternative	200 mg p.o., q.d.: $200–299.99/mo	Solution has better bioavailability than capsule; document blood levels
	Caspofungin	70 mg I.V. loading dose, then 50 mg I.V. daily	Salvage agent	50 mg I.V. q.d.: $200–299.99/day	Reduce dose for hepatic insufficiency

penia, treatment of GVHD, and treatment of threatened rejection in transplant recipients. Other factors that may predispose immunosuppressed patients to invasive infection include diminished cough reflex, impairment of mucociliary function, and ischemic damage in the perioperative period or at surgical sites. Except in outbreaks, the incidence of invasive aspergillosis should not be higher than 10% to 15%, even in high-risk patients.

Etiology

Using the bone marrow transplant recipient as a model, we see two distinct periods of onset of invasive aspergillosis. The first peak, termed early disease, occurs at a median of 16 days after transplantation, when recipients of both autologous and allogeneic bone marrow have absolute neutropenia and lymphopenia, allowing any form of silent colonization to develop rapidly into invasive and often fatal disease. The second peak, late disease, occurs at a median of 96 days. Late disease develops indolently in recipients of allogeneic bone marrow who have recovered from absolute neutropenia but remain immunosuppressed[27] [*see Figure 2*]. Risk factors for early aspergillosis include allogeneic and especially unrelated donors, male gender, summer season, and transplantation outside of laminar airflow rooms. Risk factors for late aspergillosis are construction in the vicinity of the hospital, acute GVHD, and corticosteroid therapy. The risk for both early and late disease is higher with older age and increasing severity of the underlying oncologic condition. The one-year survival estimate for bone marrow transplant patients with invasive aspergillosis is less than 10%.

Pathogenesis

Along with *A. fumigatus* and *A. flavus,* emerging species involved in invasive aspergillosis include *A. terreus, A. nidulans, A. niger, A. glaucus, A. versicolor,* and *A. ustus.* Sinusitis or pneumonia accounts for 90% of invasive disease and develops after inhalation of *Aspergillus* spores in patients with prolonged neutropenia or other intense forms of immunosuppression.[28] *Aspergillus* spores can also enter the body after direct inoculation through intact skin or ingestion. Intestinal *Aspergillus* infection has led to fatal GI bleeding in severely immunocompromised patients. For that reason, health-food supplements made from natural substances that are not quality controlled for mold spores are contraindicated in immunocompromised patients. Dissemination of invasive disease can occur either as contiguous extension (such as erosion of paranasal sinus infection into the brain) or by hematogenous spread after the organism erodes into blood vessels.

often develops in patients who are severely ill from trauma; only 50% have systemic immunocompromising disease. Conditions that increase risk for pulmonary, rhinocerebral, and disseminated zygomycosis include poorly controlled diabetes (particularly ketoacidosis) and immunosuppression (neutropenia, sustained immunosuppressive therapy, chronic prednisone use). Iron overload, as from repeated dialysis or blood transfusions, increases susceptibility to zygomycosis because iron is an essential element for the growth and metabolism of Zygomycetes. Infection may occur in patients receiving the iron chelator deferoxamine to reduce iron overload because Zygomycetes can readily use iron even when it is bound to deferoxamine.

Persons at risk for zygomycosis of the GI tract are those with some form of severe protein-calorie malnutrition, such as uremia, kwashiorkor, or chronic diarrhea. In the United States, a *Mucor* liver abscess developed in a transplant recipient who consumed health-food supplements made from natural substances that were not quality controlled for mold spores.[36]

ETIOLOGY

Cutaneous infection usually occurs by traumatic inoculation; it is preceded by skin trauma in greater than 80% of cases. Sources of trauma have included surgery, burns, motor-vehicle accidents, knives, and even insect bites. A well-publicized series of infections occurred between 1978 and 1980 from elasticized surgical dressings that were found to be contaminated with *Rhizopus*.[37]

Pulmonary, rhinocerebral, and disseminated zygomycosis are acquired via airborne spores deposited in the nasal turbinates or pulmonary alveoli. GI tract disease follows ingestion of fungal spores in moldy food.

PATHOGENESIS

Onset of cutaneous infection is usually a few days after the initiating trauma. The pace of cutaneous illness varies: Necrosis may spread slowly over weeks, resembling an arterial insufficiency ulcer, or progress rapidly over days, resembling synergistic gangrene. Secondary cutaneous dissemination is unusual, except perhaps in burn victims.

Infection that starts as colonization in the nasal turbinates or paranasal sinuses may extend contiguously. When infection extends directly along veins that drain the orbit and facial tissues, cavernous sinus thrombosis results. With posterior extension, frontal lobe necrosis with brain abscess ensues. Zygomycetes can also enter the central nervous system by hematogenous spread.

DIAGNOSIS

Clinical Manifestations

Cutaneous disease can occur anywhere on the body, but it is most often found on the extremities.[38] Cutaneous lesions are usually characterized by central dermal necrosis surrounded by a margin of red to purple edematous cellulitis, sometimes with bullae indicating epidermal necrosis. Mold may be visible on the edge of a wound. If dermal necrosis is present, pain is common. Fever may be present or absent.

Pulmonary disease typically manifests with the usual pneumonia symptoms of fever, dyspnea, pleuritic chest pain, hoarseness, and gross hemoptysis. Rhinocerebral disease may begin with fever, leukocytosis, ketoacidosis, facial pain, sinus drainage, or headache. A black eschar on the nasal or palatal mucosa should immediately raise suspicion for rhinocerebral disease. With orbital extension, clinical findings may include orbital swelling or cellulitis, extraocular muscle paresis, proptosis, and chemosis.

Rhinocerebral disease may result in cranial nerve abnormalities, most commonly a seventh-nerve palsy. In patients with cavernous sinus thrombosis, venous engorgement from outflow obstruction is noted in the retina, conjunctiva, and eyelid. Paresis of cranial nerves III, IV, and VI may result in diplopia. Less often, proptosis, meningeal irritation, epistaxis, and fifth-cranial-nerve involvement may occur.

Laboratory Tests

Most patients with pulmonary or disseminated disease will have abnormal chest x-ray results, but there is no specific radiographic appearance or lobar predilection. In neutropenic patients with early disease, chest films may show little infiltrate, perhaps because these patients may lack inflammatory cells to cause infiltrate. If pulmonary disease progresses to tissue necrosis and hemorrhage, however, those radiographic changes will become obvious.

A CT scan of the head is indicated in patients with clinical signs of rhinocerebral disease. Scans may show bone destruction, a brain infarct, or a space-occupying brain lesion and can be used to guide surgical intervention.

Definitive diagnosis is made by recovery of a zygomycete in culture. Growth occurs after 2 to 5 days of incubation. Wound surfaces can be swabbed for fungal culture, but specimens should also be taken from rapidly spreading infections, nonwound cutaneous lesions, and lesions such as a black eschar on the hard palate or nasal mucosa.

Specimens should be immediately examined with potassium hydroxide, calcofluor white stains, or both. Histologic studies should be done using hematoxylin-eosin and methenamine-silver staining. In cutaneous disease, hyphae are seen in the middle of an acute neutrophilic infiltrate. Zygomycete hyphal cells should have infrequent septations, be of variable diameter, join at 90° angles, and twist in a ribbonlike fashion upon one another. In the uncommon instance where all those histologic findings are obvious, a tentative diagnosis of zygomycete infection can be made. However, the usual situation is that the tangle of fungal hyphae cannot be distinguished from *Aspergillus*.

Histology may be the only basis for diagnosis, however, given that Zygomycetes grow less frequently in culture than other filamentous molds. One reason is that Zygomycota mold cells are large, because they have few or no septations (pauciseptate or aseptate). Consequently, when the microbiology technologist uses a razor blade to mince tissue being prepared for fungal culture, one slice through the cell wall can lead to leakage of cytoplasm and death, leaving no intact cells for growth. Homogenization of tissue submitted for culture also leads to a high rate of false negative results.

DIFFERENTIAL DIAGNOSIS

Cutaneous zygomycosis can look like ecthyma gangrenosum, which is more often caused by *Aspergillus* and *Pseudomonas*. Pulmonary zygomycosis should be differentiated from aspergillosis, pneumonia from other less common bacteria and molds, and pulmonary embolism. Rhinocerebral zygomycosis can resemble orbital tumors, cavernous sinus thrombosis from *Staphylococcus* infection, or aspergillosis.

TREATMENT

Active Infection

Zygomycosis is treated with maximal-dose intravenous amphotericin at 1.0 to 1.5 mg/kg daily for 2 to 12 weeks or for the duration of clinical disease. In addition to intravenous infusions, intracavitary or topical amphotericin may be required for CNS disease; topical amphotericin can be applied to cutaneous disease.

Treatment should include adjunctive measures such as debridement of any adherent mycelial masses at accessible sites of infection. Debridement should be repeated as often as every other day until cultures of the debrided tissues are negative. Some patients may be candidates for neutrophil transfusions or hyperbaric oxygen.

Prophylaxis

Pharmacologic prophylaxis of zygomycosis infections is unusual because the frequency of infection with this group of organisms is low even in high-risk patient groups. Additionally, the medication that would be used for prophylaxis, intravenous amphotericin, is toxic and—when the lipid formulations are used—expensive. Topical or systemic prophylaxis may be appropriate for individual patients such as burn victims in whom surveillance cultures of wounds demonstrate fungal hyphae.

PROGNOSIS

Hosts with zygomycoses may not be as immunocompromised as hosts with some of the more common opportunistic mold infections. Hence, these infections may be associated with better survival.

Fusariosis

EPIDEMIOLOGY

Fusarium is a soil-borne mold that can cause human disease if a portal of entry is available, such as skin, nails, the airways, or the eyes. Species responsible for the majority of human disease are *F. solani*, *F. moniliforme*, and *F. oxysporum*. The number of organisms and the depth of penetration may determine the course of infection. Eye infection can occur after contamination of soft-contact-lens paraphernalia through inadequate washing of soil-borne spores from the hands or contamination of the lens during use; under windy conditions, aerosolized spores can be blown into the eye.

The single most important host risk factor for invasive fusariosis in immunocompromised patients is neutropenia.[39,40] Good clinical outcomes have clearly been linked to recovery from neutropenia, and fatal relapse of disease has been linked to recurrent neutropenia.[41] Other immune system defects linked to infection include heatstroke, systemic corticosteroid use, and topical steroid use at the site of colonization.[42]

Some *Fusarium* species produce secondary metabolites called mycotoxins. Under favorable environmental conditions, those species can grow on grains and contaminate them with mycotoxins. Consumption of mycotoxin-laden foodstuffs can result in both infection and poisoning—especially in malnourished persons, who have enhanced susceptibility to the toxin. An important historical example is an outbreak of toxic alimentary aleukia that occurred in the Soviet Union at the end of World War II. Starving people harvested grains that had been left in the fields over the winter and had become heavily contaminated with *Fusarium* mycotoxin. Those who ate more than 2 kg of food made from the grains suffered an illness that progressed from mucosal inflammation to pancytopenia to mucosal necrosis with fatal bacterial infection. Hundreds of thousands of people died from the illness.

ETIOLOGY

Opportunistic *Fusarium* infection begins by colonization of broken skin, the upper airways, sinuses, or conjunctivae. Reported causes of skin-barrier breakdown include catheters (central venous and peritoneal dialysis), burns, trauma, surgical procedures (coronary bypass), and denuding of skin from infection (as from varicella). When the host has an immune system defect, tissue inflammatory reactions at the site of colonization are reduced, enabling the organism to grow and spread.

PATHOGENESIS

The mold form of *Fusarium* consists of septate hyphae with branches at acute angles. Growth of hyphae in skin lesions may result in subcutaneous granulomas. Once infection has penetrated into the lumen of blood vessels, hyphae can disseminate through the body to produce embolic infection whose hallmark is necrotic skin lesions and, less often, endophthalmitis or brain abscess.[43]

DIAGNOSIS

Clinical Manifestations

Manifestations of focal *Fusarium* infection vary with the organ involved. Keratitis presents as a corneal ulcer; if therapy is delayed, infection may progress to endophthalmitis. Primary cutaneous infections present in many forms, including ulcers, necrosis, pustules, vesicles, painful nodules, mycetomas, and panniculitis. Onychomycosis presents as a milky-white area in the nail, which may spread until the entire nail becomes opaque; the free border of the nail may become thickened.

With disseminated infection, secondary cutaneous lesions may be the first characteristic finding. These may take the form of multiple erythematous subcutaneous nodules, painful lesions with progressive central infarction, or target lesions with ecthyma gangrenosum–like centers surrounded by a rim of erythema.[44]

Laboratory Tests

Fusarium is the only opportunistic mold that can be easily recovered from the bloodstream; blood cultures will be positive in 40% to 60% of patients with disseminated infection. Many clinical laboratories identify *Fusarium* to only the genus level; speciation would not alter the prognosis or treatment. Patients with fever and neutropenia should have cultures of blood, as well as biopsy and culture from any body sites suspicious for infection. Because *Fusarium* often colonizes nonsterile tissues, the mycologic data should be combined with histopathologic data to distinguish colonization from tissue infection. Biopsies of suspicious skin lesions should be taken from the center of the lesion and should extend to subcutaneous fat, because mold organisms easily invade blood vessels of the dermis and subcutis, resulting in an overlying ischemic cone. Part of the biopsy specimen, or a second biopsy specimen, should be sent for culture.

DIFFERENTIAL DIAGNOSIS

In addition to *Fusarium,* a variety of other organisms can be responsible for new skin lesions in an immunocompromised host; these include *Aspergillus*, other molds, *Pseudomonas,* and varicella.

TREATMENT

Fusarium species are relatively resistant to treatment with antifungal agents, and sensitivity testing for *Fusarium* is not standardized. Fluconazole, itraconazole, and 5-fluorocytosine have no activity against *Fusarium* species, and amphotericin, ketoconazole, miconazole, and terbinafine have limited activity.

Active Infection

Invasive disease is usually treated with high-dose systemic amphotericin [*see Table 7*]. Topical amphotericin or nystatin cream is sometimes added to systemic amphotericin in attempts to increase local delivery of drug. Corneal ulcers caused by *Fusarium* infection are treated with topical amphotericin or natamycin.

Because outcome is clearly linked to recovery from neutropenia, adjunctive measures are essential.[41] Colony-stimulating-factor injections and neutrophil transfusions have been used to increase the neutrophil count. Further episodes of electively

Table 7 Treatment of Infections Caused by *Fusarium* Species

Infection Site	*Drug*	*Dosage*	*Relative Efficacy*	*Cost*	*Comments*
Invasive fusariosis					Surgery may be needed
	Amphotericin	1.0–1.5 mg/kg I.V. daily for 2–12 wk	First-choice agent	50 mg I.V. q.d.: $10–19.99/day	Use lipid formulation, not generic, for patients with nephrotoxicity or infusion toxicity
Keratitis/corneal ulcer	Natamycin 5% suspension	1 drop q. 1–2 hr for first 2 days, then decrease gradually over 3–6 wk	First-choice agent	15 ml: $106	May require surgery
Skin lesions (as part of invasive disease)					Treat primarily as invasive disease; continue topical therapy until lesions are dry scabs
	Nystatin	Cream twice daily to affected areas	Adjunct to I.V. amphotericin	15 g of 100 µm: $0.72	—
	Amphotericin	Topical compound twice daily to affected areas	Adjunct to I.V. amphotericin	—	Compound locally

induced myelosuppression should be avoided, because there is a high incidence of recurrence and multiple-organ failure in patients with subsequent neutropenic episodes.

Surgical treatment has an important role in the management of localized infection; examples include enucleation of an affected eye, wide excision, and nail removal. In an extreme situation, amputation of a limb can be used to cure fusarial soft tissue infections.

Prophylaxis

Prevention of primary *Fusarium* infection involves the same environmental measures that would be used to prevent other mold infections in patients at risk. In general, patients with chronic neutropenia or those about to receive myelosuppressive therapy should wash their hands regularly and avoid contact with soil or inhalation of dust. Myelosuppressive therapy should be given in an inpatient environment with air filtration to reduce the number of aerosolized spores.

Secondary prophylaxis is required when a patient with known recent *Fusarium* infection has an episode of neutropenia. A systemic antifungal agent with activity against *Fusarium* is used at treatment doses. Efforts to shorten the duration of neutropenia with colony-stimulating factors are sometimes employed. The use of neutrophil transfusions as secondary prophylaxis for patients without fever or skin lesions is difficult to justify and rarely done.

Infection by Dematiaceous Fungi

EPIDEMIOLOGY

Dematiaceous fungi live in soil and rotting wood. Current taxonomy has more than 100 species of dematiaceous fungi spread out among more than a dozen different families, falling under several classes and orders. All contain melanin pigment in the walls of hyphae or spores, resulting in a color that is dark brown, greenish gray, or black. They are an important group of opportunists, because some species have a tendency to cause CNS infection.[45] Species that appear to be particularly neurotropic include *Cladophialophora, Cladosporium, Bipolaris, Exserohilum, Dactylaria, Exophiala,* and *Fonsecaea*.

Most reports of infection by dematiaceous fungi emphasize cerebral disease in an immunocompromised patient.[46] However, there is a growing literature describing these infections in specific at-risk patient populations (such as solid-organ-transplant recipients) and in immunocompetent patients, who may experience nasal polyps and an obstructive fungal ball destroying the sinuses.[47,48]

ETIOLOGY

Injury to the skin can implant dematiaceous fungus in subcutaneous tissues; inhalation of spores can cause a minimal infection in the lung or sinuses. Sinus infection can erode through bone into the brain, or unrecognized pulmonary infection can metastasize to the brain.

PATHOGENESIS

Primary cutaneous disease usually has one of three histopathologic patterns: solid granulomas, stellate abscesses, or cavitary lesions. Cystic lesions probably start as solid granulomas, which undergo focal necrosis to form stellate abscesses. The abscesses can then coalesce into a unilocular fluctuant abscess.

DIAGNOSIS

Clinical Manifestations

Dematiaceous fungi cause primarily skin and soft tissue infections.[47] Analogous syndromes seen in tropical and subtropical areas of the world include mycetoma (tumorous growth of the skin with tissue granules) and chromoblastomycosis (verrucous skin infection with sclerotic bodies). Immunocompetent persons develop an asymptomatic initial lesion: a discrete, well-encapsulated, erythematous to flesh-colored plaque or nodule. The nodule center tends to become necrotic, forming a localized, encapsulated abscess. In immunocompromised persons, subcutaneous lesions may not encapsulate and may spread contiguously or systemically.

Systemic infections may present as unexplained fever during neutropenia that persists despite broad-spectrum antibiotics. Metastatic disease may involve the lungs, joints, esophagus, heart, peritoneum, or bone, but the favored site is the CNS.

Laboratory Tests

Histopathology and culture of a tissue specimen are generally necessary to identify an infection as dematiaceous. Fungi are visible in cells lining an abscess, in the lumen of an abscess, or free in the granulation tissue of a cyst wall. The fungi appear as yeastlike cells that can be solitary or arranged in short chains, pseudohyphal-like fungal elements, or septate hyphae of varying lengths. The hyphae may differ from *Aspergillus, Fusarium,* or the Zygomycetes by having thicker walls, irregular diameter, variable branching, or constrictions at the septations. Because the degree of visible pigment can vary between patients infected with the same species, a melanin stain such as Masson-Fontana can be used to reveal cell wall pigment in tissue sections.

In patients with CNS involvement, dematiaceous infection often presents as rim-enhancing brain abscesses on CT scan.

DIFFERENTIAL DIAGNOSIS

On histopathologic examination, the septate fungal hyphae of dematiaceous fungi bear close resemblance to *Aspergillus.* The pathologist will usually label such specimens as *Aspergillus*-like, because less than 0.1% of them will culture out as a dematiaceous fungus. The Masson-Fontana melanin stain can discriminate dematiaceous fungus from *Aspergillus* but is rarely used in histopathology laboratories, so the distinction is usually made by culture.

TREATMENT

Complete surgical excision appears critical in the management of cutaneous lesions. If the entire lesion is removed in an immunocompetent host, antifungal therapy may not be needed. Disseminated disease requires systemic antifungal medication, sometimes combined with surgery. Amphotericin, 0.8 to 1.2 mg/kg I.V. daily for 2 to 12 weeks, is typically used, but the choice of medications should be evaluated on an individual basis. The duration of therapy is determined by the immune competence of the host, the site and extent of involvement, disease responsiveness, and the susceptibility of the organism. Neutrophil transfusions may be added for patients with systemic infection and low levels of circulating neutrophils, but no controlled studies of this approach have been performed.

References

1. Fidel PL Jr, Vazquez JA, Sobel JD: *Candida glabrata*: review of epidemiology, pathogenesis, and clinical disease with comparison to *C. albicans*. Clin Microbiol Rev 12:80, 1999

2. Abi-Said D, Anaissie E, Uzun O, et al: The epidemiology of hematogenous candidiasis caused by different *Candida* species. Clin Infect Dis 24:1122, 1997

3. Wright WL, Wenzel RP: Nosocomial *Candida*: epidemiology, transmission, and prevention. Infect Dis Clin North Am 11:411, 1997

4. Lundstrom T, Sobel J: Nosocomial candiduria: a review. Clin Infect Dis 32:1602, 2001

5. Darouiche RO: Oropharyngeal and esophageal candidiasis in immunocompromised patients: treatment issues. Clin Infect Dis 26:259, 1998

6. Kontoyiannis DP, Luna MA, Samuels BI, et al: Hepatosplenic candidiasis: a manifestation of chronic disseminated candidiasis. Infect Dis Clin North Am 14:721, 2000

7. Practice guidelines for the treatment of candidiasis. Infectious Diseases Society of America. Clin Infect Dis 30:662, 2000

8. Mitchell TG, Perfect JR: Cryptococcosis in the era of AIDS—100 years after the discovery of *Cryptococcus neoformans*. Clin Microbiol Rev 8:515, 1995

9. Husain S, Wagener MM, Singh N: *Cryptococcus neoformans* infection in organ transplant recipients: variables influencing clinical characteristics and outcome. Emerg Infect Dis 7:375, 2001

10. Rex JH, Larsen RA, Dismukes WE, et al: Catastrophic visual loss due to *Cryptococcus neoformans* meningitis. Medicine (Baltimore) 72:207, 1993

11. Practice guidelines for the management of cryptococcal disease. Mycoses Study Group Subproject, Infectious Diseases Society of AmericaClin Infect Dis 30:710, 2000

12. Singh N, Barnish MJ, Berman S, et al: Low-dose fluconazole as primary prophylaxis for cryptococcal infection in AIDS patients with CD4 cell counts of ≤ 100/mm^3: demonstration of efficacy in a prospective, multicenter trial. Clin Infect Dis 23:1282, 1996

13. Diagnosis and management of increased intracranial pressure in patients with AIDS and cryptococcal meningitis. NIAID Mycoses Study Group and AIDS Cooperative Treatment Groups. Clin Infect Dis 30:47, 2000

14. Park MK, Hospenthal DR, Bennett JE: Treatment of hydrocephalus secondary to cryptococcal meningitis by use of shunting. Clin Infect Dis 28:629, 1999

15. Pappas PG, Perfect JR, Cloud GA, et al: Cryptococcosis in human immunodeficiency virus-negative patients in the era of effective azole therapy. Clin Infect Dis 33:690, 2001

16. Gordon SM, LaRosa SP, Kalmadi S, et al: Should prophylaxis for *Pneumocystis carinii* pneumonia in solid organ transplant recipients ever be discontinued? Clin Infect Dis 28:240, 1999

17. Ng VL, Yajko DM, Hadley WK: Extrapulmonary pneumocystosis. Clin Microbiol Rev 10:401, 1997

18. Predictors for failure of *Pneumocystis carinii* pneumonia prophylaxis. Multicenter AIDS Cohort Study. JAMA 273:1197, 1995

19. Consensus statement on the use of corticosteroids as adjunctive therapy for *Pneumocystis* pneumonia in the acquired immunodeficiency syndrome. National Institutes of Health-University of California Expert Panel for Corticosteroids as Adjunctive Therapy for Pneumocystis Pneumonia. N Engl J Med 323:1500, 1990

20. A randomized trial of the discontinuation of primary and secondary prophylaxis against *Pneumocystis carinii* pneumonia after highly active antiretroviral therapy in patients with HIV infection. Grupo de Estudio del SIDA. N Engl J Med 344:159, 2001

21. Dworkin MS, Williamson J, Jones JL, et al: Prophylaxis with trimethoprim-sulfamethoxazole for human immunodeficiency virus-infected patients: impact on risk for infectious diseases. Clin Infect Dis 33:393, 2001

22. Hughes WT: Use of dapsone in the prevention and treatment of *Pneumocystis carinii* pneumonia: a review. Clin Infect Dis 27:191, 1998

23. Cockrill BA, Hales CA: Allergic bronchopulmonary aspergillosis. Annu Rev Med 50:303, 1999

24. Patterson R, Greenberger PA, Radin RC, et al: Allergic bronchopulmonary aspergillosis: staging as an aid to management. Ann Intern Med 96:286, 1982

25. Nepomuceno IB, Esrig S, Moss RB: Allergic bronchopulmonary aspergillosis in cystic fibrosis: role of atopy and response to itraconazole. Chest 115:364, 1999

26. Stevens DA, Schwartz HJ, Lee JY, et al: A randomized trial of itraconazole in allergic bronchopulmonary aspergillosis. N Engl J Med 342:756, 2000

27. Wald A, Leisenring W, van Burik J-A, et al: Epidemiology of *Aspergillus* infections in a large cohort of patients undergoing bone marrow transplantation. J Infect Dis 175:1459, 1997

28. Lin S-J, Schranz J, Teutsch SM: Aspergillosis case-fatality rate: systematic review of the literature. Clin Infect Dis 32:358, 2001

29. Denning DW: Invasive aspergillosis. Clin Infect Dis 26:781, 1998

30. Yeghen T, Kibbler CC, Prentice HG, et al: Management of invasive pulmonary aspergillosis in hematology patients: a review of 87 consecutive cases at a single institution. Clin Infect Dis 31:859, 2000

31. Clarke A, Skelton J, Fraser RS: Fungal tracheobronchitis: report of 9 cases and review of the literature. Medicine (Baltimore) 70:1, 1991

32. Latge J-P: *Aspergillus fumigatus* and aspergillosis. Clin Microbiol Rev 12:310, 1999

33. Cornet M, Levy V, Fleury L, et al: Efficacy of prevention by high-efficiency particulate air filtration or laminar airflow against *Aspergillus* airborne contamination during hospital renovation. Infect Control Hosp Epidemiol 20:508, 1999

34. Offner F, Cordonnier C, Ljungman P, et al: Impact of previous aspergillosis on the outcome of bone marrow transplantation. Clin Infect Dis 26:1098, 1998

35. Hermann S, Klein SA, Jacobi V, et al: Older patients with high-risk fungal infections can be successfully allografted using non-myeloablative conditioning in combination with intensified supportive care regimens. Br J Haematol 113:446, 2001

36. Oliver MR, Van Voorhis WC, Boeckh M, et al: Hepatic mucormycosis in a bone marrow transplant recipient who ingested naturopathic medicine. Clin Infect Dis 22:521, 1996

37. Gartenberg G, Bottone EJ, Keusch GT, et al: Hospital-acquired mucormycosis (*Rhizopus rhizopodiformis*) of skin and subcutaneous tissue: epidemiology, mycology and treatment. N Engl J Med 299:1115, 1978

38. Adam RD, Hunter G, DiTomasso J, et al: Mucormycosis: emerging prominence of cutaneous infections. Clin Infect Dis 19:67, 1994

39. Gamis AS, Gudnason T, Giebink GS, et al: Disseminated infection with *Fusarium* in recipients of bone marrow transplants. Rev Infect Dis 13:1077, 1991

40. Boutati EI, Anaissie EJ: *Fusarium*, a significant emerging pathogen in patients with hematologic malignancy: ten years' experience at a cancer center and implications for management. Blood 90:999, 1997

41. Invasive *Fusarium* infections: a retrospective survey of 31 cases. French 'Groupe d'Etudes des Mycoses Opportunistes' GEMO. J Med Vet Mycol 35:107, 1997

42. Sampathkumar P, Paya CV: *Fusarium* infection after solid-organ transplantation. Clin Infect Dis 32:1237, 2001

43. Louie T, el Baba F, Shulman M, et al: Endogenous endophthalmitis due to *Fusarium*: case report and review. Clin Infect Dis 18:585, 1994

44. Prins C, Chavaz P, Tamm K, et al: Ecthyma gangrenosum–like lesions: a sign of disseminated *Fusarium* infection in the neutropenic patient. Clin Exp Dermatol 20:428, 1995

45. Rossmann SN, Cernoch PL, Davis JR: Dematiaceous fungi are an increasing cause of human disease. Clin Infect Dis 22:73, 1996

46. Osiyemi OO, Dowdy LM, Mallon SM, et al: Cerebral phaeohyphomycosis due to a novel species: report of a case and review of the literature. Transplantation 71:1343, 2001

47. Singh N, Chang FY, Gayowski T, et al: Infections due to dematiaceous fungi in organ transplant recipients: case report and review. Clin Infect Dis 24:369, 1997

48. Zieske LA, Kopke RD, Hamill R: Dematiaceous fungal sinusitis. Otolaryngol Head Neck Surg 105:567, 1991

39 Protozoan Infections

Peter F. Weller, M.D.

Toxoplasmosis

Toxoplasma gondii, the cause of toxoplasmosis, is an intracellular protozoan parasite of worldwide distribution. *T. gondii* can infect nearly all animals and birds, making it one of the most widely distributed parasites.[1] Humans acquire *T. gondii* infections by the oral and transplacental routes and, less commonly, from blood transfusion and organ transplantation. Infection via the oral route is caused by the ingestion of *T. gondii* tissue cysts in undercooked food or the ingestion of *T. gondii* oocysts, which are found in cat feces. After ingestion, bradyzoites (from tissue cysts) or sporozoites (from oocysts) invade surrounding cells and develop into tachyzoites, a rapidly dividing form that may disseminate and invade any nucleated cell type. With time and the development of immunity, the parasite will form tissue cysts containing many bradyzoites. Tissue cysts may remain viable for decades without causing disease. Loss of immunity, however, allows reactivation from the latent tissue cysts and the generation of many invasive tachyzoites.

Although toxoplasmosis is extremely common, most acquired and congenital infections are subclinical and are revealed only by the presence of antibodies. The prevalence of infection varies greatly in different population groups and geographic regions. In the United States, serologic evidence of *Toxoplasma* infection varies regionally in prevalence from 3% to 30%.

CLINICAL SYNDROMES

Toxoplasmosis can be divided into five major clinical syndromes: primary toxoplasmosis, toxoplasmosis in immunosuppression, toxoplasmosis in AIDS, congenital toxoplasmosis, and ocular toxoplasmosis.

Primary Toxoplasmosis

An immunocompetent person usually experiences subclinical illness after acquisition of a primary toxoplasmosis infection. Painless lymphadenopathy is the most common symptom. Lymphadenopathy may be localized or generalized and may persist for many months. Isolated cervical lymphadenopathy is the most frequent finding.[2] Enlarged nodes may be the only manifestation; less often, fever, malaise, myalgias, and sore throat are also present. Fatigue and weakness may be pronounced. In addition to lymphadenopathy, physical findings may include pharyngitis, maculopapular rash,[3] and, in a minority of patients, hepatosplenomegaly. Atypical lymphocytosis may be present. The major differential diagnosis includes infectious mononucleosis, cytomegalovirus infection, and lymphoma; less often, sarcoidosis, cat-scratch disease, and other infectious processes may resemble toxoplasmosis. Serologic testing is the key to diagnosis.[4]

Although symptoms of acquired lymphadenopathic toxoplasmosis can persist for weeks or months, the process is almost always self-limited and does not require specific therapy. In severe or protracted cases, pyrimethamine and sulfonamides may be helpful. Chemotherapy should also be used for the rare complications that can occur in the normal host, including chorioretinitis, pericarditis, myocarditis, pneumonitis, myositis, and meningoencephalitis.

Toxoplasmosis in Immunosuppression

In the immunosuppressed patient with defective cell-mediated immunity, *T. gondii* can cause devastating neurologic or disseminated disease. Usually this process develops from reactivation of latent infection and not from a primary infection. Seronegative recipients of organs (especially hearts) transplanted from seropositive donors are at particular risk,[5,6] as are patients with Hodgkin's disease, hairy-cell leukemia, and other malignant disorders.[7] Neurologic abnormalities predominate in at least 50% of these patients. The clinical picture is highly variable and may take the form of a diffuse encephalitis, a meningoencephalitis, or a cerebral mass lesion.[8] The cerebrospinal fluid often shows a mild lymphocytic pleocytosis and an elevation of protein levels; glucose levels, however, remain normal. Pneumonitis may occur in up to one third of immunosuppressed patients with toxoplasmosis.[9] Fever and dyspnea are present, but cough is absent and no sputum is produced. Chest radiographs typically reveal diffuse bilateral pulmonary infiltrates. In a few cases, the diagnosis has been established by finding organisms in the fluid obtained from bronchoalveolar lavage. Other manifestations of disseminated toxoplasmosis in immunosuppressed patients include myocarditis, pericarditis, peritonitis, and lymphadenitis. Many of these immunosuppressed patients have simultaneous infections with other opportunistic pathogens, especially herpesvirus and cytomegalovirus.

If appropriate serologic titers are present, they will support the diagnosis of toxoplasmosis; however, antibody levels may be low in these patients, and therefore, brain, lung, or lymph node biopsy may be required for diagnosis. An aggressive diagnostic approach is warranted because pyrimethamine and sulfonamides can be effective in these infections, which are usually fatal if left untreated.

Toxoplasmosis in AIDS

Toxoplasmosis is a particularly severe problem in patients with AIDS; clinically apparent toxoplasmosis develops in 3% to 40% of these patients.[10] Although any of the manifestations of disseminated toxoplasmosis may occur in patients with AIDS,[11] central nervous system abnormalities predominate. Most cases of toxoplasmosis in patients with AIDS result from reactivation of latent *Toxoplasma* cysts acquired before infection with HIV; reactivation is particularly likely when the $CD4^+$ T cell count falls below 100 cells/mm^3.[10] All HIV-infected persons should be tested for antibodies to *T. gondii*. All HIV-positive individuals who are *Toxoplasma* negative should be cautioned to minimize exposure by cooking meat to an internal temperature of 150° F, washing their hands after contact with raw meat or soil, washing fruits and vegetables before eating them, and avoiding contact with cat feces or contaminated litter (or wearing gloves if these materials must be handled).[12]

In AIDS patients, toxoplasmosis most often presents as necrotizing encephalitis. Symptoms include focal abnormalities (e.g., hemiparesis, sensory loss, visual abnormalities, tremor, cranial nerve palsies, and focal seizures) and generalized neurologic abnormalities (e.g., headache, personality changes, confusion, stupor or coma, and seizures). Although a CSF lymphocytic pleocytosis is consistent with the diagnosis of cerebral toxoplasmosis, computed tomographic or magnetic resonance imaging scans are the crucial diagnostic tests in most cases. Typical findings include single or multiple rounded mass lesions; when a contrast agent is administered, more than 90% of these lesions display ring or nodular enhancement. MRI scans may reveal lesions that were not visualized by CT scanning.[13] Positron emission tomography (PET) may prove useful for distinguishing lesions of toxoplasmosis (which are hypometabolic) from lymphomas (which are hypermetabolic).[14]

Serum antibody tests are useful for screening AIDS patients for cerebral toxoplasmosis; such tests are usually positive because most cases of cerebral toxoplasmosis in patients with AIDS arise from reactivation of latent infection. Although negative antibody tests suggest a diagnosis other than toxoplasmosis, a few seronegative cases have been reported. However, serum antibody tests cannot be relied on in the diagnosis of active toxoplasmosis in patients with AIDS; antibody titers do not reach the high levels typical of immunocompetent patients with toxoplasmosis, nor are IgM antibodies present in patients with AIDS.[10] Antibodies against *Toxoplasma* are present in the CSF in nearly two thirds of AIDS patients with cerebral toxoplasmosis, and their detection may assist in the diagnosis [*see* Diagnosis, *below*].[15]

In addition to toxoplasmosis, CNS lesions caused by fungi, mycobacteria, lymphomas, Kaposi's sarcoma, metastatic tumors, multifocal leukoencephalopathy, or HIV itself may develop in patients with AIDS. Despite this broad differential diagnosis of cerebral lesions in patients with AIDS, empirical treatment of toxoplasmosis is often preferable to early brain biopsy if the clinical and radiologic picture is compatible with the diagnosis and if serum anti-*Toxoplasma* antibodies are present.[16] Because toxoplasmosis is the most common and most treatable cause of cerebral lesions in patients with AIDS, empirical therapy using a combination of sulfonamides and pyrimethamine or the combination of clindamycin and pyrimethamine can be initiated; if the diagnosis is correct, clinical and radiologic improvement is often observed within 1 to 2 weeks.

If patients respond poorly to treatment and are seronegative or belong to population groups with a high risk of tuberculosis (e.g., Haitians, Africans, or intravenous drug abusers), biopsy should be strongly considered.[16]

Congenital Toxoplasmosis

Congenital toxoplasmosis arises almost exclusively when the mother develops a primary infection during gestation. Congenital infection almost never develops from latent toxoplasmosis acquired before pregnancy, and the few recognized cases have developed mainly in pregnant women with reactivation of toxoplasmosis due to immunosuppressive therapy or HIV infection.[17] The risk of fetal infection depends on when maternal infection occurs, rising from 10% during the first trimester to 60% during the third trimester.[18] The consequences of fetal infection also depend on when infection occurs: fetal infections acquired early in gestation are most likely to result in severe damage.

The clinical spectrum of congenital toxoplasmosis varies widely. About 85% of infected babies appear normal at birth; without treatment, however, about 85% of these infants will experience chorioretinitis, hearing loss, or developmental delay.[18,19] The clinical spectrum of symptomatic congenital toxoplasmosis includes fetal death, neurologic damage (cerebral calcification, seizures, retardation, hydrocephalus, or microcephaly), chorioretinitis, fever, hepatosplenomegaly, and rash. The differential diagnosis includes congenital infection with cytomegalovirus, herpes simplex, rubella, or syphilis. Congenital toxoplasmosis can be diagnosed by serologic methods, by a polymerase chain reaction (PCR) test performed on amniotic fluid,[20] or by identification of the organism in the placenta or fetal tissues. Infants with congenital toxoplasmosis may benefit from prolonged treatment with pyrimethamine and sulfonamides.[21]

The prevention of congenital toxoplasmosis is of major importance. Pregnant women should minimize contact with cats, especially strays or cats who eat raw meat; they should wash their hands after contact with cats and should have another person empty the litter box daily. In addition, pregnant women should wash all fruits and vegetables before eating them and should not eat undercooked meat. Serologic screening of pregnant women is advisable.

Ocular Toxoplasmosis

Toxoplasmosis may account for about 30% of cases of retinochoroiditis.[22] Many cases result from the reactivation of congenital infection; hence, ocular toxoplasmosis is most common in older children and young adults. Retinochoroiditis may also develop as a manifestation of primary infection.[23] Impairment of vision is the most common symptom, but pain and photophobia may accompany intense inflammation. Typical lesions appear as yellow-white fluffy exudates clustered in the posterior pole. Although a positive *Toxoplasma* serology is needed for the diagnosis of ocular toxoplasmosis, most patients have relatively low titers because the initial infection was acquired years earlier. In most cases, therefore, ocular toxoplasmosis is a clinical diagnosis that depends on the morphology of the lesions. Other conditions considered in the differential diagnosis include tuberculosis, sarcoidosis, syphilis, histoplasmosis, and candidiasis.

DIAGNOSIS

Serologic testing is important in evaluating patients with potential toxoplasmosis. Many tests are available; the most widely used are the indirect fluorescent antibody test and the Sabin-Feldman dye test. Many other tests are utilized by reference laboratories. Tests that measure IgG antibodies show positive results 1 to 3 weeks after infection and continue to show positive results for many years after infection. Diagnoses of recently acquired toxoplasmosis, especially pertinent during pregnancy, and of congenital toxoplasmosis in the newborn require assays of IgM anti-*Toxoplasma* antibodies. Some commercial IgM assays have been noted to generate false positive results and to detect IgM antibodies persisting for over 1 year, potentially confounding the reliability of these assays to detect only recent infections.[24] Positive IgM test results may necessitate confirmation by alternative testing assays.

Because tissue cysts may be present in tissues for years, definitive evidence of active toxoplasmosis within biopsied tissues requires the detection of tachyzoites. These forms are not readily seen with conventional pathologic stains. Application of immunofluorescent or peroxidase-antiperoxidase antibody staining is needed. Tachyzoites are not usually detectable in biopsied lymph nodes, although characteristic histopathologic features can support the diagnosis.[25] PCR methods are highly sensitive for detecting the organism in amniotic fluid in congenital infections,[20] but neither PCR nor direct culturing of the organisms from blood or tissues has been widely used in diagnosing other forms of toxoplasmosis.

TREATMENT

Primary and AIDS-Associated Toxoplasmosis

Although the majority of patients with primary lymphadenopathic toxoplasmosis do not require treatment, chemotherapy should be considered for patients with unusually prolonged or severe illness. Patients with active chorioretinitis, CNS involvement, or disseminated toxoplasmosis should also be treated, as should immunosuppressed patients with toxoplasmosis, including patients with AIDS.

Combined administration of pyrimethamine and sulfonamides (sulfadiazine or trisulfapyrimidines) is the treatment of choice.[26] Other sulfonamides are less active against *T. gondii* and therefore should be avoided. In adults, a loading dose of 200 mg of pyrimethamine is given on the first day of treatment, followed by the usual dosage of 50 to 75 mg/day. Sulfadiazine or trisulfapyrimidines are usually given to adults in a loading dose of 4 g, followed by a dosage of 1 to 2 g four times daily. The most common toxic effect of pyrimethamine is marrow suppression; leukocyte, red cell, and platelet counts should be monitored twice weekly, and 10 to 15 mg of folinic acid should be administered daily. Combined pyrimethamine and sulfonamide therapy is usually given for 3 to 6 weeks.

For AIDS patients who are intolerant of sulfonamides, clindamycin at a dosage of 600 mg orally or intravenously four times a day in combination with pyrimethamine has been effective in treating CNS toxoplasmosis.[27] Atovaquone plus pyrimethamine is also effective for sulfa-intolerant patients.[28]

Patients with AIDS who have been treated for toxoplasmosis and those who have not experienced active toxoplasmosis infection but have positive *Toxoplasma* serologies and CD4$^+$ T cell counts below 100/mm^3 are at risk for reactivation of toxoplasmosis and require prolonged suppressive therapy. A variety of regimens are available for patients with AIDS who have recovered from toxoplasmosis. A regimen consisting of sulfadiazine (500 to 1,000 mg four times a day) and pyrimethamine (25 to 50 mg/day) plus folinic acid (5 mg/day) is most effective.[29] Clindamycin (300 to 450 mg three times a day) is also effective for patients intolerant of sulfonamides.[30] Some regimens used for the prevention of *Pneumocystis* pneumonia also provide primary prophylaxis for toxoplasmosis; examples include trimethoprim-sulfamethoxazole, dapsone-pyrimethamine, atovaquone, and pyrimethamine alone for sulfa-intolerant patients.[31]

Congenital Toxoplasmosis

Newly acquired toxoplasmosis documented during pregnancy presents difficult choices. Pyrimethamine is teratogenic and should be avoided in the first trimester. Spiramycin—available in the United States only directly from the manufacturer, Rhône-Poulenc Rorer—given at 3 to 4 g/day, can diminish the risk of transplacental infection.[26] If in utero infection is documented, therapy with pyrimethamine and sulfadiazine should be initiated. Therapeutic abortion might be considered if infection is acquired early in pregnancy; ultrasonography can be used to detect hydrocephalus, intracranial calcifications, and other signs of fetal damage. Children who are born with serologic or clinical evidence of congenital toxoplasmosis should be treated for a year with pyrimethamine and sulfadiazine.[19]

Ocular Toxoplasmosis

Pyrimethamine and sulfonamides are the mainstays of therapy for ocular toxoplasmosis, but results are unpredictable and relapses commonly occur. In cases in which there is a threat of visual loss, the patient should receive corticosteroids in combination with antimicrobials.

Malaria

Four *Plasmodium* species cause human malaria: *P. falciparum, P. vivax, P. ovale,* and *P. malariae* [*see Table 1*]. *P. vivax* and *P. falciparum* are the most prevalent worldwide, and falciparum malaria is the one responsible for most deaths. Malaria is transmitted by anopheline mosquitoes. Although malaria transmission in the United States is highly uncommon, about 300 to 500 million malaria cases, with three million deaths, are estimated to occur annually worldwide.[32,33] Malaria is resurgent because of multiple factors, including anopheline mosquito vector resistance to insecticides, inability of governmental programs to control mosquito vector populations, increased opportunities for breeding of vector mosquitoes, and increasing resistance of malarial parasites to chemotherapeutic agents.

ETIOLOGY AND EPIDEMIOLOGY

Malaria is endemic in many countries. Most malaria in the United States is imported. In 1995, 1,167 cases of malaria, including six deaths due to malaria, were reported to the Centers for Disease Control and Prevention (CDC). Of these cases, 599 occurred in United States civilians, 461 in foreign

Table 1 Differentiating Features of Malarial *Plasmodium* Species

Species	*Global Prevalence*	*Mortality*	*Clinical Manifestations*	*Length of Erythrocytic Cycle*	*Persistence in Liver*	*Chloroquine Resistance*
P. falciparum	Common	Common (especially if untreated in nonimmune hosts)	Fever, anemia Microvascular blockade with local anoxia: brain (cerebral malaria) lungs (pulmonary edema) kidneys (acute renal failure) intestines (diarrhea) liver (tenderness, anoxia) blood (thrombocytopenia)	48 hr	No	Common
P. vivax	Common	Uncommon	Fever, anemia Splenic rupture (uncommon)	48 hr	Yes	Uncommon
P. ovale	Uncommon	Rare	Fever, anemia	48 hr	Yes	No
P. malariae	Uncommon	Rare	Mild, chronic parasitemia, often with no symptoms Immune complexes (nephrotic syndrome)	72 hr	No	No

civilians, and 12 in United States military personnel.[32] *P. vivax* and *P. falciparum* accounted for 48% and 39% of infected persons, respectively. Less commonly, malaria is transmitted by blood transfusion, by sharing of contaminated needles, by organ transplantation, and congenitally in infants who are born of infected mothers.[32,34] In addition, because species of *Anopheles* mosquitoes that are competent to transmit malaria are present in the United States, isolated cases of autochthonous malaria have developed in Americans bitten by local mosquitoes that fed on persons with imported malaria.[35] A final means of introduction of malaria into the United States is so-called airport malaria, which arises when an infected mosquito enters the country on an aircraft from a malarious area and transmits the infection in the area around the airport.

PATHOGENESIS

Infections are normally acquired by the bite of an infected female *Anopheles* mosquito, which introduces sporozoites [*see Figure 1*]. In the preerythrocytic stage of infection, all four species of *Plasmodium* infect hepatocytes. Notably, however, only two species—*P. vivax* and *P. ovale*—cause persistent infections within the liver. In the erythrocytic stage of malarial infection, merozoites released from infected hepatocytes and later from infected erythrocytes interact with specific erythrocyte membrane proteins and invade the red blood cells. (The Duffy blood group antigen is the requisite erythrocyte receptor for *P. vivax*. Individuals genetically missing the Duffy blood group antigen, such as many West Africans and their descendants, are resistant to that species of *Plasmodium*.) Within the infected cells, malarial parasites undergo schizogony to form new merozoites, which are released to reinfect other erythrocytes. A few parasites differentiate into sexual stages (gametocytes) capable of infecting mosquitoes. Male and female gametocytes transform and reproduce in the midgut of the mosquito, leading to the production of new sporozoites that localize in the mosquito's salivary glands.

Because of the capability of malarial parasites to replicate and increase their numbers within the infected human, intense infections can develop from minimal inocula of infecting sporozoites. Travelers have developed malaria after being bitten by mosquitoes during brief layovers at airports in malarious areas and during flights on airplanes that have stopped in malarious regions. Consequently, malaria prophylaxis is warranted for even the most limited exposures to mosquitoes in malarious regions.

Patients remain asymptomatic during the period between the infecting mosquito bite and the erythrocytic stage of infection, a period that may range from about 1 to 4 weeks. Because malaria chemoprophylaxis does not actually prevent malaria, but rather treats erythrocytic-stage infection, chemoprophylactic medication must be continued for the full 4 weeks after a return from a malarious area. Failure to continue weekly chemo-

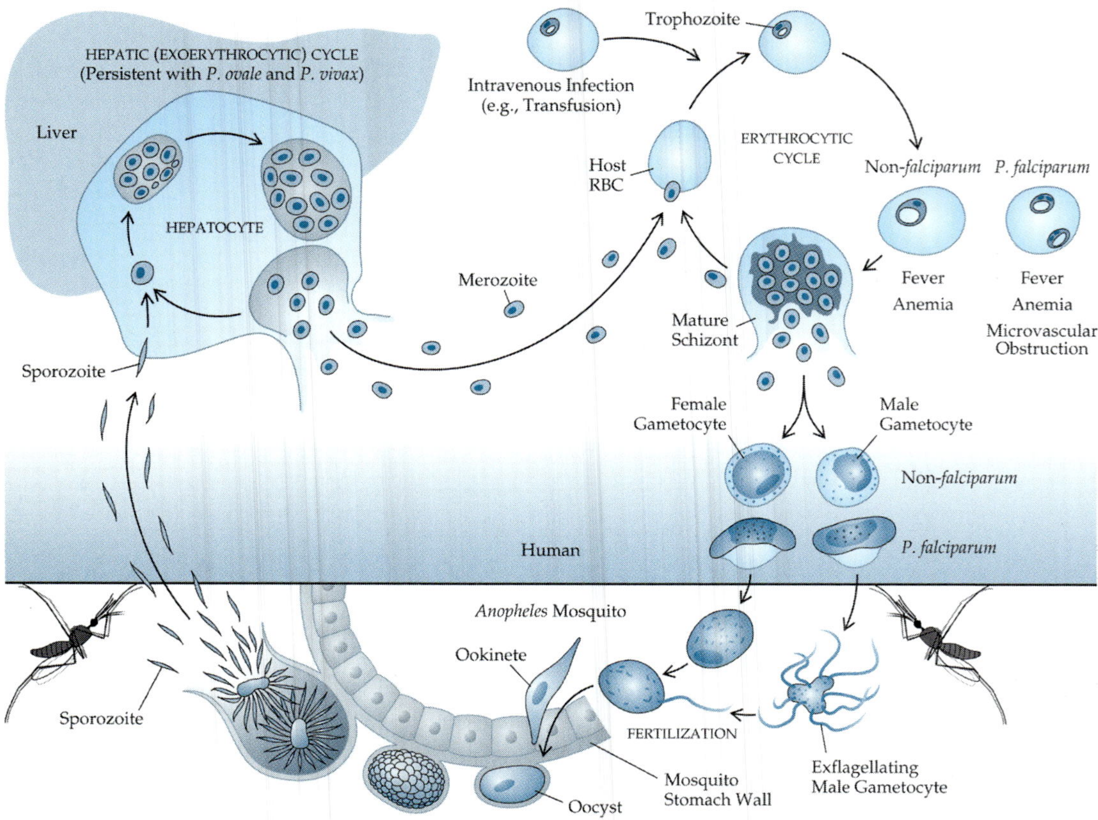

Figure 1 **All four human malaria species, *Plasmodium falciparum, P. vivax, P. ovale,* and *P. malariae,* may be transmitted by Anopheles mosquito bites or introduced by blood (e.g., congenitally, through transfusion, and by sharing of needles). Only two species, *P. vivax* and *P. ovale,* remain in the liver. Symptoms develop with infection of erythrocytes (erythrocytic cycle), about 1 or more weeks after a mosquito bite. Agents used for chemoprophylaxis or malaria therapy act on the erythrocytic cycle; only primaquine eradicates the exoerythrocytic cycles of *P. vivax* and *P. ovale.***

prophylaxis after one returns from a malarious area permits the development of malarial infection.

Immune responses develop to malarial infections. Development of antibodies to the most indolent and chronic malarial species, *P. malariae,* may lead over years to the onset of immune complex–mediated nephrotic syndrome. Repeated infections with other *Plasmodium* species can elicit a partially protective immunity that will limit the severity of infection but not prevent it. Of note, residents of malarious areas may lose their relative immunity after staying several years in a nonmalarious region; such persons may be fully susceptible to malaria infection upon their return.

DIAGNOSIS

Malaria should be considered as a cause of any febrile illness in immigrants from malarious areas and in persons who have traveled or worked in malarious areas. Recipients of transfused blood or transplanted organs and neonates of potentially infected mothers should be considered for possibly acquired malaria. Finally, even in United States residents, the diagnosis of malaria may need to be considered in febrile patients with compatible illnesses that may have developed from the uncommon autochthonous transmission of malaria.

Infections with the four human malarial species of *Plasmodium* produce distinct clinical syndromes, based in part on the interactions of each species with erythrocytes. *P. vivax* infects young red cells only, which helps limit the intensity of infection. It also explains why enlarged red cells are characteristic of *P. vivax* infections in speciation of malaria blood films. In contrast, *P. falciparum* infects erythrocytes of all ages. This capacity of falciparum malaria, the greater numbers of merozoites produced by this species, and especially the great propensity of falciparum-infected erythrocytes to adhere to the microvascular endothelium contribute to making falciparum malaria distinctly more severe than other forms of malaria. Erythrocytes infected with *P. falciparum* develop unique surface knobs that mediate binding and adherence to endothelial cells in capillaries and venules. With sequestration of infected erythrocytes in these small vessels, local anoxia develops. Severe complications, including cerebral malaria and pulmonary edema, may ensue [*see Table 1*].

Clinical Features

Clinical symptoms develop about 1 to 4 weeks after infection and typically include fever and chills. Virtually all patients with acute malaria have episodes of fever. At the outset, fever may occur daily; over time, the paroxysms may develop the typical every-other-day (*P. vivax, P. ovale, P. falciparum*) or every-third-day (*P. malariae*) pattern. The paroxysms of fever (as high as 41.5° C [106.7° F]) and chills (with or without rigors) may be irregular, however—especially in falciparum malaria. Other symptoms may be headache, increased sweating, back pain, myalgias, diarrhea, nausea, vomiting, and cough. The constellations of possible symptoms are nonspecific and may suggest diagnoses other than malaria.[36] With time, anemia and splenomegaly develop.

Because of the distinct capacity of falciparum-infected erythrocytes to cause microvascular blockade, potentially fatal organ involvement can develop rapidly in falciparum malaria. Cerebral involvement may lead to delirium, focal disorders (e.g., seizures), and coma.[37] Splanchnic involvement may cause protracted nausea, vomiting, diarrhea, melena, and abdominal pain; this syndrome can be readily mistaken for traveler's diarrhea. Lung involvement may cause pulmonary edema and the adult respiratory distress syndrome. There may be severe hypoglycemia. A rare syndrome, blackwater fever, results from massive intravascular hemolysis, which leads to hemoglobinuria and acute renal failure.

P. malariae organisms can persist in the blood as an indolent, even asymptomatic, infection for years or even decades.[38]

Laboratory Findings

The white blood cell count is usually in the normal range in malaria patients. Anemia develops but may not be prominent on presentation, especially if the patient is dehydrated. Thrombocytopenia may develop; disseminated intravascular coagulation sometimes occurs in falciparum malaria. Liver enzymes may be elevated.

The specific diagnosis and speciation of malaria depends on the recognition of parasites in properly stained smears of peripheral blood.[32] Thick smears are more sensitive than thin smears, but the layering of cells necessitates greater expertise in examining morphology. Smears should be taken repeatedly for several days because of the cyclic nature of the parasitemia. This is especially important in suspected *P. falciparum* infections, in which infected cells may be sequestered in the microvasculature. The morphologic features of the parasites (and the infected host erythrocytes) are useful in species identification and in distinguishing *Plasmodium* species from the morphologically similar *Babesia microti* organism, a cause of human babesiosis. It is very important to identify and treat *P. falciparum* infection rapidly because of its potential for swift progression if left untreated or if treated improperly.

The quantitative buffy coat (QBC) technique is sensitive in identifying plasmodial parasitemia, but it does not identify the species. Dipstick antigen-capture assays are available and have the potential to help clinicians detect falciparum infections, particularly where no specialized laboratories are available.[39] DNA probes, PCR tests, and serologic tests exist, but these are not usually immediately available for diagnosis of acute malaria at presentation. Thus, examination of blood smears is still the standard in assessing, first, whether a patient has malaria and, second, whether the malaria is caused by *P. falciparum*.

TREATMENT

Treatment of patients with acute malaria requires consideration of the species of malaria and—in cases of falciparum malaria—the likelihood of the parasite's being resistant to antimalarial medications. Chloroquine is the mainstay of treatment for all malarial species except those strains of *P. falciparum* that are resistant to the drug. Notably, chloroquine-resistant *P. falciparum* (CRPF) malaria is now widespread in all countries where *P. falciparum* is endemic except Haiti, the Dominican Republic, areas of Central America west of the Panama Canal, and parts of the Middle East. For *P. falciparum* infections acquired in countries with chloroquine-resistant strains, alternative therapies must be utilized. Mefloquine-resistant strains of *P. falciparum* have been identified at the Thailand-Myanmar border. Isolated strains of *P. vivax* resistant to chloroquine have been reported in Africa, Central and South America, and Asia.

Acute attacks caused by all species except CRPF are treated with oral chloroquine phosphate at an initial dose of 1 g (600 mg base), followed by 500 mg (300 mg base) at 6 hours and again at 24 and 48 hours.[26] For suspected CRPF malaria, several alternative regimens are available.[26] Quinine sulfate (650 mg every 8 hours for 3 to 7 days) is combined with doxycycline (100 mg b.i.d. for 7 days), pyrimethamine-sulfadoxine (Fansidar) (three tablets as a single dose on the last day of quinine treatment), or clindamycin (900 mg t.i.d. for 5 days). Alternative therapies for CRPF malaria include mefloquine (1,250 mg as a single dose), halofantrine, and atovaquone in combination with either proguanil or doxycycline.[26]

For patients who are too ill to take oral therapies, intravenous quinidine gluconate or quinine dihydrochloride are the drugs of choice for any species of malaria.[26] Quinidine is effective and well tolerated when appropriate precautions, including hemodynamic and ECG monitoring, are used. A loading dose of 10 mg/kg (maximum, 600 mg) of quinidine in normal saline is infused slowly over 1 to 2 hours, followed by continuous infusion of 0.02 mg/kg/min. Parenteral therapy should be continued until oral therapy can be tolerated; in most cases, oral therapy can be substituted within 48 to 72 hours. For fulminant falciparum malaria, exchange transfusion can be an adjunct to chemotherapy.[40]

Each of the chemotherapeutic agents mentioned above is active only in the erythrocytic stage of infection. Because *P. vivax* and *P. ovale* have persisting hepatic stages that may cause relapses of malaria after chloroquine use [*see Figure 1*], an agent that is active on the exoerythrocytic cycle should be administered after a course of chloroquine. Primaquine is the sole agent used to eradicate hepatic involvement; the dosage is 26.3 mg (15 mg base) orally every day for 2 weeks. Because primaquine may induce hemolysis in persons with glucose-6-phosphate dehydrogenase (G6PD) deficiency, patients should be screened for the disorder before treatment. If only mild G6PD deficiency is found, primaquine may be given at a dosage of 79 mg (45 mg base) orally once a week for 8 weeks.

Advice for Travelers

Most United States residents lack immunity to malaria and are at risk for the morbid and mortal consequences of the disease, especially the falciparum form, in countries where malaria transmission occurs. Of the 591 United States civilians who acquired malaria abroad in 1995, only 15.6% had followed a CDC-recommended chemoprophylactic drug regimen.[32] It is imperative that travelers receive appropriate advice on reducing their risk of acquiring malaria and on using appropriate malaria-chemoprophylaxis regimens.

Babesiosis

Babesia organisms are intraerythrocytic protozoan parasites that produce a malarialike illness. Most cases of babesiosis have been reported in the northeastern United States, but cases have also occurred in the upper Midwest, the West Coast, and other regions of the United States and in Europe and elsewhere.[41]

ETIOLOGY AND EPIDEMIOLOGY

Several species of *Babesia* have been recognized as causes of human disease. The first to be recognized was *B. divergens*, a parasite of cattle, that has caused several fatal infections in splenectomized persons, mostly in Europe, although a related species, designated MO1, has caused a fatal case in a splenectomized man in Missouri.[42]

B. microti is the principal cause of babesiosis in the United States. This parasite of white-footed mice is transmitted by deer ticks and is prevalent on the islands off Massachusetts, New York, and Rhode Island and in focal areas in Connecticut, Wisconsin, and Minnesota. Risk of *Babesia* infection is not increased by splenectomy, but the disease is more serious in persons who have undergone splenectomy, have HIV infection, or have other immunocompromising conditions.[41,43] Many infected persons have subclinical infections, as evidenced by serologic surveys in endemic areas. Because nymphal ticks are the most efficient at transmitting infection, most cases develop between May and August, when nymphal ticks are most abundant.[41]

Another form of babesiosis develops from infection with an organism found in states along the Pacific coast and designated as WA1. The vector and reservoir of this emerging *Babesia* species are not yet known. Infections have been recognized in asplenic persons and less commonly in normal hosts; serologic surveys in rural and semirural California indicate that subclinical infection with WA1 may have developed in up to 20% of the population.[41]

Babesiosis may also be acquired perinatally and through blood transfusions.[41,44]

DIAGNOSIS

Clinical Features

Many persons infected with *B. microti* or WA1 remain asymptomatic. In those who have symptoms, illness develops gradually in the weeks after tick bites or blood transfusions. Malaise, anorexia, and fatigue are followed by the onset of myalgias, fevers, and sweats. Emotional lability, depression, nausea, vomiting, and headache are common. Symptoms tend to abate over several weeks, although fatigue and malaise may persist for months. Splenomegaly is occasionally present. Infections may become more fulminant and persistent in asplenic patients, elderly patients, and patients with HIV infection or other immunocompromising conditions. Intravascular hemolysis, hemoglobinuria, and renal failure may develop. Parasitemias as high as 85% can develop; this level of infection can be fatal, especially in asplenic persons.

Laboratory Findings

Laboratory findings may include hemolytic anemia, normal to low leukocyte counts, and abnormal liver function tests. The diagnosis is based on the finding of ring forms and pleomorphic intraerythrocytic organisms on Giemsa-stained blood smears. Occasionally, extracellular merozoites are seen. Unlike malarial parasites, *Babesia* organisms do not produce pigment in red blood cells. In some patients, a parasitemia level of 5% or higher and the presence of several ring forms in a single red cell might suggest *P. falciparum* infection; the absence of gametocytes and intracellular pigmentation will help distinguish babesiosis from malaria. Serologic testing is of value for diagnosing chronic infections with *B. microti* and WA1 when parasites are not detectable on blood smears.

TREATMENT

The treatment of choice for babesiosis is a combination of clindamycin (1.2 g b.i.d., I.V., or 600 mg t.i.d., p.o., for 7 days) and quinine (650 mg t.i.d., p.o., for 7 days).[26] In a minority of patients who improve symptomatically, parasitemia may nevertheless persist.[45] Occasionally, pulmonary edema may develop after initiation of therapy for babesiosis, as also may occur with malaria. Exchange transfusion can be an adjunct to chemotherapy in cases of fulminant babesiosis. The tick vector of babesiosis may simultaneously transmit *Borrelia burgdorferi*, the agent of Lyme disease [see 25 Leptospirosis, Relapsing Fever, Rat-Bite Fever, and Lyme Disease], and *Ehrlichia* species, the agents of ehrlichiosis [see 26 Rickettsial Diseases and Q Fever]. Those coinfections may make clinical illness more severe and warrant special therapy.[46]

Intestinal Protozoan Infections

The human intestinal tract may serve as a host for several protozoan parasites. The intestinal protozoa *Entamoeba coli, Endolimax nana*, and *Iodamoeba butschlii* are nonpathogenic and do not require therapy. Pathogenic intestinal protozoan parasites include *Giardia lamblia, Entamoeba. histolytica*, coccidia, *Balantidium coli*, and *Dientamoeba fragilis*.

GIARDIASIS

G. lamblia inhabits the proximal small intestine; manifestations of *G. lamblia* infections can vary from no symptoms to profound malabsorption. *G. lamblia* and cryptosporidiosis are the most common pathogenic intestinal protozoan parasites in the United States.[47]

Etiology and Epidemiology

G. lamblia exists in two morphologic forms: the trophozoite and the cyst. The trophozoite is a pear-shaped, multiflagellated organism that measures 9 to 15 µm long, 5 to 15 µm wide, and 2 to 4 µm thick. It is bilaterally symmetrical and contains two prominent nuclei. On the ventral surface is an adhesive disk with which the trophozoite attaches to the mucosal surface of the duodenum and jejunum. During passage in the bowel, the trophozoite usually encysts. The cysts measure 8 to 12 µm long by 7 to 10 µm wide, have a well-defined outer wall, and contain four nuclei when mature.

Trophozoites may be seen in duodenojejunal fluid and in loose stools but generally are not found in formed stools [*see* Diagnosis, *below*]. Trophozoites are not resistant to external environmental stresses. In contrast, cysts are hardier and may survive in water for at least several months; decreased water temperature enhances their survival. Although infection can occur if trophozoites are ingested in quantities of food that are sufficient to buffer their transit through the stomach, the cyst stage is principally responsible for human infections. In studies, ingestion of as few as 10 cysts has resulted in human infection.

Infection derives from fecally excreted organisms and is spread by direct fecal-oral passage or by foodborne or waterborne transmission. Direct person-to-person transmission accounts for a heightened prevalence of giardiasis in several settings. In institutions where there is fecal incontinence and poor hygiene, giardiasis may be hyperendemic. Particularly in child day care centers, giardiasis can be a cause of intestinal disease.[48] The risk of acquisition and transmission is greatest for young children not yet toilet trained, who may be a source of additional secondary cases within their families.[48] Person-to-person transmission is also responsible for the prevalence of giardiasis among promiscuous male homosexuals. Sexual practices, including anilingus, can allow direct transfer of infectious cysts.

Waterborne transmission is a major source of giardiasis. Because filtration of water through soil removes *Giardia* cysts, deep well water is usually safe. In contrast, surface water, such as mountain streams and reservoirs, can harbor *Giardia* cysts, which are hardy in water and resistant to routine levels of chlorination. Coliform counts are not a reliable measure of giardial contamination. In addition, water-dwelling mammals, such as beavers, can become infected and then serve as continuing sources of water contamination. It may be difficult to recognize a water supply as the common source of giardiasis, because the resultant infection is often asymptomatic.

G. lamblia is widely distributed throughout the world. Travelers to many countries, including those in developed areas, may acquire giardiasis.

Pathogenesis

After *G. lamblia* cysts have been ingested and have passed through the stomach, they liberate trophozoites that proliferate by binary fission. Trophozoites, which localize in the duodenum and the proximal jejunum, may attach to the microvillus border of intestinal epithelial cells by means of their ventral adhesive suckers. They may also reside in the unstirred layer above the epithelium, move around in the luminal contents, or, uncommonly, invade the space between the epithelial cells. Functional changes in the absorptive capabilities of the small bowel may develop. The activities of epithelial brush-border enzymes are diminished, leading to deficiencies in disaccharidases, including lactase deficiency. Jejunal biopsies of patients with giardiasis usually reveal no pathologic findings.[49] The pathogenetic mechanisms of these functional alterations in the small bowel remain uncertain. Both types of alterations return to normal with specific antigiardial therapy—albeit slowly in some patients. Hypochlorhydria predisposes persons to infection. Giardiasis often occurs with greater severity in patients with cystic fibrosis and in those with immunoglobulin deficiencies, possibly because of deficiencies in secretory IgA.[50]

Diagnosis

Clinical features The clinical manifestations of giardiasis may be quite varied. A significant number of people with giardiasis are asymptomatic. Indeed, in one well-studied outbreak of waterborne giardiasis, two thirds of those infected were asymptomatic. In contrast, others with the infection experience typical acute giardiasis. After a 1- to 3-week incubation period, the acute onset of the illness is marked by watery diarrhea; abdominal cramping (and other, frequently epigastric, discomfort); nausea (less commonly, vomiting); and systemic symptoms. Fever may be present. Increased intestinal gas production leads to malodorous flatulence and sulfurous eructation. Impaired fat absorption and steatorrhea are common in symptomatic giardiasis. Stools are usually greasy and malodorous and float in water. Blood and mucus in stool are uncommon. These symptoms may be prominent for more than a week, diminishing in intensity over the ensuing weeks. Clinical findings that have helped identify cases of giardiasis in epidemiologic studies include a duration of illness lasting 7 or more days with at least two of the following six symptoms: diarrhea, flatulence, foul-smelling stools, nausea, abdominal cramps, and excessive fatigue.[51]

A chronic phase of giardiasis may follow the acute phase or may become manifest without an antecedent acute illness. This chronic phase is characterized by loose, but usually not diarrheic, stools that are soft and greasy. Increased abdominal gassiness with cramping, borborygmi, flatulence, and burping occurs. Fever is uncommon, but malaise, fatigue, and depression may ensue. Lactose intolerance can develop with the infection and augment intestinal symptoms after ingestion of milk products. The course can be remitting; asymptomatic periods may alternate with exacerbations of symptoms. For a small number of patients, particularly children, the persistence of infection is associated with moderate to marked malabsorption and weight loss.[52]

Uncommonly, *G. lamblia* has spread from the duodenum to the biliary and pancreatic ducts. Cases of cholecystitis, cholangitis, and granulomatous hepatitis have been reported. Impaired exocrine pancreatic function, manifested by diminished secretion of trypsin and lipase, has been noted.

Laboratory findings Leukocytosis and eosinophilia do not occur in giardiasis. Fecal fat excretion is increased (see above), and the results of other laboratory tests of malabsorption may also be abnormal. An upper GI series usually shows no significant radiologic changes.

Definitive diagnosis of giardiasis requires the morphologic identification of the cyst or trophozoite forms of the parasite. Fecal examinations are usually positive in acute giardiasis, and evaluation of three sequential daily fecal samples can detect more than 90% of infections. Cysts, which may be present in loose as well as formed stools, are hardy and do not necessitate prompt analysis of stools. In contrast, examinations to detect trophozoites should be performed on fresh stools or stools preserved in polyvinyl alcohol or merthiolate-iodine-formaldehyde (MIF). Substances that interfere with fecal microscopic evaluations, such as barium, antacids, and mineral oil, should be avoided before stool examinations. Immunologic assays detect giardial antigens in stool with greater sensitivity than a single stool examination.[53]

In chronic giardiasis, the frequency of detection of giardial forms on stool examination diminishes. If three or more stool examinations are unrevealing, the upper intestinal contents should be sampled by duodenojejunal aspiration. Alternatively, a biopsy of the small bowel can be performed. Recognition of trophozoites in biopsied material may require diligent searching of processed tissue; direct examination of mucosal imprint smears from a biopsy can increase detection.

Differential Diagnosis

Other infectious agents that cause gastroenteritis must be considered early in the course of acute giardiasis. Because most of these agents produce illness of short duration, the persistence of symptoms after a week and the prominence of symptoms of malabsorption (flatulence, lactose intolerance, burping) suggest a giardial etiology. Chronic giardiasis may resemble other diseases associated with malabsorption.

Treatment

Metronidazole, although not approved by the Food and Drug Administration for giardiasis, is the principal agent used to treat this infection[26] because quinacrine, the first effective drug for giardiasis, is no longer distributed in the United States. The usual dosage of metronidazole is 250 mg orally three times a day for 5 days, although in refractory cases, 750 mg orally three times a day for 10 days has been used. Side effects include nausea, headache, and a metallic taste in the mouth; less commonly, dark urine, paresthesias, and dizziness occur. Metronidazole may have a disulfiram-like effect, and alcohol consumption should be avoided when metronidazole is used. Although not available in the United States, tinidazole (given as a single 2 g oral dose) is highly effective.[54]

For children, furazolidone, available as a suspension, is effective and tolerated.[26] Treatment of giardiasis in pregnancy can be difficult. Metronidazole is often avoided, although studies have not documented teratogenic risks of metronidazole during pregnancy.[55] If symptoms of giardiasis are minimal, therapy can be withheld until delivery. If symptoms are bothersome, one approach is to administer a nonabsorbable aminoglycoside, paromomycin, 25 to 35 mg/kg/day orally in three divided doses for 7 days.[26] This regimen may provide at least symptomatic relief. If giardiasis in pregnancy is associated with dehydration, malabsorption, or severe symptoms, therapy with metronidazole is warranted. In any patient, resolution of malabsorptive symptoms may require months for regeneration of functioning intestinal mucosa after effective antiparasitic therapy.

Attention to hygiene is necessary to prevent person-to-person transmission of giardiasis. The risks and benefits of treating asymptomatic infected children in day care centers have not been fully defined; however, treatment of asymptomatic persons who pass cysts is indicated to prevent the spread of infection. Boiling water or heating it to at least 70°C (158° F) for 10 minutes renders water noninfectious. For hikers and campers, iodine-based water treatments are more effective than chlorine-based treatments; iodine disinfection must be carried out for at least 8 hours to be 99.9% effective. High-quality water-filtration units are effective for *Giardia* cyst removal.

AMEBIASIS

Infection with the ameba *E. histolytica* is responsible for human amebiasis. These infections may be limited primarily to the colon. Infections range in severity from asymptomatic to markedly dysenteric and may involve extraintestinal sites, of which the liver is the most common.

Etiology and Epidemiology

E. histolytica is distinguishable morphologically from the other nonpathogenic intestinal amebae, including *Escherichia coli* and *Entamoeba hartmanni*. *E. histolytica* exists in two forms: as a trophozoite and a cyst. The trophozoite, which usually measures 10 to 20 μm in diameter but may be larger in dysenteric stools, is motile and possesses a single nucleus and a granular cytoplasm. Trophozoites are passed in loose stool, but this form is not hardy and does not survive outside the body. In contrast, the cyst stage, which arises within the colon from the trophozoite, can survive environmental stresses as well as passage through the acid of the stomach. Cysts measure 10 to 20 μm in diameter and contain one to four nuclei, which have small, centric karyosomes and a pattern of fine peripheral chromatin.

It has long been recognized that not all strains of *E. histolytica* are pathogenic. Nonpathogenic strains can be isolated from asymptomatic patients and have been prevalent among promiscuous male homosexuals in the United States and England. Pathogenic and nonpathogenic strains cannot be distinguished by microscopy, except that pathogenic trophozoites often phagocytose erythrocytes. On the basis of biochemical, immunologic, and genetic data, *E. histolytica* has been redescribed. A new species, *E. dispar*, now represents the nonpathogenic isolates and is apparently never invasive in humans, whereas *E. histolytica* includes only the potentially pathogenic strains.[56] Because not all potentially pathogenic *E. histolytica* strains invariably produce disease, other processes undoubtedly influence amebic virulence.

An immunoassay to distinguish *E. histolytica* from *E. dispar* has been developed.[57] There is currently no other method available for the common diagnostic laboratory to readily distinguish one organism from the other [*see* Diagnosis, *below*].

Cysts passed in human feces are primarily responsible for human infections. Acquisition of infection represents fecal-oral contamination and may occur by waterborne or foodborne transmission as well as by person-to-person transmission. The latter accounts for the heightened prevalence of *E. histolytica* infection among promiscuous male homosexuals and in institutions where there is fecal incontinence and poor hygiene. Amebiasis is more common in lower socioeconomic groups than in the general population because of poor sanitation and overcrowding. In the United States, cases are seen in persons who have returned from international travel or have immigrated from areas where amebiasis is endemic.

Pathogenesis

Ingested cysts are carried into the intestine, where they excyst to liberate trophozoites that proliferate by binary fission within the colon. Trophozoites are cytolytic and may invade the bowel wall to produce local necrosis. The resultant ulcers are flask shaped, with a narrow neck through the mucosa and a broader submucosal base. Unless colonic involvement is extensive, intervening areas of bowel are normal. The areas most frequently affected are the cecum and the ascending colon, followed in frequency by the rectosigmoid, the appendix, the descending and transverse colon, and the terminal ileum.

The severity of colonic involvement in patients with amebiasis is quite varied and may range from mild or negligible disease to diffuse and extensive tissue invasion and necrosis. Most persons who harbor *E. histolytica* experience no significant colonic invasion. The determinants of severity are not well understood but may include the inoculum size of *E. histolytica,* the coexistent colonic microbial flora, and the nutritional and physiologic state of the host. Corticosteroid use and pregnancy both diminish host resistance. Complications of colonic involvement include hemorrhage and peritonitis, the latter developing more commonly from transmural leakage across involved colonic tissue than from frank perforation. With chronicity, a granulomatous tissue response can develop at a site of infection (most commonly in the cecum) and can produce a mass lesion termed an ameboma. Colonic strictures may also develop.

Amebiasis may spread hematogenously from the bowel to involve any organ in the body. The liver is most commonly affected, followed in frequency by the lungs, which are principally affected as a result of transdiaphragmatic spread from the liver. Trophozoites carried via the portal venous system produce necrosis in the liver and cause abscess formation. About 90% of abscesses are in the right lobe, especially in the superior and anterior aspects. Although multiple abscesses can occur, a solitary abscess ranging in size from a few centimeters to 20 cm in diameter is more common. Amebic liver abscesses are seven to nine times more common in males than in females. Uncommonly, an abscess may develop concomitantly with amebic colitis. Depending on the reported series, 50% to 70% of patients with amebic-hepatic abscesses have no history of amebic colitis. Rupture of a right lobe abscess may result in extension into the chest, producing an amebic empyema, pneumonia, or a bronchopleural fistula. Extension into the peritoneal cavity is less common. Rupture from a left lobe abscess can extend into the pericardium, frequently with fatal consequences.

Diagnosis

Clinical features Most persons with colonic amebiasis experience no symptoms. Fecal cyst excretion in these asymptomatic individuals is detected only by serendipity. In persons who do experience symptoms, the illness may range from mild diarrhea to fulminant dysentery. The former presentation is common, and most patients are able to continue daily activities as they experience mild diarrhea that may alternate with constipation. The course of illness can be remitting, with subsequent symptomatic relapses. Abdominal discomfort, tenesmus, dull sacral pain, and flatulence are common, but systemic symptoms and fever are less prominent than what is common with bacterial colitis. Blood and mucus are frequently noted in stools. Abdominal findings reflect the severity of the colonic involvement. Tenderness may be absent or mild over the involved areas. In some cases, however, prominent abdominal tenderness, together with high fever and systemic toxicity, is a consequence of extensive colonic disease.[58] Amebomas may be palpable as tender abdominal masses.

In patients with amebic liver abscess, presenting symptoms usually include malaise, fatigue, anorexia, abdominal pain, fever, and weight loss; the duration is usually 1 week to several weeks and less commonly many months. The abdominal pain is usually dull and aching and localized over the right upper quadrant or right chest. At times, there is referred pain to the right shoulder. A presentation with pleuritic chest pain, cough, and dyspnea may mistakenly suggest an intrapulmonary infection. An abscess in the left lobe may produce midepigastric or left upper quadrant pain. On examination, hepatomegaly and hepatic punch tenderness or focal tenderness over the abscess are frequent. Frank jaundice is rare. On chest examination, dullness at the right base as a result of diaphragmatic elevation and pleural effusion formation can be appreciable. Rales may be heard.

Cutaneous amebiasis, resulting in ulcerative or fungating lesions, most commonly develops on the perineum and genitalia. Lesions arise from invasion by trophozoites derived from fecal contamination or sexual transmission. The lesions can be distinguished from neoplastic, tuberculous, and syphilitic processes by the presence of trophozoites in exudate or biopsied tissue.

Laboratory findings In symptomatic amebic colitis, a mild to moderate leukocytosis may develop. Mild anemia and mild elevations of liver enzyme levels (which are not usually indicative of incipient abscess formation) may occur. Feces usually will contain frank or occult blood and eosinophil-derived Charcot-Leyden crystals.

Leukocytosis, anemia, and an elevated erythrocyte sedimentation rate are common with an amebic liver abscess. In more than two thirds of patients, alkaline phosphatase levels are one to four times higher than normal. Elevated aminotransferase levels occur in fewer than 50% of patients. Bilirubin levels may be elevated, but usually to no more than 2.5 mg/dl. Chest x-ray often shows elevation of the right diaphragm and may reveal a pleural effusion. An isotopic liver scan will reveal a space-occupying lesion; an ultrasound scan will show a round to ovoid hypoechoic lesion and can detect transdiaphragmatic pleural involvement. CT or MRI also can document the abscess and any local extension.

For intestinal amebiasis, definitive diagnosis requires morphologic identification of the cysts or trophozoites of *E. histolytica*. Unformed stool should be examined immediately for motile trophozoites. Formed stools may be examined directly or after application of concentration techniques for cysts. Stools may also be preserved in polyvinyl alcohol or MIF for subsequent examination. Fecal leukocytes and nonpathogenic amebae are easily confused with *E. histolytica*, and thus, definitive speciation should be performed on stained samples by experienced personnel. Antimicrobial agents, cathartics, antacids, and barium interfere with microscopic detection. Because the excretion rate of cysts varies daily, three or more stool samples from different days should be examined. About half of patients with symptomatic amebic colitis have rectosigmoid involvement; thus, aspirates, scrapings, or biopsies of mucosal lesions obtained at sigmoidoscopy can be examined for trophozoites. A fecal antigen detection test for *E. histolytica* has been introduced that is based on a monoclonal antibody to a specific lectin on this organism.[57]

Serologic tests for amebiasis are infrequently positive in asymptomatic cyst passers, but rates of seropositivity rise with increasing extent and duration of amebic colonic involvement. Such tests can be an adjunct to the diagnosis of acute amebic disease and can be especially helpful in the etiologic assessment of chronic colitis. Serologic tests, performed by a variety of methods, may remain positive for months to years after infection; this fact should be considered when interpreting a positive test result.

Serologic tests are positive in 90% to 95% of patients with extraintestinal amebiasis; titers increase with the duration of the disease. A positive titer, together with compatible clinical findings and tests demonstrating a cystic hepatic lesion, allows for the diagnosis of amebic hepatic abscess. Results of stool examinations, either negative or positive, are not etiologically pertinent in such cases. Trophozoites are rarely demonstrable in aspirated abscess fluid, which usually has an anchovy-sauce or chocolate-brown appearance.

Differential Diagnosis

In cases of mild intestinal amebiasis, the diagnosis of irritable bowel syndrome, diverticulitis, or regional enteritis may be suggested by the duration and symptoms of the infection. For more severe intestinal amebiasis with an acute presentation, infections with *Shigella, Salmonella, E. coli* O157, and *Campylobacter* can be distinguished by positive stool cultures and by the presence of large numbers of fecal leukocytes not found in amebic colitis. Ulcerative colitis and Crohn's disease are to be considered in the differential diagnosis for chronic amebic colitis. Lesions on sigmoidoscopy and barium enema findings may be identical in amebic colitis and ulcerative colitis. It is critical to distinguish between these two conditions because corticosteroid therapy, which may be indicated for ulcerative colitis, would aggravate amebic colitis; therefore, amebic serologic tests and examinations of feces and mucosal lesions for amebae are of cardinal importance. A therapeutic trial of metronidazole cannot be relied on to identify the etiology, because metronidazole may have a salutary effect on inflammatory bowel disease as well as on amebic colitis.

An ameboma may simulate an adenocarcinoma or another granulomatous process. A positive amebic serology and resolution of the mass with metronidazole therapy support the diagnosis of an ameboma. If resolution is not complete, a biopsy is indicated to exclude a coincidental lesion of nonamebic cause.

The differential diagnosis of amebic hepatic abscess is guided by two observations: (1) an isotopic liver scan that shows a space-occupying lesion and (2) an ultrasound, CT, or MRI scan that shows a cystic lesion. Although hepatic cysts and echinococcal cysts are usually not associated with fever and the other symptoms of an amebic lesion, they should be considered in the differential diagnosis. Pyogenic abscesses should be considered as well. A positive amebic serology supports an amebic etiology. In contrast to echinococcal cysts, amebic abscesses calcify very rarely. An amebic abscess and a pyogenic abscess may respond alike to metronidazole therapy. Amebic abscesses are uncommonly infected secondarily. If uncertainty persists about the bacterial or amebic etiology of an abscess, diagnostic aspiration of abscess fluid for bacterial cultures and Gram stain may be necessary.

Treatment

For symptomatic intestinal disease or extraintestinal disease, metronidazole (750 mg p.o., t.i.d., for 10 days) is usually highly effective and is the preferred therapy.[26] Information about the side effects of metronidazole and precautions about its use have been presented in the discussion of giardiasis. Occasional failures in the treatment of hepatic abscesses with metronidazole have been noted. Because relapses of intestinal disease may occur infrequently in the absence of reinfection, follow-up is indicated for a number of months.

Chemotherapy may be unnecessary for many asymptomatic cyst passers because they often harbor nonpathogenic *E. dispar*. If speciation of *Entamoeba* is not available, asymptomatic cyst passers should be treated if they handle food or if they are receiving corticosteroids; they should also be treated in the setting of an amebiasis outbreak.[56] In asymptomatic patients, concentrations of metronidazole in the colonic lumen may be inadequate to eradicate amebae, and one of two luminal amebicides should be used.[26] Paromomycin (25 to 35 mg/kg/day for 7 days) can be used. An alternative is iodoquinol (650 mg p.o., t.i.d., for 20 days); it is important not to exceed this dosage because of the potential for causing optic neuritis. Iodoquinol is contraindicated for patients with optic neuropathy or thyroid disease. The administration of a course of iodoquinol is recommended for patients treated for symptomatic intestinal or extraintestinal amebiasis.[26]

Therapeutic aspiration is usually not necessary for amebic hepatic abscess, although diagnostic aspiration may be useful in certain cases [*see* Differential Diagnosis, *above*]. Drainage, which can be achieved by percutaneous aspiration, is indicated for those lesions that fail to respond to initial medical therapy or that are in imminent danger of rupturing.

Prevention of amebiasis relies on personal hygiene to prevent person-to-person transmission. In areas where amebiasis is endemic, the provision and use of adequate toilet facilities can decrease the spread of disease. Avoidance of vegetables that grow in the ground is advisable because of potential contamination by human feces. Water can be rendered safe by boiling or by use of iodine-based water-treatment tablets.

COCCIDIOSIS

Coccidia, which are found in the intestines of many domestic and wild animals, are unicellular parasites that reproduce by asexual and sexual cycles in gut epithelium. Three coccidial organisms, *Isospora belli, Cryptosporidium*, and *Cyclospora cayetanensis*, have documented pathogenicity as enteric parasites for humans. Contact with infected cattle may result in infection with *Cryptosporidium*, and contaminated water sources transmit *I. belli, Cryptosporidium*, and *C. cayetanensis*.[59] All three coccidial parasites have been identified as opportunistic pathogens in patients infected with HIV.[60]

Isosporiasis

Diagnosis Infections with *I. belli* usually begin abruptly. Fever and malaise appear first, followed by abdominal pain, diarrhea, and weight loss. In most cases, the illness is self-limited, although chronic infections have lasted several weeks to several months. Severe diarrhea, steatorrhea, and hepatic involvement may ensue; in rare instances, severe disease results in death. In patients with AIDS, infection with *I. belli* causes a clinical picture of chronic watery diarrhea and weight loss that is indistinguishable from that produced by *Cryptosporidium*.

Histologic examination of mucosal lesions in patients who have isosporiasis shows shortened villi, crypt hypertrophy, and infiltration with eosinophils, neutrophils, lymphocytes, and plasma cells. Blood eosinophilia, which is not seen with other protozoan infections, may develop with *I. belli* infections. The presence of oocysts in the stool establishes the diagnosis. Although routine stool examinations may fail to detect oocysts, they can be demonstrated with acid-fast staining. If oocysts in the feces are few, incubation of stool at room temperature for 24 to 48 hours can encourage oocyst maturation and the zinc sulfate concentration technique can be used before examining the stool. Parasite forms may also be detected in biopsied intestinal tissue and in intestinal contents.

Treatment *I. belli* infections are treated with double-strength trimethoprim-sulfamethoxazole (160 mg of trimethoprim and 800 mg of sulfamethoxazole) given orally four times a day for 10 days and then twice a day for 3 weeks.[26] Because recurrences of infection are likely in patients who have AIDS, the initial 10-day course of trimethoprim-sulfamethoxazole should be followed by long-term maintenance therapy with either one double-strength tablet of trimethoprim-sulfamethoxazole three times a week or the combination of 25 mg of pyrimethamine and 500 mg of sulfadoxine once a week in those patients. In patients who are intolerant of sulfa drugs, pyrimethamine therapy (75 mg/day) has been successful; a maintenance dosage of 50 to 75 mg/day of pyrimethamine has prevented relapses of *I. belli* infections.[60]

Cryptosporidiosis

Cryptosporidium inhabits the brush border of the small intestine mucosa and can cause enterocolitis in both normal and immunocompromised hosts. Infection may be acquired by ingestion of fewer than 100 oocysts.[61] A common means of transmission is by water, including municipal drinking water supplies[62] and recreational water (pools and water slides).[47,63] Cryptosporidiosis has caused outbreaks of diarrheal disease in day care centers and may be acquired by international travelers. Because fecal oocysts are infectious, nosocomial and household spread of infection can occur.

Diagnosis In normal hosts, illness begins after a mean incubation period of about a week. It consists of watery, nonbloody diarrhea that is accompanied at times by such clinical manifestations as abdominal pain, nausea, fever, anorexia, and weight loss. Symptoms may persist for 1 to 2 weeks and are usually self-limited without therapy. By contrast, in immunocompromised patients, cryptosporidiosis can be persistent and severe. In HIV-infected patients with $CD4^+$ T cell levels greater than $180/mm^3$, cryptosporidiosis can be self-limited. However, in those individuals who are more profoundly immunocompromised, the secretory diarrhea, which is chronic and profuse, is usually unremitting. In these persons, *Cryptosporidium* organisms may also cause hepatobiliary disease, including cholecystitis, cholangitis, and papillary stenosis.

Cryptosporidium oocysts can be detected in fecal smears examined microscopically, either as an iodine wet mount or after staining with a monoclonal antibody or the modified Kinyoun acid-fast reagent [*see Figure 2a and 2b*]. In addition, direct fluorescent stains and immunoassays of fecal samples can enhance diagnostic yields of *Cryptosporidium*.

Treatment In immunocompetent patients, cryptosporidiosis is a self-limited illness and usually requires only supportive therapy. However, in immunocompromised patients, effective chemotherapy for cryptosporidiosis has not been established.[26] If immunosuppressive drugs have been administered, cessation of these agents may lead to resolution of the diarrhea. For some HIV-infected patients, paromomycin may be at least partially beneficial in treating cryptosporidiosis.[26]

Cyclosporiasis

Cyclospora appears to be widely distributed geographically; illness attributable to this protozoan has been described in the United States, Latin America, Africa, Europe, and Asia.[64] Epidemiologic studies indicate that contaminated water,[59] as well as imported raspberries,[65] have been sources of infection. Further study may delineate other modes of transmission. The incubation period is about 1 week.[66]

a

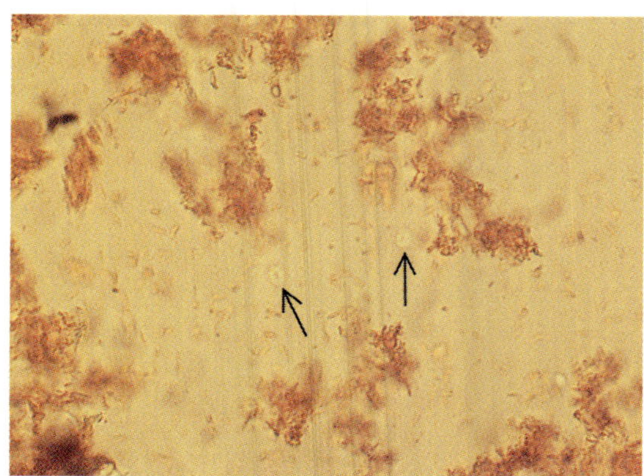

b

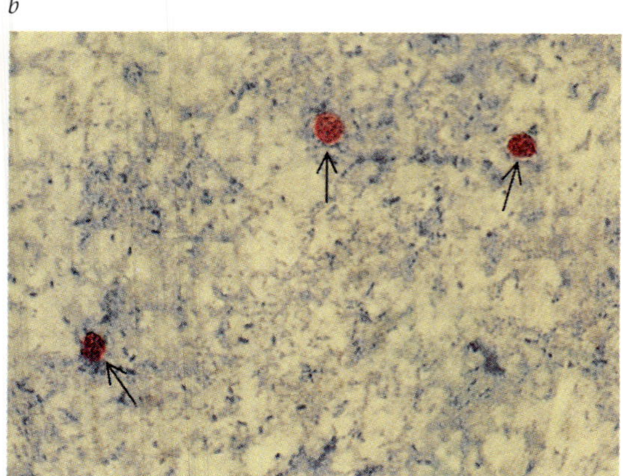

Figure 2 **(*a*) Oocysts of *Cryptosporidium* species appear in an iodine wet mount of feces as clear, unstained structures (arrows), whereas yeast and debris stain brown. (*b*) Modified Kinyoun acid-fast staining of fecal smears stains the oocysts red. Oocysts measure about 5 to 6 μm in diameter.**

Diagnosis Many patients infected with the organism have experienced diarrhea, flulike symptoms, and symptoms common to other small bowel pathogens, including flatulence and burping. The illness may be confined to a single, self-limited episode or may wax and wane, but prolonged diarrhea, anorexia, and upper GI symptoms often occur. Prolonged fatigue and weight loss are also frequent symptoms.

Small bowel biopsies can detect the parasite in epithelial cells and can detect jejunal inflammation, which is associated with increased numbers of intraepithelial lymphocytes and increased degrees of villus atrophy and crypt hyperplasia. Fecal leukocytes and blood are absent, suggesting that disease is attributable to a noninvasive mechanism. The diagnosis can be made by detection of oocysts in the stool, which, like *Cryptosporidium* oocysts, are apparent in acid-fast stains. Although *Cyclospora* oocysts, which measure 8 to 10 μm in diameter, are larger than *Cryptosporidium* oocysts, caution is needed so that diagnostic testing does not confuse the two distinct protozoan organisms. Fluorescence microscopy is a rapid and sensitive means to detect autofluorescent oocysts.[67] *Cyclospora* oocysts have been found in patients infected with HIV.[60]

Treatment Trimethoprim-sulfamethoxazole (160 mg of trimethoprim and 800 mg of sulfamethoxazole) tablets twice daily for 7 days has proved to be effective therapy for cyclosporiasis.[26] HIV-infected patients, however, may require a higher dosage (four times a day for 7 days) and may need long-term maintenance treatment (three times a week). Like cryptosporidiosis, *Cyclospora* infection must be considered in any patient with prolonged diarrhea, anorexia, and upper GI symptoms.

DIENTAMOEBA FRAGILIS INFECTION

Unlike other amebae, the large intestine parasite *D. fragilis* has only a trophozoite stage and no cyst stage. Because the trophozoite is not resistant to gastric acid, it is not clear how humans acquire infection. The eggs of the pinworm *Enterobius vermicularis* might transmit *D. fragilis* trophozoites because the two infections frequently coincide. *D. fragilis* can cause an illness characterized by abdominal pain, anorexia, and loose stools. As with *Isospora* infections, but not other protozoan infections, eosinophilia may accompany infection with *D. fragilis.*[68] The trophozoite stage is not hardy and is difficult to detect; to ensure detection, stool samples must be preserved in polyvinyl alcohol fixative, sodium acetate–acetic acid–formalin fixative, or Schaudinn's fluid and must be examined after permanent staining. *D. fragilis* infection can be treated with tetracycline (500 mg q.i.d. for 10 days), paromomycin (25 to 30 mg/kg/day in three doses for 7 days), or iodoquinol (650 mg t.i.d. for 20 days).[26]

BLASTOCYSTIS HOMINIS INFECTION

Although *B. hominis* was previously considered to be a nonpathogenic yeast, some investigators now consider this organism to be a protozoan capable of causing intestinal illness. Support for the belief that this organism may be pathogenic stems from the finding of large numbers of *B. hominis* organisms in the feces of patients with diarrhea for which no other cause has been identified. Other investigators, however, have failed to confirm this finding.[69] They have found no concordance between numbers of fecal organisms and extent of the diarrhea and no resolution of symptoms after therapy for *Blastocystis* infection. Until the issue of the pathogenicity of *B. hominis* is settled, patients with a diarrheal illness who are excreting this organism in their feces should be studied for other parasitic, bacterial, or viral infections. If diarrheal symptoms are sufficient to warrant therapy, iodoquinol, 650 mg three times a day for 20 days, or metronidazole, 750 mg three times a day for 10 days, can be used.[26]

MICROSPORIDIOSIS

Microsporidia, which are obligate intracellular, spore-forming organisms, belong to a distinct phylum of protozoans that includes many genera capable of infecting diverse vertebrate and invertebrate hosts. Human microsporidial infections have been recognized in recent years, and to date, six genera of microsporidia—*Enterocytozoon, Encephalitozoon* (including *Septata*), *Vittaforma, Trachipleistophora, Pleistophora,* and *Nosema*—have been identified as causes of human disease, especially in persons infected with HIV.[70] These microsporidia are differentiated by their size, nuclear morphology, and mode of division as well as by the intracellular site of proliferation (microsporidia multiply either freely in the cytoplasm or within membrane-bound vacuoles). Despite the ubiquity of microsporidia in other host species, how humans become infected is not known. Because almost all microsporidial infections in humans have been identified in immunocompromised hosts, it is not clear how frequently immunocompetent hosts are infected or whether infections that develop in immunocompetent hosts are symptomatic or self-limited.

The spectrum of disease attributable to microsporidia is broad, with the disease state apparently depending on the infecting species and the immune status of the host. The most commonly recognized microsporidial infections are *Enterocytozoon bieneusi* infections in HIV-infected patients. Among patients infected with HIV, intestinal *E. bieneusi* and *Encephalitozoon intestinalis* (formerly *Septata intestinalis)* infections are causes of chronic diarrhea.[71,72] In such patients, *E. bieneusi* and *E. intestinalis* may infect the biliary tract, causing cholangitis. *Encephalitozoon* species have caused keratoconjunctivitis marked by a coarse punctate epithelial keratopathy in HIV-infected patients, whereas *Vittaforma* and *Nosema* species have caused stromal keratitis in a few HIV-seronegative patients. *Encephalitozoon* microsporidia have also been associated with peritonitis and hepatitis, as well as nasal and sinus infections and infections in other diverse sites in HIV-infected patients. *Trachipleistophora* and *Pleistophora* species have caused myositis.

The small size of microsporidia, which are gram-positive organisms with mature spores that measure 0.5 to 2 μm by 1 to 4 μm, hinders detection of the parasite. Many microsporidial infections have required electron microscopic tissue evaluation for diagnosis. Intracellular spores can also be recognized by light microscopy if tissues are stained with hematoxylin-eosin, Giemsa, or Gram stain. Intestinal microsporidia appear to be spottily distributed and may not be detected on examination of biopsied tissues. Chromotrope-based and fluorochrome Uritex 2B staining methods facilitate detection of microsporidial spores in smears of either feces or duodenal aspirates.

For intestinal infections with *E. intestinalis,* oral albendazole has been beneficial and curative; *E. bieneusi* infections are less responsive, although patients may experience symptomatic improvement without eradication of the infection.[71,72] For keratoconjunctivitis caused by *Encephalitozoon hellem,* topical therapy with fumagillin suspension has been beneficial.[26]

Infections Due to Free-Living Amebae

Although amebae such as *E. histolytica* cannot survive and replicate outside of animal hosts, most amebae are free-living in soil or water. Amebae of the genera *Naegleria* and *Acanthamoeba* can cause acute meningitis, acute meningoencephalitis, and chronic granulomatous meningoencephalitis.[73]

Acanthamoeba species have also been increasingly recognized as a cause of keratitis[74] and, in a small number of HIV-infectedpatients, of disseminated disease with cutaneous manifestations.[75] *Acanthamoeba* organisms have been isolated from water, airborne dust, hot tubs, and saline solutions used to clean contact lenses. Factors associated with the development of amebic keratitis include the lack of effective disinfection of contact lenses, a history of minor corneal trauma, and exposure to soil or standing water. The lesions, which are usually chronic and severely painful, consist of variable anterior uveitis, epithelial erosion, scleritis, and an infiltrative stromal keratitis that is often ring shaped. Lesions are refractory to the usual antimicrobial medications and must be distinguished from keratitis caused by herpes simplex virus [see 29 Herpesvirus Infections]. The diagnosis can be made by microscopic examination of Giemsa- or trichrome-stained corneal scrapings and by the use of indirect immunofluorescent antibody staining of corneal scrapings. The amebae can be cultured by inoculating corneal tissue into nonnutrient agar seeded with *E. coli.* Acanthamebic keratitis has been treated with topical regimens using one or more agents, including polyhexamethylene biguanide, propamidine isethionate, and clotrimazole.[74]

Leishmaniasis

Leishmania protozoans, obligate intracellular parasites in humans, produce a wide spectrum of disease ranging from generalized visceral involvement to diffuse or circumscribed cutaneous or mucocutaneous lesions. Four species complexes of *Leishmania* may infect humans: *L. donovani, L. tropica, L. mexicana,* and *L. braziliensis*. The resulting patterns of illness arise from the tissue tropism of the leishmanial species and the host's immune response, principally the cell-mediated component of immunity.

VISCERAL LEISHMANIASIS

Etiology and Epidemiology

The *L. donovani* species complex includes several species (e.g., *L. infantum* and *L. chagasi*). These species cause visceral leishmaniasis, or kala-azar, which is endemic in areas of India, China, Central and South America, East and West Africa, and the countries surrounding the Mediterranean. Sandflies of the genus *Phlebotomus* are the insect vectors that spread *L. donovani*; the species vary in the different areas. In India, no extrahuman reservoirs are known, but in other regions, several mammals, including dogs, foxes, and wild rodents, may be infected.

Pathogenesis

The flagellated promastigotes of *L. donovani* are introduced by an insect bite. After entering macrophages of the reticuloendothelial system, these forms change into amastigotes, which multiply in phagocytic cells. Released amastigotes disseminate hematogenously and invade reticuloendothelial cells in the spleen, liver, lymph nodes, bone marrow, and skin.

Diagnosis

Clinical features Symptoms usually have a gradual onset several months after infection and include weakness, dizziness, weight loss, diarrhea, and constipation. Fever, which almost always develops, may spike twice daily and is sometimes accompanied by chills and sweating. As the disease progresses, the liver and spleen enlarge, the latter often expanding into the iliac fossa. When bone marrow macrophages are parasitized, anemia and leukopenia ensue. The thrombocytopenic patient may bleed from the gingivae, nose, or GI tract, and ecchymoses and petechiae may appear on the skin. Death can result from secondary bacterial infections, severe anemia, or uncontrolled bleeding. Latent infection can become manifest and progressive during immunosuppression, and visceral leishmaniasis can develop as an opportunistic infection in HIV-infected patients. In these patients, leishmanial parasites may localize in unusual sites, including the larynx and throughout the GI tract.

Laboratory findings Anemia, leukopenia, thrombocytopenia, hyperglobulinemia, and hypoalbuminemia suggest visceral leishmaniasis when they are observed in a patient with fever, hepatosplenomegaly, and a history of exposure in endemic areas. Definitive diagnosis requires demonstration of the organism in host tissues cultured on a Novy-MacNeal-Nicolle (NNN) or other medium or detection of Leishman-Donovan bodies (amastigotes) in stained tissue samples. In most cases, the diagnosis can be established by examining bone marrow aspirates. Splenic aspirates have the highest yields but may be risky. Liver biopsy or aspiration of enlarged lymph nodes can also provide diagnostic material.

Treatment

Sodium stibogluconate (pentavalent antimony) is the therapy of choice for treating most cases of leishmaniasis and is available as Pentostam through the CDC Drug Service (404-639-3670, days; 404-639-2888, nights and weekends) [*see Sidebar,* Protozoan Infection Information on the Internet].[26] When initial treatment of kala-azar with sodium stibogluconate fails, amphotericin B or pentamidine may be used.[26] Kala-azar resistant to sodium stibogluconate may also respond to liposomal amphotericin B.[76]

CUTANEOUS AND MUCOCUTANEOUS LEISHMANIASIS

Etiology and Epidemiology

Old World cutaneous leishmaniasis is caused by three species of *Leishmania* that belong to the *L. tropica* complex: *L. tropica* is present in the Middle East and the Mediterranean littoral; *L. major* is

Protozoan Infection Information on the Internet

Centers for Disease Control and Prevention

CDC Division of Parasitic Diseases

http://www.cdc.gov/ncidod/dod/dpd/dpd.htm

Information on parasitic diseases, including DPDx, an online interactive diagnostic service (**http://www.dpd.cdc.gov/dpdx**)

CDC Drug Service

http://www.cdc.gov/ncidod/srp/drugservice

Information on special immunobiologic agents and drugs distributed through the CDC Drug Service, Scientific Resources Program, and the Division of Quarantine of the National Center for Infectious Diseases

Emerging Infectious Diseases

http://www.cdc.gov/ncidod/eid

The online edition of the peer-reviewed journal published by the CDC's National Center for Infectious Diseases (http://www.cdc.gov/ncidod)

World Health Organization

Division of Control of Tropical Diseases

http://www.who.int/ctd

Scientific publications and other information from WHO's lead program for the control of tropical diseases

Special Programme for Research and Training in Tropical Diseases

http://www/who.int/tdr

Publications, research guidelines, grant applications, and other information from a scientific collaboration of the United Nations Development Program, the World Bank, and WHO

found in the Middle East, Arabia, the former Soviet Union, India, and sub-Saharan Africa; and *L. aethiopica* is found principally in Ethiopia and Kenya. *Phlebotomus* sandflies are the principal vectors, although direct contact with an ill person may also result in infection. Infections that are caused by *Leishmania* can be acquired by travelers as well as by military and other personnel residing in endemic areas. Military personnel in the Middle East have acquired cutaneous leishmaniasis with *L. major* as well as viscerotropic infections with *L. tropica*.

New World cutaneous leishmaniasis arises from infection with parasites belonging to the *L. mexicana* group or the *L. viannia* group. The patterns of illness vary with the nature of the infecting leishmanial organisms, which are found in different regions of North, Central, and South America [*see Table 2*]. In areas of Central and South America, infection with organisms of the *L. mexicana* group produces cutaneous leishmaniasis. A few autochthonous cases have been found in Texas. Infections with strains of *L. viannia*, which are endemic in various areas of South America, cause cutaneous leishmaniasis and may result in the later development of mucocutaneous leishmaniasis. Such mucocutaneous disease (espundia) involves the nasal or oropharyngeal mucosa, or both, and may prove fatal. All of these New World leishmanial parasites are transmitted principally by sandfly vectors,

Table 2 New World Cutaneous Leishmaniasis[80]

Parasite	*Disease in Humans*	*Geographic Areas*
Leishmania viannia group		
L. viannia braziliensis	Usually a single or few lesions but frequently very large, persistent, and disfiguring; nasopharyngeal involvement (espundia) common	Brazil, Peru, Ecuador, Bolivia, Venezuela, Paraguay, Colombia, northern Argentina, Guatemala
L. viannia guyanensis	Pian bois (bush yaws); multiple skin lesions, frequently with metastatic spread along lymphatics	Guyana, Suriname, French Guyana, northern Brazil
L. viannia panamensis	Usually a single lesion but occasional spread via lymphatics; nasopharyngeal involvement rare	Panama; possibly Costa Rica and Colombia
L. viannia peruviana	Uta; a single or few self-healing skin lesions; no nasopharyngeal involvement	Western slopes of the Peruvian Andes, the Argentinian highlands
L. mexicana group		
L. mexicana mexicana	Frequent involvement of ear pinna (chiclero's ear, bay sore); a single or few skin lesions; no nasopharyngeal lesions; diffuse cutaneous leishmaniasis rare	Mexico, Central America, southern United States
L. mexicana amazonensis	Rare human infection; a single or few skin lesions; diffuse cutaneous leishmaniasis	Amazon basin and neighboring areas, Brazil, Trinidad, Venezuela, Panama
L. mexicana pifanoi	Simple and diffuse cutaneous leishmaniasis	Venezuela
L. mexicana venezuelensis	Simple cutaneous leishmaniasis	Venezuelan Andes
L. mexicana species	Simple and diffuse cutaneous leishmaniasis	Dominican Republic

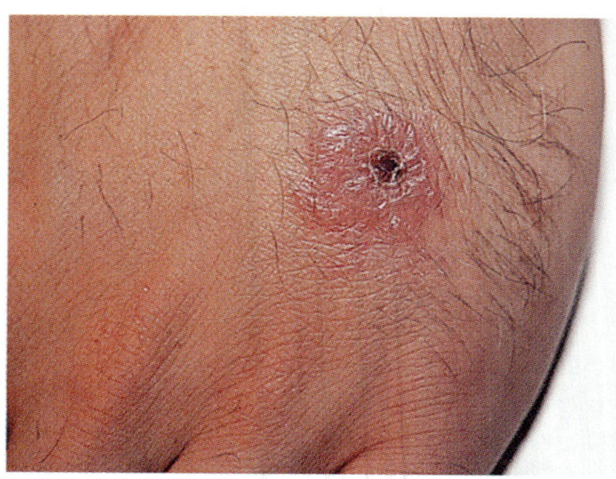

Figure 3 **A single, localized lesion of Old World cutaneous leishmaniasis that was acquired in East Africa can be seen on this patient's hand.**

although direct human contact may also bring about infection. Various mammals are naturally infected reservoirs of the organisms.

Pathogenesis

Both Old World and New World forms of leishmaniasis are initiated when the bite of an infected sandfly injects promastigotes into the human host. The organisms enter tissue macrophages and capillary endothelial cells, become amastigotes, and multiply. A granulomatous inflammatory response develops at the bite site. With local ischemia, the lesion ulcerates; bacterial infection of the necrotic area extends the ulceration.

In Old World cutaneous leishmaniasis, after an incubation period of weeks to months, a papule develops at the inoculation site. This area may resolve spontaneously. More frequently, it ulcerates and a shallow circular lesion appears that is several centimeters in diameter and has a raised margin [*see Figure 3*]. Bacterial superinfection may lead to regional lymphadenopathy. The lesions are often solitary, but multiple bites can produce several concurrent lesions. Healing of the lesions is slow, sometimes requiring more than a year.

Diagnosis

Clinical features *L. mexicana* infections either produce a single lesion or produce a few lesions on exposed surfaces of the body such as the face and ear.[77] The ulcer usually heals spontaneously over 6 months. An ulcer involving the ear, however, may cause extensive destruction of the pinna. *L. viannia* infection is associated with lesions on the skin or mucous membranes, which may be multiple and may become very large, especially when accompanied by bacterial superinfection. Cutaneous lesions caused by *L. braziliensis* are much less likely to heal spontaneously than those caused by *L. mexicana*.[77] The lesions sometimes spread up the lymphatic vessels of the arms or legs or extend locally and involve mucous membranes. Often, the infection metastasizes to the nasal or oral mucosa after an intervening period of months to years. Metastatic lesions can erode the nasal septum or the hard palate or soft palate. Some patients die of malnutrition or bacterial infection.

Diffuse cutaneous leishmaniasis occurs in parts of Ethiopia, Venezuela, Brazil, and the Dominican Republic. The initial nodule does not ulcerate; instead, multiple nodules evolve on the body. Leishmanial organisms abound in the lesions. Patients with this form of leishmaniasis have a deficiency of cell-mediated immunity, which is similar to the defective immunity that occurs in patients with lepromatous leprosy.

Laboratory findings Definitive diagnosis is made by demonstrating amastigotes on stained smears [*see Figure 4*] of a biopsy or of scrapings from the border of an ulcer. Alternatively, the diagnosis can be made by culturing amastigotes on NNN medium inoculated with lesion material. Use of DNA probes based on parasite kinetoplast DNA has allowed detection of organisms that might be missed on histologic section or culturing. Moreover, this technique serves as a rapid method for speciating *L. mexicana* and *L. viannia*. In contrast to *L. tropica* and *L. mexicana* amastigotes, which can be readily cultured and are abundant in lesions, *L. viannia* amastigotes are difficult to culture and are sparse in

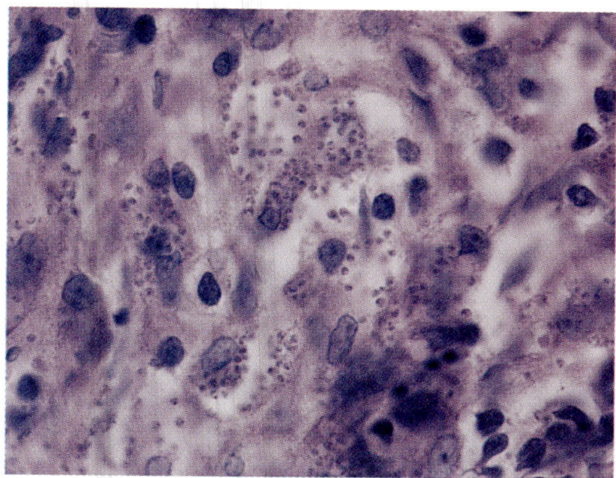

Figure 4 **Amastigotes are demonstrated on Giemsa-stained biopsied tissue from an ulcer in a patient with Old World cutaneous leishmaniasis.**

lesions, especially those of mucocutaneous leishmaniasis. Organisms of these species cannot be distinguished morphologically, and specialized immunologic, enzymatic, or nucleic acid studies may be needed for definitive speciation. Except in diffuse cutaneous leishmaniasis, the leishmanin skin test is usually positive.

Treatment

Although the pentavalent antimonial compounds, sodium stibogluconate [*see* Visceral Leishmaniasis, *above*] and meglumine antimonate (Glucantime), are the general treatments of choice for both Old World and New World cutaneous leishmaniasis,[26] optimal therapeutic regimens with these or alternative agents have not been rigorously defined. Individual species and geographic strains of *Leishmania* respond differently to treatment and have different capacities to cause mucosal disease or to heal spontaneously. Furthermore, it is difficult to distinguish infective species solely on clinical grounds. Therefore, progress in developing rational plans for appropriate treatment has been impeded. Advice on treatment of leishmaniasis is available from the CDC's Division of Parasitic Diseases [*see Sidebar*, Protozoan Infection Information on the Internet].

Trypanosomiasis

AMERICAN TRYPANOSOMIASIS (CHAGAS' DISEASE)

Infection with the protozoan hemoflagellate *Trypanosoma cruzi* produces American trypanosomiasis, or Chagas' disease, which has acute and chronic forms.[78]

Etiology and Epidemiology

Two phases of *T. cruzi* infect mammals: trypanosomes, which are carried in the blood, and amastigotes, which are found in infected cells. The parasite is transmitted by several genera of reduviid or triatomid bugs, commonly called assassin bugs because they prey on other insects or kissing bugs because of their predilection for biting the face. Nonhuman reservoirs include cats, dogs, rats, raccoons, opossums, and armadillos. The local pattern of transmission of *T. cruzi* infections depends on the species of reduviid bug, the sylvatic and domestic mammalian reservoirs, and housing conditions. Infected animals living around dwellings, usually in rural areas, are likely to transmit the organism to reduviid bugs. These infected bugs inhabit niches in walls and ceilings of poorly constructed houses. At night, they come out and feed on the blood of sleeping humans by biting exposed skin areas such as the face. During their meal, the insects excrete feces containing infective-stage metacyclic trypanosomes, which enter the host through the bite wound, cutaneous abrasions, or mucous membranes of the conjunctiva or lips.

Although reduviid vectors are present in the United States and infected mammals have been found in several states, the opportunity for transmission of infections seems limited. A few autochthonous cases of Chagas' disease have been found in the United States.[78] In rural areas of Central and South America, human infections are common where conditions favor access of infected bugs to persons. In addition, infections may be transmitted by blood transfusions, across the placenta, and, in rare instances, by ingestion of foodstuffs contaminated with the excreta of infected animals.

Pathogenesis

Both acute and chronic forms of Chagas' disease are recognized. The acute form, which develops soon after infection, principally affects children in endemic areas.[78] Within several days of infection, an indurated erythematous lesion termed a chagoma appears at the inoculation site. When this site is the conjunctiva, the characteristic constellation of unilateral conjunctivitis, periocular edema, and preauricular lymphadenopathy evolves; taken together, they constitute Romana's sign. After about 2 weeks, trypanosomes appear in the blood and invade cells, generally those of mesenchymal origin, where they multiply as leishmanial amastigote forms. The resultant intracellular pseudocysts rupture, releasing both trypanosomal and leishmanial forms.

Diagnosis

Clinical features During the acute phase, the patient may experience intermittent or continuous fever, an evanescent rubelliform rash, hepatosplenomegaly, lymphadenopathy, nonpitting edema of the face or extremities, tender subcutaneous nodules termed hematogenous chagomas, and, in infants, diarrhea. In severe cases, fatal myocarditis or meningoencephalitis can develop. The acute phase is usually self-limited: patients eventually become asymptomatic, and parasites can no longer be detected in the bloodstream.

The chronic form of Chagas' disease may become manifest either after an acute infection or more commonly after a clinically inapparent infection. It usually presents in the second or third decade of life and progresses over subsequent decades. Chronic complications of Chagas' disease result from the destruction of autonomic ganglia and from myositis; the pathogenesis of these lesions is not understood. The organ most frequently involved is the heart,[78] which develops biventricular hypertrophy and a mononuclear cell infiltrative myocarditis. Conduction disorders often include right bundle branch block, partial or complete atrioventricular block, and premature ventricular contractions. Sudden death has occurred in patients with Chagas' disease, and fatalities have also resulted from complications of congestive heart failure.

The GI tract is the second most frequently involved organ system.[78] The disease causes denervation leading to impaired motility and dilatation, which results in megaesophagus and megacolon.

Congenital infections are usually responsible for premature births. Such premature infants may have hepatosplenomegaly, abdominal distention, cardiomegaly, megaesophagus, and meningoencephalitis. In HIV-infected patients, reactivation of Chagas' disease can produce cerebral masses and, in patients with acute infections, necrotizing encephalitis.

Laboratory findings In acute Chagas' disease, the total leukocyte count often exceeds 18,000/mm^3 (70% to 90% lymphocytes), and parasites are demonstrable in the blood. On unstained blood smears, motile trypanosomes may be seen; on Giemsa-stained smears, the organisms appear as C-shaped forms. If smears do not reveal the organisms, trypanosomes may be found in stained sediment obtained by centrifuging several milliliters of blood after lysing the erythrocytes. Organisms may be cultured from blood on NNN medium or in blood broth. Alternatively, blood may be injected into a laboratory rodent, whose blood is then monitored for evidence of parasitemia. Xenodiagnosis, which is not readily available, constitutes the most sensitive diagnostic technique. In this procedure, laboratory-reared reduviid insects are allowed to feed on a patient. If the blood ingested by the insects contains trypanosomes, the insects will become infected, and such infection can be detected by subsequent examinations of the insects' feces for excreted parasites. Blood containing trypanosomes is infectious and should be handled with care. A complement fixation test, which is valuable for diagnosing acute disease, can be performed by the CDC.

In chronic Chagas' disease, a chest x-ray may reveal biventricular cardiomegaly and congestive heart failure. Electrocardiographic abnormalities are commonly seen. Methods other than xenodiagnosis are rarely capable of detecting organisms in the blood. Although the complement fixation test may be positive, this result may only reflect past infections and fail to establish a link between clinical findings and active Chagas' disease.

Treatment

Optimal therapy for *T. cruzi* infections remains to be established. Nifurtimox (available from the CDC Drug Service) eliminates parasitemia [*see Sidebar,* Protozoan Infection Information on the Internet]. It should be administered to patients with acute disease and to patients with chronic disease and demonstrated parasitemia.[26] Side effects are frequent, including hemolytic anemia in patients with G6PD deficiency; peripheral neuritis; and psychosis. The cardiovascular and GI complications of chronic Chagas' disease are managed medically, although surgical treatment may be required for megacolon.

AFRICAN TRYPANOSOMIASIS

Etiology and Epidemiology

African trypanosomiasis, or sleeping sickness, is an acute or chronic parasitic disease caused by protozoan hemoflagellates of the genus *Trypanosoma.* The disease is prevalent in a broad periequatorial belt across Africa. Two forms infect humans: West African and East African, or Rhodesian, sleeping sickness. West African trypanosomiasis is present in the tropical forests of West and Central Africa and is caused by *T. brucei gambiense,* a parasite not carried in any major animal reservoir. In contrast, *T. brucei rhodesiense,* which produces East African sleeping sickness, is prevalent in the savanna and woodlands of tropical East Africa and exists in wild animal reservoirs. Visitors to game parks are at risk for acquiring East African trypanosomiasis.[79] Both types of African trypanosomiasis are transmitted by species of tsetse flies (genus *Glossina*).

Diagnosis

Clinical features Within a few days to a couple of weeks after inoculation of organisms by a tsetse fly, a trypanosomal chancre may develop at the site of the insect bite, which is usually on exposed skin.[79] The chancre initially appears as a papule and within 2 weeks evolves into an inflamed, painful nodule that subsequently resolves spontaneously. Although a trypanosomal chancre is commonly observed in non-Africans, it usually does not develop in African patients.

During the next phase of the illness, the hemolymphatic phase, trypanosomes invade the bloodstream and lymph nodes. In Africans, the development of symptoms in this phase occurs slowly, during several months, and presenting symptoms include fever, lymphadenopathy, headache, and debility. In non-Africans, however, the onset is abrupt and early, often concomitant with the development of the chancre. In the latter group, episodes of high fever that last 1 to 7 days and recur after afebrile periods are prominent. Associated symptoms include chills, headache, malaise, and anorexia. Soft, nontender lymphadenopathy develops more prominently with West African trypanosomiasis and may include enlargement of posterior cervical nodes (Winterbottom's sign). A characteristic rash, which can be observed on light-skinned individuals, occurs about 6 to 8 weeks after infection and may appear as evanescent, circinate, erythematous patches, usually located on the trunk.

The next phase in the evolution of African trypanosomiasis is CNS invasion leading to diffuse meningoencephalitis or meningomyelitis. In West African trypanosomiasis, which is a slowly evolving illness, the symptoms of sleeping sickness may not develop until years after infection. Increasing lassitude and indifference are complicated by progressive neurologic compromise leading to coma and death by inanition or intercurrent infection. In contrast, the pace of East African trypanosomiasis is much more rapid, and CNS involvement may develop earlier. Even before CNS involvement, such manifestations as somnolence, personality changes, and an inability to concentrate may appear. Pancarditis often complicates acute East African trypanosomiasis and may cause death before the onset of CNS disease. Because East African trypanosomiasis may be acquired by visitors to game preserves and is an acute febrile illness, it may be mistaken for malaria and must be considered in the differential diagnosis of a febrile patient returning from an endemic area.

Laboratory findings The total leukocyte count is usually normal, but a mononucleosis of 50% to 70% may exist. Serum IgM levels rise 1 to 2 weeks after parasites appear in the blood and may shoot up to more than seven times the normal level. The definitive diagnosis is made by detecting trypanosomal organisms in blood, bone marrow, fluid from enlarged lymph nodes, or centrifuged CSF. Organisms stained with Wright's, Giemsa, or Leishman's stain may be found in a chancre 48 hours before they appear in the blood. If examination of peripheral blood is unrevealing, trypanosomes may be found in fluid aspirated from involved lymph nodes or among buffy coat cells. Even in cases in which neurologic symptoms are absent, CNS disease must be excluded by performing a lumbar puncture. Even if trypanosomes are not seen in centrifuged CSF, CNS involvement may still exist, as indicated by elevations of the cell count or of protein or IgM concentrations.

Treatment

Eflornithine is effective therapy for *T. brucei gambiense* infections,[2,23] even those refractory to the arsenical agent melarsoprol. Eflornithine is the treatment of choice for both the early hemolymphatic and the later CNS stages of West African trypanosomiasis.[26] Because eflornithine can cause anemias, leukopenia, and thrombocytopenia, blood cell counts should be monitored twice a week during therapy. Eflornithine has not been effective with *T. brucei rhodesiense* infections. The early stage of East African trypanosomiasis is treated with suramin, and the CNS stage is treated with melarsoprol.[26] Both of these drugs are available from the CDC Drug Service [*see Sidebar*, Protozoan Infection Information on the Internet].

Acknowledgment

Figure 1 Seward Hung.

References

1. Dubey JP, Beattie CP: Toxoplasmosis of Animals and Man. CRC Press, Boca Raton, Florida, 1988

2. McCabe RE, Brooks RG, Dorfman RF, et al: Clinical spectrum in 107 cases of toxoplasmic lymphadenopathy. Rev Infect Dis 9:754, 1987

3. Mawhorter SD, Effron D, Blinkhorn R, et al: Cutaneous manifestations of toxoplasmosis. Clin Infect Dis 14:1084, 1992

4. Montoya JG, Remington JS: Studies on the serodiagnosis of toxoplasmic lymphadenitis. Clin Infect Dis 20:781, 1995

5. Michaels MG, Wald ER, Fricker FJ, et al: Toxoplasmosis in pediatric recipients of heart transplants. Clin Infect Dis 14:847, 1992

6. Renoult E, Georges E, Biava MF, et al: Toxoplasmosis in kidney transplant recipients: report of seven cases and review. Clin Infect Dis 24:625, 1997

7. Israelski DM, Remington JS: Toxoplasmosis in patients with cancer. Clin Infect Dis 17(suppl 2):S423, 1993

8. Hunter CA, Remington JS: Immunopathogenesis of toxoplasmic encephalitis. J Infect Dis 170:1057, 1994

9. Pomeroy C, Filice GA: Pulmonary toxoplasmosis: a review. Clin Infect Dis 14:863, 1992

10. Luft BJ, Remington JS: Toxoplasmic encephalitis in AIDS. Clin Infect Dis 15:221, 1992

11. Rabaud C, May T, Amiel C, et al: Extracerebral toxoplasmosis in patients infected with HIV: a French national study. Medicine (Baltimore) 73:306, 1994

12. Richards FO Jr, Kovacs JA, Luft BJ: Preventing toxoplasmic encephalitis in persons infected with human immunodeficiency virus. Clin Infect Dis 21(suppl 1):S49, 1995

13. Knobel H, Guelar A, Graus F, et al: Toxoplasmic encephalitis with normal CT scan and pathologic MRI. Am J Med 99:220, 1995

14. Pierce MA, Johnson MD, Maciunas RJ, et al: Evaluating contrast-enhancing brain lesions in patients with AIDS by using positron emission tomography. Ann Intern Med 123:594, 1995

15. Potasman I, Resnick L, Luft BJ, et al: Intrathecal production of antibodies against *Toxoplasma gondii* in patients with toxoplasmic encephalitis and the acquired immunodeficiency syndrome (AIDS). Ann Intern Med 108:49, 1988

16. Mathews C, Barba D, Fullerton SC, et al: Early biopsy versus empiric treatment with delayed biopsy of non-responders in suspected HIV-associated cerebral toxoplasmosis: a decision analysis. AIDS 9:1243, 1995

17. Minkoff H, Remington JS, Holman S, et al: Vertical transmission of toxoplasmosis by human immunodeficiency virus-infected women. Am J Obstet Gynecol 176:555, 1997

18. Wong S, Remington JS: Toxoplasmosis in pregnancy. Clin Infect Dis 18:853, 1994

19. Guerina NG, Hsu H, Meissner C, et al: Neonatal serologic screening and early treatment for congenital *Toxoplasma gondii* infection. N Engl J Med 330:1858, 1994

20. Hohlfeld P, Daffos F, Costa J, et al: Prenatal diagnosis of congenital toxoplasmosis with a polymerase-chain-reaction test on amniotic fluid. N Engl J Med 331:695, 1994

21. McAuley J, Boyer KM, Patel D, et al: Early longitudinal evaluations of treated infants and children and untreated historical patients with congenital toxoplasmosis: the Chicago Collaborative Treatment Trial. Clin Infect Dis 18:38, 1994

22. Mets MB, Holfels E, Boyer KM, et al: Eye manifestations of congenital toxoplasmosis. Am J Ophthalmol 123:1, 1997

23. Bowie WR, King AS, Werker DH, et al: Outbreak of toxoplasmosis associated with municipal drinking water. Lancet 350:173, 1997

24. Wilson M, Remington JS, Clavet C, et al: Evaluation of six commercial kits for detection of human immunoglobulin M antibodies to *Toxoplasma gondii*. The FDA Toxoplasmosis Ad Hoc Working Group. J Clin Microbiol 35:3112, 1997

25. Frenkel JK: Toxoplasmosis. Pathology of Infectious Diseases. Connor DH, Chandler FW, Schwartz DA, et al, Eds. Appleton & Lange, Stamford, Connecticut, 1997p 1261

26. Drugs for parasitic infections. Med Lett Drugs Ther 40:1, 1998

27. Luft BJ, Harner R, Korzun AH, et al: Toxoplasmic encephalitis in patients with the acquired immunodeficiency syndrome. N Engl J Med 329:995, 1993

28. Kovacs JA: Efficacy of atovaquone in treatment of toxoplasmosis in patients with AIDS. The NIAID-Clinical Center Intramural AIDS Program. Lancet 340:637, 1992

29. Podzamczer D, Miro JM, Bolao F, et al: Twice-weekly maintenance therapy with sulfadiazine-pyrimethamine to prevent recurrent toxoplasmic encephalitis in patients with AIDS. Ann Intern Med 123:175, 1995

30. Bartlett JG: 1998 Pocket Book of Infectious Disease Therapy. Lippincott Williams & Wilkins, Baltimore, 1998

31. 1997 USPHS/IDSA guidelines for the prevention of opportunistic infections in persons infected with human immunodeficiency virus: disease-specific recommendations. Clin Infect Dis 25(suppl 3):S313, 1997

32. Williams HA, Roberts J, Kachur SP, et al: Malaria surveillance—United States, 1995. MMWR CDC Surveill Summ 48:1, 1999

33. Olliaro P, Cattani J, Wirth D: Malaria, the submerged disease. JAMA 275:230, 1996

34. Hulbert TV: Congenital malaria in the United States: report of a case and review. Clin Infect Dis 14:922, 1992

35. Zucker JR: Changing patterns of autochthonous malaria transmission in the United States: a review of recent outbreaks. Emerging Infect Dis 2:37, 1996

36. Svenson JE, MacLean JD, Gyorkos TW, et al: Imported malaria: clinical presentation and examination of symptomatic travelers. Arch Intern Med 155:861, 1995

37. White NJ: Not much progress in treatment of cerebral malaria. Lancet 352:594, 1998

38. Vinetz JM, Li J, McCutchan TF, et al: *Plasmodium malariae* infection in an asymptomatic 74-year-old Greek woman with splenomegaly. N Engl J Med 338:367, 1998

39. Jelinek T, Grobusch MP, Schwenke S, et al: Sensitivity and specificity of dipstick tests for rapid diagnosis of malaria in nonimmune travelers. J Clin Microbiol 37:721, 1999

40. Phillips P, Nantel S, Benny WB, et al: Exchange transfusion as an adjunct to the treatment of severe falciparum malaria: case report and review. Rev Infect Dis 12:1100, 1990

41. Telford SR III, Maguire JH: Babesiosis. Tropical Infectious Diseases: Principles, Pathogens, and Practice. Guerrant RL, Walker DH, Weller PF, Eds. WB Saunders Co, Philadelphia (in press)

42. Herwaldt BL, Persing DH, Precigout EA, et al: A fatal case of babesiosis in Missouri: identification of another piroplasm that infects humans. Ann Intern Med 124:643, 1996

43. Falagas ME, Klempner MS: Babesiosis in patients with AIDS: a chronic infection presenting as fever of unknown origin. Clin Infect Dis 22:809, 1996

44. Herwaldt BL, Kjemtrup AM, Conrad PA, et al: Transfusion-transmitted babesiosis in Washington State: first reported case caused by a WA1-type parasite. J Infect Dis 175:1259, 1997

45. Krause PJ, Spielman A, Telford SR III, et al: Persistent parasitemia after acute babesiosis. N Engl J Med 339:160, 1998

46. Krause PJ, Telford SR III, Spielman A, et al: Concurrent Lyme disease and babesiosis. Evidence for increased severity and duration of the disease. JAMA 275:1657, 1996

47. Levy DA, Bens MS, Craun GF, et al: Surveillance for waterborne-disease outbreaks—United States, 1995–1996. MMWR CDC Surveill Summ 47:1, 1998

48. Overturf GD: Endemic giardiasis in the United States—role of the daycare center. Clin Infect Dis 18:764, 1994

49. Oberhuber G, Kastner N, Stolte M: Giardiasis: a histologic analysis of 567 cases. Scand J Gastroenterol 32:48, 1997

50. Lai Ping So A, Mayer L: Gastrointestinal manifestations of primary immunodeficiency disorders. Semin Gastrointest Dis 8:22, 1997

51. Hopkins RS, Juranek DD: Acute giardiasis: an improved clinical case definition for epidemiologic studies. Am J Epidemiol 133:402, 1991

52. Lengerich EJ, Addiss DG, Juranek DD: Severe giardiasis in the United States. Clin Infect Dis 18:760, 1994

53. Zimmerman SK, Needham CA: Comparison of conventional stool concentration and preserved-smear methods with Merifluor Cryptosporidium/Giardia Direct Immunofluorescence Assay and ProSpecT Giardia EZ Microplate Assay for detection of *Giardia lamblia*. J Clin Microbiol 33:1942, 1995

54. Zaat JO, Mank TG, Assendelft WJ: A systematic review on the treatment of giardiasis. Trop Med Int Health 2:63, 1997

55. Burtin P, Taddio A, Ariburnu O, et al: Safety of metronidazole in pregnancy: a meta-analysis. Am J Obstet Gynecol 172:525, 1995

56. González-Ruiz A, Wright SG: Disparate amoebae. Lancet 351:1672, 1998

57. Haque R, Ali IK, Akther S, et al: Comparison of PCR, isoenzyme analysis, and antigen detection for diagnosis of *Entamoeba histolytica* infection. J Clin Microbiol 36:449, 1998

58. Chun D, Chandrasoma P, Kiyabu M: Fulminant amebic colitis: a morphologic study of four cases. Dis Colon Rectum 37:535, 1994

59. Marshall MM, Naumovitz D, Ortega Y, et al: Waterborne protozoan pathogens. Clin Microbiol Rev 10:67, 1997

60. Ackers JP: Gut coccidia—*Isospora, Cryptosporidium, Cyclospora* and *Sarcocystis*. Semin Gastrointest Dis 8:33, 1997

61. DuPont HL, Chappell CL, Sterling CR, et al: The infectivity of *Cryptosporidium parvum* in healthy volunteers. N Engl J Med 332:855, 1995

62. MacKenzie WR, Hoxie NJ, Proctor ME, et al: A massive outbreak in Milwaukee of *Cryptosporidium* infection transmitted through the public water supply. N Engl J Med 331:161, 1994

63. McAnulty JM, Fleming DW, Gonzalez AH: A community-wide outbreak of cryptosporidiosis associated with swimming at a wave pool. JAMA 272:1597, 1994

64. Ortega YR, Sterling CR, Gilman RH: Cyclospora cayetanensis. Adv Parasitol 40:399, 1998

65. Herwaldt BL, Beach MJ: The return of *Cyclospora* in 1997: another outbreak of cyclosporiasis in North America associated with imported raspberries. Ann Intern Med 130:210, 1999

66. Fleming CA, Caron D, Gunn JE, et al: A foodborne outbreak of *Cyclospora cayetanensis* at a wedding: clinical features and risk factors for illness. Arch Intern Med 158:1121, 1998

67. Eberhard ML, Pieniazek NJ, Arrowood MJ: Laboratory diagnosis of *Cyclospora* infections. Arch Pathol Lab Med 121:792, 1997

68. Cuffari C, Oligny L, Seidman EG: *Dientamoeba fragilis* masquerading as allergic colitis. J Pediatr Gastroenterol Nutr 26:16, 1998

69. Horiki N, Maruyama M, Fujita Y, et al: Epidemiologic survey of *Blastocystis hominis* infection in Japan. Am J Trop Med Hyg 56:370, 1997

70. Bryan RT, Weber R, Schwartz DA: Microsporidiosis. Tropical Infectious Diseases: Principles, Pathogens, and Practice. Guerrant RL, Walker DH, Weller PF, Eds. WB Saunders Co, Philadelphia (in press)

71. Molina JM, Chang C, Goguel J, et al: Albendazole for treatment and prophylaxis of microsporidiosis due to *Encephalitozoon intestinalis* in patients with AIDS: a randomized double-blind controlled trial. J Infect Dis 177:1373, 1998

72. Dieterich DT, Lew EA, Kotler DP, et al: Treatment with albendazole for intestinal disease due to *Enterocytozoon bieneusi* in patients with AIDS. J Infect Dis 169:178, 1994

73. Martinez AJ, Visvesvara GS: Free-living, amphizoic and opportunistic amebas. Brain Pathol 7:583, 1997

74. Illingworth CD, Cook SD: *Acanthamoeba* keratitis. Surv Ophthalmol 42:493, 1998

75. Chandrasekar PH, Nandi PS, Fairfax MR, et al: Cutaneous infections due to *Acanthamoeba* in patients with acquired immunodeficiency syndrome. Arch Intern Med 157:569, 1997

76. Berman JD: Human leishmaniasis: clinical, diagnostic, and chemotherapeutic developments in the last 10 years. Clin Infect Dis 24:684, 1997

77. Herwaldt BL, Arana BA, Navin TR: The natural history of cutaneous leishmaniasis in Guatemala. J Infect Dis 165:518, 1992

78. Kirchhoff LV: American trypanosomiasis (Chagas' disease)—a tropical disease now in the United States. N Engl J Med 329:639, 1993

79. Gear JHS, Miller GB: The clinical manifestations of Rhodesian trypanosomiasis: an account of cases contracted in the Okavango swamps of Botswana. Am J Trop Med Hyg 35:1146, 1986

80. Pearson RD, De Queiroz Sousa A: Leishmania species (kala-azar, cutaneous and mucosal leishmaniasis). Principles and Practice of Infectious Diseases, 3rd ed. Mandell GL, Douglas RG Jr, Bennett JE. Churchill Livingstone, New York, 1990, p 2067

40 Helminthic Infections

Peter F. Weller, M.D.

General Considerations

Helminthic parasites belong to two phyla: Nemathelminthes, which includes nematodes (roundworms), and Platyhelminthes, which includes cestodes (tapeworms) and trematodes (flukes). Helminthic parasites differ from protozoan parasites in several respects. First, protozoan parasites are unicellular organisms, whereas helminthic parasites are multicellular worms that possess differentiated organ systems. Second, most helminthic parasites do not replicate within the human host; rather, they develop to a certain stage within the human and mature further outside the human. During their extrahuman life cycle, helminths exist either as free-living organisms or as parasites within another host species and mature into new developmental stages capable of reinfecting humans. Thus, with only a few exceptions (i.e., those parasites capable of internal reinfection, notably *Strongyloides stercoralis* and *Capillaria philippinensis*), augmentation of the number of adult helminthic parasites that reside within the human host requires exogenous reinfection.

A third attribute characteristic of helminthic parasites but not of protozoan parasites is their tendency to elicit eosinophilia within the tissues and blood of infected humans. The magnitude of eosinophilia tends to correlate with the extent of tissue invasion by larvae or adult helminths. For example, in several helminthic infections, such as paragonimiasis, acute schistosomiasis, and *Ascaris* and hookworm infections, the elicited eosinophilia is greatest during the early phases of infection, when migrations of infecting larvae and the progression of subsequent developmental stages through the tissues are greatest. In established infections, local tissue eosinophil infiltration is often present around helminths within tissues, but blood eosinophilia may be intermittent, mild, or absent. There may be no eosinophilia in established infections that are well contained within tissues (e.g., intact echinococcal cysts) or confined within the lumen of the intestinal tract (e.g., *Ascaris* and tapeworms). For some established infections, increases in blood eosinophilia may be episodic. Intermittent leakage of fluids from echinococcal cysts can elicit transient increases in blood eosinophilia as well as symptoms attributable to allergic or anaphylactic reactions (e.g., urticaria and bronchospasm).[1] With tissue-dwelling helminths, increased eosinophilia may be associated with the migration of adult parasites, as in loiasis and gnathostomiasis. Certain established infections—including trichinellosis, anisakiasis, gnathostomiasis, visceral larva migrans, echinococcosis, and the several forms of filariasis—are capable of inducing eosinophilia but cannot be diagnosed on the basis of stool examination. In addition, some intestinal helminths may not be readily detectable on routine stool examination. The intestinal nematodes that are most likely to cause persistent eosinophilia and that may not be detected on initial stool examination are hookworms and, especially, *S. stercoralis* [*see* Intestinal Nematode Infections, *below*].[2]

Trichinellosis

Caused by several species of the nematode *Trichinella*, trichinellosis develops after ingestion of infected meat, usually pork or the meat of certain carnivores. Mild to moderate infection is usually asymptomatic or mildly symptomatic; heavy infection can cause myalgias, periorbital edema, eosinophilia, and, in rare cases, death.

ETIOLOGY AND EPIDEMIOLOGY

Five species of *Trichinella* are now recognized to infect humans. *T. spiralis*, found in many carnivorous and omnivorous animals, and *T. pseudospiralis*, found in mammals and birds, are present throughout the world. *T. nativa* is present in arctic regions and infects bears and arctic mammals; *T. nelsoni* is present in equatorial Africa, where it is common in felid predators and scavenger animals (e.g., hyenas and bush pigs); and *T. bitovi* is present in temperate areas of Europe and western Asia, where it is found in carnivores but not domestic swine.[3,4]

Trichinella is transmitted by the consumption of meat containing encysted larvae. During its sylvatic life cycle, the parasite is ingested by wild animals that eat trichinous carcasses; during its domestic life cycle, the parasite is ingested by pigs that eat contaminated meat in garbage. Most human trichinellosis is caused by ingestion of infected pork products. Although cattle are not natural hosts of the parasite, beef may be implicated in outbreaks because of adulteration with pork, either intentional or incidental, through the use of a common meat grinder. Less often, human trichinellosis is acquired from horse meat or the meat of wild animals such as bears, walrus, boars, and cougars.[5,6]

Although meat in the United States is not inspected for *Trichinella* larvae, laws proscribing the feeding of uncooked garbage to pigs have reduced the transmission of the disease. Cases in the United States are attributable to commercially obtained pork and to locally raised pigs and wild animals. About 50 cases of trichinellosis, occasionally leading to death, are reported annually in the United States, but more cases, especially mild ones, probably remain undiagnosed.

Larvae in pork may be rendered noninfective by heating to a temperature of 77° C. Freezing at –15° C for three weeks, as in a home freezer, will generally kill larvae in meat; however, arctic species of the parasite, which may be present in walrus or bear meat, are more resistant to freezing and thus may remain viable.

PATHOGENESIS AND CLINICAL FEATURES

The severity of clinical illness usually correlates with the number of ingested larvae. In most infections, there are only one to 10 larvae per gram of muscle, and prominent symptoms are absent; however, in some infections, there are more than 50 larvae per gram of muscle, and the symptoms of these heavier infections may reflect the two phases of the parasite's development (i.e., the intestinal phase and the muscle phase).

Intestinal Phase

Encysted larvae are liberated from infected meat by the action of gastric acid and peptic enzymes. The larvae mature into adult worms, which burrow into the villi of the small intestine. Within four to five days, the adult worms produce larvae, which enter the circulation. During this enteric phase, which usually lasts from one to seven days, patients may be asymptomatic or may experience nausea, vomiting, constipation, or abdominal aches. Prolonged diarrhea that lasts for weeks, as noted in patients with arctic trichinellosis, may be the result of secondary infections in previously infected and sensitized patients.[7]

Muscle Phase

After the intestinal phase, larvae are carried by the bloodstream to various organs. In the early muscle phase, periorbital and facial edema, subconjunctival and retinal hemorrhages, and subungual splinter hemorrhages commonly develop.

After about three weeks of infection, larval encystment in muscles begins. Patients experience myalgias, muscle edema and weakness, fever, and eosinophilia. Headache, cough, dyspnea, dysphagia, and macular or urticarial skin lesions develop less commonly. Although larvae encyst only in striated muscle, inflammatory lesions may develop in the heart, lungs, and central nervous system. Fatalities usually result from myocarditis. Symptoms generally abate slowly after the third week of infection. Infections with *T. pseudospiralis* may be associated with years of myositis.[8]

LABORATORY FINDINGS

Eosinophilia develops in more than 85 percent of patients with symptomatic trichinellosis.[5] Elevations of muscle enzymes (serum aspartate aminotransferase and creatine kinase) often accompany symptomatic muscle involvement. Serologic tests are positive in most patients with acute infection, but diagnostic antibody titers may not be detectable until the third week of infection.

Definitive diagnosis requires demonstration of larvae in muscle. The likelihood of obtaining a positive muscle biopsy specimen increases if the specimen is taken from a clinically involved muscle; if it is taken near a tendinous insertion, where the density of larvae is greatest; and if it is obtained after the third week of infection, when larvae are more numerous, larger, and more resistant to digestion. A portion of the biopsied muscle should be submitted for histopathological examination. In addition, another portion should be compressed between glass slides and examined microscopically for larvae. Because a larger volume of muscle can be examined by this technique, it is more sensitive than histopathological examination for detecting larvae. Differentiation of *Trichinella* species can be based on the absence of larval encystment with *T. pseudospiralis* and on DNA-based molecular biologic techniques.[4]

DIFFERENTIAL DIAGNOSIS

The triad of periorbital edema, myalgias, and eosinophilia strongly suggests the diagnosis of trichinellosis. Most patients with trichinellosis have a history of consuming pork products or meat of wild mammals. The development of symptomatic infection or eosinophilia in other persons who have eaten the meat incriminated in a case of trichinellosis provides epidemiological confirmation of the diagnosis. Persons with light infections may have minimal symptoms, or the symptoms may suggest diagnoses other than trichinellosis, such as diarrheal or influenzal syndromes or polymyositis. In rare instances, CNS involvement may suggest aseptic meningitis or encephalitis.[9]

TREATMENT

Specific therapy for trichinellosis is unsatisfactory. Most infections, however, are not life threatening and are self-limited, so that bed rest, analgesics, and antipyretics suffice to alleviate myalgias and fever. If serious cardiac, neurologic, or pulmonary involvement occurs, corticosteroid therapy with prednisone, 40 to 60 mg daily, is indicated. Prednisone is often given with mebendazole (200 to 400 mg t.i.d. for three days, increased to 400 to 500 mg t.i.d. for 10 days).[10] Limited experience suggests that *T. pseudospiralis* infection may respond to albendazole.[8]

Intestinal Nematode Infections

ROUNDWORM, PINWORM, HOOKWORM, AND WHIPWORM

In addition to *S. stercoralis* (see below), the major intestinal nematodes are roundworm, pinworm, hookworm, and whipworm [*see Table 1*]. Pinworm eggs are infectious when passed, and transmission is often on a person-to-person basis. For hookworm, roundworm, and whipworm, a soil phase is necessary for the fecally expelled eggs to develop into their infective stages. Thus, infections from these parasites usually occur in rural areas with poor sanitation; and in these areas, highly prevalent infections with these geohelminths are major contributors to malnutrition in children.[11]

Clinical Features

Infection with hookworms, either *Ancylostoma duodenale* or *Necator americanus,* is more likely where the following conditions coexist: sanitary practices that permit human fecal contamination of the soil, soil damp enough for larval survival, and human contact with contaminated soil. People at risk include children, gardeners, plumbers or electricians in contact with soil, and infantry personnel. Hookworm eggs excreted in feces hatch in the soil, releasing larvae that develop into infective larvae. Percutaneous larval penetration is the principal mode of human infection, but infections with *A. duodenale* may also be acquired by oral ingestion. Larval penetration of the skin often produces a pruritic, maculopapular eruption at each site of entry, and in persons previously infected, serpiginous tracts of intracutaneous larval migration, as in cutaneous larva migrans, can occur. From the skin, hookworm larvae travel via the bloodstream to the lungs. Like the larvae of *Ascaris,* the hookworm larvae enter the alveoli, ascend the tracheobronchial tree to the pharynx, and are swallowed. The development of *A. duodenale* larvae can be arrested for many months before the larvae proceed to the lungs for subsequent maturation. Although transpulmonary larval passage may elicit a transient eosinophilic pneumonitis, this phenomenon is much less common with hookworm infections than with roundworm infections.[12] Larvae and young adult worms in the intestinal tract may cause gastrointestinal symptoms, including nausea, diarrhea, vomiting, abdominal pain (often with postprandial accentuation), and increased flatulence. A major health impact of hookworm infection is iron loss resulting from the 0.1 to 0.4 ml of blood ingested daily by each adult worm. In malnourished hosts, such blood loss can lead to severe iron deficiency anemia.

The roundworm *Ascaris lumbricoides* is the most prevalent intestinal helminthic parasite, infecting well over one billion people worldwide. Each adult female can produce up to 200,000 eggs a day. Passed in feces, these eggs are remarkably resistant to environmental stresses and are capable of remaining viable for up to six years. With exposure to warm, humid soil, fertilized eggs become embryonated and infectious. Most transmission occurs by ingestion of fertilized eggs on dirty hands, in fecally contaminated agricultural products or other foodstuffs, or through geophagia. Infection is more common in areas with poor sanitation. In regions with large concentrations of *Ascaris* eggs in the soil, eggs may be disseminated in the air, inhaled, and swallowed later with respiratory secretions.

From swallowed eggs, larvae hatch in the intestine within one to two days and molt into second-stage larvae, which are carried hematogenously to the liver and lungs. Roughly one to two weeks

Table 1 Intestinal Nematodes

	Roundworm (Ascaris lumbricoides)	*Pinworm* (Enterobius vermicularis)	*Hookworm* (Necator americanus *or* Ancylostoma duodenale)	*Whipworm* (Trichuris trichiura)	Strongyloides stercoralis
Infective stage	Egg	Egg	Larva	Egg	Filariform larva
Route of infection	Oral	Oral	Percutaneous Oral (*A. duodenale*)	Oral	Percutaneous or internally with ongoing autoinfection
Extraintestinal penetration					
Larval stage	After egg ingestion	None	During initial infection	None	During initial infection and during ongoing autoinfection
Adult stage	With aberrant migration	Rarely via female genital tract	None	None	None
Principal symptoms	Usually none; occasionally, GI or biliary tract obstruction by adult worms	Perianal pruritus or none	Usually none; iron deficiency anemia in heavy infection	Usually none; GI symptoms or iron deficiency anemia in heavy infection	In uncomplicated infection, none or GI symptoms and skin lesions; in disseminated disease, symptoms related to involvement of GI tract, lungs, or other organs, with possible bacteremia
Diagnostic stage	Eggs in stool	Eggs from perianal skin on cellulose acetate tape	Eggs in fresh stool; larvae in old stool	Eggs in stool	Rhabditiform larvae in stool; filariform larvae in duodenal aspirate, in pulmonary secretions, in stool, or in other fluids or tissues
Indications for therapy	Presence of adult worms	Symptoms	Heavy worm burden; iron deficiency anemia	Symptoms with heavy infection	Presence of parasite
Therapy (adult dose)	Mebendazole (100 mg p.o., b.i.d., for 3 days) *or* Pyrantel pamoate (11 mg/kg p.o. in a single dose; maximum: 1 g/day) *or* Albendazole (400 mg p.o. once)	Mebendazole (100 mg p.o. in a single dose) *or* Pyrantel pamoate (11 mg/kg p.o. in a single dose; maximum: 1 g/day) *or* Albendazole (400 mg p.o. once) For each agent, repeat course after 2 wk	Mebendazole (100 mg p.o., b.i.d., for 3 days) *or* Pyrantel pamoate (11 mg/kg p.o. in a single dose; maximum: 1 g/day) *or* Albendazole (400 mg p.o. once)	Mebendazole (100 mg p.o., b.i.d., for 3 days) *or* Albendazole (400 mg p.o. once)	Ivermectin (200 µg/kg p.o. in a single dose) *or* Thiabendazole (25 mg/kg p.o., b.i.d., for 2 days or, in cases of disseminated disease, for 5 days)

after infection, larvae from the capillary bed penetrate alveoli and molt into third-stage larvae, which ascend the tracheobronchial tree, are swallowed, and return to the intestine. These larvae mature into adult male and female worms, 10 to 30 cm in length. The fertilized adult females begin producing eggs two to three months after the initial infection.

The clinical manifestations of ascariasis occur during early larval migration or with established intestinal infections. During the phase of transpulmonary migration, eosinophilic, often migratory, pulmonary infiltrates (Löffler's syndrome) can develop, especially in the previously sensitized host.[12] The large adult worms in the intestine usually elicit no symptoms, although they may contribute to malnutrition. Infrequently, adult *Ascaris* worms cause two serious complications. In heavy infections, especially in children, the mass of entangled adult worms may cause partial or complete intestinal obstruction.[13–15] The second type of complication can develop even when only a single adult worm migrates from its normal location within the intestinal lumen. Acute or recurrent migrations of one or more adult worms into the biliary tract can cause obstruction leading to acalculous cholecystitis, pyogenic cholangitis, pancreatitis, or liver abscesses.[16] Adult *Ascaris* worms do not penetrate and perforate the intestine unless the bowel wall is thinned or ulcerated by typhoid enteritis or other diseases.

Moderate infection with *Trichuris trichiura* (whipworm) provokes gastrointestinal complaints, and heavy infections (> 200 worms) cause the *Trichuris* dysentery syndrome, characterized by chronic diarrhea, anemia, and growth retardation in children.[17] The cardinal symptom of pinworm infection is perianal pruritus, but some infected patients remain asymptomatic. The pruritus often worsens at night, when the worms tend to migrate. Occasionally, migration of adult worms into or through the female genital tract results in vaginitis or peritoneal inflammation associated with granuloma formation.[17] Pinworm larvae may also cause eosinophilic enterocolitis.[18]

Laboratory Findings and Imaging Studies

Intestinal infections with roundworm, hookworm, or whipworm are usually easily diagnosed by finding the eggs of the responsible parasite in stool examinations. During the pulmonary phase of *Ascaris* or hookworm infections, the diagnosis is made by finding larvae in respiratory secretions. Results of stool examinations are usually negative at the pulmonary phase, because this phase occurs early in infection, weeks or months before adult worms have matured sufficiently to liberate eggs into the feces. Positive stool samples during the respiratory phase indicate earlier, long-standing infection. Thus, in eosinophilic pneumonitis, negative stool examination results do not exclude a parasitic etiology. Adult *Ascaris* worms can be readily detected in upper GI series; the large worms are outlined by contrast material, and in late follow-up films, the parasite's alimentary tract may be defined by a thin line of ingested contrast medium. Ultrasonography can detect adult worms in the small intestine, facilitating diagnosis of *Ascaris* as the cause of abdominal symptoms.[19] Worms in the biliary tract can be detected by ultrasonography[20] or endoscopic cholangiopancreatography.[21] At times, patients may note the passage of the large, smooth adult worms in the stool or may cough up an adult worm.

Because pinworm eggs are deposited by female worms on the perianal skin, stool examinations usually are not revealing. Pinworm infections are diagnosed by applying cellulose acetate tape to the perianal skin in the morning and microscopically examining the tape on a slide to detect the eggs. Adult pinworms may be visualized by anoscopy or colonoscopy, and adult hookworms may be visualized by endoscopy of the proximal small intestine.

Treatment

Therapy utilizes the well-tolerated broad-spectrum anthelmintic agents mebendazole, pyrantel pamoate, and albendazole (not yet FDA approved for these indications) [*see Table 1*]. Because mebendazole and albendazole may be teratogenic, they are contraindicated during pregnancy.

Therapy for *Ascaris* is mandatory to prevent unusual complications resulting from aberrant migration of the large adult worms. Adult *Ascaris* worms causing biliary and pancreatic obstruction may be removed at endoscopy.[21]

Therapy for pinworm should be repeated two weeks after the initial course; however, reinfection is common. Before treatment, hygienic measures such as frequent baths and the clipping of fingernails should be instituted to reduce the opportunity for reinfection. Because household members are often infected and can provide a source for reinfection, simultaneous treatment of all household members is indicated. Anemia caused by hookworm responds to iron supplementation.

STRONGYLOIDIASIS

Although *S. stercoralis* is the least prevalent of the intestinal nematodes in the United States, it is widely distributed within the tropics and subtropics. In the United States, *Strongyloides* infection is more prevalent in persons residing in the southern states[22]; in persons living in institutions with poor sanitation[23]; and in immigrants, military veterans, and other persons who have traveled or resided in endemic locales. *Strongyloides* is one of the few helminths capable of internal reinfection; it can multiply its numbers in the human host without reinfection by soil-dwelling larvae. As a result of ongoing internal reinfection, strongyloidiasis may persist for decades, as has been documented in some World War II and Vietnam War veterans. If

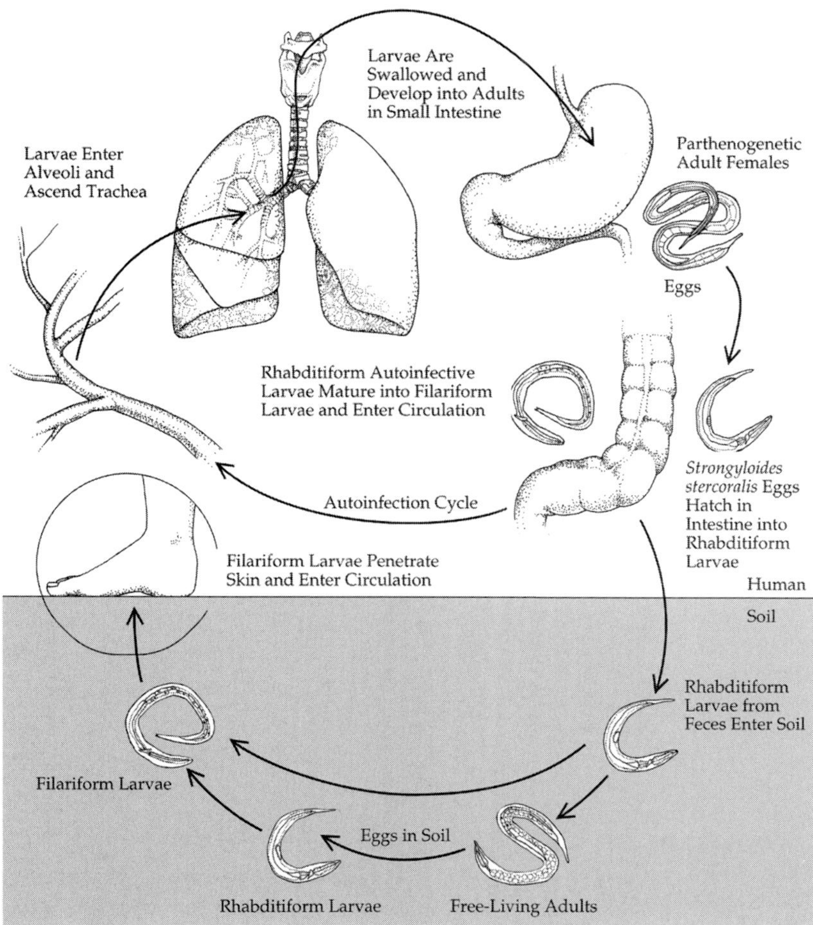

Figure 1 **Filariform larvae of the intestinal nematode *Strongyloides stercoralis* penetrate the skin or mucous membranes and enter the circulation. Larvae travel to the lungs, where they cross into the alveolar air space and ascend the tracheobronchial tree. They are then swallowed and develop into adults, which penetrate the mucosa of the proximal small bowel and lay eggs. The eggs hatch within the small intestine and develop into rhabditiform larvae, which then follow one of two paths: a soil phase or an autoinfection cycle. In the soil phase, larvae that are passed in the feces and contaminate the soil either transform directly into infectious filariform larvae or develop into free-living adults that generate new infectious larvae. In the autoinfection cycle, rhabditiform larvae penetrate the colonic wall or perianal skin and enter the circulation.**

immunity is suppressed, the internal reinfection cycle may become unbridled, leading to hyperinfection that can result in an overwhelming and frequently fatal illness.

Pathogenesis and Clinical Features

Eggs of *S. stercoralis* hatch in the intestine into rhabditiform larvae, which develop further by one of three routes [*see Figure 1*]. Two of the routes occur after stool passage: the larvae may develop in the soil into infective filariform larvae either immediately or after an intervening stage as free-living adults. The filariform larvae penetrate the skin and travel via the bloodstream to the lungs, where they enter the alveoli, ascend the trachea, and are swallowed; adult worms subsequently develop in the small intestine. The third route is the autoinfection cycle, in which the rhabditiform larvae mature directly within the intestine into filariform larvae, which penetrate the colon or the perianal skin to enter the circulation and complete the cycle of maturation into adult worms. This last route can increase the parasitic burden and permit the infection to become chronic.

Invasion of the small intestine wall by adult *S. stercoralis* worms may produce abdominal pain that is often localized to the midepigastrium; the pain is similar to that of peptic ulcer but is aggravated by food consumption. Diarrhea, nausea, and vomiting often occur; less commonly, urticaria, asthma, and weight loss may occur. In patients with heavy infection, malabsorption, gastrointestinal bleeding, and a protein-losing enteropathy may ensue. In cases of chronic infection, symptoms may be absent or may be mild and intermittent; symptoms include diarrhea, abdominal pain, and recurring episodes of urticaria, especially on the buttocks and the wrists. Less commonly, larva currens, which is a pathognomonic serpiginous, pruritic, elevated eruption, evolves along the tract of larval migration in the skin of the perianal, gluteal, or other body areas.

Disseminated strongyloidiasis may occur, especially in patients who have a malignant disorder or who are immunocompromised as a result of malnutrition or the administration of corticosteroids or other immunosuppressive medications.[22–24] Disseminated strongyloidiasis occurs but is uncommon in patients with acquired immunodeficiency syndrome (AIDS),[25] although strongyloidiasis is encountered in patients who are infected with human T cell lymphotropic virus type I (HTLV-I).[26] In immunocompromised patients, the autoinfection cycle produces large numbers of filariform larvae that may disseminate from the colon and invade any organ system. Colonic leakage or carriage of intestinal bacteria by larvae into the bloodstream often produces concomitant bacterial infection and pneumonia. This progression of events frequently results in a fatal hyperinfection syndrome in the immunocompromised host.

Laboratory Findings

Eosinophilia is elicited in strongyloidiasis but may be minimal or only episodic in chronic infection and absent in the hyperinfection syndrome. Midepigastric discomfort or unexplained eosinophilia in a patient about to receive immunosuppressive therapy should prompt a diagnostic search for the larvae of *Strongyloides*. Serial stool samples should be examined with the use of concentration techniques. About 25 percent of patients with strongyloidiasis have repeatedly negative stool examinations. An enzyme-linked immunosorbent assay (ELISA) is an especially useful diagnostic test. When hyperinfection is present, *Strongyloides* larvae may be found in other fluids, such as surgical drainage fluid and sputum, and the stool may contain filariform and rhabditiform larvae.

Treatment

Strongyloidiasis must be treated because of the potential for subsequent fatal hyperinfection. Ivermectin (200 μg/kg orally once), approved in the United States for uncomplicated infection, is safe and effective. Thiabendazole, 25 mg/kg orally twice daily to a maximum of 3 g daily, is given for two days; for disseminated disease, it is given for at least five days.[10] Thiabendazole is often associated with unpleasant side effects and is not uniformly successful. Although not approved for the treatment of strongyloidiasis in the United States, albendazole is an effective agent. Serial stool examinations should be obtained in the weeks and months after therapy to confirm eradication of the parasite.

TRICHOSTRONGYLIASIS

Humans may be infected with several species of *Trichostrongylus*. Infection is most common in Asia and is acquired by consuming food that harbors infectious larvae. Adult worms attach to the proximal small bowel and in most cases do not produce symptoms. The eggs of *Trichostrongylus* are somewhat larger and have less rounded ends than hookworm eggs. Trichostrongyliasis is treated with pyrantel pamoate (a single 11 mg/kg dose, to a maximum of 1 g), mebendazole (100 mg b.i.d. for three days), or albendazole (400 mg once).[10]

CAPILLARIASIS

Most human infection with *Capillaria* is caused by *C. philippinensis*, which is found primarily in the northern Philippines and Thailand. Humans acquire the infection by eating raw freshwater fish. The small (3 to 4 mm long) adult worms dwell in the small intestine. Symptomatic intestinal capillariasis is marked by diarrhea and abdominal pain. When infection is severe, edema, muscle wasting, fat and sugar malabsorption, and a protein-losing enteropathy may ensue.[17] If left untreated, severe infection may result in death after several months. Capillariasis is treated with mebendazole, 200 mg orally twice daily for 20 days.[10]

CANINE HOOKWORMS

In addition to *A. braziliense*, a canine hookworm that can cause cutaneous larva migrans [*see* Visceral Larva Migrans, *below*], two other canine hookworms can cause human infections. *A. ceylonicum,* a widely distributed canine and feline parasite of the tropics and subtropics, can cause intestinal infections in humans. Like human hookworm parasites, the sexually mature, egg-laying adult worms of this species can cause blood loss and consequent iron deficiency.

Most cases of *A. caninum* infection in humans[27,28] have been recognized in Australia. The clinical features have been variable, ranging from acute intestinal obstruction to subclinical infections. Eosinophilic enteritis is common, and some patients have experienced acute abdominal pain, rectal bleeding, or diarrhea. Worms, often a single worm, have been recovered at surgery or colonoscopy in most patients. The immature worms do not produce eggs and hence are not detectable by fecal examinations. An ELISA serologic test has helped with diagnosis. As in human hookworm infections [*see Table 1*], mebendazole has been effective.

Tissue Nematode Infections

ANISAKIASIS

Anisakiasis is a zoonotic infection that develops in persons who consume fish infected with anisakine or related parasites.[29] The term anisakiasis is used to denote an infection with *Anisakis* species, which are present in the muscle of mackerel, herring, and salmon. Infection caused by *Pseudoterranova* (previously termed *Phocanema*) species is referred to as codworm anisakiasis. *Pseudoterranova* parasites are found most frequently in cod, but they have also been detected in the muscle of pollack, halibut, flatfish, greenling, Pacific rockfish (Pacific red snapper), and squid. Infective third-stage larvae in fish are killed by heating to 60° C, by commercial blast freezing, or by freezing at –20° C for three days. Salting, cold smoking, and marinating do not normally kill either *Anisakis* or *Pseudoterranova* larvae.

The number of cases of anisakiasis recognized in the United States, Japan, Europe, and other countries has increased in recent years, probably as a result of three developments.[29] First, raw fish dishes, including sushi, sashimi, and lomi lomi salmon, have become increasingly popular in many regions of the world. Second, the population of marine mammals, including sea lions and seals, has increased as a result of legal protection; these marine mammals are the definitive hosts for anisakine nematodes that in a later stage of their life cycle will infect fish. Third, there has been an increased awareness of anisakiasis and, especially in Japan, greater use of endoscopy as a diagnostic modality.

In addition to anisakine nematodes, other parasites, including *Diphyllobothrium latum* [*see* Cestode Infections, Fish Tapeworm, *below*], the intestinal fluke *Nanophyetus salmincola,* and larval eustrongyloides nematodes, can be acquired by eating raw fish.[30] Eustrongyloides larvae, which have infrequently been reported to cause intestinal perforation in humans, have a distinctive bright-red coloration.[31]

Pathogenesis and Clinical Features

The clinical manifestations of infection after the ingestion of fish containing live anisakine larvae depend in part on the genus of the infecting parasite and on the anatomic localization of the larvae. Typically, in the United States, infection with *Pseudoterranova* species becomes apparent when a patient coughs up a live worm, often within 48 hours after eating raw or undercooked fish. Some patients have experienced mild epigastric pain and a tingling throat and have sensed the worm in the oropharynx or proximal esophagus. In the United States, the infection has only infrequently been associated with serious illness.[32] In Japan, by contrast, codworm anisakiasis has been associated with gastric, but usually not intestinal, invasion. Within several hours after infected fish have been consumed, the larvae can invade the stomach mucosa and produce severe epigastric pain that recurs every five to 10 minutes. Patients may experience nausea, vomiting, urticaria, and a tingling throat. Endoscopy at this time will reveal the invading larvae at a site that is swollen and hemorrhagic; often, the site is the posterior wall of the stomach.

Infections with *Anisakis* species can cause either gastric or intestinal involvement. Invasion of the gastric mucosa produces the same clinical syndrome that occurs in gastric codworm anisakiasis but without the tingling throat; the pathological findings on endoscopy are also the same.[33] Larval invasion of the intestinal mucosa can produce abdominal pain, fever, nausea, vomiting, and diarrhea. Larvae can elicit an eosinophil-rich granulomatous reaction in the submucosa and infrequently penetrate the peritoneum. The clinical presentation of intestinal anisakiasis often mimics that of acute appendicitis, but it can also be confused with gastrointestinal ulcers or neoplasms, acute Crohn's disease, or ischemic ileitis. In addition to causing invasive disease, *Anisakis* parasites may elicit allergic reactions. Patients may develop IgE-mediated reactions to *Anisakis* proteins and experience urticaria, angioedema, and anaphylactic reactions after ingesting even adequately cooked infected fish.[34]

Laboratory Findings and Imaging Studies

In gastric anisakiasis, eosinophilia is often present, and occult blood is frequently detectable in gastric fluid or stool. In intestinal anisakiasis, eosinophilia may be absent, and a leukocytosis may develop. In either form of anisakiasis, a history of recent raw fish ingestion before the onset of symptoms can strongly suggest the diagnosis. The definitive diagnosis of anisakiasis involving the stomach or proximal intestine can be made with endoscopy, which will reveal the invading larva.[32,33] The codworm larva resembles a thick piece of yellowish string, whereas the *Anisakis* larva is fine and whitish.

Treatment

Endoscopic removal of the larva is the only treatment. Radiographic studies can help identify gastric anisakiasis.[33] In intestinal anisakiasis, such studies may show thickening of the involved bowel area and may detect the larva.[35]

Although surgery for presumed appendicitis is often performed in patients with intestinal anisakiasis, surgical resection may not be needed if the correct diagnosis is considered in time. With conservative care, the illness may be self-limited, and patients may recover without surgical treatment.[35] The efficacy of anthelmintic medications against human anisakiasis has not been evaluated.

VISCERAL LARVA MIGRANS

When the nondefinitive human host is infected with nematode parasites that normally infect animals, as occasionally occurs, the parasites usually do not mature completely, but the introduced larvae may persist and induce an inflammatory reaction. For example, the syndrome of cutaneous larva migrans (creeping eruption) develops when the larvae of various parasites, including the dog or cat hookworm *A. braziliense,* penetrate human skin. Pruritic, serpiginous cutaneous lesions form along the migratory tracts of the larvae[36,37]; these lesions can be treated with oral or topical thiabendazole.[10] Analogously, the syndrome of visceral larva migrans develops when nematode larvae of animal parasites migrate in human tissues. Visceral larva migrans with fatal eosinophilic meningoencephalitis has been caused by the raccoon ascarid *Baylisascaris procyonis,*[38] but visceral larva migrans is most commonly caused by dog or cat ascarids.

Toxocara canis, the canine roundworm, is common in North American dogs. Although fewer than 20 percent of adult dogs are infected, transplacental migration of larvae from infected females results in an incidence of infection that may exceed 80 percent in their puppies at two to six months of age.[39] Both the puppies and the lactating mother shed large numbers of *T. canis* eggs in their stools within a month after parturition. The prevalence of *T. cati* in cats is generally lower than that of *T. canis* in dogs; kittens do not become infected before birth.

After *Toxocara* eggs are shed in the feces, about three weeks must elapse before the eggs develop sufficiently to become infectious; thereafter, they may remain viable for several months. Humans acquire infection principally by ingesting eggs in soil; public playgrounds have been implicated. Direct contact with infected animals is not a major source of infection because of the time required for eggs to become infectious. A history of eating soil is strongly associated with the risk of acquiring infection. Thus, visceral larva migrans is most likely to develop in children with geophagia.

Pathogenesis and Clinical Features

After infectious *Toxocara* eggs are ingested, the larvae hatch and penetrate the gastrointestinal mucosa. They are carried to the liver in the portal circulation; from there, they move into the systemic circulation. When the larvae enter vessels too small to allow their passage, they exit and migrate into the surrounding tissues. The manifestations of visceral larva migrans are a consequence of both the damage done by the migrating *Toxocara* larvae and the induced eosinophilic granulomatous inflammatory reaction.

Many infections are mild and subclinical. Clinically apparent infections may present in one of two distinct patterns: visceral and ocular.[39] In the visceral form of infection, patients are usually one to five years of age and generally have a history of geophagia. Malaise, irritability, weight loss, wheezing, cough, fever, hepatomegaly, and pruritic cutaneous eruptions are common. Neurologic involvement may produce seizures and behavioral disorders. In rare instances, death results from severe neurologic or myocardial involvement.

In the ocular form of larva migrans, patients are older: the mean age is 7.5 years, and the range includes young adults. A history of geophagia is unusual; a history of an antecedent symptomatic visceral form of the disease is rare. Common symptoms of ocular larva migrans are strabismus and failing vision. The characteristic ocular lesion is a whitish elevated granuloma measuring one to two disk diameters that is located in the posterior pole of the retina; however, the disease may also present as endophthalmitis or uveitis. The ocular lesions may be mistaken for a retinoblastoma, which can lead to unnecessary surgical enucleation of the eye.

Laboratory Findings and Imaging Studies

Usual findings in the visceral form of larva migrans are leukocytosis, prominent blood eosinophilia (generally in excess of 30 percent), and hypergammaglobulinemia (IgG, IgM, and IgE). On chest x-ray, transient pulmonary infiltrates are found in about half of the patients with pulmonary symptoms. All these findings are uncommon, however, in the ocular form of larva migrans. An ELISA serologic test has proved to be a sensitive, specific diagnostic test for both the visceral and the ocular forms; it can detect subclinical cases that may present only as an unexplained eosinophilia.[39]

Treatment

The visceral form of larva migrans is self-limited. The course is usually benign, requiring no therapy. Corticosteroids are used to treat patients with severe respiratory, myocardial, or central nervous system involvement or, in the ocular form, to suppress active inflammation. The efficacy of the anthelmintic drugs thiabendazole and diethylcarbamazine, which are sometimes given, remains uncertain for both the visceral form of the larva migrans syndrome and the ocular form.

ANGIOSTRONGYLUS CANTONENSIS INFECTION

Infection of humans with the parasite *Angiostrongylus cantonensis* may produce eosinophilic meningitis.[38] The rat is the definitive host of *A. cantonensis,* but the larval stages develop in mollusks, which serve as intermediate hosts. Humans acquire the infection either by ingesting infected mollusks (land snails or slugs) or by consuming inadequately cooked carrier hosts (freshwater shrimp, aquatic and amphibious crabs, and certain marine fish) that have previously ingested infected mollusks. In the United States, *A. cantonensis* is endemic in the Hawaiian Islands, and the parasite has been found in rats in New Orleans. *A. cantonensis* is found throughout the Pacific Basin and in Southeast Asia, Australia, and Cuba. Eosinophilic meningitis occurs in all these areas.

Pathogenesis and Clinical Features

After the larvae are ingested, they migrate to the central nervous system. There the parasites die, but their passage into the central nervous system induces an eosinophilic inflammatory reaction. The most common symptom of *A. cantonensis* infection is a severe frontal or bitemporal headache, which is usually the reason patients seek medical attention. More than half of patients experience stiffness in the neck, vomiting, or paresthesias. Extraocular muscle palsies, seizures, and significant fever are uncommon. Although some deaths have been recorded, clinical symptoms generally resolve in one to two weeks; however, paresthesias may persist for months.[38]

Laboratory Findings

Peripheral blood eosinophilia usually accompanies eosinophilic meningitis caused by *A. cantonensis;* however, the eosinophilia may be mild, and eosinophil levels may not be elevated initially. In the cerebrospinal fluid, white blood cell counts ordinarily range from 150 to 1,500 mm^3, with eosinophils accounting for more than 20 percent of the leukocytes. CSF protein is usually elevated, and sugar levels are at the low end of the normal range. On rare occasions, larvae of *A. cantonensis* are found in the CSF. No serologic tests are available for identifying the organism; diagnosis is based on a compatible epidemiological history and clinical course together with eosinophilic pleocytosis in the CSF. Eosinophils in the CSF, which are also found in other diseases,[38] may be misidentified if they are not specifically stained.

Treatment

There is no specific treatment for eosinophilic meningitis caused by *A. cantonensis;* corticosteroids and antibiotics have no effect. For most patients, the illness is self-limited and the prognosis is good.[38,40]

MAMMOMONOGAMOSIS (SYNGAMOSIS)

Nematodes of the genus *Mammomonogamus* (*Syngamus*) inhabit the trachea of cattle and other herbivores. Although the life cycle of the parasite is unknown, human infection is believed to result from the ingestion of foodstuffs that contain some intermediate host of the parasite. Of the several dozen cases recognized in humans, most have been acquired in the Caribbean area. A chronic, nonproductive cough is characteristic in such patients.[41] No blood eosinophilia is elicited, and no parenchymal lesions are seen on chest x-ray. The diagnosis is made when an adult worm is expectorated or found at bronchoscopy or when eggs are found in sputum or feces. Therapy consists of removal of the worms during bronchoscopy.

GNATHOSTOMIASIS

Nematodes of the genus *Gnathostoma* are widely distributed and usually infect the intestinal tract of

Table 2 Filarial Parasites of Humans

	Distribution	*Vector*	*Pathology*	*Localization of Adult Worms*	*Localization of Microfilariae*
Wuchereria bancrofti	Tropics worldwide	Mosquito	Lymphatic, pulmonary	Lymphatic tissues and vessels	Blood
Brugia malayi	Southeast Asia	Mosquito	Lymphatic, pulmonary	Lymphatic tissues and vessels	Blood
Brugia timori	Indonesia	Mosquito	Lymphatic	Lymphatic tissues and vessel	Blood
Onchocerca volvulus	Africa, Central and South America	Blackfly	Cutaneous, ocular	Nodules in subcutaneous tissues	Skin, subcutaneous tissues
Loa loa	Central West Africa	Horsefly	Subcutaneous	Subcutaneous tissues	Blood
Mansonella perstans	Africa, South America	Midge	Uncertain, possibly allergic	Body cavities	Blood
Mansonella ozzardi	Central and South America	Midge, blackfly	Uncertain	Body cavities	Blood, skin
Mansonella streptocerca	Africa	Midge	Cutaneous	Connective tissues	Skin

carnivorous animals. Most human infection has been reported from Asia and is caused by *G. spinigerum,* although human gnathostomiasis has also been described in South America.[42] Infectious larvae are found in the tissues of freshwater fish, eels, frogs, and snakes and in animals fed on infected fish (e.g., poultry and pigs). Humans may be infected if they ingest any infected tissues. The larvae fail to develop to maturity within humans, but acute symptoms of nausea, vomiting, and urticaria may develop one to two days after infection. Larval penetration of the liver produces inflammation and right upper quadrant pain. Subsequently, larvae may migrate within the abdominal or thoracic cavities. Eosinophilia is initially marked but diminishes after about a month, when the larvae reach subcutaneous tissues. Ensuing larval migrations produce foci of serpiginous cutaneous or migratory subcutaneous inflammation and swelling. On occasion, larvae enter the CNS and cause eosinophilic meningitis.[38] Definitive therapy requires excision of the larvae but is not always possible. Oral albendazole, 400 to 800 mg/day for 21 days, has been suggested as adjunctive therapy.[10]

DRACUNCULIASIS

Dracunculus medinensis, the guinea worm, infects persons in the Sudan and now uncommonly in India, central and West Africa, and southwestern Asia. Infection results from drinking water containing microcrustacean *Cyclops* species that harbor larvae of the parasite. Once consumed, larvae penetrate the human duodenum, where they develop into adult worms within the subcutaneous tissues. After mating, adult male worms die. Adult females, however, move into the extremities, from which they emerge after about a year. This emergence, which may be preceded by a few days of urticaria, fever, and dyspnea, occurs with the formation of a blister that becomes pruritic and painful before rupturing. Larvae are released from the ruptured blister site if the lesion is immersed in water, as occurs during wading to fetch drinking water. The life cycle is completed when larvae are ingested by and mature within the *Cyclops* intermediate host.

Clinical manifestations of dracunculiasis are usually related to emergence of the worm and include premonitory symptoms and blister formation. Secondary bacterial infection often develops at the site of the blister and may extend retrograde along the length of the worm. The conventional method of winding several centimeters of slowly emerging worm around a stick each day until the worm has fully emerged is an effective treatment, but surgical extraction is more rapid and effective.[43] An international coalition is attempting to eradicate this human infection.[44]

FILARIASIS

Several insect-transmitted filarial nematodes cause chronic infections in humans [*see Table 2*].

The major filarial nematodes are responsible for lymphatic filariasis, onchocerciasis, and loiasis. Other filarial nematodes include *Mansonella ozzardi, M. perstans* (formerly called *Tetrapetalonema perstans*), and *M. streptocerca* (formerly called *T. streptocerca*); these nematode species cause fewer cases of human infection than the major filarial nematodes and are of less certain pathogenicity.

Lymphatic Filariasis

The most common filarial infections are caused by lymphatic tissue-dwelling filarial parasites, three species of which infect humans. *Wuchereria bancrofti*, which is the most common, is broadly distributed in tropical regions. *Brugia malayi* is found in areas of Southeast Asia, and *B. timori* is found in parts of Indonesia. Mosquitoes serve as an intermediate host for all three species of filarial nematodes and introduce infectious larvae into humans by means of their bite. The larvae develop into adult worms, which reside within lymphatic vessels and tissues. Offspring of the adult worms, called microfilariae, are covered by sheaths and may circulate in the bloodstream. In most endemic regions, microfilariae of *W. bancrofti* circulate in the bloodstream in greatest numbers during the night; in the South Pacific, however, no pronounced diurnal variation occurs. Thousands of mosquito bites are probably required to produce an infection that results in patent microfilaremia. The incubation period for *W. bancrofti* ranges from three months to the more usual eight to 12 months.

Pathogenesis and clinical features Most clinical manifestations of lymphatic filariasis are attributable to inflammatory reactions caused by the adult worm; the immunopathogenesis, however, is poorly understood.[45] Many patients with microfilaremia experience no symptoms, although lymphadenopathy of the axillary, epitrochlear, and inguinal-femoral areas is common.

The more prominent clinical manifestations of lymphatic filariasis may be divided into two categories: inflammatory and obstructive. Inflammatory manifestations, which often become recurrent, include lymphadenitis, lymphangitis, funiculitis, orchitis, and epididymitis.[45] A typical presentation is the triad of lymphadenitis, lymphangitis, and fever. In contrast to bacterial ascending lymphangitis, the lymphangitis of filariasis characteristically progresses centripetally down involved extremities. Fever is variable and may be associated with frank rigors; the patient's temperature may reach 40° C (104° F). Systemic symptoms, such as nausea and vomiting, develop in many of these recurrent episodes. Urticaria and areas of cutaneous erythema commonly develop. The episodes may continue for as long as seven to 10 days before spontaneously resolving. In filariasis caused by *Brugia* species, suppurative abscesses may form in areas of involved lymphatic channels.

The obstructive phase of filariasis usually develops after decades of exposure to the parasite and reflects lymphatic compromise, the mechanism of which is poorly understood. Inflammatory features may coexist with the obstructive phase. Features of the obstructive phase include hydrocele formation, chyluria, and elephantiasis of the extremities and, less commonly, of the breast.[45]

Tropical pulmonary eosinophilia develops in some individuals infected with lymphatic tissue–dwelling filarial parasites.[46] This illness is characterized by paroxysmal asthmalike attacks that are often nocturnal; by blood and pulmonary eosinophilia; and by elevated titers of antifilarial IgG, IgM, and especially IgE. Tropical pulmonary eosinophilia should be distinguished from the transient eosinophilic pneumonitis termed Löffler's syndrome, which results from a transpulmonary migration of larval forms of *Ascaris* and, less commonly, hookworm and *Strongyloides* [*see* Intestinal Nematode Infections, *above*].

Laboratory findings Definitive diagnosis of lymphatic filariasis requires the demonstration of microfilariae in the blood. Stained blood smears may reveal microfilariae, but often, larger volumes of blood need to be examined either by centrifugational concentration after erythrocyte lysis or by filtration through Nuclepore filters. In endemic areas where *W. bancrofti* microfilariae display nocturnal periodicity, detection of microfilariae requires examination of blood obtained after midnight or one hour after daytime administration of a 100 mg provocative dose of diethylcarbamazine. Microfilariae are rarely found in patients with elephantiasis or with tropical pulmonary eosinophilia and often cannot be found in patients with inflammatory or obstructive filarial manifestations. In males, ultrasonography can detect adult filariae within scrotal lymphatics.[47] Serologic tests may be helpful in making a diagnosis. Mild eosinophilia and elevations of serum IgE are common in lymphatic filariasis.

Treatment Lymphatic filariasis can be treated with diethylcarbamazine, 2 mg/kg orally three times daily for two to three weeks. Treatment with ivermectin or a single dose of diethylcarbamazine (6 mg/kg)[48] is also effective at clearing microfilaremia.

Onchocerciasis

Onchocerca volvulus, the causative agent of onchocerciasis, is found in equatorial Africa and in elevated regions of Mexico and Guatemala, with smaller foci in Saudi Arabia, Yemen, Brazil, Ecuador, and Venezuela. *Simulium* species (blackflies) transmit the infection.

Onchocerciasis typically occurs within several kilometers of rapidly flowing rivers and streams where blackflies breed. The life cycle of *O. volvulus* is similar to that of species causing lymphatic filariasis. Adult worms, however, reside in subcutaneous tissues, often enclosed in fibrous nodules. Microfilariae, which in this species lack an enveloping sheath, are released from female adults and localize in skin and subcutaneous tissues.

Clinical features The skin is frequently involved, and pruritus is the most common clinical manifestation of onchocerciasis. With time, such complications as wrinkling, loss of elastic tissue, hypopigmentation or hyperpigmentation, papulovesicular lesions, and localized areas of eczematoid dermatitis may develop. Firm, nontender nodules containing adult worms surrounded by fibrous tissue are often palpable in subcutaneous tissues. In Central America, nodules commonly occur on the head; in Africa, nodules are more common over bony prominences of the body. Regional lymphadenopathy also develops. Ocular involvement is potentially serious and may cause blindness. Conjunctivitis with photophobia is common. Punctate keratitis, which is caused by the accumulation of inflammatory cells around dying microfilariae, may develop within the cornea and usually resolves without consequence. However, sclerosing keratitis and chorioretinal lesions may ensue and are the major causes of onchocercal blindness. Anterior uveitis, iridocyclitis, and, less frequently, optic nerve lesions may develop as well.

Laboratory findings The principal method of diagnosis involves finding microfilariae in the skin. A small piece of superficial skin obtained by excision or punch biopsy is weighed and then incubated for several hours in saline or tissue culture media. Microfilariae that exit the skin are then counted in the fluid. Care should be taken not to contaminate the skin with blood that might harbor microfilariae of other species. Skin snip sites can include scapular and gluteal areas and, in Africa, leg areas. A count of more than 100 microfilariae/mg of skin indicates a heavy infection. Another diagnostic method involves administering a 50 mg provocative dose of diethylcarbamazine; the subsequent onset of symptoms, which may include pruritus, rash, fever, and conjunctivitis, constitutes the Mazzotti reaction, which strongly suggests a diagnosis of onchocerciasis. Caution must be exercised in the use of this test because heavily infected patients may experience serious adverse reactions. Eosinophilia is often prominent during onchocerciasis.

Treatment Therapy for onchocerciasis has improved dramatically with the introduction of ivermectin. Single-dose ivermectin therapy is free of most of the immediate cutaneous, ocular, and systemic reactions that complicated therapy with diethylcarbamazine, the agent that had previously been used to treat onchocerciasis. Ivermectin, given orally in a single dose of 150 μg/kg, leads to symptomatic improvement and clearance of microfilariae from the skin. This dose is repeated every three to 12 months.[10]

Loiasis

Loiasis, which is caused by the filarial nematode *Loa loa,* occurs in the rainforest areas of central and western Africa and is transmitted by *Chrysops* species (horseflies and deerflies). Adult worms reside in subcutaneous tissues. The microfilariae, which are sheathed, circulate in the bloodstream with a diurnal periodicity in which the maximal number in the blood is reached at about noon.

Many residents of endemic areas who have loiasis have asymptomatic microfilaremia. The prominent clinical presentations are related to migrations of adult worms. In the subcutaneous tissues, migrations may produce recurrent lesions termed Calabar swellings, which are erythematous areas of swelling and edema up to 10 cm in diameter that resolve after one to three days. Infection may also present dramatically when the worm migrates subconjunctivally across the eye.

In contrast, patients who acquire loiasis after brief stays in central and West Africa exhibit different clinical and immunologic responses.[49,50] They are usually free of detectable microfilaremia but may experience more severe and pruritic episodes of angioedema and have brisk immunologic responses, including elevated antifilarial antibody titers, an elevated serum IgE level, and prominent eosinophilia—often greater than 3,000 eosinophils/mm^3.

To make a diagnosis, one must search for microfilariae in the blood by means of a Nuclepore filter concentration technique. Microfilaremia, however, may not be detectable. Eosinophilia may be marked, with elevations of 50 percent or greater. Filarial antibody titers are usually elevated. In the absence of detectable microfilaremia, the diagnosis is suggested by clinical features, history of exposure, and eosinophilia.

Therapy consists of diethylcarbamazine (6 mg/kg/day) orally for three weeks.[10] Patients with microfilaremia should be treated initially with diethylcarbamazine for three days (one 50 mg dose on the first day, three 50 mg doses on the second day, and three 100 mg doses on the third day), followed by the full three-week course. Some patients require repeated courses of therapy.[51]

Side effects are usually mild and include frequent occurrences of pruritus and the development of subcutaneous nodules soon after initiation of therapy. Patients with severe microfilaremia (> 50,000 microfilariae/ml) have acquired fatal encephalopathy after diethylcarbamazine therapy.

Diethylcarbamazine, given in a dosage of 300 mg orally once a week, is an effective chemoprophylactic agent against loiasis for persons who are planning long-term visits to areas of Africa where this infection is endemic.[52]

Zoonotic Filarial Infections

Although no human filarial parasites are indigenous to the continental United States, a variety of filarial parasites infect animals. In rare cases, these organisms may be transmitted via insect vectors to humans. Within the human host, they may develop into adult worms, which localize in the same organs in humans as in the definitive animal hosts. In this way, dog heartworm (*Dirofilaria immitis*), endemic in dogs along the Atlantic and Gulf coasts, in the Mississippi Valley, and in California, localizes to the human pulmonary arteries. A granulomatous response develops around the worm, producing a pulmonary nodule. Some patients experience chest discomfort, malaise, low-grade fever, cough, and, occasionally, hemoptysis. Typically, however, the pulmonary lesions are detected as a coin lesion on a chest x-ray.[53] Prominent blood eosinophilia is absent, and serologic tests for filariasis are negative. In the absence of reliable diagnostic tests for human pulmonary dirofilariasis, excisional biopsy serves both diagnostic and therapeutic purposes.

Other zoonotic filarial parasites include *D. repens,* which causes subcutaneous abscesses, and *B. beaveri,* which produces focal lymphadenopathy. No chemotherapy is required for these infections or for infections caused by *D. immitis.* Generalized lymphedema has developed in one immunodeficient child with a zoonotic *Brugia* infection.[54]

Trematode Infections

SCHISTOSOMIASIS

Schistosomiasis, a chronic trematode (fluke) infection of humans, constitutes a major worldwide health problem. Three major species—*Schistosoma mansoni, S. japonicum,* and *S. haematobium*—infect humans. *S. mansoni* is found in Africa, the Arabian Peninsula, South America, and parts of the Caribbean; *S. japonicum* is found in Japan, China, and the Philippines; and *S. haematobium* is found in Africa and the Middle East. Two minor species, *S. mekongi* and *S. intercalatum,* are found in mainland Indochina and central West Africa, respectively. Transmission of schistosomiasis cannot occur in the United States because of the absence of the specific freshwater snail that is a requisite intermediary host [*see Figure 2*]. However, the disease may be encountered in immigrants or travelers from endemic areas.[55]

Clinical Features

Three stages of disease may occur in schistosomiasis. The first stage, schistosomal dermatitis, may develop acutely within a day of cercarial penetration of the skin. Because this entity develops early after exposure, it usually will have subsided in patients before they are seen by physicians in the continental United States. Swimmer's itch, a similar reaction caused by exposure to animal schistosomes in fresh water and salt water, is seen in the United States.[56] The schistosomes penetrate human skin and then die, causing no further infection.

The second stage of disease, acute schistosomiasis, or Katayama fever, develops four to eight weeks after heavy, presumably primary, infection. Patients have fever, cough, hepatosplenomegaly, malaise, myalgias, urticaria, and eosinophilia.[57,58]

Chronic schistosomiasis, the third stage, is caused by the heavy deposition of eggs in the intestine or bladder and in the liver. In *S. haematobium* infection, the principal symptoms are terminal hematuria, dysuria, and frequent urination. Hydronephrosis and pyelonephritis may develop as a result of fibrosis and infection. In *S. mansoni, S. mekongi,* or *S. japonicum* infection, manifestations may include fever, malaise, abdominal pain, diarrhea, and hepatosplenomegaly. Presinusoidal hepatic trapping of *S. mansoni, S. mekongi,* or *S. japonicum* eggs and the consequent granulomatous reaction induce portal hypertension and collateral esophageal varices. Eggs may then be shunted from the liver to the lung, with the possible sequela

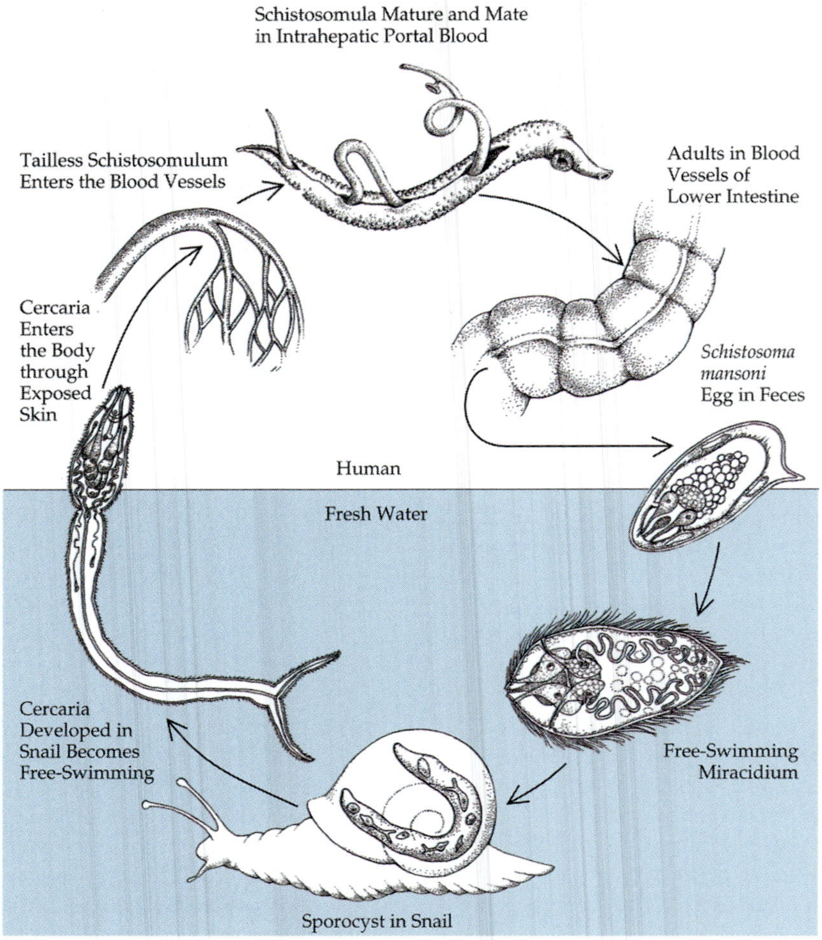

Figure 2 **Freshwater snails and the human body provide the living environment of the schistosomes *S. mansoni, S. japonicum, S. haematobium, S. mekongi,* and *S. intercalatum.* Eggs of each species hatch into schistosomal miracidia, which enter snails. Free-swimming cercariae released by the snails rapidly penetrate human skin and become tailless schistosomula, which enter the blood vessels. The schistosomula mature in the intrahepatic portal blood, form male-female pairs, and begin to mate. The pairs, still copulating, migrate to various sites: *S. mansoni, S. intercalatum,* and *S. mekongi* ultimately lodge in the blood vessels of the lower intestine; *S. japonicum* lodges in blood vessels throughout the intestine; and *S. haematobium* settles in blood vessels around the bladder. Adult worms subsequently begin laying eggs in the wall of the urinary bladder or intestine. From these sites, the eggs may be transported in the portal circulation to the liver, or they may be excreted in urine or feces.**

of pulmonary hypertension. Death may occur as a result of variceal bleeding. Hepatic encephalopathy rarely develops because the hepatic parenchyma is spared. Less common sequelae of chronic schistosomiasis include intestinal polyps, bladder carcinoma, and persistent *Salmonella* infections. Uncommonly, in both acute and chronic schistosomiasis, focal neurologic dysfunction develops from aberrant localization of eggs in CNS tissue. Embolic deposition of *S. japonicum* eggs may produce cerebral granulomas, whereas *S. haematobium* and *S. mansoni* eggs may cause transverse myelitis involving the midthoracic or lumbar spinal cord.[59]

Laboratory Findings and Imaging Studies

The diagnosis of schistosomiasis is suggested by a history of possible exposure, even exposure that occurred many years ago, along with compatible

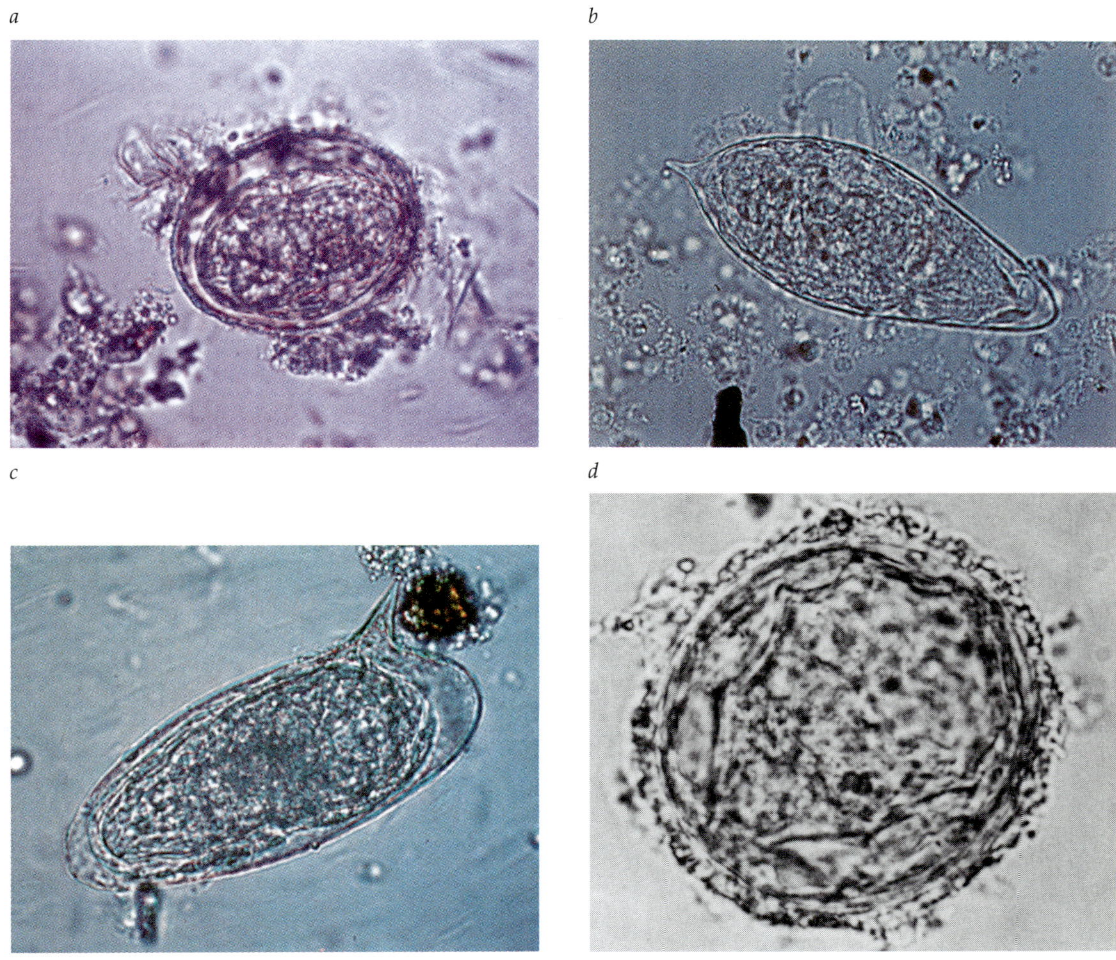

Figure 3 **Eggs of *S. japonicum* (*a*), *S. haematobium* (*b*), or *S. mansoni* (*c*) detected by microscopic examination of the stool, urine, or biopsied rectal mucosa confirm the diagnosis of schistosomiasis. The magnification is about 400 times. This *S. mekongi* egg (*d*) was found in the stool of a Laotian refugee in the United States. The magnification is about 1,000 times.**

gastrointestinal or urinary tract symptoms, hepatosplenomegaly, eosinophilia, or a combination of these findings. Computed tomography, magnetic resonance imaging, or ultrasonography may detect hepatic periportal fibrosis and calcification, colonic wall calcifications, and changes in the bladder and ureter resulting from schistosomiasis. Serologic tests can help confirm the diagnosis; an indirect immunofluorescent test for gut-associated schistosome antigens is especially sensitive for the detection of acute schistosomiasis. Stool examination should include a search for eggs of all *Schistosoma* species [*see Figure 3a, 3b, 3c, 3d*]. To find *S. haematobium*, urine should be obtained between 10:00 A.M. and 2:00 P.M. If stool and urine specimens are negative, microscopic examination of biopsy specimens of rectal mucosa may demonstrate eggs of all species.

Treatment

Praziquantel is used to treat infection caused by any of the five *Schistosoma* species. For *S. haematobium* and *S. mansoni,* two oral doses of 20 mg/kg are given in one day. For *S. japonicum* and *S. mekongi,* the dosage is 20 mg/kg given orally three times in one day. The efficacy, the paucity of side effects, and the convenience of single-day therapy make praziquantel the drug of choice for all forms of schistosomiasis.[10] In addition to praziquantel, corticosteroids are beneficial for patients with spinal cord schistosomiasis[59] and acute schistosomiasis.

PARAGONIMIASIS

Humans acquire paragonimiasis after consumption of raw, salted, or wine-soaked crustacea (freshwater crabs or crayfish) infested with the metacercarial stage of lung flukes belonging to the genus *Paragonimus. P. westermani* is endemic in parts of China, Korea, Japan, the Philippines, and Taiwan. Other *Paragonimus* species infect humans in western Africa and Central and South America. Although paragonimiasis is rare in the United States, it has developed in persons in Missouri from indigenous *Paragonimus* species.[60]

Ingested metacercariae excyst in the duodenum and migrate through the wall of the gut into the peritoneal cavity. Most pass through the diaphragm and penetrate the parenchyma of the lung. Neutrophilic and eosinophilic reactions, followed by a mononuclear leukocytic inflammatory reaction, develop around the fluke. As the lung parenchyma necrotizes, a fibrous capsule begins to surround the fluke. By about five to six weeks after ingestion, the flukes have matured and start laying eggs, which causes the capsule to enlarge and rupture, often into a bronchiole. The most common presentation of paragonimiasis is the production of brown-tinged sputum or hemoptysis, which derives from the admixture of eggs, inflammatory cells, and blood in the sputum. Patients usually appear well but may have a chronic cough, pleuritic pain, or night sweats.

Young flukes may migrate to nonpulmonary sites. Localization in the CNS produces signs and symptoms from a cerebral or spinal inflammatory mass lesion, which may calcify.[61] Less commonly, the parasites lodge in cutaneous or peritoneal sites.

During the early stages of infection, when the larvae migrate, blood eosinophilia is prominent. The chest x-ray may show transient, often basilar, infiltrations, as in Löffler's syndrome. Later in the course of the disease, blood eosinophilia commonly disappears, and the chest x-ray may show areas of cavitation; ill-defined, so-called cotton-wool and streaky densities; and bubblelike cavities.[62] Pleural reaction, with or without pleural effusion or pneumothorax, can occur. Examination of sputum, which is often gelatinous, purulent, and bloody, will reveal the diagnostic operculated eggs of *Paragonimus*. Swallowed eggs appear in the stool; therefore, examining the stool for eggs may be helpful, especially in children. Fine-needle aspiration of pulmonary lesions also yields diagnostic eggs.[63] Paragonimiasis may resemble pulmonary tuberculosis both clinically and radiographically. The diagnosis of paragonimiasis should be considered for patients from endemic areas with compatible clinical presentations.[64] Serologic tests are available.

Praziquantel, given on an investigational basis, is an effective treatment of paragonimiasis. The dosage is 25 mg/kg orally three times a day for two days.[10]

CLONORCHIASIS

Infection with *Clonorchis sinensis,* the Chinese liver fluke, is endemic in the Far East, including South China, Hong Kong, Taiwan, Japan, Korea, and Vietnam. Humans become infected with *C. sinensis,* a parasite of freshwater fish, by eating raw or undercooked fish containing encysted metacercariae. Larvae, liberated by trypsin in the duodenum, migrate to the common bile duct and then to the distal biliary tree. There they mature into adult worms, which may persist for more than 20 years. Less commonly, adult worms are found in the gallbladder and pancreatic ducts.

In the acute phase of the infection, the epithelium of the biliary tree undergoes early desquamation, which is followed by hyperplasia and increased mucin production by the epithelial cells. The hyperplasia may progress to adenomatous changes. With chronic infection, fibrosis develops around dilated bile ducts. Clinically, the syndrome of acute clonorchiasis, manifested by fever, chills, and tender hepatomegaly, may develop one week after ingestion of infected fish. Later in the course of the infection, however, most patients with light infection and many with heavy infection are asymptomatic.[65] Occasionally, adult worms block pancreatic ducts, causing pancreatitis. By occluding the biliary tract, worms may contribute to acute suppurative cholangitis. Clonorchiasis predisposes to intrahepatic bile duct stone formation and to recurrent pyogenic cholangitis; infection with *C. sinensis* has been associated with cholangiocarcinoma.

Leukocytosis, prominent eosinophilia, and elevation of alkaline phosphatase levels occur in symptomatic acute clonorchiasis. Sonography often detects diffuse dilatation of small intrahepatic bile ducts without dilatation of large intrahepatic or extrahepatic ducts. Adult flukes may be visualized in the gallbladder by ultrasonography and in the bile ducts by cholangiography.[66] In asymptomatic chronic clonorchiasis, eosinophilia is not present, and liver function tests and liver scans are normal. Egg laying begins within two to three weeks after infection; eggs may be found either in the stool or in duodenal aspirate. Diagnostic serologic tests are unavailable. The diagnosis is considered in patients who have a history of travel or residence in the Far East, have eaten undercooked fish, and have a compatible clinical syndrome.

Praziquantel, which is considered investigational for clonorchiasis, constitutes effective and well-tolerated therapy for this disease. Praziquantel is administered at a dosage of 25 mg/kg orally three times a day for one day.[10] Initially, complications of *C. sinensis* infection, including calculi, cholangitis, and pancreatitis, are managed medically, although surgical drainage procedures may be required.

OPISTHORCHIASIS

Opisthorchiasis represents infection by either *Opisthorchis felineus*, found in eastern and central Europe, Siberia, and parts of Asia, or *O. viverrini*, found in Thailand and Cambodia. Cats and wild carnivores are the definitive hosts of these species. Humans acquire infection by eating raw or undercooked fish that contains metacercariae of the parasite. Metacercariae excyst in the duodenum and migrate into the bile ducts, where they mature. Clinical features of opisthorchiasis are similar to those of clonorchiasis, and complications include the development of cholangiocarcinomas.[65,67] The diagnosis is made by finding eggs in feces or in duodenal aspirate. Therapy, which is still investigational, consists of praziquantel, 25 mg/kg orally three times in one day[10]; for complications involving biliary tract sepsis, the administration of antimicrobial agents is required.

FASCIOLIASIS

Fasciola hepatica, the liver fluke of sheep and cattle, is a major veterinary problem and can give rise to human fascioliasis.[65,68] Human infection with *F. hepatica* shows a wide geographic distribution that includes Europe, China, Africa, and Latin America.[69] Despite the prevalence of the parasite in sheep and cattle of the southern and western United States, autochthonous human cases are rare. Humans generally become infected by ingesting parasitic cysts attached to aquatic plants, most notably wild watercress.

After metacercariae are ingested, they burrow through the intestinal wall into the peritoneal cavity and then penetrate the hepatic capsule and parenchyma; they then enter the bile ducts, where they mature into adults after three to four months. Acute fascioliasis runs its course during the months of penetration and maturation. Symptoms may be minimal or include fever, upper abdominal pain, hepatomegaly, and malaise. Pruritus, urticaria, jaundice, nonproductive coughing, and anemia occur less often.[65,70]

After the flukes mature in the biliary passages, hyperplasia and dilatation of the biliary ducts as well as periductal fibrosis develop. Symptomatology in the chronic stage of infection is variable; it may include the same signs and symptoms experienced in the acute phase. Obstruction of the biliary tract, cholecystitis, and biliary cirrhosis are uncommon. In rare instances, flukes migrate to other tissues, including the lungs, muscles, and central nervous system.

Ingestion of raw sheep or goat liver containing young flukes produces halzoun, a disease recognized in the Near East. Lodging of the flukes in the pharynx produces a pharyngeal inflammatory mass lesion with attendant dysphagia and dyspnea.

In acute fascioliasis, leukocytosis, marked eosinophilia, and cholestatic-type abnormalities in liver function tests usually occur. Eggs are not found until approximately three months after infection, when they may be detected in the stool or, with a higher yield, in biliary or duodenal fluid samples. Thus, the triad of fever, marked eosinophilia, and hepatomegaly suggests acute fascioliasis. A history of ingestion of potentially infected watercress supports the diagnosis. Serologic tests are available but may reflect cross-reactions with other helminthic parasites. Nodular hepatic lesions with diminished density may be visualized by CT or MRI.[71,72] In chronic fascioliasis, the extent of the abnormalities in liver function tests and cholangiograms correlates with the magnitude of biliary tract obstruction and hepatocellular damage.

Praziquantel is not effective for fascioliasis. Bithionol, given in a dosage of 30 to 50 mg/kg on alternate days for 10 to 15 doses, is used instead for acute and chronic fascioliasis.[10]

INTESTINAL FLUKES

Fasciolopsiasis

Fasciolopsiasis results from infection with the intestinal fluke *Fasciolopsis buski*, which is found in many parts of Asia. This fluke principally parasitizes the intestine of the pig. Human infection is acquired by ingestion of water plants such as water chestnuts, which bear metacercariae of the parasite. The larvae excyst in the duodenum and develop into large adult flukes, up to 7 cm long, that attach to the mucosa of the proximal small intestine. Inflammation and ulceration may occur at these intestinal sites. Light infection is asymptomatic; heavy infection is associated with abdominal pain, ulceration, hemorrhage, intestinal obstruction, and facial and generalized edema.[73] Blood eosinophilia is common. Diagnosis is made by finding adult flukes or, more commonly, by finding in feces the eggs of *F. buski*, which are difficult to distinguish from the eggs of *Fasciola hepatica*. Fasciolopsiasis is treated, on an investigational basis, with praziquantel, 25 mg/kg orally three times in one day.[10]

Other Intestinal Flukes

Infection with two other small intestinal flukes, *Metagonimus yokogawai* (found in the Far East and Indonesia) and *Heterophyes heterophyes* (found in Tunisia, Egypt, and the Far East), occurs when humans ingest raw or undercooked fish that contains metacercariae of the parasites. The adult flukes are 2 to 3 cm long and attach to the mucosa of the small intestine. If infection is heavy, abdominal pain and diarrhea may be present.[74] Diagnosis is made by finding eggs, which resemble the eggs of *Clonorchis* species, in feces. Therapy consists of the investigational drug praziquantel, 25 mg/kg orally three times in one day.[10] More recently, human infections with *Metorchis conjunctus*, acquired near Montreal by consumption of the white sucker fish, were described. Illness consisted of upper abdominal pain, low-grade fever, eosinophilia, and raised liver enzymes. Diagnosis was made by finding eggs in the stool and by serology. Praziquantel therapy was beneficial.[75]

Cestode Infections

FISH TAPEWORM

Humans acquire fish tapeworm infection by ingestion of inadequately cooked fish containing the infective plerocercoid stage of parasitic *Diphyllobothrium* species, including *D. atum*.[76] The growing popularity of raw fish dishes, such as sushi, sashimi, seviche, and Dutch green herring, has increased the risk of acquiring diphyllobothriasis or anisakiasis. Freshwater fish, including pike and yellow perch caught in the United States, may harbor *Diphyllobothrium* species, as may anadromous salmon. *Diphyllobothrium* species other than *D. latum* are found in Pacific salmon and Alaskan blackfish.[77] Human infections are often asymptomatic, although some patients experience anorexia, nausea, or weight loss. Because *D. latum* competes with the host for vitamin B_{12}, megaloblastic anemia and neuropathy from vitamin B_{12} deficiency may develop. Diagnosis is made by finding the operculated eggs in the stool or by recovering proglottids in the stool after a saline purge. Therapy is with praziquantel (5 to 10 mg/kg, given once), which is investigational for this use.[10]

PORK TAPEWORM

Taenia solium, or pork tapeworm, causes two distinct types of disease, depending on the stage of the parasite that is ingested.[78] If cysticerci in inadequately cooked pork are ingested, the adult tapeworm develops in the intestine, causing symptoms such as abdominal pain, weight loss, and weakness. Patients may complain of passing proglottid segments of the worm. Eggs of *T. solium* are also passed in the feces. Eggs can be detected with greater frequency by applying clear cellulose acetate tape to the perianal skin and examining the tape as described for pinworm [*see* Intestinal Nematode Infections, *above*]. *T. solium* eggs are indistinguishable from eggs of *T. saginata* (beef tapeworm); diagnostic differentiation between the two species requires recovery of mature proglottids from the stool. Therapy for adults infected with intestinal pork tapeworm consists of praziquantel (5 to 10 mg/kg, given once).[10]

Cysticercosis, the second disease entity, is caused by the ingestion of *T. solium* eggs. In an uninfected person, such ingestion may occur by consumption of food contaminated by egg-containing feces from an infected person. In persons with an intestinal worm, ingestion may occur by autoinfection involving hand-to-mouth fecal carriage or by regurgitation of egg-laden proglottids into the duodenum or stomach. Most infections are encountered in developing countries, where intestinal *T. solium* infections occur frequently. Experience in the United States has demonstrated, however, that cysticercosis may develop in those who have never traveled abroad if family members, domestic workers, or others infected with *T. solium* are a source of infectious eggs.[79–81]

The ingested eggs hatch in the stomach and upper intestine, and the resultant oncospheres circulate in the blood to various tissues. Cysticerci develop most often in subcutaneous tissue, skeletal muscle, and the brain, as well as in other organs, including the eyes, heart, liver, and lungs. Developing cysticerci elicit little host reaction, but as the cysticerci begin to degenerate, usually after several years, inflammation develops. Ultimately, the cysts, which range from 0.5 to about 2.0 cm in diameter, undergo necrosis and may become calcified.

Clinical Features

Clinical signs and symptoms depend on the organ compromised by the cysticerci, the specific localization of a cysticercus within the organ, the state of inflammation surrounding the cysticerci, and the viability of the cestode. The most serious forms of cysticercosis are those with ocular, car-

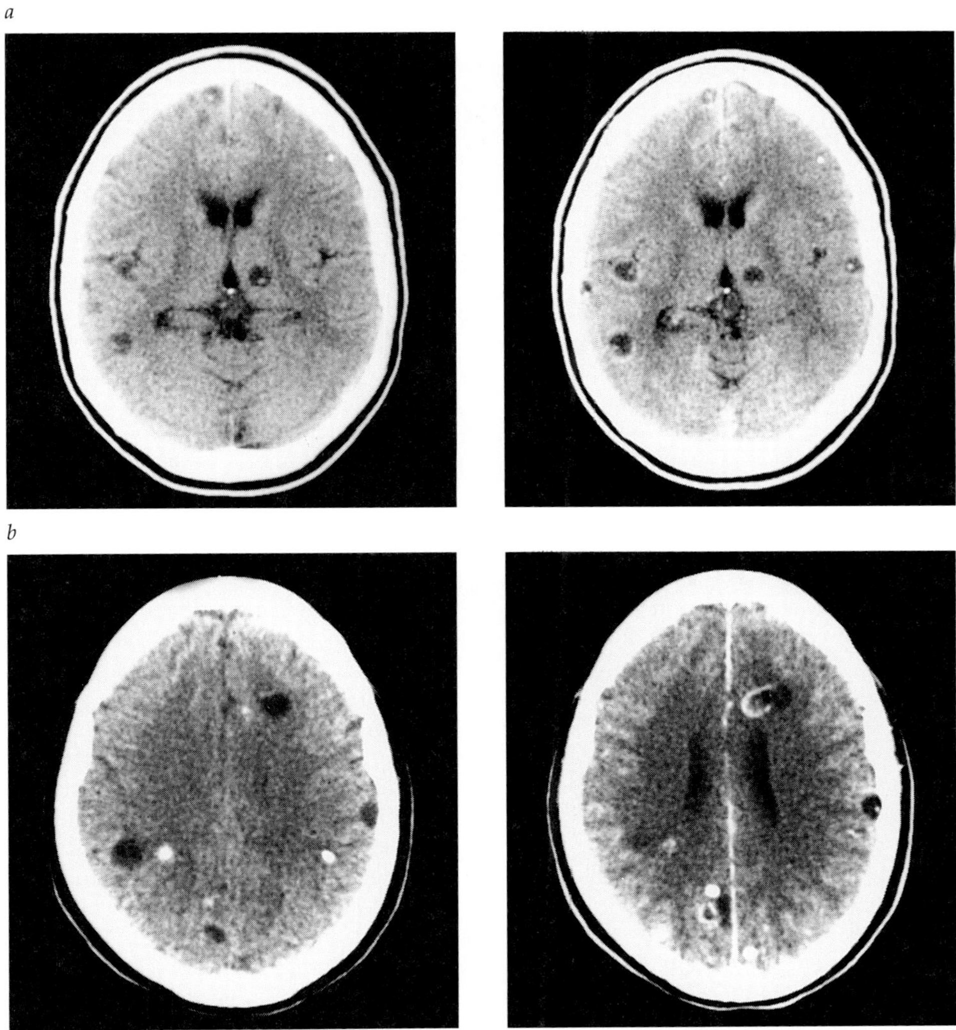

Figure 4 **Shown are CT scans of two patients (*a* and *b*) with seizures resulting from neurocysticercosis (the CT scans on the left are without contrast; those on the right are with contrast). Multiple cystic and calcified lesions are evident in both patients (the contrast agent enhances the cystic lesions). The scans from the first patient (*a*) show multiple cystic lesions with a denser central spot representing the scolex, a pathognomonic finding for neurocysticercosis.**

diac, and neurologic involvement. In endemic regions, cysticercosis is the most common cause of seizure disorders.[82]

Laboratory Findings and Imaging Studies

The use of CT and MRI has facilitated the recognition of CNS cysticercosis,[83,84] has helped delineate the various forms of neurocysticercosis,[83] and has provided a means for assessing the adequacy of therapy.[83,85] Cysticerci may be present in the brain parenchyma, within the ventricles, at the surface or the base of the brain, or within the subarachnoid space. The manifestations of neurocysticercosis, which can be quite varied, depending on the site of lesions and the evolution of inflammatory reactions, include seizure disorders and focal deficits, hydrocephalus, arachnoiditis, and intracranial hypertension.[78]

CT may miss early lesions, which have the same x-ray density as the brain, but hypodensity and contrast-enhancing ring lesions are seen with the development of inflammation around the cyst. As sclerosis occurs, a cystic lesion develops, and the cyst wall may calcify. Ultimately, degenerated cysts are replaced by small (1 to 4 mm in diameter) calcified lesions within the brain [*see Figure 4*].

The diagnosis of cysticercosis can be made with certainty only by biopsy of a cyst. Cysts in subcutaneous tissue and muscle, which have a puffed-rice appearance on radiographs after calcification, should be sought. Although the signs and symptoms of neurocysticercosis are not specific, this diagnosis is supported by the finding of characteristic multiple cystic or calcified lesions on CT scans in a patient from an endemic area. A serologic test, which should be used to test serum and CSF for antibody, is available through the Centers for Disease Control and Prevention (CDC). ELISA testing for antibody, however, may be negative in about 20 percent of patients with cysticercosis[86] and may be falsely positive in those with echinococcosis. An enzyme-linked immunoelectrotransfer blot assay for antibody is highly sensitive in patients who have several enhancing intracranial lesions; it is less sensitive in those who have only one lesion or calcified lesions.[84,87] Stool examination for *Taenia* eggs may detect concurrent infection with the tapeworm but is not directly pertinent to the diagnosis of cysticercosis.

Treatment

Therapy for cysticercosis may be medical or surgical. Patients with only calcified soft tissue or CNS lesions do not require medical therapy. Surgical excision was once the only approach for viable cysts, but praziquantel and albendazole have proved to be effective against neurocysticercosis, albendazole perhaps even more so.[83,85,88] Despite the improvements noted after medical therapy, the absence of controlled trials specifically comparing medically treated patients with untreated patients has left room for uncertainty concerning the efficacy of medical therapy for neurocysticercosis.[89] Albendazole is given in a dosage of 15 mg/kg/day in three divided doses for eight to 28 days, and praziquantel is given in a dosage of 50 mg/kg/day in three divided doses for 15 days.[10] Because treatment may cause inflammatory reactions to develop around cysticerci, ocular cysticercosis and spinal cysticercosis are not usually treated medically. For patients with neurocysticercosis, corticosteroids (e.g., dexamethasone, 4 to 16 mg/day, or prednisone, 60 to 100 mg/day) are usually given one to two days before and during treatment with albendazole or praziquantel to minimize inflammatory reactions. Patients who take anticonvulsant medications should continue to use them during treatment for cysticercosis, but many patients can stop taking antiseizure medications after cysticercosis therapy.[90] CT scanning should be repeated three to six months after therapy to determine whether any of the cysts are still viable, and therapy should be repeated if viable cysts remain.

BEEF TAPEWORM

T. saginata, or beef tapeworm, causes an intestinal infection in persons who have eaten undercooked beef containing cysticerci.[76] The infection is usually asymptomatic, although abdominal pain, weight loss, increased appetite, or passage of proglottids may be experienced. As noted, the detection of eggs in the feces or on the perianal skin is diagnostic of tapeworm infection, but differentiation between *Taenia* species requires identification of the proglottids. Therapy consists of praziquantel, as given for *T. solium* intestinal infection.[10] Infection with *T. saginata* does not lead to cysticercosis in humans.

DWARF TAPEWORM

Hymenolepis nana, a tapeworm measuring 25 to 40 mm long and 1 mm wide, has a broad geographic distribution.[76] In the United States, it is most commonly encountered in persons living in the southern states, in institutionalized patients, and in children. Unlike the other tapeworms, the larval and adult stages of *H. nana* develop in the same host. Infection is spread by the fecal-oral route and occurs when eggs, which are immediately infectious, are ingested. An oncosphere hatches from an egg and penetrates the intestinal villi, where it develops into a cerocyst; the cerocyst reenters the lumen of the small intestine and develops into an adult worm. Eggs are liberated from the distal segments of the adult worm, which lives for about one year. The eggs may cause internal reinfection. Light infection is usually asymptomatic; diarrhea and abdominal pain may accompany heavy infection. Diagnosis is made by finding eggs in feces. Therapy consists of praziquantel, which is given once in a dose of 25 mg/kg; this use of praziquantel is currently considered investigational.

OTHER TAPEWORMS

Human infection with *H. diminuta*, a tapeworm of mice and rats, occasionally occurs when humans ingest insects that harbor developing cerocysts of the tapeworm; one such insect is the flea. Infection is more common in children and is associated with few or no symptoms. Diagnosis and treatment are the same as described for the dwarf tapeworm *H. nana* (see above).

Children are also more commonly infected with the dog tapeworm *Dipylidium caninum*. Infection is acquired by consuming infected fleas or lice. Adult worms develop in the small intestine and measure 15 to 70 cm in length. Mild intestinal symptoms may or may not be present. Diagnosis is made by finding proglottids or eggs in feces. Therapy for adults consists of praziquantel (5 to 10 mg/kg once).[10]

Human infection with dog tapeworms of the genus *Multiceps* results in a syndrome termed coenurosis, which is similar to cysticercosis.[91] At present, surgical excision forms the basis of diagnosis and treatment.

Sparganosis represents infection by larval tapeworms of the genus *Spirometra,* which are closely related to tapeworms of the genus *Diphyllobothrium.* Most such infections occur in the Far East. Human infection results from drinking water containing microcrustacean *Cyclops* species that harbor procercoid larvae (spargana) of the parasite. Human infection may also be acquired by ingesting raw flesh of amphibians or snakes that contains larvae of the parasite or from applying such flesh to the skin as a poultice. After ingestion, the procercoid larvae migrate into subcutaneous tissues, where they usually present as a painless subcutaneous nodule that enlarges during the course of many months. Larvae may also migrate to the central nervous system.[92,93] Blood eosinophilia is commonly elicited. Surgical excision of larvae-containing nodules remains the basis of diagnosis and treatment.

HYDATID DISEASE

Echinococcosis in humans may result from infection with *Echinococcus granulosus,* which causes cystic hydatid disease; *E. multilocularis,* which causes alveolar hydatid disease; or *E. vogeli* or *E. oligarthus,* either of which causes polycystic hydatid disease and is found in areas of Central and South America.[94] Adult *E. granulosus* cestodes live in the intestine of dogs and wolves. Infectious eggs are passed in the feces of these animals and may be ingested by intermediate hosts such as sheep, cattle, or humans. The cycle is maintained when dogs or wolves ingest the carcasses of intermediate hosts. *E. granulosus* infection is most prevalent in sheep- and cattle-raising countries. It is also found in a number of western states, Alaska, and Canada, where autochthonous cases of human infection have been recorded.

After the eggs are ingested, oncospheres are carried in the bloodstream to the liver, lungs, and other organs. Unilocular cysts, which may contain daughter cysts, develop most commonly in the liver; the second most common site is the lungs. In children, pulmonary involvement may be more common than hepatic involvement. Unilocular hydatid cysts enlarge concentrically, increasing in diameter by about 1 to 5 cm a year, depending on the density of the organs in which they are located. A cyst may attain a large size before the initial symptoms develop; these symptoms are usually attributable to a space-occupying mass lesion. Pathological fractures or neurologic symptoms can occur with osseous or CNS localization, respectively. When cysts leak, patients may experience bronchospasm, urticaria, or anaphylaxis; blood eosinophilia, which is otherwise usually not prominent, may increase. Communicating rupture of pulmonary or hepatic cysts can lead to release of cyst contents into the bronchial or biliary systems. Because cysts contain multiple infective protoscolices, rupture of cysts can lead to dissemination of infection and the generation of new cysts from each released protoscolex.

E. multilocularis lives in the intestine of foxes and dogs. Its intermediate hosts are mice and other small mammals. *E. multilocularis* is found only in the Northern Hemisphere, including Europe, Canada, Alaska, and the north central United States.[95] Because the cysts of *E. multilocularis* lack a containing capsule, they progressively invade involved tissues and produce honeycombed alveolar hydatid cysts. The liver is most commonly affected. Severe damage caused by extensive alveolar hydatid cysts can result in jaundice and portal hypertension. The mortality in untreated alveolar disease is 90 percent.[96]

The diagnosis of hydatid disease can be strongly suggested by the results of radiographic studies.[97] Plain films detect pulmonary cysts[98] but often do not visualize cysts in other organs unless they are calcified, a process that occurs mostly in hepatic cysts. On CT and MRI,[97,99] echinococcal cysts appear as well-defined, thick- or thin-walled cysts that may have calcified rims. In older lesions, where scolices and daughter cysts form hydatid sand that settles in the dependent portion of the cyst, a layer of fluid can be visualized. A pathognomonic CT finding in intact cysts is the presence of daughter cysts that are either free within the cyst or adherent to the inner germinal layer. Separation and collapse of cyst wall layers and introduction of air into the space between the layers can be detected on plain films (as the meniscus, double arch, or water lily signs) and by CT scan.

Serologic tests can be helpful in making the diagnosis of echinococcosis but are not uniformly sensitive or specific.[94] A sensitive assay, such as

ELISA or indirect hemagglutination, is performed first. Because of the possibility of false positive results produced by cross-reacting helminthic infections, specificity is confirmed with a less sensitive but more specific assay, such as an antigen-specific immunoblot or a gel diffusion assay for the *Echinococcus*-specific arc 5 immunoprecipitin band. Even with these assays, five to 25 percent of patients with neurocysticercosis have false positive results. Conversely, negative tests do not exclude the diagnosis, because approximately 50 percent of patients with isolated pulmonary cysts and 10 to 15 percent of those with hepatic cysts lack detectable antiechinococcal antibodies. Although leakage of cyst fluid poses the risk of anaphylaxis or dissemination of infection, percutaneous aspiration of a cyst in a sero negative patient, with guidance provided by CT or ultrasonography, can yield diagnostic protoscolices or hydatid membranes.[100]

Therapeutic approaches to cystic and alveolar hydatid disease, based on current knowledge, have been recommended by the World Health Organization Informal Working Group on Echinococcosis.[96] For cystic hydatid disease, surgical resection is the first choice, offering the potential to remove the parasite totally and completely cure the patient. The former practice of injecting protoscolicidal solutions (7 to 90 percent ethanol, 0.5 percent cetrimide, or 15 to 20 percent hypertonic saline) before resection is no longer recommended, because these agents are of uncertain efficacy and are not approved for this indication and because perioperative or postoperative medical therapy is now available. For patients who are not candidates for surgical resection, there are two alternatives. The first, the PAIR procedure (percutaneous aspiration, injection of protoscolicidal agents [e.g., 95 percent ethanol or 0.5 percent cetrimide], and reaspiration), has demonstrated efficacy as an alternative to surgery.[101–103] The PAIR procedure should not be performed if hepatic cysts communicate with the biliary tract. It is more commonly associated with complications when used to treat pulmonary lesions, and it can be complicated by acute allergic reactions.[96] The second alternative involves medical therapy with mebendazole or with albendazole, which is more effective. Albendazole is given as a 400 mg dose twice a day for 28 days, often with additional 28-day courses given in subsequent months, with each course separated by 14-day treatment-free periods.[104] Neither mebendazole nor albendazole is completely effective: in 20 to 40 percent of cases, there is no improvement. Albendazole therapy results in cure in about one third of patients and leads to regression in cyst size and improvement in symptoms in another third. Both agents are contraindicated during pregnancy. Albendazole therapy also may be combined with the PAIR procedure, with improved success,[105] as well as with surgical resection to minimize dissemination of any leaked fluids containing infectious protoscolices.

Because alveolar hydatid disease is an aggressive and often fatal illness, the preferred therapy is radical resection of cysts followed by albendazole therapy for at least two years. Long-term chemotherapy can benefit patients who are not candidates for operation, as well as those who have undergone nonradical resections or liver transplantation.[96,106,107]

Acknowledgments

Figures 1 and 2 Dana Burns-Pizer.

Figures 3a through 3c Courtesy of Dr. Steve Pan, Department of Tropical Public Health, Harvard School of Public Health.

Figure 3d Courtesy of Dr. Allen W. Cheever, National Institutes of Health.

Figure 4 Courtesy of Dr. Theodore E. Nash, National Institutes of Health.

References

1. Mooraki A, Rahbar MH, Bastani B: Spontaneous systemic anaphylaxis as an unusual presentation of hydatid cyst: report of two cases. Am J Trop Med Hyg 55:302, 1996

2. Weller PF: Eosinophilia in travelers. Med Clin North Am 76:1413, 1992

3. Murrell KD, Bruschi F: Clinical trichinellosis. Prog Clin Parasitol 4: 117, 1994

4. Capo V, Despommier DD: Clinical aspects of infection with *Trichinella* Clin Microbiol Rev 9:47, 1996

5. Greenbloom SL, Martin-Smith P, Isaacs S, et al: Outbreak of trichinosis in Ontario secondary to the ingestion of wild boar meat. Can J Public Health 88:52, 1997

6. Dworkin MS, Gamble HR, Zarlenga DS, et al: Outbreak of trichinellosis associated with eating cougar jerky. J Infect Dis 174:663, 1996

7. MacLean JD, Poirier L, Gyorkos TW, et al: Epidemiologic and serologic definition of primary and secondary trichinosis in the Arctic. J Infect Dis 165:908, 1992

8. Andrews JR, Ainsworth R, Abernethy D: *Trichinella pseudospiralis* in humans: description of a case and its treatment. Trans R Soc Trop Med Hyg 88:200, 1994

9. Mawhorter SD, Kazura JW: Trichinosis of the central nervous system. Semin Neurol 13:148, 1993

10. Drugs for parasitic infections. Med Lett Drugs Ther 27:99, 1995

11. Stephenson LS: Helminth parasites, a major factor in malnutrition. World Health Forum 15:169, 1994

12. Weller PF: Parasitic pneumonias. Respiratory Infections: Diagnosis and Management, 3rd ed. Pennington JE, Ed. Raven Press, New York, 1994, p 695

13. de Silva NR, Guyatt HL, Bundy DA: Morbidity and mortality due to Ascaris-induced intestinal obstruction. Trans R Soc Trop Med Hyg 91:31, 1997

14. Wasadikar PP, Kulkarni AB: Intestinal obstruction due to ascariasis. Br J Surg 84:410, 1997

15. Villamizar E, Mendez M, Bonilla E, et al: *Ascaris lumbricoides* infestation as a cause of intestinal obstruction in children: experience with 87 cases. J Pediatr Surg 31:201, 1996

16. Khuroo MS: Ascariasis. Gastroenterol Clin North Am 25:553, 1996

17. Grencis RK, Cooper ES: *Enterobius, Trichuris, Capillaria,* and hookworm, including *Ancylostoma caninum*. Gastroenterol Clin North Am 25:579, 1996

18. Liu LX, Chi J, Upton MP, et al: Eosinophilic colitis associated with larvae of the pinworm *Enterobius vermicularis*. Lancet 346:410, 1995

19. Malde HM, Chadha D: Roundworm obstruction: sonographic diagnosis. Abdom Imaging 18:274, 1993

20. Khuroo MS, Zargar SA, Yattoo GN, et al: Sonographic findings in gallbladder ascariasis. J Clin Ultrasound 20:587, 1992

21. Khuroo MS, Zargar SA, Yattoo GN, et al: Worm extraction and biliary drainage in hepatobiliary and pancreatic ascariasis. Gastrointest Endosc 39:680, 1993

22. Woodring JH, Halfhill H 2nd, Berger R, et al: Clinical and imaging features of pulmonary strongyloidiasis. South Med J 89:10, 1996

23. Schupf N, Ortiz M, Kapell D, et al: Prevalence of intestinal parasite infections among individuals with mental retardation in New York State. Ment Retard 33:84, 1995

24. Sen P, Gil C, Estrellas B, et al: Corticosteroid-induced asthma: a manifestation of limited hyperinfection syndrome due to *Strongyloides stercoralis*. South Med J 88:923, 1995

25. Celedon JC, Mathur-Wagh U, Fox J, et al: Systemic strongyloidiasis in patients infected with the human immunodeficiency virus: a report of 3 cases and review of the literature. Medicine (Baltimore) 73: 256, 1994

26. Hayashi J, Kishihara Y, Yoshimura E, et al: Correlation between human T cell lymphotropic virus type-1 and *Strongyloides stercoralis* infections and human immunoglobulin E responses in residents of Okinawa, Japan. Am J Trop Med Hyg 56:71, 1997

27. Schad GA: Hookworms: pets to humans (editorial). Ann Intern Med 120:434, 1994

28. Croese J, Loukas A, Opdebeeck J, et al: Human enteric infection with canine hookworms. Ann Intern Med 120:369, 1994

29. Deardorff TL, Kayes SG, Fukumura T: Human anisakiasis transmitted by marine food products. Hawaii Med J 50:9, 1991

30. Schantz PM: The dangers of eating raw fish. N Engl J Med 320:1143, 1989

31. Wittner M, Turner JW, Jacquette G, et al: Eustrongylidiasis—a parasitic infection acquired by eating sushi. N Engl J Med 320:1124, 1989

32. Kakizoe S, Kakizoe H, Kakizoe K, et al: Endoscopic findings and clinical manifestations of gastric anisakiasis. Am J Gastroenterol 90:761, 1995

33. Sugimachi K, Inokuchi K, Ooiwa T, et al: Acute gastric anisakiasis: analysis of 178 cases. JAMA 53:1012, 1985

34. Fernandez de Corres L, Audicana M, Del Pozo MD, et al: *Anisakis simplex* induces not only anisakiasis: report on 28 cases of allergy caused by this nematode. J Investig Allergol Clin Immunol 6:315, 1996

35. Shirahama M, Koga T, Ishibashi H, et al: Intestinal anisakiasis: US in diagnosis. Radiology 185:789, 1992

36. Davies HD, Sakuls P, Keystone JS: Creeping eruption: a review of clinical presentation and management of 60 cases presenting to a tropical disease unit. Arch Dermatol 129:588, 1993

37. Jelinek T, Maiwald H, Nothdurft HD, et al: Cutaneous larva migrans in travelers: synopsis of histories, symptoms, and treatment of 98 patients. Clin Infect Dis 19:1062, 1994

38. Weller PF, Liu LX: Eosinophilic meningitis. Semin Neurol 13:161, 1993

39. Glickman LT, Magnaval JF: Zoonotic roundworm infections. Infect Dis Clin North Am 7:717, 1993

40. Kliks MM, Palumbo NE: Eosinophilic meningitis beyond the Pacific Basin: the global dispersal of a peridomestic zoonosis caused by *Angiostrongylus cantonensis,* the nematode lungworm of rats. Soc Sci Med 34:199, 1992

41. Nosanchuk JS, Wade SE, Landolf M: Case report of and description of parasite in *Mammomonogamus laryngeus* (human syngamosis) infection. J Clin Microbiol 33:998, 1995

42. Rusnak JM, Lucey DR: Clinical gnathostomiasis: case report and review of the English-language literature. Clin Infect Dis 16:33, 1993

43. Rohde J, Sharma BL, Patton H, et al: Surgical extraction of guinea worm: disability reduction and contribution to disease control. Am J Trop Med Hyg 48:71, 1993

44. Hopkins DR, Ruiz-Tiben E, Kaiser RL, et al: Dracunculiasis eradication: beginning of the end. Am J Trop Med Hyg 49:281, 1993

45. Lymphatic filariasis: diagnosis and pathogenesis. WHO Expert Committee on Filariasis. Bull World Health Organ 71:135, 1993

46. Ottesen EA, Nutman TB: Tropical pulmonary eosinophilia. Annu Rev Med 43:417, 1992

47. Noroes J, Addiss D, Amaral F, et al: Occurrence of living adult *Wuchereria bancrofti* Trans R Soc Trop Med Hyg 90:55, 1996

48. Kazura J, Greenberg J, Perry R, et al: Comparison of single-dose diethylcarbamazine and ivermectin for treatment of bancroftian filariasis in Papua New Guinea. Am J Trop Med Hyg 49:804, 1993

49. Klion AD, Massougbodji A, Sadeler BC, et al: Loiasis in endemic and nonendemic populations: immunologically mediated differences in clinical presentation. J Infect Dis 163:1318, 1991

50. Churchill DR, Morris C, Fakoya A, et al: Clinical and laboratory features of patients with loiasis (*Loa loa* filariasis) in the U.K. J Infect 33:103, 1996

51. Klion AD, Ottesen EA, Nutman TB: Effectiveness of diethylcarbamazine in treating loiasis acquired by expatriate visitors to endemic regions: long-term follow-up. J Infect Dis 169:604, 1994

52. Nutman TB, Miller KD, Mulligan M, et al: Diethylcarbamazine prophylaxis for human loiasis: results of a double-blind study. N Engl J Med 319:752, 1988

53. Asimacopoulos PJ, Katras A, Christie B: Pulmonary dirofilariasis: the largest single-hospital experience. Chest 102:851, 1992

54. Orihel TC, Beaver PC: Zoonotic *Brugia* infections in North and South America. Am J Trop Med Hyg 40:638, 1989

55. Cetron MS, Chitsulo L, Sullivan JJ, et al: Schistosomiasis in Lake Malawi. Lancet 348:1274, 1996

56. Gonzalez E: Schistosomiasis, cercarial dermatitis, and marine dermatitis. Dermatol Clin 7:291, 1989

57. Rocha MO, Pedroso ER, Greco DB, et al: Pathogenetic factors of acute schistosomiasis *mansoni*: correlation of worm burden, IgE, blood eosinophilia and intensity of clinical manifestations. Trop Med Int Health 1:213, 1996

58. Visser LG, Polderman AM, Stuiver PC: Outbreak of schistosomiasis among travelers returning from Mali, West Africa. Clin Infect Dis 20:280, 1995

59. Haribhai HC, Bhigjee AI, Bill PLA, et al: Spinal cord schistosomiasis: a clinical, laboratory and radiological study, with a note on therapeutic aspects. Brain 114:709, 1991

60. Pachucki CT, Levandowski RA, Brown VA, et al: American paragonimiasis treated with praziquantel. N Engl J Med 311:582, 1984

61. Cha SH, Chang KH, Cho SY, et al: Cerebral paragonimiasis in early active stage: CT and MR features. AJR Am J Roentgenol 162:141, 1994

62. Im JG, Whang HY, Kim WS, et al: Pleuropulmonary paragonimiasis: radiologic findings in 71 patients. AJR Am J Roentgenol 159:39, 1992

63. Rangdaeng S, Alpert LC, Khiyami A, et al: Pulmonary paragonimiasis: report of a case with diagnosis by fine needle aspiration cytology. Acta Cytol 36:31, 1992

64. Yee B, Hsu JI, Favour CB, et al: Pulmonary paragonimiasis in Southeast Asians living in the central San Joaquin Valley. West J Med 156:423, 1992

65. Harinasuta T, Pungpak S, Keystone JS: Trematode infections: opisthorchiasis, clonorchiasis, fascioliasis, and paragonimiasis. Infect Dis Clin North Am 7:699, 1993

66. Lim JH: Radiologic findings of clonorchiasis. AJR Am J Roentgenol 155:1001, 1990

67. Pungpak S, Viravan C, Radomyos B, et al: *Opisthorchis viverrini* infection in Thailand: studies on the morbidity of the infection and resolution following praziquantel treatment. Am J Trop Med Hyg 56:311, 1997

68. Arjona R, Riancho JA, Aguado JM, et al: Fascioliasis in developed countries: a review of classic and aberrant forms of the disease. Medicine (Baltimore) 74:13, 1995

69. Bjorland J, Bryan RT, Strauss W, et al: An outbreak of acute fascioliasis among Aymara Indians in the Bolivian Altiplano. Clin Infect Dis 21:1228, 1995

70. Price TA, Tuazon CU, Simon GL: Fascioliasis: case reports and review. Clin Infect Dis 17:426, 1993

71. Han JK, Choi BI, Cho JM, et al: Radiological findings of human fascioliasis. Abdom Imaging 18:261, 1993

72. Han JK, Han D, Choi BI, et al: MR findings in human fascioliasis. Trop Med Int Health 1:367, 1996

73. Plaut AG, Kampanart-Sanyakorn C, Manning GS: A clinical study of *Fasciolopsis buski* infection in Thailand. Trans R Soc Trop Med Hyg 63:470, 1969

74. Adams KO, Jungkind DL, Berquist EJ, et al: Intestinal fluke infection as a result of eating sushi. Am J Clin Pathol 86:688, 1986

75. MacLean JD, Arthur JR, Ward BJ, et al: Common-source outbreak of acute infection due to the North American liver fluke *Metorchis conjunctus*. Lancet 347:154, 1996

76. Schantz PM: Tapeworms (cestodiasis). Gastroenterol Clin North Am 25:637, 1996

77. Curtis MA, Bylund G: Diphyllobothriasis: fish tapeworm disease in the circumpolar north. Arctic Med Res 50:18, 1991

78. Pittella JE: Neurocysticercosis. Brain Pathol 7:681, 1997

79. Schantz PM, Moore AC, Munoz JL, et al: Neurocysticercosis in an Orthodox Jewish community in New York City. N Engl J Med 327:692, 1992

80. Kruskal BA, Moths L, Teele DW: Neurocysticercosis in a child with no history of travel outside the continental United States. Clin Infect Dis 16:290, 1993

81. Locally acquired neurocysticercosis—North Carolina, Massachusetts, and South Carolina, 1989–1991. MMWR 41:1, 1992

82. Medina MT, Rosas E, Rubio-Donnadieu F, et al: Neurocysticercosis as the main cause of late-onset epilepsy in Mexico. Arch Intern Med 150:325, 1990

83. Shandera WX, White AC Jr, Chen JC, et al: Neurocysticercosis in Houston, Texas: a report of 112 cases. Medicine (Baltimore) 73:37, 1994

84. Garcia HH, Herrera G, Gilman RH, et al: Discrepancies between cerebral computed tomography and western blot in the diagnosis of neurocysticercosis. Am J Trop Med Hyg 50:152, 1994

85. Del Brutto OH, Sotelo J, Roman GC: Therapy for neurocysticercosis: a reappraisal. Clin Infect Dis 17:730, 1993

86. Ramos-Kuri M, Montoya RM, Padilla A, et al: Immunodiagnosis of neurocysticercosis: disappointing performance of serology (enzyme-linked immunosorbent assay) in an unbiased sample of neurological patients. Arch Neurol 49:633, 1992

87. Wilson M, Bryan RT, Fried JA, et al: Clinical evaluation of the cysticercosis enzyme-linked immunoelectrotransfer blot in patients with neurocysticercosis. J Infect Dis 164:1007, 1991

88. Takayanagui OM, Jardim E: Therapy for neurocysticercosis: comparison between albendazole and praziquantel. Arch Neurol 49:290, 1992

89. Carpio A, Santillan F, Leon P, et al: Is the course of neurocysticercosis modified by treatment with antihelminthic agents? Arch Intern Med 155:1982, 1995

90. Vazquez V, Sotelo J: The course of seizures after treatment for cerebral cysticercosis. N Engl J Med 327:696, 1992

91. Pau A, Perria C, Turtas S, et al: Long-term follow-up of the surgical treatment of intracranial coenurosis. Br J Neurosurg 4:39, 1990

92. Tsai MD, Chang CN, Ho YS, et al: Cerebral sparganosis diagnosed and treated with stereotactic techniques: report of two cases. J Neurosurg 78:129, 1993

93. Moon WK, Chang KH, Cho SY, et al: Cerebral sparganosis: MR imaging versus CT features. Radiology 188:751, 1993

94. Schantz PM, Kramer HJ: Larval cestode infections: cysticercosis and echinococcosis. Curr Op Infect Dis 8:342, 1995

95. Wilson JF, Rausch RL, Wilson FR: Alveolar hydatid disease. Review of the surgical experience in 42 cases of active disease among Alaskan Eskimos. Ann Surg 221:315, 1995

96. Guidelines for treatment of cytic and alveolar echinococcosis in humans. WHO Informal Working Group on Echinococcosis. Bull World Health Organ 74:231, 1996

97. von Sinner WN: New diagnostic signs in hydatid disease: radiography, ultrasound, CT and MRI correlated to pathology. Eur J Radiol 12:150, 1991

98. Jerray M, Benzarti M, Garrouche A, et al: Hydatid disease of the lungs: study of 386 cases. Am Rev Respir Dis 146:185, 1992

99. Taourel P, Marty-Ane B, Charasset S, et al: Hydatid cyst of the liver: comparison of CT and MRI. J Comput Assist Tomogr 17:80, 1993

100. Filice C, Di Perri G, Strosselli M, et al: Parasitologic findings in percutaneous drainage of human hydatid liver cysts. J Infect Dis 161: 1290, 1990

101. Filice C, Brunetti E: Use of PAIR in human cystic echinococcosis. Acta Trop 64:95, 1997

102. Ammann RW, Eckert J: Cestodes: *Echinococcus*. Gastroenterol Clin North Am 25:655, 1996

103. Khuroo MS, Wani NA, Javid G, et al: Percutaneous drainage compared with surgery for hepatic hydatid cysts. N Engl J Med 337: 881, 1997

104. Horton RJ: Albendazole in treatment of human cystic echinococcosis: 12 years of experience. Acta Trop 64:79, 1997

105. Khuroo MS, Dar MY, Yattoo GN, et al: Percutaneous drainage versus albendazole therapy in hepatic hydatidosis: a prospective, randomized study. Gastroenterology 104:1452, 1993

106. Ammann RW, Ilitsch N, Marincek B, et al: Effect of chemotherapy on the larval mass and the long-term course of alveolar echinococcosis. Hepatology 19:735, 1994

107. Ishizu H, Uchino J, Sato N, et al: Effect of albendazole on recurrent and residual alveolar echinococcosis of the liver after surgery. Hepatology 25:528, 1997

Appendix

Summary of Recommendations for Adult Immunization*

Vaccine	CTF	USPSTF	ACP/CDC	Comments
Hepatitis A vaccine	Not reviewed	Recommended for adults at high risk; may also be considered for institutionalized persons, and workers in those institutions and in day care centers	Recommended for persons 2 yr of age and older at high risk, persons with chronic liver disease, and persons who receive clotting factor concentrates	High-risk groups include persons living in or traveling to endemic areas, men who have sex with men, injection drug users, military personnel, and certain hospital and laboratory workers; the ACIP also recommends vaccination of patients with chronic liver disease (including hepatitis B and C) and patients with clotting disorders; prevaccination serologic testing is likely to be cost-effective in persons older than 40 yr and in younger persons with a high probability of prior infection; the vaccine is given in two doses, with the second given at least 6 mo after the first
Hepatitis B vaccine	Use in adults not reviewed	Recommended for young adults who were not previously immunized and for older adults at high risk	Same as USPSTF recommendation	High-risk groups include injection drug users, persons who have more than one sex partner, men who have sex with men, patients with other sexually transmitted diseases, household and sexual contacts of HbsAg-positive persons, hemodialysis and predialysis patients, and recipients of certain blood products; vaccination is also recommended for health care workers, clients and staff of institutions for the developmentally disabled, inmates of long-term correctional facilities, patients with hepatitis C, and certain international travelers; the vaccine is given in three doses at 0, 1, and 6 mo; prevaccination and serologic testing may be cost-effective if the probability of prior infection is deemed to be high; for selected persons, postvaccination serologic testing 1–6 mo after completion of the series is recommended
Influenza vaccine	Annually for persons 65 yr of age and older and for younger persons at increased risk; insufficient evidence to recommend for or against use in healthy younger persons	Annually for persons 65 yr of age and older and for younger persons at increased risk	Recommended for persons 50 yr of age or older and younger persons at increased risk	Persons of any age at increased risk include those with cardiopulmonary disease, diabetes mellitus, renal insufficiency, hemoglobinopathies, and other conditions causing immunosuppression; influenza vaccine is also recommended for health care workers, for residents of long-term care facilities and their caregivers, for women who will be in the second or third trimester of pregnancy during influenza season, and for anyone else who desires it; protective antibodies develop 2 wk after immunization, peak at 4 to 6 wk, and wane after 6 mo; optimal time for immunization is October to mid-November, but the vaccine may be beneficial even if given as late as March or April
Measles-mumps-rubella (MMR) vaccine	Recommended for susceptible nonpregnant women of child-bearing age; not reviewed for prevention of measles or mumps in adults	Recommended for adults at high risk; may also be considered for institutionalized persons, and workers in those institutions and in day care centers	Same as USPSTF recommendation	Adults born before 1957 are likely to be immune because of natural infection; in younger persons, documentation of immunity requires serologic testing or physician records documenting live virus vaccine after the first birthday or natural infection; although children receive two doses of MMR vaccine, a single dose is considered sufficient for unimmunized adults (however, for health care workers, students entering postsecondary educational institutions, and persons traveling to an area where measles is endemic, a second dose, given no sooner than 4 wk after the first dose, is recommended); physicians must be aware of contraindications to the use of this vaccine within 3 mo of pregnancy and in some immunocompromised patients

(*continued*)

Recommendations for Adult Immunization (continued)

Vaccine	*CTF*	*USPSTF*	*ACP/CDC*	*Comments*
Pneumococcal vaccine	Once for older adults who live in an institution or live or work under crowded conditions, who have sickle cell anemia, or who have undergone splenectomy; insufficient evidence to recommend for or against use in immunocompetent adults 55 yr of age and older; not recommended for immunocompromised patients	Once for adults 65 yr of age and older and for younger adults at high risk; periodic revaccination should be considered for selected persons at high risk	Once for adults 65 yr of age and older and for younger adults at high risk; revaccination recommended at 65 yr of age if 6 yr or more have passed since initial vaccination	High-risk groups for pneumococcal infection include patients with cardiopulmonary disease, diabetes mellitus, alcoholism, cirrhosis, chronic renal failure, nephrotic syndrome, cerebrospinal fluid leaks, anatomic or functional asplenia, and other conditions causing immunosuppression; the controversy among the expert panels regarding vaccination recommendations relates to the fact that vaccine efficacy is best documented in immunocompetent adults at low risk; the ACIP has recommended a single vaccination after 5 yr or more for persons 65 yr of age or over who receive the initial vaccine before 65 yr of age, and for younger patients who are immunocompromised; revaccination increases the risk of local injection site reactions
Tetanus-diphtheria vaccine	Every 10 yr after primary immunization series	Periodically after primary immunization series	Every 10 yr after primary immunization series	Although antibody levels decline 10 yr after tetanus immunization, tetanus is unlikely to occur in persons who have received a primary immunization series; although booster immunizations every 10 yr have been recommended for adults, the focus in prevention should be to ensure that unimmunized persons are vaccinated and that wound management guidelines are followed; a primary immunization series for adults consists of a second dose 4–8 wk after the first and a third dose 6–12 months later; use of the combined adsorbed toxoid vaccine for adults is recommended
Varicella vaccine	Recommended for susceptible adolescents and adults	Recommended for healthy adults with no history of varicella or previous vaccination; strongly recommended for susceptible health care workers, family contacts of immunocompromised patients, and workers in day care centers and other sites in which transmission is likely to occur	Same as USPSTF recommendation	Adults with reliable histories of chickenpox can be assumed to be immune; in others, serologic testing may be cost-effective because most adults with a negative or uncertain history of chickenpox are immune; susceptible persons include health care workers and family contacts of immunocompromised persons, those who live or work in environments where transmission is likely (e.g., teachers of young children, day care center staff, and residents and staff in institutional settings), and international travelers who are not immune to infection; the vaccine is administered in two doses, with the second given 4–8 wk after the first; physicians must be aware of contraindications to the use of this live attenuated virus vaccine within 1 mo of pregnancy and in immunocompromised patients

*For recommendations concerning vaccinia vaccine for smallpox, see Chapter 3 Bioterrorism.

ACIP—Advisory Committee on Immunization Practices ACP—American College of Physicians CDC—Centers for Disease Control and Prevention CTF—Canadian Task Force on the Periodic Health Examination USPSTF—United States Preventive Services Task Force

Index

Note: Page numbers followed by *t* indicate tables; numbers followed by *f* indicate figures.

B

C

D

E

F

G

H

I

J

K

L

M

N

O

S

T

U

V

W

Y

Z